PRINCIPLES AND LABS FOR fitness & wellness

THIRTEENTH EDITION

Werner W.K. Hoeger
Boise State University

Sharon A. Hoeger
Fitness & Wellness, Inc.

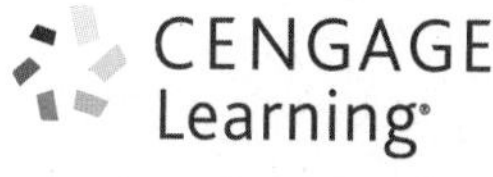

Australia • Brazil • Mexico • Singapore • United Kingdom • United States

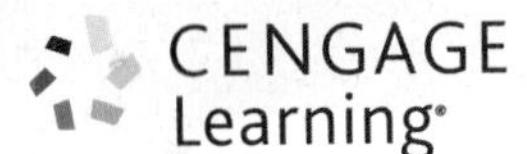

***Principles and Labs for Fitness & Wellness,* Thirteenth Edition**
Werner W.K. Hoeger, Sharon A. Hoeger

Product Director: Mary Finch

Product Manager: Aileen Berg

Content Developer: Elizabeth Momb

Associate Content Developers: Kellie Petruzzelli, Casey Lozier

Product Assistant: Chelsea Joy

Media Developer: Stefanie Chase

Marketing Manager: Julie Schuster

Content Project Manager: Tanya Nigh

Art Director: Linda May

Manufacturing Planner: Karen Hunt

Compositor and Production Service: Graphic World, Inc

IP Analyst: Christine Myaskovsky

IP Project Manager: John Sarantakis

Photo and Text Researchers: Lumina Datamatics Ltd.

Copy Editor: Graphic World, Inc

Text Designer: RHDG | Riezebos Holzbaur

Cover Designer: Ke Design

Cover Image: Bill Losh/The Image Bank/ Getty Images

Library of Congress Control Number: 2014943311

ISBN-13: 978-1-305-25107-6

ISBN-10: 1-305-25107-5

Cengage Learning
20 Channel Center Street
Boston, MA 02210
USA

Cengage Learning is a leading provider of customized learning solutions with office locations around the globe, including Singapore, the United Kingdom, Australia, Mexico, Brazil, and Japan. Locate your local office at **www.cengage.com/global.**

Cengage Learning products are represented in Canada by Nelson Education, Ltd.

To learn more about Cengage Learning Solutions, visit **www.cengage.com.**

Purchase any of our products at your local college store or at our preferred online store **www.CengageBrain.com.**

Printed in the United States of America
Print Number: 01 Print Year: 2014

chapter labs

CHAPTER 1
Physical Fitness and Wellness 1

Lab 1A Daily Physical Activity Log 33
Lab 1B Wellness Lifestyle Questionnaire 35
Lab 1C PAR-Q and Health History Questionnaire 39
Lab 1D Resting Heart Rate and Blood Pressure 41

CHAPTER 2
Behavior Modification 43

Lab 2A Exercising Control over Your Physical Activity and Nutrition Environment 71
Lab 2B Behavior Modification Plan 73
Lab 2C Setting SMART Goals 75

CHAPTER 3
Nutrition for Wellness 77

Lab 3A Nutrient Analysis 129
Lab 3B MyPlate Record Form 133

CHAPTER 4
Body Composition 135

Lab 4A Hydrostatic Weighing for Body Composition Assessment 159
Lab 4B Body Composition, Disease Risk Assessment, and Recommended Body Weight Determination 161

CHAPTER 5
Weight Management 163

Lab 5A Computing Your Daily Caloric Requirement 203
Lab 5B Weight-Loss Behavior Modification Plan 205
Lab 5C Calorie-Restricted Diet Plans 207
Lab 5D Healthy Plan for Weight Maintenance or Gain 211
Lab 5E Weight Management: Measuring Progress 213

CHAPTER 6
Cardiorespiratory Endurance 215

Lab 6A Cardiorespiratory Endurance Assessment 247
Lab 6B Caloric Expenditure and Exercise Heart Rate 249
Lab 6C Exercise Readiness Questionnaire 253
Lab 6D Cardiorespiratory Exercise Prescription 255

CHAPTER 7
Muscular Fitness: Strength and Endurance 257

Lab 7A Muscular Strength and Endurance Assessment 305
Lab 7B Strength-Training Program 307

CHAPTER 8
Muscular Flexibility 309

Lab 8A Muscular Flexibility Assessment 337
Lab 8B Posture Evaluation 339
Lab 8C Flexibility Development and Low Back Conditioning 341

CHAPTER 9
Skill Fitness and Fitness Programming 343

Lab 9A Assessment of Skill Fitness 375
Lab 9B Personal Fitness Plan 377

CHAPTER 10
Stress Assessment and Management Techniques 381

Lab 10A Stress Events Scale 409
Lab 10B Type A Personality and Hostility Assessment 411
Lab 10C Stress Vulnerability Questionnaire 413
Lab 10D Goals and Time Management Skills 415
Lab 10E Stress Management 419

CHAPTER 11
Preventing Cardiovascular Disease 421

Lab 11A Self-Assessment Coronary Heart Disease Risk Factor Analysis 453

CHAPTER 12
Cancer Prevention 455

Lab 12A Cancer Prevention Guidelines 485
Lab 12B Early Signs of Illness 487
Lab 12C Cancer Risk Profile 489

CHAPTER 13
Addictive Behavior 491

Lab 13A Addictive Behavior Questionnaires 521

Lab 13B Smoking Cessation Questionnaires 523

CHAPTER 14
Preventing Sexually Transmitted Infections 527

Lab 14A Self-Quiz on HIV and AIDS 545

CHAPTER 15
Lifetime Fitness and Wellness 547

Lab 15A Life Expectancy and Physiological Age Prediction Questionnaire 567

Lab 15B Fitness and Wellness Community Resources 571

Lab 15C Self-Evaluation and Future Behavioral Goals 573

Appendix A: Nutritive Value of Selected Foods 577

Glossary 589

Answers to Assess Your Knowledge 598

Index 599

contents

CHAPTER 1
Physical Fitness and Wellness 1

Life Expectancy 4
Leading Health Problems in the United States 6
Lifestyle as a Health Problem 7
Physical Activity and Exercise Defined 8
Importance of Increased Physical Activity 8
National Initiatives to Promote Healthy and Active Lifestyles: Federal Guidelines for Physical Activity 9
Monitoring Daily Physical Activity 11
"Sitting Disease:" A 21st Century Chronic Disease 13
Wellness 14
Wellness, Fitness, and Longevity 18
Types of Physical Fitness 19
Fitness Standards: Health versus Physical Fitness 20
Benefits of a Comprehensive Fitness Program 23
The Wellness Challenge for Our Day 26
Wellness Education: Using This Book 27
A Personalized Approach 27
Exercise Safety 27
Assessment of Resting Heart Rate and Blood Pressure 29
Mean Blood Pressure 30
Assess Your Behavior 30
Assess Your Knowledge 30
Notes 31
Suggested Readings 32
Lab 1A Daily Physical Activity Log 33
Lab 1B Wellness Lifestyle Questionnaire 35
Lab 1C PAR-Q and Health History Questionnaire 39
Lab 1D Resting Heart Rate and Blood Pressure 41

CHAPTER 2
Behavior Modification 43

Living in a Toxic Health and Fitness Environment 44
Environmental Influences on Physical Activity 46
Environmental Influence on Diet and Nutrition 48
Values and Behavior 50
Your Brain and Your Habits 51
Willpower 52
Barriers to Change 52
Self-Efficacy 54
Motivation and Locus of Control 54
Changing Behavior 56
Behavior Change Theories 57
The Process of Change 61
Techniques of Change 64
Assess Your Behavior 67
Assess Your Knowledge 67
Notes 68
Suggested Readings 69
Lab 2A Exercising Control over Your Physical Activity and Nutrition Environment 71
Lab 2B Behavior Modification Plan 73
Lab 2C Setting SMART Goals 75

CHAPTER 3
Nutrition for Wellness 77

Nutrients 81
Carbohydrates 83
Fats (Lipids) 86
Proteins 89
Vitamins 91
Minerals 91
Water 91
Balancing the Diet 92

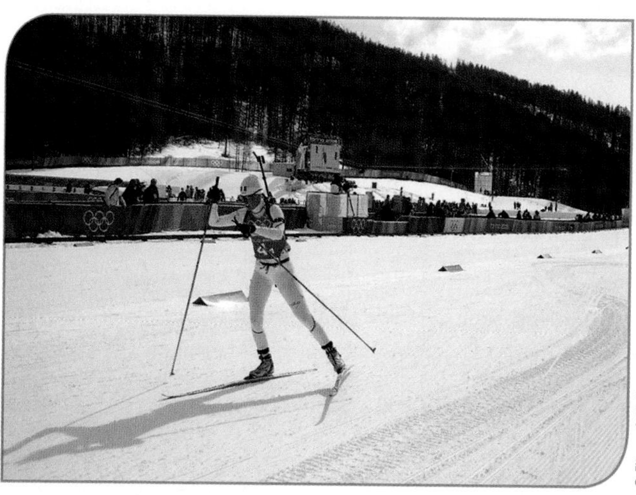

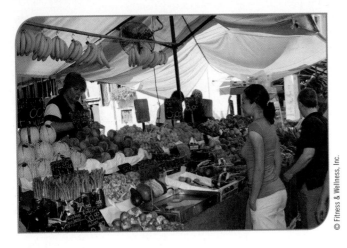
© Fitness & Wellness, Inc.

Nutrition Standards 94
Nutrient Analysis 96
Achieving a Balanced Diet 99
Choosing Healthy Foods 103
Vegetarianism 103
Nuts 105
Soy Products 106
Probiotics 106
Advanced Glycation End Products 106
Diets from Other Cultures 107
Nutrient Supplementation 109
Benefits of Foods 113
Functional Foods 114
Organic Foods 114
Genetically Modified Crops 115
Energy Substrates for Physical Activity 117
Nutrition for Athletes 117
Bone Health and Osteoporosis 120
Iron Deficiency 122
2010 Dietary Guidelines for Americans 123
Proper Nutrition: A Lifetime Prescription for Healthy Living 124
Assess Your Behavior 125
Assess Your Knowledge 125
Notes 126
Suggested Readings 127
Lab 3A Nutrient Analysis 129
Lab 3B MyPlate Record Form 133

CHAPTER 4
Body Composition 135

Essential and Storage Fat 138
Techniques to Assess Body Composition 138
Metrics Used to Determine Recommended Body Weight 148
Body Mass Index 149
Waist Circumference 150
Waist-to-Height Ratio: "Keep your waist circumference to less than half your height." 152
Determining Recommended Body Weight 154
Importance of Regular Body Composition Assessment 155
Assess Your Behavior 156
Assess Your Knowledge 156
Notes 157
Suggested Readings 158
Lab 4A Hydrostatic Weighing for Body Composition Assessment 159
Lab 4B Body Composition, Disease Risk Assessment, and Recommended Body Weight Determination 161

CHAPTER 5
Weight Management 163

Overweight versus Obese 168
Tolerable Weight 168
The Weight Loss Dilemma 169
Diet Crazes 169
Eating Disorders 174
The Physiology of Weight Loss 177
Diet and Metabolism 180
Hormonal Regulation of Appetite 181
Sleep and Weight Management 182
Monitoring Body Weight 182
Exercise and Weight Management 182
The Roles of Exercise Intensity and Duration in Weight Management 185
Overweight and Fit Debate 187
Healthy Weight Gain 188
Weight Loss Myths 188
Losing Weight the Sound and Sensible Way 188
Monitoring Your Diet with Daily Food Logs 194
Effect of Food Choices on Long-Term Weight Gain 195
Behavior Modification and Adherence to a Weight Management Program 195
The Simple Truth 196

Assess Your Behavior 199

Assess Your Knowledge 199

Notes 200

Suggested Readings 201

Lab 5A Computing Your Daily Caloric Requirement 203

Lab 5B Weight-Loss Behavior Modification Plan 205

Lab 5C Calorie-Restricted Diet Plans 207

Lab 5D Healthy Plan for Weight Maintenance or Gain 211

Lab 5E Weight Management: Measuring Progress 213

CHAPTER 6
Cardiorespiratory Endurance 215

Basic Cardiorespiratory Physiology: A Quick Survey 218

Aerobic and Anaerobic Exercise 219

Benefits of Aerobic Training 220

Physical Fitness Assessment 222

Responders versus Nonresponders 222

Assessment of Cardiorespiratory Endurance 223

Tests to Estimate VO_{2max} 224

Interpreting the Results of Your VO_{2max} 230

Predicting VO_2 and Caloric Expenditure from Walking and Jogging 230

Principles of CR Exercise Prescription 232

Guidelines for CR Exercise Prescription 233

Fitness Benefits of Aerobic Activities 240

Getting Started and Adhering to a Lifetime Exercise Program 242

A Lifetime Commitment to Fitness 245

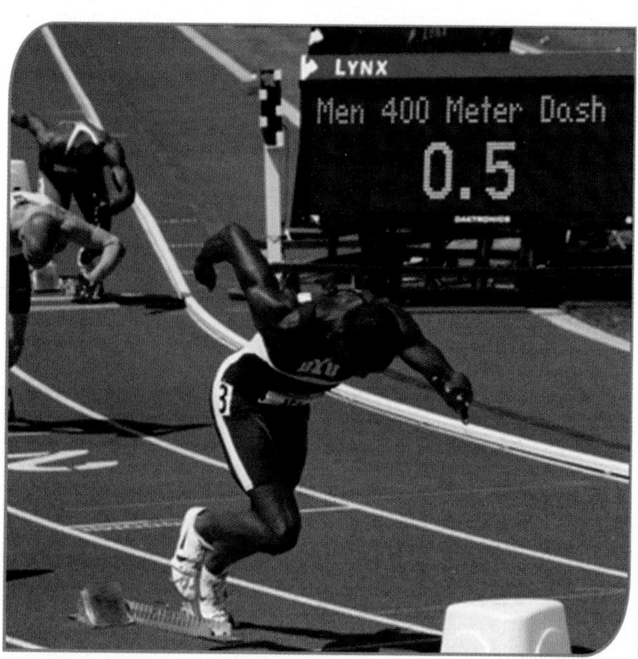

© Fitness & Wellness, Inc.

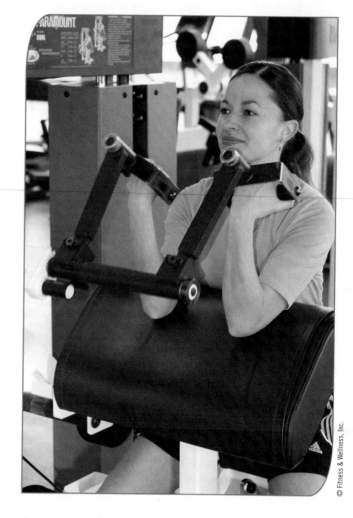

© Fitness & Wellness, Inc.

Assess Your Behavior 245

Assess Your Knowledge 245

Notes 246

Suggested Readings 246

Lab 6A Cardiorespiratory Endurance Assessment 247

Lab 6B Caloric Expenditure and Exercise Heart Rate 249

Lab 6C Exercise Readiness Questionnaire 253

Lab 6D Cardiorespiratory Exercise Prescription 255

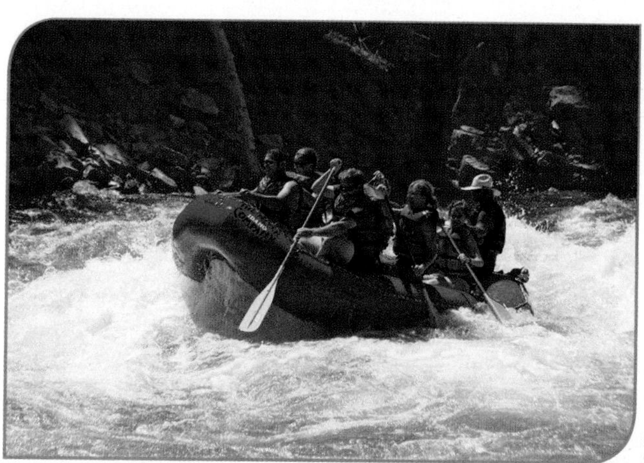

© Fitness & Wellness, Inc.

CHAPTER 7
Muscular Fitness: Strength and Endurance 257

Strength Training Benefits 260
Muscular Fitness and Aging 260
Assessment of Muscular Strength and Endurance 263
Strength-Training Prescription 268
Overload 269
Specificity of Training 270
Principles Involved in Strength Training 270
Strength-Training Exercises 277
Dietary Guidelines for Muscular and Strength Development 277
Core Strength Training 279
Pilates Exercise System 279
Stability Exercise Balls 280
Elastic-Band Resistive Exercise 280
Exercise Safety Guidelines 280
Setting Up Your Own Strength-Training Program 282
Assess Your Behavior 284
Assess Your Knowledge 284
Notes 285
Suggested Readings 285
Strength-Training Exercises without Weights 286
Strength-Training Exercises with Weights 291
Stability Ball Exercises 300
Lab 7A Muscular Strength and Endurance Assessment 305
Lab 7B Strength-Training Program 307

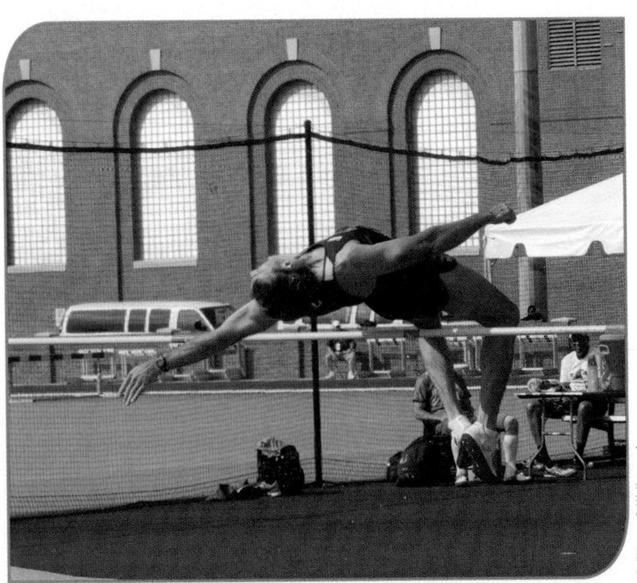

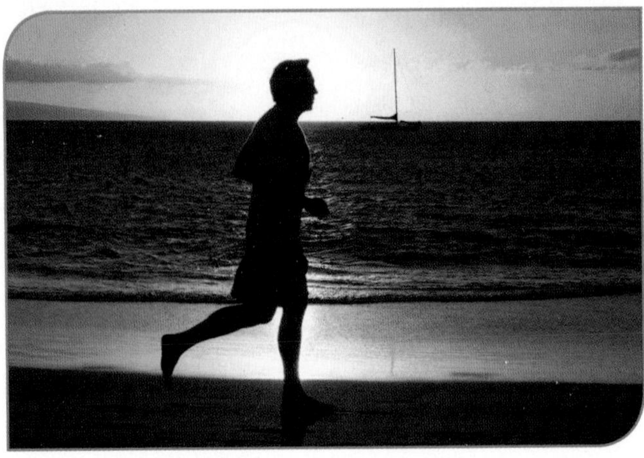

CHAPTER 8
Muscular Flexibility 309

Benefits of Good Flexibility 310
Flexibility in Older Adults 312
Factors Affecting Flexibility 312
Assessment of Flexibility 312
Interpreting Flexibility Test Results 313
Principles of Muscular Flexibility Prescription 318
Proprioceptive Neuromuscular Facilitation 318
Physiological Response to Stretching 319
Intensity 319
Repetitions 320
Frequency of Exercise 320
When to Stretch? 320
Flexibility Exercises 321
Preventing and Rehabilitating Low Back Pain 321
Effects of Stress 326
Personal Flexibility and Low Back Conditioning Program 326
Assess Your Behavior 327
Assess Your Knowledge 327
Notes 328
Suggested Readings 328
Flexibility Exercises 329
Exercises for the Prevention and Rehabilitation of Low Back Pain 332
Lab 8A Muscular Flexibility Assessment 337
Lab 8B Posture Evaluation 339
Lab 8C Flexibility Development and Low Back Conditioning 341

CHAPTER 9
Skill Fitness and Fitness Programming 343

Performance Tests for Skill-Related Fitness 346
Team Sports 350
Specific Exercise Considerations 351
Exercise-Related Injuries 359
Exercise and Aging 361
Physical Training in the Older Adult 361
Preparing for Sports Participation 362
Base Fitness Conditioning 365
Sport-Specific Conditioning 366
Overtraining 368
Periodization 369
Personal Fitness Programming: An Example 370
You Can Get It Done 372
Assess Your Behavior 372
Assess Your Knowledge 373
Notes 374
Suggested Readings 374
Lab 9A Assessment of Skill Fitness 375
Lab 9B Personal Fitness Plan 377

CHAPTER 10
Stress Assessment and Management Techniques 381

The Mind–Body Connection 382
The Brain 384
Stress and Illness 384
Sleep and Wellness 384
Stress 385
Stress Adaptation 387
Perceptions and Health 388
Self-Esteem 388
Fighting Spirit 388
Sources of Stress 388
Behavior Patterns 389
Vulnerability to Stress 392
Time Management 392
Coping with Stress 394
Physical Activity 395
Relaxation Techniques 397
Biofeedback 397
Progressive Muscle Relaxation 398
Breathing Techniques for Relaxation 399
Visual Imagery 400
Autogenic Training 402
Meditation 402
Yoga 404
Tai Chi 405
Which Technique Is Best? 405
Assess Your Behavior 406
Assess Your Knowledge 406
Notes 407
Suggested Readings 407
Lab 10A Stress Events Scale 409
Lab 10B Type A Personality and Hostility Assessment 411
Lab 10C Stress Vulnerability Questionnaire 413
Lab 10D Goals and Time Management Skills 415
Lab 10E Stress Management 419

CHAPTER 11
Preventing Cardiovascular Disease 421

Prevalence of Cardiovascular Disease 424
Stroke 424
Coronary Heart Disease 425
Coronary Heart Disease Risk Profile 425
Leading Risk Factors for CHD 425
Physical Inactivity 427
Abnormal Electrocardiograms 428
Abnormal Cholesterol Profile 429
Elevated Triglycerides 438
Elevated Homocysteine 438
Inflammation 439
Diabetes 440
Metabolic Syndrome 443
Hypertension 443
Excessive Body Fat 447
Cigarette Smoking 448
Tension and Stress 448
Personal and Family History 449
Age 449
Other Risk Factors for Coronary Heart Disease 450

Cardiovascular Risk Reduction 450
Assess Your Behavior 450
Assess Your Knowledge 450
Notes 451
Suggested Readings 452
Lab 11A Self-Assessment Coronary Heart Disease Risk Factor Analysis 453

CHAPTER 12 Cancer Prevention 455

Genetic vs Environmental Risk 459
Incidence of Cancer 460
Guidelines for Preventing Cancer 461
Dietary Changes 462
Excessive Body Weight 467
Abstaining from Tobacco 467
Avoiding Excessive Exposure to Sun 468
Monitoring Estrogen, Radiation Exposure, and Potential Occupational Hazards 469
Physical Activity 469
Early Detection 470
Other Factors 470
Warning Signals of Cancer 470
Cancer: Assessing Your Risks 471
Common Sites of Cancer 471
Skin Self-Exam 474
What Can You Do? 481
Assess Your Behavior 481
Assess Your Knowledge 482
Notes 482
Suggested Readings 483
Lab 12A Cancer Prevention Guidelines 485
Lab 12B Early Signs of Illness 487
Lab 12C Cancer Risk Profile 489

CHAPTER 13 Addictive Behavior 491

Addiction 492
Risk Factors for Addiction 494
Drugs and Dependence 495
Nonmedical Use of Prescription Drugs 495
Inhalant Abuse 496
Marijuana 496
Cocaine 497
Methamphetamine 498
MDMA (Ecstasy) 499
Heroin 500
New Psychoactive Substances (NPS) 501

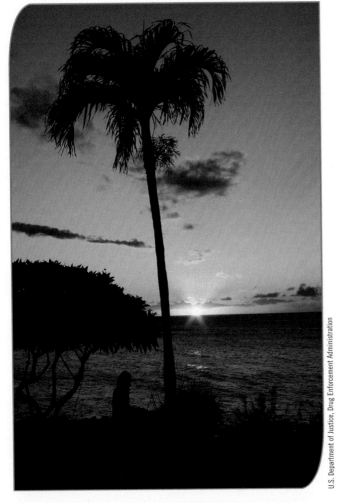

U.S. Department of Justice, Drug Enforcement Administration

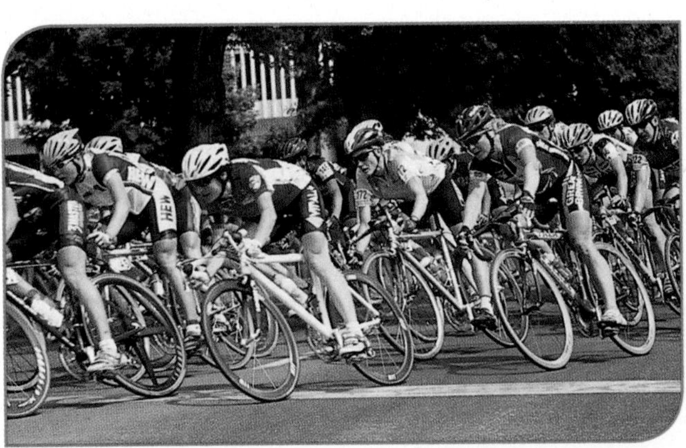

© Fitness & Wellness, Inc.

Alcohol 502
Treatment of Addictions 506
Tobacco Use 506
Why People Smoke 510
Smoking Addiction and Dependency 511
Why Do You Smoke? Test 511
Smoking Cessation 512
Do You Want to Quit? Test 512
Breaking the Habit 512
Nicotine-Substitution Products 514
Life after Cigarettes 515
Assess Your Behavior 518
Assess Your Knowledge 518
Notes 519
Suggested Readings 520
Lab 13A Addictive Behavior Questionnaires 521
Lab 13B Smoking Cessation Questionnaires 523

CHAPTER 14 Preventing Sexually Transmitted Infections 527

Types and Causes of STIs 529
Chlamydia 529
Gonorrhea 531
Syphilis 531
Trichomoniasis 532
Human Papillomavirus and Genital Warts 532
Genital Herpes 533
Hepatitis 534
HIV and AIDS 535
Trends in HIV Infection and AIDS 538
HIV Testing 539
HIV Treatment 539
Preventing STIs 540
Reducing the Risk for STIs and HIV Infection 541
Assess Your Behavior 543
Assess Your Knowledge 543
Notes 544
Suggested Readings 544
Lab 14A Self-Quiz on HIV and AIDS 545

CHAPTER 15 Lifetime Fitness and Wellness 547

Life Expectancy and Physiological Age 550
Conventional Western Medicine 550
Complementary and Alternative Medicine 552
Integrative Medicine 555
Quackery and Fraud 556
Looking at Your Fitness Future 558
Health and Fitness Club Memberships 559
Personal Trainers 560
Purchasing Exercise Equipment 561
Self-Evaluation and Behavioral Goals for the Future 561
The Fitness and Wellness Experience and a Challenge for the Future 562
Assess Your Behavior 564
Assess Your Knowledge 564
Notes 565
Suggested Readings 565
Lab 15A Life Expectancy and Physiological Age Prediction Questionnaire 567
Lab 15B Fitness and Wellness Community Resources 571
Lab 15C Self-Evaluation and Future Behavioral Goals 573

Appendix A: Nutritive Value of Selected Foods 577

Glossary 589

Answers to Assess Your Knowledge 598

Index 599

Preface

The current American way of life does not provide people with sufficient physical activity to maintain good health and improve quality of life. Actually, our way of life is such a serious threat to our health that it increases the deterioration rate of the human body and leads to premature illness and mortality.

The most recent data released by the Centers for Disease Control and Prevention (CDC) indicate that only 19.4 percent of U.S. adults 18 and over meet the Federal Physical Activity Guidelines for both aerobic and muscular fitness activities, whereas 46.1 percent meet the guidelines for aerobic fitness and just 23 percent do so for muscular fitness. Another 34 percent of Americans are completely inactive during their leisure time. Yet, most people in the United States say they believe that physical activity and positive lifestyle habits promote better health. However, many do not reap benefits because they simply do not know how to implement a sound fitness and wellness program that will yield the desired results.

The U.S. Surgeon General has determined that lack of physical activity is detrimental to good health. As a result, the importance of sound fitness and wellness programs has assumed an entirely new dimension. The Office of the Surgeon General has identified physical fitness as a top health priority by stating that the nation's top health goals in the 21st century are exercise, increased consumption of fruits and vegetables, smoking cessation, and the practice of safe sex. All four of these fundamental healthy lifestyle factors are thoroughly addressed in this book.

Furthermore, the science of behavioral therapy has established that many behaviors we adopt are a product of our environment. Unfortunately, we live in a "toxic" health and fitness environment. Becoming aware of how the environment affects our health is vital if we wish to achieve and maintain wellness. Yet, we are so habituated to this modern-day environment that we miss the subtle ways in which it influences our behaviors, personal lifestyle, and health each day.

Along with the most up-to-date health, fitness, and nutrition guidelines, the information in this book provides extensive behavior modification strategies to help you abandon negative habits and adopt and maintain healthy behaviors. As you study and assess physical fitness and wellness parameters, you need to take a critical look at your behaviors and lifestyle—and most likely make selected permanent changes to promote your overall health and wellness.

Principles and Labs for Fitness & Wellness contains 15 chapters and 42 laboratories (labs) that serve as guides to implement a complete lifetime fitness and wellness program. The book contents point out the need to go beyond the basic components of fitness to achieve total well-being.

In addition to a thorough discussion of physical fitness, including all health- and skill-related components, extensive and up-to-date information is provided on behavior modification, nutrition, weight management, stress management, cardiovascular and cancer-risk reduction, exercise and aging, prevention of sexually transmitted infections (STIs), and substance abuse control (including tobacco, alcohol, and other psychoactive drugs). The information has been written to provide you with the necessary tools and guidelines for an active lifestyle and a wellness way of life.

Scientific evidence has clearly shown that improving the quality—and most likely the longevity—of your life is a matter of personal choice. As you work through the various chapters and laboratories in the book, you will be able to develop and regularly update your healthy lifestyle program to improve physical fitness and personal wellness. The emphasis throughout the book is on teaching you how to take control of your health and lifestyle habits so that you can make a constant and deliberate effort to stay healthy and achieve the highest potential for well-being.

New in the 13th Edition

All chapters in the 13th edition of *Principles and Labs for Fitness & Wellness* have been revised and updated according to recent advances and recommendations in the field, including information reported in the literature and at professional health, fitness, and sports medicine conferences.

In this edition, we continue to provide the MyProfile feature at the beginning of each chapter for students to evaluate their current knowledge of the chapter's topic. Included also are the Confident Consumer and Diversity Considerations boxes to help students make healthier choices and be discerning fitness and wellness consumers. These features, along with the Real Life Story and FAQ sections, are intended to perk the students' interest in the chapter contents. Beyond the individual chapter updates listed in the next section, new figures and photography are included throughout the textbook.

Chapter Updates

- All statistics related to the leading causes of death, life expectancy, and health care costs have been brought up-to-date in the opening chapter, "Physical Fitness and Wellness." A new section on *Sitting Disease*, a 21st century

1

Physical Fitness and Wellness

The human body is extremely resilient during youth—not so during middle and older age. The power of prevention, nonetheless, is yours: It enables you to make healthy lifestyle choices today that will prevent disease in the future and increase the quality and length of your life.

OBJECTIVES

- Understand the health and fitness consequences of physical inactivity.
- Identify the major health problems in the United States.
- Learn how to monitor daily physical activity.
- Learn the *Physical Activity Guidelines for Americans*.
- Define wellness and list its dimensions.
- Define physical fitness and list health-related and skill-related components.
- State the differences among physical fitness, health promotion, and wellness.
- Distinguish between health fitness standards and physical fitness standards.
- Understand the benefits and significance of participating in a comprehensive wellness program.
- List key national health objectives for 2020.
- Determine whether you can safely initiate an exercise program.
- Learn to assess resting heart rate and blood pressure.

CENGAGEbrain.com
Visit **www.cengagebrain.com** to access course materials and companion resources for this text, including digital labs, quiz questions designed to check your understanding of the chapter contents, and more! See the preface on page xii for more information.

REAL LIFE STORY | Jeremy's Experience

I was a multisport athlete in high school. I played soccer, football, basketball, and ran track. I was not the best athlete on these teams, and I didn't have a chance to make a college team, but I sure loved sports and athletic competition. To earn extra money for college, I worked for a fast-food chain that summer. I was so busy that I didn't do any fitness activities or play sports that summer, and I ate too much junk food, which caused me to gain some weight. Later in college, it took some time to get used to my new surroundings and the newfound freedom from my home life. My friends kept stressing that I needed to enjoy college life as much as possible and not worry so much about academics. We went to a lot of parties and watched sporting events. There was always plenty of alcohol at these activities. I know we drank way too much, we didn't exercise, and my grades suffered as a result. I shouldn't have been so shocked when I saw my final grades. To add insult to injury, it really hit home when I signed up for the fitness and wellness class and found out I had gained more than 15 pounds since high school graduation. My fitness test results showed I was not even in an average fitness category for most components.

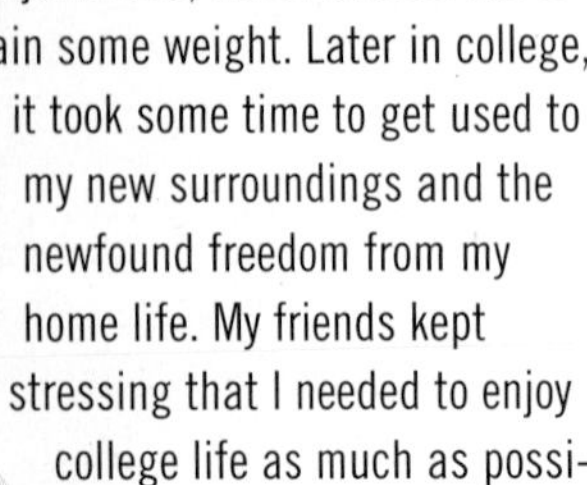

©iStockphoto.com/zhang_bo

I am so glad the fitness course was a required class, as I was able to correct my lifestyle before it spiraled out of control and I wasted more time in college. I started to exercise on an almost daily basis, and I learned so much about nutrition and healthy eating. Parties and alcohol were no longer important to me. I had a life to live and prepare for. It felt so good to once again become fit and eat a healthy/balanced diet. I rearranged my activities so that schoolwork and fitness were right at the top of my list. I stopped procrastinating on my schoolwork, and I was doing cardio five times a week and lifting twice per week. My goal is to keep this up for the rest of my life. I now understand that if I want to enjoy wellness, I have to make fitness and healthy living a top priority in my life.

Movement and physical activity are basic functions that the human organism evolved to perform with vigor and proficiency. Advances in technology, however, have almost eliminated the necessity for physical exertion in daily life. Physical activity is no longer a natural part of our existence. We live in an automated society, in which most of the activities that used to require strenuous exertion can be accomplished by machines with the simple pull of a handle or push of a button.

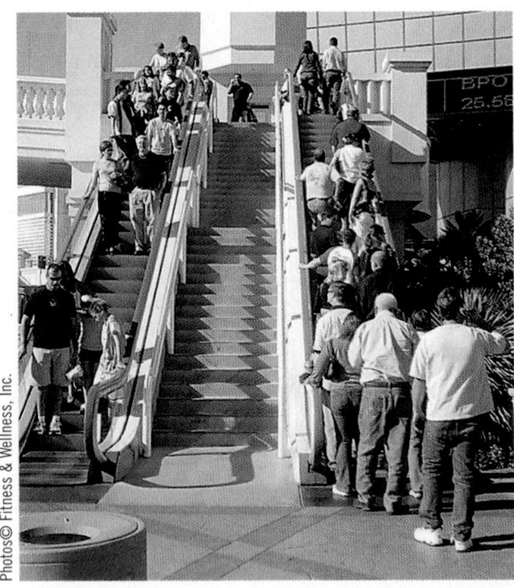

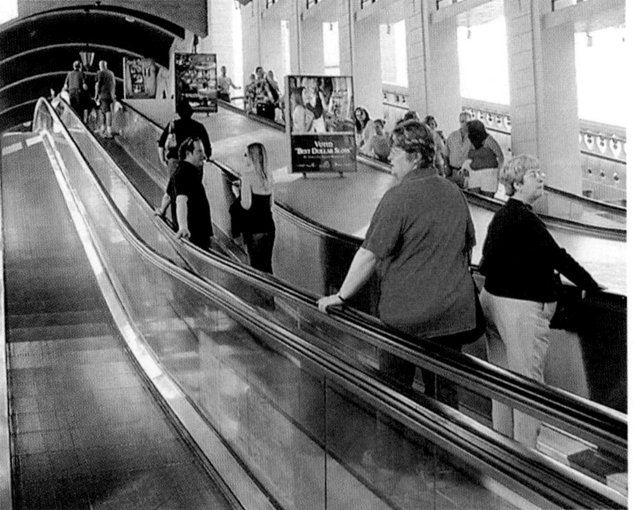

Photos© Fitness & Wellness, Inc.

Modern-day conveniences lull people into a sedentary lifestyle.

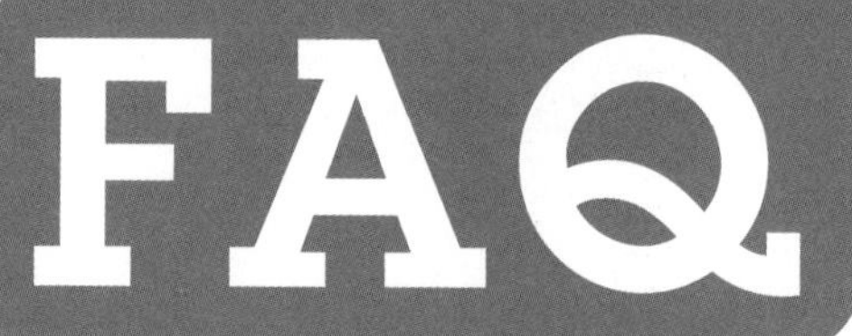

Why should I take a fitness and wellness course?

Most people go to college to learn how to make a living, but a fitness and wellness course teaches you how to *live*—truly live life to its fullest potential. Some people seem to think that success is measured by how much money they make. Making a good living does not help you unless you live a wellness lifestyle that allows you to enjoy what you earn. You may want to ask yourself: Of what value are a nice income, a beautiful home, and a solid retirement portfolio if at age 45 I suffer a massive heart attack that will seriously limit my physical capacity or end my life?

Is the attainment of good physical fitness sufficient to ensure good health?

Regular participation in a sound physical fitness program provides substantial health benefits and significantly decreases the risk of many chronic diseases. And although good fitness often motivates us toward adoption of additional positive lifestyle behaviors, to maximize the benefits for a healthier, more productive, happier, and longer life, we have to pay attention to all seven dimensions of wellness: physical, social, mental, emotional, occupational, environmental, and spiritual. These dimensions are interrelated, and one frequently affects the others. A wellness way of life requires a constant and deliberate effort to stay healthy and achieve the highest potential for well-being within all dimensions of wellness.

If a person is going to do only one thing to improve health, what would it be?

This is a common question. It is a mistake to think, though, that you can modify just one factor and enjoy wellness. Wellness requires a constant and deliberate effort to change unhealthy behaviors and reinforce healthy behaviors. Although it is difficult to work on many lifestyle changes at once, involvement in a regular physical activity program, proper nutrition, and avoidance of addictive behavior are lifestyle factors to work on first. Others should follow, depending on your current lifestyle behaviors.

MyProfile: General Understanding of Fitness and Wellness

To the best of your ability, answer the following questions. If you do not know the answer(s), this chapter will guide you through them.

I. Wellness implies making a constant and deliberate effort to stay healthy and achieve the highest potential for well-being. ___ True ___ False

II. The minimum requirement in the *U.S. Federal Physical Activity Guidelines* is that you accumulate ___ minutes of moderate-intensity aerobic activity or ___ minutes of vigorous-intensity aerobic activity weekly.

III. Cardiorespiratory endurance, strength, power, flexibility, agility, and speed are the basic components of health-related fitness. ___ True ___ False

IV. My current blood pressure is ___/___ mm Hg, which is classified as (mark one) ___ normal, ___ prehypertension, or ___ hypertension.

V. Are you aware of potential risk factors in your life and personal health family history that may increase your chances of developing disease? ___ Yes ___ No

Research findings clearly show that physical inactivity and a negative lifestyle seriously threaten health and hasten the deterioration rate of the human body. Most of the world's industrialized nations are experiencing an epidemic of physical inactivity. In the United States, physical inactivity is the second-greatest threat to public health and has been termed **sedentary death syndrome**, or **SeDS** (the number-one threat is tobacco use—the largest cause of preventable deaths).

Widespread interest in **health** and preventive medicine in recent years, nonetheless, is motivating people to participate in organized fitness and wellness programs. The growing number of participants is attributed primarily to scientific evidence linking regular physical activity and positive lifestyle habits to better health, longevity, quality of life, and overall well-being.

Sedentary death syndrome (SeDS) Cause of deaths attributed to a lack of regular physical activity.

Health State of complete well-being—not just the absence of disease or infirmity.

FIGURE 1.1 **Causes of death in the United States for selected years.**

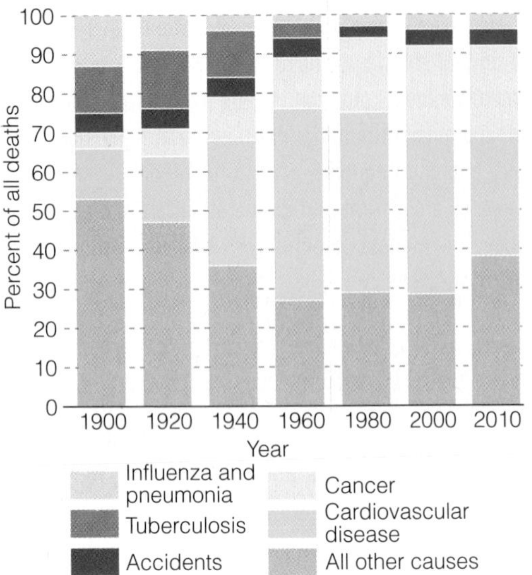

Source: National Center for Health Statistics, Division of Vital Statistics.

At the beginning of the 20th century, **life expectancy** for a child born in the United States was only 47 years. The most common health problems in the Western world were infectious diseases, such as tuberculosis, diphtheria, influenza, kidney disease, polio, and other diseases of infancy. Progress in the medical field largely eliminated these diseases. Then, as more people started to enjoy the "good life" (**sedentary** living, alcohol, fatty foods, excessive sweets, tobacco, drugs, etc.), a parallel increase appeared in the incidence of **chronic diseases** such as cardiovascular disease, cancer, diabetes, and chronic respiratory diseases (Figure 1.1). According to the World Health Organization (WHO), chronic diseases account for 60 percent of all deaths worldwide.[1]

As the incidence of chronic diseases climbed, we recognized that prevention is the best medicine. Consequently, a fitness and wellness movement developed gradually in the 1980s. We began to realize that good health is mostly self-controlled and that the leading causes of premature death and illness could be prevented by adhering to positive lifestyle habits. We all desire to live a long life, and wellness programs seek to enhance the overall quality of life—for as long as we live.

Three basic factors determine our health and longevity: genetics, the environment, and our behavior (Figure 1.2). Although we cannot change our genetic pool, we can exert control over the environment and our health behaviors so that we may reach our full physical potential based on our own genetic code. How we accomplish this goal is thoroughly discussed throughout the chapters of this book.

FIGURE 1.2 **Factors that impact health and longevity.**

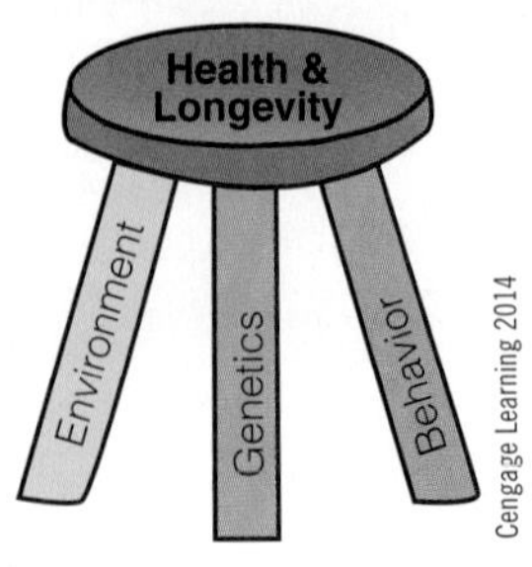

Life Expectancy

Based on the most recent data available, the average life expectancy in the United States is 78.7 years (76.3 years for men and 81.1 years for women). While in the past decade alone life expectancy has increased by 1 year, the news is not all good. The data show that people now spend an extra 1.2 years with a serious illness and an extra 2 years experiencing disability. Mortality has been postponed, because medical treatments allow people to live longer with various chronic ailments (cardiovascular disease, cancer, diabetes, etc).

Based on WHO data, the United States ranks 33rd in the world for life expectancy (Figure 1.3). Japan ranks first in the world, with an overall life expectancy of 82.6 years. While the United States was once a world leader in life expectancy, over recent years, the increase in life expectancy in the United States has not kept pace with that of other developed countries.

FIGURE 1.3 **Life expectancy at birth for selected countries: 2005–2015 projections.**

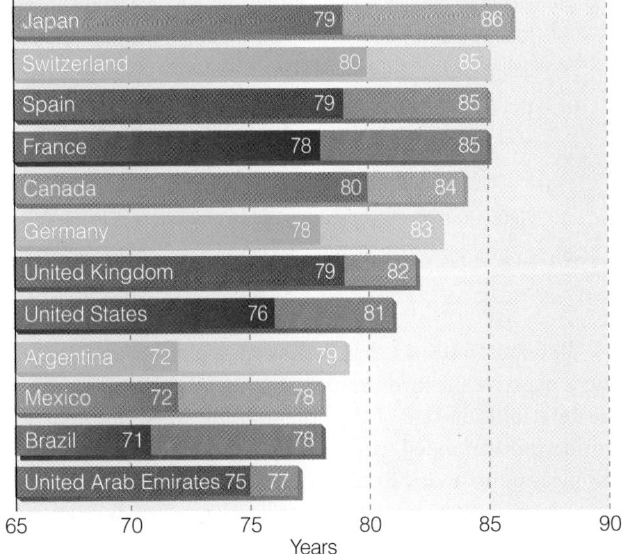

Source: United Nations, "Social Indicators: Indicators on Health," http://unstats.un.org/unsd/demographic/products/socind/health.htm, downloaded January 9, 2012.

DIVERSITY CONSIDERATIONS

Life expectancy in the United States has increased by 9 years since 1960. There is, however, a disparity among ethnic groups. Asian Americans live the longest, while African Americans have the shortest lifespan.

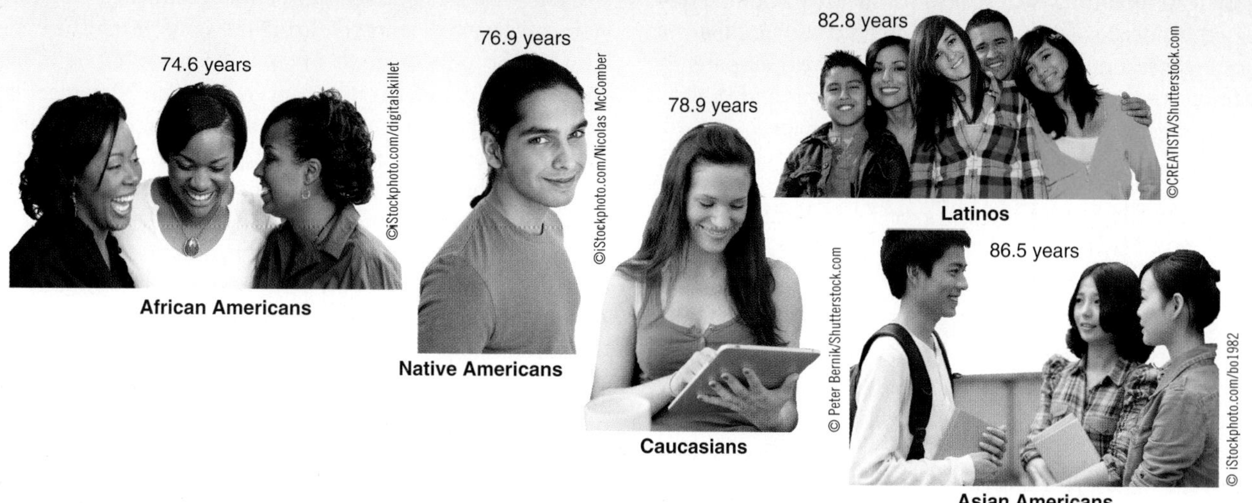

Decreasing Disparities: Improving lifestyle, how one grows up (e.g., access to health care, physical activity, good nutrition, and personal safety), work environment, and conditions under which one grows old greatly increase the chances for a longer and healthier life. Healthy choices you make *today* dictate quality of life and wellness during older age.

Several factors may account for the current U.S. life expectancy ranking: the extremely poor health of some groups (such as Native Americans, rural African Americans, and the inner-city poor), the low level of daily physical activity, the high incidence of tobacco use and coronary heart disease, fairly high levels of violence (notably homicides), and the obesity epidemic. Furthermore, a recent report by the Organisation for Economic Cooperation and Development (OECD) found that while the United States far outspent every other country in health care cost per capita, it also easily had the highest rates of obesity of all 36 OECD countries.[2]

Life expectancy for men in the United States is almost five years lower than for women. For years it has been assumed that the difference is based on biology, but most likely the gender gap is related to lifestyle behaviors most commonly observed in men. Around 1980, the gender gap in life expectancy was almost 8 years. This decrease in the gender gap is thought to be due to the fact that women are increasingly taking on jobs, habits, and stressors of men such as smoking, drinking, and employment outside the home.

Men, nonetheless, still report higher stress on the job and are less likely to engage in stress management programs. Also, 95 percent of employees in the 10 most dangerous jobs are men. Furthermore, men's health is not given the same degree of attention in terms of public health policies. Fewer programs are available that specifically target men's health issues. Thus, men need to take a more proactive role for their own health and public health policies.

"Masculinity" itself is also partially to blame. Men are less likely to visit a physician when something is wrong and are less likely to heed preventive care visits to be screened for potential risk factors such as hypertension, elevated cholesterol, diabetes, obesity, substance abuse, and depression or anxiety. Chronic diseases in men are often diagnosed at a later stage, when a cure or adequate management is more difficult to achieve.

Men typically drive faster than women and are more likely to engage in risk-taking activities. Of all road traffic fatalities among countries studied in the most recent OECD report, a disparate 74 percent of victims were men.

Although life expectancy in the United States has gradually increased by 30 years over the past century, scientists from the National Institute of Aging believe that in the coming decades, the average lifespan may decrease by as much as five years. This decrease in life expectancy will be related primarily to the growing challenges of inactivity and obesity. According to current estimates from the Centers

Life expectancy Number of years a person is expected to live based on the person's birth year.

Sedentary Description of a person who is relatively inactive and whose lifestyle is characterized by a lot of sitting.

Chronic diseases Illnesses that develop as a result of an unhealthy lifestyle and last a long time.

for Disease Control and Prevention, 35.7 percent of the adult population in the United States is obese. As a nation, we are seeing the consequences of these numbers unfold. The latest statistical update from the American Heart Association reported that the incidence of diabetes has been climbing dramatically each year in parallel step with the increased incidence of obesity.[3] If this trend continues, the current generation of children may not outlive their parents. Additional information on the obesity epidemic and its detrimental health consequences is given in Chapter 5.

Leading Health Problems in the United States

The leading causes of death in the United States today are largely lifestyle related (Figure 1.4). The U.S. Centers for Disease Control and Prevention have found that 7 of 10 Americans die of preventable chronic diseases. Specifically, about 53 percent of all deaths in the United States are caused by cardiovascular disease and cancer.[4] Almost 80 percent of the latter deaths could be prevented through a healthy lifestyle program. The third- and fourth-leading causes of death, respectively, are chronic lower respiratory disease (CLRD) and accidents.

The most prevalent degenerative diseases in the United States are those of the cardiovascular system. About 30 percent of all deaths in this country are attributed to diseases of the heart and blood vessels. According to the American Heart Association (AHA), 83.6 million people in the United States are afflicted with diseases of the cardiovascular system, including 78 million with hypertension (high blood pressure) and 15.4 million with coronary heart disease (CHD). (Many of these people have more than one type of cardiovascular disease.) More than 900,000 people suffer heart attacks each year, and close to 405,000 deaths occur from CHD and heart attacks. The yearly estimated direct and indirect cost of cardiovascular disease exceeds $204 billion.[5] A complete cardiovascular disease prevention program is outlined in Chapter 11.

The second-leading cause of death in the United States is cancer. Even though cancer is not the number-one killer, it is the number-one health fear of Americans. Twenty-three percent of all deaths in the United States are attributable to cancer. About 600,000 Americans died in 2014 from this disease (that is 1,600 each day), and an estimated 1.6 million new cases were diagnosed during the same year.[6] The major contributor to the increase in the incidence of cancer during the past five decades is lung cancer, of which 80 percent is caused by tobacco use. Furthermore, smoking accounts for almost 30 percent of all deaths from cancer. Another 33 percent of deaths are related to nutrition, physical inactivity, excessive body weight, and other faulty lifestyle habits.

The American Cancer Society maintains that the most influential factor in fighting cancer today is prevention through health education programs. Evidence indicates that as much as 80 percent of all human cancer can be prevented through positive lifestyle behaviors. A comprehensive cancer-prevention program is presented in Chapter 12.

CLRD, the third-leading cause of U.S. deaths, is a general term that includes chronic obstructive pulmonary disease, emphysema, and chronic bronchitis (all diseases of the respiratory system). Although CLRD is related mostly to tobacco use (see Chapter 13 for discussion on how to stop smoking), lifelong nonsmokers also can develop CLRD.

Precautions to prevent CLRD include consuming a low-fat, low-sodium, nutrient-dense diet; staying physically active; not smoking and not breathing cigarette smoke; getting a pneumonia vaccine if over age 50 and a current or ex-smoker; and avoiding swimming pools if sensitive to chlorine vapor.

Accidents are the fourth-leading cause of death in the United States. Even though not all accidents are preventable, many are. Fatal accidents are often related to abusing drugs and not wearing a seat belt. Furthermore, with the advent of cell phones, 1.6 million car accidents (at least 28 percent of all traffic crashes) each year are caused by drivers using cell phones or reading or sending text messages. A report by

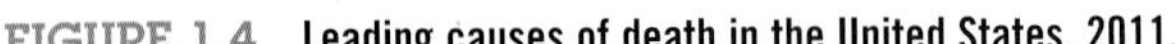

FIGURE 1.4 Leading causes of death in the United States, 2011.

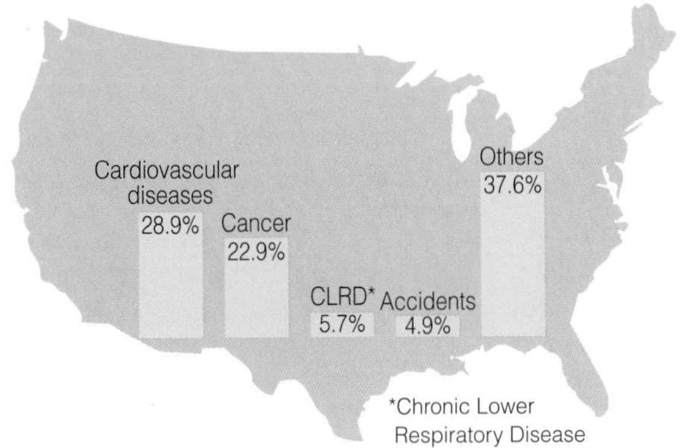

U.S. Department of Health and Human Services, Centers for Disease Control and Prevention, "Deaths: Preliminary Data for 2011," National Center for Health Statistics, National Vital Statistics Reports 61, no. 6 (October 10, 2012).

Healthy Habits That Cut Risk for Serious Disease

According to the Centers for Disease Control and Prevention, four healthy living habits can reduce your risk of chronic diseases such as heart disease, cancer, and diabetes by almost 80 percent:

- Get at least 30 minutes of daily moderate-intensity physical activity.
- Never smoke.
- Eat a healthy diet (ample fruits and vegetables, whole-grain products, and low meat consumption).
- Maintain a body mass index (BMI) under 30.

FIGURE 1.5 Death from all causes attributable to lifestyle-related risk factors for men and women in the United States.

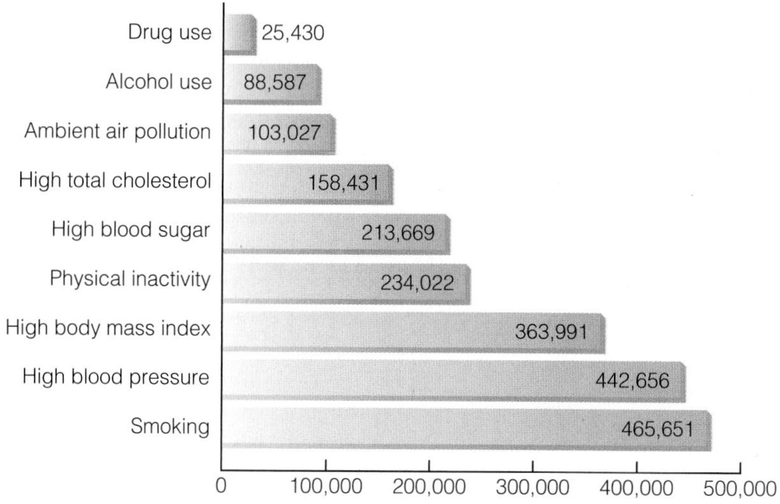

Source: Institute for Health Metrics and Evaluation News Release: July 10, 2013, "Dietary risks are leading cause of disease burden in the US and contributed to more health loss in 2010 than smoking, high blood pressure, and high blood sugar," http://www.healthmetricsandevaluation.org/news-events/news-releases, downloaded Feb. 28, 2014.

Traffic Injury Prevention indicates that texting while driving is as dangerous as driving drunk. In a simulated test, driving performance while texting was found to be at least as bad as with blood alcohol levels at or above legal driving limits. In addition to not paying attention to the road and other vehicles, the study found that people tend to increase speed and do not brake as effectively while texting.

Most people do not perceive accidents as a health problem. Even so, accidents affect the total well-being of millions of Americans each year. Accident prevention and personal safety are part of a health-enhancement program aimed at achieving better quality of life. Proper nutrition, exercise, stress management, and abstinence from cigarette smoking are of little help if the person is involved in a disabling or fatal accident as a result of distraction, a single reckless decision, or not wearing a seat belt properly.

Accidents do not just happen. We cause accidents, and we are victims of accidents. Although some factors in life, such as earthquakes, tornadoes, and airplane accidents, are beyond our control, more often than not personal safety and accident prevention are a matter of common sense. Most accidents stem from poor judgment and confused mental states, which occur when we are upset, are not paying attention to the task at hand, or are abusing alcohol or other drugs.

Alcohol abuse is the number-one cause of all U.S. accidents. About half of accidental deaths and suicides in the United States are alcohol related. Furthermore, alcohol intoxication is the nation's leading cause of fatal automobile accidents. Other commonly abused drugs alter feelings and perceptions, generate mental confusion, and impair judgment and coordination, greatly enhancing the risk for accidental **morbidity** and mortality (see Chapter 13).

The underlying causes of death attributable to leading **risk factors** in the United States (Figure 1.5) indicate that most factors are related to lifestyle choices we make. Of the approximately 2.5 million yearly deaths in the United States, the "big five" factors—tobacco smoking, high blood pressure, overweightness and obesity, physical inactivity, and high blood glucose—are responsible for almost 1.5 million deaths each year.

Lifestyle as a Health Problem

As the incidence of chronic diseases rose, it became obvious that prevention was—and remains—the best medicine. According to the U.S. Surgeon General's office, more than half of the people who die in this country each year die because of what they do. Based on estimates, more than half of disease is lifestyle related, a fifth is attributed to the environment, and a tenth is influenced by the health care the individual receives. Only 16 percent is related to genetic factors (Figure 1.6). Thus, the individual controls as much as 84 percent of his or her vulnerability to disease—and thus quality of life. The same data indicate that 83 percent of deaths before age 65 are preventable. In essence, most people in the United States are threatened by the very lives they lead today.

Because of the unhealthy lifestyles that many young adults lead, their bodies may be middle-aged or older! Many physical education programs do not emphasize the skills necessary for young people to maintain a high level of fitness and health throughout life. The intent of this book is to provide those skills and help prepare you for a lifetime of physical fitness and well-

Morbidity A condition related to or caused by illness or disease.

Risk factors Lifestyle and genetic variables that may lead to disease.

FIGURE 1.6 Estimated impact of the factors that affect health and well-being.

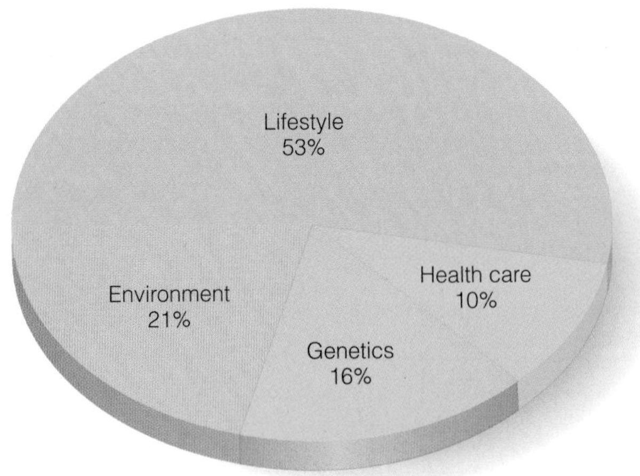

ness. A healthy lifestyle is self-controlled, and you can learn how to be responsible for your own health and fitness. Healthy choices made today influence health for decades.

Physical Activity and Exercise Defined

Abundant scientific research over the past three decades has established a distinction between physical activity and exercise. **Physical activity** is bodily movement produced by skeletal muscles. It requires energy expenditure and produces progressive health benefits. Physical activity typically requires only a low to moderate intensity of effort. Examples of physical activity include walking to and from work, taking the stairs instead of elevators and escalators, gardening, doing household chores, dancing, and washing the car by hand. Physical inactivity, by contrast, implies a level of activity that is lower than that required to maintain good health.

Exercise is a type of physical activity that requires planned, structured, and repetitive bodily movement to improve or maintain one or more components of physical fitness. Examples of exercise are walking, running, cycling, aerobics, swimming, and strength training. Exercise is usually viewed as an activity that requires vigorous-intensity effort.

Importance of Increased Physical Activity

The U.S. Surgeon General has stated that poor health as a result of lack of physical activity is a serious public health problem that must be met head-on at once. Regular **moderate physical activity** provides substantial benefits in health and well-being for the vast majority of people who are not physically active. For those who are already moderately active, even greater health benefits can be achieved by increasing the level of physical activity.

Among the benefits of regular physical activity and exercise are significantly reduced risks for developing or dying from heart disease, stroke, type 2 diabetes, colon and breast cancers, high blood pressure, osteoporotic fractures, and even dementia and Alzheimer's.[7] Regular physical activity also is important for the health of muscles, bones, and joints, and it seems to reduce symptoms of depression and anxiety, improve mood, improve memory, and enhance ability to perform daily tasks throughout life. It also can help control health care costs and maintain a high quality of life into old age.

Moderate physical activity has been defined as any activity that requires an energy expenditure of 150 calories per day, or 1,000 calories per week. The general health recommendation is that people strive to accumulate 150 minutes of moderate-intensity physical activity per week (alterna-

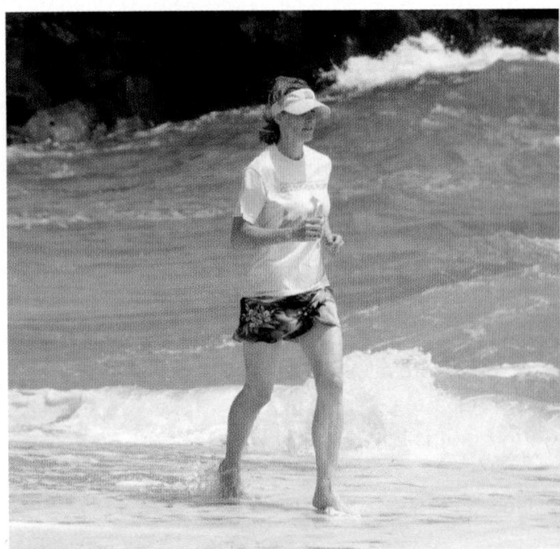

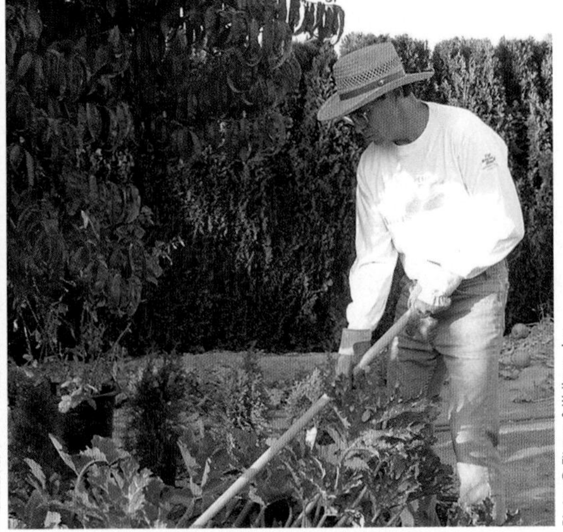

An active lifestyle increases health, quality of life, and longevity.

TABLE 1.1 Physical Activity Recommendations

Benefits	Duration	Intensity	Frequency per Week	Weekly Time
Health	30 min	MI*	≥5 times	≥150 min
Health and fitness	≥20 min	VI*	≥3 times	≥75 min
Health, fitness, and weight gain prevention	60 min	MI/VI†	5–7 times	≥300 min
Health, fitness, and weight regain prevention	60–90 min	MI/VI	5–7 times	≥450 min

*MI = moderate intensity, VI = vigorous intensity
†MI/VI = You may use MI, VI, or a combination of the two

tively 75 minutes of vigorous aerobic activity may be substituted) in addition to two strength-training sessions or activities per week. Physical activity should preferably be divided into 30-minute segments over a minimum of 5 days each week (Table 1.1). Whereas 30 minutes of continuous activity is preferred, on days when time is limited, three activity sessions of at least 10 minutes each still provide substantial health benefits. Examples of moderate physical activity are brisk walking or cycling, playing basketball or volleyball, swimming, water aerobics, fast dancing, pushing a stroller, raking leaves, shoveling snow, washing or waxing a car, washing windows or floors, and even gardening. Light-intensity activities of daily living such as casual walking, self-care, shopping, or activities lasting less than 10 minutes cannot be included as part of the moderate physical activity recommendation.

Although accumulating 30 minutes of moderate- or vigorous-intensity physical activity provide substantial health benefits, new data indicate that most of these benefits may be voided if people spend most of the rest of the day in a sedentary condition. Sitting for long periods of time seems to be an independent risk factor for premature morbidity and mortality. This topic is discussed under the heading *"Sitting Disease:" A 21st Century Chronic Disease* on page 13 in this chapter.

Because of the ever-growing epidemic of obesity in the United States and the world, adults are encouraged to increase physical activity beyond the minimum requirements and adjust caloric intake until they find their personal balance to maintain a healthy weight.[8] Individuals are also advised that additional physical activity beyond minimum thresholds is necessary for some and can provide additional health benefits for all. This recommendation goes along with evidence indicating that people who maintain healthy weight typically accumulate 1 hour of daily physical activity.[9]

In sum, although health benefits are derived from 30 minutes of physical activity performed on most days of the week, people with a tendency to gain weight need to be physically active for longer, from 60 to as many as 90 minutes daily, to prevent weight gain. This additional activity per day provides additional health benefits, including a lower risk for cardiovascular disease and diabetes.

National Initiatives to Promote Healthy and Active Lifestyles: Federal Guidelines for Physical Activity

Because of the importance of physical activity to our health, the U.S. Department of Health and Human Services issued *Physical Activity Guidelines for Americans.* These guidelines complement the current *Dietary Guidelines for Americans* (Chapter 3, pages 123–124) as well as international recommendations issued by the World Health Organization (WHO)[10] and further substantiate previous recommendations issued by the American College of Sports Medicine (ACSM) and the AHA in 2007,[11] and the U.S. Surgeon General in 1996.[12]

The federal guidelines provide science-based guidance on the importance of being physically active to promote health and reduce the risk for chronic diseases. The federal guidelines include the following recommendations:

Adults between 18 and 64 Years of Age

- Adults should do 2 hours and 30 minutes a week of moderate-intensity aerobic (cardiorespiratory) physical activity, 1 hour and 15 minutes (75 minutes) a week of vigorous-intensity aerobic physical activity, or an

Physical activity Bodily movement produced by skeletal muscles, which requires expenditure of energy and produces progressive health benefits. Examples include walking, taking the stairs, dancing, gardening, working in the yard, cleaning the house, shoveling snow, washing the car, and all forms of structured exercise.

Exercise A type of physical activity that requires planned, structured, and repetitive bodily movement with the intent of improving or maintaining one or more components of physical fitness.

Moderate physical activity Activity that uses 150 calories of energy per day, or 1,000 calories per week.

equivalent combination of moderate- and vigorous-intensity aerobic physical activity (also see Chapter 6). When combining moderate- and vigorous-intensity activities, a person could participate in moderate-intensity activity twice a week for 30 minutes and high-intensity activity for 20 minutes on another 2 days. Aerobic activity should be performed in episodes each at least 10 minutes long, preferably spread throughout the week.

- Additional health benefits are provided by increasing to 5 hours (300 minutes) a week of moderate-intensity aerobic physical activity, 2 hours and 30 minutes a week of vigorous-intensity physical activity, or an equivalent combination of both.
- Adults should also do muscle-strengthening activities that involve all major muscle groups, performing them 2 or more days per week.

Older Adults (Ages 65 and Older)

- Older adults should follow the adult guidelines. If this is not possible due to limiting chronic conditions, older adults should be as physically active as their abilities allow. They should avoid inactivity. Older adults should do exercises that maintain or improve balance if they are at risk of falling.

Children 6 Years of Age and Older and Adolescents

- Children and adolescents should do 1 hour or more of physical activity every day. Most of the 1 hour or more a day should be either moderate- or vigorous-intensity aerobic physical activity.
- As part of their daily physical activity, children and adolescents should do vigorous-intensity activity at least 3 days per week. They also should do muscle- and bone-strengthening activities at least 3 days per week.

Pregnant and Postpartum Women

- Healthy women who are not already doing vigorous-intensity physical activity should get at least 2 hours and 30 minutes (150 minutes) of moderate-intensity aerobic activity a week. Preferably, this activity should be spread throughout the week. Women who regularly engage in vigorous-intensity aerobic activity or high amounts of activity can continue their activity provided that their condition remains unchanged and they talk to their health care provider about their activity level throughout their pregnancy.

All reports agree that an amount of physical activity that exceeds the minimum recommendations provided here for adults between 18 and 64 years of age provides even greater benefits and is recommended for individuals who wish to further improve personal fitness, reduce the risk for chronic disease and disabilities, prevent premature mortality, or prevent unhealthy weight gain. College graduates are more likely to adhere to the recommendations (about 53 percent of them), followed by individuals with some college education and then high school graduates; the least likely to meet the recommendations are those with less than a high school diploma (37.8 percent).[13]

In conjunction with the preceding report, the ACSM and the American Medical Association (AMA) launched a nationwide "Exercise Is Medicine" program.[14] The goal of this initiative is to help improve the health and wellness of the nation through exercise prescriptions from physicians and health care providers. It calls on all physicians to assess and review every patient's physical activity program at every visit.

Exercise is medicine, and it's free. All physicians should be prescribing exercise to all patients and participating in exercise themselves. Exercise is considered the much-needed vaccine of our time to prevent chronic diseases. Physical activity and exercise are powerful tools for both the treatment and the prevention of chronic diseases and premature death. Additional information on this program can be obtained by consulting www.exerciseismedicine.org.

National Health Objectives for 2020 Every 10 years, the U.S. Department of Health and Human Services releases a list of objectives for preventing disease and promoting health. Since 1979, the *Healthy People* initiative has set and monitored national health objectives to meet a range of health needs, encourage collaborations across government sectors, guide individuals toward making informed health decisions, and measure the effect of prevention activity. Currently, *Healthy People* is leading the way to achieve increased quality and years of healthy life and seeking to eliminate health disparities among all groups of people. The objectives address three important points[15]:

1. *Personal responsibility for health behavior.* Individuals need to become ever more health conscious. Responsible and informed behaviors are the keys to good health.

CRITICAL THINKING

Do you consciously incorporate physical activity into your daily lifestyle? Can you provide examples? Do you think you get sufficient daily physical activity to maintain good health?

2. *Health benefits for all people and all communities.* Lower socioeconomic conditions and poor health often are interrelated. Extending the benefits of good health to all people is crucial to the health of the nation.
3. *Health promotion and disease prevention.* A shift from treatment to preventive techniques will drastically cut health care costs and help all Americans achieve better quality of life.

Developing these health objectives involves more than 10,000 people representing 300 national organizations, including the Institute of Medicine of the National Academy of Sciences, all state health departments, and the federal Office of Disease Prevention and Health Promotion. Figure 1.7 summarizes the key 2020 objectives. Living the fitness and wellness principles provided in this book will enhance the

FIGURE 1.7 Selected health objectives for the year 2020.

- Increase the proportion of persons with health insurance, a usual primary care provider, and coverage for clinical preventive services.
- Ensure that all people, including those with illnesses and chronic disability, participate daily in meaningful and freely chosen recreation, leisure, and physical activity, which directly influences well-being and quality of life.
- Reduce the proportion of adults who engage in no leisure-time physical activity.
- Increase the proportion of adolescents and adults who meet current federal physical activity guidelines.
- Increase the proportion of adults who are at a healthy weight, and reduce the proportion of children, adolescents, and adults who are overweight or obese.
- Reduce coronary heart disease and stroke deaths.
- Reduce the mean total blood cholesterol levels among adults and the proportion of persons in the population with hypertension.
- Increase the proportion of adults aged 20 years and older who are aware of, and respond to, early warning symptoms and signs of a heart attack and stroke.
- Reduce the overall cancer death rate and provide counseling about cancer prevention.
- Reduce the diabetes death rate and the annual number of new cases of diagnosed diabetes in the population.
- Reduce infections caused by key pathogens commonly transmitted through food.
- Increase the proportion of sexually active persons who use condoms.
- Reduce the rate of HIV transmission among adults and adolescents, and reduce the number of deaths resulting from HIV infection.
- Increase the proportion of substance-abuse treatment facilities that offer HIV/AIDS education, counseling, and support.
- Increase school-based health promotion programs available to youths between the ages of 14 and 22 to decrease the rate of sexually transmitted diseases and teen pregnancy and to increase the proportion of adolescents who abstain from sexual intercourse or use condoms if sexually active.
- Reduce tobacco use by adults and adolescents and reduce the initiation among children, adolescents, and young adults.
- Reduce average annual alcohol consumption and increase the proportion of adolescents who disapprove of substance abuse.
- Increase the proportion, among persons who need alcohol and/or illicit drug treatment, of those who receive specialized treatment for abuse or dependence.
- Reduce drug-induced deaths.

quality of your life and allow you to be an active participant in achieving the *Healthy People 2020* objectives.

National Physical Activity Plan Established in 2010, the *National Physical Activity Plan* calls for policy, environmental, and cultural changes to help all Americans enjoy the health benefits of physical activity. It aims to increase physical activity among all segments of the population. The plan is a comprehensive private–public sector joint effort to create a culture that supports active lifestyles and enables everyone to meet physical activity guidelines throughout life.

The vision of the plan is that one day all Americans will be physically active and will live, work, and play in environments that facilitate regular physical activity. The plan complements the federal *Physical Activity Guidelines* and the *Healthy People 2020* objectives and comprises recommendations organized in eight sectors of societal influence: education; business and industry; health care; mass media; park recreation, fitness, and sports; public health; volunteer and nonprofit; and transportation, land use, and community design. Strategies to implement the plan include the following:

- Developing and implementing policies requiring school accountability for quality and quantity of physical education and physical activity
- Encouraging early childhood education programs to have children as physically active as possible
- Providing access to and opportunities for physical activity before and after school
- Making physical activity a patient "vital sign" (tracking activity levels) that all health care providers assess and discuss with patients
- Using routine performance measures by local, state, and federal agencies to set benchmarks for active travel (walking, biking, and public transportation)
- Enhancing the existing parks and recreation infrastructure with effective policy and environmental changes to promote physical activity
- Identifying and disseminating best-practice models for physical activity in the workplace
- Providing tax breaks for building owners or employers who support active commuting and provide amenities in workplaces, including showers in buildings, secure bicycle parking, free bicycles, or transit subsidies
- Encouraging businesses to implement work policies that allow employees to get some physical activity before, during, or after work hours

The implementation of the *National Physical Activity Plan* requires cooperation among school officials, city and county council members, state legislators, corporations, and Congress.

Monitoring Daily Physical Activity

The majority of U.S. adults are not sufficiently physically active to promote good health. The most recent data released in 2013 by the Centers for Disease Control and Prevention (CDC) indicate that only 19.4 percent of U. S. adults 18 and over meet the Federal Physical Activity Guidelines for both aerobic and muscular fitness (strength and endurance) activities, whereas 46.1 percent meet the guidelines for aerobic fitness and just 23 percent do so for muscular fitness. Another 34 percent of Americans are completely inactive during their leisure time (Figure 1.8).

Other than carefully monitoring actual time engaged in activity, an excellent tool to monitor daily physical activity is a **pedometer**. A pedometer is a small mechanical device that senses vertical body motion and is used to count footsteps. Wearing a pedometer throughout the day allows you to determine the total steps you take in a day. Some pedometers also record distance, calories burned, speeds, and actual time of activity each day. A pedometer is a great motivational tool to help increase, maintain, and monitor daily physical activity that involves lower-body motion (walking, jogging, and running).

Before purchasing a pedometer, be sure to verify its accuracy. Many free and low-cost pedometers provided by corporations for promotion and advertisement purposes are inaccurate, so their use is discouraged. Pedometers also tend to lose accuracy at a very slow walking speed (slower than 30 minutes per mile) because the vertical movement of the hip is too small to trigger the spring-mounted lever arm inside the pedometer to properly record the steps taken.

You can obtain a good pedometer for about $25, and ratings are available online. The most accurate pedometer brands are Walk4Life, Yamax, Kenz, and New Lifestyles. To test the accuracy of a pedometer, follow these steps: Clip the pedometer on your waist directly above a kneecap, reset the pedometer to zero, carefully close the pedometer, walk exactly 50 steps at your normal pace, carefully open the pedometer, and look at the number of steps recorded. A reading within 10 percent of the actual steps taken (45 to 55 steps) is acceptable.

The typical male American takes about 6,000 steps per day, in comparison to the typical woman, who takes about 5,300 steps. The general recommendation for adults is 10,000 steps per day. Table 1.2 provides specific activity categories based on the number of daily steps taken.

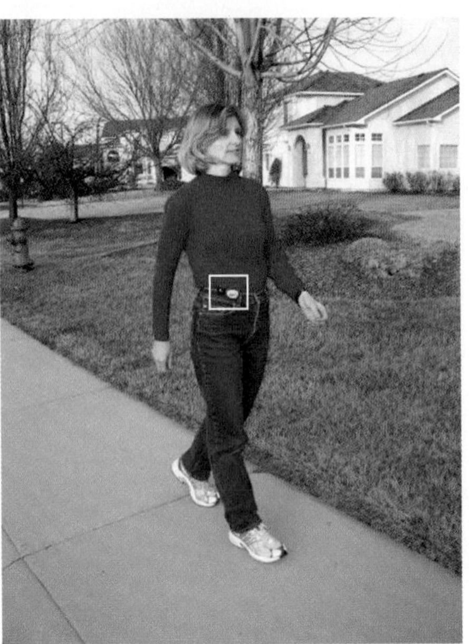

Pedometers are used to monitor daily physical activity; the recommendation is a minimum of 10,000 steps per day.

All daily steps count, but some of your steps should come in bouts of at least 10 minutes to meet the national physical activity recommendation of accumulating 30 minutes of moderate-intensity physical activity in at least three 10-minute sessions 5 days per week. A 10-minute brisk walk (a distance of about 1,200 yards at a 15-min/mile pace) is approximately 1,300 steps. A 15-min/mile (1,770 yards) walk is about 1,900 steps.[16] Thus, new pedometer brands have an aerobic steps function that records steps taken in excess of 60 steps per minute over a 10-minute period.

If you do not accumulate the recommended 10,000 daily steps, you can refer to Table 1.3 to determine the additional walking or jogging distance required to reach your goal. For example, if you are 5′8″ tall, are female, and typically accumulate 5,200 steps per day, you would need an additional 4,800 daily steps to reach your 10,000-steps goal. You can do so by jogging 3.0 miles at a 10-min/mile pace (1,602 steps × 3.0 miles = 4,806 steps) on some

FIGURE 1.8 Percentage of adults who did not meet and did meet the 2008 federal guidelines for physical activity and gender.

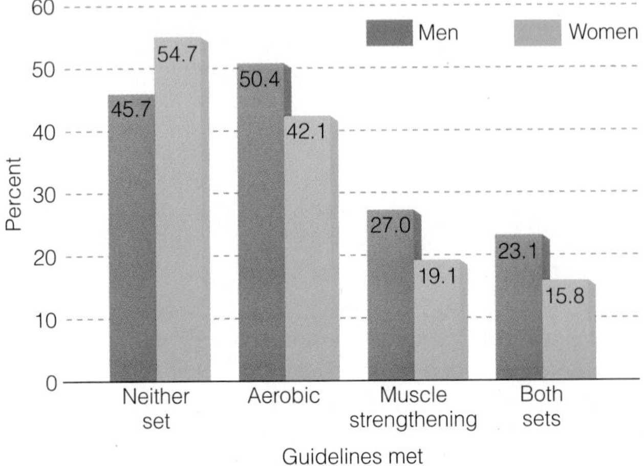

Source: http://www.cdc.gov/nchs/data/series/sr_10/sr10_257.pdf (downloaded July 9,2013)

TABLE 1.2 Adult Activity Levels Based on Total Number of Steps Taken per Day

Steps per day	Category
<5,000	Sedentary lifestyle
5,000–7,499	Low active
7,500–9,999	Somewhat active
10,000–12,499	Active
≥12,500	Highly active

Source: C. Tudor-Locke and D. R. Basset, "How Many Steps/Day Are Enough? Preliminary Pedometer Indices for Public Health," Sports Medicine 34 (2004): 1-8.

TABLE 1.3 Estimated Number of Steps to Walk, Jog, or Run a Mile Based on Pace, Height, and Gender

	Pace (min/mile)											
	Walking								Jogging/Running			
	20		18		16		15		12	10	8	6
Height	Women	Men	Women	Men	Women	Men	Women	Men	(both men and women)			
5'0"	2,371	2,338	2,244	2,211	2,117	2,084	2,054	2,021	1,997	1,710	1,423	1,136
5'2"	2,343	2,310	2,216	2,183	2,089	2,056	2,026	1,993	1,970	1,683	1,396	1,109
5'4"	2,315	2,282	2,188	2,155	2,061	2,028	1,998	1,965	1,943	1,656	1,369	1,082
5'6"	2,286	2,253	2,160	2,127	2,033	2,000	1,969	1,937	1,916	1,629	1,342	1,055
5'8"	2,258	2,225	2,131	2,098	2,005	1,872	1,941	1,908	1,889	1,602	1,315	1,028
5'10"	2,230	2,197	2,103	2,070	1,976	1,943	1,913	1,880	1,862	1,575	1,288	1,001
6'0"	2,202	2,169	2,075	2,042	1,948	1,915	1,885	1,852	1,835	1,548	1,261	974
6'2"	2,174	2,141	2,047	2,014	1,920	1,887	1,857	1,824	1,808	1,521	1,234	947

Prediction equations (pace in min/mile and height in inches):

Walking

Women: Steps/mile = 1,949 + [(63.4 x pace) – (14.1 x height)]

Men: Steps/mile = 1,916 + [(63.4 x pace) – (14.1 x height)]

Jogging

Women and Men: Steps/mile = 1,084 + [(63.4 x pace) – (14.1 x height)]

Adapted from Werner W. K. Hoeger et al., "One-Mile Step Count at Walking and Running Speeds," *ACSM's Health & Fitness Journal*, Vol 12(1):14-19, 2008.

days, and you can walk 2.5 miles at a 15-min/mile pace (1,941 steps × 2.5 miles = 4,853 steps) on other days. If you do not find a particular speed (pace) that you typically walk or jog at in Table 1.3, you can estimate the number of steps at that speed using the prediction equations at the bottom of the table.

The first practical application that you can undertake in this course is to determine your current level of daily activity. The log provided in Lab 1A will help you do this. Keep a 4-day log of all physical activities that you do daily. On this log, record the time of day, type and duration of the exercise/activity, and if possible, number of steps taken while engaged in the activity. The results will indicate how active you are and serve as a basis to monitor changes in the next few months and years.

"Sitting Disease:" A 21st Century Chronic Disease

The human body requires time to recover (sit and sleep) from labor, tasks, and other typical daily activities. Most Americans, however, sit many hours more than ever before. On *average* people spend about 8 hours per day or more of their waking time sitting. Prolonged sitting is unnatural to the body, and research now indicates that too much sitting is hazardous to human health and has a direct link to premature mortality.[17] Although not recognized by the medical community as a diagnosable illness, the scientific community has coined the term **"sitting disease"** as a chronic 21st century disease, and an entirely new field of study has emerged termed "inactivity physiology" that works to combat the detrimental effects of excessive sitting on health and well-being.

The data indicate that the risks that come with sitting are independent from those related to physical activity levels. Like the gas or the brake pedal on a car, physical activity or prolonged sitting each act upon human physiology in their own, independent ways. Therefore, even if people exercise five times per week for at least 30 minutes but otherwise spend most of the rest of the day sitting, they are accruing health risks as quickly as they are preventing them.

Our bodies are simply not designed for extended periods of sitting. As we sink into inactivity, our biological processes begin to change, down to a cellular and molecular level. Researchers are only beginning to understand all of the factors at work, but studies show, for example, that blood flow becomes sluggish and is more likely to form life-threatening clots in the lungs and legs. Blood sugar levels drop. And after meals, blood sugar levels spike due to inactive skeletal muscles, which are responsible for 80 percent of glucose disposal when active. The level of triglycerides in the blood jump during inactivity, because muscles stop producing an enzyme that usually captures this type of fat from the blood in order to turn it into fuel. Even HDL cholesterol levels (the good cholesterol) drop 20 percent after as little as one hour of uninterrupted sitting. Inactivity also appears to switch on or off dozens of genes that trigger additional risk factors.

The results of excessive sitting have a direct consequence on pre-

Pedometer An electronic device that senses body motion and counts footsteps. Some pedometers also record distance, calories burned, speed, "aerobic steps," and time spent being physically active.

mature mortality. Death rates are high for people who spend most of their day sitting, even though they meet the minimum physical activity recommendations on a weekly basis. The data show that:

- Time spent sitting correlates to overall health: The more time you spend sitting throughout the day, the greater the risk for adverse health effects.
- Sitting for more than 3 hours per day cuts off two years of life, even if you regularly exercise and avoid unhealthy habits like smoking.
- Physically inactive women and men who sit more than 6 hours a day have an almost 100 and an almost 50 percent greater chance, respectively, of dying during a span of a little over a decade than their physically active peers who sit less than 3 hours per day.
- People who spend most of their day sitting have as much as a 50 percent greater risk of dying prematurely from all causes and an 80 percent greater risk of dying from cardiovascular disease.
- Inactive adults over age 60 are at almost 50 percent greater odds of disability for each additional hour they sit per day.[18]
- Among many other conditions, excessive sitting leads to weaker muscles, a sluggish central nervous system, decreased cognitive function, increased fatigue, obesity, decreased insulin sensitivity, higher blood pressure, decreased activity of lipoprotein lipase (an enzyme that breaks down fats in the blood), and increased cholesterol, LDL cholesterol, and triglycerides.
- Excessive sitting is the "new smoking." The risk of a heart attack in people who sit most of the day is almost the same as that of smokers.
- Prolonged daily sitting time, independent of the daily physical activity/exercise routine, is an underestimated risk factor for cancer and has an effect on overall risk of premature death. Too much sitting has been estimated to cause 92,000 cancer deaths each year in the United States alone (49,000 breast cancers and 42,000 colon cancers).
- Americans who decrease their sitting time in half can expect a 2-year increase in life expectancy. Furthermore, reducing TV viewing to less than 2 hours per day adds another 1.4 years of life.

Most people do not realize how much time they spend sitting each day. On any given day, consider the amount of time that you spend driving to and from school or work (1 hour); sitting in classes or working at the office (8 hours); eating meals (1 to 1.5 hours), doing homework (2 to 4 hours), or spending a few recreational hours watching TV, at the movies, or at the computer surfing the net, checking e-mail, playing games, and visiting social networking sites (2 to 6 hours). You can easily accumulate 8 to 12 or more sitting hours.

You can fight sitting disease by taking actions to break up periods of inactivity and to become more physically active. The key is to sit less and move more. To minimize inactivity when you have limited time and space, look to enhance daily **nonexercise activity thermogenesis (NEAT)** or the energy expended doing daily activities not related to, exercise. Aim to achieve NEAT for 10 minutes every waking hour. Examples of such activities include:

- Walk instead of drive when you only need to go short distances.
- Park farther away or get off the subway, train, or bus several blocks from the campus or office.
- Take a short walk right after each meal or snack.
- Walk faster than usual.
- Move about whenever you take a break.
- Take the stairs as often as you can. Walk up and down the escalators when you don't have a choice of stairs.
- When watching TV, stand up and move during each commercial break, or even better, workout during TV time.
- Do not shy away from housecleaning chores or yard work.
- Stand more while working/studying. Place your computer on an elevated stand or shelf and stand while doing work, writing e-mails, or surfing the Internet. Standing triples the energy requirement of doing a similar activity sitting.
- Always stand while talking on the phone.
- When reading a book, get up and move after every 6 to 10 pages of the book.
- Use a stability ball for a chair. Such use enhances body stability, balance, and abdominal, low-back, and leg-strength.
- Whenever feasible, walk while conversing or holding meetings.
- Walk to classmates' homes or coworkers' offices to study or discuss matters with them instead of using the phone, e-mail, or computer.
- Take intermittent 10-minute breaks for every hour that you are at the computer or studying. Stretching, walking around, or talking to others while standing or walking is beneficial.

Wellness

Most people recognize that participating in fitness programs improves their quality of life. At the end of the 20th century, however, we came to realize that physical fitness alone was not always sufficient to lower the risk for disease and ensure better health. For example, individuals who run 3 miles (about 5 km) a day, lift weights regularly, participate in stretching exercises, and watch their body weight might be easily classified as having good or excellent fitness. Offsetting these good habits, however, might be risk factors including high blood pressure, smoking, excessive stress, drinking too much alcohol, and eating too many foods high in saturated fat. These factors place people at risk for cardiovascular disease and other chronic diseases of which they may not be aware. Thus, a new concept that is rapidly gaining popularity is **primordial prevention**, or the prevention of the development of risk factors for disease.

Even though most people are aware of their unhealthy behaviors, they seem satisfied with life as long as they are free from symptoms of disease or illness. They do not contemplate change until they incur a major health problem. Nevertheless, present lifestyle habits dictate the health and well-being of tomorrow.

Good health should not to be viewed simply as the absence of illness. The notion of good health has evolved considerably and continues to change as scientists learn more about lifestyle factors that bring on illness and affect wellness. Furthermore, once the idea took hold that fitness by itself would not always decrease the risk for disease and ensure better health, **health promotion** programs and the **wellness** concept followed.

Wellness implies a constant and deliberate effort to stay healthy and achieve the highest potential for well-being. Wellness requires implementing positive lifestyle habits to change behavior and thereby improve health and quality of life, prolong life, and achieve total well-being. Living a wellness way of life is a personal choice, but you may need additional support to achieve wellness goals. Thus, health promotion programs have been developed to educate people regarding healthy lifestyles and provide the necessary support to achieve wellness.

For example, you may be prepared to initiate an aerobic exercise program, but if you are not familiar with exercise prescription guidelines or places to exercise safely, or if you lack peer support or flexible scheduling to do so, you may have difficulty accomplishing your goal. Similarly, if you want to quit smoking but do not know how to do it and everyone else around you smokes, the chances for success are limited. To some extent, the environment limits your choices. Hence, the availability of a health promotion program provides the much-needed support to get started and implement a wellness way of life.

The Seven Dimensions of Wellness

Wellness has seven dimensions: physical, emotional, mental, social, environmental, occupational, and spiritual (Figure 1.9). These dimensions are interrelated: One frequently affects the others. For example, a person who is emotionally "down" often has no desire to exercise, study, socialize with friends, or attend church, and he or she may be more susceptible to illness and disease.

FIGURE 1.9 **Dimensions of wellness.**

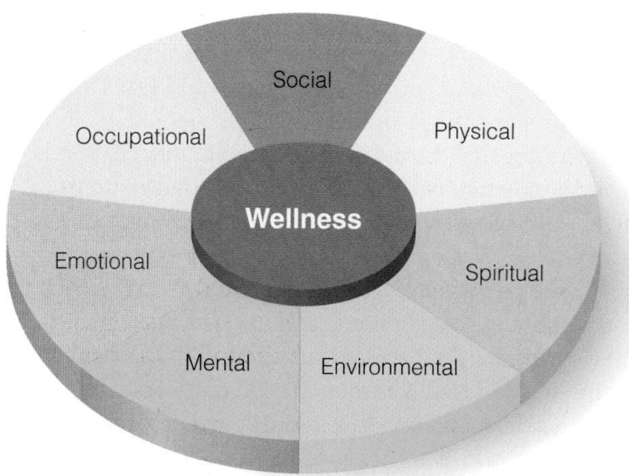

The seven dimensions show how the concept of wellness clearly goes beyond the absence of disease. Wellness incorporates factors such as adequate fitness, proper nutrition, stress management, disease prevention, spirituality, not smoking or abusing drugs, personal safety, regular physical examinations, health education, and environmental support.

For a wellness way of life, individuals must be physically fit and manifest no signs of disease. They also must be free of risk factors for disease (e.g., hypertension, hyperlipidemia, cigarette smoking, negative stress, faulty nutrition, and careless sex). The relationship between adequate fitness and wellness is illustrated in the continuum in Figure 1.10. Even though an individual tested in a fitness center may demonstrate adequate or even excellent fitness, indulging in unhealthy lifestyle behaviors still increases the risk for chronic diseases and diminishes the person's well-being.

Physical Wellness

Physical wellness is the dimension most commonly associated with being healthy. It entails confidence and optimism about the ability to protect physical health and take care of health problems.

Physically well individuals are physically active, exercise regularly, eat a well-balanced diet, maintain their recommended body weight, get sufficient sleep, practice safe sex, minimize exposure to environmental contaminants, avoid harmful drugs (including tobacco and excessive alcohol), and seek medical care and exams as needed. Physically well people also exhibit good cardiorespiratory endurance, adequate muscular strength and flexibility, proper body composition, and the ability to carry out ordinary and unusual demands of daily life safely and effectively.

Emotional Wellness

Emotional wellness involves the ability to understand your own feelings, accept your limitations, and achieve emotional stability. Furthermore, it implies the ability to express emotions appropri-

Primordial prevention Prevention of the development of risk factors for disease.

Health promotion The science and art of enabling people to increase control over their lifestyle to move toward a state of wellness.

Wellness The constant and deliberate effort to stay healthy and achieve the highest potential for well-being. It encompasses seven dimensions—physical, emotional, mental, social, environmental, occupational, and spiritual—and integrates them all into a quality life.

Physical wellness Good physical fitness and confidence in your personal ability to take care of health problems.

Emotional wellness The ability to understand your own feelings, accept your limitations, and achieve emotional stability.

FIGURE 1.10 **Wellness continuum.**

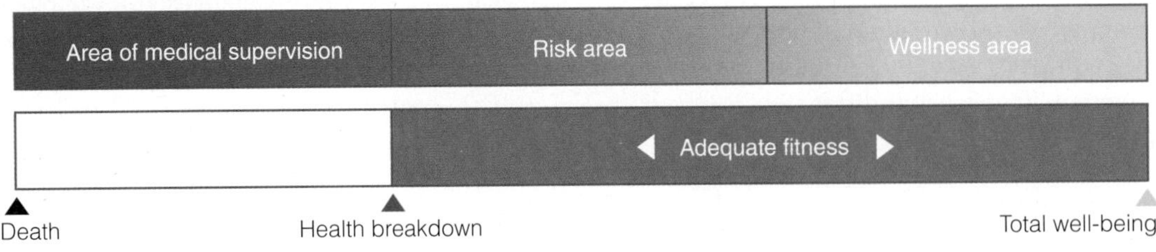

ately, adjust to change, cope with stress in a healthy way, and enjoy life despite its occasional disappointments and frustrations.

Emotional wellness brings with it a certain level of stability, an ability to look both success and failure squarely in the face and keep moving along a predetermined course. When success is evident, the emotionally well person radiates the expected joy and confidence. When failure seems evident, the emotionally well person responds by making the best of circumstances and moving beyond the failure. Wellness enables you to move ahead with optimism and energy instead of spending time and talent worrying about failure. You learn from it, identify ways to avoid it in the future, and then go on with the business at hand.

In addition, emotional wellness involves happiness—an emotional anchor that gives meaning and joy to life. Happiness is a long-term state of mind that permeates the various facets of life and influences our outlook. Although there is no simple recipe for creating happiness, researchers agree that happy people are usually participants in some category of a supportive family unit in which they feel loved. Healthy, happy people enjoy friends, work hard at something fulfilling, get plenty of exercise, and enjoy play and leisure time. They know how to laugh, and they laugh often. They give of themselves freely to others and seem to have found deep meaning in life.

An attitude of true happiness signals freedom from the tension and depression that many people endure. Emotionally well people are obviously subject to the same kinds of depression and unhappiness that occasionally plague us all, but the difference lies in the ability to bounce back. Well people take minor setbacks in stride and have the ability to enjoy life despite it all. They don't waste energy or time recounting the situation, wondering how they could have changed it, or dwelling on the past.

Mental Wellness

Mental wellness, also referred to as intellectual wellness, implies that you can apply the things you have learned, create opportunities to learn more, and engage your mind in lively interaction with the world around you. When you are mentally well, you are not intimidated by facts and figures with which you are unfamiliar; rather, you embrace the chance to learn something new. Your confidence and enthusiasm enable you to approach any learning situation with eagerness that leads to success.

Mental wellness brings with it vision and promise. More than anything else, mentally well people are open-minded and accepting of others. Instead of being threatened by people who are different from themselves, they show respect and curiosity without feeling they have to conform. They are faithful to their own ideas and philosophies and allow others the same privilege. Their self-confidence guarantees that they can take their place among others in the world without having to give up part of themselves and without requiring others to do the same.

Social Wellness

Social wellness, with its accompanying positive self-image, endows you with the ease and confidence to be outgoing, friendly, and affectionate toward others. Social wellness involves a concern for oneself and an interest in humanity and the environment as a whole.

One of the hallmarks of social wellness is the ability to relate to others and to reach out to other people, both within the family unit and outside it. Similar to emotional wellness, it involves being comfortable with your emotions and thus helps you understand and accept the emotions of others. Your own balance and sense of self allow you to extend respect and tolerance to others. Healthy people are honest and loyal. This dimension of wellness leads to the ability to maintain close relationships with other people.

Environmental Wellness

Environmental wellness refers to the effect that our surroundings have on our well-being. Our planet is a delicate ecosystem, and its health depends on the continuous recycling of its elements. Environmental wellness implies a lifestyle that maximizes harmony with Earth and takes action to protect the world around us.

Environmental threats include air pollution, chemicals, ultraviolet radiation in sunlight, water and food contamination, secondhand smoke, noise, inadequate shelter, unsatisfactory work conditions, lack of personal safety, and unhealthy relationships. Health is affected negatively when we live in a polluted, toxic, unkind, and unsafe environment.

Unfortunately, a national survey of first-year college students showed that less than 20 percent were concerned about the health of the environment.[19] To enjoy environmental wellness, we are responsible for educating and protecting ourselves against environmental hazards and protecting the environment so that we, our children, and future generations can enjoy a safe and clean environment.

Steps that you can take to live an environmentally conscious life include conserving energy (walk to your destination or ride on public transportation, do not drive unless absolutely necessary, and turn off lights and computers when not in use); not littering and politely asking others not to do it either; recycling as much as possible (paper, glass, cans, plastics, and cardboard); conserving paper and water (take shorter showers, and don't let the water run while brushing your teeth); not polluting the air, water, or earth if you can avoid doing so; not smoking; planting trees and keeping plants and shrubs alive; evaluating purchases and conveniences based on their environmental impact; donating old clothes to Goodwill, veterans' groups, or other charities; and enjoying, appreciating, and spending time outdoors in natural settings.

Occupational Wellness

Occupational wellness is not tied to high salary, prestigious position, or extravagant working conditions. Any job can bring occupational wellness if it provides rewards that are important to the individual. To one person, salary might be the most important factor, whereas another might place much greater value on creativity. Those who are occupationally well have their ideal job, which allows them to thrive.

One school of thought, developed by psychologist Fredrick Herzberg, suggests that the factors of a job that cause dissatisfaction lie on a completely separate continuum than factors that provide satisfaction. Dissatisfaction can be reduced with what Herzberg calls hygiene factors, such as a good relationship with supervisors and fair compensation; while satisfaction can be improved with motivating factors such as recognition for accomplishments or work the employee finds meaningful and satisfying. Therefore, people with occupational wellness face demands on the job, but they also have some say over demands placed on them. Any job has routine demands, but in occupational wellness, routine demands are mixed with new, unpredictable challenges that keep a job exciting. Occupationally well people are able to maximize their skills, and they have the opportunity to broaden their existing skills or gain new ones. Their occupation offers the opportunity for advancement and recognition for achievement. Occupational wellness encourages collaboration and interaction among coworkers, which fosters a sense of teamwork and support.

Spiritual Wellness

Spiritual wellness provides a unifying power that integrates all dimensions of wellness. Basic characteristics of spiritual people include a sense of meaning and direction in life and a relationship to a higher being. Pursuing these avenues may lead to personal freedom, including prayer, faith, love, closeness to others, peace, joy, fulfillment, and altruism.

Several studies have reported positive relationships among spiritual well-being, emotional well-being, and satisfaction with life. Spiritual health is somehow intertwined with physical health. People who attend church and regularly participate in religious organizations enjoy better health, have a lower incidence of chronic diseases, are more socially integrated, handle stress more effectively, and appear to live longer.[20] Other studies have shown that spirituality strengthens the immune system, is good for mental health, prevents age-related memory loss, decreases the incidence of depression, leads to fewer episodes of chronic inflammation, and decreases the risk of death and suicide.

Prayer is a signpost of spirituality at the core of most spiritual experiences. It is communication with a higher power. At least 200 studies have been conducted on the effects of prayer on health. About two-thirds of these studies have linked prayer to positive health outcomes—as long as these prayers are offered with sincerity, humility, love, empathy, and compassion. Some studies have shown faster healing time and fewer complications in patients who didn't even know they were being prayed for compared with patients who were not prayed for.[21]

Altruism, a key attribute of spiritual people, seems to enhance health and longevity. Studies indicate that people who regularly volunteer live longer. Research has found that health benefits of altruism are so powerful that doing good for others is good for oneself, especially for the immune system.

According to researchers, there seems to be a strong connection among the mind, spirit, and body: As one improves, the others follow. The relationship between spirituality and wellness is meaningful in our quest for better quality of life. As with the other dimensions, development of the spiritual dimension to its fullest potential contributes to wellness. Wellness requires a balance among all seven dimensions.

Mental wellness A state in which your mind is engaged in lively interaction with the world around you.

Social wellness The ability to relate well to others, both within and outside the family unit.

Environmental wellness The capability to live in a clean and safe environment that is not detrimental to health.

Occupational wellness The ability to perform your job skillfully and effectively under conditions that provide personal and team satisfaction and adequately reward each individual.

Spiritual wellness The sense that life is meaningful and has purpose and that some power brings all humanity together; the ethics, values, and morals that guide you and give meaning and direction to life.

Prayer Sincere and humble communication with a higher power.

Altruism Unselfish concern for the welfare of others.

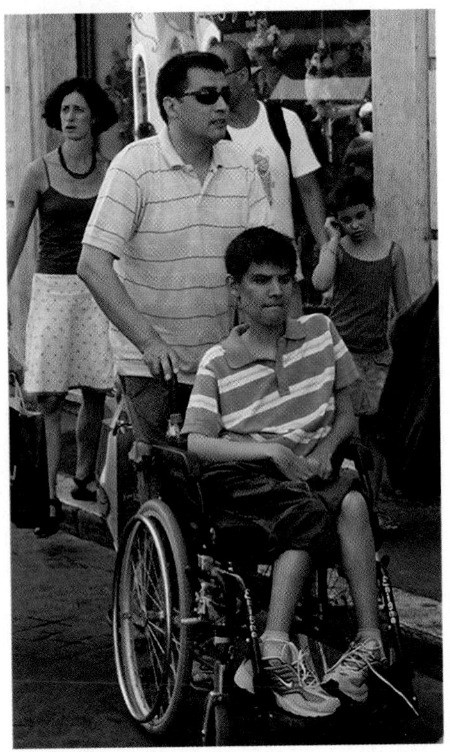

© Fitness & Wellness, Inc.

Altruism enhances health and well-being.

CRITICAL THINKING

Now that you understand the seven dimensions of wellness, rank them in order of importance to you and explain your rationale in doing so.

Wellness, Fitness, and Longevity

During the second half of the 20th century, scientists began to realize the importance of good fitness and improved lifestyle in the fight against chronic diseases, particularly those of the cardiovascular system. Because of more participation in wellness programs, cardiovascular mortality rates dropped. The decline began around 1963, and between 1960 and 2000, the incidence of cardiovascular disease dropped by 26 percent. In addition, heart attack and death rates from it have further declined by about 25 percent during the first decade of the 21st century. This decrease is credited to higher levels of wellness and better treatment modalities in the United States.

Furthermore, several studies showed an inverse relationship between physical activity and premature mortality rates. The first major study in this area was conducted in the 1980s among 16,936 Harvard alumni, and the results linked physical activity habits and mortality rates.[21] As the amount of weekly physical activity increased, the risk for cardiovascular deaths decreased. The largest decrease in cardiovascular deaths was observed among alumni who used more than 2,000 calories per week through physical activity.

A landmark study subsequently conducted at the Aerobics Research Institute in Dallas upheld the findings of the Harvard alumni study.[22] Based on data from 13,344 people followed over an average of eight years, the study revealed a graded and consistent inverse relationship between physical activity levels and mortality, regardless of age and other risk factors. As illustrated in Figure 1.11, the higher the level of physical activity, the longer the lifespan.

During the eight-year study, the death rate from all causes for the low-fit men was 3.4 times higher than that for the high-fit men. For the low-fit women, the death rate was 4.6 times higher than that for the high-fit women. A significant finding of this landmark study was the large drop in all-cause, cardiovascular, and cancer mortality when individuals went from low fitness to moderate fitness—a clear indication that moderate-intensity physical activity, achievable by most adults, provides considerable health benefits and extends life. The data also revealed that the participants attained more protection by combining higher fitness levels with reduction in other risk factors, such as hypertension, serum cholesterol, cigarette smoking, and excessive body fat.

A 2013 study looked to specifically compare the efficacy of commonly prescribed drugs against the impact of regular exercise. The data is based on more than 14,000 patients recovering from stroke, being treated for heart failure, or looking to prevent Type 2 diabetes or a second episode of coronary heart disease. The study looked at the effectiveness of exercise versus drugs on health outcomes. The results were revealing: Exercise programs were more effective than medical treatment in stroke patients and equally effective as medical treatment in patients of diabetes and coronary heart disease; only in the prevention of heart failure were diuretic drugs more effective in preventing mortality than exercise.[23]

Two additional studies reported in 2009 confirm that fitness improves wellness, quality of life, and longevity. The first study included 4,384 subjects, and the results showed that the least-fit group had an almost twofold greater risk of all-cause and cardiovascular mortalities compared with the moderately fit groups and a fourfold increased risk in comparison to the most-fit group.[24] The researchers concluded that the mortality rates between the least-fit and the other groups was most likely related to their sedentary lifestyle rather than differences in other health parameters.

The second study looked at four health-related factors among a group of more than 23,000 people.[25] These factors included lifetime nonsmoker, not considered obese (body mass index, or BMI, below 30), engaging in a minimum of 3.5 hours of weekly physical activity, and adherence to healthy nutrition principles (high consumption of whole-grain breads, fruits, and vegetables and low consumption of red meat). Those who adhered to all four health habits were 78 percent less likely to develop chronic diseases (diabetes, heart disease, stroke, and cancer) during the almost-eight-year study. Furthermore, the risk for developing a chronic disease progressively increased as the number of health factors decreased.

FIGURE 1.11 **Death rates by physical fitness groups.**

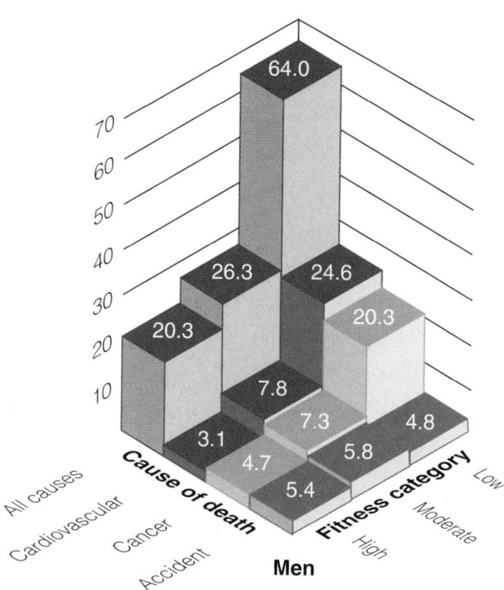

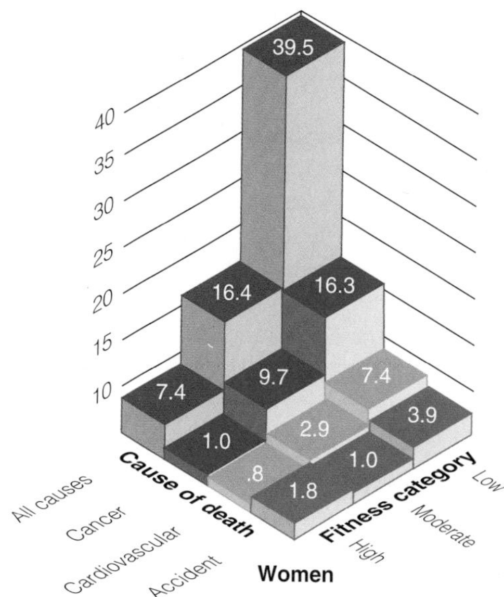

Numbers on top of the bars are all-cause death rates per 10,000 person-years of follow-up for each cell; 1 person-year indicates one person who was followed up 1 year later.
Source: Based on Data from S. N. Blair, H. W. Kohl III, R. S. Paffenbarger, Jr., G. G. Clark, K. H. Cooper, and L. W. Gibbons, "Physical Fitness and All-cause Mortality: A Prospective Study of Healthy Men and Women," Journal of the American Medical Association 262 (1989):2395-2401.

A series of studies published in 2012 in the British medical journal *The Lancet* further substantiate the importance of regular physical activity worldwide. In one of the studies, it was determined that 1 in 10 deaths is caused by physical inactivity, accounting for more than 5.3 million deaths worldwide.[26] If the inactivity rate were to go down by only 20 percent, more than 1 million lives could be saved on a yearly basis and global life expectancy would increase by almost a year.[27]

Research on the benefits of physical activity and exercise on health and longevity is too impressive to be ignored. A 2010 analysis of 33 studies involving more than 180,000 people clearly concluded that better aerobic fitness is associated with a substantially lower risk of all-cause mortality and cardiovascular disease.[28] In today's society, a person cannot afford not to participate in a lifetime physical fitness program.

While it is clear that moderate-intensity exercise provides substantial health benefits, research data also show a dose–response relationship between physical activity and health. That is, greater health and fitness benefits occur at higher duration, intensity, or both of physical activity. **Vigorous activity** and longer duration to the extent of a person's capabilities are preferable because they are most clearly associated with better health and longer life.

Vigorous-intensity exercise seems to provide the best benefits.[29] Compared with prolonged moderate-intensity activity, vigorous-intensity exercise has been shown to provide the best improvements in aerobic capacity, CHD risk reduction, and overall cardiovascular health.[30]

Furthermore, a comprehensive review of research studies found a lower rate of heart disease in vigorous-intensity exercisers compared with those who exercised at moderate intensity.[31] While no differences were found in weight loss between the two groups, greater improvements were seen in cardiovascular risk factors in the vigorous-intensity groups, including aerobic fitness, blood pressure, and blood glucose control.

A word of caution, however, is in order: Vigorous exercise should be reserved for healthy individuals who have been cleared to do so (Lab 1C) and who have been participating regularly in at least moderate-intensity activities.

Types of Physical Fitness

As the fitness concept grew at the end of the past century, it became clear that several specific components contribute to an individual's overall level of fitness. **Physical fitness** is classified into health-related and skill-related categories.

Health-related fitness relates to the ability to perform activities of daily living without undue fatigue and is conducive to a low risk of

Vigorous activity Any exercise that requires a metabolic equivalent task (MET) level equal to or greater than 6 METs (21 mL/kg/min). One MET is the energy expenditure at rest (3.5 mL/kg/min), and METs are defined as multiples of this resting metabolic rate (examples of activities that require a 6-MET level include aerobics, walking uphill at 3.5 mph, cycling at 10 to 12 mph, playing doubles in tennis, and vigorous strength training).

Physical fitness The ability to meet the ordinary, as well as unusual, demands of daily life safely and effectively without being overly fatigued and still have energy left for leisure and recreational activities.

Health-related fitness Fitness programs prescribed to improve the individual's overall health.

premature **hypokinetic diseases**. The health-related fitness components are cardiorespiratory (aerobic) endurance, muscular fitness (muscular strength and endurance), muscular flexibility, and body composition (Figure 1.12).

Skill-related fitness components consist of agility, balance, coordination, reaction time, speed, and power (Figure 1.13). These components are related primarily to successful sports and motor skill performance. Participating in skill-related activities contributes to physical fitness, but in terms of general health promotion and wellness, the main emphasis of physical fitness programs should be on the health-related components.

CRITICAL THINKING

What role do the four health-related components of physical fitness play in your life? Rank them in order of importance to you, and explain the rationale you used.

FIGURE 1.12 **Health-related components of physical fitness.**

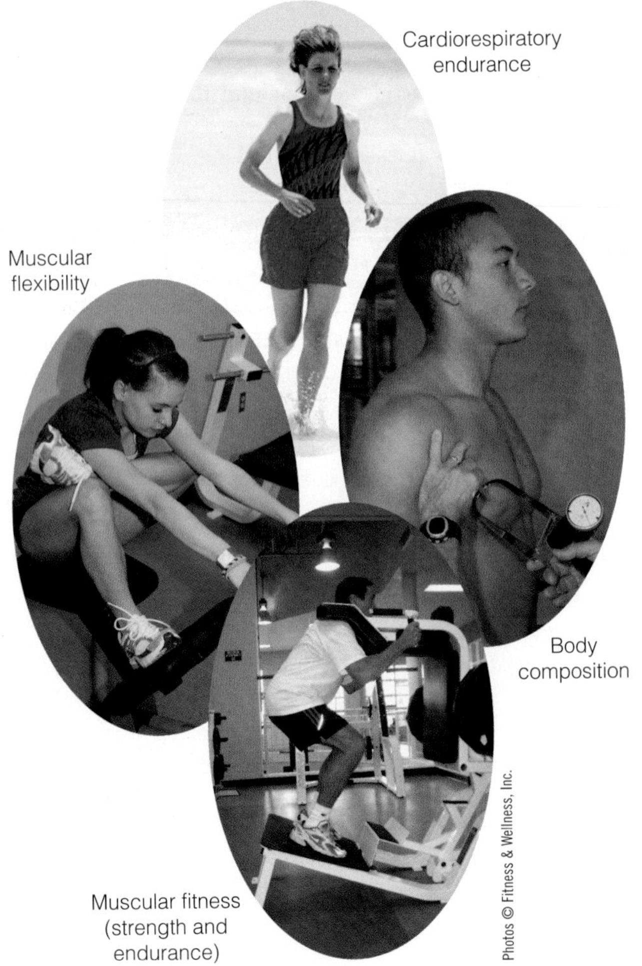

FIGURE 1.13 **Motor skill–related components of physical fitness.**

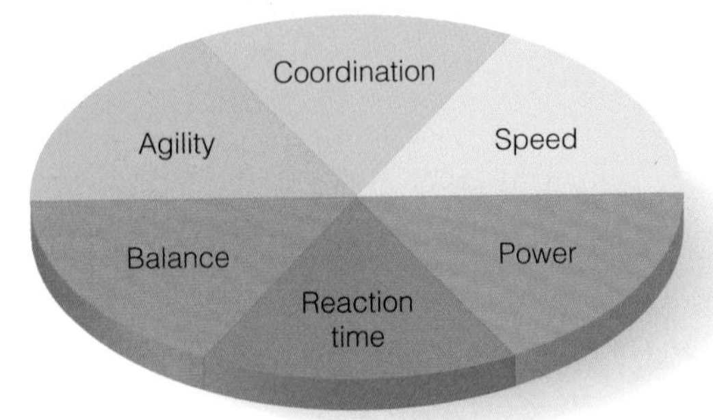

© Cengage Learning

Fitness Standards: Health versus Physical Fitness

A meaningful debate regarding age- and gender-related fitness standards has resulted in two standards: health fitness (also referred to as *criterion referenced*) and physical fitness. Both are discussed here. The assessment of health-related fitness is presented in Chapters 4, 6, 7, and 8; where appropriate, physical fitness standards are included for comparison.

Health Fitness Standards The **health fitness standards** proposed here are based on data linking minimum fitness values to disease prevention and health. Attaining health fitness standards requires only moderate physical activity. For example, a 2-mile walk in less than 30 minutes, five or six times a week, seems to be sufficient to achieve the health fitness standard for cardiorespiratory endurance.

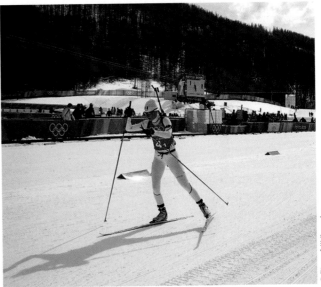

Good health-related fitness and skill-related fitness are required to participate in highly skilled activities.

As illustrated in Figure 1.14, significant health benefits can be reaped with such a program, although fitness improvements, expressed in terms of maximum oxygen uptake, or VO_{2max} (explained next and in Chapter 6), are not as notable. Nevertheless, health improvements are quite striking. These benefits include reduction in blood lipids, lower blood pressure, weight loss, stress release, less risk for diabetes, and lower risk for disease and premature mortality.

More specifically, improvements in **metabolic profile** (measured by insulin sensitivity, glucose tolerance, and improved cholesterol levels) can be notable despite little or no weight loss or improvement in aerobic capacity. Metabolic fitness can be attained through an active lifestyle and moderate-intensity physical activity.

An assessment of health-related fitness uses **cardiorespiratory endurance** measured in terms of the maximal amount of oxygen the body is able to utilize per minute of physical activity (VO_{2max})—essentially, a measure of how efficiently the heart, lungs, and muscles can operate during aerobic exercise (see Chapter 6). VO_{2max} is commonly expressed in milliliters (mL) of oxygen (volume of oxygen) per kilogram (kg) of body weight per minute (mL/kg/min). Individual values can range from about 10 mL/kg/min in cardiac patients to more than 80 mL/kg/min in world-class runners, cyclists, and cross-country skiers.

Research data from the study presented in Figure 1.11 reported that achieving VO_{2max} values of 35 and 32.5 mL/kg/min for men and women, respectively, may be sufficient to lower the risk for all-cause mortality significantly. Although greater improvements in fitness yield an even lower risk for premature death, the largest drop is seen between the least fit and the moderately fit. Therefore, the 35 and 32.5 mL/kg/min values could be selected as health fitness standards.

Physical Fitness Standards

Physical fitness standards are set higher than health fitness standards and require a more intense exercise program. Physically fit people of all ages have the freedom to enjoy most of life's daily and recreational activities to their fullest potentials. Current health fitness standards may not be enough to achieve these objectives.

Sound physical fitness gives the individual a degree of independence throughout life that many people in the United States no longer enjoy. Most adults should be able to carry out activities similar to those they conducted in their youth, though not with the same intensity. These standards do not require being a championship athlete, but activities such as changing a tire, chopping wood, climbing several flights of stairs, playing basketball, mountain biking, playing soccer with children or grandchildren, walking several miles around a lake, and hiking through a national park require more than the current average fitness level of most Americans.

Hypokinetic diseases *Hypo* denotes "lack of"; therefore, illnesses related to lack of physical activity.

Skill-related fitness Fitness components important for success in skillful activities and athletic events; encompasses agility, balance, coordination, reaction time, speed, and power.

Health fitness standards The lowest fitness requirements for maintaining good health, decreasing the risk for chronic diseases, and lowering the incidence of muscular–skeletal injuries.

Metabolic profile A measurement of plasma insulin, glucose, lipid, and lipoprotein levels to assess risk for diabetes and cardiovascular disease.

Cardiorespiratory endurance The ability of the lungs, heart, and blood vessels to deliver adequate amounts of oxygen to the cells to meet the demands of prolonged physical activity.

Physical fitness standards A fitness level that allows a person to sustain moderate-to-vigorous physical activity without undue fatigue and the ability to closely maintain this level throughout life.

FIGURE 1.14 Health and fitness benefits based on type of lifestyle and physical activity program.

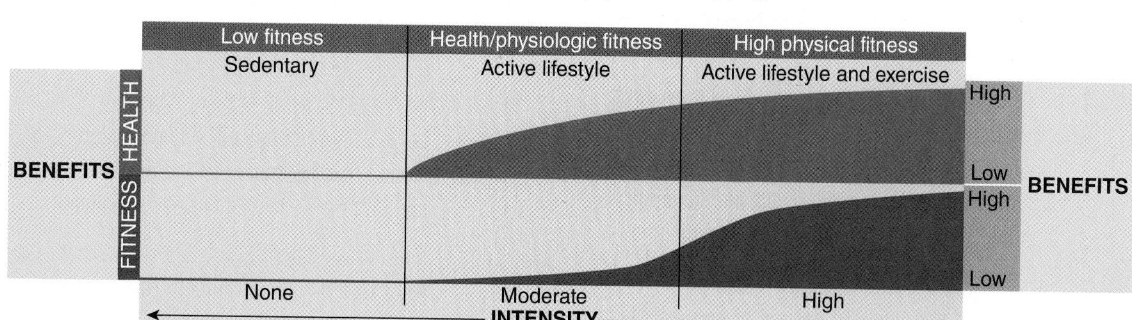

Source: Fitness & Wellness, Inc.

BEHAVIOR MODIFICATION PLANNING

Financial Fitness Prescription

Although not one of the components of physical fitness, taking control of your personal finances is critical for your success and well-being. The sooner you start working on a lifetime personal financial plan, the more successful you will be in becoming financially secure and being able to retire early, in comfort, if you choose to do so. Most likely, you have not been taught basic principles to improve personal finance and enjoy "financial fitness." Thus, start today using the following strategies:

I PLAN TO	I DID IT	
❑	❑	1. Develop a personal financial plan. Set short-term and long-term financial goals for yourself. If you do not have financial goals, you cannot develop a plan or work toward that end.
❑	❑	2. Subscribe to a personal finance magazine or newsletter. In the same way that you should regularly read reputable fitness/wellness journals or newsletters, you should regularly peruse a "financial fitness" magazine. If you don't enjoy reading financial materials, then find a periodical that is quick and to the point; there are many available. You don't have to force yourself to read the *Wall Street Journal* to become financially knowledgeable. Many periodicals have resources to help you develop a financial plan. Educate yourself and stay current on personal finances and investment matters.
❑	❑	3. Set up a realistic budget and live on less than you make. Pay your bills on time and keep track of *all* expenses. Then develop your budget so that you spend less than you earn. Your budget may require that you either cut back on expenses and services or figure out a way to increase your income. Balance your checkbook regularly and do not overdraft your checking account. Remind yourself that satisfaction comes from being in control of the money you earn.
❑	❑	4. Learn to differentiate between wants and needs. It is fine to reward yourself for goals that you have achieved (see Chapter 2), but limit your spending to items that you truly need. Avoid simple impulse spending because "it's a bargain" or something you just want to have.
❑	❑	5. Pay yourself first; save 10 percent of your income each month. Before you take any money out of your paycheck, put 10 percent of your income into a retirement or investment account. If possible, ask for an automatic withdrawal at your bank from your paycheck to avoid the temptation to spend this money. This strategy may allow you to have a solid retirement fund or even provide for an early retirement. If you start putting away $100 a month at age 20, and earn an average 6 percent interest rate, at age 65 you will have more than $275,000.
❑	❑	6. Set up an emergency savings fund. Whether you ultimately work for yourself or for someone else, there may be uncontrollable financial setbacks or even financial disasters in the future. So, as you are able, start an emergency fund equal to three to six months of normal monthly earnings. Additionally, start a second savings account for expensive purchases such as a car, a down payment on a home, or a vacation.
❑	❑	7. Use credit, gas, and retail cards responsibly and sparingly. As soon as you receive new cards, sign them promptly and store them securely. Due to the prevalence of identity theft (someone stealing your creditworthiness), cardholders should even consider a secure post office box, rather than a regular mailbox, for all high-risk mail. Shred your old credit cards, monthly statements, and any and all documents that contain personal information to avoid identity theft. Pay off all credit card debt monthly and do not purchase on credit unless you have the cash to pay it off when the monthly statement arrives. Develop a plan at this very moment to pay off your debt if you have such. Credit card balances, high interest rates, and frequent credit purchases lead to financial disaster. Credit card debt is the worst enemy to your personal finances!
❑	❑	8. Understand the terms of your student loans. Do not borrow more money than you absolutely need for actual educational expenses. Student loans are not for wants but for needs (see item 4). Remember, loans must be repaid, with interest, once you leave college. Be informed regarding the repayment process and do not ever default on your loan. If you do, the entire balance (principal, interest, and collection fees) is due immediately and serious financial and credit consequences will follow.
❑	❑	9. Eat out infrequently. Besides saving money that you can then pay to yourself, you will eat healthier and consume fewer calories.

BEHAVIOR MODIFICATION PLANNING

❑ ❑ 10. Make the best of tax "motivated" savings and investing opportunities available to you. For example, once employed, your company may match your voluntary 401(k) contributions (or other retirement plan), so contribute at least up to the match (you may use the 10 percent you "pay yourself first"—see item 5—or part of it). Also, under current tax law, maximize your Roth IRA contribution personally. Always pay attention to current tax rules that provide tax incentives for investing in retirement plans. If at all possible, ***never*** cash out a retirement account early. You may pay penalties in addition to tax, in most situations. As you are able, employ a tax professional or financial planner to avoid serious missteps in your tax planning.

❑ ❑ 11. Stay involved in your financial accumulations. You may seek professional advice, but stay in control. Ultimately, no one will look after your interests as well as you. Avoid placing all your trust (and assets) in one individual or institution. Spreading out your assets is one way to diversify your risk.

❑ ❑ 12. Protect your assets. As you start to accumulate assets, get proper insurance coverage (yes, even renter's insurance) in case of an accident or disaster. You have disciplined yourself and worked hard to obtain those assets; now make sure they are protected.

❑ ❑ 13. Review your credit report. The best way to ensure that your credit "identity" is not stolen and ruined is to regularly review your credit report, at least once a year, for accuracy.

❑ ❑ 14. Contribute to charity and the needy. Altruism (doing good for others) is good for heart health and emotional well-being. Remember the less fortunate, donate regularly to some of your favorite charitable organizations, and volunteer time to worthy causes.

The Power of Investing Early

Jon and Jim are both 20 years old. Jon begins investing $100 a month starting on his 20th birthday. He stops investing on his 30th birthday (he has set aside a total of $12,000). Jim does not start investing until he's 30. He chooses to invest $100 a month as Jon had done, but he does so for the next 30 years (Jim invests a total of $36,000). Although Jon stopped investing at age 30, assuming an 8 percent annual rate of return in a tax-deferred account, by the time both Jon and Jim are 60, Jon will have accumulated $199,035, whereas Jim will have $150,029. At a 6 percent rate of return, they would both accumulate about $100,000, but Jim invested three times as much as Jon did.

Try It

Post these principles of financial fitness in a visible place at home where you can review them often. Start implementing these strategies as soon as you can and watch your financial fitness level increase over the years.

Which Program Is Best? Your personal objectives will determine the fitness program you decide to use. If the main objective of your fitness program is to lower the risk for disease, attaining health fitness standards provides substantial health benefits. If, however, you want to participate in vigorous fitness activities, achieving high physical fitness standards is recommended. This book gives both health fitness and physical fitness standards for each fitness test so that you can personalize your approach.

Benefits of a Comprehensive Fitness Program

An inspiring story illustrating what fitness can do for a person's health and well-being is that of George Snell from Sandy, Utah. At age 45, Snell weighed approximately 400 pounds, his blood pressure was 220/180, he was blind because of undiagnosed diabetes, and his blood glucose level was 487.

Snell had determined to do something about his physical and medical condition, so he started a walking and jogging program. After about 8 months of conditioning, he had lost almost 200 pounds, his eyesight had returned, his glucose level was down to 67, and he was taken off medication. Just 2 months later—less than 10 months after beginning his personal exercise program—he completed his first marathon, a running course of 26.2 miles!

Health Benefits Most people exercise because it improves their personal appearance and makes them feel good about themselves. Although many benefits accrue from participating in a regular fitness and wellness program and active people generally live longer, *the greatest benefit of all is* *that physically fit individuals enjoy better quality of life.* These people live life to its fullest and experience far fewer health problems than do inactive individuals.

The benefits derived by regularly participating in exercise are so extensive that it is difficult to compile an all-inclusive list. As far back as 1982, the AMA indicated, "There is no drug in current or prospective use that holds as much promise for sustained health as a lifetime program of physical exercise." Furthermore, researchers and sports medicine leaders have stated that *if the benefits of exercise could be packaged in a pill, it would be the most widely prescribed medication throughout the world today.*

While most chronic (long-term) benefits of exercise are well established, what many people fail to realize is that there are immediate benefits derived by participating in just one bout of exercise. Most of these benefits dissipate within 48 to 72 hours following exercise. The immediate benefits, summarized in Table 1.4, are so striking that it prompted Dr. William L. Haskell of Stanford University to state, "Most of the health benefits of exercise are relatively short term, so people should think of exercise as a medication and take it on a daily basis." As you regularly exercise a minimum of 30 minutes five times per week, you will realize the impressive long-term benefits listed in Table 1.5.

Exercise and Brain Function If the previous benefits of exercise still have not convinced you to start a regular exercise program, you may want to consider the effects of exercise on brain function and academic performance. Physical activity is related to better cognitive health and effective functioning across the lifespan.

While much of the research is still in its infancy, as long ago as 400 BC, the Greek philosopher Plato stated, "In order for man to succeed in life, God provided him with two means, education and physical activity. Not separately, one for the soul and the other for the body, but for the two together. With these two means, man can attain perfection."

Data on more than 2.4 million students in the state of Texas showed consistent significant associations between physical fitness and various indicators of academic achievement; in particular, higher levels of fitness were associated with better academic grades. Cardiorespiratory fitness was shown to have a dose–response association with academic performance (better fitness, better grades), independent of other sociodemographic and fitness variables.[32] Another analysis looked at the short-term boost of exercise on academics. After reviewing the results from 19 different studies of children to young adults, researchers found that students who had 20 minutes of exercise immediately preceding a test or giving a speech had higher academic performance and better focus than those who did not exercise.[33]

Emerging research shows that exercise allows the brain to function at its best through a combination of biological reactions. First, exercise increases blood flow to the brain, providing oxygen, glucose, and other nutrients and improving the removal of metabolic waste products. The increased blood and oxygen flow also prompt the release of the protein brain-derived neurotrophic factor (BDNF). This protein works by strengthening connections between brain cells and repairing any damage within them. BDNF stimulates the growth of new neurons in the hippocampus, the portion of the brain involved in memory, planning, learning, and decision-making. The hippocampus is one of only two parts of the adult brain where new cells can be generated. These connections are critical for learning to take place and for memories to be stored. Exercise provides the necessary stimulus for brain neurons to interconnect, creating the perfect environment in which the brain is ready, willing, and able to learn.[34]

The hippocampus tends to shrink in late adulthood, leading to memory impairment. In older adults, regular aerobic

TABLE 1.4 Immediate (Acute) Benefits of Exercise

You can expect a number of benefits as a result of a single exercise session. Some of these benefits last as long as 72 hours following your workout. Exercise:

- increases heart rate, stroke volume, cardiac output, pulmonary ventilation, and oxygen uptake.
- begins to strengthen the heart, lungs, and muscles.
- enhances metabolic rate or energy production (burning calories for fuel) during exercise and recovery (for every 100 calories you burn during exercise, you can expect to burn another 15 during recovery).
- uses blood glucose and muscle glycogen.
- improves insulin sensitivity (decreasing the risk of type 2 diabetes).
- immediately enhances the body's ability to burn fat.
- lowers blood lipids.
- improves joint flexibility.
- reduces low-grade (hidden) inflammation (see page 427 in Chapter 11).
- increases endorphins (hormones), which are naturally occurring opioids that are responsible for exercise-induced euphoria.
- increases fat storage *in muscle,* which can then be burned for energy.
- improves endothelial function (endothelial cells line the entire vascular system, which provides a barrier between the vessel lumen and surrounding tissue–endothelial dysfunction contributes to several disease processes, including tissue inflammation and subsequent atherosclerosis).
- enhances mood and self-worth.
- provides a sense of achievement and satisfaction.
- decreases blood pressure the first few hours following exercise.
- decreases arthritic pain.
- leads to muscle relaxation.
- decreases stress.
- improves brain function.
- promotes better sleep (unless exercise is performed too close to bedtime).
- improves digestion.
- boosts energy levels.
- improves resistance to infections.

TABLE 1.5 Long-Term Benefits of Exercise

Regular participation in exercise:

- improves and strengthens the cardiorespiratory system.
- maintains better muscle tone, muscular strength, and endurance.
- improves muscular flexibility.
- enhances athletic performance.
- helps maintain recommended body weight.
- helps increase or preserve lean body tissue.
- increases resting metabolic rate.
- improves the body's ability to use fat during physical activity.
- improves posture and physical appearance.
- improves functioning of the immune system.
- lowers the risk for chronic diseases and illnesses (including heart disease, stroke, and certain cancers).
- decreases the mortality rate from chronic diseases.
- thins the blood so that it doesn't clot as readily, thereby decreasing the risk for CHD and stroke.
- helps the body manage cholesterol levels more effectively.
- prevents or delays the development of high blood pressure and lowers blood pressure in people with hypertension.
- helps prevent and control type 2 diabetes.
- helps achieve peak bone mass in young adults and maintain bone mass later in life, thereby decreasing the risk for osteoporosis.
- helps people sleep better.
- helps prevent chronic back pain.
- relieves tension and helps in coping with life stresses.
- raises levels of energy and job productivity.
- extends longevity and slows the aging process.
- improves and helps maintain cognitive function.
- promotes psychological well-being, including higher morale, self-image, and self-esteem.
- reduces feelings of depression and anxiety.
- encourages positive lifestyle changes (improving nutrition, quitting smoking, controlling alcohol and drug use).
- speeds recovery time following physical exertion.
- speeds recovery following injury or disease.
- regulates and improves overall body functions.
- improves physical stamina and counteracts chronic fatigue.
- reduces disability and helps maintain independent living, especially in older adults.
- enhances quality of life: People feel better and live a healthier and happier life.

exercise has been shown to increase the size of the hippocampus and decrease the rate of brain shrinkage, dramatically minimizing declines in thinking and memory skills.

The strongest data from research so far show that regular physical activity is the most important lifestyle change a person can make to prevent dementia and Alzheimer's later in life. Aerobics, strength training, and even stretching and toning are all beneficial, and researchers have been surprised by the strength of the association between exercise and these conditions. An emerging set of new studies is finding that along the entire age spectrum, subjects improve brain function with physical activity and exercise. Additionally, maintaining a high level of physical fitness in mid-life can reduce a person's chances of developing Alzheimer's by half and dementia by 60 percent.[35]

Keeping the mind engaged with proactive cognitive challenges like reading, studying, playing games, and doing puzzles is critical (but not passive TV watching). Physical activity and exercise, nonetheless, provide better protection than intellectual challenges themselves. Even light-intensity activities of daily living appear to provide protection against cognitive impairment. The research further shows that as the amount of activity increases, the rate of cognitive decline decreases. And the amount of daily activity performed appears to be more important than the intensity itself in terms of warding off dementia. Of course, greater protection is obtained by combining both physical and cognitive challenges.

Exercise also increases the neurotransmitters dopamine, glutamate, norepinephrine, and serotonin, all of which are vital in the generation of thought and emotion. Low levels of serotonin have been linked to depression, and exercise has repeatedly been shown to be effective in treating depression.

Economic Benefits Sedentary living can have a strong effect on a nation's economy. As the need for physical exertion in Western countries decreased steadily during the past century, health care expenditures increased dramatically. Health care costs in the United States rose from

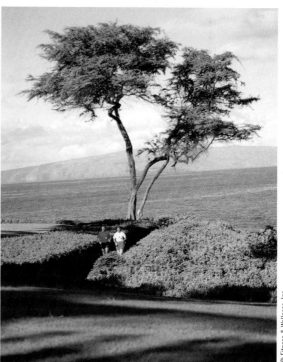

No current drug or medication provides as many health benefits as a regular physical activity program.

$12 billion in 1950 to $2.7 trillion in 2011 (Figure 1.15), or about 17.7 percent of the country's gross domestic product (GDP). This ratio far outpaces the spending of all other countries in the Organisation for Economic Co-operation and Development (OECD). The next closest country is the Netherlands, at 11.9 percent, and Canada ranks fifth, at 11.2 percent of GDP (Figure 1.16). In 1980, health care costs in the United States represented 8.8 percent of the U.S. GDP, and if the current trend continues, they are projected to reach almost 20 percent by 2019.

In terms of yearly health care costs per person, the United States spends more than any other industrialized nation. Per capita U.S. health care costs are over $8,500 per

FIGURE 1.15 U.S. health care cost increments since 1950.

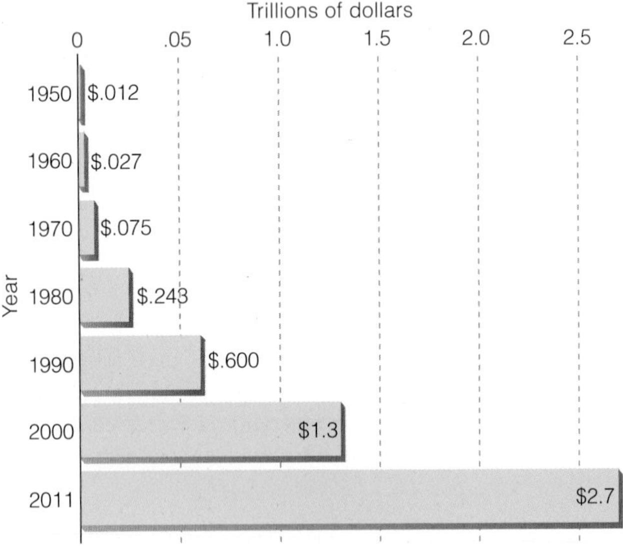

FIGURE 1.16 Health care expenditures for selected countries as a percentage of the GDP, 2011.

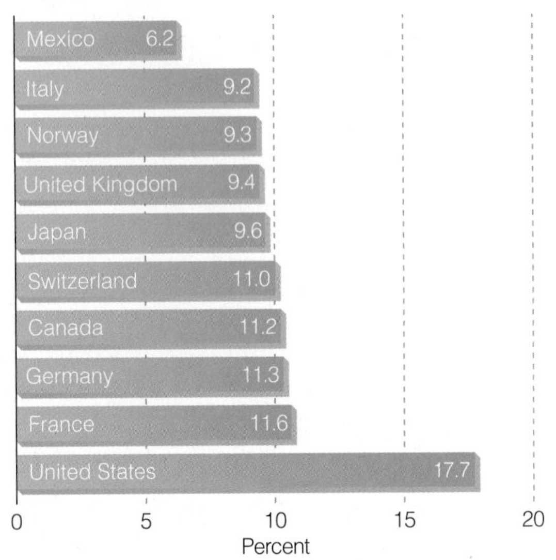

Source: Organisation for Economic Co-operation and Development, 2013.

FIGURE 1.17 Health care expenditure per capita for selected countries, 2011.

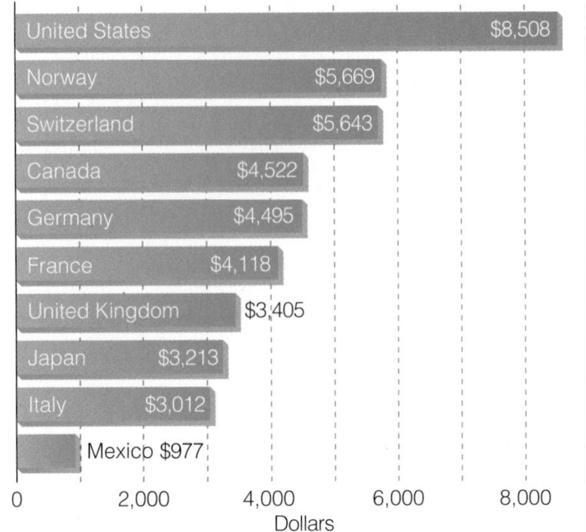

year. These costs are about 2.5 times the OECD average (Figure 1.17).

One of the reasons for the low overall ranking of the United States is the overemphasis on state-of-the-art cures instead of prevention programs. The United States is the best place in the world to treat people once they are sick, but the system does a poor job of keeping people healthy initially. Ninety-five percent of U.S. health care dollars are spent on treatment strategies, and less than 5 percent are spent on prevention.

Unhealthy behaviors also contribute to the staggering U.S. health care costs. Risk factors for disease such as obesity and smoking carry a heavy price tag. An estimated 1 percent of the people account for 30 percent of health care costs.[36] Half of the people use about 97 percent of health care dollars. Without reducing the current burden of disease, real health care reform will most likely be impossible. True health care reform requires a nationwide call for action by everyone against chronic disease.

Scientific evidence links participation in fitness and wellness programs to better health, in addition to lower medical costs and higher job productivity. As a result of the staggering rise in medical costs, many organizations offer health promotion programs, because keeping employees healthy costs less than treating them once they are sick.

The Wellness Challenge for Our Day

Because a better and healthier life is something that every person should strive for, the biggest health challenge today is to teach people how to take control of their personal health habits and adhere to a positive lifestyle. A wealth of information on the benefits of fitness and wellness programs indicates that improving the quality and possible length of your life is a matter of personal choice.

Even though people in the United States believe a positive lifestyle has a great effect on health and longevity, most people do not reap the benefits because they simply do not know how to implement a safe and effective fitness and wellness program. Others are exercising incorrectly and therefore are not reaping the full benefits of their program. How, then, can we meet the health challenges of the 21st century? That is the focus of this book—to provide the necessary tools that will enable you to write, implement, and regularly update your personal lifetime fitness and wellness program.

CRITICAL THINKING

What are your thoughts about lifestyle habits that enhance health and longevity? How important are they to you? What obstacles keep you from adhering to these habits or incorporating new habits into your life?

Wellness Education: Using This Book

Although everyone would like to enjoy good health and wellness, most people don't know how to reach this objective. Lifestyle is the most important factor affecting personal well-being. Granted, some people live long because of genetic factors, but quality of life during middle age and the "golden years" is more often related to wise choices initiated during youth and continued throughout life. In a few short years, lack of wellness can lead to loss of vitality and gusto for life, as well as premature morbidity and mortality.

A Personalized Approach

Because fitness and wellness needs vary significantly from one individual to another, all exercise and wellness prescriptions must be personalized to obtain the best results. The wellness lifestyle questionnaire in Lab 1B provides an initial rating of your current efforts to stay healthy and well. Subsequent chapters of this book and their respective labs discuss the components of a wellness lifestyle and set forth the necessary guidelines that will allow you to develop a personal lifetime program to improve fitness and promote your own preventive health care and personal wellness.

The labs in this book have been prepared on tear-out sheets so that they can be turned in to class instructors. As you study this book and complete the labs, you will learn to

- implement motivational and behavior modification techniques to help you adhere to a lifetime fitness and wellness program.
- determine whether medical clearance is needed for your safe participation in exercise.
- conduct nutritional analyses and follow the recommendations for adequate nutrition.
- write sound diet and weight control programs.
- assess the health-related and motor skill-related components of fitness.
- write exercise prescriptions for cardiorespiratory endurance, muscular fitness, and muscular flexibility.
- understand the relationship between fitness and aging.
- determine your levels of tension and stress, reduce your vulnerability to stress, and implement a stress management program, if necessary.
- determine your potential risk for cardiovascular disease and implement a risk-reduction program.
- follow a cancer risk–reduction program.
- implement a smoking cessation program, if applicable.
- avoid chemical dependency and know where to find assistance, if needed.
- learn the health consequences of sexually transmitted infections (STIs), including human immunodeficiency virus (HIV)/acquired immune deficiency syndrome (AIDS), and guidelines for preventing STIs.
- write goals and objectives to improve your fitness and wellness and learn how to chart a wellness program for the future.
- differentiate myths from facts about exercise and health-related concepts.

Exercise Safety

Even though testing and participation in exercise are relatively safe for most apparently healthy individuals, the reaction of the cardiovascular system to higher levels of physical activity cannot be totally predicted. Consequently, a small but real risk exists for exercise-induced abnormalities in people with a history of cardiovascular problems, with certain chronic conditions, and at higher risk for disease. Among the exercise-induced abnormalities are abnormal blood pressure, irregular heart rhythm, fainting, and, in rare instances, heart attack or cardiac arrest.

Before you engage in an exercise program or participate in any exercise testing, as a minimum you should fill out the PAR-Q found in Lab 1C. Additional information can be obtained by filling out the health history questionnaire, also given in Lab 1C. Exercise testing and participation are not wise under some conditions listed in this activity and may require a medical evaluation, including a stress electrocardiogram (ECG) test for a few individuals. If you have questions regarding your current health status, consult your doctor before initiating, continuing, or increasing your level of physical activity.

BEHAVIOR MODIFICATION PLANNING

Healthy Lifestyle Habits

Research indicates that adherence to the following 12 lifestyle habits significantly improves health and extends life:

1. **Participate in a lifetime physical activity program.** Attempt to accumulate 60 minutes of moderate-intensity physical activity most days of the week. The 60 minutes should include 20 to 30 minutes of aerobic exercise (vigorous intensity) at least three times per week, along with strengthening and stretching exercises two to three times per week. Furthermore, keep moving throughout the day. Do not sit for more than an hour at a time without getting up to move or stretch for five to ten minutes.
2. **Do not smoke cigarettes.** Cigarette smoking is the largest preventable cause of illness and premature death in the United States. If we include all related deaths, smoking is responsible for more than 480,000 unnecessary deaths each year.
3. **Eat right.** Eat a good breakfast and two additional well-balanced meals every day. Avoid eating too many calories, processed foods, and foods with a lot of sugar, fat, and salt. Increase your daily consumption of fruits, vegetables, and whole-grain products.
4. **Avoid snacking.** Refrain from frequent high-sugar snacks between meals. Insulin is released to remove sugar from the blood, and frequent spikes in insulin may contribute to the development of heart disease.
5. **Maintain recommended body weight through adequate nutrition and exercise.** This is important in preventing chronic diseases and in developing a higher level of fitness.
6. **Sleep 7 to 8 hours each night.**
7. **Lower your stress levels.** Reduce your vulnerability to stress and practice stress management techniques as needed.
8. **Be wary of alcohol.** Drink alcohol moderately or not at all. Alcohol abuse leads to mental, emotional, physical, and social problems.
9. **Surround yourself with healthy friendships.** Unhealthy friendships contribute to destructive behaviors and low self-esteem. Associating with people who strive to maintain good fitness and health reinforces a positive outlook in life and encourages positive behaviors. Mortality rates are much higher among people who are socially isolated.
10. **Be informed about the environment.** Seek clean air, clean water, and a clean environment. Be aware of pollutants and occupational hazards: asbestos fibers, nickel dust, chromate, uranium dust, and so on. Take precautions when using pesticides and insecticides.
11. **Increase education.** Data indicate that people who are more educated live longer. As education increases, so does the number of connections between nerve cells. An increased number of connections helps the individual make better survival (healthy lifestyle) choices.
12. **Take personal safety measures.** Although not all accidents are preventable, many are. Taking simple precautionary measures—such as using seat belts and keeping electrical appliances away from water—lessens the risk for avoidable accidents.

Try It

Look at the preceding list and indicate which habits are already a part of your lifestyle. What changes could you make to incorporate some additional healthy habits into your daily life?

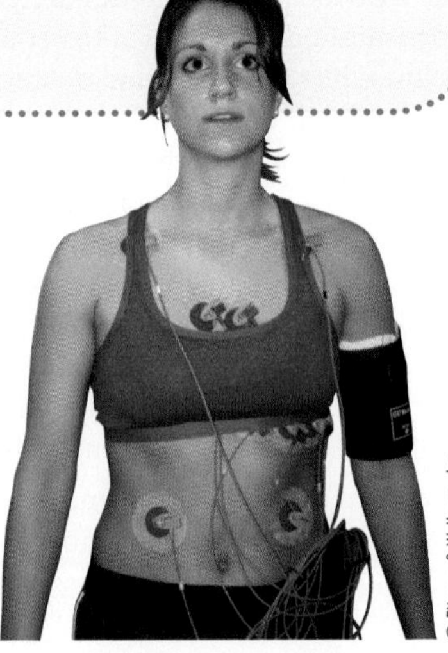

An exercise tolerance test with 12-lead ECG monitoring may be required of some individuals prior to initiating an exercise program.

Assessment of Resting Heart Rate and Blood Pressure

Heart rate can be obtained by counting your pulse either on the wrist over the radial artery or over the carotid artery in the neck (see Chapter 6, page 225). In Lab 1D, you have an opportunity to determine your heart rate and blood pressure and calculate the extra heart rate life-years an increase in exercise may produce.

You may count your pulse for 30 seconds and multiply by 2 or take it for a full minute. The heart rate usually is at its lowest point (resting heart rate) late in the evening after you have been sitting quietly for about half an hour, watching a relaxing TV show or reading in bed, or early in the morning just before you get out of bed. Your pulse should have a consistent (regular) rhythm. A pulse that misses beats or speeds up or slows down may be an indication of heart problems and should be followed up by a physician.

Unless you have a pathological condition, a lower resting heart rate indicates a stronger heart. To adapt to cardiorespiratory or aerobic exercise, blood volume increases, the heart enlarges, and the muscle gets stronger. A stronger heart can pump more blood with fewer strokes.

Resting heart rate categories are given in Table 1.6. Although resting heart rate decreases with training, the extent of **bradycardia** depends not only on the amount of training but also on genetic factors. Although most highly trained athletes have a resting heart rate around 40 beats per minute, occasionally one of these athletes has a resting heart rate in the 60s or 70s, even during peak training months of the season. For most individuals, however, the resting heart rate decreases as the level of cardiorespiratory endurance increases.

Blood pressure is assessed using a **sphygmomanometer** and a stethoscope. Use a cuff of the appropriate size to get accurate readings. Size is determined by the width of the inflatable bladder, which should be about 80 percent of the circumference of the midpoint of the arm.

Blood pressure usually is measured while the person is in the sitting position, with the forearm and the manometer at the same level as the heart. The arm should be flexed slightly and placed on a flat surface. The pressure is recorded from each arm first and then from the arm with the highest reading.

TABLE 1.6 **Resting Heart Rate Ratings**

Heart Rate (beats/min)	Rating
≤59	Excellent
60–69	Good
70–79	Average
80–89	Fair
≥90	Poor

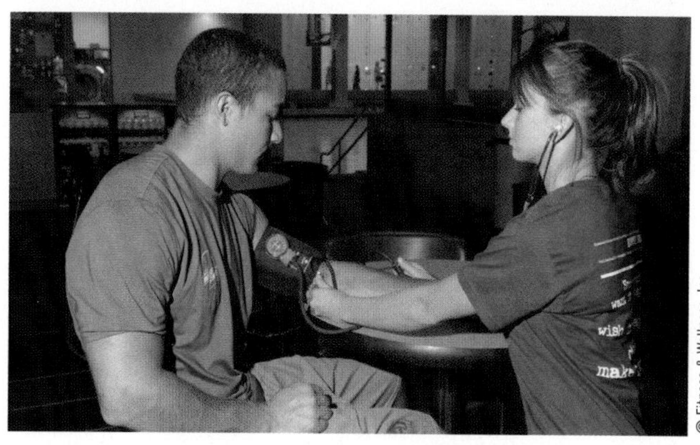

Assessment of resting blood pressure with an aneroid manometer.

TABLE 1.7 **Resting Blood Pressure Guidelines (in mm Hg)**

Rating	Systolic	Diastolic
Normal	≤120	≤80
Prehypertension	120–139	80–89
Hypertension	≥140	≥90

Source: National Heart, Lung and Blood Institute.

The cuff should be applied approximately an inch above the antecubital space (natural crease of the elbow), with the center of the bladder directly over the medial (inner) surface of the arm. The stethoscope head should be applied firmly, but with little pressure, over the brachial artery in the antecubital space.

To determine how high the cuff should be inflated, the person recording the blood pressure monitors the subject's radial pulse with one hand and, with the other hand, inflates the manometer's bladder to about 30 to 40 mm Hg above the point at which the feeling of the pulse in the wrist disappears. Next, the pressure is released, followed by a wait of about 1 minute, and then the bladder is inflated to the predetermined level to take the blood pressure reading. The cuff should not be overinflated, because this may cause blood vessel spasm, resulting in higher blood pressure readings. The pressure should be released at a rate of 2 to 4 mm Hg per second.

As the pressure is released, **systolic blood pressure (SBP)** is recorded as the point where the sound of the pulse becomes audible. **Diastolic blood pressure (DBP)** is the point where the sound disap-

Bradycardia Slower heart rate than normal.

Sphygmomanometer Inflatable bladder contained within a cuff and a mercury gravity manometer (or aneroid manometer) from which blood pressure is read.

Systolic blood pressure (SBP) Pressure exerted by blood against walls of arteries during forceful contraction (systole) of the heart.

Diastolic blood pressure (DBP) Pressure exerted by the blood against the walls of the arteries during the relaxation phase (diastole) of the heart.

pears. The recordings should be expressed as systolic over diastolic pressure—for example, 124/80.

If you take more than one reading, be sure the bladder is deflated between readings and allow at least a full minute before making the next recording. The person measuring the pressure also should note whether the pressure was recorded from the left or the right arm. Resting blood pressure ratings are given in Table 1.7.

In some cases, the pulse sounds become less intense (point of muffling sounds) but still can be heard at a lower pressure (50 or 40 mm Hg) or even all the way down to zero. In this situation, the diastolic pressure is recorded at the point of a clear, definite change in the loudness of the sound (also referred to as fourth phase) and at complete disappearance of the sound (fifth phase) (e.g., 120/78/60 or 120/82/0).

Mean Blood Pressure

During a normal resting contraction/relaxation cycle of the heart, the heart spends more time in the relaxation (diastolic) phase than in the contraction (systolic) phase. Accordingly, mean blood pressure (MBP) cannot be computed by taking an average of SBP and DBP blood pressures. The equations used to determine MBP are shown in Lab 1D.

When measuring blood pressure, be aware that a single reading may not be an accurate value because of the various factors (rest, stress, physical activity, food) that can affect blood pressure. Thus, if you are able, ask different people to take several readings at different times of the day, to establish the real values. You can record the results of your resting heart rate and your SBP, DBP, and MBP assessments in Lab 1D. You can also calculate the effects of aerobic activity on resting heart rate in this activity.

ASSESS YOUR BEHAVIOR

CENGAGE brain.com To access course materials, including companion resources, please visit **www.cengagebrain.com**.

1. Are you aware of your family health history and lifestyle factors that may negatively affect your health?
2. Do you accumulate at least 150 minutes of moderate-intensity physical activity or 75 minutes of vigorous-intensity physical activity on a weekly basis?
3. Do you make a constant and deliberate effort to stay healthy and achieve the highest potential for well-being?

ASSESS YOUR KNOWLEDGE

1. Advances in modern technology
   a. help people achieve higher fitness levels.
   b. have led to a decrease in chronic diseases.
   c. have almost completely eliminated the necessity for physical exertion in daily life.
   d. help fight hypokinetic disease.
   e. make it easier to achieve good aerobic fitness.
2. Most activities of daily living in the United States help people
   a. get adequate physical activity regularly.
   b. meet health-related fitness standards.
   c. achieve good levels of skill-related activities.
   d. Choices a, b, and c are correct.
   e. None of the choices are correct.
3. The federal guidelines for physical activity recommend that every adult should do
   a. 150 minutes a week of moderate-intensity aerobic activity.
   b. 75 minutes a week of vigorous-intensity aerobic activity.
   c. an equivalent combination of choices a and b.
   d. Choices a, b, and c above are correct.
   e. None of the choices are correct.
4. Bodily movement produced by skeletal muscles is called
   a. physical activity.
   b. kinesiology.
   c. exercise.
   d. aerobic exercise.
   e. muscle strength.
5. Among the long-term benefits of regular physical activity and exercise are significantly reduced risks for developing or dying from
   a. heart disease.
   b. type 2 diabetes.
   c. colon and breast cancers.
   d. osteoporotic fractures.
   e. All of the choices are correct.

6. To be ranked in the "active" category, an adult has to take between
   a. 3,500 and 4,999 steps per day.
   b. 5,000 and 7,499 steps per day.
   c. 7,500 and 9,999 steps per day.
   d. 10,000 and 12,499 steps per day.
   e. 12,500 and 15,000 steps per day.

7. The constant and deliberate effort to stay healthy and achieve the highest potential for well-being is defined as
   a. health.
   b. physical fitness.
   c. wellness.
   d. health-related fitness.
   e. physiological fitness.

8. Research on the effects of fitness on mortality indicates that the largest drop in premature mortality is seen between
   a. the average and excellent fitness groups.
   b. the low and moderate fitness groups.
   c. the high and excellent fitness groups.
   d. the moderate and good fitness groups.
   e. The drop is similar among all fitness groups.

9. Metabolic fitness can be achieved through
   a. a moderate-intensity exercise program.
   b. a vigorous-intensity speed-training program.
   c. an increased basal metabolic rate.
   d. anaerobic training.
   e. an increase in lean body mass.

10. What is the greatest benefit of being physically fit?
   a. absence of disease
   b. higher quality of life
   c. improved sports performance
   d. better personal appearance
   e. maintenance of recommended body weight

Correct answers can be found at the back of the book.

NOTES

1. World Health Organization, "2008-2013 Action plan for the global strategy for the prevention and control of noncommunicable diseases," http://www.who.int/nmh/**publications/en/**, downloaded February 24, 2014.
2. OECD (2013), Health at a Glance 2013: OECD Indicators, OECD Publishing, http://www.oecd-ilibrary.org/social-issues-migration-health/health-at-a-glance-2013_health_glance-2013-en, downloaded February 28, 2014.
3. American Heart Association, "Heart Disease and Stroke Statistics—2014 Update," http://circ.ahajournals.org/content/129/3/e28.extract, downloaded February 28, 2014.
4. U.S. Department of Health and Human Services, Centers for Disease Control and Prevention, "Deaths: Preliminary Data for 2011," *National Center for Health Statistics, National Vital Statistics Reports* 60, no. 4 (January 11, 2012).
5. See note 3.
6. American Cancer Society, *2014 Cancer Facts and Figures* (New York: ACS, 2014).
7. American College of Sports Medicine, *ACSM's Guidelines for Exercise Testing and Prescription* (Philadelphia: Wolters Kluwer/Lippincott Williams & Wilkins, 2010).
8. U.S. Department of Health and Human Services and U.S. Department of Agriculture, *Dietary Guidelines for Americans 2010* (Washington, DC: DHHS, 2010).
9. National Academy of Sciences, Institute of Medicine, *Dietary Reference Intakes for Energy, Carbohydrates, Fiber, Fat, Fatty Acids, Cholesterol, Protein and Amino Acids (Macronutrients)* (Washington, DC: National Academy Press, 2005).
10. World Health Organization, "Global Recommendations on Physical Activity for Health," http://www.who.int/dietphysicalactivity/leaflet-physical-activity-recommendations.pdf?ua=1, downloaded February 28, 2014.
11. W. L. Haskell et al., "Physical Activity and Public Health: Updated Recommendation for Adults from the American College of Sports Medicine and the American Heart Association," *Medicine & Science in Sports & Exercise* 39 (2007): 1423–1434.
12. U.S. Department of Health and Human Services, *Physical Activity and Health: A Report of the Surgeon General* (Atlanta, GA: Centers for Disease Control and Prevention, National Center for Chronic Disease Prevention and Health Promotion, 1996).
13. U.S. Department of Health and Human Services, "2008 Physical Activity Guidelines for Americans," http://health.gov/paguidelines, downloaded October 15, 2008.
14. American College of Sports Medicine, "Exercise Is Medicine," http://www.exerciseismedicine.org/, downloaded January 10, 2012.
15. U.S. Department of Health and Human Services, *Healthy People 2020* (Washington, DC: DHHS, 2010).
16. W. W. K. Hoeger, L. Bond, L. Ransdell, J. M. Shimon, and S. Merugu, "One-Mile Step Count at Walking and Running Speeds," *ACSM's Health & Fitness Journal* 12, no. 1 (2008): 14–19.
17. E. G. Wilmot, C. L. Edwardson, F. A. Achana, M. J. Davies, T. Gorely, L. J. Gray, K. Khunti, T. Yates, S. J. H. Biddle. "Sedentary Time in Adults and the Association with Diabetes, Cardiovascular Disease and Death: Systematic Review and Meta-Analysis," *Diabetologia* 55 (2012): 2895–2905.
18. D. Dunlop et al. "Sedentary Time in U.S. Older Adults Associated With Disability in Activities of Daily Living Independent of Physical Activity," *Journal of Physical Activity and Health,* February 5, 2014, http://www.ncbi.nlm.nih.gov/pubmed/24510000, downloaded April 30, 2014.
19. L. Sax et al., *The American Freshman: National Norms for Fall 2000* (Los Angeles:

University of California–Los Angeles, Higher Education Research Institute, 2000).

20. L. Dossey, "Can Spirituality Improve Your Health?" *Bottom Line/Health* 15 (July 2001): 11–13.
21. R. S. Paffenbarger Jr., R. T. Hyde, A. L. Wing, and C. H. Steinmetz, "A Natural History of Athleticism and Cardiovascular Health," *Journal of the American Medical Association* 252 (1984): 491–495.
22. S. N. Blair, H. W. Kohl III, R. S. Paffenbarger Jr., D. G. Clark, K. H. Cooper, and L. W. Gibbons, "Physical Fitness and All-Cause Mortality: A Prospective Study of Healthy Men and Women," *Journal of the American Medical Association* 262 (1989): 2395–2401.
23. H. Naci, J. P. A. Ioannidis, "Comparative Effectiveness of Exercise and Drug Interventions on Mortality Outcomes: Metaepidemiological Study," *BMJ* (2013); 347:f5577.
24. S. Mandic et al., "Characterizing Differences in Mortality at the Low End of the Fitness Spectrum," *Medicine & Science in Sports & Exercise* 41 (2009): 1573–1579.
25. E. S. Ford et al., "Healthy Living Is Better Revenge," *Archives of Internal Medicine* 169 (2009): 1355–1362.
26. Lee et al., "Effect of Physical Inactivity on Major Non-communicable Diseases Worldwide: An Analysis of Burden of Disease and Life Expectancy," *The Lancet* 380 (2012): 219–229.
27. P. C. Hallal et al., "Global Physical Activity Levels: Surveillance, Progress, Pitfalls, and Prospects," *The Lancet* 380 (2012): 247–257.
28. S. Kodama et al., "Cardiorespiratory Fitness as a Quantitative Predictor of All-Cause Mortality and Cardiovascular Events in Healthy Men and Women," *Journal of the American Medical Association* 301 (2010): 2024–2035.
29. D. P. Swain, "Moderate- or Vigorous-Intensity Exercise: What Should We Prescribe?" *ACSM's Health & Fitness Journal* 10, no. 5 (2007): 7–11.
30. P. T. Williams, "Physical Fitness and Activity as Separate Heart Disease Risk Factors: A Meta-analysis," *Medicine & Science in Sports & Exercise* 33 (2001): 754–761.
31. D. P. Swain and B. A. Franklin, "Comparative Cardioprotective Benefits of Vigorous vs. Moderate Intensity Aerobic Exercise," *American Journal of Cardiology* 97 (2006): 141–147.
32. Cooper Institute, "Texas Youth Fitness Study (Dallas, TX)," http://www.cooperinstitute.org/youth/documents/Texas%20Youth%20Fitness%20Study%20—%20Charts.pdf, downloaded March 9, 2011.
33. L. Verburgh, M. Konigs, E. J. A. Scherder, and J. Oosterlaan, "Physical Exercise and Executive Functions in Preadolescent Children, Adolescents and Young Adults: A Meta-Analysis," *British Journal of Sports Medicine,* March 6, 2013, http://bjsm.bmj.com/content/early/2013/02/13/bjsports-2012-091441, downloaded April 30, 2014.
34. J. J. Ratey and E. Hagerman, *Spark: The Revolutionary New Science of Exercise and the Brain* (New York: Little, Brown and Company, 2008).
35. P. Elwood et al. "Healthy Lifestyles Reduce the Incidence of Chronic Diseases and Dementia: Evidence from the Caerphilly Cohort Study," *PLOS ONE,* December 09, 2013, http://www.plosone.org/article/info%3Adoi%2F10.1371%2Fjournal.pone.0081877, downloaded April 30, 2014.
36. See note 27.

SUGGESTED READINGS

Bouchard, C., S. N. Blair, and W. Haskell. *Physical Activity and Health.* Champaign, IL: Human Kinetics, 2007.

Haskell, W. L. et al. "Physical Activity and Public Health: Updated Recommendation for Adults from the American College of Sports Medicine and the American Heart Association," *Medicine & Science in Sports & Exercise* 39 (2007): 1423-1434.

Hoeger, W. W. K., and S. A. Hoeger. *Fitness and Wellness.* Belmont, CA: Wadsworth/Cengage Learning, 2015.

Hoeger, W. W. K., and S. A. Hoeger. *Lifetime Physical Fitness and Wellness: A Personalized Program.* Belmont, CA: Wadsworth/Cengage Learning, 2015.

Hoeger, W. W. K., L. W. Turner, and B. Q. Hafen. *Wellness: Guidelines for a Healthy Lifestyle.* Belmont, CA: Wadsworth/Thomson Learning, 2007.

National Academy of Sciences, Institute of Medicine. *Dietary Reference Intakes for Energy, Carbohydrates, Fiber, Fat, Fatty Acids, Cholesterol, Protein and Amino Acids (Macronutrients).* Washington, DC: National Academy Press, 2005.

Schroeder S. A. "Shattuck Lecture. We Can Do Better—Improving the Health of the American People," *New England Journal of Medicine,* 357, no. 12 (2007): 1221-1228.

U.S. Department of Health and Human Services. "2008 Physical Activity Guidelines for Americans," available at http://www.health.gov/paguidelines.

U.S. Department of Health and Human Services. "Healthy People 2020," available at http://www.healthypeople.gov.

Lab 1A: Daily Physical Activity Log

Name ______________________ Date __________ Grade __________

Instructor ______________________ Course __________ Section __________

NECESSARY LAB EQUIPMENT

None.

OBJECTIVE

To indicate how active you are and serve as a basis to monitor future changes.

INSTRUCTIONS

Record the time of day, type and duration of the exercise/activity, and if possible, steps taken while engaged in the activity.

Date: __________ Day of the Week: __________

Time of Day	Exercise/Activity	Duration	Number of steps	Comments
	Totals:			

Activity category based on steps per day (use Table 1.2, page 12): __________

Date: __________ Day of the Week: __________

Time of Day	Exercise/Activity	Duration	Number of steps	Comments
	Totals:			

Activity category based on steps per day (use Table 1.2, page 12): __________

Date: ______ Day of the Week: ______

Time of Day	Exercise/Activity	Duration	Number of steps	Comments
	Totals:			

Activity category based on steps per day (use Table 1.2, page 12): ______

Date: ______ Day of the Week: ______

Time of Day	Exercise/Activity	Duration	Number of steps	Comments
	Totals:			

Activity category based on steps per day (use Table 1.2, page 12): ______

Briefly evaluate your current activity patterns, discuss your feelings about the results, and provide a goal for the weeks ahead.

Lab 1B: Wellness Lifestyle Questionnaire

Name ______________________ **Date** __________ **Grade** __________

Instructor ______________________ **Course** __________ **Section** __________

NECESSARY LAB EQUIPMENT

None.

OBJECTIVE

To analyze current lifestyle habits and help determine changes necessary for future health and wellness.

INSTRUCTIONS

Check the appropriate answer to each question and obtain a final score according to the guidelines provided at the end of the questionnaire.

	ALWAYS	NEARLY ALWAYS	OFTEN	SELDOM	NEVER
1. I participate in vigorous-intensity aerobic activity for 20 minutes on 3 or more days per week, and I accumulate at least 30 minutes of moderate-intensity physical activity on a minimum of 2 additional days per week.	5	4	3	2	1
2. I avoid uninterrupted sitting for more than an hour at a time and accumulate less than 6 hours of sitting time in a 24-hour time period.	5	4	3	2	1
3. I participate in strength-training exercises, using a minimum of eight different exercises, 2 or more days per week.	5	4	3	2	1
4. I perform flexibility exercises a minimum of 2 days per week.	5	4	3	2	1
5. I maintain recommended body weight (includes avoidance of excessive body fat, excessive thinness, or frequent fluctuations in body weight).	5	4	3	2	1
6. Every day, I eat three regular meals that include a wide variety of foods.	5	4	3	2	1
7. I limit the amount of saturated fat and trans fats in my diet on most days of the week.	5	4	3	2	1
8. I eat a minimum of five servings of fruits and vegetables and six servings from grain products daily.	5	4	3	2	1
9. I regularly avoid snacks, especially those that are high in calories and fat and low in nutrients and fiber.	5	4	3	2	1
10. I avoid cigarettes or tobacco in any other form.	5	4	3	2	1
11. I avoid alcoholic beverages. If I drink, I do so in moderation (one daily drink for women and two for men), and I do not combine alcohol with other drugs.	5	4	3	2	1
12. I avoid addictive drugs and needles that have been used by others.	5	4	3	2	1
13. I use prescription drugs and over-the-counter drugs sparingly (only when needed), and I follow all directions for their proper use.	5	4	3	2	1
14. I readily recognize and act on it when I am under excessive tension and stress (distress).	5	4	3	2	1
15. I am able to perform effective stress-management techniques.	5	4	3	2	1
16. I have close friends and relatives with whom I can discuss personal problems and approach for help when needed, and with whom I can express my feelings freely.	5	4	3	2	1
17. I spend most of my daily leisure time in wholesome recreational activities.	5	4	3	2	1
18. I sleep 7 to 8 hours each night.	5	4	3	2	1
19. I floss my teeth every day and brush them at least twice daily.	5	4	3	2	1

	ALWAYS	NEARLY ALWAYS	OFTEN	SELDOM	NEVER
20. I get "safe sun" exposure (that is, 10–20 minutes unprotected sun exposure to the face, neck, and arms, on most days of the week between hours of 10:00 a.m. and 4:00 p.m.), I avoid overexposure to the sun, and I use sunscreen and appropriate clothing when I am out in the sun for an extended time.	5	4	3	2	1
21. I avoid using products that have not been shown by science to be safe and effective. (This includes drugs and unproven nutrient and weight loss supplements.)	5	4	3	2	1
22. I stay current with the warning signs for heart attack, stroke, and cancer.	5	4	3	2	1
23. I practice monthly breast/testicle self-exams, get recommended screening tests (blood lipids, blood pressure, Pap tests), and seek a medical evaluation when I am not well or disease symptoms arise.	5	4	3	2	1
24. I have a dental checkup at least once a year, and I get regular medical exams according to age recommendations.	5	4	3	2	1
25. I am not sexually active. / I practice safe sex.	5	4	3	2	1
26. I can deal effectively with disappointments and temporary feelings of sadness, loneliness, and depression. If I am unable to deal with these feelings, I seek professional help.	5	4	3	2	1
27. I can work out emotional problems without turning to alcohol, other drugs, or violent behavior.	5	4	3	2	1
28. I associate with people who have a positive attitude about life.	5	4	3	2	1
29. I respond to temporary setbacks by making the best of the circumstances and by moving ahead with optimism and energy. I do not spend time and talent worrying about failures.	5	4	3	2	1
30. I wear a seat belt whenever I am in a car, I ask others in my vehicle to do the same, and I make sure that children are in an infant seat or wear a shoulder harness.	5	4	3	2	1
31. I do not drive under the influence of alcohol or other drugs, and I make an effort to keep others from doing the same.	5	4	3	2	1
32. I avoid being alone in public places, especially after dark; I seek escorts when I visit or exercise in unfamiliar places.	5	4	3	2	1
33. I seek to make my living quarters accident-free, and I keep doors and windows locked, especially when I am home alone.	5	4	3	2	1
34. I try to minimize environmental pollutants, and I support community efforts to minimize pollution.	5	4	3	2	1
35. I use energy conservation strategies and encourage others to do the same.	5	4	3	2	1
36. I study and/or work in a clean environment (including avoidance of secondhand smoke).	5	4	3	2	1
37. I participate in recycling programs for paper, cardboard, glass, plastic, and aluminum.	5	4	3	2	1

How to Score

Enter the score you have marked for each question in the spaces provided below. Next, total the score for each specific wellness lifestyle category and obtain a rating for each category according to the criteria provided below.

	Health-Related Fitness	Nutrition	Avoiding Chemical Dependency	Stress Manage-ment	Personal Hygiene/ Health	Disease Prevention	Emotional Well-being	Personal Safety	Environmental Health & Protection
	1.	6.	10.	14.	18.	22.	26.	30.	34.
	2.	7.	11.	15.	19.	23.	27.	31.	35.
	3.	8.	12.	16.	20.	24.	28.	32.	36.
	4.	9.	13.	17.	21.	25.	29.	33.	37.
	5.								
Total:									
Rating:									

Category Rating

Excellent (E) = ≥17 Your answers show that you are aware of the importance of this category to your health and wellness. You are putting your knowledge to work for you by practicing good habits. As long as you continue to do so, this category should not pose a health risk. You are also setting a good example for family and friends to follow. Because you got a very high score on this part of the test, you may want to consider other categories in which your score indicates room for improvement.

Good (G) = 13–16 Your health practices in this area are good, but you have room for improvement. Look again at the items you answered with a 4 or lower and identify changes that you can make to improve your lifestyle. Even small changes often can help you achieve better health.

Needs Improvement (NI) = ≤12 Your health risks are showing. You may be taking serious and unnecessary risks with your health. Perhaps you are not aware of the risks or what to do about them. Most likely you need additional information and help in deciding how to successfully make the changes you desire. You can easily get the information that you need to improve, if you wish. The next step is up to you.

Please note that no final overall rating is provided for the entire questionnaire, because it may not be indicative of your overall wellness. For example, an excellent rating in most categories will not offset the immediate health risks and life-threatening consequences of using addictive drugs or not wearing a seat belt.

Lab 1C: PAR-Q and Health History Questionnaire

Name ______________________ **Date** __________ **Grade** __________

Instructor ______________________ **Course** __________ **Section** __________

NECESSARY LAB EQUIPMENT
None.

OBJECTIVE
To determine the safety of exercise participation.

Physical Activity Readiness
Questionnaire - PAR-Q
(revised 2002)

PAR-Q & YOU

(A Questionnaire for People Aged 15 to 69)

Regular physical activity is fun and healthy, and increasingly more people are starting to become more active every day. Being more active is very safe for most people. However, some people should check with their doctor before they start becoming much more physically active.

If you are planning to become much more physically active than you are now, start by answering the seven questions in the box below. If you are between the ages of 15 and 69, the PAR-Q will tell you if you should check with your doctor before you start. If you are over 69 years of age, and you are not used to being very active, check with your doctor.

Common sense is your best guide when you answer these questions. Please read the questions carefully and answer each one honestly: check YES or NO.

YES	NO	
☐	☐	**1. Has your doctor ever said that you have a heart condition and that you should only do physical activity recommended by a doctor?**
☐	☐	**2. Do you feel pain in your chest when you do physical activity?**
☐	☐	**3. In the past month, have you had chest pain when you were not doing physical activity?**
☐	☐	**4. Do you lose your balance because of dizziness or do you ever lose consciousness?**
☐	☐	**5. Do you have a bone or joint problem (for example, back, knee or hip) that could be made worse by a change in your physical activity?**
☐	☐	**6. Is your doctor currently prescribing drugs (for example, water pills) for your blood pressure or heart condition?**
☐	☐	**7. Do you know of any other reason why you should not do physical activity?**

If you answered YES to one or more questions

Talk with your doctor by phone or in person BEFORE you start becoming much more physically active or BEFORE you have a fitness appraisal. Tell your doctor about the PAR-Q and which questions you answered YES.

- You may be able to do any activity you want — as long as you start slowly and build up gradually. Or, you may need to restrict your activities to those which are safe for you. Talk with your doctor about the kinds of activities you wish to participate in and follow his/her advice.
- Find out which community programs are safe and helpful for you.

NO to all questions

If you answered NO honestly to all PAR-Q questions, you can be reasonably sure that you can:

- start becoming much more physically active – begin slowly and build up gradually. This is the safest and easiest way to go.
- take part in a fitness appraisal – this is an excellent way to determine your basic fitness so that you can plan the best way for you to live actively. It is also highly recommended that you have your blood pressure evaluated. If your reading is over 144/94, talk with your doctor before you start becoming much more physically active.

DELAY BECOMING MUCH MORE ACTIVE:

- if you are not feeling well because of a temporary illness such as a cold or a fever – wait until you feel better; or
- if you are or may be pregnant – talk to your doctor before you start becoming more active.

PLEASE NOTE: If your health changes so that you then answer YES to any of the above questions, tell your fitness or health professional. Ask whether you should change your physical activity plan.

Informed Use of the PAR-Q: The Canadian Society for Exercise Physiology, Health Canada, and their agents assume no liability for persons who undertake physical activity, and if in doubt after completing this questionnaire, consult your doctor prior to physical activity.

No changes permitted. You are encouraged to photocopy the PAR-Q but only if you use the entire form.

NOTE: If the PAR-Q is being given to a person before he or she participates in a physical activity program or a fitness appraisal, this section may be used for legal or administrative purposes.

"I have read, understood and completed this questionnaire. Any questions I had were answered to my full satisfaction."

NAME ______________________

SIGNATURE ______________________ DATE __________

SIGNATURE OF PARENT ______________________ WITNESS __________
or GUARDIAN (for participants under the age of majority)

Note: This physical activity clearance is valid for a maximum of 12 months from the date it is completed and becomes invalid if your condition changes so that you would answer YES to any of the seven questions.

continued on other side...

HEALTH HISTORY QUESTIONNAIRE

INTRODUCTION

Although exercise testing and exercise participation are relatively safe for most apparently healthy individuals, the reaction of the cardiovascular system to increased levels of physical activity cannot always be totally predicted. Consequently, there is a small but real risk of certain changes occurring during exercise testing and participation. Some of these changes may be abnormal blood pressure, irregular heart rhythm, fainting, and in rare instances a heart attack or cardiac arrest. Therefore, you must provide honest answers to this questionnaire. Exercise may be contraindicated under some of the conditions listed below; others may simply require special consideration. **If any of the conditions apply, consult your physician before you participate in an exercise program.** Also, promptly report to your instructor any exercise-related abnormalities that you may experience during the course of the semester.

A. Have you ever had or do you now have any of the following conditions?

- ☐ 1. A myocardial infarction
- ☐ 2. Coronary artery disease
- ☐ 3. Congestive heart failure
- ☐ 4. Elevated blood lipids (cholesterol and triglycerides)
- ☐ 5. Chest pain at rest or during exertion
- ☐ 6. Shortness of breath
- ☐ 7. An abnormal resting or stress electrocardiogram
- ☐ 8. Uneven, irregular, or skipped heartbeats (including a racing or fluttering heart)
- ☐ 9. A blood embolism
- ☐ 10. Thrombophlebitis
- ☐ 11. Rheumatic heart fever
- ☐ 12. Elevated blood pressure
- ☐ 13. A stroke
- ☐ 14. Diabetes
- ☐ 15. A family history of coronary heart disease, syncope, or sudden death before age 60
- ☐ 16. Any other heart problem that makes exercise unsafe

B. Do you have any of the following conditions?

- ☐ 1. Arthritis, rheumatism, or gout
- ☐ 2. Chronic low back pain
- ☐ 3. Any other joint, bone, or muscle problems
- ☐ 4. Any respiratory problems
- ☐ 5. Obesity (more than 30 percent overweight)
- ☐ 6. Anorexia
- ☐ 7. Bulimia
- ☐ 8. Mononucleosis
- ☐ 9. Any physical disability that could interfere with safe participation in exercise

C. Do any of the following conditions apply?

- ☐ 1. Do you smoke cigarettes?
- ☐ 2. Are you taking any prescription drugs?

D. Do you have any other concern regarding your ability to safely participate in an exercise program? If so, explain:

____

____

____

Student's Signature: ______________________________ **Date:** ____________

Lab 1D: Resting Heart Rate and Blood Pressure

Name ______________________ Date ____________ Grade ____________

Instructor ______________________ Course ____________ Section ____________

NECESSARY LAB EQUIPMENT
Stopwatches, stethoscopes, and blood pressure sphygmomanometers.

OBJECTIVE
To determine resting heart rate and blood pressure.

PREPARATION
The instructions to determine heart rate and blood pressure are given on pages 29–30. Many factors can affect heart rate and blood pressure. Factors such as excitement, nervousness, stress, food, smoking, pain, temperature, and physical exertion all can alter heart rate and blood pressure significantly. Therefore, whenever possible, readings should be taken in a quiet, comfortable room following a few minutes of rest in the recording position. Avoid any form of exercise several hours prior to the assessment. Wear exercise clothing, including a shirt with short or loose-fitting sleeves to allow for placement of the blood pressure cuff around the upper arm.

I. Resting Heart Rate and Blood Pressure

Determine your resting heart rate and blood pressure in the right and left arms while sitting comfortably in a chair.

Resting Heart Rate: ________ bpm Rating (see Table 1.6, page 29): ________

Blood Pressure:	Right Arm	Rating (from Table 1.7, page 29)	Left Arm	Rating (from Table 1.7, page 29)
Systolic				
Diastolic				

II. Standing, Walking, Jogging Heart Rate and Blood Pressure

Have one individual measure your heart rate and another individual your blood pressure immediately after standing for one minute, after walking for one minute, and after jogging in place for one minute. For blood pressure assessment use the arm that showed the highest reading in the sitting position (in Part I, above).

Activity	Heart Rate (bpm)	Systolic/Diastolic Blood Pressure (mm Hg)
Standing		/
Walking		/
Jogging		/

III. Effects of Aerobic Activity on Resting Heart Rate

Using your actual resting heart rate (RHR) from Part I of this lab, compute the total number of times your heart beats each day and each year:

A. Beats per day = ________ (RHR bpm) × 60 (min per hour) × 24 (hours per day) = ________ beats per day

B. Beats per year = ________ (heart rate in beats per day, use item A) × 365 = ________ beats per year

If your RHR dropped 20 bpm through an aerobic exercise program, determine the number of beats that your heart would save each year at that lower RHR:

C. Beats per day = ________ (your current RHR − 20) × 60 × 24 = __________ beats per day

D. Beats per year = ________ (heart rate in beats per day, use item C) × 365 = ____________ beats per year

E. Number of beats saved per year (B − D) __________ − ____________ = ____________ beats saved per year

Assuming that you will reach the average U.S. life expectancy of 80 years for women or 75 for men, determine the additional number of "heart rate life years" available to you if your RHR were 20 bpm lower:

F. Years of life ahead = ______ (use 80 for women and 75 for men) − ______ (current age) = ______ years

G. Number of beats saved = __________ (use item E) × ______ (use item F) = ____________ beats saved

H. Number of heart rate life years based on the lower RHR = ____________ (use item G) ÷ ______ (use item D) = ______ years

IV. Mean Blood Pressure Computation

During a normal resting contraction/relaxation cycle of the heart, the heart spends more time in the relaxation (diastolic) phase than in the contraction (systolic) phase. Accordingly, mean blood pressure (MBP) cannot be computed by taking an average of the systolic (SBP) and diastolic (DBP) blood pressures. The following equations are, therefore, used to determine MBP:

MBP = DBP + ⅓ PP Where PP = pulse pressure or the difference between the systolic and diastolic pressures.

A. Compute your MBP using your own blood pressure results:

PP = ________ (systolic) − ________ (diastolic) = ________ mm Hg

MBP = ________ (DBP) + $\frac{\text{\_\_\_\_\_\_\_\_ (PP)}}{3}$ = ________ mm Hg

B. Determine the MBP for a person with a BP of 130/80 and a second person with a BP of 120/90.

____

____

____

____

Which subject has the lower MBP? ______________________________

V. What I Learned

Draw conclusions based on your observed resting and activity heart rates and blood pressures. Discuss the importance of a lower resting heart rate to your health and comment on the effects of a higher systolic versus diastolic blood pressure on the mean arterial blood pressure.

____

____

____

____

____

____

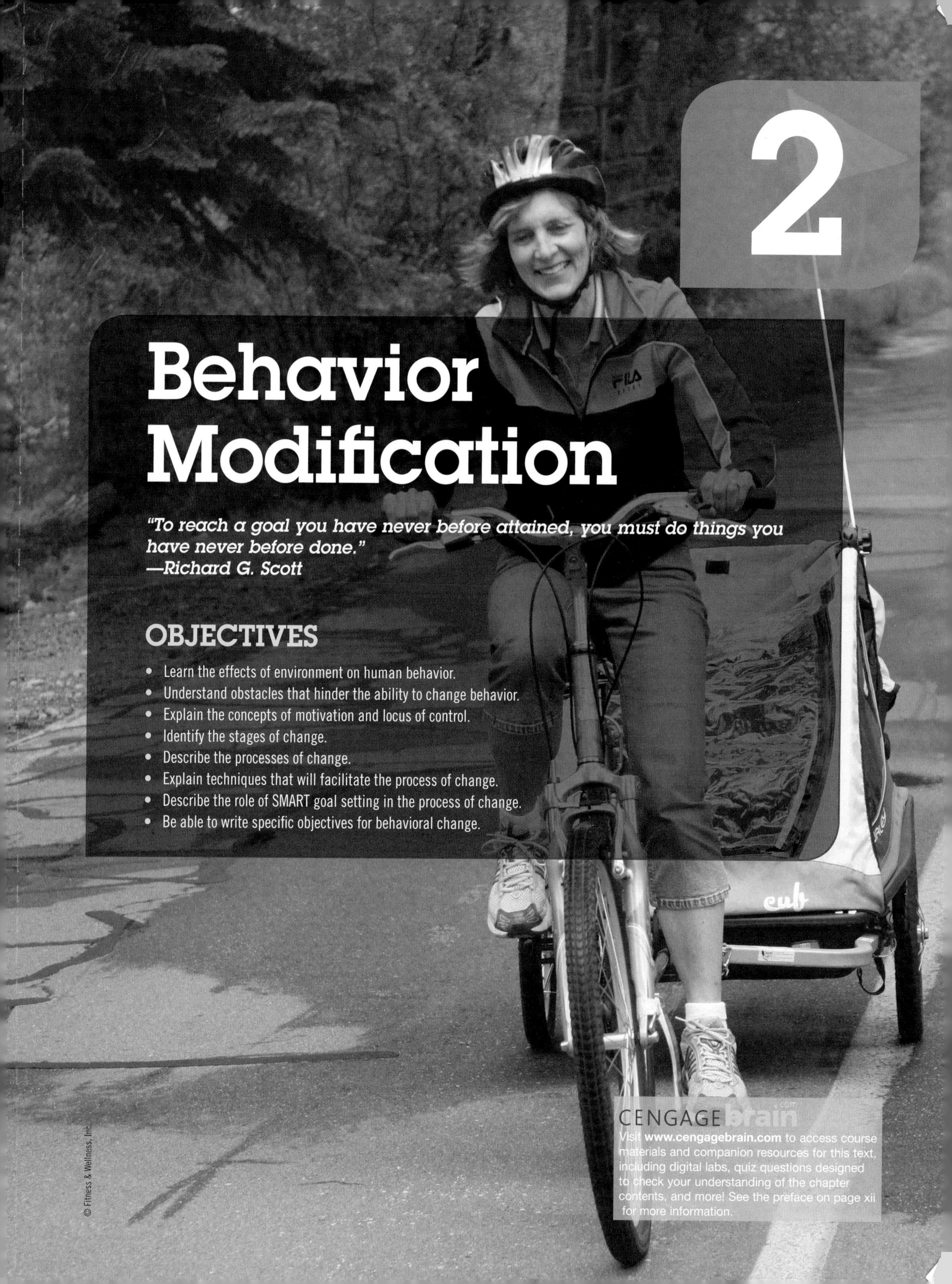

2

Behavior Modification

"To reach a goal you have never before attained, you must do things you have never before done."
—Richard G. Scott

OBJECTIVES

- Learn the effects of environment on human behavior.
- Understand obstacles that hinder the ability to change behavior.
- Explain the concepts of motivation and locus of control.
- Identify the stages of change.
- Describe the processes of change.
- Explain techniques that will facilitate the process of change.
- Describe the role of SMART goal setting in the process of change.
- Be able to write specific objectives for behavioral change.

CENGAGEbrain.com

Visit **www.cengagebrain.com** to access course materials and companion resources for this text, including digital labs, quiz questions designed to check your understanding of the chapter contents, and more! See the preface on page xii for more information.

REAL LIFE STORY | Sharon's Experience

Prior to my marriage, I had never really tried jogging. But then I became convinced that aerobic exercise would improve my fitness and help me maintain a healthy weight. My fiancé was really serious about fitness and had been jogging regularly for several years. We wrote out an exercise prescription and started jogging together. Exercise helped me to accomplish my health goals through my first two pregnancies. The feeling of being physically fit was a reward in itself, but jogging two consecutive miles was rarely truly enjoyable. With young children at home, my husband and I were forced to take turns jogging so that one of us would always be home. My jogging program consisted of a 20-minute jog: 1 mile out and 1 mile back, five to six times per week. Five years later, on one particular day, 25 minutes went by and I wasn't ready to stop jogging. At 30 minutes, I went and knocked on the door: "Honey, I feel great—I'll be back in 10 minutes." I did this again at 40 and 50 minutes. I ended up jogging for a full 60 minutes for the first time in my life, and the experience was genuinely joyful! That day, I finally reached "the top of the mountain" (the termination/adoption stage of change) and truly experienced the joy of being physically fit. Jogging became as easy as a "bird in flight." I have not stopped jogging in more than 35 years! It wasn't easy at first, but knowledge, commitment, support, action, and perseverance paid off.

Fitness also was the factor that led to improvements in other wellness components in our lives (continuing health education, good nutrition, stress reduction, and chronic disease prevention). Fitness is the daily "bread and butter" that enhances our quality of life. Our five children now also follow our active lifestyle. We always said: "A family that exercises together stays together."

The benefits of regular physical activity and living a healthy lifestyle to achieve wellness are well documented. Nearly all Americans accept that exercise is beneficial to health and see a need to incorporate it into their lives. Seventy percent of new and returning exercisers, however, are at risk for early dropout.[1] As the scientific evidence continues to mount each day, most people still are not adhering to a healthy lifestyle program.

Let's look at an all-too-common occurrence on college campuses. Most students understand that they should be exercising, and they contemplate enrolling in a fitness course. The motivating factor might be improved physical appearance, health benefits, or simply fulfillment of a college requirement. They sign up for the course, participate for a few months, finish the course, and stop exercising! They offer a wide array of excuses: too busy, no one to exercise with, already have the grade, inconvenient open-gym hours, job conflicts, and so on. A few months later, they realize once again that exercise is vital, and they repeat the cycle (Figure 2.1).

The information in this book will be of little value to you if you are unable to abandon your negative habits and adopt and maintain healthy behaviors. Before looking at any physical fitness and wellness guidelines, you will need to take a critical look at your behaviors and lifestyle, and most likely make some permanent changes to promote your overall health and wellness.

FIGURE 2.1 **Exercise/exercise dropout cycle.**

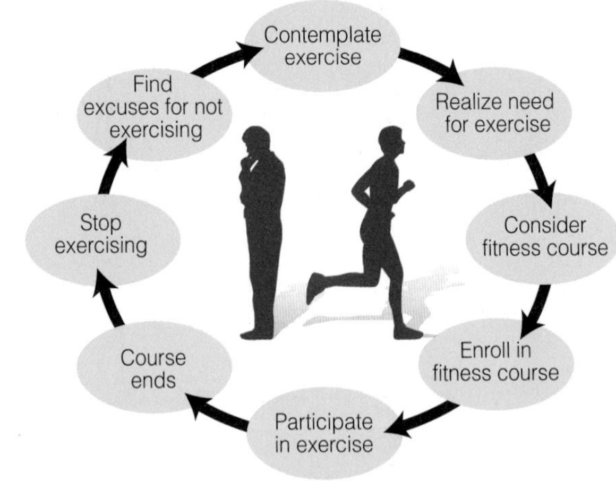

Living in a Toxic Health and Fitness Environment

Most of the behaviors we adopt are a product of our environment—the forces of social influences we encounter and the thought processes we go through (also see self-efficacy on pages 12–15). This environment includes fami-

FAQ

Why is it so hard to change?

Change is incredibly difficult for most people. Our behaviors are based on our core values and actions that are rewarded. Whether we are trying to increase physical activity, quit smoking, change unhealthy eating habits, or reverse heart disease, it is human nature to resist change that isn't immediately rewarded, even when we know that change will provide substantial benefits in the near future. Furthermore, Dr. Richard Earle, managing director of the Canadian Institute of Stress and the Hans Selye Foundation, explains that people have a tendency toward pessimism. This tendency, commonly referred to as a "negativity bias," is hardwired into our biology. In every spoken language, there is a ratio of three pessimistic adjectives to one positive adjective. Thus, linguistically, psychologically, and emotionally, we focus on what can go wrong and we lose motivation before we even start. That's why we have the saying, "The only person who truly welcomes a change is a baby with a full diaper."

What triggers the desire to change?

Motivation comes from within. In most instances, no amount of pressure, reasoning, or fear will inspire people to take action. Change in behavior is most likely to occur when people either receive instant gratification for their actions or when people's feelings are addressed. People may pursue change when it's rewarded (for example, lower health care premiums if you quit smoking) or they may start contemplating change when there is a shift in core values that will make them feel uncomfortable with the present behavior(s) or lack thereof (e.g., a long and healthy life is more important than smoking). Core values change when feelings are addressed. The challenge is to find ways that will help people understand the problems and solutions in a manner that will influence emotions and not just the thought process. Once the problem behavior is understood and "felt," the person may become uncomfortable with the situation and will be more inclined to address the problem behavior or adopt a healthy behavior.

Dr. Jan Hill, a Toronto based life skills specialist, stated that discomfort is a great motivator. People tolerate any situation until it becomes too uncomfortable for them: "Then they have to take steps to make changes in their lives." It is at this point that the skills presented in this chapter will help you implement a successful plan for change. Keep in mind that as you make lifestyle changes, your relationships and friendships also need to be addressed. You need to distance yourself from those individuals who share your bad habits (e.g., smoking, drinking, sedentary lifestyle) and associate with people who practice healthy habits. Are you prepared to do so?

SOURCE: Adapted from K. Jenkins, "Why Is Change So Hard?" http://www.healthnexus.ca/projects/articles/change.htm, downloaded March 12, 2011.

MyProfile: Personal Behavior Modification Profile

Are you able to answer the following questions regarding behavior change? If you are unable to do so, the chapter contents will help you.

I. Can you identify behavioral changes that you have consciously made in your life and the process that you went through to do so? ______________________________

II. Would you categorize yourself as having an internal or external locus of control? ______

III. Can you identify your current stage of change for the following? Physical activity: ______ exercise: ______ nutrition: ______ weight management: ______

IV. A person precontemplating a change in behavior is said to be ready to start the process of change.
___ True ___ False

V. SMART goals enhance the odds of success.
___ True ___ False

VI. Can you list the processes of change that most helped Sharon adhere to her fitness program? ______

lies, friends, peers, homes, schools, workplaces, television, radio, and movies, as well as our communities, country, and culture in general. Unfortunately, when it comes to fitness and wellness, we live in a "toxic" environment. Becoming aware of how the environment affects us is vital if we wish to achieve and maintain wellness. Yet, we are so habituated to the environment that we miss the subtle ways it influences our behaviors, personal lifestyle, and health each day.

From a young age, we observe, we learn, we emulate, and without realizing it, we incorporate into our own lifestyle the behaviors of people around us. Social norms have a way of affecting nearly every decision we make. A recent group of studies carried out in the United Kingdom, for example, found that something as simple as informing diners of what their fellow diners were choosing changed eating behavior. Participants chose to eat larger or smaller portions and make lower- or higher-calorie food choices to conform to what they were told their fellow diners were eating.[2]

Consider the endless ways our social and physical environment affect us each day. We are transported by parents and friends who drive us nearly any place we need to go. We watch them drive short distances to run errands. We see them take escalators and elevators and ride moving sidewalks at malls and airports. They use remote controls and cell phones. We observe them choosing food for convenience and price point over nutritional value, and we watch as they stop at fast-food restaurants and pick up supersized, calorie-dense, high-fat snacks and meals. They watch television and surf the net for hours at a time. Some smoke, some drink heavily, and some have hard-drug addictions. Others engage in risky behaviors by not wearing seat belts, by drinking and driving, and by having unprotected sex. All of these unhealthy habits can be passed along, unquestioned, to the next generation.

Environmental Influences on Physical Activity

Among the leading underlying causes of death in the United States are physical inactivity and poor diet. This is partially because most activities of daily living, which a few decades ago required movement or physical activity, now require almost no effort and negatively affect health, fitness, and body weight. Small movements that have been streamlined out of daily life quickly add up, especially when we consider these over 7 days a week and 52 weeks a year.

Consider the decrease in the required daily energy (caloric) expenditure as a result of modern-day conveniences that lull us into physical inactivity. For example, short automobile trips that replace walking or riding a bike decrease energy expenditure by 50 to 300 calories per day; automatic car window and door openers represent about 1 calorie at each use; automatic garage door openers, 5 calories; drive-through windows at banks, fast-food restaurants, dry cleaners, and pharmacies add up to about 5 to 10 calories each time; elevators and escalators, 3 to 10 calories per trip; food processors, 5 to 10 calories; riding lawnmowers, about 100 calories; automatic car washes, 100 calories; hours of computer use to e-mail, surf the net, text, and conduct Internet transactions represent another 50 to 300 calories of lost opportunity for everyday physical activity, not to mention the additional risks of uninterrupted sitting; and excessive television viewing can add up to 200 or more calories. Little wonder that we have such a difficult time maintaining a healthy body weight.

With the advent of now-ubiquitous cell phones, people are moving even less. Shopping and banking can be done from the couch. Family members call each other on the phone even within the walls of their own home. Some people don't get out of the car anymore to ring a doorbell. Instead, they wait in front and send a text message to have the person come out.

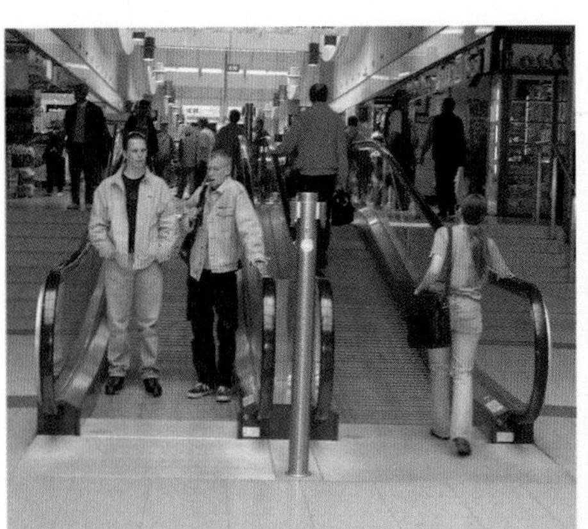
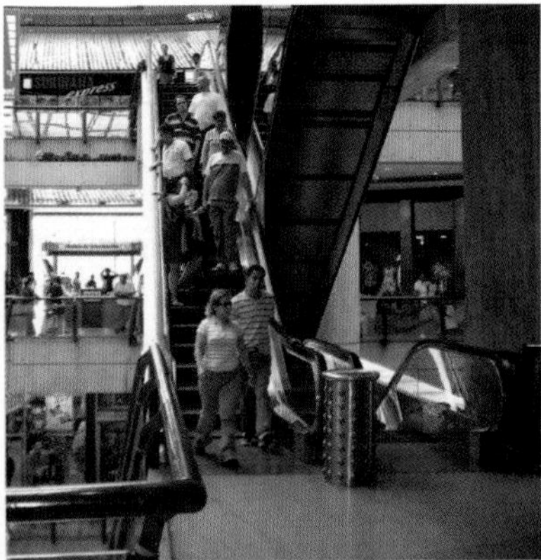
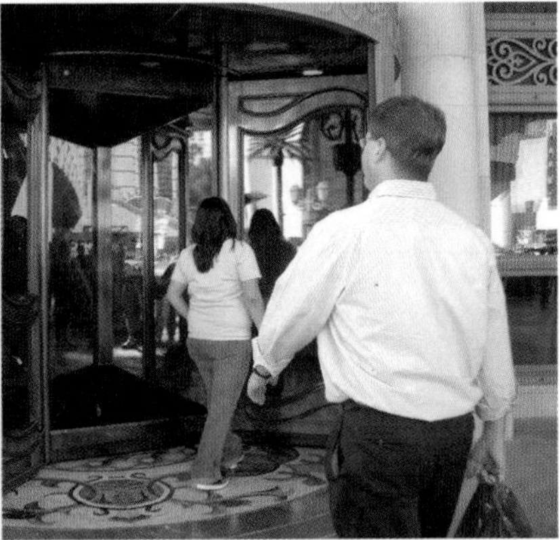
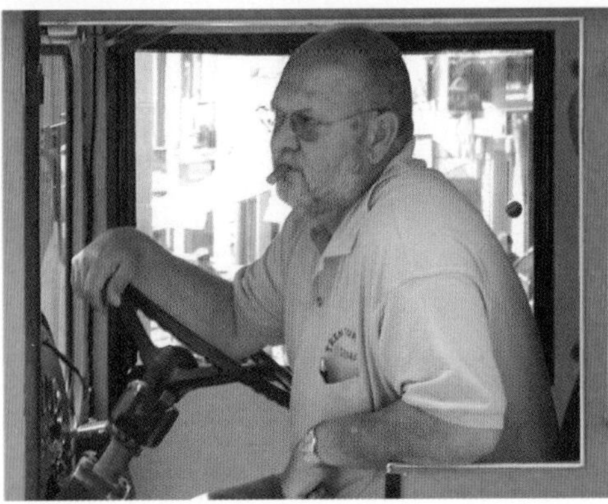
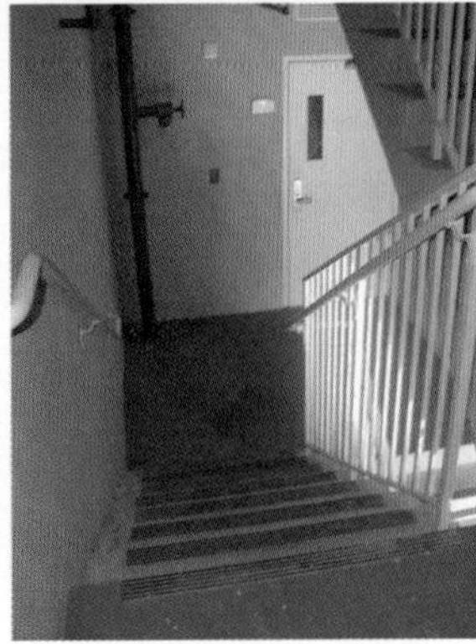
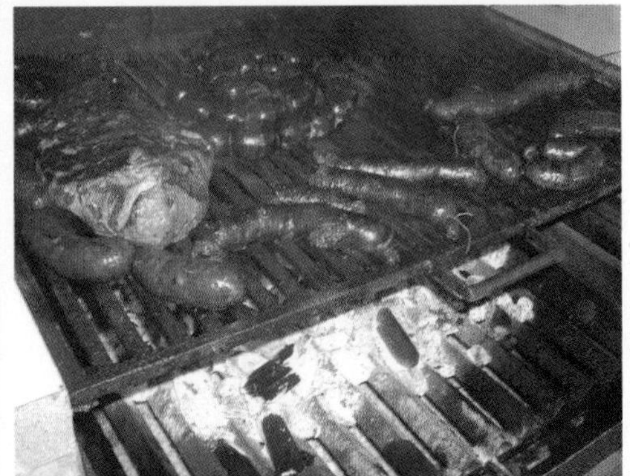

Our environment is not conducive to a healthy, physically active lifestyle.

Even modern-day architecture reinforces unhealthy behaviors. Elevators and escalators are often of the finest workmanship and located conveniently. Many of our newest, showiest shopping centers and convention centers don't provide accessible stairwells, so people are all but forced to ride escalators. If they want to walk up the escalator, they can't because the people in front of them obstruct the way. Entrances to buildings provide electric sensors and automatic door openers. Without a second thought, people walk through automatic doors instead of taking the time to push a door open.

At work, most people have jobs that require them to sit most of the day. We don't even get up and walk a short distance to talk to coworkers. Instead, we use e-mail, IM, texting, and phone calls.

Health experts recommend five to six miles of walking per day. This level of activity equates to about 10,000 to 12,000 daily steps. If you have never clipped on a pedometer, try to do so. When you look at the total number of steps it displays at the end of the day, you may be shocked by how few steps you took.

As indicated in Chapter 1, an excessive amount of daily time spent sitting (riding in a car, sitting at a desk, watching TV and movies, playing computer games, surfing the Internet), directly correlates with an increased risk for all-cause and cardiovascular disease mortality, independent of leisure-time physical activity and excessive body weight.[3] The greater the amount of sitting time per day, the greater the risk of disability, disease, and premature mortality. As expected, the highest mortality rates were seen in obese individuals who sit almost all of the time.

Of particular interest, studies have shown that death rates were still high for people who spent a large portion of their day sitting, even though they met the current minimum moderate-physical activity recommendations (30 minutes, at least five times per week). The researchers concluded that for better health and a longer life people should break up periods of uninterrupted sitting, avoid sedentarism, and most importantly, decrease total daily sitting time.Not surprisingly then, other data have linked excessive TV watching and earlier death.[4] A total of 8,800 adults with no history of heart disease were followed for more than six years. As compared to individuals who only watched two hours of TV per day, those who watched four or more daily hours were 80 percent more likely to die from heart disease and 46 percent more likely to die from all causes. The authors indicated that, as with excessive sitting, exercise does not make up for long TV sessions. Sitting is the "default position" for TV viewing, and such an action minimizes tasks such as standing, walking, and moving about during the course of the day. Excessive TV viewing may also be more detrimental than other sedentary activities such as reading, studying, or doing homework. A subsequent study concluded that for every hour of sedentary TV watching per day, life expectancy decreases 22 minutes.[5] Thus, a 25-year-old individual who watches TV six hours per day reduces life expectancy by almost 5 years. Both excessive TV viewing and excessive sitting appear to be associated with a loss of life that is as severe as other disease risk factors such as physical inactivity, smoking, and obesity.

When people find a few free minutes during the day or arrive home after work, they turn to a screen. Americans spend an average of 4.4 hours of their leisure time each day on a screen.[6] The average American school child, when graduating from high school, will have spent more time watching TV and viewing screens than they will have spent in school.[7] And it is no wonder. The first thing people consider when setting up a family room is where to put the television. This little (or big-screen) box has truly lulled us into inactivity.

Television viewing is more than just a sedentary activity. Think about people's habits before they sit down to watch a favorite show. They turn on the television, then stop by the kitchen for a box of crackers and processed cheese. They return to watch the show, start snacking, and are bombarded with commercials about soft drinks, beer, and unhealthy foods. Viewers are enticed to purchase and eat unhealthy, calorie-dense foods in an unnecessary and mindless "snacking setting." Television viewing has been shown to reduce the number of fruits and vegetables some people consume, most likely because people are eating the unhealthy foods advertised on television.[8] A similar result has been observed in those playing video games. Calorie intake has been found to go up regardless of the individual's hunger cues.[9]

In addition to sitting most of the day at work and at home, we also sit in our cars. We are transported or we drive everywhere we have to go. Safety concerns also keep people in cars instead of on sidewalks and in parks. And communities are designed around the automobile. City

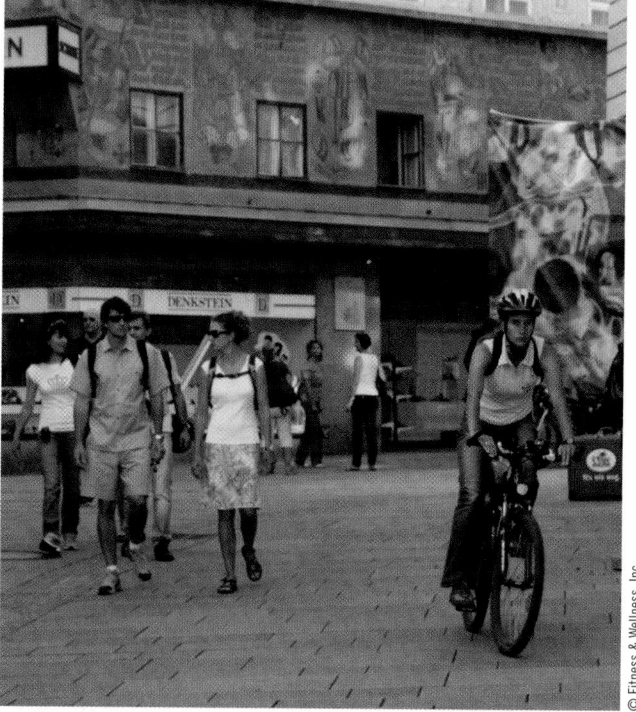

Walking and cycling are priority activities in many European communities.

streets make driving convenient and walking or cycling difficult, impossible, or dangerous. Streets typically are rated by traffic engineers according to their "level of service"—that is, based on how well they facilitate motorized traffic. A wide, straight street with few barriers to slow motorized traffic gets a high score. According to these guidelines, pedestrians are "obstructions." Only recently have a few local governments and communities started to devise standards to determine how useful streets are for pedestrians and bicyclists and to measure communities by their "walkability score." Neighborhoods where walking is safe, inviting, and a practical means to reach a nearby destination are healthier for their residents. In one large-scale study, the average man in a walkable neighborhood weighed 10 pounds less and the average woman 6 pounds less than their counterparts in less walkable neighborhoods.[10]

Many people drive because the distances to cover are on a vast scale. We live in bedroom communities and commute to work. When people live near frequently visited destinations, they are more likely to walk or bike for transportation. In the United States, the automobile is used about half of the time for distances shorter than 500 yards, whereas it is used more than 90 percent of the time for distances greater than two-thirds of a mile. Neighborhoods that mix commercial and residential land use encourage walking over driving because of the short distances among home, shopping, and work.

Children also walk or cycle to school today less frequently than in the past. The reasons? Distance, traffic, weather, perceived crime, and school policy. Distance is a significant barrier because the trend during the past few decades has been to build larger schools on the outskirts of communities instead of small schools within neighborhoods.

For each car in the United States, there are seven parking spaces.[11] Drivers can almost always find a parking spot, but walkers often run out of sidewalks and crosswalks in modern streets. Sidewalks and walkability features have simply not been a priority in city, suburban, or commercial development. Whereas British street design manuals recommend sidewalks on both sides of the street, American manuals recommend sidewalks on one side of the street only.

One measure that encourages activity is the use of "traffic-calming" strategies: intentionally slowing traffic to make the pedestrian's role easier. These strategies were developed and are widely used in Europe. Examples include narrower streets, rougher pavement (cobblestone), pedestrian islands, and raised crosswalks.

Many European communities place a high priority on walking, cycling, and the use of public transit (the latter requires walking or cycling to the transit stops), which makes up 40 to 67 percent of all daily trips taken by people in Germany, Austria, Spain, the Netherlands, Switzerland, and Latvia. By contrast, in the United States, walking, cycling, and public transit account for 9 percent of daily trips, whereas the automobile accounts for 85 percent.[12]

Environmental Influence on Diet and Nutrition

The present obesity epidemic in the United States and other developed countries has been getting worse every year. In the United States thirty years ago, the state with the highest obesity rate was still lower than the state today with the lowest obesity rate. Indeed we have adopted a new norm. We are becoming a nation of overweight and obese people. You may ask why. Let's examine the evidence.

Let's begin with the amount of calories available to us as a nation. According to the U.S. Department of Agriculture, the American food supply contains a surplus of 500 calories per day, per person, after wastage. This is a surplus that did not exist in the 1970 food supply, which means that we have taken the amount of food available to us and tossed in a Big Mac's worth of calories per day for every person in the country. The nutritional quality of the U.S. food supply does not brighten the outlook. Indeed, if we set about to align the food available in the U.S. with nutritional guidelines, major changes would be in order. The supply of vegetables would need to rise by 70 percent, the supply of fruit would need to double, and as for the grain supply, four times as much of our grain would need to remain whole instead of being refined.[13]

The overabundance of food and the need for profits increases pressure on food suppliers to advertise and try to convince consumers to buy their products. As explained by a former executive of a large food company who left after feeling uncomfortable with industry ethics, "Over the years, relentless efforts were made to increase the number of 'eating occasions' people indulged in and the amount of food they consumed at each."[14] It is perhaps illuminating to imagine a world in which other industries successfully carried out the same campaigns of increase. Imagine the results if, for example, the cosmetics industry successfully urged customers toward the same consumption pattern of more occasions for use and higher quantities consumed at each use. Yet we follow this pattern with food consumption, which affects our very mortality. The food industry spends more than $33 billion each year on advertising and promotion, and most of this money goes toward highly processed foods. The few ads and campaigns promoting healthy foods and healthful eating simply cannot compete. Most of us would be hard-pressed to recall a jingle for brown rice or kale. It is not unusual for the money spent advertising a single food product across the United States to be 10 to 50 times more than the money the federal government spends promoting MyPlate or encouraging us to eat fruits and vegetables.[15]

Coupled with our sedentary lifestyle, many activities of daily living in today's culture are associated with eating. We seem to be eating all the time. We eat during coffee breaks, when we socialize, when we play, when we watch sports, at the movies, during television viewing, and when the clock tells us it's time for a meal. Our lives seem to be centered on food, a nonstop string of occasions to eat and overeat. And much of the overeating is done without a second thought.

For instance, when people rent a video, they usually end up in line with the video and also with popcorn, candy, and soft drinks. Do we really have to eat while watching a movie? These "eating occasions" are a major contribution to our growing waistlines, and have made a notable jump from an average of 3.8 daily occasions thirty years ago to 4.9 daily occasions today.[16] You may take a moment to reflect on your typical day and consider your own average number of eating occasions. Also, consider how long it has been since the last time you were hungry; that is, *really hungry.*

As a nation, we now eat out more often than in the past, portion sizes are larger, and we snack more than ever before as we have an endless variety of foods to choose from. Unhealthy food is relatively inexpensive and is sold in places where it was not available in the past. Current food prices and shopping trends show that, while the overall cost of food has made a steady decline in the United States, shoppers must be willing to spend extra for good nutrition. However, passing over some opportunities to eat out is often enough to compensate for the cost difference, and choosing nutrition over a low price point can pay big dividends in future health costs, not to mention quality of life. *You can pay for healthy food now or spend a much higher amount in health care later.* Also, eating dinner at home around the table accompanied by meaningful conversation (as compared to watching TV) has been linked to a lower BMI.[17]

Unfortunately, people have decided that they no longer require special occasions to eat out. Mother's Day, a birthday, or someone's graduation are no longer reasons to eat at a restaurant. Eating out is part of today's lifestyle. In the 1970s, Americans ate out an average of two times per week, nowadays people in the United States average five meals per week. Almost half of the money Americans spend on food today is on meals away from home.[18]

Eating out would not be such a problem if portion sizes were reasonable or if restaurant food were similar to food prepared at home. Compared with home-cooked meals, restaurant and fast-food meals are higher in calories, fat, saturated fat, and sodium and lower in vitamins, minerals, and fiber. Today, the average restaurant meal contains more than half of an entire day's caloric and fat allowance and a day and a half's worth of the recommended amount of sodium.

Food portions in restaurants have increased substantially in size. Patrons consume huge amounts of food, almost as if this were the last meal they would ever have. They drink entire pitchers of soda pop or beer instead of the traditional 8-ounce cup sizes. Some restaurant menus may include selections that are called "healthy choices," but these items may not provide nutritional information, including calories. In all likelihood, the menu has many other choices that look delicious but provide larger serving sizes with more fat and calories and fewer fruits and vegetables. Making a healthy selection is difficult, because people tend to choose food for its taste, convenience, and cost instead of nutrition.

Restaurant food is often less healthy than we think. Indeed, restaurant patrons often underestimate the number of calories they consume during a meal. One recent study of fast-food patrons found two-thirds of study participants underestimated their calorie intake by hundreds of calories in many cases.[19] Another study asked trained dietitians to estimate nutrition information for five restaurant meals. The results showed that the dietitians underestimated the number of calories and amount of fat by 37 and 49 percent, respectively.[20] Findings such as these do not offer much hope for the average consumer who tries to make healthy choices when eating out.

We can also notice that most restaurants are pleasurable places to be: colorful, well lit, and thoughtfully decorated. These intentional features are designed to enhance comfort, appetite, and length of stay, with the intent to entice more eating. Employees are formally trained in techniques that urge patrons to eat more and spend more. Servers are prepared to approach the table and suggest specific drinks, with at least one from the bar. When the drink is served, they recommend selected appetizers. Drink refills are often free while dining out. Following dinner, the server offers desserts and coffee. A person could literally get a full day's worth of calories in one meal without ever ordering an entrée, and often without realizing their calorie consumption.

Even as the awareness of the need for healthful eating habits has grown, few changes have been made in fast food. One recent study found that in a period of 14 years, the nutritional rating of fast food offerings as measured by the USDA's Healthy Eating Index has improved by only 3 percent. A study looking at a similar time period found that the overall sodium levels had increased by 2.6 percent.[21] If changes are going to be made for the better, they will need to be spurred from both the company and the consumer. When a fast-food chain recently added its latest salad selections to the menu, sales of their extra-large burgers rose as well. The reason for this rise was that customers imagined themselves ordering more healthy options in the future and felt justified in ordering a less healthy option during their current visit. Menu items at many fast food restaurants frequently are introduced at one size and, over time, popular items are increased in size by two to five times.[22] Large portion sizes are a major problem because people tend to eat what they are served. A study by the American Institute for Cancer Research found that with bigger portion sizes, 67 percent of Americans ate the larger amount of food they were served.[23] The tendency of most patrons is to "clean the plate."

Individuals seem to have the same disregard for hunger cues when snacking. Participants in one study were randomly given an afternoon snack of potato chips in different bag sizes. The participants received bags from 1 to 20 ounces for 5 days. The results showed that the larger the bag, the more the person ate. Men ate 37 percent more chips from the largest than the smallest bag. Women ate 18 percent more. Of significant interest, the size of the snack did not change the amount of food the person ate during the next meal. Another study found no major difference in reported hunger or fullness after participants ate different sizes of sandwiches that were served to them, even though they ate more when they were given larger sandwiches.[24]

Other researchers set out to see if the size of the package—not just the amount of food—affects how much people eat. Study participants received two different-sized packages with the same number of spaghetti strands. The larger package was twice the size of the smaller package. When participants were asked to take out enough spaghetti to prepare a meal for two adults, they took out an average of 234 strands from the small package versus 302 strands from the larger package.[25] In our own kitchens, and in restaurants, we seem to have taken away from our internal cues the decision of how much to eat. Instead we have turned that choice over to businesses that profit from our overindulgence.

Also working against our hunger cues is our sense of thrift. Many of us consider cost ahead of nutrition when we choose foods. Restaurants and grocery stores often appeal to this sense of thrift by using "value marketing," meaning that they offer us a larger portion for only a small price increase. Customers think they are getting a bargain, and the food providers turn a better profit because the cost of additional food is small compared with the cost of marketing, production, and labor.

The National Alliance for Nutrition has further shown that a little more money buys a lot more calories. Ice cream upsizing from a kid's scoop to a double scoop, for example, adds an extra 390 calories for only an extra $1.62. A medium-size movie theater popcorn (unbuttered) provides 500 additional calories over a small-size popcorn for just an extra 71 cents. Equally, king-size candy bars provide about 230 additional calories for just another 33 cents over the standard size.[26] We often eat more simply because we get more for our money without taking into consideration the detrimental consequences to our health and waistline.

Another example of financial but not nutritional sense is free soft-drink refills. When people choose a high-calorie drink over diet soda or water, the person does not compensate by eating less food later that day.[27] Liquid calories seem to be difficult for people to account for. A 20-ounce bottle of regular soda contains the equivalent of one-third cup of sugar. One extra can of soda (160 calories) per day represents an extra 16.5 pounds of fat per year (160 calories × 365 days ÷ 3,500 calories). Even people who regularly drink diet sodas tend to gain weight. In their minds, they may rationalize that a calorie-free drink allows them to consume more food.

A larger variety of food also entices overeating. Think about your own experiences at parties that have a buffet of snacks. Do you eat more when everyone brings something to contribute to the snack table? When unhealthy choices outnumber healthy choices, people are less likely to follow their natural cues to choose healthy food.

The previously mentioned environmental factors influence our thought processes and hinder our ability to determine what constitutes an appropriate meal based on actual needs. The result: On average, American women consume 335 more daily calories than they did 20 years ago, and men an additional 170 calories.[28]

Now you can analyze and identify the environmental influences on your behaviors. Lab 2A provides you with the opportunity to determine whether you control your environment or the environment controls you.

Living in the 21st century, we have all the modern-day conveniences that lull us into overconsumption and sedentary living. By living in America, we adopt behaviors that put our health at risk. And though we understand that lifestyle choices affect our health and well-being, we still have an extremely difficult time making changes.

Let's look at weight gain. Most people do not start life with a weight problem. By age 20, a man may weigh 160 pounds. After a year or two, the weight climbs and he may reach 170 pounds. He now adapts and accepts 170 pounds as his weight. He may go on a diet but not make the necessary lifestyle changes. Gradually his weight climbs to 180, 190, 200 pounds. Although he may not like it and would like to weigh less, once again he adapts and accepts 200 pounds as his stable weight.

The time comes, usually around middle age, when values change, that people want to make changes in their lives but find this difficult to accomplish, illustrating the adage that "old habits die hard." Acquiring positive behaviors that will lead to better health and well-being is a long-term process and requires continual effort. Understanding why so many people are unsuccessful at changing their behaviors and are unable to live a healthy lifestyle may increase your readiness and motivation for change. Next we will examine barriers to change, what motivates people to change, behavior change theories, the transtheoretical or stages-of-change model, the process of change, techniques for change, and **actions** required to make permanent changes in behavior.

Values and Behavior

To understand human behavior, or why people do what they do, we need to understand values. Values are defined as the core beliefs and ideals that people have. Values govern behavior as people look to conduct themselves in a manner that is conducive to living and attaining goals consistent with their beliefs and what's important to them. A person's values reflect who they are.

Values are established through experience and learning, and their development is a lifelong process that influences all aspects of life. Personal values are developed within family circles, schools, the media, and the culture where people grow up and live; according to what is acceptable or unacceptable, desirable or undesirable, good or bad, and rewarded or ignored/punished. Educational experiences play a key role in the establishment of values (see Figure 2.2). Education is power: It provides people with knowledge to form opinions, allows them to better grasp future outcomes from today's choices, and forces them to question issues and take stands.

Values are also learned through examples and role models. People tend to emulate and adopt behaviors from people they admire, look up to, or view as heroes. Role models are most often parents, life heroes, siblings, classmates, sports figures, or people one sees on television or in movies, or reads and hears about through books or other media sources. As people look to develop values, they typically search for and emulate people of high ethical values

FIGURE 2.2 **Values and behavior.**

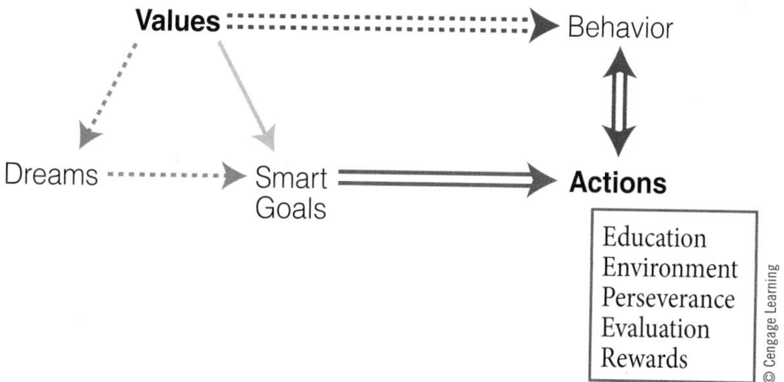

and accomplishments that make them feel positive both about the people whose behaviors they are trying to emulate and themselves. Subsequently, the constant and habitual repetition of similar actions, behaviors, and expectations has a powerful conditioning effect on the mind and the role of the value for success in life.

Core values change throughout life based on education and the environment in which people live. Learning and gaining a belief about a particular issue is most critical in the establishment of values. For example, individuals who lead a sedentary lifestyle and never exercise lack an understanding of and don't experience the myriad benefits and vibrant quality of life obtained through fitness participation. Through a book, a class, sports participation, or a friend, the person may first be exposed to exercise and an active lifestyle. The individual may then seek an environment wherein he/she can learn and actively participate in a physical activity or exercise program. The feelings of well-being and increased health, functional capacity, quality of life, and the education gained about the benefits of fitness in turn become the reward for program participation and lead to the development of the value that daily activity is vital for health and wellness. The person, often subconsciously, learns to analyze the feelings experienced through participation that lead to the development of a new value. The value now sways the person's actions to live according to what is important to achieve wellness (Figure 2.2). This feeling of "fitness" often snowballs into the adoption of other healthy behaviors that further improve the individual's state of well-being. Of utmost importance in the maintenance of core values is to live the principles involved to reap the benefits. Thus, a constant and deliberate effort is required to be in an environment that rewards the behavior(s) the individual is trying to live.

Your Brain and Your Habits

Habits are a necessary tool for everyday brain function. Our minds learn to use familiar cues to carry out automatic behavior that has worked successfully in the past. While we carry out these automatic behaviors, we allow our minds to spend energy working on other tasks and puzzling through other problems. If you've ever found yourself driving a familiar route when you had intended to turn off and drive elsewhere, you are performing a habit. In fact, researchers who study victims with brain damage that prevents habit formation have found that these people are unable to process the multitude of information they encounter in everyday life.

Habits happen in familiar environments and not in new environments. Habits, however, can be changed by deliberate choice. During times of stress or when our minds are preoccupied with other problems, we are much more prone to return to and rely on habits, good or bad, and we are less likely to consider deliberate choice, core values, and long-term goals. There is a biological explanation for the way habits go from planned to automatic behavior. The area of our brain where habits are formed is known as the basal ganglia, composed of a cluster of nuclei. The basal ganglia are situated where they can communicate with both the forebrain, involved in decision making, and the midbrain, which controls motor movement. The largest nucleus of the basal ganglia, known as the striatum (corpus striatum), plays a key role in habit formation. The striatum is activated by events that are rewarding, exciting, unexpected, and intense, as well as by cues from the environment that are associated with those events. The striatum then memorizes events that are pleasurable and rewarding. For example, most people love cake because its taste is much more pleasurable (immediate reward) than that of a green salad, even though the latter provides better nutrition and is conducive to weight management (long-term gratification).

The neurotransmitter dopamine is abundant in the striatum. Dopamine has many functions in the brain, including cognition, learning, behavior, motivation, and reward and punishment. As such, it plays a key role in habit formation. Any activity that links an action to a reward involves dopamine. Following repeated pairings with a reward, the behavior becomes a conditioned response that is now hard-wired in the brain. This behavior is triggered by a familiar environmental cue, upon which the brain automatically responds by performing the habit. As these behaviors become "ingrained" in the brain, we lose awareness as they are carried out. Once we recognize the familiar trigger, we often perform the

Actions Steps required to reach a goal.

habit whether it is helpful or detrimental, and therefore often sabotage the desire for willful change.

There are probably some habits you'd like to break or some triggers you'd rather not respond to as you usually do. Perhaps there are positive habits you'd like to create so that in times of pressure and stress you fall into that set of positive habits.

There are steps you can take to change unwanted behaviors ingrained in the brain or to create helpful behaviors. First, recognize that there are biological processes that lead to behavioral habits. Take note of the situational cues or stressful experiences that trigger a habit. Researchers have found that 45 percent of our behaviors are conducted in uniform contexts and location from day to day.[29]

As you are adopting a new habit, repetition is critical. The more you repeat a new behavior under similar circumstances, the more likely you will be to develop the required circuitry in the striatum to make it a habit. For example, exercising at the same time of day helps develop the exercise habit. In due time, when you fail to exercise, the striatum will let you know that that specific time of the day is exercise time. Or perhaps, when you get in your car, you wait to put on your seatbelt until you are well on your way. Work to use the cue of getting in your car as a signal to immediately strap on your seatbelt and note how long it takes to become a new habit.

You must also consciously prepare to eliminate bad habits, such as not eating while watching television. Better yet, exercise or stretch while viewing television! Finally, realize that excessive stress (distress—see Chapter 10) often triggers old bad habits. For example, an argument with a roommate may lead to excessive TV viewing while eating unhealthy calorie-dense foods. You must prepare for an adequate response in these situations. If you made a mistake and did not adequately respond to that specific situation, chalk it up to experience, use it as a learning tool, and next time come back with the proper response.

Understanding how to create and break habits through mindfulness and repetition is a powerful tool. Fortunately, there are also greater forces at work in behavioral change that go beyond changing pathways of automatic behavior. Those greater forces are our core values and our understanding of who we are and what greater long-term desires we hold. Change in core values often overrules instant rewards as we seek long-term gratification. This ability to change according to values also has a biological explanation.

An entirely separate portion of the brain, the prefrontal cortex, is responsible for reminding us of who we are and of our long-term goals. The prefrontal cortex is also responsible for personality expression; social behavior; and complex thought processing, such as predicting likely outcomes based on prior experience and weighing competing thoughts. When you find yourself getting out of bed in the morning to go to work or stopping yourself from checking a new text message because you are driving, you are experiencing your prefrontal cortex at work, placing long-term desires ahead of your short-term urges.

As you work to change behavior you will notice competing desires, especially as you begin change. Human resilience, nonetheless, should not be underestimated. We can look all around us for proof of success. In the United States, for example, there are more people who have quit smoking than there are current smokers.[30]

Find ways to guide yourself toward new behaviors by understanding and visualizing the reward you are seeking and educating yourself about the best way to obtain it. Remind yourself often of your core values and look for opportunities throughout the day to align your behaviors with those core values.

Willpower

Understanding the concept of willpower, or self-control, is helpful in the process of behavioral change. Scientists have found that self-restraint against impulses can be built, like a muscle, if built slowly and gradually. Start with something small. If you feel you need to read every text message the moment it arrives, you may try to learn to wait a few minutes and finish the activity you are working on and then read your text message. As you do so, your ability to exert self-control increases. Studies have found that willpower is a limited resource. It is highest in the morning and is depleted as we use it throughout the day, primarily when confronted with difficult challenges and stress. When you are planning to take on a significant task, help yourself be successful by doing it at a time when you can put aside as many other demands and stressors as possible.

Studies indicate that willpower reserve can be increased through exercise, balanced nutrition, a good night's sleep, and quality time spent with important people in your life. Willpower decreases, on the other hand, in times of depression, anxiety, anger, and loneliness.

Researchers have found an actual growth in gray matter in the prefrontal cortex as individuals build self-control. Daily meditation, too, has been proven to develop the self-control "muscle".[31]

Barriers to Change

In spite of the best intentions, people make unhealthy choices daily. The most common reasons are:

1. **Lack of core values.** Most people recognize the benefits of a healthy lifestyle but are unwilling or unable to trade convenience (sedentary lifestyle, unhealthy eating, substance abuse) for health or other benefits.

   Tip to initiate change. Educate yourself regarding the benefits of a healthy lifestyle and subscribe to several reputable health, fitness, and wellness newsletters (see Chapter 15). The more you read, understand, and then start living a wellness lifestyle, the more your core values will change. At this time you should also break relationships with individuals who are unwilling to change with you.

2. **Procrastination.** People seem to think that tomorrow, next week, or after the holiday is the best time to start change.

Tip to initiate change. Ask yourself: Why wait until tomorrow when you can start changing today? Lack of motivation is a key factor in procrastination (motivation is discussed later in this chapter).

3. **Preconditioned cultural beliefs**. If we accept the idea that we are a product of our environment, our cultural beliefs and our physical surroundings pose significant barriers to change. In Salzburg, Austria, people of both genders and all ages use bicycles as a primary mode of transportation. In the United States, few people other than children ride bicycles.

   Tip to initiate change. Find a like-minded partner. In the pre-Columbian era, people thought the world was flat. Few dared to sail long distances for fear that they would fall off the edge. If your health and fitness are at stake, preconditioned cultural beliefs shouldn't keep you from making changes. Finding people who are willing to "sail" with you will help overcome this barrier.

4. **Gratification.** People prefer instant gratification to long-term benefits. Therefore, they will overeat (instant pleasure) instead of using self-restraint to eat moderately to prevent weight gain (long-term satisfaction). We like tanning (instant gratification) and avoid paying much attention to skin cancer (long-term consequence).

   Tip to initiate change. Think ahead and ask yourself: How did I feel the last time I engaged in this behavior? How did it affect me? Did I really feel good about myself or about the results? In retrospect, was it worth it?

5. **Risk complacency.** Consequences of unhealthy behaviors often don't manifest themselves until years later. People tell themselves, "If I get heart disease, I'll deal with it then. For now, let me eat, drink, and be merry."

   Tip to initiate change. Ask yourself: How long do I want to live? How do I want to live the rest of my life and what type of health do I want to have? What do I want to be able to do when I am 60, 70, or 80 years old? Visualize long-term goals that align with your own true core values.

6. **Complexity.** People think the world is too complicated, with too much to think about. If you are living the typical lifestyle, you may feel overwhelmed by everything that seems to be required to lead a healthy lifestyle, such as:
   - getting exercise
   - decreasing intake of saturated and trans fats
   - eating high-fiber meals and cutting total calories
   - controlling use of substances
   - managing stress
   - wearing seat belts
   - practicing safe sex
   - getting annual physicals, including blood tests, Pap smears, and so on
   - fostering spiritual, social, and emotional wellness

   Tip to initiate change. Take it one step at a time. Work on only one or two behaviors at a time so the task won't seem insurmountable.

7. **Indifference and helplessness.** A defeatist thought process often takes over, and we may believe that the way we live won't really affect our health, that we have no control over our health, or that our destiny is all in our genes (also see discussion of locus of control, pages 54–55).

   Tip to initiate change. As much as 83 percent of the leading causes of death in the United States are preventable. Realize that only you can take control of your personal health and lifestyle habits and affect the quality of your life. Implementing many of the behavioral modification strategies and programs outlined in this book will get you started on a wellness way of life.

8. **Rationalization.** Even though people are not practicing healthy behaviors, they often tell themselves that they do get sufficient exercise, that their diet is fine, that they have good, solid relationships, or that they don't smoke/drink/get high enough to affect their health.

   Tip to initiate change. Learn to recognize when you're glossing over or minimizing a problem. You'll need to face the fact that you have a problem before you can commit to change. Your health and your life are at stake. Monitoring lifestyle habits through daily logs and then analyzing the results can help you change self-defeating behaviors.

9. **Illusions of invincibility.** At times people believe that unhealthy behaviors will not harm them. Young adults often have the attitude that "I can smoke now, and in a few years I'll quit before it causes any damage." Unfortunately, nicotine is one of the most addictive drugs known to us, so quitting smoking is not an easy task. Health problems may arise before you quit, and the risk of lung cancer lingers for years after you quit. Another example is drinking and driving. The feeling of "I'm in control" or "I can han-

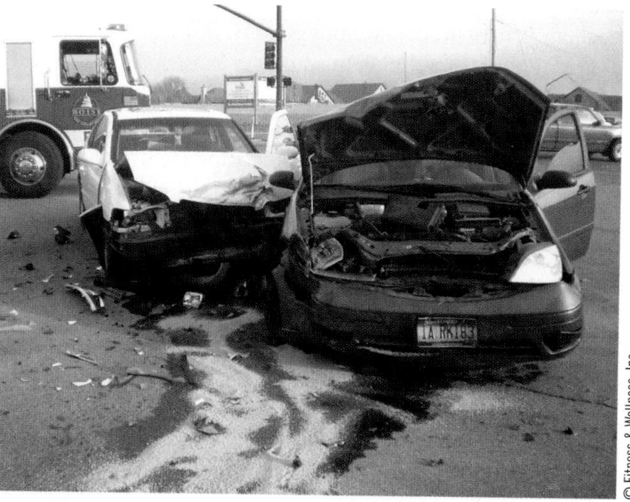

Feelings of invincibility are a strong barrier to change that can bring about life-threatening consequences.

dle it" while under the influence of alcohol is a deadly combination. Others perceive low risk when engaging in negative behaviors with people they like (for example, sex with someone you've recently met and feel attracted to) but perceive themselves at risk just by being in the same classroom with an HIV-infected person.

Tip to initiate change. No one is immune to sickness, disease, and tragedy. The younger you are when you implement a healthy lifestyle, the better are your odds to attain a long and healthy life. Thus, initiating change right now will help you enjoy the best possible quality of life for as long as you live.

CRITICAL THINKING

What barriers to exercise do you encounter most frequently? How about barriers that keep you from managing your daily caloric intake?

When health and appearance begin to deteriorate—usually around middle age—people seek out health care professionals in search of a "magic pill" to reverse and cure the many ills they have accumulated during years of abuse and overindulgence. The sooner we implement a healthy lifestyle program, the greater will be the health benefits and quality of life that lie ahead.

Self-Efficacy

At the heart of behavior modification is the concept of **self-efficacy**, or the belief in one's own ability to perform a given task. Self-efficacy exerts a powerful influence on people's behaviors and touches virtually every aspect of their lives. It determines how you feel, think, behave, motivate yourself, make choices, set goals, and pursue courses of action, as well as the effort you put into all of your tasks or activities. It also influences your vulnerability to stress and depression. Furthermore, your confidence in your coping skills determines how resilient you are in the face of adversity. Possessing high self-efficacy enhances wellness in countless ways, including your desire to learn, be productive, be fit, and be healthy.

The knowledge and skills you possess and further develop determine your goals and what you do and choose not to do. Mahatma Gandhi once stated, "If I have the belief that I can do it, I shall surely acquire the capacity to do it even if I may not have it at the beginning." Likewise, Teilhard de Chardin, a French paleontologist and philosopher, stated, "It is our duty as human beings to proceed as though the limits of our capabilities do not exist." With this type of attitude, how can you not strive to be the best that you can possibly be?

As you have already learned in this chapter, the environment has a tremendous effect on our behaviors. We can therefore increase self-efficacy by the type of environment we choose. Experts agree that four different sources affect self-efficacy (discussed next). If you understand these sources and learn from them, you can use them to improve your degree of efficacy. Subsequently, you can apply the concepts for change provided in this chapter to increase confidence in your abilities to master challenging tasks and succeed at implementing change.

Sources of Self-Efficacy The best contributors to self-efficacy are mastery experiences, or personal experiences that one has had with successes and failures. Successful past performances greatly enhance self-efficacy: "Nothing breeds success like success." Failures, on the other hand, can undermine confidence, in particular if they occur before a sense of efficacy is established.

You should structure your activities in such ways that they will bring success. Don't set your goals too high or make them too difficult to achieve. Your success at a particular activity increases your confidence in being able to repeat that activity. Once strong self-efficacy is developed through successful mastery experiences, an occasional setback does not have a significant effect on one's beliefs.

Vicarious experiences provided by role models or those one admires also influence personal efficacy. This involves the thought process of your belief that you can also do it. When you observe a peer of similar capabilities master a task, you are more likely to develop a belief that you too can perform that task—"If he can do it, so can I." Here you imitate the model's skill or you follow the same approach demonstrated by your model to complete the task. You may also visualize success. Visual imagery of successful personal performance, that is, watching yourself perform the skill in your mind, also increases personal efficacy.

Although not as effective as past performances and vicarious experiences, verbal persuasion of one's capabilities to perform a task also contributes to self-efficacy. When you are verbally persuaded that you possess the capabilities, you will be more likely to try the task and believe that you can get it done. The opposite is also true. Negative verbal persuasion has a far greater effect in lowering efficacy than positive messages do to enhance it. If you are verbally persuaded that you lack the skills to master a task, you will tend to avoid the activity and will be more likely to give up without giving yourself a fair chance to succeed.

The least significant source of self-efficacy beliefs are physiological cues that people experience when facing a challenge. These cues in turn affect performance. For example, feeling calm, relaxed, and self-confident enhances self-efficacy. Anxiety, nervousness, perspiration, dryness of the mouth, and a rapid heart rate are cues that may adversely affect performance. You may question your competence to successfully complete the task.

Motivation and Locus of Control

The explanation given for why some people succeed and others do not is often **motivation**. Motivation is the drive that dictates human behavior by providing direction, energy,

confidentconsumer

Developing self-confidence and becoming a confident consumer often require behavioral-change techniques to enhance the rate of success. The current market is saturated with fraudulent products and services intended to deceive the consumer with unproven claims for profit. Not even the fitness and wellness industry is immune to fraudulent scams. Deceit is all around us, on radio and television, the Internet, newspapers, magazines, trade books, and social media. Some advertisements are based on testimonials, unproven and secret research, half-truths, myths, and quick-fix statements intended to lure the consumer into a purchase. To protect yourself and become a confident consumer you should:

1. Educate yourself as much as possible about the product/service you are looking to purchase. Consult reputable books, magazines, the Internet, and professionals who do not stand to make a profit from the transaction.
2. Know who you are dealing with. You can go to the Better Business Bureau website (BBB.org) and use it to search for companies you can trust. If you shop using an iPhone or iPad, download the free app "BBB Search" from the App Store to look into the product.
3. Take your time and don't rush into your purchase. Only do so after you have had a chance to research the product, think about it, and make an informed decision.
4. Read the fine print. Most disputes can be avoided by reading the small print, frequently used so as to be easily overlooked by the consumer. Furthermore, when a contract is involved, get all stipulations in writing and carefully review the document before you sign and turn over any money.
5. For significant financial commitments or purchases, always compare costs by visiting different stores/businesses or searching various Internet sites.
6. Be aware of your consumer rights. Know the necessary steps required to resolve disputes, billing errors, and unwanted telemarketing calls (access www.DoNotCall.gov).
7. Become aware of your mental habits. Some individuals are much more susceptible to impulse buying. If you have done so in the past and regretted the choice you made, use the experience to prevent such actions in the future.
8. Remember that if it seems to be too good to be true, it probably is. Be sure to look into the matter before making a decision.
9. Protect your personal information. Use credit cards and share personal information only with companies that you *absolutely* trust.
10. Review your credit report. The Fair Credit Reporting Act (FCRA) requires nationwide consumer reporting companies to provide a free copy of your credit report once a year. To request a copy, visit www.annualcreditreport.com or call 1-877-322-8228.

Additional information can be obtained from How to be an Informed Consumer from the Federal Trade Commission at www.ftc.gov.

and persistence. Although motivation comes from within, external factors trigger the inner desire to accomplish a given task. These external factors, then, control behavior.

When studying motivation, understanding locus of control is helpful. People who believe they have control over events in their lives are said to have an internal locus of control. People with an external **locus of control** believe that what happens to them is a result of chance or the environment and is unrelated to their behavior. People with an internal locus of control generally are healthier and have an easier time initiating and adhering to a wellness program than those who perceive that they have no control and think of themselves as powerless and vulnerable. The latter people also are at greater risk for illness. When illness does strike a person, establishing a sense of control is vital to recovery.

Few people have either a completely external or a completely internal locus of control. They fall somewhere along a continuum. The more external one's locus of control is, the greater is the challenge to change and adhere to exercise and other healthy lifestyle behaviors. Fortunately, people can develop a more internal locus of control. Understanding that most events in life are not determined genetically or environmentally helps people pursue goals and gain control over their lives. Three impediments, however, can keep people from taking action: lack of competence, of confidence, and of motivation.[32]

1. **Problems of competence**. Lacking the skills to get a given task done leads to reduced competence. If your friends play basketball regularly but you don't know how to play, you might be inclined not to participate. The solution to this problem of competence is to master the skills you required to par-

Self-efficacy One's belief in the ability to perform a given task.

Motivation The desire and will to do something.

Locus of control A concept examining the extent to which a person believes he or she can influence the external environment.

ticipate. Most people are not born with all-inclusive natural abilities, including playing sports.

Another alternative is to select an activity in which you are skilled. It may not be basketball, but it well could be aerobics. Don't be afraid to try new activities. Similarly, if your body weight is a problem, you could learn to cook healthy, low-calorie meals. Try different recipes until you find foods that you like.

2. **Problems of confidence.** Problems with confidence arise when you have the skill but don't believe you can get it done. Fear and feelings of inadequacy often interfere with the ability to perform the task. You shouldn't talk yourself out of something until you have given it a fair try. If you have the skills, the sky is the limit. Initially, try to visualize yourself doing the task and getting it done. Repeat this several times, then actually try it. You will surprise yourself.

   Sometimes, lack of confidence arises when the task seems insurmountable. In these situations, dividing a goal into smaller, more realistic objectives helps to accomplish the task. You might know how to swim but may need to train for several weeks to swim a continuous mile. Set up your training program so you swim a little farther each day until you are able to swim the entire mile. If you don't meet your objective on a given day, try it again, reevaluate, cut back a little, and, most important, don't give up.

3. **Problems of motivation.** With problems of motivation, both the competence and the confidence are there but individuals are unwilling to change because the reasons to change are not important to them. For example, people begin contemplating a smoking-cessation program only when the reasons for quitting outweigh the reasons for smoking. The primary causes of unwillingness to change are lack of values, knowledge, and lack of goals. Knowledge determines values and goals, and goals determine motivation. How badly you want something dictates how hard you'll work at it.

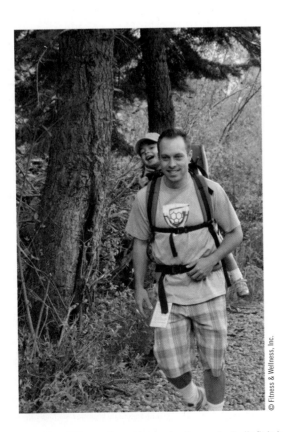

The higher quality of life experienced by people who are physically fit is hard to explain to someone who has never achieved good fitness.

Many people are unaware of the magnitude of benefits of a wellness program. When it comes to a healthy lifestyle, however, you may not get a second chance. A stroke, a heart attack, or cancer can have irreparable or fatal consequences. Greater understanding of what leads to disease can help initiate change. Joy, however, is a greater motivator than fear. Even fear of dying often doesn't instigate change.

Two years following coronary bypass surgery (heart disease), most patients' denial returns, and surveys show that they have not done much to alter their unhealthy lifestyle. The motivating factor for the few who do change is the "joy of living." Rather than dwelling on the "fear of dying" and causing patients to live in emotional pain, point out the fact that change will help them feel better. They will be able to enhance their quality of life by carrying out activities of daily living without concern for a heart attack, go for a walk without chest pain, play with children, and even resume an intimate relationship.

Also, feeling physically fit is difficult to explain to people unless they have experienced it themselves. Feelings of fitness, self-esteem, confidence, health, and better quality of life cannot be conveyed to someone who is constrained by sedentary living. In a way, wellness is like reaching the top of a mountain. The quiet, the clean air, the lush vegetation, the flowing water in the river, the wildlife, and the majestic valley below are difficult to explain to someone who has spent a lifetime within city limits.

Changing Behavior

The first step in addressing behavioral change is to recognize that you indeed have a problem. The five general categories of behaviors addressed in the process of willful change are:

1. Stopping a negative behavior
2. Preventing relapse to a negative behavior
3. Developing a positive behavior
4. Strengthening a positive behavior
5. Maintaining a positive behavior

Most people do not change all at once. Thus, psychotherapy has been used successfully to help people change their behavior. But most people do not seek professional help. They usually attempt to change by themselves with limited or no knowledge of how to achieve change. In essence, the process of change moves along a continuum from being not willing to change to recognizing the need for change to taking action and implementing change.

The simplest model of change is the two-stage model of unhealthy behavior and healthy behavior. This model states that either you do it or you don't. Most people who use this model attempt self-change but end up asking themselves why they're unsuccessful. They just can't do it (exercise, perhaps, or quit smoking). Their intent to change may be good, but to accomplish it, they need knowledge about how to achieve change.

Behavior Change Theories

For most people, changing chronic/unhealthy behaviors to stable/healthy behaviors is challenging. The "do it or don't do it" approach seldom works when attempting to implement lifestyle changes. Thus, several theories or models have been developed over the years. Among the most accepted are learning theories, the problem-solving model, social cognitive theory, the relapse prevention model, humanistic theory of change, and the transtheoretical model.

Learning Theories **Learning theories** maintain that most behaviors are learned and maintained under complex schedules of reinforcement and anticipated outcomes. The process involved in learning a new behavior requires modifying many small behaviors that shape the new pattern behavior. For example, a previously inactive individual who wishes to accumulate 10,000 steps per day may have to gradually increase the number of steps daily, park farther away from the office and stores, decrease television and Internet use, take stairs instead of elevators and escalators, and avoid the car and telephone when running errands that are only short distances away. The outcomes are better health and body weight management and feelings of well-being.

Problem-Solving Model The **problem-solving model** proposes that many behaviors are the result of making decisions as we seek to change the problem behavior. The process of change requires conscious attention, the setting of goals, and a design for a specific plan of action. For instance, to quit smoking cigarettes, one has to understand the reasons for smoking, know under what conditions each cigarette is smoked, decide that one will quit, select a date to do so, and then draw up a plan of action to reach the goal (a complete smoking-cessation program is outlined in Chapter 13).

Social Cognitive Theory In **social cognitive theory**, behavior change is influenced by the environment, self-efficacy, and characteristics of the behavior itself. You can increase self-efficacy by educating yourself about the behavior, developing the skills to master the behavior, performing smaller mastery experiences successfully, and receiving verbal reinforcement and vicarious experiences. If you desire to lose weight, for example, you need to learn the principles of proper weight management, associate with people who are also losing weight or who have lost weight, eat less, shop and cook wisely, be more active, set small weight-loss goals of 1 to 2 pounds per week, praise yourself for your accomplishments, and visualize losing the weight as others you admire have done.

Relapse Prevention Model In the **relapse prevention model**, people are taught to anticipate high-risk situations and develop action plans to prevent **lapses** and **relapses**. Examples of factors that disrupt behavior change include negative physiological or psychological states (stress, illness), social pressure, lack of support, limited coping skills, change in work conditions, and lack of motivation. For example, if the weather turns bad for your evening walk, you can choose to walk around an indoor track (or at the mall), do water aerobics, swim, or play racquetball.

Humanistic Theory of Change Humanists believe in the basic goodness of humanity and respect for mankind. At the core of the theory is the belief that people are unique in the development of personal goals—with the ultimate goal being self-actualization. Self-actualized people are independent, are creative, set their own goals, and accept themselves. Humanists also propose that people are motivated by a hierarchy of needs that include approval, recognition, achievement, and the fulfillment of each person's potential. In this hierarchy, each need requires fulfillment before the next need becomes relevant. The present is the most important time for any person rather than the past or the future. For instance, a person will not exercise unless he or she has had something to eat within a reasonable amount of time. Similarly, a person who uses cigarette smoking to maintain weight will not give up smoking unless proper weight management is accomplished by other means (healthy eating habits and increased physical activity). The challenge, then, is to identify basic

Learning theories Behavioral modification perspective stating that most behaviors are learned and maintained under complex schedules of reinforcement and anticipated outcomes.

Problem solving model Behavioral modification model proposing that many behaviors are the result of making decisions as the individual seeks to solve the problem behavior.

Social cognitive theory Behavioral modification model holding that behavior change is influenced by the environment, self-efficacy, and characteristics of the behavior itself.

Relapse prevention model Behavioral modification model based on the principle that high-risk situations can be anticipated through the development of strategies to prevent lapses and relapses.

Lapse (v.) To slip or fall back temporarily into unhealthy behavior(s); (n.) short-term failure to maintain healthy behaviors.

Relapse (v.) To slip or fall back into unhealthy behavior(s) over a longer time; (n.) longer-term failure to maintain healthy behaviors.

needs at the core of the hierarchy (acceptance, independence, recognition) before other healthy behaviors (exercise, stress management, altruism) are considered.

Transtheoretical Model The **transtheoretical model**, developed by psychologists James Prochaska, John Norcross, and Carlo DiClemente, is based on the theory that change is a gradual process that involves several stages.[33] The model is used most frequently to change health-related behaviors such as physical inactivity, smoking, poor nutrition, weight problems, stress, and alcohol abuse.

An individual goes through five stages in the process of willful change. The stages describe underlying processes that people go through to change problem behaviors and replace them with healthy behaviors. A sixth stage (termination/adoption) was subsequently added to this model. The six stages of change are precontemplation, contemplation, preparation, action, maintenance, and termination/adoption (see Figure 2.3).

After years of study, researchers indicate that applying specific behavioral-change processes during each stage of the model increases the success rate for change (the specific processes for each stage are shown in Table 2.1). Understanding each stage of this model will help you determine where you are in relation to your personal healthy lifestyle behaviors. It also will help you identify processes to make successful changes. The discussion in the remainder of the chapter focuses on the transtheoretical model, with the other models integrated as applicable with each stage of change.

1. Precontemplation

Individuals in the **precontemplation stage** are not considering change or do not want to change a given behavior. They typically deny having a problem and have no intention of changing in the immediate future. These people are usually unaware or underaware of the problem. Other people around them, including family, friends, health care practitioners, and coworkers, however, identify the problem clearly. Precontemplators do not care about the problem behavior and may even avoid information and materials that address the issue. They tend to avoid free screenings and workshops that might help identify and change the problem, even if they receive financial compensation for attending. Often they actively resist change and seem resigned to accepting the unhealthy behavior as their "fate."

Precontemplators are the most difficult people to inspire toward behavioral change. Many think that change isn't even a possibility. At this stage, knowledge is power. Educating them about the problem behavior is critical to help them start contemplating the process of change. The challenge is to find ways to help them realize that they are ultimately responsible for the consequences of their behavior. Typically, they initiate change only when their values change or when people whom they respect or job requirements pressure them to do so.

2. Contemplation

In the **contemplation stage**, individuals acknowledge that they have a problem and begin to think seriously about overcoming it. Although they are not quite ready for change,

FIGURE 2.3 Stages of change model.

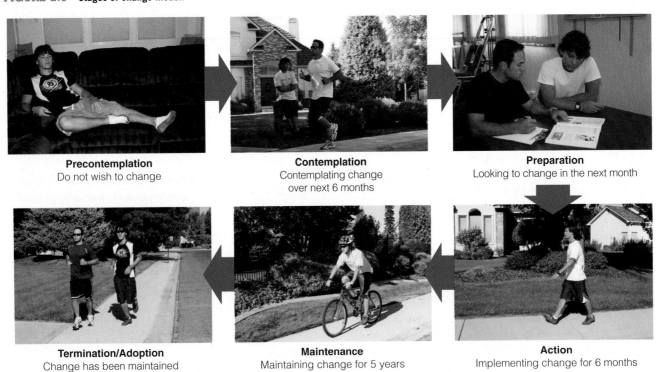

Photos © Fitness & Wellness, Inc.

TABLE 2.1 Applicable Processes of Change During Each Stage of Change

Precontemplation	Contemplation	Preparation	Action	Maintenance	Termination/ Adoption
Consciousness-raising	Consciousness-raising	Consciousness-raising			
Social liberation	Social liberation	Social liberation	Social liberation		
	Self-analysis	Self-analysis			
	Emotional arousal	Emotional arousal			
	Positive outlook	Positive outlook	Positive outlook		
		Commitment	Commitment	Commitment	Commitment
		Behavior analysis	Behavior analysis		
			Mindfulness	Mindfulness	Mindfulness
		Goal setting	Goal setting	Goal setting	
		Self-reevaluation	Self-reevaluation	Self-reevaluation	
			Countering	Countering	
			Monitoring	Monitoring	Monitoring
			Environmental control	Environmental control	Environmental control
			Helping relationships	Helping relationships	Helping relationships
			Rewards	Rewards	Rewards

Source: Adapted from J. O. Prochaska, J. C. Norcross, and C. C. DiClemente, Changing for Good *(New York: William Morrow, 1994); and W. W. K. Hoeger and S. A. Hoeger,* Lifetime Physical Fitness & Wellness *(Belmont, CA: Wadsworth/Cengage, 2009).*

they are weighing the pros and cons of changing. Core values are starting to change. Even though they may remain in this stage for years, in their minds they are planning to take some action within the next six months. Education and peer support remain valuable during this stage. In Lab 2B, you will be able to list under the processes of change self-defeating and constructive habits (pros and cons) that work against and for you when attempting to accomplish that specific behavior.

3. Preparation

In the **preparation stage**, individuals are seriously considering change and planning to change a behavior within the next month. They are taking initial steps for change and may even try the new behavior for a short while, such as stopping smoking for a day or exercising a few times during the month. During this stage, people define a general goal for behavioral change (for example, to quit smoking by the last day of the month) and write specific actions (or strategies) to accomplish this goal. The discussion on goal setting later in this chapter will help you write SMART goals and plan specific actions to reach your goal. Continued peer and environmental support is helpful during the preparation stage.

A key concept to keep in mind during the preparation stage is that in addition to being prepared to address the behavioral change or goal you are attempting to reach, you must prepare to address the specific actions (supportive behaviors) required to reach that goal (Figure 2.4). For example, you may be willing to give weight loss a try, but are you prepared to start eating less, eating out less often, eating less calorie-dense foods, shopping and cooking wisely, exercising more, watching television less, and becoming much more active? Achieving goals generally requires changing these supportive behaviors, and you must be prepared to do so.

4. Action

The **action stage** requires the greatest commitment of time and energy. Here, the individual is actively doing things to change or modify the problem behavior or to adopt a new, healthy behavior. The action stage requires that the person follow the specific guidelines set forth for that behavior. For example, a person has actually stopped smoking completely, is exercising aerobically three times a week according to

Transtheoretical model Behavioral modification model proposing that change is accomplished through a series of progressive stages in keeping with a person's readiness to change.

Precontemplation stage Stage of change in the transtheoretical model in which an individual is unwilling to change behavior.

Contemplation stage Stage of change in the transtheoretical model in which the individual is considering changing behavior within the next six months.

Preparation stage Stage of change in the transtheoretical model in which the individual is getting ready to make a change within the next month.

Action stage Stage of change in the transtheoretical model in which the individual is actively changing a negative behavior or adopting a new, healthy behavior.

FIGURE 2.4 **Goal setting and supportive behaviors.**

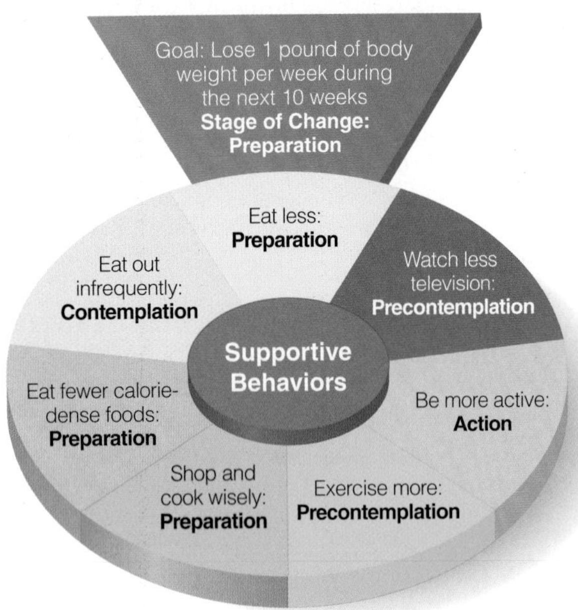

Note: This example may not lead to goal achievement. All supportive behaviors should be in the preparation stage to enhance success in the action stage.

exercise prescription guidelines, or is maintaining a healthy diet.

Relapse is common during this stage, and the individual may regress to a previous stage. If unsuccessful, a person should reevaluate his or her readiness to change supportive behaviors as required to reach the overall goal. Problem solving that includes identifying barriers to change and specific actions (strategies) to overcome supportive behaviors is useful during relapse. Once people are able to maintain the action stage for six consecutive months, they move into the maintenance stage.

5. Maintenance

During the **maintenance stage**, the person continues the new behavior for up to five years. This stage requires the person to continue to adhere to the specific guidelines that govern the behavior (such as complete smoking cessation, exercising aerobically three times a week, or practicing proper stress management techniques). At this time, the person works to reinforce the gains made through the various stages of change and strives to prevent lapses and relapses.

6. Termination/Adoption

Once a person has maintained a behavior more than five years, he or she is said to be in the **termination or adoption stage** and exits from the cycle of change without fear of relapse. In the case of negative behaviors that are terminated, the stage of change is referred to as termination. If a positive behavior has been adopted successfully for more than five years, this stage is designated as adoption.

Many experts believe that once an individual enters the termination/adoption stage, former addictions, problems, or lack of compliance with healthy behaviors no longer presents an obstacle in the quest for wellness. The change has become part of one's lifestyle. This phase is the ultimate goal for all people searching for a healthier lifestyle.

For addictive behaviors such as alcoholism and hard drug use, however, some health care practitioners believe that the individual never enters the termination stage. Chemical dependency is so strong that most former alcoholics and hard-drug users must make a lifetime effort to prevent relapse. Similarly, some behavioral scientists suggest that the adoption stage might not be applicable to health behaviors such as exercise and weight control because the likelihood of relapse is always high.

Use the guidelines provided in Lab 2B to determine where you stand in respect to behaviors you want to change or new ones you wish to adopt. As you follow the guidelines, you will realize that you might be at different stages for different behaviors. For instance, you might be in the preparation stage for aerobic exercise and smoking cessation, in the action stage for strength training, but only in the contemplation stage for a healthy diet. Realizing where you are with respect to different behaviors will help you design a better action plan for a healthy lifestyle.

Relapse After the precontemplation stage, relapse may occur at any level of the model. Even individuals in the maintenance and termination/adoption stages may regress to any of the first three stages of the model (Figure 2.5). Relapse, however, does not mean failure. Failure comes only to those who give up and don't use prior experiences as a building block for future success.

FIGURE 2.5 **Model of progression and relapse.**

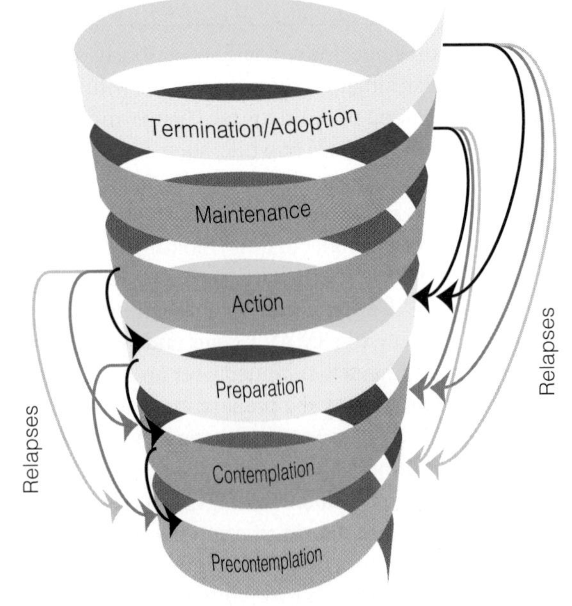

When relapse is viewed as a useful learning experience, the individual should be able to consider the circumstances that led to that relapse and will be better prepared to prevent such in the future. Relapses tend to follow short-term frustrations or underlying difficulties that have been building up to a critical level. A relapse may be a cue that the person should evaluate the stressors they are facing and build the resources and support needed to reach the goal. The chances of moving back up to a higher stage of the model are far better for someone who has previously made it into one of those stages.

The Process of Change

Using the same plan for everyone who wishes to change a behavior will not work. With exercise, for instance, we provide different prescriptions to people of varying fitness levels (Chapter 6). The same prescription would not provide optimal results for a person who has been inactive for 20 years, compared with one who already walks regularly three times each week. This principle also holds true for individuals who are attempting to change their behaviors.

Timing is also important in the process of willful change. People respond more effectively to selected **processes of change** in keeping with the stage of change they have reached at any given time. Thus, applying appropriate processes at each stage of change enhances the likelihood of changing behavior permanently. The following description of 14 of the most common processes of change will help you develop a personal plan for change. The respective stages of change in which each process works best are summarized in Table 2.1.

Consciousness-Raising The first step in a **behavior modification** program is consciousness-raising. This step involves obtaining information about the problem so you can make a better decision about the problem behavior. For example, the problem could be physical inactivity. Learning about the benefits of exercise or the difference in benefits between physical activity and exercise (Chapter 1) can help you decide the type of fitness program (health or high fitness) that you want to pursue. Possibly, you don't even know that a certain behavior is a problem, such as being unaware of saturated and total fat content in many fast-food items. Consciousness-raising may continue from the precontemplation stage through the preparation stage.

Social Liberation Social liberation stresses external alternatives that make you aware of problem behaviors and make you begin to contemplate change. Examples of social liberation include pedestrian-only traffic areas, nonsmoking areas, health-oriented cafeterias and restaurants, advocacy groups, civic organizations, policy interventions, and self-help groups. Social liberation often provides opportunities to get involved, stir up emotions, and enhance self-esteem—helping you gain confidence in your ability to change.

Self-Analysis The next process in modifying behavior is developing a decisive desire to do so, called self-analysis. If you have no interest in changing a behavior, you won't do it. You will remain a precontemplator or a contemplator. A person who has no intention of quitting smoking will not quit, regardless of what anyone may say or how strong the evidence in favor of quitting may be. In your self-analysis, you may want to prepare a list of reasons for continuing or discontinuing the behavior. When the reasons for changing outweigh the reasons for not changing, you are ready for the next stage—either the contemplation stage or the preparation stage.

Emotional Arousal In emotional arousal, a person experiences and expresses feelings about the problem and its solutions. Also referred to as "dramatic release," this process often involves deep emotional experiences. Watching a loved one die from lung cancer caused by cigarette smoking may be all that is needed to make a person quit smoking. As in other examples, emotional arousal might be prompted by a dramatization of the consequences of drug use and abuse, a film about a person undergoing open-heart surgery, or a book illustrating damage to body systems as a result of unhealthy behaviors.

Positive Outlook Having a positive outlook means taking an optimistic approach from the beginning and believing in yourself. Following the guidelines in this chapter will help you design a plan so you can work toward change and remain enthused about your progress. Also, you may become motivated by looking at the outcome—how much healthier you will be, how much better you will look, or how far you will be able to jog. Studies of individuals who are trying to quit an addictive behavior have found that asking that person to reconnect with positive and meaningful goals in their life greatly improves chances for success. In many cases, goals that will bring the person enjoyment and purpose will be incompatible with the undesired behaviors.

Commitment Upon making a decision to change, you accept the responsibility to change and believe in your ability to do so. During the commitment process, you engage in preparation and may draw up a specific plan of action. Write down your goals and, preferably, share them with others. In essence, you are signing a behav-

Maintenance stage Stage of change in the transtheoretical model in which the individual maintains behavioral change for up to five years.

Termination/adoption stage Stage of change in the transtheoretical model in which the individual has eliminated an undesirable behavior or maintained a positive behavior for more than five years.

Processes of change Actions that help you achieve change in behavior.

Behavior modification The process of permanently changing negative behaviors to positive behaviors that will lead to better health and well-being.

ioral contract for change. You will be more likely to adhere to your program if others know you are committed to change.

Behavior Analysis How you determine the frequency, circumstances, and consequences of the behavior to be altered or implemented is known as behavior analysis. If the desired outcome is to consume less trans and saturated fats, you first must find out what foods in your diet are high in these fats, when you eat them, and when you don't eat them—all part of the preparation stage. Knowing when you don't eat them points to circumstances under which you exert control over your diet and will help as you set goals.

Mindfulness The simple act of being aware of thoughts and choices is a powerful tool. A person should not feel that because they have an urge they need to act on it. A common technique of mindfulness is referred to as "urge surfing," and it directs the person to notice the urge, pay attention to the way the urge feels as it builds, and then simply continue noticing as the urge subsides. Professional behavioral therapists have found that having some kind of preemptive strategy for coping with urges, no matter how simple, greatly improves an individual's chance of success for overcoming and choosing the desired behavior.

Goals Goals motivate change in behavior. The stronger the goal or desire, the more motivated you'll be either to change unwanted behaviors or to implement new, healthy behaviors. The discussion on goal setting (beginning on page 64) will help you write goals and prepare an action plan to achieve them. This will aid with behavior modification.

Written Goals For a goal to be effective, it must be written down. An unwritten goal is simply a wish. When you write it down it becomes "real" and a contract with yourself. You should also share your goal with a family member, a friend, or an instructor. You can have this person witness the contract you have made with yourself by signing alongside your signature. This simple strategy enhances your success rate because you are now accountable to that person. People who are accountable for their actions are much more likely to complete the task.

Self-Reevaluation During the process of self-reevaluation, individuals analyze their feelings about a problem behavior. The pros and cons or advantages and disadvantages of a certain behavior can be reevaluated at this time. For example, you may decide that strength training will help you get stronger and tone up, but implementing this change will require you to stop watching an hour of TV three times per week. If you presently have a weight problem and are unable to lift certain objects around the house, you may feel good about weight loss and enhanced physical capacity as a result of a strength-training program. You also might visualize what it would be like if you were successful at changing.

Countering The process whereby you substitute healthy behaviors for a problem behavior, known as countering, is critical in changing behaviors as part of the action and maintenance stages. You need to replace unhealthy behaviors with new, healthy ones. You can use exercise to combat sedentary living, smoking, stress, or overeating. Or you may use exercise, diet, yard work, volunteer work, or reading to prevent overeating and achieve recommended body weight.

Monitoring During the action and maintenance stages, continuous behavior monitoring increases awareness of the desired outcome. It focuses your attention on the task at hand. Sometimes this process of monitoring is sufficient in itself to cause change. For example, keeping track of daily food

BEHAVIOR MODIFICATION PLANNING

Steps for Successful Behavior Modification

1. Acknowledge that you have a problem.
2. Describe the behavior to change (increase physical activity, stop overeating, quit smoking).
3. List advantages and disadvantages of changing the specified behavior.
4. Decide positively that you will change.
5. Identify your stage of change.
6. Set a realistic goal (SMART goal) and a completion date and sign a behavioral contract.
7. Define your behavioral change plan: List processes of change, techniques of change, and actions that will help you reach your goal.
8. Implement the behavior change plan.
9. Monitor your progress toward the desired goal.
10. Periodically evaluate and reassess your goal.
11. Reward yourself when you achieve your goal.
12. Maintain the successful change for good.

Try It

In your Online Journal or class notebook, record your answers to the following questions: Have you consciously attempted to incorporate a healthy behavior into or eliminate a negative behavior from your lifestyle? If so, what steps did you follow, and what helped you achieve your goal?

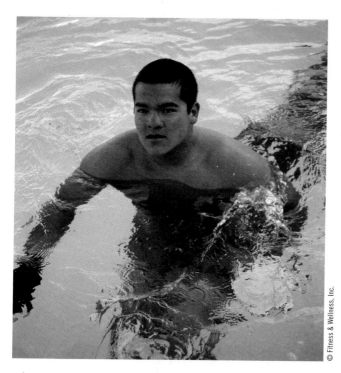

Countering: Substituting healthy behaviors for problem behaviors facilitates change.

intake reveals sources of excessive calories and fat in the diet. This can help you gradually cut down or completely eliminate calorie-dense and high-fat foods. Also, people who weigh themselves daily are more successful at maintaining recommended body weight than those who only do so once in a while. If the goal is to increase daily intake of fruits and vegetables, keeping track of the number of servings consumed each day raises awareness and can help increase intake.

Studies have also documented that carefully monitoring behavior in writing makes a significant difference in goal achievement. Individuals who log each workout are three times more likely to workout at least five times per week. Similarly, individuals who log daily caloric intake lose twice as much weight as those who don't. Further, it has been shown that choosing your own method of record keeping (paper, iPad, smartphone, computer), as opposed to being told what system to use, greatly enhances your recording/logging capability and subsequent goal achievement.

Furthermore, monitoring allows you to evaluate what is taking place and your progress toward the goal. Don't be reluctant to change the plan if you are failing to meet your goal.

Environment Control In environment control, the person restructures the physical surroundings to avoid problem behaviors and decrease temptations. If you don't buy alcohol, you can't drink any. If you shop on a full stomach, you can reduce impulse-buying of junk food.

Similarly, you can create an environment in which exceptions become the norm, and then the norm can flourish. You may leave yourself reminders or prompts that you are likely to see as you are making healthy choices. Such reminders, also referred to as "point-of-decision-prompts," have been used successfully on a public level. For example, reminders on soda machines that "calories count" encourage consumers to look at the calories listed by each soda selection prior to making a choice. You can also place notes to yourself on the refrigerator and pantry to avoid unnecessary snacking. Put baby carrots or sugarless gum where you used to put cigarettes. Post notes around the house to remind you of your exercise time. Leave exercise shoes and clothing by the door so they are visible as you walk into your home. Instead of bringing home cookies for snacks, bring fruit. Put an electric timer on the TV so it will shut off automatically at 7:00 p.m. All of these tactics will be helpful throughout the action, maintenance, and termination/adoption stages.

Helping Relationships Surrounding yourself with people who will work toward a common goal with you or those who care about you and will encourage you along the way. "Helping relationships" will be supportive during the action, maintenance, and termination/adoption stages.

Attempting to quit smoking, for instance, is easier when a person is around others who are trying to quit as well. The person also could get help from friends who have quit smoking already. One particular research study examined a social network of 12,000 people to understand the smoking habits of individuals who personally knew someone who had quit. They found out that smokers quit in social clusters. If an individual knew someone who had quit smoking, their own likelihood of quitting was better than the average. People were 67 percent less likely to be a smoker than the national average if the person who had quit was their spouse, 36 percent if it was a friend, and 25 percent if it was a sibling. Researchers found that, consistently, it was the closeness of the relationship, and not geographical closeness, that made the difference in health behaviors.[34]

Losing weight is difficult if meal planning and cooking are shared with roommates who enjoy foods that are high in fat and sugar. This situation can be even worse if a roommate also has a weight problem but does not wish to lose weight.

Peer support is a strong incentive for behavioral change. Thus, the individual should avoid people who will not be supportive and associate with those who will. Friends who have no desire to quit smoking or to lose weight, or whatever behavior a person is trying to change, may tempt one to smoke or overeat and encourage relapse into unwanted behaviors.

In some cases, people who have achieved the same goal already may not be supportive either. For instance, someone may say, "I can do six consecutive miles." Your response should be, "I'm proud that I can jog three consecutive miles."

Rewards People tend to repeat behaviors that are rewarded and to disregard those that are not rewarded or are punished. Rewarding oneself or being rewarded by others is a powerful tool during the process of change in all stages. If you have successfully cut down your caloric intake during the week, reward yourself by going to a movie or buying a new pair of shoes. Do not reinforce yourself with destructive

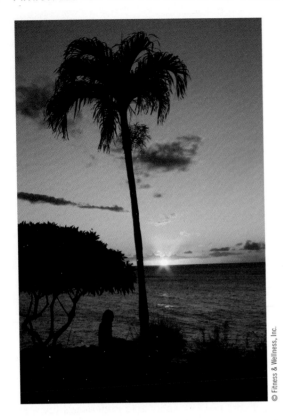

Rewarding oneself when a goal is achieved, such as scheduling a weekend getaway, is a powerful tool during the process of change.

behaviors such as eating a high-fat/calorie-dense dinner. If you fail to change a desired behavior (or to implement a new one), you may want to put off buying those new shoes you had planned for that week. When a positive behavior becomes habitual, give yourself an even better reward. Treat yourself to a weekend away from home or buy a new bicycle.

CRITICAL THINKING

Your friend John is a 20-year-old student who is not physically active. Exercise has never been a part of his life, and it has not been a priority in his family. He has decided to start a jogging and strength-training course in two weeks. Can you identify his current stage of change and list processes and techniques of change that will help him maintain a regular exercise behavior?

Techniques of Change

Not to be confused with the processes of change, you can apply any number of **techniques of change** within each process to help you through it (Table 2.2). For example, following dinner, people with a weight problem often can't resist continuous snacking during the rest of the evening until it is time to retire for the night. In the process of countering, for example, you can use various techniques to avoid unnecessary snacking. Examples include going for a walk, flossing and brushing your teeth immediately after dinner, going for a drive, playing the piano, going to a show, or going to bed earlier.

As you develop a behavior modification plan, you need to identify specific techniques that may work for you within each process of change. A list of techniques for each process is provided in Table 2.2. This is only a sample list; dozens of other techniques could be used as well. For example, a discussion of behavior modification and adhering to a weight management program starts on page 61; getting started and adhering to a lifetime exercise program is presented on page 242; stress management techniques are provided in Chapter 10; and tips to help stop smoking are offered on pages 516–517. Some of these techniques also can be used with more than one process. Visualization, for example, is helpful in emotional arousal and self-reevaluation.

Now that you are familiar with the stages of change in the process of behavior modification, use Figure 2.6 and Lab 2B to identify two problem behaviors in your life. In this activity, you will be asked to determine your stage of change for two behaviors according to six standard statements. Based on your selection, determine the stage of change classification according to the ratings provided in Table 2.3. Next, develop a behavior modification plan according to the processes and techniques for change that you have learned in this chapter. (Similar exercises to identify stages of change for other fitness and wellness behaviors are provided in activities for subsequent chapters.)

Goal Setting and Evaluation To initiate change, **goals** are essential, as goals motivate behavioral change. One cannot achieve a goal without changing behavior. A person's behavior either facilitates or interferes with the ability to accomplish a goal.

Whatever you decide to accomplish, setting goals will provide the road map to help make your dreams a reality. Setting goals, however, is not as simple as it looks. Setting goals is more than just deciding what you want to do. A vague statement such as "I will lose weight" is not sufficient to help you achieve this goal.

SMART Goals Only a well-conceived action plan will help you attain goals. Determining what you want to accomplish is the starting point, but to reach your goal you need to write **SMART goals**. These goals are **S**pecific, **M**easurable, **A**cceptable, **R**ealistic, and **T**ime specific. In Lab 2C, you have an opportunity to set SMART goals for two behaviors that you wish to change or adopt.

1. **Specific.** When writing goals, state exactly and in a positive manner what you would like to accomplish. For example, if you are overweight at 150 pounds and at 27 percent body fat, to simply state, "I will lose weight" is not a specific goal. Instead, rewrite your goal to state, "I will reduce my body fat to 20 percent (137 pounds) in 12 weeks." This strategy was confirmed by the National Weight Control Registry upon studying people who successfully lost weight and maintained weight-loss. These individuals were found to have highly specific goals,

TABLE 2.2 Sample Techniques for Use with Processes of Change

Process	Techniques
Consciousness-Raising	Become aware that there is a problem, read educational materials about the problem behavior or about people who have overcome this same problem, find out about the benefits of changing the behavior, watch an instructional program on television, visit a therapist, talk and listen to others, ask questions, take a class.
Social Liberation	Seek out advocacy groups (Overeaters Anonymous, Alcoholics Anonymous), join a health club, buy a bike, join a neighborhood walking group, work in nonsmoking areas.
Self-Analysis	Become aware that there is a problem, question yourself on the problem behavior, express your feelings about it, analyze your values, list advantages and disadvantages of continuing (smoking) or not implementing a behavior (exercise), take a fitness test, do a nutrient analysis.
Emotional Arousal	Practice mental imagery of yourself going through the process of change, visualize yourself overcoming the problem behavior, do some role-playing in overcoming the behavior or practicing a new one, watch dramatizations (a movie) of the consequences or benefits of your actions, visit an auto salvage yard or a drug rehabilitation center.
Positive Outlook	Believe in yourself, know that you are capable, know that you are special, draw from previous personal successes.
Commitment	Just do it, set New Year's resolutions, sign a behavioral contract, set start and completion dates, tell others about your goals, work on your action plan.
Behavior Analysis	Prepare logs of circumstances that trigger or prevent a given behavior, look for patterns that prompt the behavior or cause you to relapse.
Goal Setting	Write goals and objectives, design a specific action plan.
Self-Reevaluation	Determine accomplishments and evaluate progress, rewrite goals and objectives, list pros and cons, weigh sacrifices (can't eat out with others) versus benefits (weight loss), visualize continued change, think before you act, learn from mistakes, prepare new action plans accordingly.
Countering	Seek out alternatives: Stay busy, walk (don't drive), read a book (instead of snacking), attend alcohol-free socials, carry your own groceries, mow your yard, dance (don't eat), go to a movie (instead of smoking), practice stress management.
Monitoring	Use exercise logs (days exercised, sets and resistance used in strength training), keep journals, conduct nutrient analyses, count grams of saturated and trans fats, count number of consecutive days without smoking, list days and type of relaxation technique(s) used.
Environment Control	Rearrange your home (no TVs, ashtrays, large-sized cups), get rid of unhealthy items (cigarettes, junk food, alcohol), avoid unhealthy places (bars, happy hour), avoid relationships that encourage problem behaviors, use reminders to control problem behaviors or encourage positive ones (post notes indicating "don't snack after dinner" or "lift weights at 8 p.m."), frequent healthy environments (a clean park, a health club, restaurants with low-fat/low-calorie/nutrient-dense menus, friends with goals similar to yours).
Helping Relationships	Associate with people who have and want to overcome the same problem, form or join self-help groups, join community programs specifically designed to deal with your problem.
Rewards	Go to a movie, buy a new outfit or shoes, buy a new bike, go on a weekend getaway, reassess your fitness level, use positive self-talk ("good job," "that felt good," "I did it," "I knew I'd make it," "I'm good at this").

they envisioned themselves obtaining a specific percent body fat or fitting into a certain piece of clothing.

Once you have identified and written down a specific goal, write the specific **actions** that will help you reach that goal. These actions are necessary steps. For example, a goal might be to achieve recommended body weight. Several specific actions could be to:

a. lose an average of 1 pound (or 1 fat percentage point) per week
b. monitor body weight before breakfast every morning
c. assess body composition at three-week intervals

TABLE 2.3 Stage of Change Classification

Selected Statements (see Figure 2.6 and Lab 2B)	Classification
1	Precontemplation
2	Contemplation
3	Preparation
4	Action
5	Maintenance
6	Termination/Adoption

Techniques of change Methods or procedures used during each process of change.

Goals The ultimate aims toward which effort is directed.

SMART (goals) An acronym used in reference to specific, measurable, attainable, realistic, and time-specific goals.

FIGURE 2.6 **Stage of change identification.**

Please indicate which response most accurately describes your current __________ behavior (in the blank space identify the behavior: smoking, physical activity, stress, nutrition, weight control). Next, select the statement below (select only one) that best represents your current behavior pattern. To select the most appropriate statement, fill in the blank for one of the first three statements if your current behavior is a problem behavior. (For example, you may say, "I currently smoke, and I do *not* intend to change in the foreseeable future," or "I currently *do not* exercise, but I am contemplating changing in the next 6 months.") If you have already started to make changes, fill in the blank in one of the last three statements. (In this case, you may say: "I currently *eat a low saturated/trans fat diet*, but I have only done so within the last 6 months," or "I currently *practice adequate stress management techniques*, and I have done so for over 6 months.") As you can see, you may use this form to identify your stage of change for any type of health-related behavior.

1. I currently __________, and I do not intend to change in the foreseeable future.
2. I currently __________, but I am contemplating changing in the next 6 months.
3. I currently __________ regularly, but I intend to change in the next month.
4. I currently __________, but I have done so only within the last 6 months.
5. I currently __________, and I have done so for more than 6 months.
6. I currently __________, and I have done so for more than 5 years.

d. limit fat intake to less than 25 percent of total daily caloric intake (fat is calorie-dense and during a weight-loss program can lead to caloric overconsumption)

e. eliminate all pastries from the diet during this time

f. walk/jog in the proper target zone for 60 minutes, 6 times a week

2. **Measurable.** Whenever possible, goals and **objectives** should be measurable. For example, "I will lose weight" is not measurable, but "reduce body fat to 20 percent" is measurable. Also note that all of the sample-specific actions (a) through (f) under "Specific" are measurable. For instance, you can figure out easily whether you are losing a pound or a percentage point per week; you can conduct a nutrient analysis to assess your average fat intake; or you can monitor your weekly exercise sessions to make sure you are meeting this specific objective.

3. **Acceptable.** Goals that you set for yourself are more motivational than goals that someone else sets for you. These goals will motivate and challenge you and should be consistent with your other goals. As you set an acceptable goal, ask yourself: Do I have the time, commitment, and necessary skills to accomplish this goal? If not, you need to restate your goal so it is acceptable to you.

   When successful completion of a goal involves others, such as an athletic team or an organization, an acceptable goal must be compatible with those of the other people involved. If a team's practice schedule is set Monday through Friday from 4:00 to 6:00 p.m., it is unacceptable for you to train only three times per week or at a different time of the day.

   Acceptable goals also embrace positive thoughts. Visualize and believe in your success. As difficult as some tasks may seem, where there's a will, there's a way. A plan of action, prepared according to the guidelines in this chapter, will help you achieve your goals.

4. **Realistic.** Goals should be within reach. On the one hand, if you currently weigh 190 pounds and your target weight is 140 pounds, setting a goal to lose 50 pounds in a month would be unsound, if not impossible. Such a goal does not allow you to implement adequate behavior modification techniques or ensure weight maintenance at the target weight. Unattainable goals only set you up for failure, discouragement, and loss of interest. On the other hand, do not write goals that are too easy to achieve and do not challenge you. If a goal is too easy, you may lose interest and stop working toward it.

   You can write both short-term and long-term goals. If the long-term goal is to attain recommended body weight and you are 53 pounds overweight, you might set a short-term goal of losing 10 pounds and write specific objectives to accomplish this goal. Then the immediate task will not seem as overwhelming and will be easier.

   At times, problems arise even with realistic goals. Try to anticipate potential difficulties as much as possible, and plan for ways to deal with them. If your goal is to jog for 30 minutes on six consecutive days, what are the alternatives if the weather turns bad? Possible solutions are to jog in the rain, find an indoor track, jog at a different time of day when the weather is better, or participate in a different aerobic activity such as stationary cycling, swimming, zumba, or step aerobics.

   Monitoring your progress as you move toward a goal also reinforces behavior. Keeping an exercise log or doing a body composition assessment periodically enables you to determine your progress at any given time.

FIGURE 2.7 SMART goals.

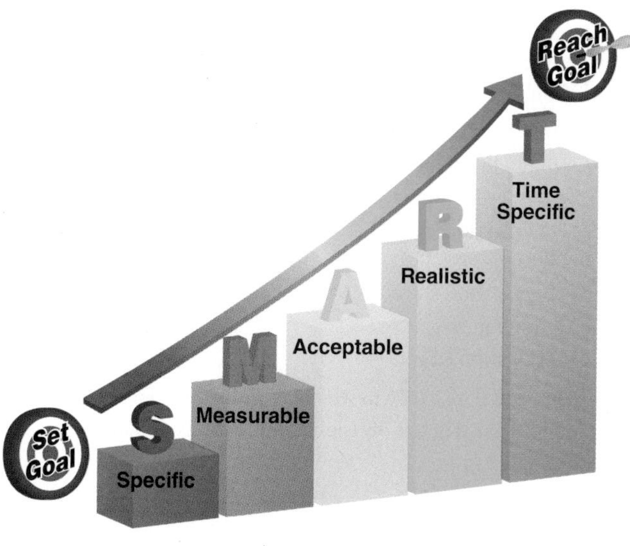

5. **Time specific.** A goal should always have a specific date set for completion. The example to reach 20 percent body fat in 12 weeks is time specific. The chosen date should be realistic but not too distant in the future. Allow yourself enough time to achieve the goal, but not too much time, as this could affect your performance. With a deadline, a task is much easier to work toward.

Goal Evaluation In addition to the SMART guidelines provided, you should conduct periodic evaluations of your goals. Reevaluations are vital to success. You may find that after you have fully committed and put all your effort into a goal, that goal may be unreachable. If so, reassess the goal.

Also, if you are failing to meet a goal, make a list with two columns: *helpful behaviors* and *damaging behaviors*. The first set includes behaviors that actually help you reach your goal. The latter lists the behaviors that interfere with your ability to achieve the goal. Work on the damaging behaviors and make the necessary changes to overcome them. Meeting your goal will become easier once you are able to eliminate damaging behaviors.

Recognize that you will face obstacles and you will not always meet your goals. Use your setbacks and learn from them. Rewrite your goal and create a plan that will help you get around self-defeating behaviors in the future. Once you achieve a goal, set a new one to improve upon or maintain what you have achieved. Goals keep you motivated.

ASSESS YOUR BEHAVIOR

CENGAGE brain.com To access course materials, including companion resources, please visit **www.cengagebrain.com**.

1. What are your feelings about the science of behavior modification and how its principles may help you on your journey to health and wellness?
2. Can you accept that for various healthy lifestyle factors (e.g. regular exercise, healthy eating, not smoking, stress management, and prevention of sexually transmitted infections) you are in either the precontemplation or the contemplation stage of change? As such, are you willing to learn what is required to change and eliminate unhealthy behaviors and adopt healthy lifestyle behaviors?
3. Are you now in the action (or a higher) phase for exercise and healthy eating? If not, what barriers keep you from doing so?

ASSESS YOUR KNOWLEDGE

1. Most of the behaviors that people adopt in life are
   a. a product of their environment.
   b. learned early in childhood.
   c. learned from parents.
   d. genetically determined.
   e. the result of peer pressure.
2. Instant gratification is
   a. a barrier to change.
   b. a factor that motivates change.
   c. one of the six stages of change.
   d. the end result of successful change.
   e. a technique in the process of change.

3. The desire and will to do something is referred to as
   a. invincibility.
   b. confidence.
   c. competence.
   d. external locus of control.
   e. motivation.

4. People who believe they have control over events in their lives
   a. tend to rationalize their negative actions.
   b. exhibit problems of competence.
   c. often feel helpless over illness and disease.
   d. have an internal locus of control.
   e. often engage in risky lifestyle behaviors.

5. A person who is unwilling to change a negative behavior because the reasons for change are not important enough is said to have problems of
   a. competence.
   b. conduct.
   c. motivation.
   d. confidence.
   e. risk complacency.

6. Which of the following is a stage of change in the transtheoretical model?
   a. recognition
   b. motivation
   c. relapse
   d. preparation
   e. goal setting

7. A precontemplator is a person who
   a. has no desire to change a behavior.
   b. is looking to make a change in the next 6 months.
   c. is preparing for change in the next 30 days.
   d. willingly adopts healthy behaviors.
   e. is talking to a therapist to overcome a problem behavior.

8. An individual who is trying to stop smoking and has not smoked for 3 months is in the
   a. maintenance stage.
   b. action stage.
   c. termination stage.
   d. adoption stage.
   e. evaluation stage.

9. The process of change in which an individual obtains information to make a better decision about a problem behavior is known as
   a. behavior analysis.
   b. self-reevaluation.
   c. commitment.
   d. positive outlook.
   e. consciousness-raising.

10. A goal is effective when it is
   a. specific.
   b. measurable.
   c. realistic.
   d. time specific.
   e. all of the above.

Correct answers can be found at the back of the book.

NOTES

1. J. Annesi, "Using Emotions to Empower Members for Long-Term Exercise Success," *Fitness Management* 17 (2001): 54–58.
2. E. Robinson, J. Thomas, P. Aveyard, and S. Higgs, "What Everyone Else Is Eating: A Systematic Review and Meta-Analysis of the Effect of Informational Eating Norms on Eating Behavior," *Journal of the Academy of Nutrition and Dietetics* 114, no. 3 (2014): 414–429.
3. P. T. Katzmarzyk et al., "Sitting Time and Mortality from All Causes, Cardiovascular Disease, and Cancer," *Medicine and Science in Sports and Exercise* 41 (2009): 998–1005.
4. D. W. Dunstan et al., "Television Viewing Time and Mortality: The Australian Diabetes, Obesity, and Lifestyle Study (AusDiab)," *Circulation* 121 (2010): 384–391.
5. J. L. Veerman et al., "Television Viewing Time and Reduced Life Expectancy: A Life Table Analysis," *British Journal of Sports Medicine* (August 15 2011), doi:10.1136/bjsm.2011.085662.
6. Google, "The New Multi-screen World: Understanding Cross-platform Consumer Behavior, August 2012," http://services.google.com/fh/files/misc/multiscreenworld_final.pdf, downloaded March 30, 2014.
7. American Academy of Child and Adolescent Psychiatry, "Children and Watching TV," http://www.aacap.org/AACAP/Families_and_Youth/Facts_for_Families/Facts_for_Families_Pages/Children_And_Wat_54.aspx, downloaded March 20, 2014.
8. R. Boynton-Jarret, T. N. Thomas, K. E. Peterson, J. Wiecha, A. M. Sobol, and S. L. Gortmaker, "Impact of Television Viewing Patterns on Fruit and Vegetable Consumption among Adolescents," *Pediatrics* 113 (2003): 1321–1326.
9. J. P. Chaput et al., "Video Game Playing Increases Food Intake in Adolescents: a randomized crossover study," *American Journal of Clinical Nutrition* 93, no. 6 (2011): 1196–1203.
10. K. R. Smith et al., "Walkability and Body Mass Index Density, Design, and New Diversity Measures," *American Journal of Preventative Medicine* 35, no. 3 (2008): 237–244.
11. League of California Cities Planners Institute, Pasadena Conference Center (April 13-15, 2005).
12. J. Pucher and C. Lefevre, *The Urban Transport Crisis in Europe and North America* (London: Macmillan Press Ltd., 1996).
13. S. M. Krebs-Smith, J. Reedy, C. Bosire, "Healthfulness of the U.S. Food Supply: Little Improvement Despite Decades of Dietary Guidance," *American Journal of Preventative Medicine* 38, no. 5 (2010):472–477, available online at http://nccor.org/downloads/roundtable/Krebs-Smith%20-%20Healthfulness%20of%20the%20US%20Food%20Supply.pdf.
14. M. Mudd, "How to Force Ethics on the Food Industry," *The New York Times* (March 16, 2013).
15. M. Nestle, *Food Politics, Revised and Expanded 10th Anniversary Edition*, (Berkeley: University of California Press, 2013), 1–22.

16. K. J. Duffey and B. M. Popkin, "Energy Density, Portion Size, and Eating Occasions: Contributions to Increased Energy Intake in the United States, 1977–2006," *PLoS Medicine* (2011): 8.

17. B. Wansink and E. van Kleef, "Dinner Rituals That Correlate with Child and Adult BMI," *Obesity*. doi: 10.1002/oby.20629 (December 19, 2013).

18. "Food Prepared Away from Home Is Increasing and Found to Be Less Nutritious," *Nutrition Research Newsletter* 21, no. 8 (August 2002): 10 (2); USDA "2012 Food Prices and Spending," http://www.ers.usda.gov/data-products/ag-and-food-statistics-charting-the-essentials/food-prices-and-spending, downloaded March 20, 2014.

19. J. P. Block et al., "Consumers' Estimation of Calorie Content at Fast Food Restaurants: cross sectional observational study," *British Medical Journal* (2013); 346:f2907.

20. "A Diner's Guide to Health and Nutrition Claims on Restaurant Menus" (Washington, DC: Center for Science in the Public Interest, 1997), available at http://www.cspinet.org/reports/dinersgu.html, accessed March 20, 2014.

21. M. O. Hearst et al., "Nutritional Quality at Eight U.S. Fast-Food Chains 14-Year Trends," *Medical Journal of Preventative Medicine* 44, no. 6 (2013): 589–594.

22. "How to Make Healthy Lifestyle Changes," *Tufts University Health & Nutrition Newsletter* (June 2013): 5.

23. J. A. Ello-Martin, L. S. Roe, J. S. Meengs, D. E. Wall, and B. J. Rolls, "Increasing the Portion Size of a Unit Food Increases Energy Intake" *Appetite* 39 (2002): 74.

24. American Institute for Cancer Research, "As Restaurant Portions Grow, Vast Majority of Americans Still Belong to 'Clean Plate Club,' New Survey Finds," AICR News Release, January 15, 2001.

25. B. Wansink, "Can Package Size Accelerate Usage Volume?" *Journal of Marketing* 60 (1996): 1–14.

26. National Alliance for Nutrition and Activity (NANA), "From Wallet to Waistline: The Hidden Costs of Super Sizing," available at http://www.preventioninstitute.org/portionsizerept.html (accessed March 20, 2014).

27. S. H. A. Holt, N. Sandona, and J. C. Brand-Miller, "The Effects of Sugar-Free vs. Sugar-Rich Beverages on Feelings of Fullness and Subsequent Food Intake," *International Journal of Food Sciences and Nutrition* 51, no. 1 (January 2000): 59.

28. Wellness Facts, "*University of California at Berkeley Wellness Letter,*" (Palm Coast, FL: The Editors, May 2004).

29. W. Wood, L. Tam, and M. Guerrero Witt, "Changing Circumstances, Disrupting Habits," *Journal of Personality and Social Psychocogy,* 83, 1281–1297, as sited in David T. Neal, Wendy Wood, and Jeffry M. Quinn, "Habits—A Repeat Performance," *Current Directions in Psychocolgical Science* 15, no. 4: 198.

30. K. McGowan, "The New Quitter," *Psychology Today,* (July/August 2010): 54.

31. K. McGonigal, *The Willpower Instict: How Self-Control Works, Why It Matters, and What You Can Do to Get More of It,* (New York: Avery, 2012): 25.

32. G. S. Howard, D. W. Nance, and P. Myers, *Adaptive Counseling and Therapy* (San Francisco: Jossey–Bass, 1987).

33. J. O. Prochaska, J. C. Norcross, and C. C. DiClemente, *Changing for Good* (New York: William Morrow, 1994).

34. N. A. Christakis and J. Fowler, "Social Networks Exert Key Influences on Decision to Quit Smoking," *New England Journal of Medicine* (May 22, 2008): 25.

SUGGESTED READINGS

Brehm, B. *Successful Fitness Motivation Strategies*. Champaign, IL: Human Kinetics, 2004.

Burgand, M., and K. Gallagher. "Self-Monitoring: Influencing Effective Behavior Change in Your Clients." *ACSM's Health & Fitness Journal* 10, no 1 (2006): 14-19.

Hagger, M. S., and N. L. D. Chatzisarantis, editors. *Intrinsic Motivation and Self-Determination in Exercise and Sport*. Champaign, IL: Human Kinetics, 2007.

Prochaska, J. O., J. C. Norcross, and C. C. DiClemente. *Changing for Good*. New York: William Morrow, 1994.

Rodgers, W. M., and C. C, Loitz. *The Role of Motivation in Behavior* Change. *ACSM's Health & Fitness Journal* 13, no 1 (2009): 7-12.

White, M. W., E. L. Mailey., and E. McAuley. Leading a Physically Active Lifestyle. *ACSM's Health & Fitness Journal* 14, no 1 (2010): 8-15.

McGonigal, K., *The Willpower Instict: How Self-Control Works, Why It Matters, and What You Can Do to Get More of It,* (New York: Avery, 2012).

Krebs-Smith, S. M., J. Reedy, and C. Bosire, "Healthfulness of the U.S. Food Supply: Little Improvement Despite Decades of Dietary Guidance," *Am J Prev Med* 38 no. 5 (2010):472-477, available online at http://nccor.org/downloads/roundtable/Krebs-Smith%20-%20Healthfulness%20of%20the%20US%20Food%20Supply.pdf.

Lab 2A: Exercising Control over Your Physical Activity and Nutrition Environment

Name ______________________ Date ____________ Grade ____________

Instructor ______________________ Course ____________ Section ____________

OBJECTIVE

To aid in the identification of environmental factors that have an effect on your physical activity and nutrition habits.

INSTRUCTIONS

Select the appropriate answer to each question and obtain a final score for each section. Then rate yourself according to the guidelines at the end of the lab.

I. Physical Activity

Note: Based on the definitions of *physical activity* and *exercise*, as you take this questionnaire, keep in mind that you can be physically active without exercising, but you cannot exercise without being physically active.

	NEARLY ALWAYS	OFTEN	SELDOM	NEVER
1. Do you identify daily time slots to be *physically active?*	4	3	2	1
2. Do you seek additional opportunities to be active each day (walk, cycle, park farther away, do yard work/gardening)?	4	3	2	1
3. Do you avoid labor-saving devices/activities (escalators, elevators, self-propelled lawn mowers, snow blowers, drive through windows)?	4	3	2	1
4. Does physical activity improve your health and well-being?	4	3	2	1
5. Does physical activity increase your energy level?	4	3	2	1
6. Do you seek professional and/or medical (if necessary) advice prior to starting an exercise program or when increasing the intensity, duration, and frequency of exercise?	4	3	2	1
7. Do you identify time slots to *exercise* most days of the week?	4	3	2	1
8. Do you schedule exercise during times of the day when you feel most energetic?	4	3	2	1
9. Do you have an alternative plan to be active or exercise during adverse weather conditions (walk at the mall, swim at the health club, climb stairs, skip rope, dance)?	4	3	2	1
10. Do you cross-train (participate in a variety of activities)?	4	3	2	1
11. Do you surround yourself with people who support your physical activity/exercise goals?	4	3	2	1
12. Do you let family and friends know of your physical activity/exercise interests?	4	3	2	1
13. Do you invite family and friends to exercise with you?	4	3	2	1
14. Do you seek new friendships with people who are physically active?	4	3	2	1
15. Do you select friendships with people whose fitness and skill levels are similar to yours?	4	3	2	1
16. Do you plan social activities that involve physical activity?	4	3	2	1
17. Do you plan activity/exercise when you are away from home (during business and vacation trips)?	4	3	2	1
18. When you have a desire to do so, do you take classes to learn new activity/sport skills?	4	3	2	1
19. Do you limit daily television viewing and Internet and computer game time?	4	3	2	1
20. Do you spend leisure hours being physically active?	4	3	2	1

Physical Activity Score: ____________

Total number of daily steps: [ ]

II. Nutrition

	NEARLY ALWAYS	OFTEN	SELDOM	NEVER
1. Do you prepare a shopping list prior to going to the store?	4	3	2	1
2. Do you select food items primarily from the perimeter of the store (site of most fresh/unprocessed foods)?	4	3	2	1
3. Do you limit the unhealthy snacks you bring into the home and the workplace?	4	3	2	1
4. Do you plan your meals and is your pantry well stocked so you can easily prepare a meal without a quick trip to the store?	4	3	2	1
5. Do you help cook your meals?	4	3	2	1
6. Do you pay attention to how hungry you are before and during a meal?	4	3	2	1
7. When reaching for food, do you remind yourself that you have a choice about what and how much you eat?	4	3	2	1
8. Do you eat your meals at home?	4	3	2	1
9. Do you eat your meals at the table only?	4	3	2	1
10. Do you include whole-grain products in your diet each day (whole-grain bread/cereal/crackers/rice/pasta)?	4	3	2	1
11. Do you make a deliberate effort to include a variety of fruits and vegetables in your diet each day?	4	3	2	1
12. Do you limit your daily saturated fat and trans fat intake (red meat, whole milk, cheese, butter, hard margarines, luncheon meats, baked goods, processed foods)?	4	3	2	1
13. Do you avoid unnecessary/unhealthy snacking (at work or play, during TV viewing, at the movies or socials)?	4	3	2	1
14. Do you plan caloric allowances prior to attending social gatherings that include food and eating?	4	3	2	1
15. Do you limit alcohol consumption to two drinks a day if you are a man or one drink a day if you are a woman?	4	3	2	1
16. Are you aware of strategies to decrease caloric intake when dining out (resist the server's offerings for drinks and appetizers, select a low-calorie/nutrient-dense item, drink water, resist cleaning your plate, ask for a doggie bag, share meals, request whole-wheat substitutes, get dressings on the side, avoid cream sauces, skip desserts)?	4	3	2	1
17. Do you avoid ordering larger meal sizes because you get more food for your money?	4	3	2	1
18. Do you avoid buying food when you hadn't planned to do so (gas stations, convenience stores, video rental stores)?	4	3	2	1
19. Do you fill your time with activities that will keep you away from places where you typically consume food (kitchen, coffee room, dining room)?	4	3	2	1
20. Do you know what situations trigger your desire for unnecessary snacking and overeating (vending machines, TV viewing, food ads, cookbooks, fast-food restaurants, buffet restaurants)?	4	3	2	1

Nutrition Score: ________

Ratings (Check the appropriate box.)

		Physical Activity	Nutrition
≥71	You have good control over your environment	☐	☐
51–70	There is room for improvement	☐	☐
31–50	Your environmental control is poor	☐	☐
≤30	You are controlled by your environment	☐	☐

Lab 2B: Behavior Modification Plan

Name ______________________ **Date** ____________ **Grade** ____________

Instructor ______________________ **Course** ____________ **Section** ____________

NECESSARY LAB EQUIPMENT
None.

OBJECTIVE
To help you identify the stage of change for two problem behaviors and the processes and techniques for change.

INSTRUCTIONS
Chapter 2 must be read prior to this lab.

I. Stages of Change Instructions

Please indicate which response most accurately describes your current ______________________ behavior (in the blank space identify the behavior: smoking, physical activity, stress, nutrition, weight control). Next, select the statement below (select only one) that best represents your current behavior pattern. To select the most appropriate statement, fill in the blank for one of the first three statements if your current behavior is a problem behavior. For example, you may say:

"I currently smoke, and I do not intend to change in the foreseeable future" or

"I currently do not exercise, but I am contemplating changing in the next 6 months."

If you have already started to make changes, fill in the blank in one of the last three statements. In this case you may say:

"I currently eat a low-fat diet, but I have only done so within the last 6 months" or

"I currently practice adequate stress management techniques, and I have done so for over 6 months."

You may use this form to identify your stage of change for any health-related behavior. After identifying two problem behaviors, look up your stage of change for each one using Table 2.3 (on page 65).

Behavior #1. Fill in only one blank.

☐ 1. I currently ______________________, and do not intend to change in the foreseeable future.

☐ 2. I currently ______________________, but I am contemplating changing in the next 6 months.

☐ 3. I currently ______________________ regularly, but I intend to change in the next month.

☐ 4. I currently ______________________, but I have only done so within the last 6 months.

☐ 5. I currently ______________________, and I have done so for over 6 months.

☐ 6. I currently ______________________, and I have done so for over 5 years.

Stage of change: ______________ (see Table 2.3 on page 65).

Behavior #2. Fill in only one blank.

☐ 1. I currently ______________________, and do not intend to change in the foreseeable future.

☐ 2. I currently ______________________, but I am contemplating changing in the next 6 months.

☐ 3. I currently ______________________ regularly, but I intend to change in the next month.

☐ 4. I currently ______________________, but I have only done so within the last 6 months.

☐ 5. I currently ______________________, and I have done so for over 6 months.

☐ 6. I currently ______________________, and I have done so for over 5 years.

Stage of change: ______________ (see Table 2.3 on page 65).

II. Processes of Change

According to your stage of change for the two behaviors you have identified, list the processes of change that apply to each behavior (see Table 2.1 on page 59).

Behavior #1: ____________________

____

Behavior #2: ____________________

____

III. Techniques for Change

List a minimum of three techniques that you will use with each process of change (see Table 2.2 on page 65).

Behavior #1: 1. ____________________

2. ____________________

List:	Self-Destructive Behaviors	Constructive Behaviors
	______	______
	______	______
	______	______
	______	______

3. ____________________

Behavior #2: 1. ____________________

2. ____________________

List:	Self-Destructive Behaviors	Constructive Behaviors
	______	______
	______	______
	______	______
	______	______

3. ____________________

Today's date: __________ Completion date: __________ Signature: ____________________

Lab 2C: Setting SMART Goals

Name ______________________ Date ____________ Grade ____________

Instructor ______________________ Course ____________ Section ____________

OBJECTIVE

To learn to write SMART goals.

INSTRUCTIONS

In Lab 2B you identified two behaviors that you wish to change. Using SMART goal guidelines, write goals and actions that will provide a road map for behavioral change. In the spaces provided in this lab, indicate how your stated goals meet each one of the SMART goal guidelines.

I. SMART Goals

Goal 1:

____

____

Indicate what makes your goal specific.

____

How is your goal measurable?

____

____

Why is this an acceptable goal?

____

____

State why you consider this goal realistic.

____

____

How is this goal time-specific?

____

____

Goal 2:

____

____

Indicate what makes your goal specific.

____

How is your goal measurable?

____

____

Why is this an acceptable goal?

____

____

State why you consider this goal realistic.

____

____

How is this goal time-specific?

____

____

II. Specific Actions

Write a minimum of five specific objectives that will help you reach your two SMART goals.

Goal 1: ____

Actions:

1. ____
2. ____
3. ____
4. ____
5. ____

Goal 2: ____

Actions:

1. ____
2. ____
3. ____
4. ____
5. ____

3

Nutrition for Wellness

Preparing most meals at home is one of the surest ways to eat healthier and enjoy a longer, more productive, and better life. If you feel that you don't have time to cook healthy meals, or you don't care to cook healthy meals, sooner or later you will have to make time to treat and care for illness and disease.

OBJECTIVES

- Define nutrition and describe its relationship to health and well-being.
- Learn to use the U.S. Department of Agriculture MyPlate guidelines for healthier eating.
- Describe the functions of carbohydrates, fiber, fats, proteins, vitamins, minerals, and water in the human body.
- Define the various energy production mechanisms of the human body.
- Be able to conduct a comprehensive nutrient analysis and implement changes to meet the Dietary Reference Intakes.
- Identify myths and fallacies regarding nutrition.
- Become aware of guidelines for nutrient supplementation.
- Learn the *Dietary Guidelines for Americans 2010*.

REAL LIFE STORY | Gunther's Experience

I have never been a morning person. I always got up late and just grabbed a caffè mocha with whipped cream, grande sized, to get some calories before class. Following my first class or two, I would stop at the student union and get a couple of doughnuts or a bagel with cream cheese. In the early afternoon, I would typically have some type of a burger, often with cheese, a soda, and a candy bar. A quick snack from the candy machine on my afternoon trips to the library had become a part of my daily routine. School-day dinners usually consisted of pizza or some other processed food that wouldn't take long to prepare. Fruits, grains, and vegetables were practically nonexistent in my diet. Eating out on weekends, junk food at school games or at parties, often including a fair amount of alcohol, was not uncommon my first semester in college. I had gained eight pounds, and I was definitely not happy with how I felt. I enrolled in the *Wellness for Life* course during the winter semester. We were given extra credit for having a blood test done, as long as we were able to interpret the results, look into our health family history, and explain lifestyle choices we could make to improve or maintain recommended values. Being so out of shape, I figured I could use all the extra credit I could get. Man, was I in for a shock! Both my LDL cholesterol and triglycerides were in the high categories, meaning high risk for heart disease, and I was just 19 years old. Thanks to the work I had to do to get the extra credit, the subsequent nutrition discussions, and my exercise program, I was able to make drastic lifestyle changes that paid off big dividends in just three months. I literally took the advice to heart. My blood lipids are now in the normal range, and my weight is back where it should be. It wasn't easy, but my teacher, roommates, and friends were very supportive. I earned an A in the course, but most importantly, I feel that I have added quality and healthy years to my life.

MyProfile: Personal Nutrition Habits

To the best of your ability, answer the following questions. If you do not know the answer(s), this chapter will guide you through them.

I. Are you aware of the average daily caloric intake and macronutrient content of your diet? ___ Yes ___ No

II. If you answered "yes," please indicate your average daily caloric intake (_______ calories) and your daily percentage of total calories for carbohydrates (___ percent), fat (___ percent), and protein (___ percent).

III. According to nutritional guidelines, the daily average caloric intake should be distributed so that ___ to ___ percent of the total daily calories come from carbohydrates, ___ to ___ percent come from fat, and ___ to ___ percent come from protein.

IV. Nutrient supplements are encouraged for most people to achieve a balanced diet. ___ True ___ False

V. Current *Dietary Guidelines for Americans* encourage people to balance calories with physical activity to sustain healthy weight and focus on consuming nutrient-dense foods and beverages. ___ True ___ False

VI. As a "pediatric disease," osteoporosis can be prevented early in life by making sure that the diet has sufficient calcium and by participating in weight-bearing activities. ___ True ___ False

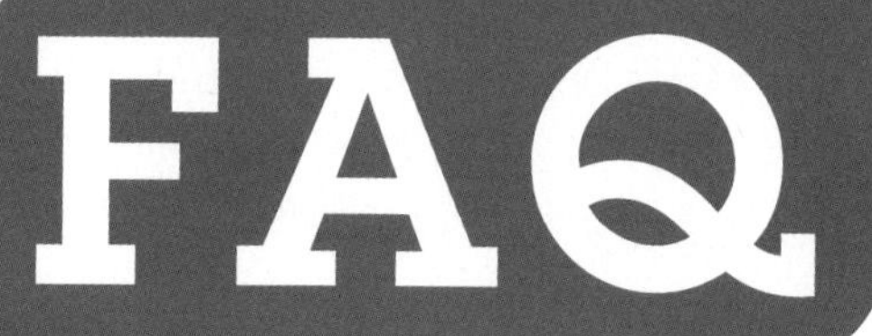

Do I have to follow a diet 24/7 to derive health benefits?

A sound diet is vital for good health and wellness. An extreme approach, however, is not the best advice when it comes to proper nutrition. Health experts believe that such an approach may lead to "orthorexia nervosa," a new category of eating disorder characterized by an unhealthy compulsion over food choices. Moderation and common sense in all things is solid advice when it comes to healthy diet and nutrition. Healthy eating patterns that can be maintained for a lifetime include small and occasional treats from time to time.

Should I be concerned about antibiotics in meat?

The use of antibiotics in animals in the United States is a common practice to increase animal growth and prevent chronic livestock illness in overcrowded farms with unsanitary living conditions. The concern is that overuse may lead to antibiotic resistance in humans. The World Health Organization, the American Medical Association, and the National Resources Defense Council consider non-therapeutic antibiotic use in livestock as a significant public health risk. As a consumer, you are encouraged to minimize the use of meats anyway, for overall health reasons (see page 90), and when you do eat meats, search for products from companies that certify antibiotic use in animals for therapeutic purposes only.

What is gluten sensitivity?

Gluten sensitivity falls under an umbrella of adverse effects on the body caused by gluten, a protein found in wheat, barley, rye, malts, and triticale. Gluten is also used as an additive for flavoring and stabilizing food or as a thickening agent.

About 1 percent of Americans suffer from celiac disease, an autoimmune disorder in genetically predisposed people of all ages that damages the lining of the small intestine and the ability to absorb nutrients. The disease is caused by a reaction to gluten, leading to an inflammatory reaction that induces a series of symptoms, including vomiting, severe abdominal pain, diarrhea, and fatigue. A gluten-free diet is the accepted treatment for individuals with celiac disease.

Many people test negative for celiac disease but appear to be gluten sensitive. They indicate that they feel better when they eliminate gluten from the diet. A gluten-free diet, however, is not completely free of gluten; rather, it contains a low, harmless level. Switching to a healthy diet often helps gluten-sensitive individuals because processed and junk foods tend to have high amounts of gluten. Some gluten in the diet may not affect these people much.

How much should I worry about sugar in my diet?

Traditionally, the most significant health concerns regarding excessive sugar intake included increased caloric intake, weight gain, obesity, tooth decay, and lower nutrient intake ("empty" or "discretionary" calories with no nutritional benefit). But following a 24-year study of almost 90,000 women published in the *American Journal of Clinical Nutrition*, the dada indicated that consumption of one or two sugar-sweetened beverages per day increased coronary heart disease risk by 23 or 35 percent, respectively. Regular soft-drink consumers have about an 80 percent greater risk for developing type 2 diabetes. Excessive body weight increases the risk for metabolic syndrome and heart disease. Excessive added sugar (any sugar removed from its natural product and added to another food) in the diet also raises blood fats known as triglycerides, which along with cholesterol clog up the arteries. People who consume a sugar-heavy diet run a greater risk for pancreatic cancer. Other data indicate that sugar overconsumption leads to liver cirrhosis and dementia and individuals who drink more than five sugary soft drinks per week have reduced bone density in the hips and more than double joint-cushioning cartilage loss in the knees. An estimated 25,000 deaths annually are attributed to excessive sugar intake. Furthermore, 2013 research indicates that the hardest dietary habit for post heart attack victims to change is drinking sugary drinks, with soft drink consumption being the most difficult habit to kick.

You do not have to eliminate all sugar from your diet. Data indicate that the typical American consumes about 475 daily calories from added sugar, the equivalent of 30 teaspoons per day. Most people simply cannot afford those extra daily empty calories. People should strive for a "nutrient-rich" diet—that is, a high nutrient-to-calorie ratio. The American Heart Association recommends no more than six and nine daily teaspoons of added sugar for women and men, respectively. Data also indicate that liquid calories (soft drinks) do not result in less food consumption during a meal. Adults who drink one or more sodas per day are 27 percent more likely to be overweight or obese.

Unfortunately, as of early 2014, food labels do not differentiate between natural and added sugars, making it difficult to determine the quantity added to foods and drinks. Natural sugars in food (fructose and lactose) are acceptable, because these foods contain many other healthy substances. Among others, added sugars listed on food labels include ordinary table sugar (sucrose), raw sugar, cane sugar, brown sugar, invert sugar, high-fructose corn syrup

(HFCS), corn syrup, corn sweetener, glucose, dextrose, fructose, lactose, maltose, maltodextrin, molasses, honey, agave syrup, maple syrup, malt syrup, fruit juice concentrate, and sorghum. You can estimate the number of teaspoons of sugar in processed food by dividing the total grams of sugar on the label by 4.

The American Diabetic Association indicates that soft drinks and sweetened drinks are the biggest source of added sugar in the diet, accounting for 38 percent of all added sugar intake (each 12-ounce can of soft drink contains about 10 teaspoons of sugar). Soda consumption in the United States has increased by 500 percent over the past 50 years. The soda industry generates about 47 gallons of soft drink per year for each American. Other drinks loaded with added sugar include fruit drinks, iced teas, sports drinks, and energy drinks. Soft drinks and other sugar-sweetened beverages are the most significant source of added sugars in the American diet. Plain sugar, candy, and desserts account for another 34 percent of Americans' added sugar intake.

Currently, energy drinks are a major health concern in the United States. Besides added sugar, the caffeine content in these drinks can be five times (250 to 500 mg) what's in a cup of coffee (40 to 90 mg). Five deaths have been attributed to these energy drinks, most likely due to an irregular heartbeat caused by the excess caffeine. Some of the most detrimental health effects of overconsumption of energy drinks include tachycardia (rapid heart rate), chest pain, tremors, restlessness, gastrointestinal discomfort, dizziness, syncope, headaches, respiratory distress, and insomnia. Furthermore, energy drinks such as Red Bull and sports beverages like Gatorade, because of their high acidity, cause irreversible erosion of the teeth's enamel, with energy drinks being twice as damaging. If you occasionally drink them, rinse your mouth properly with water following their consumption and do not brush your teeth within an hour as such can worsen the damage caused by the acids. The same can be said about soft drinks and fruit drinks, but to a slightly lesser damaging extent.

Many researchers have expressed particular concern over HFCS, a liquid sweetener made from cornstarch but greatly enhanced with fructose. HFCS is used in many products, including soft drinks, candies, baked goods, and breakfast cereals. HFCS is thought to be a major contributor to obesity, cardiovascular disease, and type 2 diabetes and possibly high blood pressure, liver and kidney disease, and systemic inflammation.

Only athletes who participate in vigorous-intensity exercise for longer than 60 minutes at a time can benefit from sports drinks as an additional source of energy. Sports drinks contain between 70 and 100 calories (four to six teaspoons of added sugar) per 12 ounces. Most individuals who participate in 30 to 60 minutes of physical activity or exercise for health and fitness purposes do not need or benefit from sports drinks. For proper weight management and healthy living, moderation is a sound principle regarding added sugar consumption.

Fish is known to be heart healthy, but should we have mercury toxicity concerns?

Fish and shellfish contain high-quality protein, omega-3 fatty acids, and other essential nutrients. Fish is lower in saturated fat and cholesterol than meat or poultry. Data indicate that eating as little as six ounces of fatty fish per week can reduce the risk of premature death from heart disease by one-third and overall death rates by about one-sixth. Fish also appears to have anti-inflammatory properties that can help treat chronic inflammatory kidney disease, osteoarthritis, rheumatoid arthritis, Crohn's disease, and autoimmune disorders like asthma and lupus. Data indicate that consuming fish at least twice per week adds about two years of life to an already 65-year-old person. Thus, fish is one of the healthiest foods we can consume.

Potential contaminants in fish, particularly mercury, have created concerns among some people. Mercury cannot be removed from food. As it accumulates in the body, it harms the brain and nervous system. Mercury is a naturally occurring trace mineral that can be released into the air from industrial pollution. As mercury falls into streams and oceans, it accumulates in the aquatic food chain. Larger fish accumulate larger amounts of mercury because they eat medium-sized and small fish. Of particular concern are shark, swordfish, king mackerel, pike, bass, and tilefish, which have higher levels of the mineral. Farm-raised salmon also have slightly higher levels of polychlorinated biphenyls, which the U.S. Environmental Protection Agency lists as a "probable human carcinogen."

The American Heart Association recommends consuming fish twice a week. The risk for adverse effects from eating fish is extremely low and primarily theoretical in nature. For most people, eating two servings (up to six ounces) of fish per week poses no health threat. Pregnant and nursing women and young children, however, should avoid mercury in fish. The best recommendation is to balance the risks against the benefits. If you are still concerned, consume no more than 12 ounces per week of a variety of fish and shellfish that are lower in mercury, including canned light tuna, wild salmon, shrimp, pollack, catfish, and scallops. And check local advisories about the safety of fish caught by family and friends in local streams, rivers, lakes, and coastal areas. Many preventive medicine experts now think that fish is likely the most important food an individual can consume for good health.

What do the terms "glycemic index" and "glycemic load" mean?

The glycemic index (GI) provides a numeric value that measures the blood glucose (sugar) response following ingestion of individual carbohydrate foods. Carbohydrates that are quickly absorbed and cause a rapid rise in blood glucose are said to have a high GI. Those that break down slowly and gradually release glucose into the blood have a low GI. Consumption of high glycemic foods in combination with some fat and protein, nonetheless, brings down the average index. The glycemic load (GL) is calculated by multiplying the GI of a particular food by its carbohydrate content in grams and dividing by 100. The usefulness of the glycemic load is based on the theory that a high-glycemic index food eaten in small quantities provides a similar effect in blood sugar rise as consumption of a larger quantity of a low-glycemic food. Research also indicates that a low-GL diet significantly reduces inflammatory conditions that lead to chronic diseases in the human body. The most accurate source of the GI and glycemic load of 750 foods has been published in the *Journal of Clinical Nutrition.* Additional information on the GI is also provided in Chapter 5 on pages 170–172.

What is the difference between antioxidants and phytonutrients?

Antioxidants, comprising vitamins, minerals, and phytonutrients, help prevent damage to cells from highly reactive and unstable molecules known as oxygen free radicals (see page 110). Antioxidants are found both in plant and animal foods, whereas phytonutrients (also known as phytochemicals) are found in plant foods only, including fruits, vegetables, beans, nuts, and seeds. Thousands of these bioactive compounds found in plants offer an array of health benefits ranging from cardiovascular disease and cancer prevention to vision health. The actions of phytonutrients go beyond those of most antioxidants. In particular, they appear to have powerful anti-cancer properties. For example, at almost every stage of cancer, phytonutrients can block, disrupt, slow, or even reverse the process. In terms of heart disease, they may reduce inflammation, inhibit blood clots, or prevent the oxidation of low-density lipoprotein cholesterol. People should consume ample amounts of plant-based foods to obtain a healthy supply of antioxidants, including a wide array of phytonutrients.

Proper **nutrition** is essential to overall health and wellness. Good nutrition means that a person's diet supplies all essential nutrients for healthy body functioning, including normal tissue growth, repair, and maintenance. The diet should also provide enough **substrates** to produce the energy necessary for work, physical activity, and relaxation.

Nutrients should be obtained from a variety of sources. Figure 3.1 shows MyPlate nutrition guidelines and recommended daily food amounts according to various caloric requirements. To lower the risk for chronic disease, an effective wellness program must incorporate healthy eating guidelines. These guidelines are discussed throughout this chapter and in later chapters.

Too much or too little of any nutrient can precipitate serious health problems. The typical U.S. diet is too high in calories, sugar, saturated fat, and sodium and not high enough in **whole grains**, fruits, and vegetables—factors that undermine good health. On a given day, nearly half of the people in the United States eat no fruit and almost one fourth eat no vegetables.

Food availability is not a problem. The problem is overconsumption of the wrong foods. Diseases of dietary excess and imbalance are among the leading causes of death in many developed countries throughout the world, including the United States.

Diet and nutrition often play a crucial role in the development and progression of chronic diseases. A diet high in saturated fat, trans fat, and cholesterol increases the risk for diseases of the cardiovascular system, including atherosclerosis, coronary heart disease (CHD), and strokes. In sodium-sensitive individuals, high salt intake has been linked to high blood pressure. Up to 50 percent of all cancers may be diet related. Obesity, diabetes, and osteoporosis also have been associated with faulty nutrition.

Nutrients

The essential nutrients that the human body requires are carbohydrates, fat, protein, vitamins, minerals, and water. The first three are called *fuel nutrients,* because they are the only substances that the body uses to supply the energy (commonly measured in calories) needed for work and normal body functions. The three others—vitamins, minerals, and water—are regulatory nutrients. They have no caloric value but are still necessary for a person to function normally and maintain good

Nutrition Science that studies the relationship of foods to optimal health and performance.

Substrates Substances acted upon by an enzyme (e.g., carbohydrates and fats).

Nutrients Substances found in food that provide energy, regulate metabolism, and help with growth and repair of body tissues.

Whole grains Foods that contain all three major parts of a seed grain: the germ, the bran, and the endosperm. Each part contains essential nutrients and plant chemicals that work in synergy to provide optimal health and prevent disease.

FIGURE 3.1 MyPlate food plan.

Switch to fat-free or low-fat (1%) milk.

Make half your plate fruits and vegetables.

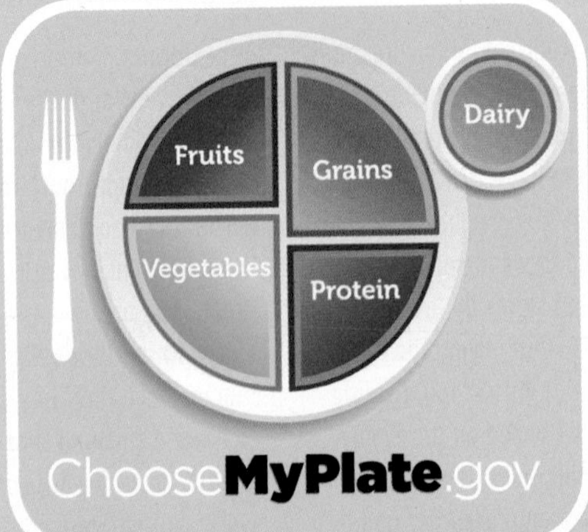

Make at least half your grains whole grains.

Choose fish and lean or low-fat meat and poultry.

VEGETABLES	FRUITS	GRAINS	PROTEIN	DAIRY
Any vegetable or 100% vegetable juice counts as a member of the Vegetable Group. Vegetables may be raw or cooked; fresh, frozen, canned, or dried/dehydrated; and may be whole, cut-up, or mashed. Vegetables are organized into 5 subgroups, based on their nutrient content: Dark green vegetables, red and orange vegetables, beans and peas, starchy vegetables, and other vegetables.	Any fruit or 100% fruit juice counts as part of the Fruit Group. Fruits may be fresh, canned, frozen, or dried, and may be whole, cut-up, or pureed.	Any food made from wheat, rice, oats, cornmeal, barley, or another cereal grain is a grain product. Bread, pasta, oatmeal, breakfast cereals, tortillas, and grits are examples of grain products. Grains are divided into 2 subgroups: whole grains and refined grains.	All foods made from meat, poultry, seafood, beans, and peas, eggs, processed soy products, nuts, and seeds are considered part of the Protein Foods Group (beans and peas are also part of the Vegetable Group). Select at least 8 ounces of cooked seafood per week. Meat and poultry choices should be lean or low-fat. Young children need less, depending on their age and calorie needs. The advice to consume seafood does not apply to vegetarians. Vegetarian options in the Protein Foods Group include beans and peas, processed soy products, and nuts and seeds.	All fluid milk products and many foods made from milk are considered part of this food group. Most Dairy Group choices should be fat-free or low-fat. Foods made from milk that retain their calcium content are part of the group. Foods made from milk that have little to no calcium, such as cream cheese, cream, and butter, are not. Calcium-fortified soymilk (soy beverage) is also part of the Dairy Group.

Recommended Daily Amounts

Women	Vegetables	Fruits	Grains	Protein	Dairy
19–30 years old	2½ cups	2 cups	6 oz. equivalents	5½ oz. equivalents	3 cups
31–50 years old	2½ cups	1½ cups	6 oz. equivalents	5 oz. equivalents	3 cups
51+ years old	2 cups	1½ cups	5 oz. equivalents	5 oz. equivalents	3 cups
Men					
19–30 years old	3 cups	2 cups	8 oz. equivalents	6½ oz. equivalents	3 cups
31–50 years old	3 cups	2 cups	7 oz. equivalents	6 oz. equivalents	3 cups
51+ years old	2½ cups	2 cups	6 oz. equivalents	6½ oz. equivalents	3 cups

Source: http://www.choosemyplate.gov/. Additional information can be obtained on this site, including an online individualized MyPlate eating plan (Plan a Healthy Menu option on the site) based on your age, gender, weight, height, and activity level.

health. Many nutritionists add to this list a seventh nutrient: fiber. This nutrient is vital for good health. Recommended amounts seem to provide protection against several diseases, including cardiovascular disease and some cancers.

Carbohydrates, fats, proteins, and water are termed "macronutrients," because we need them in proportionately large amounts daily. Vitamins and minerals are required in only small amounts—grams, milligrams, and micrograms instead of, say, ounces—and nutritionists refer to them as micronutrients.

Depending on the amount of nutrients and number of calories they contain, foods can be classified by their **nutrient density**. Foods that contain few or a moderate number of calories but are packed with nutrients are said to have high nutrient density. Foods that have a lot of calories but few nutrients are of low nutrient density and are commonly called *junk food*.

A **calorie** is the unit of measure indicating the energy value of food to the person who consumes it. It also is used to express the amount of energy a person expends in physical activity. Technically, a kilocalorie (kcal), or large calorie, is the amount of heat necessary to raise the temperature of one kilogram of water by one degree Celsius (1°C). For simplicity, people also call it a calorie rather than a kilocalorie. For example, if the caloric value of a food is 100 calories (i.e., 100 kcal), the energy in this food would raise the temperature of 100 kilograms of water by 1°C. Similarly, walking one mile would burn about 100 calories (again, 100 kcal).

FIGURE 3.2 **Major types of carbohydrates.**

Simple carbohydrates

Monosaccharides	Disaccharides
Glucose	Sucrose (glucose+fructose)
Fructose	Lactose (glucose+galactose)
Galactose	Maltose (glucose+glucose)

Complex carbohydrates

Polysaccharides	Fiber
Starches	Cellulose
Dextrins	Hemicellulose
Glycogen	Pectins
	Gums
	Mucilages

Carbohydrates

Carbohydrates constitute the major source of calories that the body uses to provide energy for work, maintain cells, and generate heat. They are necessary for brain, muscle, and nervous system function and help regulate fat and metabolize protein. Each gram of carbohydrate provides the human body with four calories. The major sources of carbohydrates are breads, cereals, fruits, vegetables, and milk and other dairy products. Carbohydrates are classified as simple carbohydrates or complex carbohydrates (Figure 3.2).

Simple Carbohydrates

Often called *sugars*, **simple carbohydrates** have little nutritive value. Examples are candy, soda, and cakes. Simple carbohydrates are divided into monosaccharides and disaccharides. These carbohydrates—whose names end in "ose"—often take the place of more nutritive foods in the diet.

Monosaccharides

The simplest sugars are **monosaccharides**. The three most common monosaccharides are glucose, fructose, and galactose.

1. Glucose is a natural sugar found in food and produced in the body from other simple and complex carbohydrates. It is used as a source of energy, or it may be stored in the muscles and liver in the form of glycogen (a long chain of glucose molecules hooked together). Excess glucose in the blood is converted to fat and stored in **adipose tissue**.
2. Fructose, or fruit sugar, occurs naturally in fruits and honey and is converted to glucose in the body. Galactose is produced from milk sugar in the mammary glands of lactating animals and is converted to glucose in the body.

Disaccharides

There are three major **disaccharides**:

1. Sucrose or table sugar (glucose + fructose)
2. Lactose (glucose + galactose)
3. Maltose (glucose + glucose)

These disaccharides are broken down in the body, and the resulting simple sugars (monosaccharides) are used as indicated previously.

Nutrient density A measure of the amount of nutrients and calories in various foods.

Calorie The amount of heat necessary to raise the temperature of one gram of water 1°C; used to measure the energy value of food and cost (energy expenditure) of physical activity.

Carbohydrates A classification for nutrients containing carbon, hydrogen, and oxygen; the major source of energy for the human body.

Simple carbohydrates Formed by simple or double sugar units with little nutritive value; divided into monosaccharides and disaccharides.

Monosaccharides The simplest carbohydrates (sugars), formed by five-or six-carbon skeletons. The three most common monosaccharides are glucose, fructose, and galactose.

Adipose tissue Fat cells in the body.

Disaccharides Simple carbohydrates formed by two monosaccharide units linked together, one of which is glucose. The major disaccharides are sucrose, lactose, and maltose.

Complex Carbohydrates **Complex carbohydrates** are also called polysaccharides. Anywhere from about 10 to thousands of monosaccharide molecules can unite to form a single polysaccharide. Examples of complex carbohydrates are starches, dextrins, and **glycogen**.

1. Starch is the storage form of glucose in plants that is needed to promote their earliest growth. Starch is commonly found in grains, seeds, corn, nuts, roots, potatoes, and legumes. In a healthful diet, grains, the richest source of starch, should supply most of the body's energy. Once eaten, starch is converted to glucose for the body's own energy use.
2. Dextrins are formed from the breakdown of large starch molecules exposed to dry heat, such as in baking bread or producing cold cereals. These complex carbohydrates of plant origin provide many valuable nutrients and can be an excellent source of fiber.
3. Glycogen is the animal polysaccharide synthesized from glucose and is found in only tiny amounts in meats. In essence, we manufacture it; we don't consume it. Glycogen constitutes the body's reservoir of glucose. Thousands of glucose molecules are linked, to be stored as glycogen in the liver and muscles. When a surge of energy is needed, enzymes in the muscles and the liver break down glycogen and thereby make glucose readily available for energy transformation. (This process is discussed under "Nutrition for Athletes," starting on page 117.)

Fiber

Fiber is a form of complex carbohydrate. A high-fiber diet gives a person a feeling of fullness without adding too many calories to the diet. **Dietary fiber** is present mainly in plant leaves, skins, roots, and seeds. Processing and refining foods removes almost all of their natural fiber. In the human diet, the main sources of fiber are whole-grain cereals and breads, fruits, vegetables, and legumes.

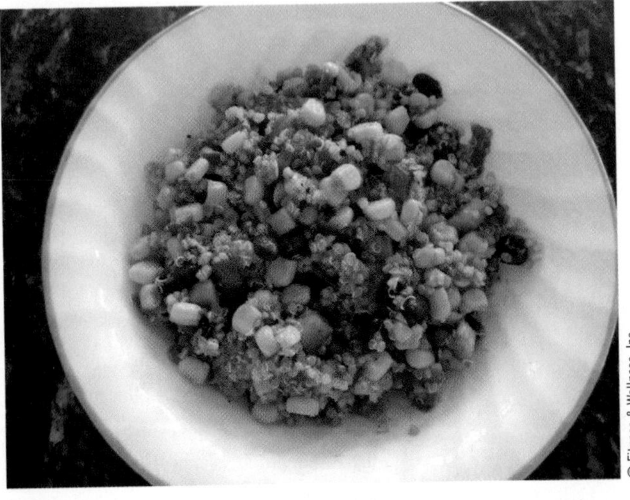

High-fiber foods are essential in a healthy diet.

Fiber is important in the diet because it decreases the risk for disease, in particular cardiovascular disease. Increased fiber intake may lower the risk for CHD, because saturated fats and trans fats often take the place of fiber in the diet, increasing the absorption and formation of cholesterol. Other health disorders that have been tied to low intake of fiber are infections, respiratory diseases, constipation, diverticulitis, hemorrhoids, gallbladder disease, and obesity. Data from 2011 showed that individuals who eat the most dietary fiber have a 22 percent lower mortality rate from any cause compared to those who eat the least amount of fiber.[1]

TABLE 3.1 Dietary Fiber Content of Selected Foods

Food	Serving Size	Dietary Fiber (g)
Almonds (shelled)	¼ cup	3.9
Apple	1 medium	3.7
Banana	1 small	1.2
Beans, red kidney	½ cup	8.2
Beets, red, canned (cooked)	½ cup	1.4
Blackberries	½ cup	4.9
Brazil nuts	1 oz	2.5
Broccoli (cooked)	½ cup	3.3
Brown rice (cooked)	½ cup	1.7
Carrots (cooked)	½ cup	3.3
Cauliflower (cooked)	½ cup	5.0
Cereal		
All-Bran	1 oz	8.5
Cheerios	1 oz	1.1
Corn Flakes	1 oz	0.5
Fruit 'n Fibre	1 oz	4.0
Fruit Wheats	1 oz	2.0
Just Right	1 oz	2.0
Wheaties	1 oz	2.0
Corn (cooked)	½ cup	2.2
Eggplant (cooked)	½ cup	3.0
Lettuce (chopped)	½ cup	0.5
Orange	1 medium	4.3
Parsnips (cooked)	½ cup	2.1
Pear	1 medium	4.5
Peas (cooked)	½ cup	4.4
Popcorn (plain)	1 cup	1.2
Potato (baked)	1 medium	4.9
Strawberries	½ cup	1.6
Summer squash (cooked)	½ cup	1.6
Watermelon	1 cup	0.1

BEHAVIOR MODIFICATION PLANNING

Tips to Increase Fiber in Your Diet

I PLAN TO	I DID IT	
❑	❑	Eat more vegetables, either raw or steamed
❑	❑	Eat salads daily that include a wide variety of vegetables
❑	❑	Eat more fruit, including the skin
❑	❑	Choose whole-wheat and whole-grain products
❑	❑	Choose breakfast cereals with more than 3 grams of fiber per serving
❑	❑	Sprinkle a teaspoon or two of unprocessed bran or 100 percent bran cereal on your favorite breakfast cereal
❑	❑	Add high-fiber cereals to casseroles and desserts
❑	❑	Add beans to soups, salads, and stews
❑	❑	Add vegetables to sandwiches: sprouts, green and red pepper strips, diced carrots, sliced cucumbers, red cabbage, onions
❑	❑	Add vegetables to spaghetti: broccoli, cauliflower, sliced carrots, mushrooms
❑	❑	Experiment with unfamiliar fruits and vegetables: collards, kale, broccoflower, asparagus, papaya, mango, kiwi, star fruit
❑	❑	Blend fruit juice with small pieces of fruit and crushed ice
❑	❑	When increasing fiber in your diet, drink plenty of fluids

Try It

Do you know your average daily fiber intake? If you do not know, keep a 3-day record of daily fiber intake. How do you fare against the recommended guidelines? If your intake is low, how can you change your diet to increase your daily fiber intake?

The recommended fiber intake for adults age 50 years and younger is 25 grams per day for women and 38 grams per day for men. As a result of decreased food consumption in people older than 50 years, an intake of 21 and 30 grams of fiber per day, respectively, is recommended.[2] Most people in the United States eat only 15 grams of fiber per day, putting them at increased risk for disease.

A person can increase fiber intake by eating more fruits, vegetables, legumes, and whole grains. Research provides evidence that increasing fiber intake to 30 grams per day leads to a significant reduction in heart attacks, cancer of the colon, breast cancer, diabetes, and diverticulitis. Table 3.1 provides the fiber content of selected foods. A practical guideline to obtain your fiber intake is to eat at least five (preferably nine) daily servings of fruits and vegetables and three servings of whole-grain foods (whole-grain bread, cereal, and rice). Think of your servings of these food items as servings of absolute goodness to your taste and health.

Fiber is typically classified according to its solubility in water:

- Soluble fiber dissolves in water and forms a gel-like substance that encloses food particles. This property allows soluble fiber to bind and excrete fats from the body. This type of fiber has been shown to lower blood cholesterol and blood sugar levels. Soluble fiber is found primarily in oats, fruits, barley, legumes, and psyllium (an ancient Indian grain added to some breakfast cereals).
- Insoluble fiber is not easily dissolved in water, and the body cannot digest it. This type of fiber is important because it binds water, causing a softer and bulkier stool that increases **peristalsis**, the involuntary muscle contractions of intestinal walls that force the stool through the intestines and enable quicker excretion of food residues. Speeding the passage of food residues through the intestines seems to lower the risk for colon cancer, mainly because it reduces the amount of time that cancer-causing agents are in contact with the intestinal wall. Insoluble fiber is also thought to bind with carcinogens (cancer-producing substances), and more water in the stool may dilute the cancer-causing agents, lessening their potency. Sources of insoluble fiber include wheat, cereals, vegetables, and skins of fruits.

The following are the most common types of fiber:

1. Cellulose, the water-insoluble fiber found in plant cell walls

Complex carbohydrates Carbohydrates formed by three or more simple sugar molecules linked together; also referred to as polysaccharides.

Glycogen Form in which glucose is stored in the body.

Dietary fiber A complex carbohydrate in plant foods that is not digested but is essential to digestion.

Peristalsis Involuntary muscle contractions of intestinal walls that facilitate excretion of wastes.

2. Hemicellulose, the water-insoluble fiber found in cereal fibers
3. Pectins, the water-soluble fiber found in vegetables and fruits
4. Gums and mucilages, water-soluble fibers found in small amounts in foods of plant origin

Surprisingly, excessive fiber intake can be detrimental to health. It can produce loss of calcium, phosphorus, and iron, to say nothing of gastrointestinal discomfort. If your fiber intake is below the recommended amount, increase your intake gradually over several weeks to avoid gastrointestinal disturbances. While increasing your fiber intake, be sure to drink more water to avoid constipation and even dehydration. Excellent complex carbohydrate choices include beans, sweet potatoes, and quinoa. Quinoa, one of the best whole grains you can eat, is also high in protein; it is a complete protein that contains all essential amino acids.

Fats (Lipids)

The human body uses **fats** as a source of energy. Also called lipids, fats are the most concentrated energy source, with each gram of fat supplying 9 calories to the body (in contrast to 4 calories for carbohydrates). Fats are part of the human cell structure. Deposits of fat cells are used as stored energy and as an insulator to preserve body heat. They absorb shock, supply essential fatty acids, and carry the fat-soluble vitamins A, D, E, and K. Fats can be divided into three main groups: simple, compound, and derived (Figure 3.3). The most familiar sources of fat are whole milk and other dairy products, meats, and meat alternatives such as eggs and nuts.

Simple Fats A simple fat consists of a glyceride molecule linked to one, two, or three units of fatty acids. Depending on the number of fatty acids attached, simple fats are divided into monoglycerides (one fatty acid), diglycerides (two fatty acids), and triglycerides (three fatty acids). More than 90 percent of the weight of fat in foods and more than 95 percent of the stored fat in the human body are in the form of triglycerides.

FIGURE 3.3 **Major types of fats (lipids).**

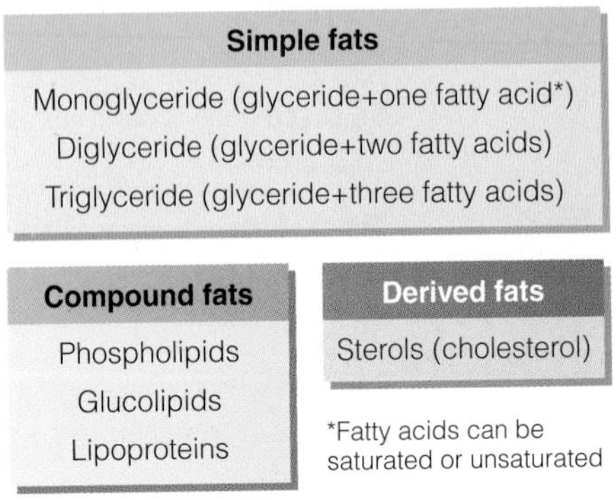

Simple fats
Monoglyceride (glyceride+one fatty acid*)
Diglyceride (glyceride+two fatty acids)
Triglyceride (glyceride+three fatty acids)

Compound fats
Phospholipids
Glucolipids
Lipoproteins

Derived fats
Sterols (cholesterol)

*Fatty acids can be saturated or unsaturated

The length of the carbon atom chain and the amount of hydrogen saturation (i.e., the number of hydrogen molecules attached to the carbon chain) in fatty acids vary. Based on the extent of saturation, fatty acids are said to be saturated or unsaturated. Unsaturated fatty acids are further classified as monounsaturated or polyunsaturated. Saturated fatty acids are mainly of animal origin, and unsaturated fats are found mostly in plant products.

Saturated Fats

In saturated fatty acids (or saturated fats), the carbon atoms are fully saturated with hydrogen atoms; only single bonds link the carbon atoms on the chain (Figure 3.4). Foods high in saturated fatty acids are meats, animal fat, lard, whole milk, cream, butter, cheese, ice cream, hydrogenated oils (hydrogenation saturates fat with hydrogens, also known as trans fats), coconut oil, and palm oils. Saturated fats typically do not melt at room temperature. Coconut and palm oils are exceptions. In general, saturated fats raise a person's blood cholesterol level. The data on coconut and palm oils are controversial, because some research indicates that these oils may be neutral in terms of their effects on cholesterol. Thus, some individuals promote the use of coconut oil as a health food, but the scientific evidence to support the claim is not strong. Coconut oil might be better than saturated animal fats, but it is not a good choice as compared to extra virgin olive and canola oils. Until more definite studies become available, coconut oils is to be used sparingly.

Although saturated fats raise the "bad" low-density lipoprotein (LDL) cholesterol (in particular, the less damaging

FIGURE 3.4 **Chemical structure of saturated and unsaturated fats.**

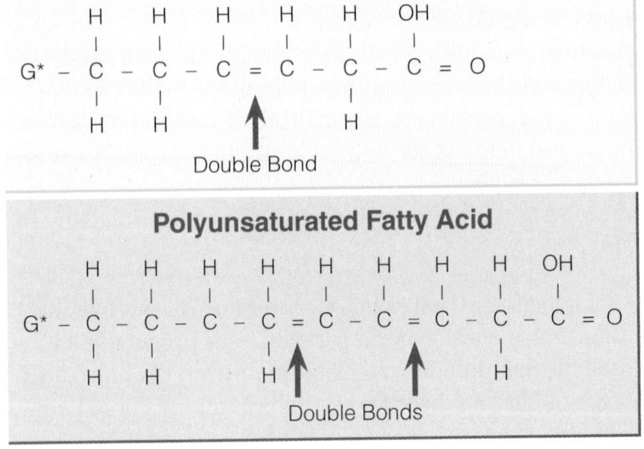

Saturated Fatty Acid

```
       H   H   H   H   H   OH
       |   |   |   |   |   |
G* -   C - C - C - C - C - C = O
       |   |   |   |   |
       H   H   H   H   H
```

Monounsaturated Fatty Acid

```
       H   H   H   H   H   OH
       |   |   |   |   |   |
G* -   C - C - C = C - C - C = O
       |   |           |
       H   H   ↑       H
          Double Bond
```

Polyunsaturated Fatty Acid

```
       H   H   H   H   H   H   H   H   OH
       |   |   |   |   |   |   |   |   |
G* -   C - C - C - C = C - C = C - C - C = O
       |   |       |               |
       H   H       H ↑       ↑     H
                   Double Bonds
```

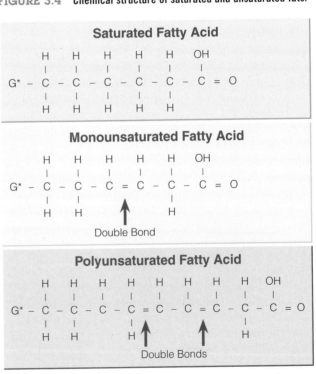

*Glyceride component

larger LDL particles) and daily intake should be limited, data indicate that people who replace saturated fat in their diet with refined carbohydrates, such as white bread and pasta and low-fat sweetened baked goods, are at greater risk for cardiovascular disease, because the latter tend to decrease the "good" high-density lipoprotein (HDL) cholesterol and increase triglycerides (blood fats) and the more dangerous smaller LDL particles.[3] Individuals who replace saturated fats with polyunsaturated fats (see the discussion that follows) derive significant health benefits. A more thorough discussion on this topic is provided in Chapter 11 (page 421).

Unsaturated Fats

In unsaturated fatty acids (or unsaturated fats), double bonds form between unsaturated carbons. These healthy fatty acids include monounsaturated and polyunsaturated fats, which are usually liquid at room temperature. Other shorter fatty acid chains also tend to be liquid at room temperature. Unsaturated fats help lower blood cholesterol. When unsaturated fats replace saturated fats in the diet, the former stimulate the liver to clear cholesterol from the blood.

In monounsaturated fatty acids (MUFA), only one double bond is found along the chain. Monounsaturated fatty acids are found in olive, canola, peanut, and sesame oils. They are also found in avocados, peanuts, and cashews.

Olive oil is considered the healthiest oil because of the nutrients it contains. Extra virgin olive oil contains antioxidants, polyphenols, and omega-3 fatty acids, all of which promote cardiovascular health, improved cognitive function, and a healthier immune system. Olive oil may even help prevent or reverse type 2 diabetes because it helps the body produce adiponectin, a hormone that aids with blood sugar regulation. Olive oil even has anti-inflammatory properties that protect against chronic diseases.

Extra virgin olive oil is produced from the first pressing of the olives and as such holds the most nutrients. Virgin olive oil is derived from the second pressing. Juices collected from subsequent olive pressings are then used to manufacture light and pure olive oils.

Canola oil is also extremely healthy. Its composition is the closest to the optimum requirements of fatty acids by the human body and it contains a nearly ideal mix of unsaturated fatty acids that promote cardiac health. The omega-3s in canola oil also counteract fibrinogen, a compound in the blood that has been linked to thrombosis (blood clot formation in the blood vessels) and inflammation.

Extra virgin and virgin olive oils retain to a greater extent the flavor of the olives, thus they are best used to make tasty dish toppings and salad dressings, but may not be the most ideal for cooking or baking. Because olive oil is more expensive than canola oil, you can use canola oil for cooking, and reserve olive oil for toppings, dips, and dressings.

Polyunsaturated fatty acids (PUFA) contain two or more double bonds between unsaturated carbon atoms along the chain. Corn, cottonseed, safflower, walnut, sunflower, and soybean oils are high in polyunsaturated fatty acids and are found in fish, almonds, and pecans.

Trans-Fatty Acids

Hydrogen often is added to monounsaturated and polyunsaturated fats to increase shelf life and to solidify them so that they are more spreadable. During this process, called partial hydrogenation, the position of hydrogen atoms may be changed along the carbon chain, transforming the fat into a **trans-fatty acid**. Some margarine spreads, shortening, pastries, nut butters, crackers, cookies, frozen breakfast foods, dairy products, snacks and chips, cake mixes, meats, **processed foods**, and fast foods contain trans-fatty acids.

Trans-fatty acids are not essential and provide no known health benefit. Health-conscious people minimize their intake of these types of fats, because diets high in trans-fatty acids increase LDL cholesterol and decrease HDL cholesterol, increase rigidity of the coronary arteries, contribute to the formation of blood clots that may lead to heart attacks and strokes, and increase visceral fat (fat around the abdomen) by redistributing fat tissue from other parts of the body. According to 2013 research published in the *American Journal of Clinical Nutrition*, high trans-fatty acid intake has been associated with an increased risk of all-cause mortality, accounting for an estimated 7 percent of all death in the United States in recent years.[4]

Paying attention to food labels is important because the words "partially hydrogenated" and "trans-fatty acids" indicate that the product carries a health risk just as high as or higher than that of saturated fat. Since 2006, the U.S. Food and Drug Administration (FDA) requires food labeling of products that contain more than half a gram of trans-fats per serving, so that consumers can make healthier choices. Subsequently, the Institute of Medicine indicated that there is no safe level of consumption. In 2013, the FDA further proposed regulation to ban trans-fats from all products by stating that they are not safe for human health and ordered that they be removed from the "generally recognized as safe" (GRAS) list of food additives.

Polyunsaturated Omega Fatty Acids

Omega fatty acids have been named based on where the first double bond appears in the carbon chain—starting from the end of the chain; hence, the term "omega" from the end of the Greek alphabet. Accordingly, omega fats are classified as omega-3, omega-6, and omega-9. **Omega-3 fatty acids** and

Fats A classification for nutrients containing carbon, hydrogen, some oxygen, and sometimes other chemical elements.

Trans-fatty acid Solidified fat formed by adding hydrogen to monounsaturated and polyunsaturated fats to increase shelf life.

Processed foods Includes all agricultural commodities that undergo processing (cooking, canning, freezing, dehydration, or milling) or addition of another ingredient.

Omega-3 fatty acids Polyunsaturated fatty acids found primarily in cold-water seafood, flaxseed, and flaxseed oil and thought to lower blood cholesterol and triglycerides.

omega-6 fatty acids have gained considerable attention in recent years. These fatty acids are essential to human health and cannot be manufactured by the body; they have to be consumed in the diet. Omega-9 fatty acids are defined as nonessential because the body can synthesize them from other foods we eat, and we don't have to depend on direct dietary sources to obtain them.

Maintaining a balance between omega-3 and omega 6 fatty acids is important for good health. Some leaders in the field maintain that excessive intake of omega-6 fatty acids contributes to low-grade body inflammation, a risk factor for heart disease, cancer, asthma, arthritis, and depression. They recommend a four-to-one ratio of omega-6 to omega-3 fatty acids to maintain and improve health. At present, however, there is no good evidence to substantiate this recommendation. The guideline to maintain healthy weight, a diet high in vegetable polyunsaturated fats, omega-3 fatty acids, slow-digesting carbohydrates (low-glycemic loads), antioxidant-rich foods, probiotic foods, and less animal saturated fat, trans fats, and reduced intake of red meat is the best advice to prevent low-grade body inflammation.

Most critical in the diet are omega-3 fatty acids, which provide substantial health benefits. Omega-3 fatty acids tend to decrease cholesterol, triglycerides, inflammation, blood clots, abnormal heart rhythms, and high blood pressure. They also decrease the risk for heart attack, abnormal heart rhythms, stroke, Alzheimer's disease, dementia, macular degeneration, and joint degeneration.

Unfortunately, only 25 percent of the U.S. population consumes the recommended amount (approximately 500 milligrams) of omega eicosapentaenoic acid (EPA) and docosahexaenoic acid (DHA) on any given day. These are two of the three major types of omega-3 fatty acids, along with alpha-linolenic acid (ALA). The evidence is strongest for EPA and DHA being cardioprotective. Once consumed, the body converts ALA to EPA and then to DHA, but the process is not efficient. It is best to increase consumption of EPA and DHA to obtain the greatest health benefit.

Individuals at risk for heart disease are encouraged to get an average of .5 to 1.8 grams (500 to 1,800 milligrams) of EPA and DHA per day.[5] These fatty acids protect against irregular heartbeats and blood clots, reduce triglycerides and blood pressure, and defend against inflammation.[6]

Fish—especially fresh or frozen salmon, mackerel, herring, tuna, and rainbow trout—are high in EPA and DHA. Table 3.2 lists total EPA plus DHA content of selected species of fish. Canned fish is best when packed in water. In oil-packed fish, the oil mixes with some of the natural fat in fish. When the oil is drained, some omega-3 fatty acids are lost as well. Good sources of omega-3 ALA include flaxseeds, canola oil, walnuts, wheat germ, and green leafy vegetables.

The oil in flaxseeds is high in ALA and has been shown to reduce abnormal heart rhythms and prevent blood clots. Flaxseeds are also high in fiber and plant chemicals known as lignans. Studies are being conducted to investigate the potential cancer-fighting ability of lignans. In one report, the addition of a daily ounce (three to four tablespoons) of ground flaxseeds to the diet seemed to lead to a decrease in the onset of tumors, preventing their formation and even leading to their shrinkage.[7] Excessive flaxseed in the diet is not recommended; high doses actually may be detrimental to health. Pregnant and lactating women, especially, should not consume large amounts of flaxseed.

Because flaxseeds have a hard outer shell, they should be ground to obtain the nutrients; whole seeds pass through the body undigested. Flavor and nutrients are best preserved by grinding the seeds just before use. Preground seeds should be kept sealed and refrigerated. Ground flaxseeds can be mixed with salad dressings, salads, wheat flour, pancakes, muffins, cereals, rice, cottage cheese, and yogurt. Flaxseed oil also may be used, but the oil has little or no fiber and lignans and must be kept refrigerated because it spoils quickly. The oil cannot be used for cooking either, because it scorches easily.

Most polyunsaturated fatty acid consumption in the United States comes from omega-6 fatty acids. Once viewed as healthy fats, excessive intake may be detrimental to health. Omega-6 fatty acids include linoleic acid (LA), gamma-linolenic acid (GLA), and arachidonic acid (AA). The typical American diet contains 10 to 20 times more omega-6 than omega-3 fatty acids. Most omega-6 fatty acids come in the form of LA from vegetable oils, the primary oil ingredient added to most processed foods, including salad dressing. LA-rich oils include corn, soybean, sunflower, safflower, and cottonseed oils.

Although more research is required, the imbalance between omega-3 and omega-6 fatty acids is thought to be responsible for the increased rate of inflammatory conditions

TABLE 3.2 Omega-3 Fatty Acid Content (EPA + DHA) per 100 Grams (3.5 oz) of Fish

Type of Fish	Total EPA + DHA (g)
Anchovy	1.4
Bluefish	1.2
Halibut	0.4
Herring	1.7
Mackerel	2.4
Sardine	1.4
Salmon, Atlantic	1.0
Salmon, Chinook	1.9
Salmon, Coho	1.2
Salmon, pink	1.0
Salmon, Sockeye	1.3
Shrimp	0.3
Trout, lake	1.6
Trout, rainbow	0.6
Tuna, light (water canned)	0.3
Tuna, white (Albacore)	0.8

seen in the United States today. Furthermore, in terms of heart health, while omega-6 fatty acids lower the "bad" LDL cholesterol, they also lower the "good" HDL cholesterol; thus, their overall effect on cardiac health is neutral. To decrease your intake of LA, watch for corn, soybean, sunflower, and cottonseed oils in salad dressings, mayonnaise, and margarine.

The best source of omega-3 EPA and DHA, the fatty acids that provide the most health benefits, is fish. Data suggest that the amount of fish oil obtained by eating two servings of fish weekly lessens the risk for CHD and may contribute to brain, joint, and vision health. A word of caution: People who have diabetes or a history of hemorrhaging or strokes, are on aspirin or blood-thinning therapy, or are presurgical patients should not consume fish oil except under a physician's instruction.

Omega-9 fatty acids are from a family of polyunsaturated fats generally found in vegetable oils (canola, olive, peanut, safflower, and sunflower oils), but they are also found in avocados, olives, and nuts (almonds, cashews, macadamias, peanuts, pecans, pistachios, and walnuts). These fatty acids are uniquely high in monounsaturated fat, low in saturated fat, and contain zero trans fat. Omega-9 fatty acids are protective against metabolic syndrome and cardiovascular disease as they have been shown to increase HDL cholesterol and decrease LDL cholesterol.

Compound Fats Compound fats are a combination of simple fats and other chemicals. Examples include the following:

1. Phospholipids, which are similar to triglycerides except that choline (or another compound) and phosphoric acid take the place of one of the fatty acid units
2. Glucolipids, a combination of carbohydrates, fatty acids, and nitrogen
3. Lipoproteins, water-soluble aggregates of protein and triglycerides, phospholipids, or cholesterol

Lipoproteins (a combination of lipids and proteins) are especially important because they transport fats in the blood. The major forms of lipoproteins are HDL, LDL, and very low-density lipoprotein (VLDL). Lipoproteins play a large role in developing or preventing heart disease. High HDL cholesterol levels have been associated with lower risk for CHD, whereas high levels of LDL cholesterol have been linked to increased risk. HDL is more than 50 percent protein and contains little cholesterol. LDL is approximately 25 percent protein and nearly 50 percent cholesterol. VLDL contains about 50 percent triglycerides, only about 10 percent protein, and 20 percent cholesterol.

Derived Fats Derived fats combine simple and compound fats. **Sterols** are an example. Although sterols contain no fatty acids, they are considered lipids because they do not dissolve in water. The sterol mentioned most often is cholesterol, which is found in many foods or can be manufactured in the body—primarily from saturated fats and trans fats.

In the 1980s and 1990s, people were concerned with overall fat intake. As a result, they cut back on fats and started to overconsume refined carbohydrates. Nowadays, people understand that healthy unsaturated fats and caloric balance are essential to good health. The latter is important because overconsumption of even healthy fats leads to weight gain. Keep in mind that as you add something healthy to your diet, you need to remove an equal amount of calories from a different food item, preferably a less healthy item.

Proteins

Proteins are the main substances the body uses to build and repair tissues such as muscles, blood, internal organs, skin, hair, nails, and bones. They form a part of hormone, antibody, and enzyme molecules. **Enzymes** play a key role in all of the body's processes. Because all enzymes are formed by proteins, this nutrient is necessary for normal functioning. Proteins also help maintain the normal balance of body fluids.

Proteins can be used as a source of energy too, but only if sufficient carbohydrates are not available. Each gram of protein yields four calories of energy (the same as carbohydrates). The main sources of protein are meats and meat alternatives, milk, and other dairy products. Excess proteins may be converted to glucose or fat or even excreted in the urine.

The human body uses 20 **amino acids** to form various types of protein. Amino acids contain nitrogen, carbon, hydrogen, and oxygen. Of the 20 amino acids, 9 are called essential amino acids because the body cannot produce them. The other 11, termed nonessential amino acids, can be manufactured in the body if food proteins in the diet provide enough nitrogen (see Table 3.3). For the body to function normally, all amino acids shown in Table 3.3 must be present in the diet.

Proteins that contain all the es-

Omega-6 fatty acids Polyunsaturated fatty acids found primarily in corn and sunflower oils and most oils in processed foods.

Lipoproteins Lipids covered by proteins, which transport fats in the blood. Types are LDL, HDL, and VLDL.

Sterols Derived fats, of which cholesterol is the best-known example.

Proteins A classification for nutrients consisting of complex organic compounds containing nitrogen and formed by combinations of amino acids; the main substances used in the body to build and repair tissues.

Enzymes Catalysts that facilitate chemical reactions in the body.

Amino acids Chemical compounds that contain nitrogen, carbon, hydrogen, and oxygen; the basic building blocks the body uses to build different types of protein.

TABLE 3.3 **Amino Acids**

Essential Amino Acids*	Nonessential Amino Acids
Histidine	Alanine
Isoleucine	Arginine
Leucine	Asparagine
Lysine	Aspartic acid
Methionine	Cysteine
Phenylalanine	Glutamic acid
Threonine	Glutamine
Tryptophan	Glycine
Valine	Proline
	Serine
	Tyrosine

*Must be provided in the diet because the body cannot manufacture them.

sential amino acids, known as "complete" or "higher-quality" proteins, are usually of animal origin. If one or more of the essential amino acids are missing, the proteins are termed incomplete or lower-quality protein. The essential amino acid that is missing in an incomplete protein is called the limiting amino acid. All plant products, including grains, fruits, vegetables, grains, beans, nuts, and seeds are incomplete proteins. The only exceptions of complete proteins found in plant products are soy and quinoa (a grain-like crop grown for its edible seed).

Individuals have to take in enough protein to ensure nitrogen for adequate production of all amino acids. On a vegetarian diet, consumption of a variety of food sources is required so that the diet supplies all the essential amino acids within a meal or a given day. When different foods are consumed, the limiting amino acid in one food can be obtained from another food source. This principle is referred to as complementing proteins (also see page 105). For example, consumption of grains and legumes complement each other. Legumes and nuts also complement each other. Nuts and grains, however, are not complementary proteins. Soy and quinoa can also be used to complement the limiting amino acids in grains, legumes, nuts, and seeds.

Protein deficiency is not a problem in the typical U.S. diet. Two glasses of skim milk combined with about four ounces of poultry or fish meet the daily protein requirement. But too much animal protein can cause health problems. Some people eat twice as much protein as they need. Protein foods from animal sources are often high in fat, saturated fat, and cholesterol, which can lead to cardiovascular disease and cancer.

Importance of Adequate Daily Protein Intake The role of protein in the American diet, nonetheless, is gaining relevance as *adequate protein intake with each meal* is crucial for satiety, weight management, and to help build, repair, and maintain lean tissue. The latter has even greater relevance for people who are physically active. Loss of lean tissue with sedentary living, aging, exhaustive exercise training, and while dieting (negative caloric balance) without proper energy and protein intake is inevitable. Loss of lean tissue is never desirable because of the decrease in functional physical capacity (the ability to perform ordinary and unusual tasks of daily living), as well as in the resting metabolic rate.

As an individual, you can prevent or even completely reverse such a loss. The recommendation is that we distribute our protein intake in equal parts throughout the day. To do so, determine your daily intake in grams (see Table 3.4) and divide by three (meals per day). For example, if you weigh 141 pounds (64 kg) and you are physically active, your total protein intake should be between 64 and 77 grams per day (64 × 1.0 and 64 × 1.2 or the equivalent of 256 to 308 calories derived from protein each day—each gram of protein supplies the body with 4 calories) or 21 to 26 grams of protein per meal.

Limiting Red Meat Consumption Several recent research articles provide strong evidence that excessive red meat consumption increases the risk of premature death, primarily from heart disease, stroke, some cancers, and type 2 diabetes. Both, unprocessed read meat (beef, pork, and lamb) and processed red meat (cold cuts, ham, bacon, bologna, sausage, hot dogs) consumption lead to this outcome.

Researchers believe that it is not just the saturated fat and cholesterol that are the culprits, but L-carnitine, a compound abundant in red meat, feed intestinal bacteria that turn it into trimethylamine-N-oxide (TMAO), a compound believed to cause atherosclerosis (obstruction of the arteries). Red-meat eaters also have a higher incidence of pancreatic, prostate, and esophageal cancers. Nitrites, chemical compounds used to cure (preserve) meats, are believed to increase the risk. Processed meats labeled as "no nitrite added," most likely are not nitrite free because nitrite and nitrate (which the body can convert to nitrite) occur naturally in meats.

Eating less red meat also protects the environment by requiring less cattle feed and water, decreasing the production of methane gas and solid waste by the animals, decreasing the requirement of nitrous oxide used in fertilizers to grow the feed, and leading to less deforestation to make pasture and farmland.

Table 3.4 **Recommended Daily Protein Intake**

Activity Level	Grams/kg of Body Weight
Sedentary	0.8 g/kg
Physically active	1.0–1.2 g/kg
Athlete	1.2–2.0 g/kg
Weight gain/loss	1.5–2.0 g/kg

SOURCE: Adapted from H. H. Fink, A. E. Mikesky, and L. A. Burgoon, *Practical Applications in Sports Nutrition.* (Sudbury, MA: Jones & Bartlet Learning, 2015).

The most compelling evidence comes from a 2012 study of more than 120,000 people at the Harvard School of Public Health showing a 30 percent increased risk of premature death among people who eat the most red meat as compared to those who eat the least (about a half a serving per day).[8] In the study, three ounces of unprocessed red meat were considered as one serving, but only one ounce of processed red meat was viewed as a serving. The mortality rate was highest among processed read meat eaters. Eating just one serving per day increased the risk between 13 percent (unprocessed) and 20 percent (processed).

The data also indicated that replacing one serving a day of red meat with fish, poultry, nuts, beans, low-fat dairy, or whole grains decreased the chances of premature death in the range of 7 percent to 19 percent. The researchers concluded that "*The message we want to communicate is it would be great if you could reduce your intake of red meat consumption to half a serving a day or two to three servings a week, and severely limit processed red meat intake.*"

A 2013 study involving almost a half a million people from 10 European countries found that individuals eating 5.7 ounces of processed meats (the equivalent of two daily sausages and a slice of bacon) had a 44 percent greater risk of dying during the 13-year study. One in every 17 people followed during this time died, and almost twice as many from cancer as from heart disease.[9] A subsequent study that included almost 150,000 health professionals found that people who increase red meat consumption by more than a half a serving per day, have a 48 percent greater risk of developing type 2 diabetes over the next four years.[10] In contrast, people who cut their daily intake in half had a 14 percent lower risk of type 2 diabetes.

As mentioned earlier, a well-balanced diet contains a variety of foods from all five basic food groups, including a wise selection of foods from animal sources (see also "Balancing the Diet" in this chapter). Based on current nutrition data, meat (poultry and fish included) should be replaced by grains, legumes, vegetables, and fruits as main courses. Meats should be used more for flavoring than for volume. Daily consumption of beef, poultry, or fish should be limited to three to six ounces (about the size of one to two decks of cards).

Vitamins

Vitamins are necessary for normal bodily metabolism, growth, and development. Vitamins are classified into two types based on their solubility:

1. Fat soluble (A, D, E, and K)
2. Water soluble (B complex and C)

The body does not manufacture most vitamins, so they can be obtained only through a well-balanced diet. To decrease loss of vitamins during cooking, natural foods should be microwaved or steamed rather than boiled in water that is thrown out later.

A few exceptions, such as vitamins A, D, and K, are formed in the body. Vitamin A is produced from beta-carotene, found mainly in yellow foods such as carrots, pumpkin, and sweet potatoes. Vitamin D is found in certain foods and is created when ultraviolet light from the sun transforms 7-dehydrocholesterol, a compound in human skin. Vitamin K is created in the body by intestinal bacteria. The major functions of vitamins are outlined in Table 3.5.

Vitamins C and E and beta-carotene also function as antioxidants, which are thought to play a key role in preventing chronic diseases. (The specific functions of these antioxidant nutrients and of the mineral selenium, also an antioxidant, are discussed under "Antioxidants," page 110.)

Minerals

Approximately 25 minerals have important roles in body functioning. **Minerals** are inorganic substances contained in all cells, especially those in hard parts of the body (bones, nails, and teeth). Minerals are crucial to maintaining water balance and the acid–base balance. They are essential components of respiratory pigments, enzymes, and enzyme systems, and they regulate muscular and nervous tissue impulses, blood clotting, and normal heart rhythm. The four minerals mentioned most often are calcium, iron, sodium, and selenium. Calcium deficiency may result in osteoporosis, and low iron intake can induce iron-deficiency anemia (see page 122). High sodium intake may contribute to high blood pressure. Selenium has been shown to prevent some tumors in laboratory animals, but its effect in humans has been disappointing. Specific functions of some of the most important minerals are given in Table 3.6.

Water

The most important nutrient is **water**, because it is involved in almost every vital body process: in digesting and absorbing food, in producing energy, in the circulatory process, in regulating body heat, in removing waste products, in building and rebuilding cells, and in transporting other nutrients. In men, about 61 percent of total body weight is water. The proportion of body weight in women is 56 percent (Figure 3.5). The difference is primarily because of the higher amount of muscle mass in men.

Almost all foods contain water, but it is found primarily in liquid foods, fruits, and vegetables. People obtain about 80 percent of the daily water needs from beverages and the remainder 20 percent from foods. Although for decades the

Vitamins Organic nutrients essential for normal metabolism, growth, and development of the body.

Minerals Inorganic nutrients essential for normal body functions and found in the body and in food.

Water The most important classification for essential body nutrients, involved in almost every vital body process.

TABLE 3.5 **Major Functions of Vitamins**

Nutrient	Good Sources	Major Functions	Deficiency Symptoms
Vitamin A	Milk, cheese, eggs, liver, yellow and dark-green fruits and vegetables	Required for healthy bones, teeth, skin, gums, and hair; maintenance of inner mucous membranes, thus increasing resistance to infection; adequate vision in dim light.	Night blindness; decreased growth; decreased resistance to infection; rough, dry skin
Vitamin D	Fortified milk, cod liver oil, salmon, tuna, egg yolk	Necessary for bones and teeth; needed for calcium and phosphorus absorption.	Rickets (bone softening), fractures, muscle spasms
Vitamin E	Vegetable oils, yellow and green leafy vegetables, margarine, wheat germ, whole-grain breads and cereals	Related to oxidation and normal muscle and red blood cell chemistry.	Leg cramps, red blood cell breakdown
Vitamin K	Green leafy vegetables, cauliflower, cabbage, eggs, peas, potatoes	Essential for normal blood clotting.	Hemorrhaging
Vitamin B_1 (Thiamin)	Whole-grain or enriched bread, lean meats and poultry, fish, liver, pork, poultry, organ meats, legumes, nuts, dried yeast	Assists in proper use of carbohydrates, normal functioning of nervous system, maintenance of good appetite.	Loss of appetite, nausea, confusion, cardiac abnormalities, muscle spasms
Vitamin B_2 (Riboflavin)	Eggs, milk, leafy green vegetables, whole grains, lean meats, dried beans and peas	Contributes to energy release from carbohydrates, fats, and proteins; needed for normal growth and development, good vision, and healthy skin.	Cracking of the corners of the mouth, inflammation of the skin, impaired vision
Vitamin B_6 (Pyridoxine)	Vegetables, meats, whole-grain cereals, soybeans, peanuts, potatoes	Necessary for protein and fatty acids metabolism and for normal red blood cell formation.	Depression, irritability, muscle spasms, nausea
Vitamin B_{12}	Meat, poultry, fish, liver, organ meats, eggs, shellfish, milk, cheese	Required for normal growth, red blood cell formation, nervous system and digestive tract functioning.	Impaired balance, weakness, drop in red blood cell count
Niacin	Liver and organ meats, meat, fish, poultry, whole grains, enriched breads, nuts, green leafy vegetables, dried beans and peas	Contributes to energy release from carbohydrates, fats, and proteins; normal growth and development; and formation of hormones and nerve-regulating substances.	Confusion, depression, weakness, weight loss
Biotin	Liver, kidney, eggs, yeast, legumes, milk, nuts, dark-green vegetables	Essential for carbohydrate metabolism and fatty acid synthesis.	Inflamed skin, muscle pain, depression, weight loss
Folic Acid	Leafy green vegetables, organ meats, whole grains and cereals, dried beans	Needed for cell growth and reproduction and for red blood cell formation.	Decreased resistance to infection
Pantothenic Acid	All natural foods, especially liver, kidney, eggs, nuts, yeast, milk, dried peas and beans, green leafy vegetables	Related to carbohydrate and fat metabolism.	Depression, low blood sugar, leg cramps, nausea, headaches
Vitamin C (Ascorbic acid)	Fruits, vegetables	Helps protect against infection; required for formation of collagenous tissue, normal blood vessels, teeth, and bones.	Slow-healing wounds; loose teeth; hemorrhaging; rough, scaly skin; irritability

recommendation was to consume at least eight cups of water per day, a panel of scientists at the Institute of Medicine of the National Academy of Sciences (NAS) indicated that people are getting enough water from the liquids (milk, juices, sodas, and coffee) and the moisture content of solid foods. Most Americans and Canadians remain well hydrated simply by using thirst as their guide. Caffeine-containing drinks also are acceptable as a water source, because data indicate that people who regularly consume such beverages do not have more 24-hour urine output than those who don't.

An exception to not waiting for the thirst signal to replenish water loss is when an individual exercises in the heat or does so for an extended time (see Chapter 9, pages 356–358). Water lost under these conditions must be replenished regularly. If you wait for the thirst signal, you may have lost too much water already. At 2 percent of body weight lost, a person is dehydrated. At 5 percent, the person may become dizzy and disoriented, have trouble with cognitive skills and heart function, and even lose consciousness.

Balancing the Diet

One of the fundamental ways to enjoy good health and live life to its fullest is through a well-balanced diet. Several guidelines have been published to help you accomplish this. As illustrated in Table 3.7, the most recent recommended guidelines by the NAS state that daily caloric intake should be distributed so that 45 to 65 percent of total calories come from carbohydrates (mostly complex carbohydrates and less than 25 percent from sugar), 20 to 35 percent (for certain individuals) from fat, and 10 to 35 percent from protein.[11] The recommended ranges allow for flexibility in planning diets according to individual health and physical activity needs.

In addition to the macronutrients, the diet must include all essential vitamins, minerals, and water. The source of fat calories is also critical. The National Cholesterol Education Program recommends that of total calories, saturated fat should constitute less than 7 percent, polyunsaturated fat up to 10 percent, and monounsaturated fat up to 20 percent. Rating a particular diet accurately is difficult without a complete nutrient analysis. You have an opportunity to perform this analysis in Lab 3A.

The NAS guidelines vary slightly from those previously issued by major national health organizations, which recommend 50 to 60 percent of total calories from carbohydrates, less than 30 percent from fat, and about 15 percent from protein. These percentages are within the ranges recommended by the NAS. The most drastic difference appears in the NAS allowed range of fat intake: up to 35 percent of total calories. This higher percentage, however, was included to accommodate individuals with metabolic syndrome (see Chapter 11, page 443), who have an abnormal insulin re-

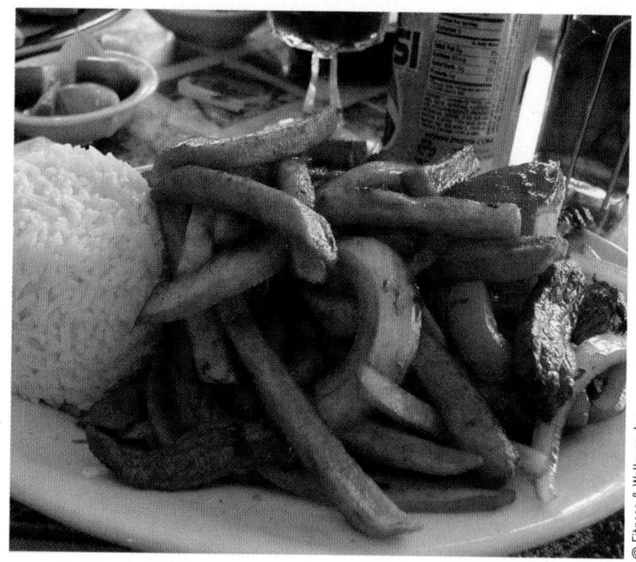

The typical American diet is too high in calories and saturated fat.

TABLE 3.6 **Major Functions of Minerals**

Nutrient	Good Sources	Major Functions	Deficiency Symptoms
Calcium	Milk, yogurt, cheese, green leafy vegetables, dried beans, sardines, salmon	Required for strong teeth and bone formation and maintenance of good muscle tone, heartbeat, and nerve function.	Bone pain and fractures, periodontal disease, muscle cramps
Copper	Seafood, meats, beans, nuts, whole grains	Helps with iron absorption and hemoglobin formation; required to synthesize the enzyme cytochrome oxidase.	Anemia (although deficiency is rare in humans)
Iron	Organ meats, lean meats, seafood, eggs, dried peas and beans, nuts, whole and enriched grains, green leafy vegetables	Major component of hemoglobin; aids in energy utilization.	Nutritional anemia, overall weakness
Phosphorus	Meats, fish, milk, eggs, dried beans and peas, whole grains, processed foods	Required for bone and teeth formation and for energy release regulation.	Bone pain and fracture, weight loss, weakness
Zinc	Milk, meat, seafood, whole grains, nuts, eggs, dried beans	Essential component of hormones, insulin, and enzymes; used in normal growth and development.	Loss of appetite, slow-healing wounds, skin problems
Magnesium	Green leafy vegetables, whole grains, nuts, soybeans, seafood, legumes	Needed for bone growth and maintenance, carbohydrate and protein utilization, nerve function, temperature regulation.	Irregular heartbeat, weakness, muscle spasms, sleeplessness
Sodium	Table salt, processed foods, meat	Needed for body fluid regulation, transmission of nerve impulses, heart action.	Rarely seen
Potassium	Legumes, whole grains, bananas, orange juice, dried fruits, potatoes	Required for heart action, bone formation and maintenance, regulation of energy release, acid–base regulation.	Irregular heartbeat, nausea, weakness
Selenium	Seafood, meat, whole grains	Component of enzymes; functions in close association with vitamin E.	Muscle pain, possible heart muscle deterioration, possible hair loss and nail loss

FIGURE 3.5 Approximate proportions of nutrients in the human body.

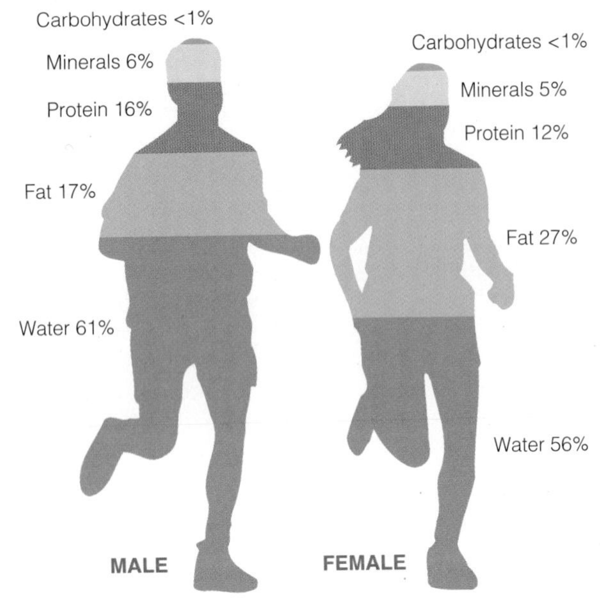

TABLE 3.7 The American Diet: Current and Recommended Carbohydrate, Fat, and Protein Intake Expressed as a Percentage of Total Calories

	Current Percentage	Recommended Percentage*
Carbohydrates	50	45–65
Simple	26	<25
Complex	24	20–40
Fat	34	20–30**
Monounsaturated	11	≤20
Polyunsaturated	10	≤10
Saturated	13	<7
Protein	16	10–35

*Adapted from the 2002 recommended guidelines by the National Academy of Sciences.
**Less than 30% is recommended by most major national health organizations. Up to 35% is allowed for individuals with metabolic syndrome who may need additional fat in the diet.

sponse to carbohydrates and may need additional fat in the diet.

The NAS recommendations are effective only if people consistently replace saturated and trans-fatty acids with unsaturated fatty acids. This requires changes in the typical "unhealthy" American diet, which is generally high in red meats, whole-milk dairy products, and fast foods—all of which are high in saturated fats, trans-fatty acids, or both.

Diets in most developed countries changed significantly in the 20th century. Today, we eat more calories and unhealthy fats, fewer complex carbohydrates, and about the same amount of protein. Furthermore, Americans eat too much junk, processed, and refined foods. And as a group we weigh more than we did in 1900, an indication that we are eating more calories and are not as physically active as our forebearers.

Surveys indicate that on average people now eat out one meal per day compared to only two per week in the 1970s. Not only do Americans eat more when they eat out, but they also eat far fewer healthy foods than at home. Among the most popular foods ordered at restaurants and fast-food places today are French fries, hamburgers, and pizza. About one-fifth of all restaurant meals are purchased at drive-throughs, with almost one-half of young people and a third of baby boomers indicating that they eat full meals in the car. In contrast, whenever possible, healthy eating implies consuming primarily whole, fresh, or locally grown food items made with few ingredients and minimal processing and packaging.

Nutrition Standards

Nutritionists use a variety of nutrient standards, the most widely known of which is **Recommended Dietary Allowance (RDA)**. Others are the **Dietary Reference Intakes (DRIs)** and the **Daily Values (DVs)** on food labels. Each standard has a different purpose and utilization in dietary planning and assessment.

Dietary Reference Intakes To help people meet dietary guidelines, the NAS developed the DRIs for healthy people in the United States and Canada. The DRIs are based on a review of the most current research on nutrient needs of healthy people. The DRI reports are written by the Food and Nutrition Board of the NAS in cooperation with scientists from Canada.

The DRIs encompass four types of reference values, including the RDA, for planning and assessing diets and for establishing adequate amounts and maximum safe nutrient intakes in the diet. The other three reference values are the **Estimated Average Requirement (EAR)**, **Adequate Intake (AI)**, and **Tolerable Upper Intake Level (UL)**. The type of reference value used for a given nutrient and a specific age and gender group is determined according to available scientific information and the intended use of the dietary standard.

Nutrients for which a daily DRI has been set are given in Table 3.8.

Estimated Average Requirement

The EAR is the amount of a nutrient that is estimated to meet the nutrient requirement of half the healthy people in specific age and gender groups. At this nutrient intake level, the nutritional requirements of 50 percent of the people are not met. For example, looking at 300 healthy women at age 26, the EAR would meet the nutritional requirement for only half of these women.

Recommended Dietary Allowance

The RDA is the daily amount of a nutrient that is considered adequate to meet the known nutrient needs of nearly all healthy people in the United States. RDAs of nutrients are determined by a committee of the Food and Nutrition Board of the NAS. Because the committee must decide what level of intake to recommend for everybody, the RDA is set

Table 3.8 Dietary Reference Intakes (DRIs): Recommended Dietary Allowances (RDA) and Adequate Intakes (AI) for Selected Nutrients

	Recommended Dietary Allowances (RDA)															Adequate Intakes (AI)			
	Thiamin (mg)	Riboflavin (mg)	Niacin (mg NE)	Vitamin B_6 (mg)	Folate (μg)	Vitamin B_{12} (μg)	Phosphorus (mg)	Magnesium (mg)	Vitamin A (μg)	Vitamin C (mg)	Vitamin D (μg)	Vitamin E (mg)	Selenium (mcg)	Iron (mg)	Calcium (mg)	Fluoride (mg)	Panthothenic acid (mg)	Biotin (mg)	Choline (mg)
Males																			
14–18	1.2	1.3	16	1.3	400	2.4	1,250	410	900	75	15	15	55	11	1,300	3	5.0	25	550
19–30	1.2	1.3	16	1.3	400	2.4	700	400	900	90	15	15	55	8	1,000	4	5.0	30	550
31–50	1.2	1.3	16	1.3	400	2.4	700	420	900	90	15	15	55	8	1,000	4	5.0	30	550
51–70	1.2	1.3	16	1.7	400	2.4	700	420	900	90	15	15	55	8	1,000	4	5.0	30	550
>70	1.2	1.3	16	1.7	400	2.4	700	420	900	90	20	15	55	8	1,200	4	5.0	30	550
Females																			
14–18	1.0	1.0	14	1.2	400	2.4	1,250	360	700	65	15	15	55	15	1,300	3	5.0	25	400
19–30	1.1	1.1	14	1.3	400	2.4	700	310	700	75	15	15	55	18	1,000	3	5.0	30	425
31–50	1.1	1.1	14	1.3	400	2.4	700	320	700	75	15	15	55	18	1,000	3	5.0	30	425
51–70	1.1	1.1	14	1.5	400	2.4	700	320	700	75	15	15	55	8	1,200	3	5.0	30	425
>70	1.1	1.1	14	1.5	400	2.4	700	320	700	75	20	15	55	8	1,200	3	5.0	30	425
Pregnant (19–30)	1.4	1.4	18	1.9	600	2.6	*	+40	770	85	15	15	60	27	1,000	3	6.0	30	450
Lactating (19–30)	1.4	1.6	17	2.0	500	2.8	*	*	1,300	120	15	19	70	9	1,000	3	7.0	35	550

*Values for these nutrients do not change with pregnancy or lactation. Use the value listed for women of comparable age.

SOURCE: Reprinted with permission from "Dietary Reference Intakes: Recommended Dietary Allowances and Adequate Intakes, Elements," and "Dietary Reference Intakes for Calcium and Vitamin D," 2011 by the National Academy of Sciences, Courtesy of the National Academics Press, Washington D.C.

well above the EAR and covers about 98 percent of the population. Stated another way, the RDA for any nutrient is well above almost everyone's actual requirement. The RDA could be considered a goal for adequate intake. The process for determining the RDA depends on being able to set an EAR, because RDAs are determined statistically from the EAR values. If an EAR cannot be set, no RDA can be established.

Adequate Intake

When data are insufficient or inadequate to set an EAR, an AI value is determined instead of the RDA. The AI value is derived from approximations of observed nutrient intakes by a group or groups of healthy people. The AI value for children and adults is expected to meet or exceed the nutritional requirements of a corresponding healthy population.

CRITICAL THINKING

What do the nutrition standards mean to you? How much of a challenge would it be to apply those standards in your daily life?

Recommended Dietary Allowance (RDA) The daily amount of a nutrient (statistically determined from the EAR) that is considered adequate to meet the known nutrient needs of almost 98 percent of all healthy people in the United States.

Dietary Reference Intakes (DRIs) A general term that describes four types of nutrient standards that establish adequate amounts and maximum safe nutrient intakes in the diet: EAR, RDA, AI, and UL.

Daily Values (DVs) Reference values for nutrients and food components used in food labels.

Estimated Average Requirement (EAR) The amount of a nutrient that meets the dietary needs of half the people in a specific age and gender group.

Adequate Intake (AI) The recommended amount of a nutrient intake when sufficient evidence is not available to calculate the EAR and subsequent RDA.

Tolerable Upper Intake Level (UL) The highest level of nutrient intake that seems safe for most healthy people, beyond which exists an increased risk of adverse effects.

Tolerable Upper Intake Level

The UL establishes the highest level of nutrient intake that seems to be safe for most healthy people, beyond which exists an increased risk for adverse effects. As intakes increase above the UL, so does the risk for adverse effects. Established UL values are presented in Table 3.9.

Daily Values The DVs are reference values for nutrients and food components listed on food-packaging labels. The DVs include measures of fat, saturated fat, and carbohydrates (as a percentage of total calories); cholesterol, sodium, and potassium (in milligrams); and fiber and protein (in grams). The DVs for total fat, saturated fat, and carbohydrates are expressed as percentages for a 2,000-calorie diet and therefore may require adjustments depending on an individual's daily **estimated energy requirement (EER)** in calories. For example, for a 2,000-calorie diet (the EER), the recommended carbohydrate intake is about 300 grams (about 60 percent of the EER), and the recommendation for fat is 65 grams (about 30 percent of the EER). The vitamin, mineral, and protein DVs were adapted from the RDA. The DVs are not as specific for age and gender groups as the DRIs. Both the DRIs and the DVs apply only to healthy adults. They are not intended for people who are ill, because these individuals may require additional nutrients. Figure 3.6 shows a food label with U.S. recommended DVs.

In early 2014, the FDA proposed the first major food label change since 1994. The proposed revision includes a major update to present caloric value per serving bigger and bolder and make the serving size more realistic to reflect the amount people typically eat. These changes are proposed to emphasize the need for adequate daily caloric balance. Added sugar information, along with DV information for sodium, potassium fiber, and vitamin D are also recommended. The listing of calories from fat on the label is to be removed because the emphasis needs to be on the type of fat consumed (unsaturated) rather than the total amount itself.

Nutrient Analysis

The first step in evaluating your diet is to conduct a nutrient analysis. This can be quite educational, because most people do not realize how harmful and non-nutritious many common foods are.

The top sources of calories in the American diet are soft drinks, sweet rolls, pastries, doughnuts, cakes, hamburgers, cheeseburgers, meatloaf, pizza,

Estimated Energy Requirement (EER) The average dietary energy (caloric) intake that is predicted to maintain energy balance in a healthy adult of defined age, gender, weight, height, and level of physical activity, consistent with good health.

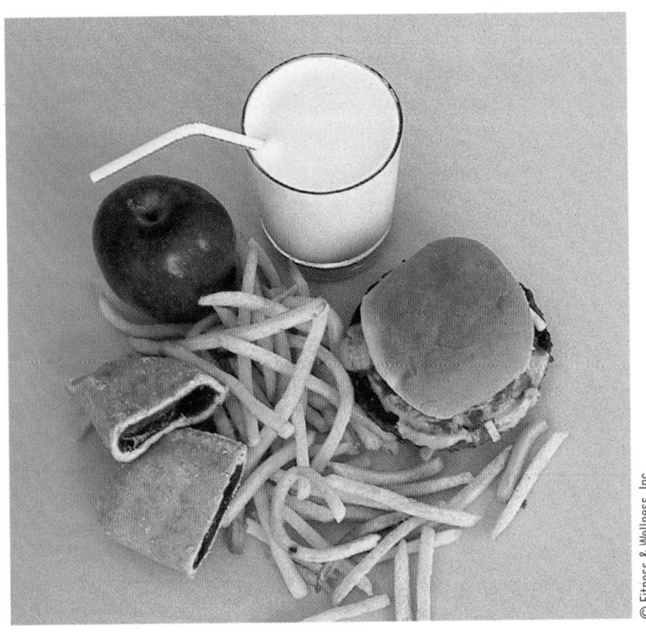

An apple a day will not keep the doctor away if most meals come from processed foods and are high in saturated fat and trans fat content.

TABLE 3.9 Tolerable Upper Intake Levels (ULs) of Selected Nutrients for Adults (19–70 years)

Nutrient	UL per Day	Nutrient	UL per Day
Calcium	2.5 g	Vitamin B_6	100 mg
Phosphorus	4.0 g*	Folate	1,000 mcg
Magnesium	350 mg	Choline	3.5 g
Vitamin D	100 mcg	Vitamin A	3,000 mcg
Fluoride	10 mg	Vitamin C	2,000 mg
Niacin	35 mg	Vitamin E	1,000 mg
Iron	45 mg	Selenium	400 mcg

*3.5 g per day for pregnant women.

FIGURE 3.6 Food label with U.S. recommended Daily Values.

1 Better by Design
to recognize the new food labels

The new food labels feature a revamped nutrition panel titled "Nutrition Facts," with nutrient listings that reflect current health concerns. Now you'll be able to find information on fat, fiber, and other food components fundamental to lowering your risk of cancer and other chronic diseases. Listings for nutrients like thiamin and riboflavin will no longer be required, because Americans generally eat enough of them these days.

2 Size Up the Situation
All serving sizes are created equal

Now you can compare similar products and know that their serving sizes are basically identical. So when you realize how much fat is packed into that carton of double-dutch-chocolate-caramel-chew ice cream you're eyeing, you might opt for low-fat frozen yogurt instead. Serving sizes will also be standardized, so manufacturers can't make nutrition claims for unrealistically small portions. That means a chocolate cake, for example, must be divided into 8 servings sized to satisfy the average person—not 16 servings sized to satisfy the average munchkin.

3 Look Before You Leap
Use the Daily Values

You will find the Daily Values on the bottom half of the "Nutrition Facts" panel. Some represent maximum levels of nutrients that should be consumed each day for a healthful diet (as with fat) while others refer to minimum levels that can be exceeded (as with carbohydrates). They are based on both a 2,000 and 2,500 calorie diet. Your own needs may be more or less, but these figures give you a point from which to compare. For example, the sample label indicates that someone with a 2,000 calorie diet should eat no more than 65 grams of fat per day. This is based on a diet getting 30 percent of calories as fat. If you normally eat fewer calories, or want to eat less than 30 percent of calories as fat, your daily fat consumption will be lower.

4 Rate It Right
Scan the % Daily Values

The % Daily Values make judging the nutritional quality of a food a snap. For instance, you can look at the % Daily Value column and find that a food has 25 percent of the Daily Value for fiber. This means the product will give you a substantial portion of the recommended amount of fiber for the day. You can also use this column to compare nutrients in similar products. The % Daily Values are based on a 2,000 calorie diet.

5 Trust Adjectives
Descriptors have legal definitions

Terms like "low," "high," and "free" have long been used on food labels. What these words actually mean, however, could vary. Thanks to the new labeling laws, such descriptions must now meet legal definitions. For example, you may be shopping for foods high in vitamin A, which has been linked to lower risk of certain cancers. Under the new label laws, a food described as "high" in a particular nutrient must contain 20 percent or more of the Daily Value for that nutrient. So if the bottle of juice you're thinking of buying says "high in vitamin A," you can now feel confident that it really is a good source of the vitamin.

6 Read Health Claims with Confidence
The nutrient link to disease prevention

You can also expect to see food packages with health claims linking certain nutrients to reduced risk of cancer and other diseases. The federal government has approved three health claims dealing with cancer prevention: a low-fat diet may reduce your risk for cancer; high fiber foods may reduce your risk for cancer; and fruits and vegetables may reduce your risk for cancer. A food may not make such a health claim for one nutrient if it contains other nutrients that undermine its health benefits. A high fiber, but high fat, jelly doughnut cannot carry a health claim!

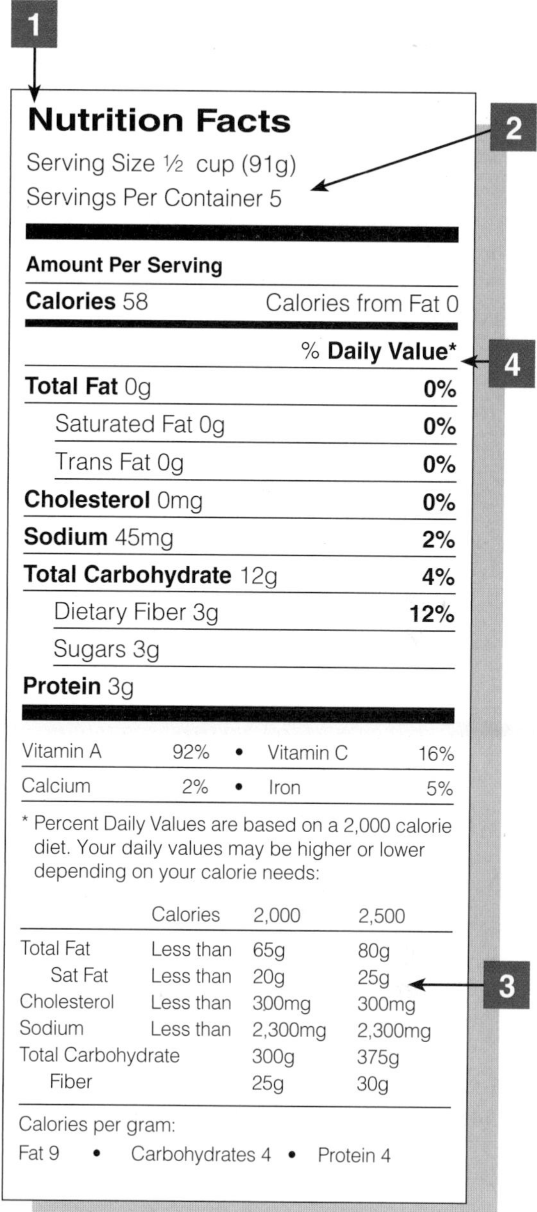

1
Nutrition Facts
Serving Size ½ cup (91g)
Servings Per Container 5
2
Amount Per Serving
Calories 58 Calories from Fat 0
% Daily Value*
4
Total Fat 0g 0%
Saturated Fat 0g 0%
Trans Fat 0g 0%
Cholesterol 0mg 0%
Sodium 45mg 2%
Total Carbohydrate 12g 4%
Dietary Fiber 3g 12%
Sugars 3g
Protein 3g
Vitamin A 92% • Vitamin C 16%
Calcium 2% • Iron 5%
* Percent Daily Values are based on a 2,000 calorie diet. Your daily values may be higher or lower depending on your calorie needs:
Calories 2,000 2,500
Total Fat Less than 65g 80g
Sat Fat Less than 20g 25g
Cholesterol Less than 300mg 300mg
Sodium Less than 2,300mg 2,300mg
Total Carbohydrate 300g 375g
Fiber 25g 30g
3
Calories per gram:
Fat 9 • Carbohydrates 4 • Protein 4

Many factors affect cancer risk. Eating a diet low in fat and high in fiber may lower risk of this disease. 6

- GOOD SOURCE OF FIBER
- LOWFAT 5

Reprinted with permission from the American Institute for Cancer Research.

potato and corn chips, and buttered popcorn, all of which are low in essential nutrients and high in unhealthy fats, sugar, and calories, or all three.

Most nutrient analyses cover calories, carbohydrates, fats, cholesterol, and sodium, as well as eight essential nutrients: protein, calcium, iron, vitamin A, thiamin, riboflavin, niacin, and vitamin C. If the diet has enough of these eight nutrients, the foods consumed in natural form to provide these nutrients typically contain all other nutrients the human body needs.

To do your own nutrient analysis, keep a three-day record of everything you eat using Figure 3A.1 in Lab 3A (make additional copies of this form as needed). At the end of each day, look up the nutrient content for those foods in the "Nutritive Value of Selected Foods" list (Appendix A). Record this information on the form in Lab 3A. If you do not find a food in Appendix A, the information may be on the food container.

When you have recorded the nutritive values for each day, add up each column and write the totals at the bottom of the chart. After the third day, fill in your totals in Figure 3A.2 in Lab 3A and compute an average for the three days. To rate your diet, compare your figures with those in the RDA (Table 3.8). The results will give a good indication of areas of strength and deficiency in your current diet.

Some of the most revealing information learned in a nutrient analysis is the source of fat and saturated fat intake in the diet. The average daily fat consumption in the U.S. diet is about 34 percent of total caloric intake, much of it from saturated fats, which increases the risk for chronic diseases such as cardiovascular disease, cancer, diabetes, and obesity. Although fat provides a smaller percentage of total daily caloric intake compared with two decades ago (37 percent), the decrease in percentage is simply because Americans now eat more calories than 20 years ago (335 additional daily calories for women and 170 for men).

As illustrated in Figure 3.7, one gram of carbohydrates or protein supplies the body with four calories, and fat provides nine calories per gram consumed (alcohol yields seven

Behavior Modification Planning

Caloric and Fat Content of Selected Fast Food Items

	Calories	Total Fat (grams)	Saturated Fat (grams)	Percent Fat Calories
Burgers				
McDonald's Big Mac	590	34	11	52
McDonald's Big N' Tasty with Cheese	590	37	12	56
McDonald's Quarter Pounder with Cheese	530	30	13	51
Burger King Whopper	760	46	15	54
Burger King Bacon Double Cheeseburger	580	34	18	53
Burger King BK Smokehouse Cheddar Griller	720	48	19	60
Burger King Whopper with Cheese	850	53	22	56
Burger King Double Whopper	1,060	69	27	59
Burger King Double Whopper with Cheese	1,150	76	33	59
Wendy's Baconator	830	51	22	55
Sandwiches				
Arby's Regular Roast Beef	350	16	6	41
Arby's Super Roast Beef	470	23	7	44
Arby's Roast Chicken Club	520	28	7	48
Arby's Market Fresh Roast Beef & Swiss	810	42	13	47
McDonald's Crispy Chicken	430	21	8	43
McDonald's Filet-O-Fish	470	26	5	50
McDonald's Chicken McGrill	400	17	3	38
Wendy's Chicken Club	470	19	4	36
Wendy's Breast Fillet	430	16	3	34
Wendy's Grilled Chicken	300	7	2	21
Burger King Specialty Chicken	560	28	6	45
Subway Veggie Delight*	226	3	1	12
Subway Turkey Breast	281	5	2	16
Subway Sweet Onion Chicken Teriyaki	374	5	2	12
Subway Steak & Cheese	390	14	5	32
Subway Cold Cut Trio	440	21	7	43
Subway Tuna	450	22	6	44
Mexican				
Taco Bell Crunchy Taco	170	10	4	53
Taco Bell Taco Supreme	220	14	6	57
Taco Bell Soft Chicken Taco	190	7	3	33

Behavior Modification Planning

Taco Bell Bean Burrito	370	12	4	29
Taco Bell Fiesta Steak Burrito	370	12	4	29
Taco Bell Grilled Steak Soft Taco	290	17	4	53
Taco Bell Double Decker Taco	340	14	5	37
French Fries				
Wendy's, biggie (5½ oz)	440	19	7	39
McDonald's, large (6 oz)	540	26	9	43
Burger King, large (5½ oz)	500	25	13	45
Shakes				
Wendy's Frosty, medium (16 oz)	440	11	7	23
McDonald's McFlurry, small (12 oz)	610	22	14	32
Burger King, Old Fashioned Ice Cream Shake, medium (22 oz)	760	41	29	49
Hash Browns				
McDonald's Hash Browns (2 oz)	130	8	4	55
Burger King, Hash Browns, small (2½ oz)	230	15	9	59

*6-inch sandwich with no mayo

Try It

Using the information in the table, record in your Online Journal or class notebook ways you can restructure fast-food consumption to decrease caloric value and fat and saturated fat content in your diet.

SOURCE: Adapted from *Restaurant Confidential 2002 by the Center for Science in the Public Interest.*

calories per gram). Therefore, looking at only the total grams consumed for each type of food can be misleading.

For example, a person who eats 160 grams of carbohydrates, 100 grams of fat, and 70 grams of protein has a total intake of 330 grams of food. This indicates that 30 percent of the total grams of food are in the form of fat (100 grams of fat ÷ 330 grams of total food = .30; .30 × 100 = 30 percent)—and in reality, almost half of that diet is in the form of fat calories.

In the sample diet, 640 calories are derived from carbohydrates (160 grams × 4 calories per gram), 280 calories from protein (70 grams × 4 calories per gram), and 900 calories from fat (100 grams × 9 calories per gram), for a total of 1,820 calories. If 900 calories are derived from fat, almost half of the total caloric intake is in the form of fat (900 ÷ 1,820 × 100 = 49.5 percent).

Each gram of fat provides 9 calories—more than twice the calories of a gram of carbohydrate or protein. When figuring out the percentage of fat calories of individual foods, you may find Figure 3.8 to be a useful guideline. Multiply the total fat grams by 9, and divide by the total calories in that particular food (per serving). Then multiply that number by 100 to get the percentage. For example, the food label in Figure 3.8 lists a total of 120 calories and five grams of fat, and the equation below it shows the fat content to be 38 percent of total calories. This simple guideline can help you decrease the fat in your diet.

The fat content of selected foods, given in grams and as a percentage of total calories, is presented in Figure 3.9. The percentage of fat is further subdivided into saturated, monounsaturated, polyunsaturated, and other fatty acids.

FIGURE 3.7 **Caloric value of food (fuel nutrients).**

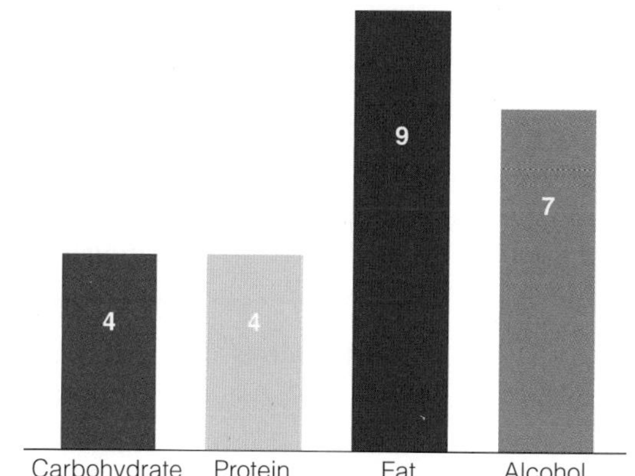

Achieving a Balanced Diet

Anyone who has completed a nutrient analysis and has given careful attention to Tables 3.3 (vitamins) and 3.4 (minerals) probably realizes that a well-balanced diet entails eating a variety of nutrient-dense foods and monitoring total daily caloric intake. The MyPlate healthy food plan in Figure 3.1 (page 82) contains five major food groups. The food groups are vegetables, fruits, grains, protein, and dairy. A Healthy Eating Plate, based on the MyPlate guidelines, was subsequently developed by the Harvard School of

FIGURE 3.8 Computation for fat content in food.

Nutrition Facts
Serving Size 1 cup (240 ml)
Servings Per Container 4

Amount Per Serving	
Calories 120	Calories from Fat 45
	% **Daily Value***
Total Fat 5g	8%
Saturated Fat 3g	15%
Trans Fat 0g	0%
Cholesterol 20mg	7%
Sodium 120mg	5%
Total Carbohydrate 12g	4%
Dietary Fiber 0g	0%
Sugars 12g	
Protein 8g	

Vitamin A 10%	Vitamin C 4%
Calcium 30%	Iron 0%

* Percent Daily Values are based on a 2,000 calorie diet. Your daily values may be higher or lower depending on your calorie needs:

	Calories	2,000	2,500
Total Fat	Less than	65g	80g
Sat Fat	Less than	20g	25g
Cholesterol	Less than	300mg	300mg
Sodium	Less than	2,300mg	2,300mg
Total Carbohydrate		300g	375g
Fiber		25g	30g

Calories per gram:
Fat 9 • Carbohydrate 4 • Protein 4

Percent fat calories = (grams of fat × 9) ÷ calories per serving × 100

5 grams of fat × 9 calories per grams of fat = 45 calories from fat

45 calories from fat ÷ 120 calories per serving × 100 = 38% fat

Public Health to offer specific recommendations for healthier food choices within the various food groups (Figure 3.10).

For most meals, three quarters of the plate should be taken up by fruits, vegetables, and grains, as they provide the nutritional base for a healthy diet. When increasing the intake of these food groups, it is important to decrease the intake of low-nutrient foods to effectively balance caloric intake with energy needs.

In addition to providing nutrients crucial to health, fruits and vegetables are the sole source of **phytonutrients** ("phyto" comes from the Greek word for plant). These compounds show promising results in the fight against cancer and heart disease. More than 4,000 phytonutrients have been identified. The main function of phytonutrients in plants is to protect them from sunlight. In humans, phytonutrients seem to have a powerful ability to block the formation of cancerous tumors. Their actions are so diverse that at almost every stage of cancer, phytonutrients have the ability to block, disrupt, slow, or even reverse the process. In terms of heart disease, they may reduce inflammation, inhibit blood clots, or prevent the oxidation of LDL cholesterol.

The consistent message is to eat a diet with ample fruits and vegetables. The daily recommended amount of fruits and vegetables has absolutely no substitute. A large number of scientific studies has linked fruit and vegetable consumption with many health benefits, including a substantial decrease in the risk for cardiovascular disease, cancer, diabetes mellitus, obesity, high blood pressure, metabolic syndrome, osteoporosis, and cognitive function among many others. And research states that, on average, people who consume five servings per day live three years longer than people who seldom or never eat fruits and vegetables. Science has not yet found a way to allow people to eat a poor diet, pop a few pills, and derive the same benefits.

Whole grains are a major source of fiber, as well as of other nutrients. Whole grains contain the entire grain kernel (the bran, germ, and endosperm). Examples include whole-wheat flour, whole cornmeal, oatmeal, cracked wheat (bulgur), and brown rice. Refined grains have been milled—a process that removes the bran and germ. The process also removes fiber, iron, and many B vitamins. Refined grains include white flour, white bread, white rice, and degermed cornmeal. Refined grains are often enriched to add back B vitamins and iron. Fiber, however, is not added back.

Milk and milk products (select low-fat or nonfat) can decrease the risk of low bone mass (osteoporosis) throughout life. Besides calcium, other nutrients from milk are potassium, vitamin D, and protein.

Foods in the protein group consist of poultry, fish, eggs, nuts, legumes, and seeds. Nutrients in this group include protein, B vitamins, vitamin E, iron, zinc, and magnesium. Choose low-fat or lean meats and poultry, and bake, grill, or broil them at low temperature (to prevent the formation of advanced glycation end products; see page 106). Most Americans eat sufficient food in this group but need to choose leaner foods and a greater variety of fish, dry beans, nuts, and seeds. In terms of meat, poultry, and fish, the recommendation is to consume about three ounces and not to exceed six ounces daily. All visible fat and skin should be trimmed off meats and poultry before cooking.

Oils are fats that come from different plants and fish and are liquid at room temperature. Choose carefully and avoid oils that have trans or saturated fats (check the food label). Solid fats at room temperature come from animal sources or can be made from vegetable oils through the process of hydrogenation (trans fats).

As an aid to balancing your diet, the form in Figure 3B.1 in Lab

Phytonutrients Compounds thought to prevent and fight cancer and found in large quantities in fruits and vegetables.

FIGURE 3.9 Fat content of selected foods.

Food	Calories	Total fat (grams)	% fat calories
Avocado/Florida (1)	340	27	71.5
Bacon (3 pieces)	109	9	74.3
Beef/ground/lean/broiled (4 oz)	318	20	56.6
Beef/sirloin (4 oz)	320	21	59.1
Beef/T-bone (4 oz)	338	24	63.9
Butter (1 tbs)	102	11	97.1
Cheese/American (1 oz)	93	7	67.7
Cheese/cheddar (1 oz)	114	9	71.1
Cheese/cottage 4% (1 cup)	216	9	37.5
Cheese/cream (1 oz)	99	10	90.9
Cheese/Parmesan (1 oz)	129	9	62.8
Cheese/Swiss (1 oz)	106	8	67.9
Cheeseburger (1)	305	13	38.4
Chicken/breast/no skin (4 oz)	188	4	19.1
Chicken/thigh/no skin (4 oz)	232	13	50.4
Egg/hard-cooked (1)	77	5	58.4
Frankfurter/beef & pork (1)	182	17	84.1
Halibut/baked (4 oz)	159	3	17.0
Hamburger (1)	255	9	31.8
Ice cream/vanilla (1 cup)	267	15	50.6
Ice milk/vanilla (1 cup)	182	6	29.7
Lamb/lean & fat (4 oz)	293	19	58.4
Margarine (1 tbs)	101	11	98.0
Mayonnaise (1 tbs)	99	11	100.0
Milk/2% (1 cup)	121	5	37.2
Milk/skim (1 cup)	85	.5	5.3
Milk/whole (1 cup)	149	8	48.3
Nuts/cashew/oil roasted (1 oz)	163	14	77.3
Nuts/peanuts/oil roasted (1 oz)	165	14	76.4
Oil/canola (1 tbs)	126	14	100.0
Oil/olive (1 tbs)	124	14	100.0
Salmon/baked (4 oz)	245	12	44.1
Sherbet (1 cup)	266	4	13.5
Shrimp/boiled (3 oz)	85	1	10.6
Tuna/oil/drained (3 oz)	167	7	37.7
Tuna/water/drained (3 oz)	99	1	9.1
Turkey/dark meat/no skin (4 oz)	212	8	34.0
Turkey/light meat/no skin (4 oz)	117	4	30.8

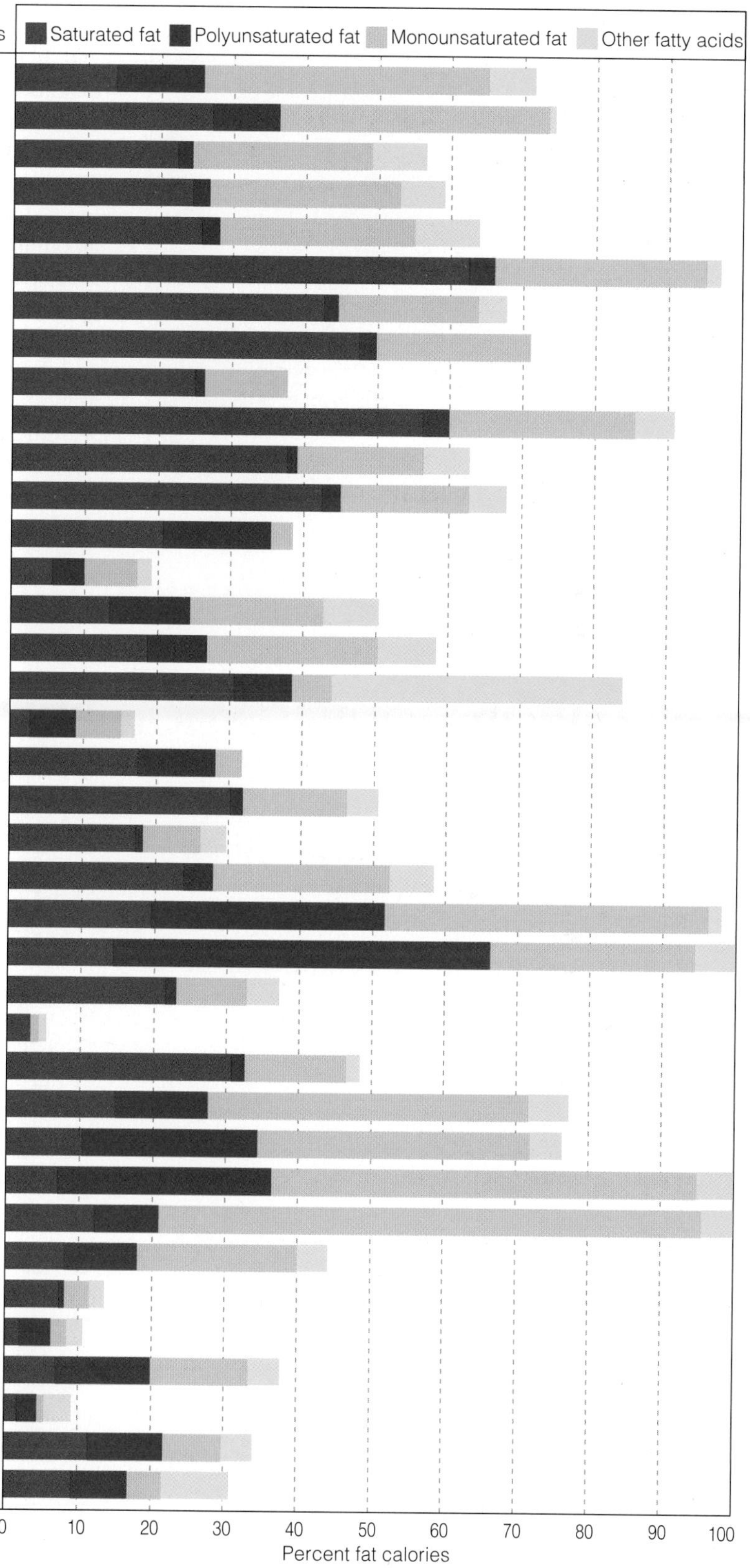

Saturated fat | Polyunsaturated fat | Monounsaturated fat | Other fatty acids

0 10 20 30 40 50 60 70 80 90 100

Percent fat calories

FIGURE 3.10 Healthy Eating Plate

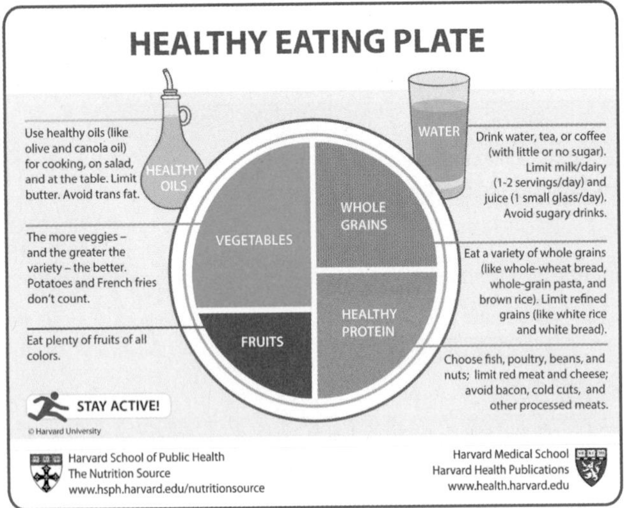

3B enables you to record your daily food intake. This record is much easier to keep than the complete dietary analysis in Lab 3A. Make one copy for each day you wish to record.

To start the activity, go to www.choosemyplate.gov and establish your personal MyPlate plan (SuperTracker option on the website) based on your age, sex, weight, height, and activity level. Record this information on the form provided in Lab 3B. Next, whenever you have something to eat, record the food and the amount eaten according to the MyPlate standard amounts (ounce, cup, or teaspoon—Figure 3.1). Do this immediately after each meal to keep track of your actual food intake more easily. At the end of the day, evaluate your diet by checking whether you ate the minimum required amounts for each food group. If you meet the minimum required servings at the end of each day and your caloric intake is in balance with the recommended amount, you are taking good steps to a healthier you.

BEHAVIOR MODIFICATION PLANNING

"Super" Foods

The following "super" foods that fight disease and promote health should be included often in the diet. Are you eating these foods regularly?

I PLAN TO	I DID IT	
❑	❑	Avocados
❑	❑	Bananas
❑	❑	Beans
❑	❑	Beets
❑	❑	Blueberries
❑	❑	Broccoli
❑	❑	Butternut squash
❑	❑	Carrots
❑	❑	Grapes
❑	❑	Kale
❑	❑	Kiwifruit
❑	❑	Flaxseeds
❑	❑	Nuts (Brazil, walnuts)
❑	❑	Salmon (wild)
❑	❑	Soy
❑	❑	Oats and oatmeal
❑	❑	Olives and olive oil
❑	❑	Onions
❑	❑	Oranges
❑	❑	Peppers
❑	❑	Pomegranates
❑	❑	Spinach
❑	❑	Strawberries
❑	❑	Tea (green, black, red)
❑	❑	Tomatoes
❑	❑	Watermelon
❑	❑	Yogurt

Try It

Using the above list, make a list of which super foods you can add to your diet and when you can eat them (snacks/meals). List meals that you can add these foods to.

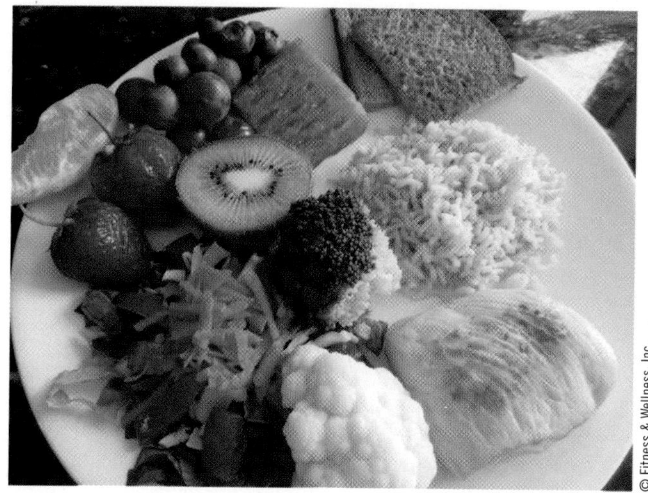

© Fitness & Wellness, Inc.

You can restructure your meals so that rice, pasta, beans, breads, and vegetables are in the center of the plate; meats are on the side and added primarily for flavoring; fruits are used for desserts; and low- or nonfat milk products are used.

Choosing Healthy Foods

Once you have completed the nutrient analysis and the MyPlate record form (Labs 3A and 3B), you may conduct a self-evaluation of your current nutritional habits. In Lab 3B, you can also assess your current stage of change regarding healthy nutrition and list strategies to help you improve your diet.

Initially, developing healthy eating habits requires a conscious effort to select nutritious foods (see the box on page 115). You must learn the nutritive value of typical foods that you eat. You can do so by reading food labels and looking up the nutritive values using listings such as the one provided in Appendix A or by using computer software available for such purposes.

Although not a major concern, be aware that in a few cases there is label misinformation. Whether it is a simple mistake or outright deception is difficult to determine, because there is little testing of food products and limited risks (penalties) if label misrepresentation occurs. The FDA simply does not have adequate staffing to regularly check food labels.

A limited number of organizations are trying to help. For example, the Florida Department of Agriculture and Consumer Services has found a 10 percent violation rate in food products tested. As a consumer, you may never know which products are mislabeled, although in a few cases you may be able to discern the truth by yourself. If a product claims to be low in calories and fat but tastes "too good to be true," that may indeed be the case. For example, an independent analysis of Rising Dough Bakery cookies found that the oatmeal cranberry cookie (the size of a compact disc) had more than twice as many calories as those listed on the label.

In most cases, when monitoring caloric intake, doing your own food preparation using healthy cooking methods is a better option than eating out or purchasing processed foods. Healthy eating requires proper meal planning and adequate coping strategies when confronted with situations that encourage unhealthy eating and overindulgence. Additional information on these topics is provided in the weight management chapter (Chapter 5).

Vegetarianism

About 7.5 million people in the United States are vegetarians, and another 23 million people follow a vegetarian-inclined diet. **Vegetarians** rely primarily on foods from the bread, cereal, rice, pasta, and fruit and vegetable groups and avoid most foods from animal sources in the dairy and protein groups. The basic types of vegetarians are as follows:

1. **Vegans** eat no animal products.
2. **Ovovegetarians** allow eggs in their diet.
3. **Lactovegetarians** consume foods from the milk group.
4. **Ovolactovegetarians** include egg and milk products in their diet.
5. **Semivegetarians** do not eat red meat but include fish (pescetarian) and/or poultry, in addition to milk products and eggs, in their diet.

Vegetarian diets are very healthy and can be consistent with the *Dietary Guidelines for Americans 2010* and can meet the DRIs for nutrients. Vegetarians who do not select their food combinations properly, however, can develop nutritional deficiencies of protein, vitamins, minerals, and even calories. Even greater attention should be paid when planning vegetarian diets for infants and children. Unless carefully planned, a strict plant-based diet prevents proper growth and development.

Nutrient Concerns

In some vegetarian diets, protein deficiency can be a concern. Vegans in particular must be careful to eat foods that provide a balanced distribution of essential amino acids, such as grain products and legumes. Strict vegans also need a supplement of vitamin B_{12}. This vitamin is not

Vegetarians Individuals whose diet is of vegetable or plant origin.

Vegans Vegetarians who eat no animal products.

Ovovegetarians Vegetarians who allow eggs in their diet.

Lactovegetarians Vegetarians who consume foods from the milk group.

Ovolactovegetarians Vegetarians who include eggs and milk products in their diet.

Semivegetarians Vegetarians who include milk products, eggs, and fish and poultry in their diet.

BEHAVIOR MODIFICATION PLANNING

Selecting Nutritious Foods

Do you regularly follow the habits below?

To select nutritious foods:

I PLAN TO | I DID IT

❏ ❏ Given the choice between whole foods and refined, processed foods, choose the former (apples rather than apple pie, potatoes rather than potato chips). No nutrients have been refined out of the whole foods, and they contain less fat, salt, and sugar.

❏ ❏ Choose the leaner cuts of meat. Select fish or poultry often, beef seldom. Ask for broiled, not fried, to control your fat intake.

❏ ❏ Use both raw and cooked vegetables and fruits. Raw foods offer more fiber and vitamins, such as folate and thiamin that are destroyed by cooking. Cooking foods frees other vitamins and minerals for absorption.

❏ ❏ Include milk, milk products, or other calcium sources for the calcium you need. Use low-fat or nonfat items to reduce fat and calories.

❏ ❏ Learn to use margarine, butter, and oils sparingly. A little gives flavor; a lot overloads you with fat and calories and increases disease risk.

❏ ❏ Vary your choices. Eat broccoli today, carrots tomorrow, and corn the next day. Eat Chinese today, Italian tomorrow, and broiled fish with brown rice and steamed vegetables the third day.

❏ ❏ Load your plate with vegetables and unrefined starchy foods. A small portion of meat or cheese is all you need for protein.

❏ ❏ When choosing breads and cereals, choose the whole-grain varieties.

To select nutritious fast foods:

❏ ❏ Choose the broiled sandwich with lettuce, tomatoes, and other goodies—and hold the mayo—rather than the fish or chicken patties coated with breadcrumbs and cooked in fat.

❏ ❏ Select a salad—and use more plain vegetables than those mixed with oily or mayonnaise-based dressings.

❏ ❏ Order chili with more beans than meat. Choose a soft bean burrito over tacos with fried shells.

❏ ❏ Drink low-fat milk rather than soft drinks (soda).

When choosing from a vending machine:

❏ ❏ Choose cracker sandwiches over chips and pork rinds (virtually pure fat). Choose peanuts, pretzels, and unbuttered popcorn over cookies and candy.

❏ ❏ Choose milk and juices over cola beverages.

Try It

Based on what you have learned, list strategies you can use to increase food variety, enhance the nutritive value of your diet, and decrease fat and caloric content in your meals.

SOURCE: Adapted from W. W. K. Hoeger, L. W. Turner, & B. Q. Hafen. *Wellness: Guidelines for a Healthy Lifestyle* (Wadsworth Thomson Learning, 2007).

found in plant foods; its only source is animal foods. Deficiency of this vitamin can lead to anemia and nerve damage.

The key to a healthful vegetarian diet is to eat foods that possess complementary proteins, because most plant-based products lack one or more essential amino acids in adequate amounts. For example, both grains and legumes are good protein sources, but neither provides all essential amino acids. Grains and cereals are low in the amino acid lysine, and legumes lack methionine. Foods from these two groups—such as combinations of tortillas and beans, rice and beans, rice and soybeans, or wheat bread and peanuts—complement each other and provide all required protein nutrients. Complementing protein foods include grains with legumes; legumes with nuts and seeds; or soy and quinoa with either grains, legumes, or nuts and seeds. These complementary proteins may be consumed over the course of one day, but it is best if they are consumed during the same meal (also see discussion under Proteins on pages 89–91).

Other nutrients likely to be deficient in vegetarian diets—and ways to compensate—are as follows:

- Vitamin D can be obtained from moderate exposure to the sun or by taking a supplement.
- Riboflavin can be found in green leafy vegetables, whole grains, and legumes.
- Calcium can be obtained from fortified soybean milk or fortified orange juice, calcium-rich tofu, and selected cereals. A calcium supplement is also an option.

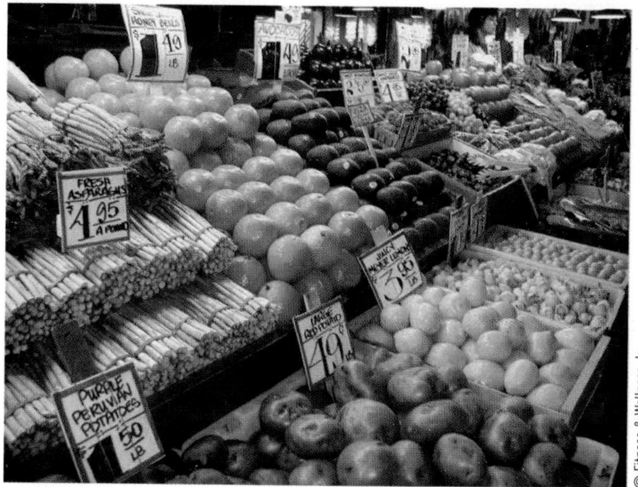

© Fitness & Wellness, Inc.

Most fruits and vegetables contain large amounts of cancer-preventing phytonutrients.

- Iron can be found in whole grains, dried fruits and nuts, and legumes. To enhance iron absorption, a good source of vitamin C should be consumed with these foods (calcium and iron are the most difficult nutrients to consume in sufficient amounts in a strict vegan diet).
- Zinc can be obtained from whole grains, wheat germ, beans, nuts, and seeds.

MyPlate also can be used as a guide for vegetarians. The key is food variety. Most vegetarians today eat dairy products and eggs. They can replace meat with legumes, nuts, seeds, eggs, and meat substitutes (tofu, tempeh, soy milk, and commercial meat replacements such as veggie burgers and soy hot dogs). To learn additional MyPlate healthy eating tips for vegetarians and how to get enough of the previously mentioned nutrients, go to www.choosemyplate.gov. Those interested in vegetarian diets are encouraged to consult additional resources, because special vegetarian diet planning cannot be covered adequately in a few paragraphs.

Nuts

Consumption of nuts, commonly used in vegetarian diets, has received considerable attention in recent years. Although nuts are 70 to 90 percent fat, most of this is healthy unsaturated fats. Nuts are known to be nutrient powerhouses. They are an excellent source of vitamin E and magnesium, and provide selenium, folate, vitamin K, beta-carotene, phosphorus, copper, potassium, zinc, and many phytonutrients.

A large Harvard study of some 119,000 health care professionals indicated that people who eat a handful of nuts each day had a 20 percent lower incidence of death during the 30-year study.[12] The results showed a reduction in premature mortality, heart disease, cancer, and respiratory disease. Previous research had already shown that people who eat nuts several times a week have a lower incidence of heart disease and enjoy beneficial effects on cholesterol, blood pressure, blood glucose control, and they decrease inflammation and the risk for dementia.

The research indicates that people who eat nuts several times a week have a lower incidence of heart disease. Eating two to three ounces (about one-half cup) of almonds, walnuts, or peanuts a day may decrease high LDL cholesterol by about 7 percent. Nuts can even enhance the cholesterol-lowering effects of the Mediterranean diet. Other data indicate that consumption of one daily serving of mixed nuts decreases oxidized LDL cholesterol concentrations. LDL cholesterol causes even greater damage when it is oxidized, inflaming the arteries, promoting atherosclerosis, and increasing the risk of a heart attack and stroke. Furthermore, studies have shown that nut consumption is associated with lower concentrations of other circulating inflammatory molecules. Daily substitution of 200 grams of carbohydrates with 22 ounces of nuts also helps control blood glucose in type 2 diabetics.

Heart-health benefits are attributed not only to the unsaturated fats but also to other nutrients found in nuts, including vitamin E and folic acid. Nuts are also packed with

FIGURE 3.11 Complementing Proteins for Vegetarians.

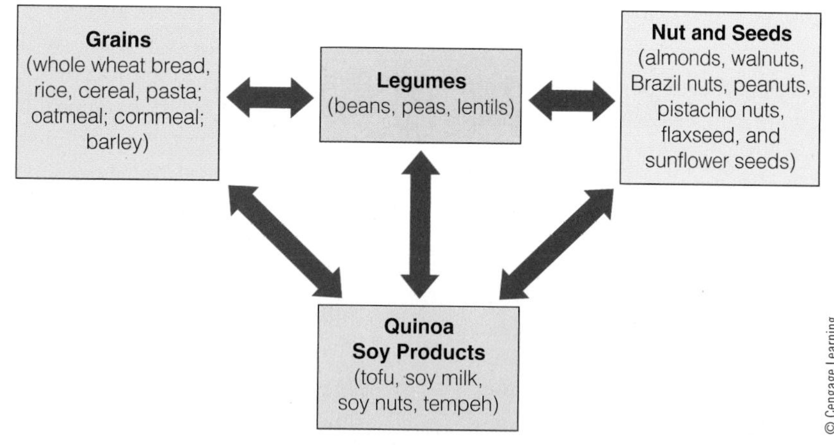

© Cengage Learning

B vitamins, calcium, copper, potassium, magnesium, fiber, and phytonutrients. Many of these nutrients are cancer- and cardioprotective, help lower homocysteine levels, and act as antioxidants (discussed in "Antioxidants," page 110, and "Folate," page 113).

Nuts do have a drawback: They are high in calories. A handful of nuts provides as many calories as a piece of cake, so nuts should be avoided as a snack. Excessive weight gain is a risk factor for cardiovascular disease. Nuts are recommended for use in place of high-protein foods such as meats, bacon, and eggs or as part of a meal in fruit or vegetable salads, homemade bread, pancakes, casseroles, yogurt, and oatmeal. Peanut butter is also healthier than cheese or some cold cuts in sandwiches. Nuts with a meal increase satiety, helping your meal last a little longer and thus helping you avoid snacks between meals. Women who eat two or more servings of nuts per week have a slightly lower risk of obesity. Nuts are also an excellent choice for a snack instead of simple carbohydrates, soda, candy bars, or other junk food. Limit the size of your snack to filling the palm of your hand.

Soy Products

The popularity of soy foods, including use in vegetarian diets, is attributed primarily to Asian research that points to less heart disease and fewer hormone-related cancers in people who regularly consume soy foods. A benefit of eating soy is that it replaces unhealthy animal products high in saturated fat. Soy is rich in plant protein, unsaturated fat, and fiber, and some soy is high in calcium.

The benefits of soy lie in its high protein content and plant chemicals, known as isoflavones that act as antioxidants and are thought to protect against estrogen-related cancers (breast, ovarian, and endometrial). The compound genistein, one of many phytonutrients in soy, may reduce the risk for breast cancer, and soy consumption may lower the risk for prostate cancer. Limited animal studies have suggested an actual increase in breast cancer risk. Human studies are still inconclusive but tend to favor a slight protective effect in premenopausal women.

Until more data become available, the *University of California at Berkeley Wellness Letter* has issued the following recommendations[13]:

1. Do not exceed three servings of soy per day (a serving constitutes one-half cup of tofu, edamame, or tempeh; one-fourth cup of roasted soy nuts; or one cup of soy yogurt or soy milk).
2. Limit soy intake to just a few servings per week if you have or have had breast cancer.
3. Avoid soy supplements, because they may contain higher levels of isoflavones than those found in soy foods. Individuals with a history of breast cancer and women who are pregnant or lactating should not use such supplements.

Probiotics

Yogurt is rated in the "super foods" category because, in addition to being a good source of calcium, potassium, riboflavin, and protein, it contains **probiotics**. The latter are friendly "for life" microbes that are thought to rebalance the naturally present intestinal bacteria. These microorganisms help break down foods and are thought to prevent disease-causing organisms from settling in. Although low-fat or nonfat yogurt is an excellent choice, you should not consume yogurt expecting miraculous medical benefits. Probiotics have been found to offer protection against gastrointestinal infections and boost immune activity. Nonetheless, additional research is needed to further investigate probiotic benefits.

Yogurts are cultured with *Lactobacillus delbrueckii bulgaricus* and *Streptococcus salivarius thermophilus* probiotics. When selecting yogurt, it is preferable to look for low-fat or nonfat products that also contain *Lactobacillus acidophilus, Lactobacillus bifidus*, and the prebiotic (substances on which probiotics feed) inulin. The latter, a soluble fiber, appears to enhance calcium absorption. Avoid yogurt with added fruit jam, sugar, and candy. Most yogurts have lots of added sugar and limited fruit. Thus, it is best to buy plain yogurt and add fresh fruit.

Advanced Glycation End Products

A new area of research in nutrition has to do with **advanced glycation end products (AGEs)**, compounds that have been implicated in aging, adverse effects, and chronic diseases by increasing oxidation and inflammation. AGEs are thought to contribute to the development of atherosclerosis, heart disease, diabetes and diabetes-related complications, kidney disease, osteoarthritis, rheumatoid arthritis, and Alzheimer's disease, among others. These compounds are produced when glucose combines with proteins, lipids, and other ingredients in foods.

AGEs are found primarily in foods cooked in dry heat, cooked at high temperatures, that are processed, and that have high fat content. Broiling, grilling, and frying create the highest levels of AGEs, whereas braising, steaming, stewing, roasting, boiling, and poaching decrease the levels. French-fried potatoes have about eight times the amount of AGEs compared with the amount in a baked potato. Fast-food restaurants take advantage of the flavor-enhancing effects of AGEs by adding these toxic compounds to their foods to increase the foods' appeal to the consumer. The take-home message to the consumer is again moderation. You do not have to eliminate grilling, frying, and fast foods, but common sense is vital to maintaining good health.

The following guidelines can help you decrease AGEs in your diet:

1. Limit cooking of meats at high temperatures.
2. Avoid high-fat foods (whole-milk products and meats).
3. Increase intake of fruits, vegetables, grains, fish, and low-fat milk products.

4. Choose unprocessed over processed foods by cooking fresh foods from scratch.
5. Eat at home most of the time and avoid prepackaged and fast foods as much as possible.
6. Avoid browning (the process of browning sugars and proteins on food surfaces increases the formation of AGEs).

Diets from Other Cultures

Increasingly, Americans eat foods reflecting the ethnic composition of people from other countries. Learning how to wisely select from the wide range of options is the task of those who seek a healthy diet.

Mediterranean Diet The **Mediterranean diet** receives much attention because people in that region have notably lower rates of diet-linked diseases and a longer life expectancy. The diet focuses on minimally processed (whole) foods. It features an abundance of fresh fruits and vegetables, olive oil, whole grains, legumes; in moderation, fish, red wine, nuts, and dairy products (mostly yogurt and cheese); and limits refined grains, sweets, and red and processed meats. Although it is a semivegetarian diet, up to 40 percent of the total daily caloric intake may come from fat—mostly monounsaturated fat from olive oil. Moderate intake of red wine is included with meals. The dietary plan also encourages regular physical activity (Figure 3.12).

More than a "diet," the Mediterranean diet is a dietary pattern that has existed for centuries. According to the largest and most comprehensive **observational study** on this dietary pattern, the health benefits and decreased mortality are not linked to any specific component of the diet (such as olive oil or red wine) but are achieved through the interaction of all the components of the pattern.[14] Those who adhere most closely to the dietary pattern have a lower incidence of heart disease (33 percent) and deaths from cancer (24 percent). A subsequent study published in 2013, the first randomized **clinical study** on the diet, was terminated early because individuals on a Mediterranean diet had an almost 30 percent decreased risk of heart disease.[15] The Mediterranean diet has also been linked to lower risk for metabolic syndrome and stroke, improved brain health and cognitive function, and lower risk for Alzheimer's disease. Although most people in the United States focus on the olive oil component of the diet, olive oil is used mainly as

FIGURE 3.12 The Traditional Healthy Mediterranean Diet Pyramid.

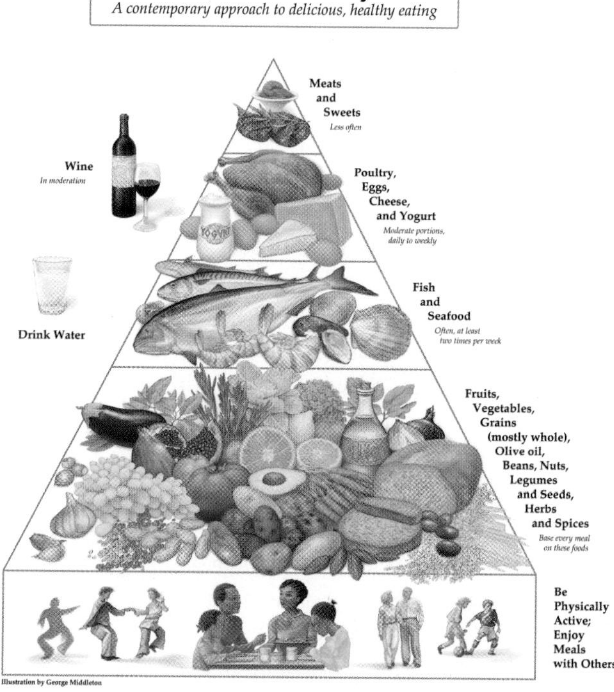

DIVERSITY CONSIDERATIONS

Large disparities exist in health risk factors, obesity rates, and chronic diseases across racial and ethnic groups in the United States. The question has been raised: Are racial differences in nutrition, exercise, and body weight related to better knowledge about healthy nutrition and exercise, or are they more closely related to differences in socioeconomic status? Study findings suggest that disparities in obesity may be more affected by the person's social and economic conditions. The research finds that people with lower economic resources are more likely to have a weight problem, regardless of racial or ethnic background. Poor-quality retail-food environments in disadvantaged neighborhoods, in conjunction with low economic resources, lead to increased obesity risk within ethnic minorities and socioeconomically disadvantaged populations.

Probiotics Healthy microbes (bacteria) that help break down foods and prevent disease-causing organisms from settling in the intestines.

Advanced glycation end products (AGEs) Derivatives of glucose–protein and glucose–lipid interactions that are linked to aging and chronic diseases.

Mediterranean diet Typical diet of people around the Mediterranean region, focusing on olive oil, red wine, fish, grains, legumes, vegetables, and fruits, with limited amounts of red meat, fish, milk, and cheese.

Observational study A research study in which the investigator does not intervene to make changes but only observes the outcomes based on a particular lifestyle pattern.

Clinical study A research study in which the investigator intervenes (makes certain changes or uses certain interventions or programs) to prevent or treat a disease.

a means to increase consumption of vegetables because vegetables sautéed in oil taste better than steamed vegetables.

Ethnic Diets As people migrate, they take their dietary practices with them. Many ethnic diets are healthier than the typical American diet, because they emphasize consumption of complex carbohydrates and limit fat intake. The predominant minority ethnic groups in the United States are African American, Hispanic American, and Asian American. Unfortunately, the generally healthier ethnic diets quickly become Americanized when these groups adapt to the United States. Often, they cut back on vegetables and add meats and salt to the diet to conform to the expectations of the American consumer.

Ethnic dishes can be prepared at home. They are easy to make and healthier when they use the typical (original) variety of vegetables, corn, rice, spices, and condiments. Ethnic health recommendations also encourage daily physical activity and suggest no more than two alcoholic drinks per day for men and one per day for women (research indicates that even one drink per week in women increases breast-cancer risk, three to six alcoholic drinks per week increases the risk by 15 percent, while heavier drinking increases risk 50 percent). Three typical ethnic diets are as follows:

- The African American diet ("soul food") is based on the regional cuisine of the American South. Soul food includes yams, black-eyed peas, okra, and peanuts. The latter have been combined with American foods such as corn products and pork. Today, most people think of soul food as meat, fried chicken, sweet potatoes, and chitterlings.
- Hispanic foods in the United States arrived with the conquistadores and evolved through combinations with other ethnic diets and local foods available in Latin America. For example, Cuban cuisine combined Spanish, Chinese, and native foods; Puerto Rican cuisine developed from

BEHAVIOR MODIFICATION PLANNING

Strategies for Healthier Restaurant Eating

On average, Americans eat out six times per week. Research indicates that when dining out, most people consume too many calories and too much fat. Such practice is contributing to the growing obesity epidemic and chronic conditions afflicting most Americans in the 21st century. Below are strategies that you can implement to eat healthier when dining out.

I PLAN TO | I DID IT

- ❑ ❑ Plan ahead. Decide before you get to the restaurant that you will select a healthy meal. Then stick to your decision. If you are unfamiliar with the menu, you may be able to access the menu at the restaurant's website beforehand, or you can obtain valuable nutrition information at www.healthydiningfinder.com. This website is maintained by registered dietitians and provides information on many restaurant chains located in your area.
- ❑ ❑ Be aware of calories in drinks. You can gulp down several hundred extra calories through drinks alone. Restaurants and beverage industries are eager to get your money, and servers wouldn't mind a larger tip by having you consume additional items on the menu. Water, sparkling soda water, or unsweetened teas are good choices.
- ❑ ❑ Avoid or limit appetizers, regardless of how tempting they might be. Ask your server not to bring to the table high-fat premeal free foods such as tortilla chips, bread and butter, or vegetables to be dipped in high-fat salad dressings. If you munch on food freebies or appetizers (or make a meal out of them), have your server box up half or the entire meal for you to take home. If you box up an entire meal, you now have two additional meals that you can consume at home; most restaurant meals can be split into two meals.
- ❑ ❑ Request a half-size or a child's portion. If you are unable to do so, split the meal with your dining partner or box up half the meal before you start to eat.
- ❑ ❑ Inquire about ingredients and cooking methods. Don't be afraid to ask for healthy substitutes. For example, you may request that meat be sautéed instead of deep fried or that canola or olive oil be used instead of other oil choices. You can also request a baked potato or brown rice instead of french fries or white rice. Ask for dressing, butter, or sour cream on the side. Request whole-wheat bread for sandwiches. Furthermore, avoid high-fat foods or ingredients such as creamy or cheese sauces, butter, oils, and fatty, fried, or crispy meats. When in doubt, ask the server for additional information. If the server can't answer your questions, select a different meal.

Try It

Implement as many of the above strategies every time you dine out. Take pride in your healthy choices. Your long-term health and well-being are at stake. You will feel much better about yourself following a healthy meal than you would otherwise.

TABLE 3.10 **Ethnic Eating Guide**

	Choose Often	Choose Less Often
Chinese	Beef with broccoli Chinese greens Steamed rice, brown or white Steamed beef with pea pods Stir-fry dishes Teriyaki beef or chicken Wonton soup	Crispy duck Egg rolls Fried rice Kung pao chicken (fried) Peking duck Pork spareribs
Japanese	Chiri nabe (fish stew) Grilled scallops Sushi, sashimi (raw fish) Teriyaki Yakitori (grilled chicken)	Tempura (fried chicken, shrimp, or vegetables) Tonkatsu (fried pork)
Italian	Cioppino (seafood stew) Minestrone (vegetarian soup) Pasta with marinara sauce Pasta primavera (pasta with vegetables) Steamed clams	Antipasto Cannelloni, ravioli Fettuccini alfredo Garlic bread White clam sauce
Mexican	Beans and rice Black bean/vegetable soup Burritos, bean Chili Enchiladas, bean Fajitas Gazpacho Taco salad Tamales Tortillas, steamed	Chili relleno Chimichangas Enchiladas, beef or cheese Flautas Guacamole Nachos Quesadillas Tostadas Sour cream (as topping)
Middle Eastern	Tandoori chicken Curry (yogurt-based) Rice pilaf Lentil soup Shish kebab	Falafel
French	Poached salmon Spinach salad Consommé Salad niçoise	Beef Wellington Escargot French onion soup Sauces in general
Soul Food	Baked chicken Baked fish Roasted pork (not smothered or "etouffe") Sauteed okra Baked sweet potato	Fried chicken Fried fish Smothered pork tenderloin Okra in gumbo Sweet potato casserole or pie
Greek	Gyros Pita Lentil soup	Baklava Moussaka

Source: Adapted from P. A. Floyd, S. E. Mimms, and C. Yelding-Howard. *Personal Health: Perspectives & Lifestyles* (Belmont, CA: Wadsworth Thomson Learning, 1998).

Spanish, African, and native products; and Mexican diets evolved from Spanish and native foods. Prominent in all of these diets were corn, beans, squash, chili peppers, avocados, papayas, and fish. The colonists later added rice and citrus foods. Today, the Hispanic diet incorporates a variety of foods, including red meat and cheese, but the staples still consist of rice, corn, and beans.

- Asian American diets are characteristically rich in vegetables and use minimal meat and fat. The Okinawan diet in Japan, where some of the healthiest and oldest people in the world live, is high in fresh (versus pickled) vegetables, high in fiber, and low in fat and salt. Chinese cuisine includes more than 200 vegetables, and fat-free sauces and seasonings are used to enhance flavor. The Chinese diet varies by region in China. The lowest in fat is that of southern China, with most meals containing fish, seafood, and stir-fried vegetables. Chinese food in American restaurants contains a much higher percentage of fat and protein than traditional Chinese cuisine.

Table 3.10 provides a list of healthier foods to choose from when dining at selected ethnic restaurants. In addition, you can consult the box on the previous page for strategies that you can use for healthy dining out.

All healthy diets have similar characteristics: They are high in fruits, vegetables, and grains and low in fat and saturated fat. Healthy diets also use low-fat or fat-free dairy products, and they emphasize portion control—essential in a healthy diet plan.

Many people think that if a food item is labeled "low fat" or "fat free," they can consume it in large quantities. "Low fat" or "fat free" does not imply "calorie free." Many people who consume low-fat diets eat more (and thus increase their caloric intake), which in the long term leads to obesity and its associated health problems.

Nutrient Supplementation

The Academy of Nutrition and Dietetics states that consuming a wide variety of nutrient-dense foods is more effective for good health and chronic disease prevention than taking vitamin and mineral supplements. Approximately half of all adults in the United States, nonetheless, take daily nutrient **supplements**. Nutrient requirements for the body normally can be met by consuming as few as 1,500 calories per day, as long as the diet contains the recommended amounts of food from the different food groups. Still, many people consider it necessary to take vitamin supplements.

It's true that the body cannot retain water-soluble vitamins as long as fat-soluble vitamins. The body excretes excessive intakes readily, although it can retain small amounts for weeks or months in various organs and tissues. Fat-soluble vitamins, by contrast, are stored in fatty tissue. Therefore, daily intake of these vitamins is not as crucial.

People should not take a **megadose** of vitamins

Supplements Tablets, pills, capsules, liquids, or powders containing vitamins, minerals, antioxidants, amino acids, herbs, or fiber that individuals take to increase their intake of these nutrients.

Megadose For most vitamins, 10 times the RDA or more; for vitamin A, five times the RDA.

and minerals. For some nutrients, a dose of five times the RDA taken over several months may create problems. For other nutrients, it may not pose a threat to human health. Vitamin and mineral doses should not exceed the UL (with the possible exception of vitamin D; see page 112). For nutrients that do not have an established UL, one day's dose should be no more than three times the RDA.

Iron deficiency (determined through blood testing) is more common in women than in men. Iron supplementation is frequently recommended for women who have a heavy menstrual flow. Pregnant and lactating women also may require supplements. The average pregnant woman who eats an adequate amount of a variety of foods should take a low dose of an iron supplement daily. Women who are pregnant with more than one baby may need additional supplements. Folate supplements also are encouraged prior to and during pregnancy to prevent certain birth defects (see the following discussions of antioxidants and folate). In the preceding instances, individuals should take supplements under a physician's supervision.

Adults over the age of 60 may need to supplement their nutrient intake with a daily multivitamin. Aging may decrease the body's ability to absorb and utilize certain nutrients. Nutrients sometimes deficient in older adults include vitamins C, D, B_6, and B_{12}; folate; and the minerals calcium, zinc, and magnesium. Iron needs, however, decrease with age; thus, a supplement with lower levels of iron is recommended.

Other people who may benefit from supplementation are those with nutrient deficiencies, alcoholics and street-drug users who do not have a balanced diet, smokers, vegans (strict vegetarians), individuals on low-calorie diets (fewer than 1,500 calories per day), and people with disease-related disorders or who are taking medications that interfere with proper nutrient absorption.

Although supplements may help a small group of individuals, most supplements do not provide benefits to healthy people who eat a balanced diet. A supplement cannot replace the array of nutrients found in whole foods. These nutrients often work in synergy; that is, the interaction of the nutrients when combined is greater than the sum of their individual effects. Studies published as recent as December 2013 show that there is no clear health benefit to most vitamin and mineral supplements. Supplements do not appear to prevent chronic diseases (including heart disease and cancer) or help people run faster, jump higher, relieve stress, improve sexual prowess, cure a common cold, or boost energy levels. A multivitamin supplement may act as an "insurance policy" for people with unhealthy diets, but it is quite clear that it will never replace the benefits of a well-balanced diet. If you choose to take a multivitamin, you are encouraged to pick one that does not exceed 100 percent of the Daily Values for most vitamins and minerals (men and postmenopausal women are advised to select one without iron, as such is not necessary).

Antioxidants Much research and discussion are taking place regarding the effectiveness of **antioxidants** in thwarting several chronic diseases. Although foods probably contain more than 4,000 antioxidants, the four most studied antioxidants are vitamins E and C, beta-carotene (a precursor to vitamin A), and the mineral selenium (technically not an antioxidant but a component of antioxidant enzymes).

Oxygen is used during metabolism to change carbohydrates and fats into energy. During this process, oxygen is transformed into stable forms of water and carbon dioxide. A small amount of oxygen, however, ends up in an unstable form, referred to as **oxygen free radicals**. A free radical molecule has a normal proton nucleus with a single unpaired electron. Having only one electron makes the free radical extremely reactive, and it looks constantly to pair its electron with one from another molecule. When a free radical steals a second electron from another molecule, that other molecule in turn becomes a free radical. This chain reaction goes on until two free radicals meet to form a stable molecule.

Free radicals attack and damage proteins and lipids—in particular, cell membranes and DNA. This damage is thought to contribute to the development of conditions such as cardiovascular disease, cancer, emphysema, cataracts, Parkinson's disease, and premature aging. Solar radiation, cigarette smoke, air pollution, radiation, some drugs, injury, infection, chemicals (e.g., pesticides), and other environmental factors also seem to encourage the formation of free radicals. Antioxidants are thought to offer protection by absorbing free radicals before they can cause damage and by interrupting the sequence of reactions once damage has begun, thwarting certain chronic diseases (Figure 3.13).

The body's own defense systems typically neutralize free radicals so that they don't cause damage. When free radicals are produced faster than the body can neutralize them, they can damage the cells. Research, however, indicates that the body's antioxidant defense system improves as fitness improves.[16] That is, physically fit people have greater protection against free radicals.

Antioxidants are found abundantly in food, especially in fruits and vegetables. Unfortunately, most Americans do not eat the minimum recommended amounts of fruits and vegetables.

Antioxidants work best in the prevention and progression of disease, but they cannot repair damage that has already occurred or cure people who have disease. The benefits are obtained primarily from food sources, and controversy surrounds the benefits of antioxidants taken in supplement form.

For years, people believed that taking antioxidant supplements could further prevent free radical damage. Then, adding to the controversy, a report published in the *Journal of the American Medical Association* indicated that antioxidant supplements increase the risk of death.[17] Vitamin E, beta-carotene, and vitamin A increased the risk for mortality by 4 percent, 7 percent, and 16 percent, respectively. Vitamin C had no effect on mortality, while selenium decreased the risk by 9 percent. Some researchers, however, have questioned the design and conclusions of this report. More research is required to settle the controversy.

FIGURE 3.13 Antioxidant protection: blocking and absorbing oxygen free radicals to prevent chronic disease.

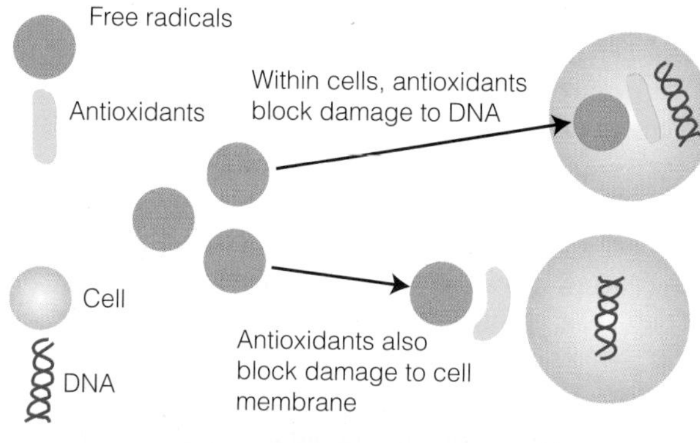
Free radicals
Antioxidants
Within cells, antioxidants block damage to DNA
Cell
DNA
Antioxidants also block damage to cell membrane

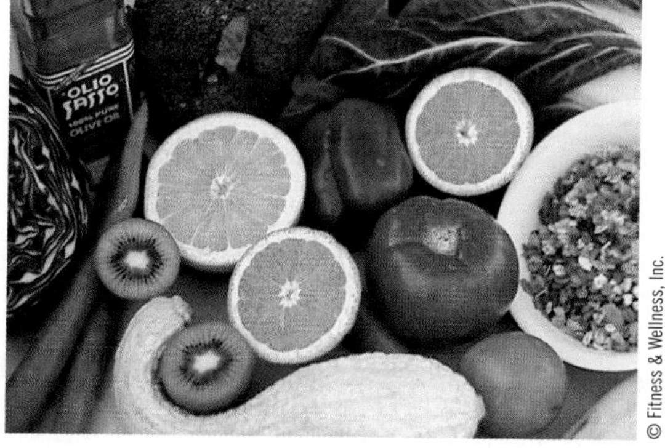
OLIO SASSO

© Fitness & Wellness, Inc.

Vitamin E The RDA for vitamin E for almost everyone is 15 milligrams or 22 **international units**, abbreviated **IU**. Although no evidence indicates that vitamin E supplementation below the UL of 1,000 milligrams per day is harmful, little or no clinical research supports any health benefits. Vitamin E is found primarily in oil-rich seeds and vegetable oils. Foods high in vitamin E include almonds, hazelnuts, peanuts, canola oil, safflower oil, cottonseed oil, kale, sunflower seeds, shrimp, wheat germ, sweet potato, avocado, and tomato sauce. You should incorporate some of these foods regularly in your diet to obtain the RDA.

Vitamin C Studies have shown that vitamin C may offer benefits against heart disease, cancer, and cataracts. People who consume the recommended amounts of daily fruits and vegetables need no supplementation, because they obtain their daily vitamin C requirements through their diet alone.

Vitamin C is water soluble, and the body eliminates it in about 12 hours. For best results, consume food rich in vitamin C twice a day. High intake of a vitamin C supplement, above 500 milligrams per day, is not recommended. The body absorbs little vitamin C beyond the first 200 milligrams per serving or dose. Foods high in vitamin C include oranges and other citrus fruit, kiwifruit, cantaloupe, guava, bell peppers, strawberries, broccoli, kale, cauliflower, and tomatoes.

Beta-Carotene Obtaining the daily recommended dose of beta-carotene (20,000 IU) from food sources rather than supplements is preferable. Clinical trials have found that beta-carotene supplements do not offer protection against heart disease or cancer or provide other health benefits. Therefore, the recommendation is to "skip the pill and eat the carrot." One medium raw carrot contains about 20,000 IU of beta-carotene. Other foods high in beta-carotene include sweet potatoes, pumpkin, cantaloupe, squash, kale, broccoli, tomatoes, peaches, apricots, mangoes, papaya, turnip greens, and spinach.

Selenium Research on individuals who took 200 micrograms (mcg) of selenium daily indicates that it decreased the risk for prostate, colorectal, and lung cancers by about 50 percent and may have decreased the risk for cancers of the breast, liver, and digestive tract. More recent research, however, has failed to confirm such benefits, and experts recommend caution with selenium supplements. One report indicated that men and women taking 200 mcg per day for eight years were almost three times more likely to suffer from diabetes than those taking a placebo.[18]

At present, the best recommendation available is not to exceed a daily supplement that contains more than 100 mcg of selenium. Based on the current body of research, 100 to 200 mcg of selenium per day seems to provide the necessary amount of antioxidant for this nutrient. Although the UL for selenium has been set at 400 mcg, a person has no reason to take more than 200 mcg daily. Too much selenium can damage cells rather than protect them.

One Brazil nut that you crack yourself provides about 100 mcg of selenium. Shelled nuts found in supermarkets average only about 20 mcg each. Other foods high in selenium include red snapper, salmon, cod, tuna, noodles, whole grains, and meats.

Multivitamins Although much interest has been generated in the previously mentioned individual supplements, Americans prefer multivitamins as supplements. Study after study has found little or no long-lasting benefit from taking multivitamin-and-mineral supplements. At present, there is no solid scientific evidence that they decrease the risk for either cardiovascular disease or cancer. The most convincing data came in a 2009 study on more than 161,000 postmenopausal women taking multivitamin pills.[19] The results showed no benefits in terms of cardiovascular, cancer, or premature mortality risk reduction in women taking a

Antioxidants Compounds such as vitamins C and E, beta-carotene, and selenium that prevent oxygen from combining with other substances in the body to form harmful compounds.

Oxygen free radicals Substances formed during metabolism that attack and damage proteins and lipids, in particular the cell membrane and DNA, leading to diseases such as heart disease, cancer, and emphysema.

International unit (IU) Measure of nutrients in food.

multivitamin complex for an average of eight years compared with those who did not. A panel of experts from the National Institutes of Health has indicated that there aren't enough data to support the use of multivitamins.

If you take a multivitamin for general health reasons, it doesn't grant you a license to eat carelessly. Multivitamin-and-mineral supplements are not magic pills. They don't provide energy, fiber, or phytonutrients. People who eat a healthy diet, with ample amounts of fruits, vegetables, and grains, have a low risk of cardiovascular disease and cancer compared with people with deficient diets who take a multivitamin complex.

Vitamin D Vitamin D is attracting a lot of attention because research suggests that the vitamin possesses anticancer properties, especially against breast, colon, and prostate cancers and possibly lung and digestive cancers. It also decreases inflammation, fighting cardiovascular disease, periodontal disease, and atherosclerosis. Furthermore, vitamin D strengthens the immune system, controls blood pressure, helps maintain muscle strength, decreases the risk for arthritis and dementia, prevents birth defects, and may help deter diabetes and fight depression. In addition, it is necessary for absorption of calcium, a nutrient critical for building and maintaining bones to prevent osteoporosis and for ensuring dental health.

The theory that vitamin D protects against cancer is based on studies showing that people who live farther north (who have less sun exposure during the winter months) have a higher incidence of cancer. Furthermore, people diagnosed with breast, colon, or prostate cancer during the summer months, when vitamin D production by the body is at its highest, are 30 percent less likely to die from cancer, even 10 years following the initial diagnosis. Researchers think that vitamin D level at the time of cancer onset affects survival rates.

Technically, vitamin D is a prohormone. Its metabolic product, calcitriol, is a secosteroid hormone that influences more than 2,000 genes affecting health and well-being. During the winter months, most people in the United States living north of a 35-degree latitude (above the states of Georgia and Texas) and in Canada are not getting enough vitamin D. The body uses ultraviolet B (UVB) rays to generate vitamin D. UVB rays are shorter than ultraviolet A rays, so they penetrate the atmosphere at higher angles. During the winter season, the sun is too far south for the UVB rays to get through.

In 2010, the Institute of Medicine of the NAS increased the DRI of vitamin D to 600 IU (15 mcg) for children and adults up to 70 years of age. Older adults should get 800 IU (20 mcg) per day. Vitamin D experts had hoped for higher levels, considering amounts to be too low for most individuals, especially during the winter months. Preliminary evidence suggests that people should get between 1,000 and 2,000 IU (25 to 50 mcg) of vitamin D per day.[20] For now, the UL has been set at 2,000 IU (50 mcg).

The most accurate test to measure how much vitamin D is in the body is the 25-hydroxyvitamin D test. Blood levels should remain between 50 and 80 ng/mL all year long. To increase your levels, the Vitamin D Council recommends that all adults supplement their diets with 5,000 IU of vitamin D daily for three months and then take a 25-hydroxyvitamin D test.[21] You may then adjust your supplement dosage based on your test results, your daily sun exposure, and the season of the year.

Depending on skin tone and sun intensity, about 15 minutes of unprotected sun exposure (without sunscreen) of the face, arms, hands, and lower legs during peak daylight hours (10:00 a.m. and 4:00 p.m.—when your shadow is shorter than your actual height) generates between 2,000 and 5,000 IU of vitamin D. Thus, it makes no sense that the UL is set at 2,000 IU when the human body manufactures more than that in just 15 minutes of unprotected sun exposure. The UL of 2,000 IU will most likely be revised in the next update of the DRI reports. Experts have reported no data implicating toxic effects up to 10,000 IU (250 mcg) a day.

Good sources of vitamin D in the diet include salmon, mackerel, tuna, and sardines. Fortified milk, yogurt, orange juice, margarines, and cereals are also good sources. To obtain up to 2,000 IU per day from food sources alone, however, is difficult (Table 3.11). Thus, daily safe sun exposure, supplementation (especially during the winter months), or both are highly recommended.

The best source of vitamin D is sunshine. UVB rays lead to the production on the surface of the skin of inactive, oil-soluble vitamin D_3. The inactive form is then transformed by the liver, and subsequently the kidneys, into the active form of vitamin D. Sun-generated vitamin D is better than that obtained from foods or supplements.

Vitamin D_3 generated on the surface of the skin, however, doesn't immediately penetrate into the blood. It takes up to 48 hours to absorb most of the vitamin. Because it is an oil-soluble compound, experts recommend that you

TABLE 3.11 **Good Sources of Vitamin D**

Food	Amount	IU*
Multivitamins (most brands)	daily dose	400
Salmon	3.5 oz	360
Mackerel	3.5 oz	345
Sardines, oil (drained)	3.5 oz	250
Shrimp	3.5 oz	200
Orange juice, D-fortified	8 oz	100
Milk, any type/D-fortified	8 oz	100
Margarine, D-fortified	1 tbsp	60
Yogurt, D-fortified	6–8 oz	60
Cereal, D-fortified	¾–1 cup	40
Egg	1	20

*IU = international unit

avoid using soap following safe sun exposure, because it washes off most of the vitamin. You may use soap for your armpits, groin area, and feet, but avoid using soap on newly sun-exposed skin.

Excessive sun exposure can lead to skin damage and skin cancer. It is best to strive for daily *safe sun* exposure, that is, 10 to 20 minutes (based on skin tone and sun intensity) of unprotected sun exposure during peak hours of the day a few times a week. Generating too much vitamin D from the sun is impossible because the body generates only what it needs. If you have sensitive skin, you may want to start with 5 minutes and progressively increase sun exposure by 1 minute per day. If your skin turns a slight pink following exposure, you have overdone it and need to cut back on the time that you are out in the sun.

People at the highest risk for low vitamin D levels are older adults, those with dark skin (they make less vitamin D), and individuals who spend most of their time indoors and get little sun exposure. Two studies have found that over a span of six to seven years, individuals 65 and over with low blood levels of vitamin D are two and a half times more likely to die in that time frame than those with high levels. People with darker skin also need 5 to 10 times the sun exposure of lighter-skinned people to generate the same amount of vitamin D. The skin's dark pigment reduces the ability of the body to synthesize vitamin D from the sun by up to 95 percent.

In the United States and Canada, most of the population does not make vitamin D from the sun during the winter months, when UVB rays do not get through; most people's time is spent indoors, and extra clothing is worn to protect against the cold. According to the National Health and Nutrition Examination Survey published in 2011, 41.6 percent of the U.S. population doesn't have a 25-hydroxyvitamin D level of even 20 ng/mL. The highest deficiency rate is seen in Blacks and Hispanics, with 82.1 percent and 69.2 percent deficiency rates respectively. During periods of limited sun exposure, you should consider a daily vitamin D_3 supplement of up to 2,000 IU per day (some supplements contain vitamin D_2, which is a less potent form of the vitamin).

Folate Although it is not an antioxidant, 400 mcg of **folate** (a B vitamin) are recommended. In women, folate helps prevent some birth defects and seems to offer protection against colon and cervical cancers. Women who might become pregnant should plan to take a folate supplement, because studies have shown that folate before and during pregnancy can prevent serious birth defects (in particular, spina bifida). Some of these defects occur during the first few days and weeks of pregnancy. Adequate folate intake can also prevent congenital heart defects, early miscarriages, and premature birth. Thus, women who may become pregnant need to have adequate folate levels before conception and throughout pregnancy.

Some evidence also indicates that adequate intake of folate, along with vitamins B_6 and B_{12}, prevents heart attacks by reducing homocysteine levels in the blood (see Chapter 11). High concentrations of homocysteine accelerate the process of plaque formation (atherosclerosis) in the arteries. Five servings of fruits and vegetables per day usually meet the needs for these nutrients. Almost 9 of 10 adults in the United States do not obtain the recommended 400 mcg of folate per day and less than 8 percent eat the recommended daily servings of fruits and vegetables.

With the possible exception of women of childbearing age, obtaining your daily folate RDA from natural foods is preferable to getting it from supplements. The UL for folate has been set at 1,000 mcg per day. Evidence suggests that exceeding 1,000 mcg through a combination of diet and supplements may fuel the progression of precancerous growths and cancer.[22] A daily multivitamin or a serving of a highly fortified cereal provides 400 mcg of folate. In combination with a supplement, you can easily exceed the UL of 1,000 mcg per day. To date, no data have linked folate obtained from natural foods to increased cancer risk. On the contrary, natural foods have been found to have a cancer-protective effect.

Benefits of Foods

In its latest position statement on nutrient supplements, the American Dietetic Association stated, "The best nutrition-based strategy for promoting optimal health and reducing the risk of chronic disease is to wisely choose a wide variety of foods." Additional nutrients from supplements can help some people meet their nutrient needs as specified by science-based nutrition standards such as the Dietary Reference Intakes.[23]

Fruits and vegetables are the richest sources of antioxidants and phytonutrients. For example, researchers at the U.S. Department of Agriculture (USDA) compared the antioxidant effects of vitamins C and E with those of various common fruits and vegetables. The results indicated that three-fourths of a cup of cooked kale (which contains only 11 IU of vitamin E and 76 milligrams of vitamin C) neutralized as many free radicals as did approximately 800 IU of vitamin E or 600 milligrams of vitamin C. A list of the top antioxidant foods is presented in Table 3.12.

Many people who eat unhealthily think that they need supplementation to balance their diets. This is a fallacy about nutrition. The problem here is not necessarily a lack of vitamins and minerals but, rather, a diet too high in calories, saturated fat, trans fats, and sodium. Vitamin, mineral, and fiber supplements do not supply all of the nutrients and other beneficial substances present in food and needed for good health.

Wholesome foods contain vitamins, minerals, carbohydrates, fiber, proteins, fats, and phytonutrients, along with other substances not yet discovered. Researchers think that in most cases the protective effects are caused by a combination of

Folate One of the B vitamins.

antioxidants with other nutrients or simply by some other substances in food that have not been investigated yet. Furthermore, many nutrients work in **synergy**, enhancing chemical processes in the body. For example, broccoli, a cruciferous vegetable, contains healthful substances that protect against cancer, but they are activated by enzymes also found in broccoli. Most likely, only by eating the respective substances in broccoli do people reap all benefits of these compounds. Other research confirms that eating the "entire whole grain" provides more benefits than eating wheat germ, bran, or supplements of other nutrients found in grain foods.

Supplementation does not offset poor eating habits. Pills are no substitute for common sense. If you think your diet is not balanced, you first need to conduct a nutrient analysis (see Lab 3A) to determine which nutrients you lack in sufficient amounts. Eat more of them, as well as foods that are high in antioxidants and phytonutrients. Following a nutrient assessment, a **registered dietitian (RD)** can help you decide what supplement or supplements, if any, might be necessary.

Furthermore, the American Heart Association does not recommend antioxidant supplements until more definite research is available. If an RD recommends that you take supplements in pill form, look for products that say they meet the disintegration standard of the U.S. Pharmacopoeia (USP) on the bottle. The USP standard suggests that the supplement should completely dissolve in 45 minutes or less. Supplements that do not dissolve, of course, cannot get into the bloodstream.

CRITICAL THINKING

Do you take supplements? If so, for what purposes are you taking them—and do you think you could restructure your diet so that you could do without them?

TABLE 3.12 Top Antioxidant Foods

Food
Red beans
Wild blueberries
Red kidney beans
Pinto beans
Blueberries
Cranberries
Artichokes
Blackberries
Kale
Prunes
Raspberries

Source: U. S. Department of Agriculture.

Functional Foods

Functional foods are foods or food ingredients that offer specific health benefits beyond those supplied by the traditional nutrients they contain. Many functional foods come in their natural forms. A tomato, for example, is a functional food because it contains the phytonutrient lycopene, thought to reduce the risk for prostate cancer. Other examples of functional foods are kale, broccoli, blueberries, red grapes, and green tea.

The term "functional food," however, has been used primarily as a marketing tool by the food industry to attract consumers. Unlike **fortified foods**, which have been modified to help prevent nutrient deficiencies, functional foods are created by the food industry by the addition of ingredients aimed at treating or preventing symptoms or disease. In functional foods, the added ingredient(s) is typically not found in the food item in its natural form but is added to allow manufacturers to make appealing health claims.

In most cases, only one extra ingredient is added (a vitamin, mineral, phytonutrient, or herb). An example is calcium added to orange juice to make the claim that this brand offers protection against osteoporosis. Food manufacturers now offer cholesterol-lowering margarines (enhanced with plant stanol), cancer-protective ketchup (fortified with lycopene), memory-boosting candy (with ginkgo added), calcium-fortified chips, and corn chips containing kava kava (to enhance relaxation).

The use of some functional foods, however, may undermine good nutrition. Margarines still may contain saturated fats or partially hydrogenated oils. Regularly consuming ketchup on top of large orders of fries adds many calories and fat to the diet. Sweets are also high in calories and sugar. Chips are high in calories, salt, and fat. In all of these cases, the consumer would be better off taking the specific ingredient in a supplement form rather than consuming functional foods with their extra calories, sugar, salt, and/or fat.

Functional foods can provide added benefits if used in conjunction with a healthful diet. You may use nutrient-dense functional foods in your overall wellness plan as an adjunct to health-promoting strategies and treatments.

Organic Foods

Concerns over food safety have led many people to turn to organic foods. Currently, there's no solid evidence that organic food is more nutritious than conventional food, but pesticide residues in organic foods are substantially lower than in conventionally grown foods. Health risks from pesticide exposure from foods are relatively small for healthy adults. The health benefits of pesticide-treated produce far outweigh the risks. Children, older adults, pregnant and lactating women, and people with weak immune systems, however, may be vulnerable to some types of pesticides.

Organic foods, including crops, meat, poultry, eggs, and dairy products, are produced under strict government regu-

BEHAVIOR MODIFICATION PLANNING

Guidelines for a Healthy Diet

I PLAN TO	I DID IT	
❑	❑	Use portion control by keeping them small to moderate.
❑	❑	Base your diet on a large variety of foods.
❑	❑	Consume ample amounts of green, yellow, and orange fruits and vegetables.
❑	❑	Eat foods high in complex carbohydrates, including at least three 1-ounce servings of whole-grain foods per day.
❑	❑	Obtain most of your vitamins and minerals from food sources.
❑	❑	Eat foods rich in vitamin D.
❑	❑	Maintain adequate daily calcium intake and consider a bone supplement with vitamin D_3.
❑	❑	Consume protein in moderation.
❑	❑	Limit daily fat, trans fat, and saturated fat intake.
❑	❑	Limit cholesterol consumption to less than 300 mg per day.
❑	❑	Limit sodium intake to 2,300 mg per day.
❑	❑	Limit sugar intake.
❑	❑	If you drink alcohol, do so in moderation (one daily drink for women and two for men).
❑	❑	Consider taking a daily multivitamin (preferably one that includes vitamin D_3).

Try It

Carefully analyze the above guidelines and note the areas where you can improve your diet. Work on one guideline each week until you are able to adhere to all of the above guidelines.

lations in the way they are grown, handled, and processed. Organic crops have to be grown without the use of conventional pesticides, artificial fertilizers, human waste, or sewage sludge and have been processed without ionizing radiation or food additives. Harmful microbes in manure must also be destroyed prior to use, and genetically modified organisms (GMOs) may not be used. Organic livestock are raised under certain grazing conditions, using organic feed but not using antibiotics and growth hormones.

Organic foods can just as easily be contaminated with bacteria, pathogens, and heavy metals that pose major health risks as nonorganic foods. Soil may become contaminated. If produce comes in contact with feces of grazing cattle, wild animals or birds, farmworkers, or any other source, potentially harmful microorganisms can contaminate the produce. Recently, *Escherichia coli*–contaminated spinach, sold nationwide, was grown in a field that was in transition from conventional to organic crops. The best safeguard to protect yourself is to follow the food safety guidelines provided in the box on page 116.

Genetically Modified Crops

In a **genetically modified (GM) food**, the DNA (or basic genetic material) is manipulated to obtain certain results. This is done by inserting genes with desirable traits from one plant, animal, or microorganism into another one to either introduce new traits or enhance existing traits.

Crops are modified in this way to make them better resist disease and extreme environmental conditions (e.g., heat and frost), require fewer fertilizers and pesticides, last longer, and improve their nutrient content and taste. GMOs could help save billions of dollars by producing more crops and helping feed the hungry in developing countries around the world.

Concern over the safety of GM foods has led to heated public debates in Europe and, to a lesser extent, in the United States. The concern is that genetic modifications create "transgenic" organisms that have not previously existed and that have potentially unpredictable effects on the environment and on humans. Also,

Synergy A reaction in which the result is greater than the sum of its two parts.

Registered dietitian (RD) A person with a college degree in dietetics who meets all certification and continuing education requirements of the American Dietetic Association or Dietitians of Canada.

Functional foods Foods or food ingredients containing physiologically active substances that provide specific health benefits beyond those supplied by basic nutrition.

Fortified foods Foods that have been modified by the addition or increase of nutrients that either were not present or were present in insignificant amounts, with the intent of preventing nutrient deficiencies.

Genetically modified (GM) food Food whose basic genetic material (DNA) is manipulated by inserting genes with desirable traits from one plant, animal, or microorganism into another one to either introduce new traits or enhance existing ones.

BEHAVIOR MODIFICATION PLANNING

Minimizing the Risk of Food Contamination and Pesticide Residues

Most food is safe to eat, but there is no 100 percent guarantee that all produce is free of contamination. Follow the tips below to minimize risk.

I PLAN TO | I DID IT

- ❑ ❑ Wash your hands thoroughly before and after touching raw produce.
- ❑ ❑ Do not place raw fruits and vegetables next to uncooked meat, poultry, or fish.
- ❑ ❑ Trim all visible fat from meat, remove the skin from poultry and fish prior to cooking (pesticides concentrate in animal fat).
- ❑ ❑ Rinse, scrub, and peel. Use a scrub brush to wash fresh produce under running water. Pay particular attention to crevices in the produce. Washing fresh produce reduces pesticide levels but does not completely eliminate them. Eat a variety of foods to decrease exposure to any given pesticide.
- ❑ ❑ Select produce that is free of dirt and does not have holes or cuts or other signs of spoilage.
- ❑ ❑ Discard the outermost leaves of leafy vegetables such as lettuce and cabbage.
- ❑ ❑ Cut your own fruits and vegetables instead of getting them precut. Wash all produce thoroughly before cutting, even melons and avocados. Cutting into potentially contaminated (unwashed) inedible rinds of fruit can contaminate the inside of the fruit. Always use a knife to remove orange peels instead of biting into them. Peel waxed fruits and vegetables, and other produce as necessary (cucumbers, carrots, peaches, apples).
- ❑ ❑ Store produce in the refrigerator in clean containers or clean plastic bags (previously used bags that are not kept cold can grow harmful bacteria).
- ❑ ❑ For some produce, consider buying certified organic foods. Look for the "USDA Organic" seal. According to data from the Environmental Working Group, a nonprofit consumer activist organization, conventional produce with the most pesticide residue include apples, celery, cherry tomatoes, collard greens, cucumbers, grapes, imported grapes, kale, nectarines, peaches, potatoes, spinach, strawberries, summer squash, and sweet bell peppers. Among the least contaminated are asparagus, avocados, bananas, cabbage, cantaloupe, eggplant, frozen sweet peas, kiwifruit, mangoes, mushrooms, onions, pineapples, sweet corn, and sweet potatoes (list of foods downloaded from www.foodnews.org).

Try It

Lifestyle behavior patterns are difficult to change. The above recommendations can minimize your risk of food contamination and ingestion of pesticide residues. Make a copy of the above recommendations and determine how many of these suggestions you are able to include in daily life over the course of the next seven days.

there is some concern that GM foods may cause illness or allergies in humans and that cross-pollination may destroy other plants or create "superweeds" with herbicide-resistant genes. Some researchers believe that GM crops have increased usage of harmful herbicides, causing an overall negative impact on the environment.

GM crops were first introduced into the United States in 1996. This technology is moving forward so rapidly that the USDA already has approved more than 50 GM crops. Today, more than 40 percent of U.S. cropland produces GM foods. About 70 percent of processed foods in the United States contain at least one GM ingredient and more than 94 percent of soybeans, 90 percent of cotton, 90 percent of canola, and 88 percent of corn come from GM crops.

Avoiding GM foods is difficult, because more than 75 percent of processed foods on the market today contain GMOs. Americans have been consuming GM foods for almost two decades now with no apparent detrimental health consequences. If people do not wish to consume GM foods, organic foods are an option, because organic trade organizations do not certify foods with genetic modifications. Produce bought at the local farmers' market also may be an option, because small farmers are less likely to use this technology.

At this point, the World Health Organization, the American Medical Association, and the National Academy of Sciences have indicated that there is no evidence of any hazards from GM foods. Many questions remain, and much research is required in this field. As a consumer, you must continue educating yourself as more evidence becomes available in the next few years.

Energy Substrates for Physical Activity

The two main fuels that supply energy for physical activity are glucose (sugar) and fat (fatty acids). The body uses amino acids, derived from proteins, as an energy substrate when glucose is low, such as during fasting, prolonged aerobic exercise, or a low-carbohydrate diet.

Glucose is derived from foods that are high in carbohydrates, such as breads, cereals, grains, pasta, beans, fruits, vegetables, and sweets. Glucose is stored as glycogen in muscles and the liver. Fatty acids (discussed on pages 86–89) are the product of the breakdown of fats. Unlike glucose, an almost unlimited supply of fatty acids, stored as fat in the body, can be used during exercise.

Energy (Adenosine Triphosphate) Production The energy derived from food is not used directly by human cells. It is first transformed into **adenosine triphosphate (ATP)**. The subsequent breakdown of this compound provides the energy used by all energy-requiring processes of the body (Figure 3.14).

ATP must be recycled continually to sustain life and work. ATP can be resynthesized in three ways:

1. **ATP-CP system.** The body stores small amounts of ATP and creatine phosphate (CP). These stores are used during all-out activities such as sprinting, long jumping, and weight lifting. The amount of stored ATP provides energy for just one or two seconds. During brief all-out efforts, ATP is resynthesized from CP, another high-energy phosphate compound. This is the ATP-CP, or phosphagen, system. Depending on the amount of physical training, the concentration of CP stored in cells is sufficient to allow maximum exertion for up to 10 seconds. Once the CP stores are depleted, the person is forced to slow down or rest to allow ATP to form through anaerobic and aerobic pathways.
2. **Anaerobic or lactic acid system.** During maximal-intensity exercise that is sustained for 10 to 180 seconds, ATP is replenished primarily from the breakdown of glucose through a series of chemical reactions that do not require oxygen (hence the term "anaerobic"). In the process, though, **lactic acid** is produced. As lactic acid accumulates, it leads to muscle fatigue.

   Because of the accumulation of lactic acid with high-intensity exercise, the formation of ATP during anaerobic activities is limited to about three minutes. A recovery period of several minutes then is necessary to allow for the removal of lactic acid. Formation of ATP through the anaerobic system requires glucose (carbohydrates).
3. **Aerobic system.** The production of energy during slow, sustained exercise is derived primarily through aerobic metabolism. Glucose (carbohydrates), fatty acids (fat), and oxygen (hence the term "aerobic") are required to form ATP using this process. Under steady-state exercise conditions, lactic acid accumulation is minimal or nonexistent.

Because oxygen is required, a person's capacity to utilize oxygen is crucial for successful athletic performance in aerobic events. The higher an individual's maximal oxygen uptake (VO_{2max}) (see pages 220–221), the greater the capacity to generate ATP through the aerobic system—and the better that person's athletic potential in long-distance events. From the previous discussion, it becomes evident that for optimal performance, both recreational and highly competitive athletes make the required nutrients part of their diet.

FIGURE 3.14 Contributions of the energy formation mechanisms during various forms of physical activity.

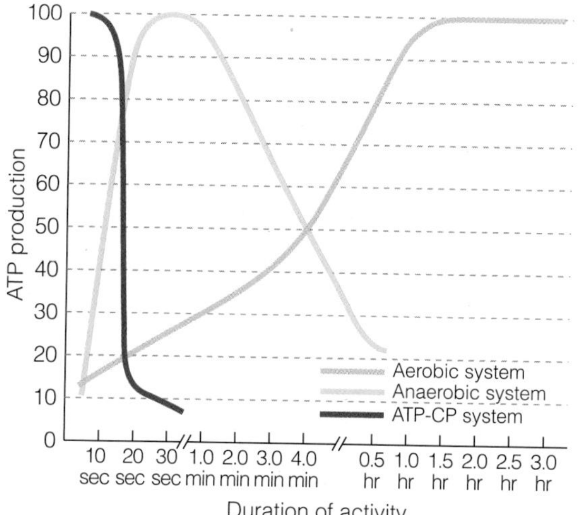

Nutrition for Athletes

During resting conditions, fat supplies about two-thirds of the energy to sustain the body's vital processes. During exercise, the body uses both glucose (glycogen) and fat in combination to supply the energy demands. The proportion of fat to glucose changes with the intensity of exercise. When a person is exercising below 60 percent of his or her maximal work capacity (VO_{2max}), fat is used as the primary energy substrate. As the intensity of exercise increases, so does the percentage of glucose utilization—up to 100 percent during maximal work that can be sustained for only two to three minutes.

In general, athletes do not require supplementation or a special

Adenosine triphosphate (ATP) A high-energy chemical compound that the body uses for immediate energy.

Lactic acid End product of anaerobic glycolysis (metabolism).

type of diet. Unless the diet is deficient in basic nutrients, no secret or magic diet helps people perform better or develop faster as a result of what they eat. As long as they eat a balanced diet—that is, based on a large variety of nutrients from all basic food groups—athletes do not require supplements. Even in strength training and bodybuilding, protein in excess of 20 percent of total daily caloric intake is not necessary. The recommended daily protein intake ranges from .8 gram per kilogram of body weight for sedentary people to 2.0 grams per kilogram for extremely active individuals (Table 3.4).

The main difference between a sensible diet for a sedentary person and a sensible diet for a highly active individual is the total number of calories required daily and the amount of carbohydrate intake needed during prolonged physical activity. People in training consume more calories because of their greater energy expenditure—which is required as a result of intense physical training.

Carbohydrate Loading On a regular diet, the body is able to store between 1,500 and 2,000 calories in the form of glycogen. About 75 percent of this glycogen is stored in muscle tissue. This amount, however, can be increased greatly through **carbohydrate loading**.

A regular diet should be altered during several days of heavy aerobic training or when a person is going to participate in a long-distance event of more than 90 minutes (e.g., marathon, triathlon, or road cycling). For events shorter than 90 minutes, carbohydrate loading does not seem to enhance performance.

During prolonged exercise, glycogen is broken down into glucose, which then is readily available to the muscles for energy production. In comparison with fat, glucose frequently is referred to as "high-octane fuel," because it provides about 6 percent more energy per unit of oxygen consumed.

Heavy training over several consecutive days leads to depletion of glycogen faster than it can be replaced through the diet. Glycogen depletion with heavy training is common in athletes. Signs of depletion include chronic fatigue, difficulty in maintaining accustomed exercise intensity, and lower performance.

On consecutive days of exhaustive physical training (several hours daily), a carbohydrate-rich diet—70 percent of total daily caloric intake or 8 grams of carbohydrate per kilogram (2.2 pounds) of body weight—is recommended. This diet often restores glycogen levels in 24 hours. Along with the high-carbohydrate diet, a day of rest often is needed to allow the muscles to recover from glycogen depletion following days of intense training. For people who exercise less than an hour a day, a 60 percent carbohydrate diet, or 6 grams of carbohydrate per kilogram of body weight, is enough to replenish glycogen stores.

Following an exhaustive workout, eating a combination of carbohydrates and protein (e.g., a tuna sandwich) within 30 minutes of exercise seems to speed up glycogen storage even more. Protein intake increases insulin activity, thereby enhancing glycogen replenishment. A 70 percent carbohydrate intake then should be maintained throughout the rest of the day.

By following a special diet and exercise regimen on five days before a long-distance event, highly (aerobically) trained individuals are capable of storing two to three times the amount of glycogen found in the average person. Athletic performance may be enhanced for long-distance events of more than 90 minutes by eating a regular balanced diet (50 to 60 percent carbohydrates), along with intensive physical training on the fifth and fourth days before the event, followed by a diet high in carbohydrates (about 70 percent) and a gradual decrease in training intensity over the last three days before the event.

The amount of glycogen stored as a result of a carbohydrate-rich diet does not seem to be affected by the proportion of complex and simple carbohydrates. The intake of simple carbohydrates (sugars) can be raised while on a 70 percent carbohydrate diet, as long as it doesn't exceed 25 percent of the total calories. Complex carbohydrates provide more nutrients and fiber, making them a better choice for a healthier diet.

On the day of the long-distance event, carbohydrates are still the recommended choice of substrate. As a general rule, athletes should consume one gram of carbohydrate for each kilogram (2.2 pounds) of body weight one hour prior to exercise. If you weigh 160 pounds (73 kg), you should consume 72 grams. If the pre-event meal is eaten earlier, the amount of carbohydrate can be increased to two, three, or

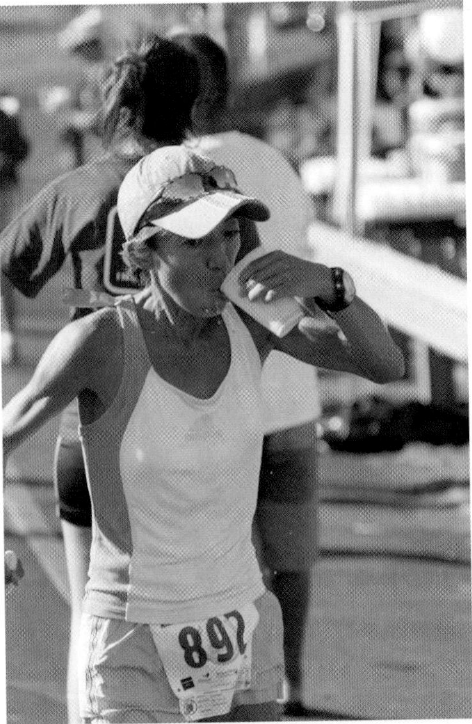

Fluid and carbohydrate replenishment during exercise are essential when participating in long-distance aerobic endurance events, such as a marathon or a triathlon.

four grams per kilogram of weight two, three, or four hours, respectively, before exercise.

During the long-distance event, researchers recommend that the athlete consume 30 to 60 grams of carbohydrates (120 to 240 calories) every hour. This is best accomplished by drinking 8 ounces of a 6 to 8 percent carbohydrate sports drink every 15 minutes (check labels to ensure proper carbohydrate concentration). This also lessens the chance of dehydration during exercise, which hinders performance and endangers health. The percentage of the carbohydrate drink is determined by dividing the amount of carbohydrate (in grams) by the amount of fluid (in milliliters) and then multiplying by 100. For example, 18 grams of carbohydrate in 240 milliliters (8 ounces) of fluid yields a drink that is 7.5 percent (18 ÷ 240 × 100) carbohydrate.

Strenuous Exercise and Strength Training

Meeting your protein needs close to your training time is critical during high-intensity aerobic workouts and in strength training. Minute tears in muscle tissue occur during intense training. The availability of protein to the muscles promote faster repair, development, and may even prevent damage from taking place in the first place. Thus, consuming a light carbohydrate/protein snack 30 to 60 minutes prior to intense exercise and immediately following exercise (10 to 20 g of protein) is beneficial to repair and maintain muscle and further promote muscle growth. Additional protein taken with meals throughout the day is needed for optimal development. More information on this topic is provided in Chapter 9 under "Dietary Guidelines for Muscular and Strength Development" (page 277).

Hyponatremia In some cases, athletes participating in long- or ultra–long-distance races may suffer from **hyponatremia**, or low sodium concentration in the blood. The longer the race, the greater the risk of hyponatremia. This condition occurs as lost sweat, which contains salt and water, is replaced by only water (no salt) during a very long-distance race. Although the athlete is overhydrated, blood sodium is diluted and hyponatremia occurs. Typical symptoms are similar to those of heat illness and include fatigue, weakness, disorientation, muscle cramps, bloating, nausea, dizziness, confusion, slurred speech, fainting, and even seizures and coma in severe cases.

Based on estimates, about 30 percent of the participants in the Hawaii Ironman Triathlon suffer from hyponatremia. The condition, however, is rare in the everyday exerciser. To help prevent hyponatremia, athletes should ingest extra sodium prior to the event and then adequately monitor fluid intake during the race to prevent overhydration. Sports drinks that contain sodium should be used during the race (ingest about one gram of sodium per hour) to replace **electrolytes** lost in sweat and to prevent blood sodium dilution.

Creatine Supplementation

Creatine is an organic compound obtained in the diet primarily from meat and fish. In the human body, creatine combines with inorganic phosphate and forms **creatine phosphate (CP)**, a high-energy compound. CP then is used to resynthesize ATP during short bursts of all-out physical activity. Individuals on a normal mixed diet consume an average of one gram of creatine per day. Each day, one additional gram is synthesized from various amino acids. One pound of meat or fish provides approximately two grams of creatine.

Creatine supplementation is popular among individuals who want to increase muscle mass and improve athletic performance. Creatine monohydrate—a white, tasteless powder that is mixed with fluids prior to ingestion—is the form most popular among people who use the supplement. Supplementation can result in an approximate 20 percent increase in the amount of creatine that is stored in muscles. Most of this creatine binds to phosphate to form CP, and 30 to 40 percent remains as free creatine in the muscles. Increased creatine storage is thought to enable individuals to train more intensely—thereby building more muscle mass and enhancing performance in all-out activities of very short duration (less than 30 seconds).

Creatine supplementation has two phases: the loading phase and the maintenance phase. During the loading phase, the person consumes between 20 and 25 grams (one teaspoonful is about 5 grams) of creatine per day for five to six days, divided into four or five doses of 5 grams each throughout the day (this amount represents the equivalent of consuming 10 or more pounds of meat per day). Research also suggests that the amount of creatine stored in muscles is enhanced by taking creatine in combination with a high-carbohydrate food. Once the loading phase is complete, taking 2 grams per day seems to be sufficient to maintain the increased muscle stores.

To date, no serious side effects have been documented in people who take up to 25 grams of creatine per day for five days. Stomach distress and cramping have been reported only in rare instances. The 2 grams taken per day during the maintenance phase is just slightly above the average intake in a daily diet. Long-term effects of creatine supplementation on health, however, have not been established.

A frequently documented re-

Carbohydrate loading Increasing intake of carbohydrates during heavy aerobic training or prior to aerobic endurance events that last longer than 90 minutes.

Hyponatremia A low sodium concentration in the blood caused by excessive perspiration during exercise overhydration with plain water.

Electrolytes Substances that become ions in solution and are critical for proper muscle and neuron activation (include sodium, potassium, chloride, calcium, magnesium, phosphate, and bicarbonate).

Creatine An organic compound derived from meat, fish, and amino acids that combines with inorganic phosphate to form CP.

Creatine phosphate (CP) A high-energy compound that the cells use to resynthesize ATP during all-out activities of very short duration.

sult following five to six days of creatine loading is an increase of two to three pounds in body weight. This increase appears to be related to the increased water retention necessary to maintain the additional creatine stored in muscles. Some data, however, suggest that the increase in stored water and CP stimulates protein synthesis, leading to an increase in lean body mass.

The benefits of elevated creatine stores may be limited to high-intensity and short-duration activities, such as sprinting, strength training (weight lifting), and sprint cycling. Supplementation is most beneficial during exercise training, rather than as an aid to enhance athletic performance a few days before competition.

Enhanced creatine stores do not benefit athletes competing in aerobic endurance events, because CP is not used in energy production for long-distance events. Actually, the additional weight can be detrimental in long-distance running and swimming events, because the athlete must expend more energy to carry the extra weight during competition.

Bone Health and Osteoporosis

Osteoporosis, literally meaning "porous bones," is a condition in which bones lack the minerals required to keep them strong. In osteoporosis, bones—primarily of the hip, wrist, and spine—become so weak and brittle that they fracture readily. The process begins slowly in the third and fourth decades of life. Women are especially susceptible after menopause because of the accompanying loss of **estrogen**, which increases the rate at which bone mass is broken down.

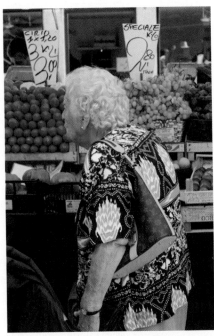

Osteoporosis is the leading cause of serious morbidity and functional loss in the elderly.

According to the National Osteoporosis Foundation, 10 million Americans (8 million women and 2 million men) already have the disease and another 43 million have low bone density, placing them at increased risk for osteoporosis and bone fractures. About 30 percent of postmenopausal women have osteoporosis, but only about 2 percent are actually diagnosed and treated for this condition.

Osteoporosis is the leading cause of serious morbidity and functional loss in the elderly population. One of every two women and up to one in four men over age 50 will have an osteoporotic-related fracture at some point in their lives. The chances of a postmenopausal woman developing osteoporosis are much greater than her chances of developing breast cancer or incurring a heart attack or stroke. Up to 20 percent of people who have a hip fracture die within a year because of complications related to the fracture. As alarming as these figures are, they do not convey the pain and loss of quality of life in people who suffer the crippling effects of osteoporotic fractures.

Although osteoporosis is viewed primarily as a woman's disease, more than 30 percent of all men will be affected by age 75. About 100,000 of the yearly 300,000 hip fractures in the United States occur in men.

Despite the strong genetic component, osteoporosis is preventable. Maximizing bone density at a young age and subsequently decreasing the rate of bone loss later in life are critical factors in preventing osteoporosis.

Normal hormone levels prior to menopause and adequate calcium intake and physical activity throughout life cannot be overemphasized. These factors are all crucial in preventing osteoporosis. The absence of any one of these three factors leads to bone loss for which the other two factors never completely compensate. Smoking and excessive use of alcohol and corticosteroid drugs also accelerate the rate of bone loss in women and men alike. And osteoporosis is more common in whites, Asians, and people with small frames. Figure 3.15 depicts these variables.

Bone health begins at a young age. Some experts have called osteoporosis a "pediatric disease." Bone density can be promoted early in life by making sure the diet has sufficient calcium and participating in weight-bearing activities. Adequate calcium intake in women and men alike is also associated with a reduced risk for colon cancer. The RDA for calcium is between 1,000 and 1,300 mg per day (see Table 3.13).

To obtain your daily calcium requirement, get as much calcium as possible from calcium-rich foods, including calcium-fortified foods. If you don't get enough, you need to make a conscious and deliberate effort to reach the RDA through foods in the diet. Calcium supplements are no longer recommended because they may cause more harm than good, including a modest increase in risk of heart attacks, kidney stones in both men and women, and possibly increased risk of prostate cancer in men. Calcium obtained from food has not been linked to these negative health risks. Supplements are only warranted in extreme cases, when dietary intake from food absolutely does not supply the need.

FIGURE 3.15 **Threats to bone health (osteoporosis).**

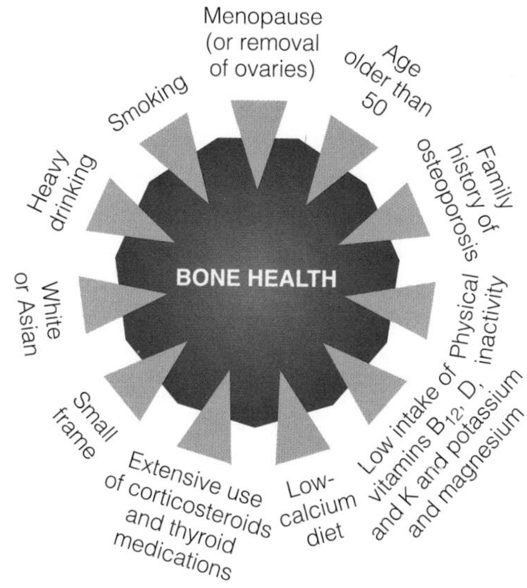

Table 3.13 **Recommended Daily Calcium Intake**

Age	Amount (mg)
9–18	1,300
19–50	1,000
51–70 Men	1,000
51–70 Women	1,200
>70	1,200

Pregnant and lactating women should follow the recommendation for their respective age group.

TABLE 3.14 **Low-Fat Calcium-Rich Foods**

Food	Amount	Calcium (mg)	Calories
Beans, red kidney (cooked)	1 cup	70	218
Beet, greens (cooked)	½ cup	82	19
Bok choy (Chinese cabbage)	1 cup	158	20
Broccoli (cooked, drained)	1 cup	72	44
Burrito, bean (no cheese)	1	57	225
Cottage cheese, 2% low-fat	½ cup	78	103
Ice milk, vanilla	½ cup	102	100
Instant Breakfast, nonfat milk	1 cup	407	216
Kale (cooked, drained)	1 cup	94	36
Milk, nonfat (powdered)	1 tbsp	52	15
Milk, skim	1 cup	296	88
Oatmeal, instant, fortified (plain)	½ cup	109	70
Okra (cooked, drained)	½ cup	74	23
Orange juice, fortified	1 cup	300	110
Soy milk, fortified, fat-free	1 cup	400	110
Spinach (raw)	1 cup	56	12
Turnip greens (cooked)	1 cup	197	29
Tofu, some types	½ cup	138	76
Yogurt, fruit	1 cup	372	250
Yogurt, low-fat (plain)	1 cup	448	155

Table 3.14 provides a list of selected foods and their calcium content. Along with having an adequate calcium intake, taking a minimum of 400 to 800 IU of vitamin D daily is recommended for optimal calcium absorption (for overall health benefits, 1,000 to 2,000 IU of vitamin D is preferable). Close to half of people over 50 are also vitamin D deficient. Without vitamin D, it is practically impossible for the body to absorb sufficient calcium to protect the bones.

Protein is also necessary for the continuous rebuilding of bones. Excessive protein, however, is detrimental to bone health because it makes the blood more acidic. To neutralize the acid, calcium is taken from the bones and released into the bloodstream. The more protein we eat, the higher the calcium content in the urine (i.e., the more calcium excreted). This might be the reason that countries with a high protein intake, including the United States, also have the highest rates of osteoporosis. Individuals should aim to achieve the RDA for protein nonetheless, because people who consume too little protein (less than 35 grams per day) lose more bone mass than those who eat too much (more than 100 grams per day). The RDA for protein is about 50 grams per day for women and 63 grams for men.

Vitamin B_{12} may also be a key nutrient in the prevention of osteoporosis. Several reports have shown an association between low vitamin B_{12} and lower bone mineral density in both men and women. Vitamin B_{12} is found primarily in dairy products, meats, poultry, fish, and some fortified cereals. Other nutrients vital for bone health are potassium (also neutralizes acid), vitamin K (works with bone-building proteins), and magnesium (also keep bone from becoming too brittle).

Soft drinks and alcoholic beverages also can contribute to a loss in bone density if consumed in large quantities. Although they may not cause the damage directly, they often take the place of dairy products in the diet.

Exercise plays a key role in preventing osteoporosis by decreasing the rate of bone loss following the onset of menopause. Active people are able to maintain bone density

Osteoporosis A condition of softening, deterioration, or loss of bone mineral density that leads to disability, bone fractures, and even death from medical complications.

Estrogen Female sex hormone essential for bone formation and conservation of bone density.

much more effectively than their inactive counterparts. A combination of weight-bearing exercises, such as walking or jogging and weight training, is especially helpful.

The benefits of exercise go beyond maintaining bone density. Exercise strengthens muscles, ligaments, and tendons—all of which provide support to the bones (skeleton). Exercise also improves balance and coordination, which can help prevent falls and injuries.

People who are active have higher bone mineral density than inactive people do. Similar to other benefits of participating in exercise, there is no such thing as "bone in the bank." To have good bone health, people need to participate in a regular lifetime exercise program.

Prevailing research also tells us that estrogen is the most important factor in preventing bone loss. Lumbar bone density in women who have always had regular menstrual cycles exceeds that of women with a history of **oligomenorrhea** and **amenorrhea** interspersed with regular cycles. Furthermore, the lumbar density of these two groups of women is higher than that of women who have never had regular menstrual cycles.

For instance, athletes with amenorrhea (who have lower estrogen levels) have lower bone mineral density than even nonathletes with normal estrogen levels. Studies have shown that amenorrheic athletes at age 25 have the bones of women older than 50. It has become clear that sedentary women with normal estrogen levels have better bone mineral density than active amenorrheic athletes. Many experts believe the best predictor of bone mineral content is the history of menstrual regularity.

As a baseline, women age 65 and older should have a bone density test to establish the risk for osteoporosis. Younger women who are at risk for osteoporosis should discuss a bone density test with their physician at menopause. The test also can be used to monitor changes in bone mass over time and to predict the risk of future fractures. The bone density test is a painless scan requiring only a small amount of radiation to determine bone mass of the spine, hip, wrist, heel, or fingers. The amount of radiation is so low that technicians administering the test can sit next to the person receiving it. The procedure often takes less than 15 minutes.

Various therapy modalities available to prevent and/or treat osteoporosis should be discussed with a physician. If you have osteoporosis, lifestyle changes may be required and you may also need medication to prevent future fractures. A calcium-rich diet, adequate vitamin D, daily exercise, and drug therapy are all treatment options.

New medical treatments have been developed and continue to evolve to prevent and treat bone loss. The newer medications can be classified into two categories: antiresorptive and anabolic. Antiresorptive medications slow bone loss, but the body still makes new bone at the same rate, so bone density may increase. The drugs that fall into this category include bisphosphonates, calcitonin, denosumab, estrogen agonists/antagonists (also referred to as selective estrogen receptor modulators or SERMs), and menopausal hormone therapy (MHT). Anabolic medications increase the rate of bone formation. The only FDA-approved drug in this category is teriparatide, a form of parathyroid hormone.

Menopausal hormone therapy (MHT) may be the most effective treatment to relieve acute (short-term) symptoms of menopause, such as hot flashes, mood swings, sleep difficulties, and vaginal dryness. Due to potential health risks, experts recommend that women on MHT use the lowest dose that still provides benefits and use it for the shortest time needed. Regardless of the treatment modality, women should always work with a physician to determine the best course of action.

Iron Deficiency

Iron is a key element of **hemoglobin** in blood. The daily RDA for iron for adult, nonpregnant, premenopausal women is between 15 and 18 milligrams and for postmenopausal women is 8 milligrams (8 to 11 milligrams for men). Inadequate iron intake is often seen in children, teenagers, women of childbearing age, and endurance athletes. If iron absorption does not compensate for losses or if dietary intake is low, iron deficiency develops. As many as 50 percent of American women have an iron deficiency. Over time, excessive depletion of iron stores in the body leads to iron-deficiency anemia, a condition in which the concentration of hemoglobin in the red blood cells is lower than it should be.

Physically active individuals, in particular women, have a greater-than-average need for iron. Heavy training creates a demand for iron that is higher than the recommended intake, because small amounts of iron are lost through sweat, urine, and stools. Mechanical trauma, caused by the pounding of the feet on the pavement during extensive jogging, may also lead to destruction of iron-containing red blood cells.

A large percentage of female endurance athletes are reported to have iron deficiency. The blood **ferritin** levels of women who participate in intense physical training should be checked frequently.

The rates of iron absorption and iron loss vary from person to person. In most cases, though, people can get enough iron by eating more iron-rich foods, such as beans, peas, green leafy vegetables, enriched grain products, egg yolks, fish, and lean meats. Although organ meats, such as liver, are especially good sources of iron, they also are high in cholesterol. A list of foods high in iron is given in Table 3.15.

If you are iron-deficient, be aware that calcium interferes with iron absorption. Thus, try not to include dietary sources of calcium with your main iron-rich meal. The intake of these two minerals should be separated as much as possible. This is particularly critical in young menstruating women who need the iron, and calcium can be detrimental with the absorption of iron.

2010 Dietary Guidelines for Americans

The secretaries of the U.S. Department of Health and Human Services and the USDA appoint an expert Dietary Guidelines Advisory Committee every five years to issue a report and make recommendations concerning U.S. dietary guidelines. The guidelines should be used as a goal to help people achieve a healthier life.

The *Dietary Guidelines for Americans 2010* are intended for healthy people two years and older. Due to the dramatic increase in obesity, eating and physical activity patterns focused on consuming fewer calories, making informed food choices, and being physically active are emphasized to help people attain and maintain a healthy weight, reduce their risk of chronic disease, and promote overall health. The improved recommendations give individuals the information necessary to make thoughtful choices of healthier foods in the right portions and complement those choices with physical activity. Two key concepts are emphasized in the 2010 guidelines:

- Balance calories with physical activity to sustain a healthy weight.
- Focus on consuming nutrient-dense foods and beverages. This includes greater consumption of certain foods and nutrients, such as fruits, vegetables, whole grains, fat-free and low-fat dairy products, and seafood, and decreased consumption of foods with saturated fats, trans fats, cholesterol, sodium (salt), refined grains, and added sugars.

The 2010 dietary guidelines include 20 key recommendations for the general population and 9 additional recommendations for specific population groups.[24] The recommendations are intended to help people choose an overall healthy diet.

Additional information on the following guidelines is posted at www.dietaryguidelines.gov.

Oligomenorrhea Irregular menstrual cycles.

Amenorrhea Cessation of regular menstrual flow.

Hemoglobin Protein-iron compound in red blood cells that transports oxygen in the blood.

Ferritin Iron stored in the body.

TABLE 3.15 Iron-Rich Foods

Food	Amount	Iron (mg)	Calories	% Calories from Fat
Beans, red kidney (cooked)	1 cup	3.2	218	4
Beef, ground lean (21% fat)	3 oz	2.1	237	57
Beef, sirloin, lean only	3 oz	2.9	171	36
Beef, liver (fried)	3 oz	5.3	184	33
Beet, greens (cooked)	½ cup	1.4	19	—
Broccoli (cooked, drained)	1 cup	1.3	44	—
Burrito, bean (no cheese)	1	2.3	225	28
Egg (hard-cooked)	1	.7	77	58
Farina (Cream of Wheat) (cooked)	½ cup	5.2	65	—
Instant Breakfast, nonfat milk	1 cup	4.8	216	4
Peas (frozen, cooked, drained)	½ cup	1.3	62	—
Shrimp (boiled)	3 oz	2.7	87	10
Spinach (raw)	1 cup	1.5	12	—
Vegetables, mixed (cooked)	1 cup	1.5	108	—

Specific Nutrition Recommendations in the *Dietary Guidelines for Americans 2010*

Increase consumption of

- Fruits and vegetables
- Whole grains
- Low-fat dairy products
- Various lean protein choices
- Seafood
- Healthy fats
- Foods high in fiber, calcium, potassium, and vitamin D

Decrease intake of

- Saturated fats
- Trans fats
- Dietary cholesterol
- Sodium
- Refined grains
- Alcohol

Balancing Calories to Manage Weight

1. Prevent and/or reduce overweightness and obesity through improved eating and physical activity behaviors.
2. Control total caloric intake to manage body weight. For people who are overweight or obese, this means consuming fewer calories from foods and beverages.
3. Increase physical activity and reduce time spent in sedentary behaviors.
4. Maintain appropriate caloric balance during each stage of life—childhood, adolescence, adulthood, pregnancy and breastfeeding, and older age.
5. Reduce daily sodium intake to less than 2,300 milligrams and further reduce intake to 1,500 milligrams among people who are 51 and older and those of any age who are African American or have hypertension, diabetes, or chronic kidney disease. The 1,500-milligram recommendation applies to about half of the U.S. population, including children and the majority of adults.
6. Consume less than 10 percent of calories from saturated fatty acids by replacing them with monounsaturated and polyunsaturated fatty acids.
7. Consume less than 300 milligrams per day of dietary cholesterol.
8. Keep trans-fatty acid consumption as low as possible by limiting foods that contain synthetic sources of trans fats, such as partially hydrogenated oils, and by limiting other solid fats.
9. Reduce intake of calories from solid fats and added sugars.
10. Limit consumption of foods that contain refined grains, especially refined-grain foods that contain solid fats, added sugars, and sodium.
11. If alcohol is consumed, it should be consumed in moderation—up to one drink per day for women and two drinks per day for men—and only by adults of legal drinking age.

Foods and Nutrients to Increase

Individuals should meet the following recommendations as part of a healthy eating pattern while staying within their caloric needs:

1. Increase vegetable and fruit intake.
2. Eat a variety of vegetables, especially dark-green, red, and orange vegetables; beans; and peas.
3. Consume at least half of all grains as whole grains. Increase whole-grain intake by replacing refined grains with whole grains.
4. Increase intake of fat-free or low-fat milk and milk products, such as milk, yogurt, cheese, or fortified soy beverages.
5. Choose a variety of protein foods, which include seafood, lean meat and poultry, eggs, beans and peas, soy products, and unsalted nuts and seeds.
6. Increase the amount and variety of seafood consumed by choosing seafood in place of some meat and poultry.
7. Replace protein foods that are higher in solid fats with choices that are lower in solid fats and calories and/or are sources of oils.
8. Use oils to replace solid fats where possible.
9. Choose foods that provide more potassium, dietary fiber, calcium, and vitamin D, which are nutrients of concern in American diets. These foods include vegetables, fruits, whole grains, and milk and milk products.

Recommendations for Specific Population Groups

Women Capable of Becoming Pregnant

1. Choose foods that supply heme iron, which is more readily absorbed by the body; additional iron sources; and enhancers of iron absorption such as vitamin C–rich foods.
2. Consume 400 mcg per day of synthetic folic acid (from fortified foods and/or supplements), in addition to food forms of folate from a varied diet.

Pregnant or Breastfeeding Women

1. Consume 8 to 12 ounces of seafood per week from a variety of seafood types.
2. Due to their high methyl mercury content, limit white (albacore) tuna to 6 ounces per week and do not eat the following four types of fish: tilefish, shark, swordfish, and king mackerel.
3. If pregnant, take an iron supplement as recommended by an obstetrician or other health care provider.

Individuals 50 Years and Older

- Consume foods fortified with vitamin B_{12}, such as fortified cereals, or dietary supplements.

Building Healthy Eating Patterns

1. Select an eating pattern that meets nutrient needs over time at an appropriate caloric level.
2. Account for all foods and beverages consumed and assess how they fit within a total healthy eating pattern.
3. Follow food safety recommendations when preparing and eating foods to reduce the risk of foodborne illnesses.

Additional information on these guidelines is posted at www.DietaryGuidelines.gov/

Proper Nutrition: A Lifetime Prescription for Healthy Living

The three factors that do the most for health, longevity, and quality of life are proper nutrition, a sound exercise program, and quitting (or never starting) smoking. Achieving and maintaining a balanced diet is not as difficult as most people think. If everyone were more educated about their nutrition habits and the nutrition habits of their children, the current magnitude of nutrition-related health problems would be smaller. Although treatment of obesity is important, we should place far greater emphasis on preventing obesity in youth and adults in the first place.

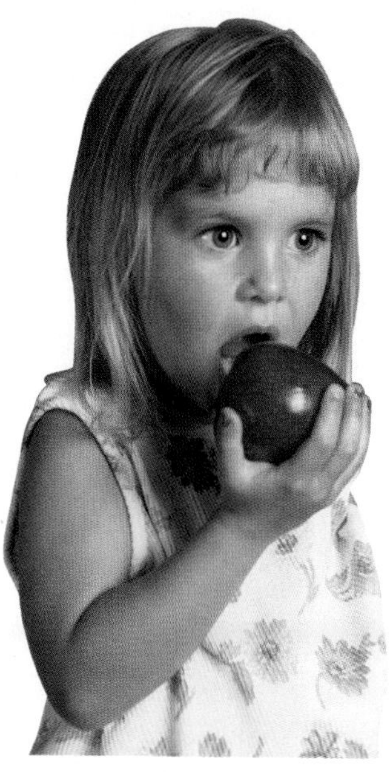

© Fitness & Wellness, Inc.

Positive nutrition habits should be taught and reinforced in early youth.

CRITICAL THINKING

What factors in your life and the environment have contributed to your current dietary habits? Do you need to make changes? What may prevent you from doing so?

Children tend to eat the way their parents do. If parents adopt a healthy diet, children most likely will follow. The difficult part for most people is to retrain themselves—starting by closely examining the eating habits they learned from their parents—to follow a lifetime healthy nutrition plan that includes lots of grains, legumes, fruits, vegetables, and low-fat dairy products, with moderate use of animal protein, junk food, sodium, and alcohol.

Despite the ample scientific evidence linking poor dietary habits to early disease and mortality rates, many people remain precontemplators: They are not willing to change their eating patterns. Even when faced with obesity, elevated blood lipids, hypertension, and other nutrition-related conditions, people do not change. The motivating factor to change personal eating habits seems to be a major health breakdown, such as a heart attack, a stroke, or cancer—by which time the damage has been done. In many cases it is irreversible and, for some, fatal.

An ounce of prevention is worth a pound of cure. The sooner you implement the dietary guidelines presented in this chapter, the better your chances of preventing chronic diseases and reaching a higher state of wellness.

ASSESS YOUR BEHAVIOR

CENGAGE brain .com To access course materials, including companion resources, please visit **www.cengagebrain.com**.

1. Are whole grains, fruits, and vegetables the staples of your diet? Have you considered actions to help you increase consumption of these foods?
2. Are you meeting your personal MyPlate recommendations for daily fruits, vegetables, grains, meat (or substitutes) and legumes, and milk? If not, what changes do you need to make?
3. Are there dietary changes that you feel you need to implement to meet energy, nutrition, and disease risk-reduction guidelines and improve health and wellness? If so, list these changes and indicate what it will take to make them happen.

ASSESS YOUR KNOWLEDGE

1. The science of nutrition studies the relationship of
   a. vitamins and minerals to health.
   b. foods to optimal health and performance.
   c. carbohydrates, fats, and proteins to the development and maintenance of good health.
   d. macronutrients and micronutrients to physical performance.
   e. kilocalories to calories in food items.
2. Faulty nutrition often plays a crucial role in the development and progression of which disease?
   a. cardiovascular disease
   b. cancer
   c. osteoporosis
   d. diabetes
   e. All of the choices are correct.

3. According to MyPlate, daily vegetable consumption is measured in
   a. servings.
   b. ounces.
   c. cups.
   d. calories.
   e. All of the choices are correct.

4. The recommended amount of fiber intake for adults 50 years and younger is
   a. 10 grams per day for women and 12 grams for men.
   b. 21 grams per day for women and 30 grams for men.
   c. 28 grams per day for women and 35 grams for men.
   d. 25 grams per day for women and 38 grams for men.
   e. 45 grams per day for women and 50 grams for men.

5. Unhealthy fats include
   a. unsaturated fatty acids.
   b. monounsaturated fats.
   c. polyunsaturated fatty acids.
   d. saturated fats.
   e. All of the choices are correct.

6. The daily recommended carbohydrate intake is
   a. 45 to 65 percent of total calories.
   b. 10 to 35 percent of total calories.
   c. 20 to 35 percent of total calories.
   d. 60 to 75 percent of total calories.
   e. 35 to 50 percent of total calories.

7. The amount of a nutrient that is estimated to meet the nutrient requirement of half the healthy people in specific age and gender groups is known as the
   a. Estimated Average Requirement.
   b. Recommended Dietary Allowance.
   c. Daily Value.
   d. Adequate Intake.
   e. Dietary Reference Intake.

8. The percentage of fat intake for an individual who on a given day consumes 2,385 calories with 106 grams of fat is
   a. 44 percent of total calories.
   b. 17.7 percent of total calories.
   c. 40 percent of total calories.
   d. 31 percent of total calories.
   e. 22.5 percent of total calories.

9. Carbohydrate loading is beneficial for
   a. endurance athletes.
   b. people with diabetes.
   c. strength athletes.
   d. sprinters.
   e. All of the choices are correct.

10. Osteoporosis is
   a. a crippling disease.
   b. more prevalent in women.
   c. more prevalent in people who were calcium deficient at a young age.
   d. linked to heavy drinking and smoking.
   e. All of the choices are correct.

Correct answers can be found at the back of the book.

NOTES

1. A. Park, F. Subar, A. Hollenbeck, and A. Schatzkin, "Dietary Fiber Intake and Mortality in the NIH-AARP Diet and Health Study," *Online Archives of Internal Medicine* (February 14, 2011).
2. National Academy of Sciences, Institute of Medicine, *Dietary Reference Intakes for Energy, Carbohydrates, Fiber, Fat, Protein and Amino Acids (Macronutrients)* (Washington, DC: National Academy Press, 2002).
3. "Saturated Fat: Not Quite so Bad After All?" *University of California at Berkeley Wellness Letter* 26, no. 6 (June 2010): 1–2.
4. J. N. Kiage, et al., "Intake of trans fat and all-cause mortality in the Reasons for Geographical and Racial Differences in Stroke (REGARDS) cohort," *The American Journal of Clinical Nutrition* 97 (2013): 1121–1128.
5. Editors of *Environmental Nutrition, Healthy Eating: Essential Information for Living Longer and Living Better* (Norwalk, CT: Belvoir Media Group, 2008).
6. J. L. Breslow, "n-3 Fatty Acids and Cardiovascular Disease," *American Journal of Clinical Nutrition* 83 (2006): 1477S–1482S.
7. P. E. Bowen, "Evaluating the Health Claim of Flaxseed and Cancer Prevention," *Nutrition Today* 36 (2001): 144–158; "Flax Facts," *University of California at Berkeley Wellness Letter* 18, no. 5 (May 2002): 1.
8. A. Pan, et al., "Red Meat Consumption and Mortality: Results from 2 Prospective Cohort Studies," *Archives of Internal Medicine* 172 (2012): 555–563.
9. S. Rohrmann, et al., "Meat Consumption and Mortality—Results from the European prospective Investigation into Cancer and Nutrition," *BMC Medicine* 11(2013): 63. doi:10.1186/1741-7015-11-63
10. A. Pan, et al., "Changes in Red Meat Consumption and Subsequent Risk of Type 2 Diabetes Mellitus," *Journal of the American Medical Association Internal Medicine* 173 (2013): 1328–1335.
11. See note 2.
12. Y. Bau, et al., "Association of nut consumption with total and cause-specific mortality," *New England Journal of Medicine* 369 (2013): 2001–2011.
13. "Soy and Breast Cancer," *University of California at Berkeley Wellness Letter* 23, no. 6 (June 2007): 1–2.
14. A. Trichopoulou et al., "Adherence to a Mediterranean Diet and Survival in a Greek Population," *New England Journal of Medicine* 348 (2003): 2599–2608.
15. R. Estrutch, "Primary Prevention of Cardiovascular Disease with a Mediterranean Diet," *New England Journal of Medicine* 368 (2013): 1279–1290.
16. G. Kojda and R. Hambrecht, "Molecular Mechanism of Vascular Adaptations to Exercise: Physical Activity as an Effective Antioxidant Therapy?" *Cardiovascular Research* 67 (2005): 187–197.
17. G. Bjelakovic et al., "Mortality in Randomized Trials of Antioxidant Supplements for Primary and Secondary Prevention," *Journal*

of the American Medical Association 297 (2007): 842–857.

18. S. Saverio et al., "Effects of Long-Term Selenium Supplementation on the Incidence of Type 2 Diabetes: A Randomized Trial," *Annals of Internal Medicine* 147 (2007): 217–223.

19. M. L. Neuhouser et al., "Multivitamin Use and Risk of Cancer and Cardiovascular Disease in the Women's Health Initiative Cohorts," *Archives of Internal Medicine* 169 (2009): 294–304.

20. H. Wright, "Vitamin D May Help You Dodge Cancer: How to Be Sure You Get Enough," *Environmental Nutrition* 30, no. 6 (2007): 1, 4.

21. Vitamin D Council, "Understanding Vitamin D Cholecalciferol," http://www.vitamindcouncil.org, downloaded June 19, 2009.

22. American Dietetic Association, "Position of the American Dietetic Association: Nutrient Supplementation," *Journal of the American Dietetic Association* 109 (2009): 2073–2085.

23. Writing Group for the Women's Health Initiative, "Risks and Benefits of Combined Estrogen and Progestin in Healthy Postmenopausal Women: Principal Results from the Women's Health Initiative Randomized Controlled Trial," *Journal of the American Medical Association* 288 (2002): 321–333.

24. U.S. Department of Health and Human Services and U.S. Department of Agriculture, *Dietary Guidelines for Americans 2010* (Washington, DC: U.S. Government Printing Office, 2010).

SUGGESTED READINGS

Clark, N. *Nancy Clark's Sports Nutrition Guidebook.* Champaign, IL: Human Kinetics, 2014.

McArdle, W. D., F. I. Katch, and V. L. Katch. *Sports & Exercise Nutrition.* Baltimore: Lippincott Williams & Wilkins, 2012.

National Academy of Sciences, Institute of Medicine. *Dietary Reference Intakes for Energy, Carbohydrates, Fiber, Fat, Protein and Amino Acids (Macronutrients).* Washington, DC: National Academy Press, 2002.

Rolfes, S. R., K. Pinna, and E. N. Whitney. *Understanding Normal and Clinical Nutrition.* Belmont, CA: Wadsworth/Cengage Learning, 2015.

Sizer, F. S., and E. N. Whitney. *Nutrition: Concepts and Controversies.* Belmont, CA: Wadsworth/Cengage Learning, 2014.

Whitney, E. N., and S. R. Rolfes. *Understanding Nutrition.* Belmont, CA: Wadsworth/Cengage Learning, 2013.

Lab 3A: Nutrient Analysis

Name ______________________ Date ____________ Grade ____________

Instructor ______________________ Course ____________ Section ____________

NECESSARY LAB EQUIPMENT

Appendix A (Nutritive Value of Selected Foods) and a small calculator.

OBJECTIVE

To evaluate your present diet using the Recommended Dietary Allowances (RDA).

INSTRUCTIONS

To conduct the nutrient analysis, record all the foods eaten during a 3-day period using the list of Nutritive Value of Selected Foods provided in Appendix A. Record this information prior to this lab session in the form provided in Figure 3A.1 (make additional copies for a 3-day record). After recording the nutritive values for each day, add up the values in each column and record the totals at the bottom of the form. During your lab, proceed to compute an average for the 3 days. The percentages of carbohydrates, fat, saturated fat, and the protein requirements can be computed by using the instructions at the bottom of Figure 3A.2. The results can then be compared against the Recommended Dietary Allowances.

FIGURE 3A.1 Daily nutrient intake

Foods	Amount	Calories	Protein (g)	Fat (total g)	Sat. Fat (g)	Cho-lesterol (mg)	Carbo-hydrates (g)	Dietary Fiber (g)	Calcium (mg)	Iron (mg)	Sodium (mg)	Vit. E (mg)	Folate (mcg)	Vit. C (mg)	Selenium (mcg)
Totals															

FIGURE 3A.2 Daily nutrient intake

Day	Calories	Protein (g)	Fat (g)	Sat. Fat (g)	Cho-lesterol (mg)	Carbo-hydrates (g)	Dietary Fiber (g)	Calcium (mg)	Iron (mg)	Sodium (mg)	Vit. E (mg)	Folate (mcg)	Vit. C (mg)	Selenium (mcg)
One														
Two														
Three														
Totals														
Average[a]														
Percentages[b]														
Recommended Dietary Allowances*														
Men 14–18 yrs.	See below[c]	See below[d]	20–30%[e]	7%	<300	45–65%	38	1,300	12	2,300	15	400	75	55
19–30 yrs.	↓	↓	20–30%[e]	7%	<300	45–65%	38	1,000	10	2,300	15	400	90	55
31–50 yrs.	↓	↓	20–30%[e]	7%	<300	45–65%	38	1,000	10	2,300	15	400	90	55
51 + yrs.	↓	↓	20–30%[e]	7%	<300	45–65%	30	1,000	10	2,300	15	400	90	55
Women 14–18 yrs.	↓	↓	20–30%[e]	7%	<300	45–65%	25	1,300	15	2,300	15	400	65	55
19–30 yrs.	↓	↓	20–30%[e]	7%	<300	45–65%	25	1,000	15	2,300	15	400	75	55
31–50 yrs.	↓	↓	20–30%[e]	7%	<300	45–65%	25	1,000	15	2,300	15	400	75	55
51 + yrs.	↓	↓	20–30%[e]	7%	<300	45–65%	21	1,200	15	2,300	15	400	75	55
Pregnant	↓	↓	20–30%[e]	7%	<300	45–65%	25	1,200	30	2,300	15	600	85	60
Lactating	↓	↓	20–30%[e]	7%	<300	45–65%	25	1,200	15	2,300	15	500	120	70

[a] Divide totals by 3 or number of days assessed.
[b] Percentages: Protein and carbohydrates = multiply average by 4, divide by average calories, and multiply by 100.
Fat and saturated fat = multiply average by 9, divide by average calories, and multiply by 100.
[c] Use Table 5.5 (page 180) for all categories.
[d] Protein intake should be .8 grams per kilogram of body weight. Pregnant women should consume an additional 15 grams of daily protein, and lactating women should have an extra 20 grams.
[e] Based on recommendations by nutrition experts. Up to 35% is allowed for individuals who suffer from metabolic syndrome.
*Adapted from *Recommended Dietary Allowances,* 10th Edition, and the Dietary Reference Intakes series, National Academy Press, © National Academy of Sciences 1989, 1997, 1998, 2000, 2001. Washington, DC.

Lab 3B: MyPlate Record Form

Homework Assignment

Name ______________________ Date ____________ Grade ____________

Instructor ______________________ Course ____________ Section ____________

ASSIGNMENT
This laboratory experience should be carried out as a homework assignment to be completed over the next 7 days.

LAB RESOURCES Figure 3.1, page 82, and MyPlate at http://choosemyplate.gov.

OBJECTIVE
To meet the minimum daily required amounts of the basic food groups and monitor total daily fat intake.

INSTRUCTIONS
Go to www.choosemyplate.gov and select SuperTracker. Near the top right, click on Create Profile, type in the required information, and click Submit. Next, click on My Plan near the top left, and record your Daily Food Targets on the next page of this lab. Now, keep a 7-day record of your food consumption using the MyPlate guidelines. Whenever you have something to eat, record the food item, the number of calories, the grams of fat (use the Nutritive Value of Selected Foods list given in Appendix A), and the amounts eaten based on the MyPlate guidelines. If a particular food item is not listed in the Nutritive Value of Selected Foods list, the information can be obtained from the food container itself.

Record all information immediately after each meal, because it will be easier to keep track of foods and amounts eaten. If twice the amount of a particular serving is eaten, the calories, grams of fat, and amounts must be doubled as well.

At the end of the day, evaluate the diet by checking whether the minimum required amounts for each food group were met, and by total amount of calories and fat consumed. If you meet the required food group amounts and your daily caloric intake recommendation, you are well on your way to achieving a well-balanced diet. In addition, fat intake should not exceed 30 percent of the daily caloric consumption (may be up to 35 percent for individuals who suffer from metabolic syndrome—see Table 3.7, page 94). If you are on a diet, you may want to reduce fat intake to less than 20 percent of total daily calories (see Table 5.5, page 193).

I. Nutrition Stage of Change

Using Figure 2.6 (page 66) and Table 2.3 (page 65) identify your current stage of change for nutrition (healthy diet):

[ ]

II. What I Learned and What I Can Do to Improve My Nutrition:

Based on the nutrient analysis conducted in Lab 3A and your daily diet analysis conducted in this lab, explain what these experiences have taught you and list specific changes and strategies that you can use to improve your present nutrition habits. Use an extra blank sheet of paper as needed.

I have learned the following about myself/my current diet: ______________________

____

Specific changes I plan to make: ______________________

____

Strategies I will use: ______________________

____

III. Current number of daily steps: [ ]

Category (Use Table 1.2, page 12): ______________________

Name: ______________________ Date: __________

Course: __________ Section: __________ Gender: __________ Age: ______

No.	Food*	Calories	Fat (gm)	Food Groups Daily Goals (see Figure 3.1)					
				Grains (oz.)	Vegetables (cups)	Fruits (cups)	Dairy (cups)	Protein Foods (oz.)	Oils (tsp.)
1									
2									
3									
4									
5									
6									
7									
8									
9									
10									
11									
12									
13									
14									
15									
16									
17									
18									
19									
20									
21									
22									
23									
24									
25									
26									
27									
28									
29									
30									
Totals									
Recommended Amount: Obtain online at www.choosemyplate.gov based on age, gender, weight, height, and activity level			**						
Deficiencies/Excesses									

*See "List of Nutritive Value of Selected Foods" in Appendix A.

**Multiply the recommended amount of calories by .30 (30%) and divide by 9 to obtain the daily recommended amount of grams of fat.

4

Body Composition

Achieving recommended body weight improves health parameters, but most importantly, it improves quality of life by allowing you to pursue tasks of daily living along with leisure and recreational activities without functional limitations.

OBJECTIVES

- Define body composition and understand its relationship to assessment of recommended body weight.
- Explain the difference between essential fat and storage fat.
- Describe various techniques used to assess body composition.
- Be able to assess body composition using skinfold thickness and girth measurements.
- Understand the importance of body mass index (BMI), waist-to-height ratio (WHtR), and waist circumference (WC) in the assessment of risk for disease.
- Be able to determine recommended weight according to recommended percent body fat values and BMI.

CENGAGEbrain.com

Visit **www.cengagebrain.com** to access course materials and companion resources for this text, including digital labs, quiz questions designed to check your understanding of the chapter contents, and more! See the preface on page xii for more information.

REAL LIFE STORY | Camille's Experience

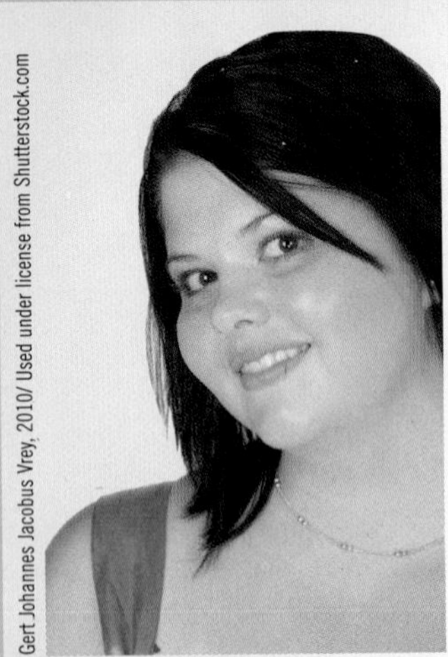

Gert Johannes Jacobus Vrey, 2010/ Used under license from Shutterstock.com

I took the Fit for Life class at my school only because it was required. For someone who was dramatically overweight, I thought the class would just make me feel bad about how unfit I was. When I heard that we were all going to do body composition testing, I wanted to cry. I really didn't want to know what my body composition was. I had been avoiding even getting onto a scale, but to actually assess my body composition was even worse—it meant that I couldn't just excuse it all away by saying, I'm big boned! However, now that I look back on it, the body composition assessment we did in that class was actually what jump-started my journey toward fitness. We took our skinfold measurements and used those numbers to calculate our percent body fat. Then we also calculated our recommended body weight. So finally, after hiding from knowing my weight for so long and just trying to ignore the issue, I now had really specific information about where I was and how far I needed to go to get to a healthy weight. It was hard for me to hear how high my current body fat was, but I did feel that it was a breakthrough for me to be brave enough to even find out. So armed with that momentum, and with the specific information on exactly how much weight I needed to lose, I began to make a plan for change. I had a specific goal, and the ability to measure my progress. As the class went on, I followed the advice that I learned, began an exercise program, and made changes to what I ate. Now, a year and a half later, I have lost about fifty pounds, and I am continuing to lose weight. I consider the body composition assessment the first step of my weight management process, because before you go on a journey, it helps to know where you are starting from, and where you want to go!

MyProfile: Personal Body Composition Profile

Please answer the following questions to the best of your ability. If you cannot answer all of them at this time, you will be able to do so as you work through the chapter contents.

I. Do you understand the concept of body composition and its relationship to recommended body weight, proper weight management, and good health? ___ Yes ___ No

II. Current values

Body weight: _____ lbs
Percent body fat: _____% Classification: __________
Lean body mass: _____ lbs
Body Mass Index (BMI): ____________
Disease risk: ____________
Classification: ____________
Waist Circumference (WC): ____________
Disease risk: ____________
Classification: ____________

III. Goals for the end of the term:

Body weight: _____ lbs Percent body fat: _____%
BMI: _____ WC: _____

IV. Can you relate to Camille's experience and what can you do in your life to avoid the same pitfalls?

To understand the concept of **body composition**, we must recognize that the human body consists of fat and non-fat components. The fat component is called fat mass or **percent body fat**. The non-fat component is termed **lean body mass.**

To determine **recommended body weight**, we need to find out what percent of total body weight is fat and what amount is lean tissue; in other words, assess body composition. Body composition should be assessed by a well-trained technician who understands the procedure being used.

Once the fat percentage is known, recommended body weight can be calculated from recommended body fat. Rec-

Body composition The fat and non-fat components of the human body; important in assessing recommended body weight.

Percent body fat Proportional amount of fat in the body based on the person's total weight; includes both essential fat and storage fat; also termed fat mass.

Lean body mass Body weight without body fat.

Recommended body weight Body weight at which there seems to be no harm to human health; healthy weight.

FAQ

What constitutes ideal body weight?

There is no such thing as ideal body weight. Health/fitness professionals prefer to use the terms recommended or healthy body weight. Let's examine the question in more detail. For instance, 25 percent body fat is the recommended health fitness standard for a 40-year-old man. For the average apparently healthy individual, this body fat percentage does not constitute a threat to good health. Due to genetic and lifestyle conditions, however, if a person this same age at 25 percent body fat is prediabetic, prehypertensive, and with abnormal blood lipids (cholesterol and triglycerides—see Chapter 10), weight (fat) loss and a lower percent body fat may be recommended. Thus, what will work as recommended weight for most individuals may not be the best standard for individuals with disease risk factors. The current recommended or healthy weight standards (based on percent body fat or BMI) are established at the point where there appears to be a lower incidence for overweight-related conditions for most people. Individual differences have to be taken into consideration when making a final recommendation, especially in people with risk factors or a personal and family history of chronic conditions.

How accurate are body composition assessments?

Most of the techniques to determine body composition require proper training on the part of the technician administering the test (skinfolds, hydrostatic weighing, DXA) and, in the case of hydrostatic weighing, proper performance on the part of the person being tested. As detailed in this chapter, body composition assessment is not a precise science. Some of the procedures are more accurate than others. Before undergoing body composition testing, make sure that you understand the accuracy of the technique (see standard error of estimates [SEEs] included under the description of each technique); and even more important, inquire about the training and experience of the person administering the test. We often encounter individuals who have been tested elsewhere by any number of assessments, particularly skinfolds, who come to our laboratory in disbelief (and rightfully so) because of the results that were given to them. To obtain the best possible results, look for trained and experienced technicians.

Is there a future trend in body composition assessment?

Data indicate that the area of the body where people store fat is more critical than how much is stored. Individuals with a higher amount of intra-abdominal or abdominal visceral fat (located around internal organs), as opposed to primarily abdominal subcutaneous fat (fat stored directly beneath the skin), are at greater risk for disease. Thus, to increase disease risk evaluation, future body composition tests will be designed to get a clearer view of where the abdominal fat lies.

Additionally, although not body composition assessments, metrics such as body mass index (BMI), waist circumference (WC), and waist-to-height ratio (WHtR) are simple and free to measure and are an excellent starting point for detecting disease risk as well as thinness and excessive fatness in an individual (see Metrics Used to Determine Recommended Body Weight, page 148). The latest research has found that using these indicators in conjunction with one another offers a better picture of individual health. Researchers are suggesting that recording abdominal girth along with height and weight become a routine part of every healthcare visit, and that worldwide guidelines be developed for evaluating abdominal girth within an individual's BMI category. That way both overall weight and distribution of that weight will be accounted for. Guidelines may also better accommodate individual differences by adding adjustments for age, gender, physical activity patterns, and possibly ethnicity. For example, BMIs of 25 or greater are not accurate predictors of excessive fatness in younger people and in athletic populations or in people who are quite physically active. Furthermore, because of differences in essential fat between men and women, the same standard may not apply for both genders alike.

ommended body weight, also called healthy weight, implies the absence of any medical condition that would improve with weight loss and a fat distribution pattern that is not associated with higher risk for illness.

Formerly, people relied on simple height/weight charts to determine their recommended body weight, but these tables can be highly inaccurate and fail to identify critical fat values associated with higher risk for disease. Standard height/weight tables, first published in 1912, were based on average weights (including shoes and clothing) for men and women who obtained life insurance policies between 1888 and 1905—a notably unrepresentative population. The recommended body weight on these tables was obtained according to gender, height, and frame size. Because no scientific guidelines were given to determine frame size, most people chose their frame size based on the column in which the weight came closest to their own!

The best way to determine whether people are truly **overweight** or falsely at recommended body weight is through assessment of body composition. **Obesity** is an excess of body fat. If body weight is the only criterion, an individual might easily appear to be overweight according to height/weight charts, yet not have too much body fat. Typical examples are football players, body builders, weight lifters, and other athletes with large muscle size. Some athletes who appear to be 20 or 30 pounds overweight really have little body fat.

The inaccuracy of height/weight charts was illustrated clearly when a young man who weighed about 225 pounds applied to join a city police force but was turned down without having been granted an interview. The reason? He was too fat, according to the height/weight charts. When this young man's body composition was assessed at a preventive medicine clinic, it was determined that only 5 percent of his total body weight was in the form of fat—considerably less than the recommended standard. In the words of the director of the clinic, "The only way this fellow could come down to the chart's target weight would have been through surgical removal of a large amount of his muscle tissue."

At the other end of the spectrum, some people who weigh very little (and may be viewed as skinny or underweight) actually can be classified as overweight because of their high body fat content. People who weigh as little as 120 pounds but are more than 30 percent fat (about one-third of their total body weight) are not rare. These cases are found more readily in the sedentary population and among people who are always dieting. Physical inactivity and a constant negative caloric balance both lead to a loss in lean body mass (see Chapter 5). These examples illustrate that body weight alone clearly does not tell the whole story.

Essential and Storage Fat

Total fat in the human body is classified into two types: **essential fat** and **storage fat**. Essential fat is needed for normal physiological function. Without it, human health and physical performance deteriorate. This type of fat is found within tissues such as muscles, nerve cells, bone marrow, intestines, heart, liver, and lungs. Essential fat constitutes about 3 percent of the total weight in men and 12 percent in women (see Figure 4.1). The percentage is higher in women because it includes sex-specific fat, such as that found in the breast tissue, the uterus, and other sex-related fat deposits.

Storage fat is the fat stored in adipose tissue, mostly just beneath the skin (subcutaneous fat) and around major organs in the body (visceral fat). This fat serves three basic functions:

1. As an insulator to retain body heat
2. As energy substrate for metabolism
3. As padding against physical trauma to the body

FIGURE 4.1 Typical body composition of an adult man and an adult woman.

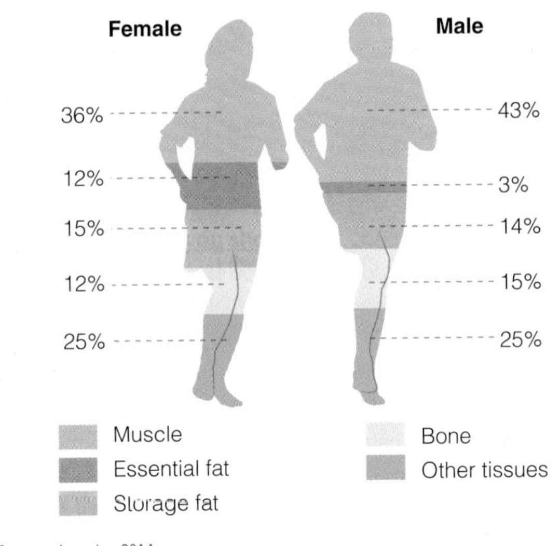

The amount of storage fat does not differ between men and women, except that men tend to store fat around the waist and women around the hips and thighs.

Techniques to Assess Body Composition

Body composition can be estimated through the several procedures described in the following pages. Each procedure includes a standard error of estimate (SEE), a measure of the accuracy of the prediction made through the regression equation for that specific technique. For example, if the SEE for a given technique is ±3.0 percent and the individual tests at a fat percentage of 18.0, the actual fat percentage may range from 15 to 21 percent.

Dual Energy X-ray Absorptiometry

Dual energy x-ray absorptiometry (DXA) is a method to assess body composition that is used most frequently in research and by medical facilities. A radiographic technique, DXA uses very low-dose beams of x-ray energy (hundreds of times lower than a typical body x-ray) to measure total body fat mass, fat distribution pattern (see "Waist Circumference" on page 150), and bone density. Bone density is measured to assess the risk for osteoporosis. The procedure itself is simple and takes less than 15 minutes to administer. Many exercise scientists consider DXA to be the standard technique to assess body composition. The SEE for this technique is ±1.8 percent.

Due to costs, DXA is not readily available to most fitness participants. Thus, other methods to estimate body composition are used. The most common of these follow:

1. Hydrostatic or underwater weighing
2. Air displacement
3. Skinfold thickness

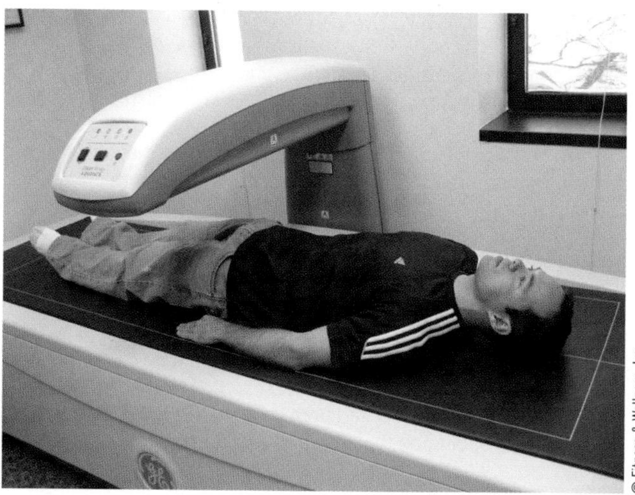

The dual energy x-ray absorptiometry (DXA) technique is used to assess body composition and bone density.

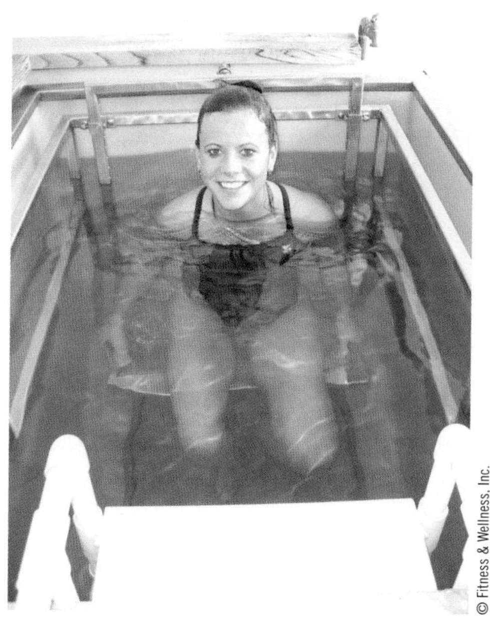

Hydrostatic or underwater weighing technique.

4. Girth measurements
5. Bioelectrical impedance

Because these procedures yield estimates of body fat, each technique may yield slightly different values. Therefore, when assessing changes in body composition, be sure to use the same technique for pre- and post-test comparisons.

The most accurate technique presently available in fitness laboratories is still hydrostatic weighing. Other techniques to assess body composition are available, but the equipment is costly and not easily accessible to the general population. In addition to percentages of lean tissue and body fat, some of these methods also provide information on total body water and bone mass. These techniques include air displacement, magnetic resonance imaging (MRI), computed tomography (CT), and total body electrical conductivity (TOBEC). In terms of predicting percent body fat, these techniques are not more accurate than hydrostatic weighing.

Hydrostatic Weighing For decades, **hydrostatic weighing** has been the most common technique used in determining body composition in exercise physiology laboratories. In essence, a person's "regular" weight is compared with a weight taken underwater. Because fat is more buoyant than lean tissue, comparing the two weights can determine a person's percent of fat. Almost all other indirect techniques to assess body composition have been validated against hydrostatic weighing. The procedure requires a considerable amount of time, skill, space, and equipment and must be administered by a well-trained technician. The SEE for hydrostatic weighing is ±0.5 percent.

This technique has several drawbacks. First, because each individual assessment can take as long as 30 minutes, hydrostatic weighing is not feasible when testing a lot of people. Furthermore, the person's residual lung volume (amount of air left in the lungs following complete forceful exhalation) should be measured before testing. If residual volume cannot be measured, as is the case in some laboratories and health/fitness centers, it is estimated using the predicting equations—which may decrease the accuracy of hydrostatic weighing. Also, the requirement of being completely under water makes hydrostatic weighing difficult to administer to **aquaphobic** people. For accurate results, the individual must be able to perform the test properly.

As described in Figure 4.2 and in Lab 4A, for each underwater weighing trial, the person has to (a) force out all of the air in the lungs, (b) lean forward and completely submerge underwater for about 5 to 10 seconds (long enough to get the underwater weight), and (c) remain as calm as possible (chair movement makes

Overweight An excess amount of weight against a given standard, such as height or recommended percent body fat.

Obesity An excessive accumulation of body fat, usually at least 30 percent above recommended body weight.

Essential fat Minimal amount of body fat needed for normal physiological functions; constitutes about 3 percent of total weight in men and 12 percent in women.

Storage fat Body fat in excess of essential fat; stored in adipose tissue.

Dual energy x-ray absorptiometry (DXA) Method to assess body composition that uses very low-dose beams of x-ray energy to measure total body fat mass, fat distribution pattern, and bone density.

Hydrostatic weighing Underwater technique to assess body composition; considered the most accurate of the body composition assessment techniques.

Aquaphobic Having a fear of water.

FIGURE 4.2 Hydrostatic weighing procedure.

A small tank or pool, an autopsy scale, and a submersible chair are needed. The scale should measure up to about 10 kilograms (kg) and should be readable to the nearest .01 kilogram. The chair is suspended from the scale and submerged in a tank of water or pool measuring at least 5 × 5 × 5 feet. A swimming pool can be used in place of the tank.

The procedure for the technician is

1. Ask the person to be weighed to fast for approximately 6 to 8 hours and to have a bladder and bowel movement prior to underwater weighing.

2. Measure the individual's residual lung volume (RV, or amount of air left in the lungs following complete exhalation). If no equipment (spirometer) is available to measure the residual volume, estimate it using the following predicting equations* (to convert inches to centimeters, multiply inches by 2.54):

   Men: $RV = [(0.027 \times \text{height in centimeters}) + (0.017 \times \text{age})] - 3.447$

   Women: $RV = [(0.032 \times \text{height in centimeters}) + (0.009 \times \text{age})] - 3.9$

3. Have the person remove all jewelry prior to weighing. Weigh the person on land in a swimsuit and subtract the weight of the suit. Convert the weight from pounds to kilograms (divide pounds by 2.2046).

4. Record the water temperature in the tank in degrees centigrade. Use that temperature to obtain the water density factor provided below, which is required in the formula to compute body density.

Temp (°C)	Water Density (g/ml)	Temp (°C)	Water Density (g/ml)
28	0.99626	35	0.99406
29	0.99595	36	0.99371
30	0.99567	37	0.99336
31	0.99537	38	0.99299
32	0.99505	39	0.99262
33	0.99473	40	0.99224
34	0.99440		

5. After the person is dressed in the swimsuit, have him or her enter the tank and completely wipe off all air clinging to the skin. Have the person sit in the chair with the water at about chin level (raise or lower the chair as needed). If you do not have a system that uses computerized electronic sensors, make sure the water and scale remain as still as possible during the entire procedure, because this allows for a more accurate reading. (During underwater weighing, you can decrease scale movement by holding and slowly releasing the neck of the scale until the subject is floating freely in the water.)

6. Now have the person forcefully exhale all of the air out of the lungs. The individual then totally submerges underwater. Make sure that all the air is exhaled from the lungs prior to submerging. Record the reading on the scale. Repeat this procedure 8 to 10 times, because practice and experience increase the accuracy of the underwater weight. Use the average of the three heaviest underwater weights as the gross underwater weight.

7. Because tare weight (the weight of the chair and chain or rope used to suspend the chair) accounts for part of the gross underwater weight, subtract this weight to obtain the person's net underwater weight. To determine tare weight, place a clothespin on the chain or rope at the water level when the person is submerged completely. After the person comes out of the water, lower the chair into the water to the pin level. Now record tare weight. Determine the net underwater weight by subtracting the tare weight from the gross underwater weight.

8. Compute body density and percent fat using the following equations:

$$\text{Body density} = \frac{BW}{\frac{BW - UW}{WD} - RV - .1}$$

$$\text{Percent fat}^{**} = \frac{495}{BD} - 450$$

Where:
BW = body weight in kg
UW = net underwater weight
WD = water density (determined by water temperature)
RV = residual volume
BD = body density

A sample computation for body fat assessment according to hydrostatic weighing is provided in Lab 4A.

*From H. L. Goldman and M. R. Becklake, "Respiratory Function Tests: Normal Values at Medium Altitudes and the Prediction of Normal Results," *American Review of Tuberculosis* 79 (1959): 457–467.
**From W. E. Siri, *Body Composition from Fluid Spaces and Density* (Berkeley, CA: University of California, Donner Laboratory of Medical Physics, March 19, 1956).

reading the scale difficult). This procedure is repeated 8 to 10 times.

Forcing all of the air out of the lungs is not easy for everyone but is important to obtain an accurate reading. Leaving additional air (beyond residual volume) in the lungs makes a person more buoyant. Because fat is less dense than water, overweight individuals weigh less in water. Additional air in the lungs makes a person lighter in water, yielding a false, higher body fat percentage.

Air Displacement **Air displacement** (also known as air displacement plethysmography) is a technique that holds considerable promise. With this method, an individual sits inside a small chamber, commercially known as the **Bod Pod.** Computerized pressure sensors determine the amount of air displaced by the person inside the chamber. Body volume is calculated by subtracting the air volume with the person inside the chamber from the volume of the empty chamber. The amount of air in the person's lungs also is taken into consideration when determining the actual body volume. Body density and percent body fat then are calculated from the obtained body volume.

The procedure to assess body composition according to air displacement takes only about 15 minutes. Initial re-

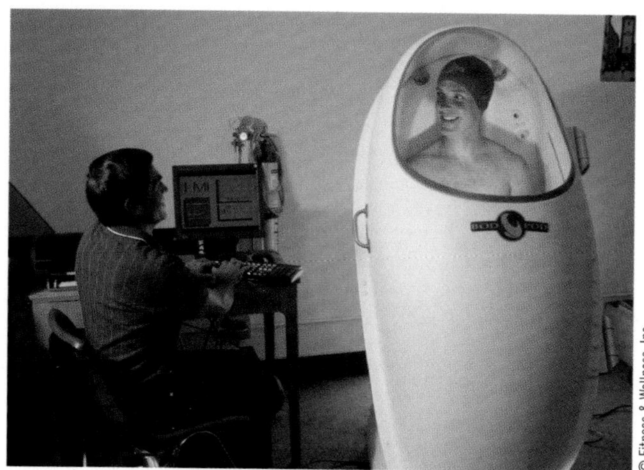

© Fitness & Wellness, Inc.

Bod Pod used for assessment of body composition.

FIGURE 4.3 **Anatomical landmarks for skinfold measurements.**

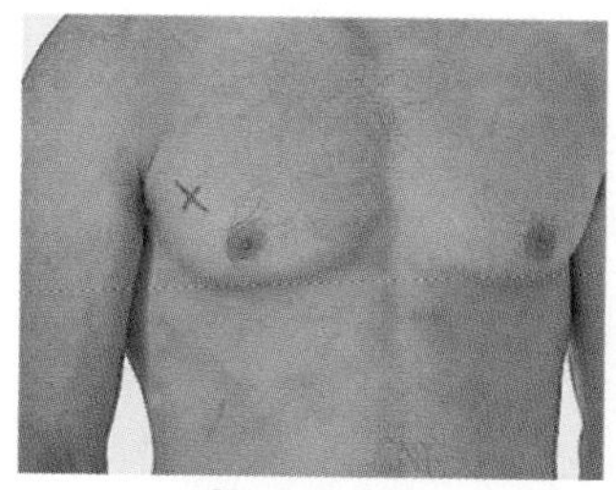

Chest (men)

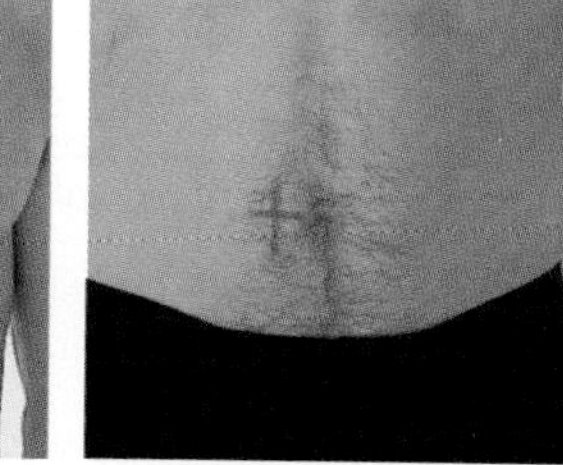

Abdomen (men)

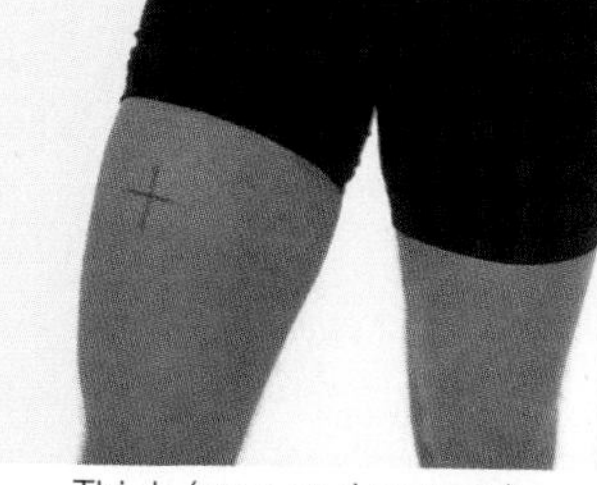

Thigh (men and women)

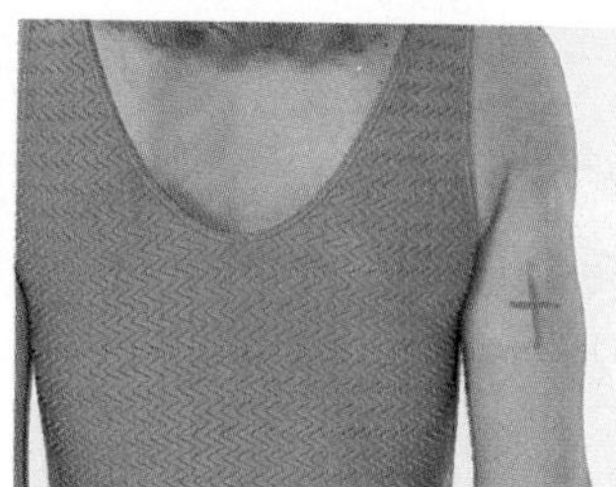

Triceps (women)

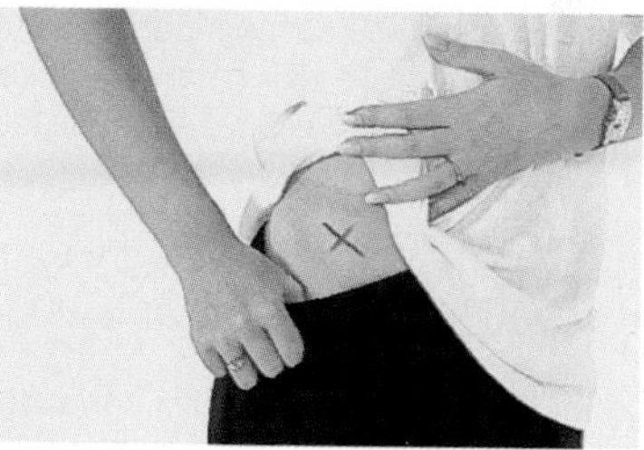

Suprailium (women)

Photos © Fitness & Wellness, Inc.

search showed that this technique compared favorably with hydrostatic weighing, and it is less cumbersome to administer. The published SEE for air displacement as compared with hydrostatic weighing was approximately ±2.2 percent; however, the SEE may actually be higher. Recent research has determined that percent body fat is about 5 percentage points higher with air displacement as compared to hydrostatic weighing.[1] The strong positive correlations found between the two techniques are due to the fact that air displacement consistently overestimates percent body fat. The researchers concluded that further technical work is required to make air displacement an acceptable technique to determine body composition. Other investigators have also found this method to overestimate percent body fat.[2] Furthermore, research is required to determine its accuracy among different age groups, ethnic backgrounds, and athletic populations. At present, the Bod Pod is not readily available in most fitness centers and exercise laboratories.

Skinfold Thickness Because of the cost, time, and complexity of hydrostatic weighing and the expense of Bod Pod equipment, most health and fitness programs use **anthropometric measurement** techniques. These techniques, primarily skinfold thickness and girth measurements, allow quick, simple, and inexpensive estimates of body composition.

Assessing body composition using **skinfold thickness** is based on the principle that the amount of **subcutaneous fat** is proportional to total body fat. Valid and reliable measurements of this tissue give a good indication of percent body fat. The SEE for skinfold analysis is ±3.5 percent.

The skinfold test is done with the aid of pressure calipers. Several techniques requiring measurement of three to seven sites have been developed. The following three-site procedure is the most commonly used technique. The sites measured are as follows (also see Figure 4.3):

Women: triceps, suprailium, and thigh skinfolds

Men: chest, abdomen, and thigh

All measurements should be taken on the right side of the body (see Figure 4.4).

With the skinfold technique, training is necessary to obtain accurate measurements. In addition, different technicians may produce slightly different measurements of the same person. Therefore, the same technician should take pre- and post-test measurements.

Measurements should be done at the same time of the day—preferably in the morning—because changes in water hydration from activity

Air displacement Technique to assess body composition by calculating the body volume from the air replaced by an individual sitting inside a small chamber.

Bod Pod Commercial name of the equipment used to assess body composition through the air displacement technique.

Anthropometric measurement Techniques to measure body girths at different sites.

Skinfold thickness Technique to assess body composition by measuring a double thickness of skin at specific body sites.

Subcutaneous fat Deposits of fat directly under the skin.

FIGURE 4.4 Procedure for body fat assessment using the skinfold thickness technique.

1. Select the proper anatomical sites. For men, use chest, abdomen, and thigh skinfolds. For women, use triceps, suprailium, and thigh skinfolds. Take all measurements on the right side of the body with the person standing. The correct anatomical landmarks for skinfolds are

Chest:	a diagonal fold halfway between the shoulder crease and the nipple.
Abdomen:	a vertical fold taken about one inch to the right of the umbilicus.
Triceps:	a vertical fold on the back of the upper arm, halfway between the shoulder and the elbow.
Thigh:	a vertical fold on the front of the thigh, midway between the knee and the hip.
Suprailium:	a diagonal fold above the crest of the ilium (on the side of the hip).

2. Measure each site by grasping a double thickness of skin firmly with the thumb and forefinger, pulling the fold slightly away from the muscular tissue. Hold the calipers perpendicular to the fold and take the measurement ½ inch below the finger hold. Measure each site three times and read the values to the nearest .1 to .5 mm. Record the average of the two closest readings as the final value. Take the readings without delay to avoid excessive compression of the skinfold. Releasing and refolding the skinfold is required between readings.
3. When doing pre- and post-assessments, conduct the measurement at the same time of day. The best time is early in the morning to avoid hydration changes resulting from activity or exercise.
4. Obtain percent fat by adding the three skinfold measurements and looking up the respective values on Table 4.1 for women, Table 4.2 for men under age 40, and Table 4.3 for men over 40.

For example, if the skinfold measurements for an 18-year-old female are (a) triceps = 16, (b) suprailium = 4, and (c) thigh = 30 (total = 50), the percent body fat is 20.6%.

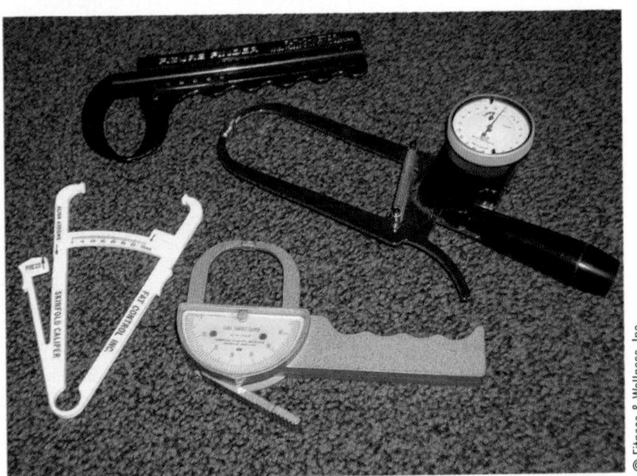

Various calipers used to assess skinfold thickness.

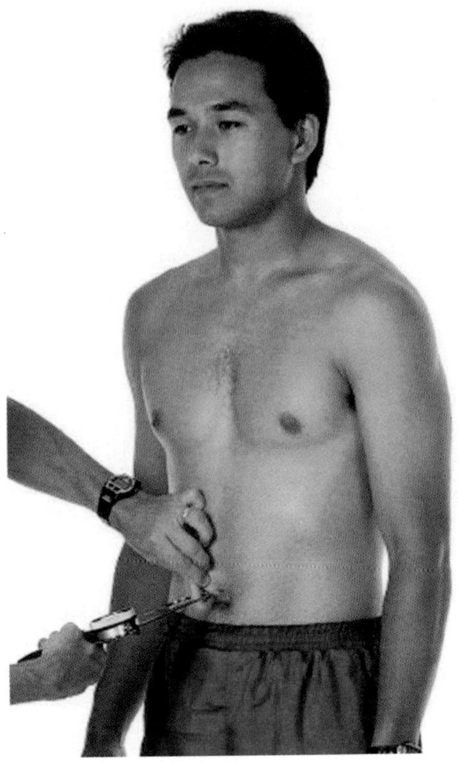

Skinfold thickness technique.

and exercise can affect skinfold girth. The procedure is given in Figure 4.4. If skinfold calipers are available, you may assess your percent body fat with the help of your instructor or an experienced technician (also see Lab 4A). Then locate the percent fat estimates in Table 4.1, 4.2, or 4.3, as appropriate.

Girth Measurements Another method that is frequently used to estimate body fat is to measure circumferences, or **girth measurements**, at various body sites. This technique requires only a standard measuring tape. The limitation is that it may not be valid for athletic individuals (men or women) who participate actively in strenuous physical activity or for people who can be classified visually as thin or obese. The SEE for girth measurements is approximately ±4 percent.

The required procedure for girth measurements is given in Figure 4.5; conversion factors are in Tables 4.4 and 4.5. Measurements for women are the upper arm, hip, and wrist; for men, the waist and wrist.

Bioelectrical Impedance The **bioelectrical impedance** technique is much simpler to administer, but its accuracy is questionable. In this

Girth measurements Technique to assess body composition by measuring circumferences at specific body sites.

Bioelectrical impedance Technique to assess body composition by running a weak electrical current through the body.

TABLE 4.1 Skinfold Thickness Technique: Percent Fat Estimates for Women Calculated from Triceps, Suprailium, and Thigh

	Age at Last Birthday								
Sum of 3 Skinfolds	22 or Under	23 to 27	28 to 32	33 to 37	38 to 42	43 to 47	48 to 52	53 to 57	58 and Over
23–25	9.7	9.9	10.2	10.4	10.7	10.9	11.2	11.4	11.7
26–28	11.0	11.2	11.5	11.7	12.0	12.3	12.5	12.7	13.0
29–31	12.3	12.5	12.8	13.0	13.3	13.5	13.8	14.0	14.3
32–34	13.6	13.8	14.0	14.3	14.5	14.8	15.0	15.3	15.5
35–37	14.8	15.0	15.3	15.5	15.8	16.0	16.3	16.5	16.8
38–40	16.0	16.3	16.5	16.7	17.0	17.2	17.5	17.7	18.0
41–43	17.2	17.4	17.7	17.9	18.2	18.4	18.7	18.9	19.2
44–46	18.3	18.6	18.8	19.1	19.3	19.6	19.8	20.1	20.3
47–49	19.5	19.7	20.0	20.2	20.5	20.7	21.0	21.2	21.5
50–52	20.6	20.8	21.1	21.3	21.6	21.8	22.1	22.3	22.6
53–55	21.7	21.9	22.1	22.4	22.6	22.9	23.1	23.4	23.6
56–58	22.7	23.0	23.2	23.4	23.7	23.9	24.2	24.4	24.7
59–61	23.7	24.0	24.2	24.5	24.7	25.0	25.2	25.5	25.7
62–64	24.7	25.0	25.2	25.5	25.7	26.0	26.2	26.4	26.7
65–67	25.7	25.9	26.2	26.4	26.7	26.9	27.2	27.4	27.7
68–70	26.6	26.9	27.1	27.4	27.6	27.9	28.1	28.4	28.6
71–73	27.5	27.8	28.0	28.3	28.5	28.8	29.0	29.3	29.5
74–76	28.4	28.7	28.9	29.2	29.4	29.7	29.9	30.2	30.4
77–79	29.3	29.5	29.8	30.0	30.3	30.5	30.8	31.0	31.3
80–82	30.1	30.4	30.6	30.9	31.1	31.4	31.6	31.9	32.1
83–85	30.9	31.2	31.4	31.7	31.9	32.2	32.4	32.7	32.9
86–88	31.7	32.0	32.2	32.5	32.7	32.9	33.2	33.4	33.7
89–91	32.5	32.7	33.0	33.2	33.5	33.7	33.9	34.2	34.4
92–94	33.2	33.4	33.7	33.9	34.2	34.4	34.7	34.9	35.2
95–97	33.9	34.1	34.4	34.6	34.9	35.1	35.4	35.6	35.9
98–100	34.6	34.8	35.1	35.3	35.5	35.8	36.0	36.3	36.5
101–103	35.2	35.4	35.7	35.9	36.2	36.4	36.7	36.9	37.2
104–106	35.8	36.1	36.3	36.6	36.8	37.1	37.3	37.5	37.8
107–109	36.4	36.7	36.9	37.1	37.4	37.6	37.9	38.1	38.4
110–112	37.0	37.2	37.5	37.7	38.0	38.2	38.5	38.7	38.9
113–115	37.5	37.8	38.0	38.2	38.5	38.7	39.0	39.2	39.5
116–118	38.0	38.3	38.5	38.8	39.0	39.3	39.5	39.7	40.0
119–121	38.5	38.7	39.0	39.2	39.5	39.7	40.0	40.2	40.5
122–124	39.0	39.2	39.4	39.7	39.9	40.2	40.4	40.7	40.9
125–127	39.4	39.6	39.9	40.1	40.4	40.6	40.9	41.1	41.4
128–130	39.8	40.0	40.3	40.5	40.8	41.0	41.3	41.5	41.8

Body density is calculated based on the generalized equation for predicting body density of women developed by A. S. Jackson, M. L. Pollock, and A. Ward and published in *Medicine and Science in Sports and Exercise* 12 (1980): 175–182. Percent body fat is determined from the calculated body density using the Siri formula.

technique, sensors are applied to the skin and a weak (totally painless) electrical current is run through the body to measure its electrical resistance which is then used to estimate body fat, lean body mass, and body water.

The technique is based on the principle that fat tissue is a less efficient conductor of electrical current than is lean

TABLE 4.2 Skinfold Thickness Technique: Percent Fat Estimates for Men Calculated from Chest, Abdomen, and Thigh

	Age at Last Birthday							
Sum of 3 Skinfolds	19 or Under	20 to 22	23 to 25	26 to 28	29 to 31	32 to 34	35 to 37	38 to 40
8–10	.9	1.3	1.6	2.0	2.3	2.7	3.0	3.3
11–13	1.9	2.3	2.6	3.0	3.3	3.7	4.0	4.3
14–16	2.9	3.3	3.6	3.9	4.3	4.6	5.0	5.3
17–19	3.9	4.2	4.6	4.9	5.3	5.6	6.0	6.3
20–22	4.8	5.2	5.5	5.9	6.2	6.6	6.9	7.3
23–25	5.8	6.2	6.5	6.8	7.2	7.5	7.9	8.2
26–28	6.8	7.1	7.5	7.8	8.1	8.5	8.8	9.2
29–31	7.7	8.0	8.4	8.7	9.1	9.4	9.8	10.1
32–34	8.6	9.0	9.3	9.7	10.0	10.4	10.7	11.1
35–37	9.5	9.9	10.2	10.6	10.9	11.3	11.6	12.0
38–40	10.5	10.8	11.2	11.5	11.8	12.2	12.5	12.9
41–43	11.4	11.7	12.1	12.4	12.7	13.1	13.4	13.8
44–46	12.2	12.6	12.9	13.3	13.6	14.0	14.3	14.7
47–49	13.1	13.5	13.8	14.2	14.5	14.9	15.2	15.5
50–52	14.0	14.3	14.7	15.0	15.4	15.7	16.1	16.4
53–55	14.8	15.2	15.5	15.9	16.2	16.6	16.9	17.3
56–58	15.7	16.0	16.4	16.7	17.1	17.4	17.8	18.1
59–61	16.5	16.9	17.2	17.6	17.9	18.3	18.6	19.0
62–64	17.4	17.7	18.1	18.4	18.8	19.1	19.4	19.8
65–67	18.2	18.5	18.9	19.2	19.6	19.9	20.3	20.6
68–70	19.0	19.3	19.7	20.0	20.4	20.7	21.1	21.4
71–73	19.8	20.1	20.5	20.8	21.2	21.5	21.9	22.2
74–76	20.6	20.9	21.3	21.6	22.0	22.2	22.7	23.0
77–79	21.4	21.7	22.1	22.4	22.8	23.1	23.4	23.8
80–82	22.1	22.5	22.8	23.2	23.5	23.9	24.2	24.6
83–85	22.9	23.2	23.6	23.9	24.3	24.6	25.0	25.3
86–88	23.6	24.0	24.3	24.7	25.0	25.4	25.7	26.1
89–91	24.4	24.7	25.1	25.4	25.8	26.1	26.5	26.8
92–94	25.1	25.5	25.8	26.2	26.5	26.9	27.2	27.5
95–97	25.8	26.2	26.5	26.9	27.2	27.6	27.9	28.3
98–100	26.6	26.9	27.3	27.6	27.9	28.3	28.6	29.0
101–103	27.3	27.6	28.0	28.3	28.6	29.0	29.3	29.7
104–106	27.9	28.3	28.6	29.0	29.3	29.7	30.0	30.4
107–109	28.6	29.0	29.3	29.7	30.0	30.4	30.7	31.1
110–112	29.3	29.6	30.0	30.3	30.7	31.0	31.4	31.7
113–115	30.0	30.3	30.7	31.0	31.3	31.7	32.0	32.4
116–118	30.6	31.0	31.3	31.6	32.0	32.3	32.7	33.0
119–121	31.3	31.6	32.0	32.3	32.6	33.0	33.3	33.7
122–124	31.9	32.2	32.6	32.9	33.3	33.6	34.0	34.3
125–127	32.5	32.9	33.2	33.5	33.9	34.2	34.6	34.9
128–130	33.1	33.5	33.8	34.2	34.5	34.9	35.2	35.5

Body density is calculated based on the generalized equation for predicting body density of men developed by A. S. Jackson, M. L. Pollock, and A. Ward and published in *British Journal of Nutrition* 40 (1978): 497–504. Percent body fat is determined from the calculated body density using the Siri formula.

TABLE 4.3 Skinfold Thickness Technique: Percent Fat Estimates for Men over 40 Calculated from Chest, Abdomen, and Thigh

	Age at Last Birthday							
Sum of 3 Skinfolds	41 to 43	44 to 46	47 to 49	50 to 52	53 to 55	56 to 58	59 to 61	62 and Over
8–10	3.7	4.0	4.4	4.7	5.1	5.4	5.8	6.1
11–13	4.7	5.0	5.4	5.7	6.1	6.4	6.8	7.1
14–16	5.7	6.0	6.4	6.7	7.1	7.4	7.8	8.1
17–19	6.7	7.0	7.4	7.7	8.1	8.4	8.7	9.1
20–22	7.6	8.0	8.3	8.7	9.0	9.4	9.7	10.1
23–25	8.6	8.9	9.3	9.6	10.0	10.3	10.7	11.0
26–28	9.5	9.9	10.2	10.6	10.9	11.3	11.6	12.0
29–31	10.5	10.8	11.2	11.5	11.9	12.2	12.6	12.9
32–34	11.4	11.8	12.1	12.4	12.8	13.1	13.5	13.8
35–37	12.3	12.7	13.0	13.4	13.7	14.1	14.4	14.8
38–40	13.2	13.6	13.9	14.3	14.6	15.0	15.3	15.7
41–43	14.1	14.5	14.8	15.2	15.5	15.9	16.2	16.6
44–46	15.0	15.4	15.7	16.1	16.4	16.8	17.1	17.5
47–49	15.9	16.2	16.6	16.9	17.3	17.6	18.0	18.3
50–52	16.8	17.1	17.5	17.8	18.2	18.5	18.8	19.2
53–55	17.6	18.0	18.3	18.7	19.0	19.4	19.7	20.1
56–58	18.5	18.8	19.2	19.5	19.9	20.2	20.6	20.9
59–61	19.3	19.7	20.0	20.4	20.7	21.0	21.4	21.7
62–64	20.1	20.5	20.8	21.2	21.5	21.9	22.2	22.6
65–67	21.0	21.3	21.7	22.0	22.4	22.7	23.0	23.4
68–70	21.8	22.1	22.5	22.8	23.2	23.5	23.9	24.2
71–73	22.6	22.9	23.3	23.6	24.0	24.3	24.7	25.0
74–76	23.4	23.7	24.1	24.4	24.8	25.1	25.4	25.8
77–79	24.1	24.5	24.8	25.2	25.5	25.9	26.2	26.6
80–82	24.9	25.3	25.6	26.0	26.3	26.6	27.0	27.3
83–85	25.7	26.0	26.4	26.7	27.1	27.4	27.8	28.1
86–88	26.4	26.8	27.1	27.5	27.8	28.2	28.5	28.9
89–91	27.2	27.5	27.9	28.2	28.6	28.9	29.2	29.6
92–94	27.9	28.2	28.6	28.9	29.3	29.6	30.0	30.3
95–97	28.6	29.0	29.3	29.7	30.0	30.4	30.7	31.1
98–100	29.3	29.7	30.0	30.4	30.7	31.1	31.4	31.8
101–103	30.0	30.4	30.7	31.1	31.4	31.8	32.1	32.5
104–106	30.7	31.1	31.4	31.8	32.1	32.5	32.8	33.2
107–109	31.4	31.8	32.1	32.4	32.8	33.1	33.5	33.8
110–112	32.1	32.4	32.8	33.1	33.5	33.8	34.2	34.5
113–115	32.7	33.1	33.4	33.8	34.1	34.5	34.8	35.2
116–118	33.4	33.7	34.1	34.4	34.8	35.1	35.5	35.8
119–121	34.0	34.4	34.7	35.1	35.4	35.8	36.1	36.5
122–124	34.7	35.0	35.4	35.7	36.1	36.4	36.7	37.1
125–127	35.3	35.6	36.0	36.3	36.7	37.0	37.4	37.7
128–130	35.9	36.2	36.6	36.9	37.3	37.6	38.0	38.5

Body density is calculated based on the generalized equation for predicting body density of men developed by A. S. Jackson, M. L. Pollock, and A. Ward and published in *British Journal of Nutrition* 40 (1978): 497–504. Percent body fat is determined from the calculated body density using the Siri formula.

TABLE 4.4 Girth Measurement Technique: Conversion Constants to Calculate Body Density for Women

Upper Arm (cm)	Constant A	Age (years)	Constant B	Hip (cm)	Constant C	Hip (cm)	Constant C	Wrist (cm)	Constant D
20.5	1.0966	17	.0086	79	.0957	114.5	.1388	13.0	.0819
21	1.0954	18	.0091	79.5	.0963	115	.1394	13.2	.0832
21.5	1.0942	19	.0096	80	.0970	115.5	.1400	13.4	.0845
22	1.0930	20	.0102	80.5	.0976	116	.1406	13.6	.0857
22.5	1.0919	21	.0107	81	.0982	116.5	.1412	13.8	.0870
23	1.0907	22	.0112	81.5	.0988	117	.1418	14.0	.0882
23.5	1.0895	23	.0117	82	.0994	117.5	.1424	14.2	.0895
24	1.0883	24	.0122	82.5	.1000	118	.1430	14.4	.0908
24.5	1.0871	25	.0127	83	.1006	118.5	.1436	14.6	.0920
25	1.0860	26	.0132	83.5	.1012	119	.1442	14.8	.0933
25.5	1.0848	27	.0137	84	.1018	119.5	.1448	15.0	.0946
26	1.0836	28	.0142	84.5	.1024	120	.1454	15.2	.0958
26.5	1.0824	29	.0147	85	.1030	120.5	.1460	15.4	.0971
27	1.0813	30	.0152	85.5	.1036	121	.1466	15.6	.0983
27.5	1.0801	31	.0157	86	.1042	121.5	.1472	15.8	.0996
28	1.0789	32	.0162	86.5	.1048	122	.1479	16.0	.1009
28.5	1.0777	33	.0168	87	.1054	122.5	.1485	16.2	.1021
29	1.0775	34	.0173	87.5	.1060	123	.1491	16.4	.1034
29.5	1.0754	35	.0178	88	.1066	123.5	.1497	16.6	.1046
30	1.0742	36	.0183	88.5	.1072	124	.1503	16.8	.1059
30.5	1.0730	37	.0188	89	.1079	124.5	.1509	17.0	.1072
31	1.0718	38	.0193	89.5	.1085	125	.1515	17.2	.1084
31.5	1.0707	39	.0198	90	.1091	125.5	.1521	17.4	.1097
32	1.0695	40	.0203	90.5	.1097	126	.1527	17.6	.1109
32.5	1.0683	41	.0208	91	.1103	126.5	.1533	17.8	.1122
33	1.0671	42	.0213	91.5	.1109	127	.1539	18.0	.1135
33.5	1.0666	43	.0218	92	.1115	127.5	.1545	18.2	.1147
34	1.0648	44	.0223	92.5	.1121	128	.1551	18.4	.1160
34.5	1.0636	45	.0228	93	.1127	128.5	.1558	18.6	.1172
35	1.0624	46	.0234	93.5	.1133	129	.1563		
35.5	1.0612	47	.0239	94	.1139	129.5	.1569		
36	1.0601	48	.0244	94.5	.1145	130	.1575		
36.5	1.0589	49	.0249	95	.1151	130.5	.1581		
37	1.0577	50	.0254	95.5	.1157	131	.1587		
37.5	1.0565	51	.0259	96	.1163	131.5	.1593		
38	1.0554	52	.0264	96.5	.1169	132	.1600		

continued

TABLE 4.4 Girth Measurement Technique: Conversion Constants to Calculate Body Density for Women *(Continued)*

Upper Arm (cm)	Constant A	Age (years)	Constant B	Hip (cm)	Constant C	Hip (cm)	Constant C	Wrist (cm)	Constant D
38.5	1.0542	53	.0269	97	.1176	132.5	.1606		
39	1.0530	54	.0274	97.5	.1182	133	.1612		
39.5	1.0518	55	.0279	98	.1188	133.5	.1618		
40	1.0506	56	.0284	98.5	.1194	134	.1624		
40.5	1.0495	57	.0289	99	.1200	134.5	.1630		
41	1.0483	58	.0294	99.5	.1206	135	.1636		
41.5	1.0471	59	.0300	100	.1212	135.5	.1642		
42	1.0459	60	.0305	100.5	.1218	136	.1648		
42.5	1.0448	61	.0310	101	.1224	136.5	.1654		
43	1.0434	62	.0315	101.5	.1230	137	.1660		
43.5	1.0424	63	.0320	102	.1236	137.5	.1666		
44	1.0412	64	.0325	102.5	.1242	138	.1672		
		65	.0330	103	.1248	138.5	.1678		
		66	.0335	103.5	.1254	139	.1685		
		67	.0340	104	.1260	139.5	.1691		
		68	.0345	104.5	.1266	140	.1697		
		69	.0350	105	.1272	140.5	.1703		
		70	.0355	105.5	.1278	141	.1709		
		71	.0360	106	.1285	141.5	.1715		
		72	.0366	106.5	.1291	142	.1721		
		73	.0371	107	.1297	142.5	.1728		
		74	.0376	107.5	.1303	143	.1733		
		75	.0381	108	.1309	143.5	.1739		
				108.5	.1315	144	.1745		
				109	.1321	144.5	.1751		
				109.5	.1327	145	.1757		
				110	.1333	145.5	.1763		
				110.5	.1339	146	.1769		
				111	.1345	146.5	.1775		
				111.5	.1351	147	.1781		
				112	.1357	147.5	.1787		
				112.5	.1363	148	.1794		
				113	.1369	148.5	.1800		
				113.5	.1375	149	.1806		
				114	.1382	149.5	.1812		
						150	.1818		

TABLE 4.5 Girth Measurement Technique: Estimated Percent Body Fat for Men

Waist Minus Wrist Girth Measurement (inches)

Body Weight (pounds)	22	22.5	23	23.5	24	24.5	25	25.5	26	26.5	27	27.5	28	28.5	29	29.5	30	30.5	31	31.5	32	32.5	33	33.5	34	34.5	35	35.5	36	36.5	37	37.5	38	38.5	39	39.5	40	40.5	41	41.5	42	42.5	43	43.5	44	44.5	45	45.5	46	46.5	47	47.5	48	48.5	49	49.5	50
120	4	6	8	10	12	14	16	18	20	21	23	25	27	29	31	33	35	37	39	41	43	45	47	49	50	52	54	56	58																												
125	4	6	7	9	11	13	15	17	19	20	22	24	26	28	30	32	33	35	37	39	41	43	45	46	48	50	52	54	56	58																											
130	3	5	7	9	11	12	14	16	18	20	21	23	25	27	28	30	32	34	36	37	39	41	43	44	46	48	50	52	53	55	57																										
135	3	5	7	8	10	12	13	15	17	19	20	22	24	26	27	29	31	32	34	36	38	39	41	43	44	46	48	50	51	53	55	56																									
140	3	5	6	8	10	11	13	15	16	18	19	21	23	24	26	28	29	31	33	34	36	38	39	41	43	44	46	48	49	51	53	54	56																								
145	3	4	6	7	9	11	12	14	15	17	19	20	22	23	25	27	28	30	31	33	35	36	38	39	41	43	44	46	47	49	51	52	54	55																							
150	2	4	6	7	9	10	12	13	15	16	18	19	21	23	24	26	27	29	30	32	33	35	36	38	40	41	43	44	46	47	49	50	52	53	55																						
155	2	4	5	7	8	10	11	13	14	16	17	19	20	22	23	25	26	28	29	31	32	34	35	37	38	40	41	43	44	46	47	49	50	52	53	55																					
160	2	4	5	6	8	9	11	12	14	15	17	18	19	21	22	24	25	27	28	30	31	33	34	35	37	38	40	41	43	44	46	47	48	50	51	53	54																				
165	2	3	5	6	8	9	10	12	13	15	16	17	19	20	22	23	24	26	27	29	30	31	33	34	36	37	38	40	41	43	44	45	47	48	50	51	52	54																			
170	2	3	4	6	7	9	10	11	13	14	15	17	18	19	21	22	24	25	26	28	29	30	32	33	34	36	37	39	40	41	43	44	45	47	48	49	51	52	54																		
175	2	3	4	6	7	8	10	11	12	13	15	16	17	19	20	21	23	24	25	27	28	29	31	32	33	35	36	37	39	40	41	43	44	45	47	48	49	51	52	53																	
180		3	4	5	7	8	9	10	12	13	14	16	17	18	19	21	22	23	25	26	27	28	30	31	32	34	35	36	37	39	40	41	43	44	45	47	48	49	50	52	53																
185		3	4	5	6	8	9	10	11	13	14	15	16	18	19	20	21	23	24	25	26	28	29	30	31	33	34	35	36	38	39	40	41	43	44	45	46	48	49	50	51	53															
190		2	4	5	6	7	8	10	11	12	13	15	16	17	18	19	21	22	23	24	26	27	28	29	30	32	33	34	35	37	38	39	40	41	43	44	45	46	48	49	50	51	52														
195		2	3	5	6	7	8	9	11	12	13	14	15	16	18	19	20	21	22	24	25	26	27	28	30	31	32	33	34	35	37	38	39	40	41	43	44	45	46	47	49	50	51	52													
200		2	3	4	6	7	8	9	10	11	12	14	15	16	17	18	19	21	22	23	24	25	26	28	29	30	31	32	33	35	36	37	38	39	40	41	43	44	45	46	47	48	50	51	52												
205		2	3	4	5	6	8	9	10	11	12	13	14	15	17	18	19	20	21	22	23	25	26	27	28	29	30	31	32	34	35	36	37	38	39	40	41	43	44	45	46	47	48	49	51	52											
210		2	3	4	5	6	7	8	9	11	12	13	14	15	16	17	18	19	21	22	23	24	25	26	27	28	29	30	32	33	34	35	36	37	38	39	40	42	43	44	45	46	47	48	49	50	51										
215		2	3	4	5	6	7	8	9	10	11	12	13	15	16	17	18	19	20	21	22	23	24	25	26	28	29	30	31	32	33	34	35	36	37	38	39	40	42	43	44	45	46	47	48	49	50	51									
220			2	3	4	6	7	8	9	10	11	12	13	14	15	16	17	18	19	20	22	23	24	25	26	27	28	29	30	31	32	33	34	35	36	37	38	39	41	42	43	44	45	46	47	48	49	50	51								
225			2	3	4	6	7	8	9	10	11	12	13	14	15	16	17	18	19	20	21	22	23	24	25	26	27	28	29	30	31	32	33	34	35	36	37	38	40	41	42	43	44	45	46	47	48	49	50	51							
230			2	3	4	5	6	7	8	9	10	11	12	13	14	15	16	17	18	19	20	21	22	23	24	25	26	27	28	30	31	32	33	34	35	36	37	38	39	40	41	42	43	44	45	46	47	48	49	50	51						
235			2	3	4	5	6	7	8	9	10	11	12	13	14	15	16	17	18	19	20	21	22	23	24	25	26	27	28	29	30	31	32	33	34	35	36	37	38	39	40	41	42	43	44	45	46	47	48	49	50	51					
240			2	3	4	5	6	7	8	9	10	11	12	13	14	15	16	17	17	18	19	20	21	22	23	24	25	26	27	28	29	30	31	32	33	34	35	36	37	38	39	40	41	42	43	44	45	46	46	47	48	49	50				
245			2	3	4	5	6	7	8	9	9	10	11	12	13	14	15	16	17	18	19	20	21	22	23	24	25	26	27	27	28	29	30	31	32	33	34	35	36	37	38	39	40	41	42	43	44	44	45	46	47	48	49	50			
250			2	3	4	5	6	6	7	8	9	10	11	12	13	14	15	16	17	18	18	19	20	21	22	23	24	25	26	27	28	29	30	31	31	32	33	34	35	36	37	38	39	40	41	42	43	44	44	45	46	47	48	49	50		
255			2	3	3	4	5	6	7	8	9	10	11	12	13	14	14	15	16	17	18	19	20	21	22	23	24	24	25	26	27	28	29	30	31	32	33	34	34	35	36	37	38	39	40	41	42	43	44	44	45	46	47	48	49	50	
260			2	2	3	4	5	6	7	8	9	10	10	11	12	13	14	15	16	17	18	19	19	20	21	22	23	24	25	26	27	27	28	29	30	31	32	33	34	35	35	36	37	38	39	40	41	42	43	43	44	45	46	47	48	49	50
265				2	3	4	5	6	7	8	8	9	10	11	12	13	14	15	15	16	17	18	19	20	21	22	22	23	24	25	26	27	28	29	29	30	31	32	33	34	35	36	36	37	38	39	40	41	42	43	43	44	45	46	47	48	49
270				2	3	4	5	6	7	7	8	9	10	11	12	13	13	14	15	16	17	18	19	19	20	21	22	23	24	25	25	26	27	28	29	30	31	31	32	33	34	35	36	37	37	38	39	40	41	42	43	43	44	45	46	47	48
275				2	3	4	5	5	6	7	8	9	10	11	11	12	13	14	15	16	16	17	18	19	20	21	22	22	23	24	25	26	27	27	28	29	30	31	32	32	33	34	35	36	37	38	38	39	40	41	42	43	43	44	45	46	47
280				2	3	4	4	5	6	7	8	9	9	10	11	12	13	14	14	15	16	17	18	19	19	20	21	22	23	24	24	25	26	27	28	29	29	30	31	32	33	33	34	35	36	37	38	38	39	40	41	42	43	43	44	45	46
285				2	3	4	4	5	6	7	8	8	9	10	11	12	12	13	14	15	16	17	17	18	19	20	21	21	22	23	24	25	26	26	27	28	29	30	30	31	32	33	34	34	35	36	37	38	39	39	40	41	42	43	43	44	45
290				2	3	3	4	5	6	7	7	8	9	10	11	11	12	13	14	15	15	16	17	18	19	19	20	21	22	23	23	24	25	26	27	27	28	29	30	31	31	32	33	34	35	35	36	37	38	39	39	40	41	42	43	43	44
295				2	2	3	4	5	6	6	7	8	9	10	10	11	12	13	14	14	15	16	17	17	18	19	20	21	21	22	23	24	25	25	26	27	28	28	29	30	31	32	32	33	34	35	36	36	37	38	39	39	40	41	42	43	43
300				2	2	3	4	5	5	6	7	8	9	9	10	11	12	12	13	14	15	16	16	17	18	19	19	20	21	22	22	23	24	25	26	26	27	28	29	29	30	31	32	33	33	34	35	36	36	37	38	39	39	40	41	42	43

FIGURE 4.5 Procedure for body fat assessment according to girth measurements.

Girth Measurements for Women*

1. Using a regular tape measure, determine the following girth measurements in centimeters (cm):

   Upper arm: Measure halfway between the shoulder and the elbow.

   Hip: Measure at the point of largest circumference.

   Wrist: Take the girth in front of the bones where the wrist bends.

2. Obtain the person's age.

3. Using Table 4.4, find the subject's age, girth measurement for each site in the left column, then look up the constant values for each. These values will allow you to derive body density (BD) by substituting the constants in the following formula:

   BD = A − B − C + D

4. Using the derived body density, calculate percent body fat (%F) according to the following equation:

   %F = (495 ÷ BD) − 450**

Example: Jane is 20 years old and the following girth measurements were taken: biceps = 27 cm, hip = 99.5 cm, wrist = 15.4 cm.

Data		Constant
Upper arm	= 27 cm	A = 1.0813
Age	= 20	B = .0102
Hip	= 99.5 cm	C = .1206
Wrist	= 15.4 cm	D = .0971

BD = A − B − C + D
BD − 1.0813 − .0102 − .1206 + .0971 = 1.0476

%F = (495 ÷ BD) − 450
%F = (495 ÷ 1.0476) − 450 = 22.5

Girth Measurements for Men***

1. Using a regular tape measure, determine the following girth measurements in inches (the men's measurements are taken in inches, as opposed to centimeters for women):

   Waist: Measure at the umbilicus (belly button).

   Wrist: Measure in front of the bones where the wrist bends.

2. Subtract the wrist from the waist measurement.
3. Obtain the weight of the subject in pounds.
4. Look up the percent body fat (%F) in Table 4.5 by using the difference obtained in number 2 above and the person's body weight.

Example: John weighs 160 pounds, and his waist and wrist girth measurements are 36.5 and 7.5 inches, respectively.

Waist girth = 36.5 inches
Wrist girth = 7.5 inches
Difference = 29.0 inches
Body weight = 160.0 lbs.
%F = 22

*From R. B. Lambson, "Generalized Body Density Prediction Equations for Women Using Simple Anthropometric Measurements." Unpublished doctoral dissertation, Brigham Young University, Provo, UT, August 1987. Reproduced by permission.
**From W. E. Siri, *Body Composition from Fluid Spaces and Density* (Berkeley, CA: University of California, Donner Laboratory of Medical Physics, March 19, 1956).
***From A. G. Fisher and P. E. Allsen, Jogging, Dubuque, IA: "Generalized Body Composition Equation for Men Using Simple Measurement Techniques;" by K. W. Penrouse, A. G. Nelson, and A. G. Fisher, *Medicine and Science in Sports and Exercise* 17, no. 2 (1985): 189. © American College of Sports Medicine, 1985.

tissue. The easier the conductance, the leaner the individual. Specialized equipment or simple body weight scales with sensors on the surface can be used to perform this procedure.

The accuracy of equations used to estimate percent body fat with this technique is questionable. A single equation cannot be used for everyone, but rather valid and accurate equations to estimate body fat for the specific population (age, gender, and ethnicity) being tested are required. Several factors can affect the results, including hydration and body temperature. Following all manufacturers' instructions will ensure the most accurate result, but even then percent body fat may be off—typically on the higher end—by as much as 10 percentage points (or even more on some scales).

Metrics Used to Determine Recommended Body Weight

Knowing your body composition and percent body fat is an important step towards taking control of your health and lifestyle. As you evaluate your body weight and the weight you would like to reach and maintain throughout life, there are a few other metrics that can help you do so. These metrics provide an estimate of healthy and unhealthy body weight. These commonly used techniques include body mass index (BMI), waist circumference (WC), and waist-to-height ratio (WHtR). These assessments re-

TABLE 4.6 Determination of Body Mass Index (BMI)

Determine your BMI by looking up the number where your weight and height intersect on the table. According to the results, look up your disease risk in Tables 4.7 and 4.9.

	Weight																												
Height	**110**	**115**	**120**	**125**	**130**	**135**	**140**	**145**	**150**	**155**	**160**	**165**	**170**	**175**	**180**	**185**	**190**	**195**	**200**	**205**	**210**	**215**	**220**	**225**	**230**	**235**	**240**	**245**	**250**
5′0″	21	22	23	24	25	26	27	28	29	30	31	32	33	34	35	36	37	38	39	40	41	42	43	44	45	46	47	48	49
5′1″	21	22	23	24	25	26	26	27	28	29	30	31	32	33	34	35	36	37	38	39	40	41	42	43	43	44	45	46	47
5′2″	20	21	22	23	24	25	26	27	27	28	29	30	31	32	33	34	35	36	37	37	38	39	40	41	42	43	44	45	46
5′3″	19	20	21	22	23	24	25	26	27	27	28	29	30	31	32	33	34	35	35	36	37	38	39	40	41	42	43	43	44
5′4″	19	20	21	21	22	23	24	25	26	27	27	28	29	30	31	32	33	33	34	35	36	37	38	39	39	40	41	42	43
5′5″	18	19	20	21	22	22	23	24	25	26	27	27	28	29	30	31	32	32	33	34	35	36	37	37	38	39	40	41	42
5′6″	18	19	19	20	21	22	23	23	24	25	26	27	27	28	29	30	31	31	32	33	34	35	36	36	37	38	39	40	40
5′7″	17	18	19	20	20	21	22	23	23	24	25	26	27	27	28	29	30	31	31	32	33	34	34	35	36	37	38	38	39
5′8″	17	17	18	19	20	21	21	22	23	24	24	25	26	27	27	28	29	30	30	31	32	33	33	34	35	36	36	37	38
5′9″	16	17	18	18	19	20	21	21	22	23	24	24	25	26	27	27	28	29	30	30	31	32	32	33	34	35	35	36	37
5′10″	16	17	17	18	19	19	20	21	22	22	23	24	24	25	26	27	27	28	29	29	30	31	32	32	33	34	34	35	36
5′11″	15	16	17	17	18	19	20	20	21	22	22	23	24	24	25	26	26	27	28	29	29	30	31	31	32	33	33	34	35
6′0″	15	16	16	17	18	18	19	20	20	21	22	22	23	24	24	25	26	26	27	28	28	29	30	31	31	32	33	33	34
6′1″	15	15	16	16	17	18	18	19	20	20	21	22	22	23	24	24	25	26	26	27	28	28	29	30	30	31	32	32	33
6′2″	14	15	15	16	17	17	18	19	19	20	21	21	22	22	23	24	24	25	26	26	27	28	28	29	30	30	31	31	32
6′3″	14	14	15	16	16	17	17	18	19	19	20	21	21	22	22	23	24	24	25	26	26	27	27	28	29	29	30	31	31
6′4″	13	14	15	15	16	16	17	18	18	19	19	20	21	21	22	23	23	24	24	25	26	26	27	27	28	29	29	30	30

quire only a scale and a measuring tape, are quick and easy to obtain, and offer a realistic way for you to track your body weight throughout the years. While BMI has become a familiar standard, the waist metrics of WHtR and WC are an important compliment to BMI. Researchers are finding that these seemingly simple measurements, when used in conjunction with one another, are appropriate risk assessment tools for individuals and entire populations.

Body Mass Index

The most common technique to determine thinness and excessive fatness is the **body mass index (BMI)**. BMI incorporates height and weight to estimate critical fat values at which the risk for disease increases.

BMI is calculated by either (a) dividing the weight in kilograms by the square of the height in meters or (b) multiplying body weight in pounds by 705 and dividing this figure by the square of the height in inches. For example, the BMI for an individual who weighs 172 pounds (78 kg) and is 67 inches (1.7 m) tall would be 27: $[78 \div (1.7)^2]$ or $[172 \times 705 \div (67)^2]$. You also can look up your BMI in Table 4.6 according to your height and weight.

Because of its simplicity and measurement consistency across populations, BMI is the most widely used method to determine overweight and obesity. Due to the various limitations of previously mentioned body composition techniques—including cost, availability to the general population, lack of consistency among technicians and laboratories, inconsistent results between techniques, and standard error of measurement of the procedures—BMI is used almost exclusively to determine health risks and mortality rates associated with excessive body weight.

Scientific evidence indicates that the risk for disease starts to increase when BMI exceeds 25.[3] Although a BMI index between 18.5 and 25 is considered normal (see Tables 4.7 and 4.9), the lowest risk for chronic disease is in the 22-to-25 range.[4] Individuals are classified as overweight if their indexes lie between 25 and 30. BMIs above 30 are defined as obese, and those below 18.5 as **underweight**. Scientific evidence has shown that even though the risk for premature illness and death is greater for those who are overweight, the risk is also increased for individuals who are underweight[5] (see Figure 4.6).

Compared with individuals with BMIs between 22 and 25, people with BMIs

Body mass index (BMI) Technique to determine thinness and excessive fatness that incorporates height and weight to estimate critical fat values at which the risk for disease increases.

Underweight Extremely low body weight.

between 25 and 30 (overweight) exhibit mortality rates up to 25 percent higher; rates for those with BMIs above 30 (obese) are 50 to 100 percent higher.[6] Table 4.7 provides disease risk categories when BMI is used as the sole criterion to identify people at risk. Currently, more than one-third of the U.S. adult population has a BMI of 30 or more. Overweight and obesity trends starting in 1960 according to BMI are given in Figure 4.7. Additionally, the prevalence of obesity by classification (obesity I, II, and III) is provided in Figure 4.8. Furthermore, the yearly direct health-related costs of obesity, that is, those that result from outpatient and inpatient health services (including surgery), laboratory tests, and drug therapy, are estimated to be $170 billion or about 17 percent of all medical costs. These costs are expected to rise to a staggering $319 billion by 2020. Surveys also indicate that per capita medical spending is 42 percent higher for obese individuals as compared to normal weight people.

BMI is a useful tool to screen and compare large populations, but its one weakness is that it fails to differentiate fat from lean body mass or note where most of the fat is located (waist circumference and waist-to-height ratio—see discussion that follows). Using BMI, athletes with a large amount of muscle mass (such as body builders and football players) can easily fall in the moderate- or even high-risk categories.

Waist Circumference

Scientific evidence suggests that the way people store fat affects their risk for disease. The total amount of body fat by itself is not the best predictor of increased risk for

FIGURE 4.7 Overweight and obesity trends in the United States, 1960–2010.

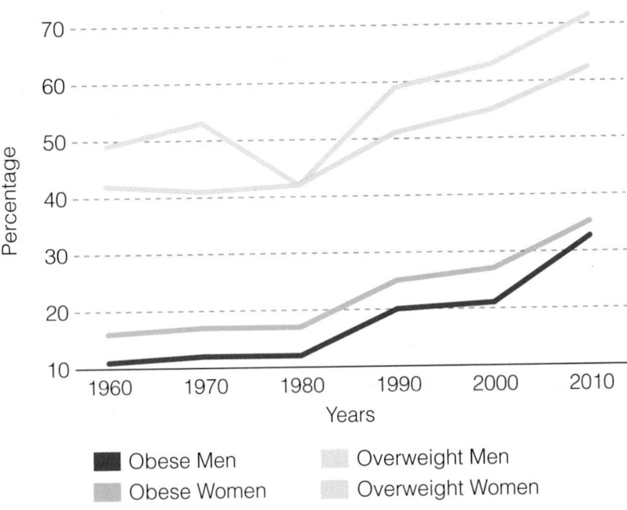

Source: Adapted from the National Center for Health Statistics, Centers for Disease Control and Prevention, and the Journal of the American Medical Association.

TABLE 4.7 Disease Risk According to Body Mass Index (BMI)

BMI	Disease Risk	Classification
<18.5	Increased	Underweight
18.5–21.99	Low	Acceptable
22.0–24.99	Very low	Acceptable
25.0–29.99	Increased	Overweight
30.0–34.99	High	Obesity I
35.0–39.99	Very high	Obesity II
≥40.0	Extremely high	Obesity III

FIGURE 4.6 Morbidity and mortality risk versus BMI.

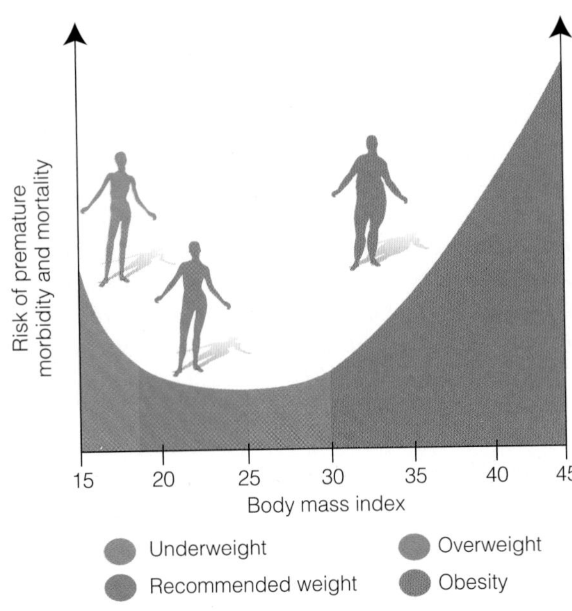

FIGURE 4.8 Obesity prevalence by classification in U.S. adults (>20 years of age), 2008.

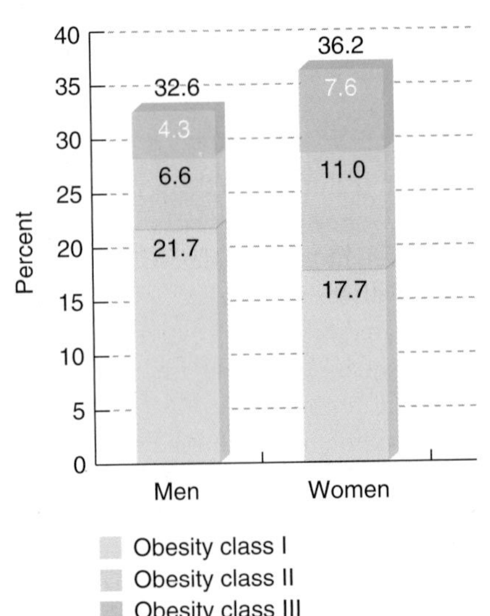

FIGURE 4.9 Visceral (VSC) fat is a greater risk factor for heart disease, stroke, hypertension, diabetes, and cancer than subcutaneous (SBC) or retroperitoneal (RTP) fat.

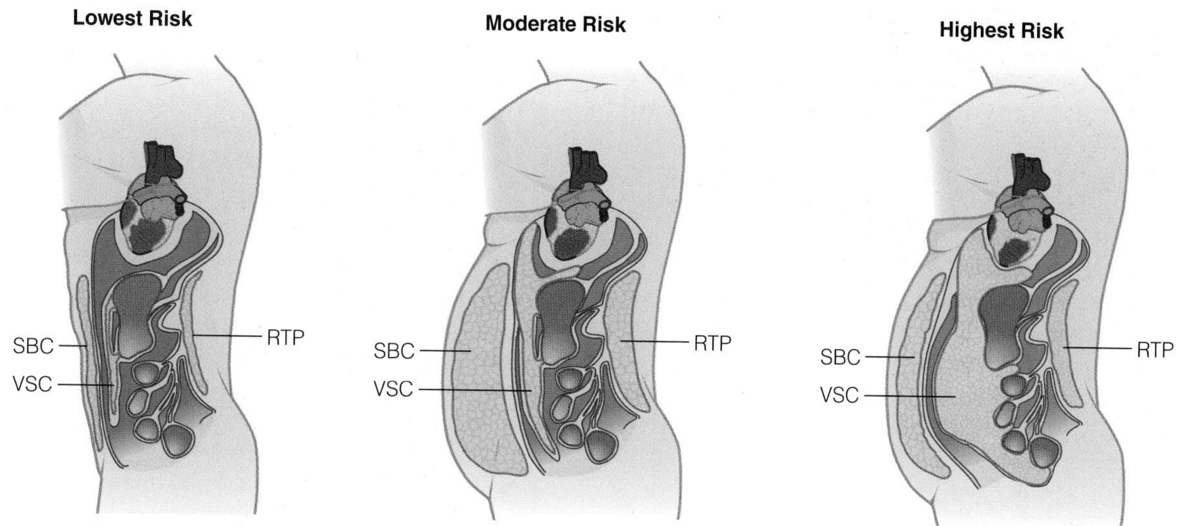

disease but, rather, the location of the fat. **Android obesity** is seen in individuals who tend to store fat in the trunk or abdominal area (which produces the "apple" shape). **Gynoid obesity** is seen in people who store fat primarily around the hips and thighs (which creates the "pear" shape).

Compared with people whose body fat is stored primarily in the hips and thighs, an increasing amount of evidence is showing that obese individuals with abdominal fat are clearly at higher risk for heart disease, hypertension, type 2 diabetes ("non-insulin-dependent" diabetes), stroke, some types of cancer, kidney disease, dementia, migraines, and diminished lung function. Evidence also indicates that among individuals with a lot of abdominal fat, those whose fat deposits are located around internal organs (intra-abdominal or visceral fat) rather than subcutaneously or retroperitoneally (see Figure 4.9) have an even greater risk for disease than those with fat mainly just beneath the skin (subcutaneous fat).[7] Of even greater significance, the results of a study that followed more than 350,000 people over almost 10 years concluded that even when body weight is viewed as "normal," individuals with a large waist circumference nearly double the risk for premature death.[8] Researchers believe that visceral fat is more metabolically active than subcutaneous fat and secretes harmful inflammatory substances that contribute to chronic conditions.

Complex scanning techniques used to identify individuals at risk because of high intra-abdominal fatness are costly, so a simple **waist circumference (WC)** measure, designed by the National Heart, Lung, and Blood Institute, is used to assess this risk.[9] WC seems to predict abdominal visceral fat as accurately as the DXA technique.[10] A waist circumference of more than 40 inches in men and 35 inches in women indicates a higher risk for cardiovascular disease, hypertension, stroke, and type 2 diabetes (Table 4.8). Weight loss is encouraged when individuals exceed these measurements.

TABLE 4.8 Disease Risk According to Waist Circumference (WC)

Men	Women	Disease Risk
<35.5	<32.5	Low
35.5–40.0	32.5–35.0	Moderate
>40.0	>35.0	High

Research indicates that WC is a better predictor than BMI of the risk for disease.[11] Even better is using the two measurements in conjunction to identify individuals at higher risk resulting from excessive body fat. Table 4.9 provides guidelines to identify people at risk according to BMI and WC.

Android obesity Obesity pattern seen in individuals who tend to store fat in the trunk or abdominal area.

Gynoid obesity Obesity pattern seen in people who store fat primarily around the hips and thighs.

Waist circumference (WC) A waist girth measurement to assess potential risk for disease based on intra-abdominal fat content.

TABLE 4.9 **Disease Risk According to Body Mass Index (BMI) and Waist Circumference (WC)**

		Disease Risk Relative to Normal Weight and WC	
Classification	BMI (kg/m²)	Men ≤40″ (102 cm) Women ≤35″ (88 cm)	Men >40″ (102 cm) Women >35″ (88 cm)
Underweight	<18.5	Increased	Low
Normal	18.5–24.9	Very low	Increased
Overweight	25.0–29.9	Increased	High
Obesity class I	30.0–34.9	High	Very high
Obesity class II	35.0–39.9	Very high	Very high
Obesity class III	≥40.0	Extremely high	Extremely high

Adapted from Expert Panel, Executive Summary of the Clinical Guidelines on the Identification, Evaluation, and Treatment of Overweight and Obesity in Adults, *Archives of Internal Medicine* 158:1855–1867, 1998.

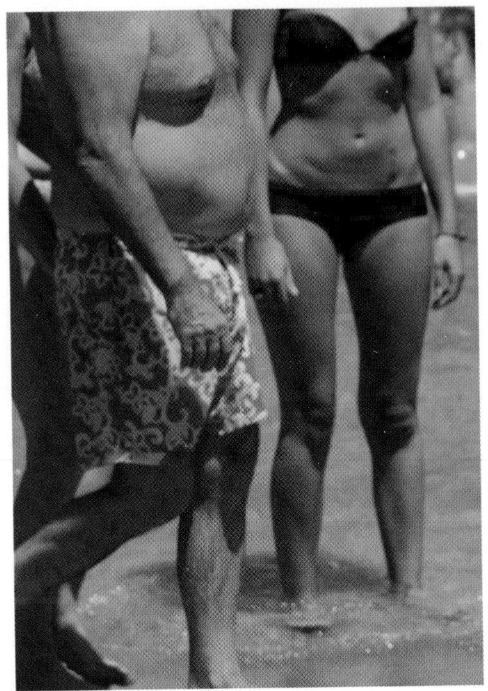

Individuals who accumulate body fat around the midsection are at greater risk for disease than those who accumulate body fat in other areas.

Waist-to-Height Ratio: "Keep your waist circumference to less than half your height."

The waist-to-height ratio (WHtR) is a new health risk assessment also used to ascertain the health risks of obesity. The ratio is rapidly gaining popularity in the scientific community as research indicates that it is a better predictor of health outcomes, including multiple coronary heart disease risk factors, than BMI or WC.[12] While WC is superior to BMI, two individuals with a similar WC (e.g., 43) but of different heights may not be at the same risk for disease. The new WHtR method takes height into account and is therefore more accurate across all ethnicities. Like WC, however, it does not consider overall weight, and therefore it is an important compliment to BMI.

A systematic review of the literature that included 31 research studies, including more than 300,000 adults of several ethnic groups, showed that WHtR has significantly greater discriminatory power in predicting cardiac and metabolic complications as compared to BMI and WC.[13] This has proven to be true even for WHtR measured in school-age children and teenagers.[14] Another study presented at the 2013 European Congress on Obesity compared the effect of abdominal obesity on life expectancy in terms of years of life lost. The data showed that a 30-year-old man with a BMI over 40 has a years-of-life-lost value of 10.5 years as compared to 16.7 years using the most severe category of the WHtR. A 30-year-old woman in these same categories loses 5.3 years of life through BMI as compared to 9.5 years using WHtR.[15]

WHtR is determined by simply dividing the waist circumference in inches by the height in inches. As illustrated in Figure 4.10, a ratio of .4 to .5 indicates the lowest risk for disease, whereas less than .4 or between .5 and .7 require "care" to decrease health risks, and a ratio of .7 or above require "action" to conform to the lowest health risk category of .4 to .5. An example of the WHtR for a person with a WC of 32 inches and a height of 68 inches (5′ 8″) would be (32 ÷ 68). The findings of many of these studies have prompted researchers to promote a public health message: "Keep your waist circumference to less than half your height." The simplicity of the message, and the fact that WHtR can be easily determined and used with any other assessment, makes it all the more plausible that WHtR may become a standard worldwide health index. Table 4.10 lists the various risk categories according to WHtR.

Before WHtR can be implemented on a global scale and used to compare risk factors across populations, worldwide health organizations will need to agree on precisely where

TABLE 4.10 **Health Categories According to Waist-to-Height Ratio (WHtR)**

Category	WHtR (Waist/Height)	Disease Risk
Take Care	<.4	Increased
Acceptable (OK)	.4-.5	Very low
Take Care	.5-.7	Increased
Take Action	>.7	High

FIGURE 4.10 **The Ashwell® Shape Chart (waist-to-height ratio).**

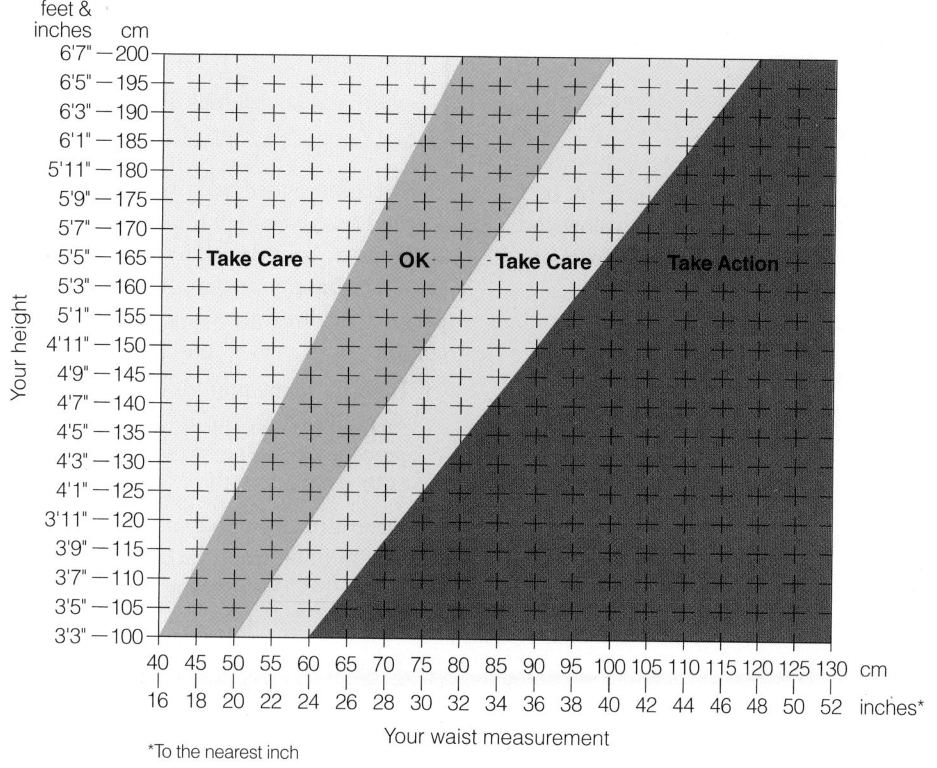

TABLE 4.11 **Body Composition Classification According to Percent Body Fat**

			MEN			
Age	**Underweight**	**Excellent**	**Good**	**Moderate**	**Overweight**	**Obese**
≤19	<3	12.0	12.1–17.0	17.1–22.0	22.1–27.0	≥27.1
20–29	<3	13.0	13.1–18.0	18.1–23.0	23.1–28.0	≥28.1
30–39	<3	14.0	14.1–19.0	19.1–24.0	24.1–29.0	≥29.1
40–49	<3	15.0	15.1–20.0	20.1–25.0	25.1–30.0	≥30.1
≥50	<3	16.0	16.1–21.0	21.1–26.0	26.1–31.0	≥31.1
			WOMEN			
Age	**Underweight**	**Excellent**	**Good**	**Moderate**	**Overweight**	**Obese**
≤19	<12	17.0	17.1–22.0	22.1–27.0	27.1–32.0	≥32.1
20–29	<12	18.0	18.1–23.0	23.1–28.0	28.1–33.0	≥33.1
30–39	<12	19.0	19.1–24.0	24.1–29.0	29.1–34.0	≥34.1
40–49	<12	20.0	20.1–25.0	25.1–30.0	30.1–35.0	≥35.1
≥50	<12	21.0	21.1–26.0	26.1–31.0	31.1–36.0	≥36.1

High physical fitness standard *Health fitness standard*

(how high or low on the waist) the measurement should be taken. An abdominal measurement, for example, could be taken at the naval or at the narrowest point of the waist, as no clear landmark has been set. Taking the measurement just below the rib cage may provide the best estimation of visceral fat, but that measurement site is not widely used as of yet. It is important when recording your own abdominal measurements to note the site where the measurement was taken and to be consistent with future measurements.

The following guidelines are recommended to get an accurate and repeatable waist measurement:

1. Stand in front of a mirror while taking the measurement to insure the measuring tape is horizontal.
2. Use a measuring tape that is not elastic and hold it snug against the skin, but do not compress the waist.
3. Choose a site on the waist and be sure to consistently measure at the same site.

4. When the tape is in place, relax, exhale, and then take the reading.

WHtR results can provide an early warning sign of potential risk for disease and morbidity, including in children and low-income populations where more specialized tools may not be available. This metric can be used worldwide as an opportunity to promote better health and to empower health-care practitioners to intervene before the onset of disease and prescribe positive lifestyle changes to slow and even reverse the trend of growing mortality rates from preventable chronic disease.

Determining Recommended Body Weight

After finding out your percent body fat, you can determine your current body composition classification by consulting Table 4.11, which presents percentages of fat according to both the health fitness standard and the high physical fitness standard (see discussion in Chapter 1).

For example, the recommended health fitness fat percentage for a 20-year-old female is 28 percent or less. Although there are no clearly identified percent body fat levels at which the risk for disease definitely increases, the health fitness standard in Table 4.11 is currently the best estimate of the point at which there seems to be no harm to health.

According to Table 4.11, the high physical fitness range for this same 20-year-old woman would be between 18 and 23 percent. The high physical fitness standard does not mean that you cannot be somewhat below this number. Many highly trained male athletes are as low as 3 percent, and some female distance runners have been measured at 6 percent body fat (which may not be healthy).

Scientists generally agree that the mortality rate is higher for obese people, and some evidence indicates that the same is true for underweight people. "Underweight" and "thin" do not necessarily mean the same thing. The body fat of a healthy thin person is near the high physical fitness standard, whereas an underweight person has extremely low body fat, even to the point of compromising the essential fat.

The 3 percent essential fat for men and 12 percent for women seem to be the lower limits for people to maintain good health. Below these percentages, normal physiological functions can be seriously impaired. Some experts point out that a little storage fat (in addition to the essential fat) is better than none at all. As a result, the health and high fitness standards for percent fat in Table 4.11 are set higher than the minimum essential fat requirements, at a point beneficial to optimal health and well-being. Finally, because lean tissue decreases with age, one extra percentage point is allowed for every additional decade of life.

CRITICAL THINKING

Do you think you have a weight problem? Do your body composition results make you feel any different about the way you perceive your current body weight and image?

Your recommended body weight is computed based on the selected health or high fitness fat percentage for your age and gender. Your decision to select a "desired" fat percentage should be based on your current percent body fat and your personal health/fitness objectives. Following are steps to compute your own recommended body weight:

1. Determine the pounds of body weight that are fat (FW) by multiplying your body weight (BW) by the current percent fat (%F) expressed in decimal form (FW = BW × %F).
2. Determine lean body mass (LBM) by subtracting the weight in fat from the total body weight (LBM = BW − FW). (Anything that is not fat must be part of the lean component.)
3. Select a desired body fat percentage (DFP) based on the health or high fitness standards given in Table 4.11.
4. Compute recommended body weight (RBW) according to the formula RBW = LBM ÷ (1.0 − DFP).

As an example of these computations, a 19-year-old female who weighs 160 pounds and is 30 percent fat would like to know what her recommended body weight would be at 22 percent:

Sex: female
Age: 19
BW: 160 lbs
%F: 30% (.30 in decimal form)

1. FW = BW × %F
   FW = 160 × .30 = 48 lbs
2. LBM = BW − FW
   LBM = 160 − 48 = 112 lbs
3. DFP: 22% (.22 in decimal form)
4. RBW = LBM ÷ (1.0 − .DFP)
   RBW = 112 ÷ (1.0 − .22)
   RBW = 112 ÷ .78 = 143.6 lbs

In Lab 4A, you will have the opportunity to determine your own body composition and recommended body weight. A second column is provided in the activity for a follow-up assessment at a future date. The disease risk according to BMI and WC and recommended body weight according to BMI also are determined in Lab 4B.

Other than hydrostatic weighing, skinfold thickness seems to be the most practical and valid technique to estimate body fat, unless the person is significantly overweight and an accurate skinfold cannot be measured. If skinfold calipers are available, use this technique to assess your percent body fat. If none of these techniques is available to you, estimate your percent fat according to girth measurements

BEHAVIOR MODIFICATION PLANNING

Tips for Lifetime Weight Management

Maintenance of recommended body composition is one of the most significant health issues of the 21st century. If you are committed to lifetime weight management, the following strategies will help:

I PLAN TO | I DID IT

- ❑ ❑ Accumulate 60 to 90 minutes of physical activity daily.
- ❑ ❑ Exercise at a vigorous aerobic pace (high intensity) for a minimum of 20 minutes three times per week.
- ❑ ❑ Strength train two to three times per week.
- ❑ ❑ Use common sense and moderation in your daily diet.
- ❑ ❑ Consume primarily a nutrient dense/low calorie diet (fruits, vegetables, whole grains, moderate protein, and low fat products—see chapter 5).
- ❑ ❑ "Junior-size" instead of "super-size."
- ❑ ❑ Regularly monitor body weight, body composition, body mass index, and waist circumference.
- ❑ ❑ Do not allow increases in body weight (percent fat) to accumulate; deal immediately with the problem through moderate reductions in caloric intake and maintenance of physical activity and exercise habits.

Try It

In your Online Journal or your class notebook, note which of these tips you are already using and which ones you can incorporate into your daily habits right away.

(or another technique available to you). You also may wish to use several techniques and compare the results.

CRITICAL THINKING

How do you feel about your current body weight and what influence does society have on the way you perceive yourself in terms of your weight?

Importance of Regular Body Composition Assessment

Children in the United States do not start with a weight problem. Although a few struggle with weight throughout life, most are not overweight in the early years of life.

Trends indicate that adults in the United States gain one to two pounds per year. Thus, during a span of 40 years, the average American will have gained 40 to 80 pounds. Because of the typical reduction in physical activity in our society, however, the average person also loses a half pound of lean tissue each year. Therefore, this span of 40 years has produced an actual fat gain of 60 to 100 pounds accompanied by a 20-pound loss of lean body mass (Figure 4.11). These changes cannot be detected without assessing body composition periodically.

If you are on a diet/exercise program, you should repeat your percent body fat assessment and recommended weight computations about once a month. This is important because lean body mass is affected by weight-reduction programs and amount of physical activity. As lean body mass changes, so will your recommended body weight. To make valid comparisons, use the same technique for both pre- and post-program assessments. Knowing your percent body fat also is useful to identify fad diets that promote water loss and loss of lean body mass, especially muscle mass.

Changes in body composition resulting from a weight control/exercise program were illustrated in a co-ed aerobic dance course taught during a six-week summer term. Students participated in a 60-minute aerobics routine four times a week. On the first and last days of class, several physiological parameters, including body composition, were assessed. Students also were given information on diet and nutrition, but they followed their own dietary program.

At the end of the six weeks, the average weight loss for the entire class was three pounds (Figure 4.12). But, because body composition was assessed, class members were surprised to find that the average fat loss was actually six pounds, accompanied by a three-pound increase in lean body mass.

When dieting, have your body composition reassessed periodically because of the effects of negative caloric balance on lean body mass. As discussed in Chapter 5, dieting does decrease lean body mass. This loss of lean body mass can be offset or eliminated by combining a sensible diet with exercise.

FIGURE 4.11 Typical body composition changes for adults in the United States.

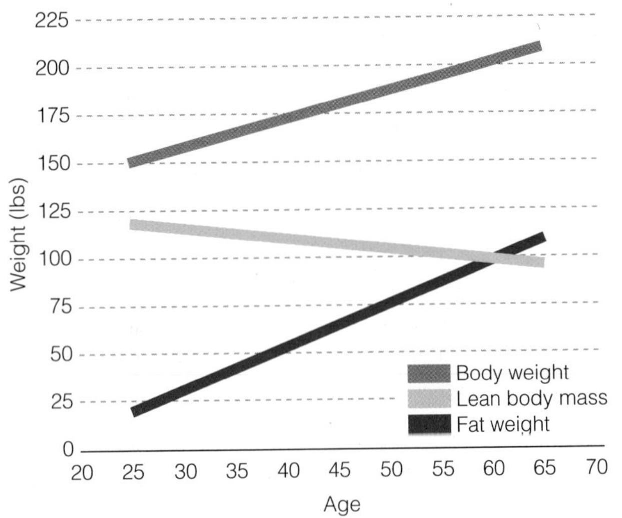

FIGURE 4.12 Effects of a 6-week aerobics exercise program on body composition.

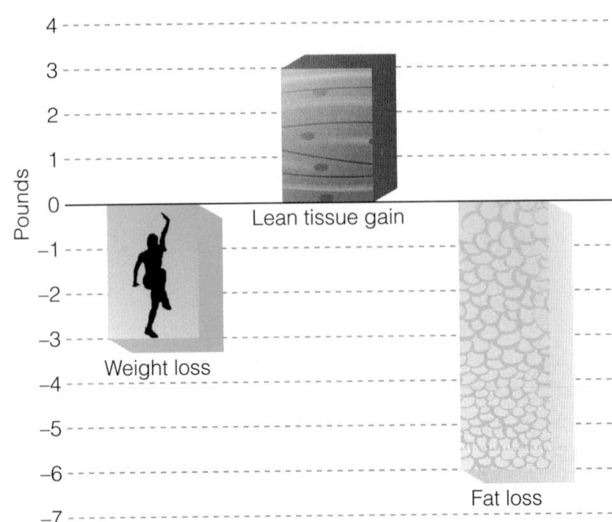

Source: W. W. K. Hoeger, data collected at the University of Texas of the Permian Basin, 1985.

Assess Your Behavior

CENGAGE brain .com To access course materials, including companion resources, please visit **www.cengagebrain.com**.

1. Do you know what your percent body fat is according to a reliable body composition assessment technique administered by a qualified technician?
2. Do you know your disease risk according to BMI, WC, and WHtR parameters?
3. Have you been able to maintain your body weight at a stable level during the past 12 months?

Assess Your Knowledge

1. Body composition incorporates
   a. a fat component.
   b. a non-fat component.
   c. percent body fat.
   d. lean body mass.
   e. all of the four components above.
2. Recommended body weight can be determined through
   a. body mass index.
   b. body composition analysis.
   c. BMI and waist circumference.
   d. waist circumference.
   e. all of the above.
3. Essential fat in women is
   a. 3 percent.
   b. 5 percent.
   c. 8 percent.
   d. 12 percent.
   e. 17 percent.
4. Which of the following is *not* a technique to assess body fat?
   a. body mass index
   b. skinfold thickness
   c. hydrostatic weighing
   d. circumference measurements
   e. air displacement
5. Which of the following sites is used to assess percent body fat according to skinfold thickness in men?
   a. suprailium
   b. chest
   c. scapular
   d. triceps
   e. All four sites are used.

6. Which variable is *not* used to assess percent body fat in women according to girth measurements?
  a. age
  b. hip
  c. wrist
  d. upper arm
  e. height

7. Waist circumference can be used to
  a. determine percent body fat.
  b. assess risk for disease.
  c. measure lean body mass.
  d. identify underweight people.
  e. All of the above are correct.

8. An acceptable BMI is between
  a. 15 and 18.49.
  b. 18.5 and 24.99.
  c. 25 and 29.99.
  d. 30 and 34.99.
  e. 35 and 39.99.

9. The health fitness percent body fat for women of various ages is in the range of
  a. 3 to 7 percent.
  b. 7 to 12 percent.
  c. 12 to 20 percent.
  d. 20 to 27 percent.
  e. 27 to 31 percent

10. When a previously inactive individual starts an exercise program, the person may
  a. lose weight.
  b. gain weight.
  c. improve body composition.
  d. lose more fat pounds than total weight pounds.
  e. do all of the above.

Correct answers can be found at the back of the book.

NOTES

1. W. W. K. Hoeger, D. Gonzalez, L. B. Ransdell, and J. Gao, "A Comparison of Air Displacement Plethysmography and Hydrostatic Weighing Techniques for Assessment of Percent Body Fat in Adults By Gender and BMI Category," *International Journal of Body Composition Research* 9 (2010): 89–94.
2. E. W. Demerath, et al., "Comparison of Percent Body Fat Estimates Using Air Displacement Plethysmography and Hydrodensitometry in Adults and Children," *International Journal of Obesity* 26 (2002): 389–397.
3. J. Stevens, J. Cai, E. R. Pamuk, D. F. Williamson, M. J. Thun, and J. L. Wood, "The Effect of Age on the Association Between Body Mass Index and Mortality," *New England Journal of Medicine* 338 (1998): 1–7.
4. E. E. Calle, M. J. Thun, J. M. Petrelli, C. Rodriguez, and C. W. Heath, "Body-Mass Index and Mortality in a Prospective Cohort of U.S. Adults," *New England Journal of Medicine* 341 (1999): 1097–1105.
5. K. M. Flegal, et al., "Cause-Specific Excess Deaths Associated with Underweight, Overweight, and Obesity," *Journal of the American Medical Association* 298 (2007): 2028–2037.
6. K. M. Flegal, M. D. Carrol, R. J. Kuczmarski, and C. L. Johnson, "Overweight and Obesity in the United States: Prevalence and Trends, 1960–1994," *International Journal of Obesity and Related Metabolic Disorders* 22 (1998): 39–47.
7. C. Bouchard, G. A. Bray, and V. S. Hubbard, "Basic and Clinical Aspects of Regional Fat Distribution," *American Journal of Clinical Nutrition* 52 (1990): 946–950; G. Hu, et al., "Joint Effects of Physical Activity, Body Mass Index, Waist Circumference, and Waist-to-Hip Ratio on the Risk of Heart Failure," *Circulation* 121 (2010): 237–244; D. Canoy, et al., "Body Fat Distribution and Risk of Coronary Heart Disease in Men and Women in the European Prospective Investigation Into Cancer and Nutrition in Norfolk Cohort," *Circulation* 116 (2007): 2933–2943; J. P. Després, I. Lemieux, and D. Prud-homme, "Treatment of Obesity: Need to Focus on High Risk Abdominally Obese Patients," *British Medical Journal* 322 (2001): 716–720; Kwakernaak, AJ et al., "Central Body Fat Distribution Associates with Unfavorable Renal Hemodynamics Independent of Body Mass Index." *Journal of the American Society of Nephrology* 24 (2013).
8. T. Pischon, et al., "General and Abdominal Adiposity and Risk of Death in Europe," *New England Journal of Medicine* 359 (2008): 2105–2120.
9. National Heart, Lung, and Blood Institute, National Institutes of Health, *The Practical Guide: Identification, Evaluation, and Treatment of Overweight and Obesity in Adults* (NIH Publication no. 00-4084) (Washington, DC: Government Printing Office, 2000).
10. M. B. Snijder, et al., "The Prediction of Visceral Fat by Dual-Energy X-ray Absorptiometry in the Elderly: A Comparison with Computed Tomography and Anthropometry," *International Journal of Obesity* 26 (2002): 984–993.
11. I. Janssen, P. T. Katzmarzyk, and R. Ross, "Waist Circumference and Not Body Mass Index Explains Obesity-Related Health Risk," *American Journal of Clinical Nutrition* 79 (2004): 379–384.
12. M. Ashwell, "Charts Based on Body Mass Index and Waist-to-Height Ratio to Assess the Health Risks of Obeisity," The Open Obesity Journal 3 (2011): 78–84. S. C. Savva, D. Lamnisos, and A. G. Kafatos, "Predicting Cardiometabolic Risk: Waist-to-Height Ratio or BMI. A Meta-Analysis," *Diabetes Metab Syndr Obes.* 6 (2013): 403–419.
13. M Ashwell, P. Gunn, and S. Gibson, "Waist-to-Height ratio is a Better Screening Tool than Waist Circumference and BMI for Adult Cardiometabolic Risk Factors: Systematic Review and Meta-Analysis," *Obesity Review* 13 (2012): 275–286; S.C. Savva, D. Lamnisos, and A. G. Kafatos, "Predicting Cardiometabolic Risk: Waist-to-Height Ratio or BMI. A Meta-analysis," *Diabetes Metab Syndr Obes* 6 (2013): 403–419.
14. H. Schröder, et al., "Prevalence of Abdominal Obesity in Spanish Children and Adolescents. Do We Need Waist Circumference Measurements in Pediatric Practice?" *PLoS One* 9(1) (2014): e87549. Published online 2014 January 27. doi: 10.1371/journal.pone.0087549; T. Nawarycz, et al. "Waist

Circumference and Waist-to-Height Ratio Distributions in Polish and German Schoolchildren: Comparative Analysis," *International Journal of Preventative Medicine* 4(7) (2013 July): 786–796.

15. M. Ashwell, et al., "Waist-to-Height Ratio Is More Accurate than Body Mass Index to Quantify Reduced Life Expectancy," European Congress on Obesity 2013; Abstract T3T4:P.013.

SUGGESTED READINGS

Heymsfield, S. B., T. G. Lohman, Z. Wang, and S. B. Going. *Human Body Composition*. Champaign, IL: Human Kinetics, 2005.

Heyward, V. H., and D. Wagner. *Applied Body Composition Assessment*. Champaign, IL: Human Kinetics, 2004.

Parr, R., and S. Haight. "Abdominal Visceral Fat: The New Direction in Body Composition," *ACSM's Health & Fitness Journal* 10, no. 4 (2006): 26-30.

Serviente, C., and G. Sforzo. "A Simple Yet Complicated Tool: Measuring Waist Circumference to Determine Cardiometabolic Risk," *ACSM's Health & Fitness Journal* 17, no. 6 (2013): 29-34.

Lab 4A: Hydrostatic Weighing for Body Composition Assessment

Name ______________________ **Date** __________ **Grade** __________

Instructor ______________________ **Course** __________ **Section** __________

NECESSARY LAB EQUIPMENT

Hydrostatic or underwater weighing tank and residual volume spirometer (if no spirometer is available, predicting equations can be used to determine this volume—see Figure 4.2, page 140).

OBJECTIVE

To determine body density and percent body fat according to hydrostatic weighing.

LAB PREPARATION

Bring a swimsuit and towel to this lab. A 6- to 8-hour fast and bladder and bowel movements are recommended prior to underwater weighing.

INSTRUCTIONS

Follow the procedure outlined in Figure 4.2. If time is a factor, assess only the body composition of one or two participants in the course and compute the results using the form provided below. A sample of the computations is provided on the back of this page.

I. Hydrostatic Weighing

Name: ______________________ Age: __________ Weight: __________ lbs

Height: __________ inches × 2.54 = __________ cm Water temperature: __________ °C Water density (WD): _______ gr/ml

Residual volume (RV): _______ lt (See Figure 4.2)

Body weight (BW) in kg = weight in pounds ÷ 2.2046

BW in kg = __________ ÷ 2.2046 = __________ kg

Gross underwater weights:

1. __________ kg 2. __________ kg 3. __________ kg 4. __________ kg 5. __________ kg

6. __________ kg 7. __________ kg 8. __________ kg 9. __________ kg 10. __________ kg

Average of three heaviest underwater weights (AUW): __________ kg

Tare weight (TW): __________ kg

Net underwater weight (UW) = AUW − TW

Net underwater weight (UW) = __________ − __________ = __________ kg

Body density (BD):

$$BD = \frac{BW}{\frac{BW - UW}{WD} - RV - .1}$$

$$BD = \frac{\_\_\_\_\_\_}{\frac{\_\_\_ - \_\_\_}{\_\_\_} - \_\_\_ - .1} =$$

Percent body fat (%Fat):

$$\%Fat = \frac{495}{BD} - 450 = \frac{495}{\_\_\_\_\_\_} - 450 = \_\_\_\_\_\_ \%$$

Follow-up percent body fat: __________ %

Sample computation for percent body fat according to hydrostatic weighing

Name: Jane Doe Age: 20 Weight: 148.5 lbs

Height: 67 inches × 2.54 = 170.2 cm Water temperature: 33 °C Water density (WD): .99473 gr/ml

Residual volume (RV): 1.73 lt (See Figure 4.2)

Body weight (BW) in kg = weight in pounds ÷ 2.2046

BW in kg = 148.5 ÷ 2.2046 = 67.36 kg

Gross underwater weights:

1. 6.15 kg 2. 6.12 kg 3. 6.24 kg 4. 6.26 kg 5. 6.21 kg
6. 6.26 kg 7. 6.29 kg 8. 6.28 kg 9. 6.24 kg 10. 6.27 kg

Average of three heaviest underwater weights (AUW): 6.28 kg

Tare weight (TW): 5.154 kg

Net underwater weight (UW) = AUW − TW

Net underwater weight (UW) = 6.28 − 5.154 = 1.126 kg

Body density (BD):

$$BD = \frac{BW}{\frac{BW - UW}{WD} - RV - .1}$$

$$BD = \frac{67.36}{\frac{67.36 - 1.126}{1.73} - 1.73 - .1} = 1.0402301$$

Percent body fat (%Fat):

$$\%Fat = \frac{495}{BD} - 450 = \frac{495}{1.0402301} - 450 = 25.9\%$$

Follow-up percent body fat: ______ %

II. What I learned from the underwater weighing procedure.

Describe the experience of being weighed underwater. Do you feel that the results of the test were accurate?

____

____

____

____

____

____

____

____

____

____

____

Lab 4B: Body Composition, Disease Risk Assessment, and Recommended Body Weight Determination

Name ______________________ Date ____________ Grade ____________

Instructor ______________________ Course ____________ Section ____________

NECESSARY LAB EQUIPMENT
Skinfold calipers and standard measuring tapes.

OBJECTIVE
To assess percent body fat according to skinfold thickness or girth measurements; disease risk according to body mass index and waist circumference; and recommended body weight.

INSTRUCTIONS
If skinfold calipers are available, use this technique to assess your percent body fat (see Figure 4.4, page 142). Otherwise, estimate the percent fat according to the girth measurements technique. You may wish to use both techniques and compare the results. Next, compute your recommended body weight according to your current percent body fat and the recommended percent body fat guidelines provided in Table 4.11, page 153. Determine also your waist circumference, body mass index, and recommended weight using the guidelines provided in this lab.

I. Percent Body Fat According to Skinfold Thickness

Men	
Chest (mm):	________
Abdomen (mm):	________
Thigh (mm):	________
Total (mm):	________
% Fat:	________

Women	
Triceps (mm):	________
Suprailium (mm):	________
Thigh (mm):	________
Total (mm):	________
% Fat:	________

Follow-up

Date ____________

% Fat ____________ %

II. Percent Fat According to Girth Measurements (Follow the instructions in Figure 4.5 on page 148 to obtain percent body fat, using Table 4.4 (women) or 4.5 (men).)

Men Waist (in): [ ] Wrist (in): [ ] Body weight: [ ] lb Percent body fat: [ ] %

Women Upper arm (cm): [ ] Hip (cm): [ ] Wrist (cm): [ ] Age: [ ]

Percent body fat: [ ] %

III. Recommended Body Weight Determination

A. Body weight (BW): [ ] lb

B. Current %F*: [ ] %

C. Fat weight (FW) = BW × %F

FW = [ ] × [ ] = [ ] lb

D. Lean body mass (LBM) = BW − FW = [ ] − [ ] = [ ] lb

E. Age: [ ]

F. Desired fat percent (DFP − see Table 4.10, page 142): [ ] %

G. Recommended body weight (RBW) = LBM ÷ (1.0 − DFP*)

RBW = [ ] ÷ (1.0 − [ ]) = [ ] lb

*Express percentages in decimal form (for example, 25% = .25).

Follow Up

Date:	[ ]	
A. BW:	[ ]	lbs
B. %F:	[ ]	%
C. FW:	[ ]	
D. LBM:	[ ]	lbs
E. Age:	[ ]	
F. DFP:	[ ]	%
G. RBW:	[ ]	lbs

IV. Body Mass Index

Weight: ______ lb ______ kg

Height: ______ in ______ m

BMI = Weight (lb) × 705 ÷ Height (in) ÷ Height (in)

BMI = ______ (lb) ÷ 705 ÷ ______ (in) ÷ ______ (in)

BMI = ______ Disease Risk: (use Table 4.7, page 150): ______

Follow-up Date: ______ BMI: ______ Disease Risk (use Table 4.7, page 150): ______

V. Waist Circumference

Waist (in): ______

Disease Risk (use Table 4.8, page 151): ______

Follow Up

______

______

VI. Disease Risk According to BMI and WC (use Table 4.9, page 152): ______

VII. Recommended Body Weight (RBW) According to BMI

RBW based on BMI = Desired BMI × height (in) × height (in) ÷ 705

RBW at BMI of 25 = 25 × ______ × ______ ÷ 705 = ______ lb

RBW at BMI of 22 = 22 × ______ × ______ ÷ 705 = ______ lb

VIII. Disease Risk According to Waist-to-Height Ratio (WHtR)

WHtR ______ Category: ______ Disease Risk: ______

IX. Determining Body Composition Results and Goals

Briefly state your feelings about your body composition results and your recommended body weight using both percent body fat and BMI. Do you plan to reduce your percent body fat and increase your lean body mass? Write the goal(s) you want to achieve by the end of the term and indicate how you plan to achieve them.

______

______

______

______

______

______

______

______

______

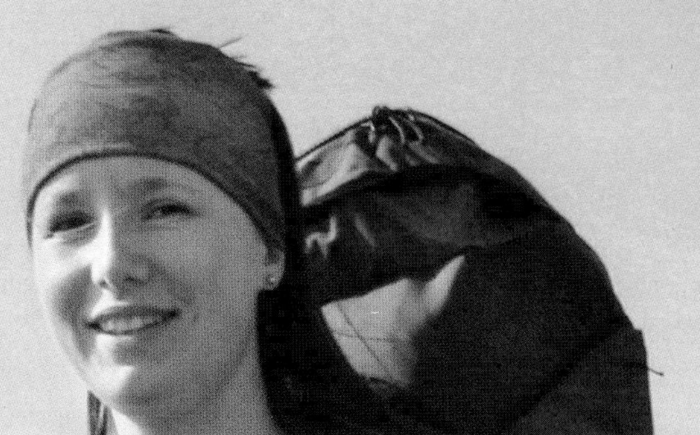

5

Weight Management

Physical activity is the cornerstone of any sound weight management program. If you are unwilling to increase daily physical activity, you might as well not even attempt to lose weight, because in all likelihood you won't be able to keep it off.

OBJECTIVES

- Describe the health consequences of obesity.
- Expose some popular fad diets and myths and fallacies regarding weight control.
- Describe eating disorders and their associated medical problems and behavior patterns, and outline the need for professional help in treating these conditions.
- Explain the physiology of weight loss, including the setpoint theory and effects of diet on basal metabolic rate.
- Explain the key role of a lifetime exercise program in a successful weight loss and weight maintenance program.
- Be able to implement a physiologically sound weight reduction and weight maintenance program.
- Describe behavior modification techniques that help support adherence to a lifetime weight maintenance program.

REAL LIFE STORY | David's Experience

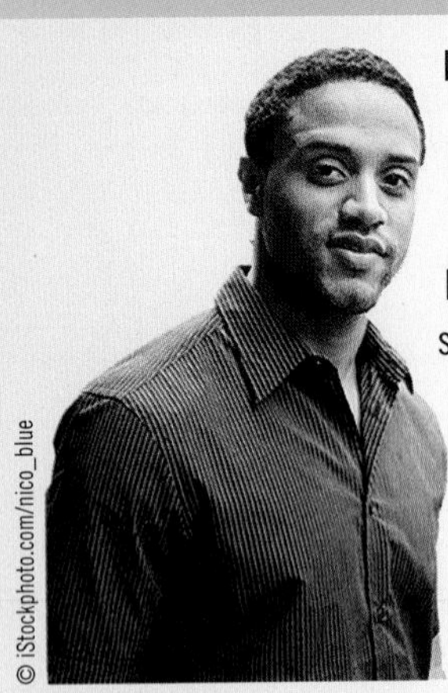

I played high school football, and I knew I was in real good shape and had a lot of muscle. After high school, my football days were over. My freshman year in college took some adjustment, even more so being away from home and all my buddies. I wasn't exercising and gained 12 pounds that year. At 192 pounds, I still thought I was in pretty good shape. My sophomore year I stopped at the school's annual health and fitness fair during the fall semester. There I had my body fat checked. It turned out to be 26.5 percent. I always thought I was pretty fit and I wasn't happy to be rated "overweight." That one body fat test motivated me to enroll in the fitness and wellness course. In class, I learned how to set up a good aerobic and strength-training exercise program, eat better, and the value of increasing daily physical activity. At the end of the semester I had only lost 8 pounds, but I was pleasantly surprised to find out that I had also gained 7 pounds of lean body mass (in essence, I lost 15 pounds of body fat) and my body fat decreased to 19.6 percent.

Obesity is a health hazard of epidemic proportions in most developed countries around the world. According to the World Health Organization, an estimated 35 percent of the adult population in industrialized nations is obese. Obesity has been defined as a body mass index (BMI) of 30 or higher. The obesity level is the point at which excess body fat can lead to significant health problems.

The current 21st century environment in which we live is rich in cues to overeat high-calorie, high-fat, sugary foods 24/7. Food overconsumption coupled with advances in modern technology that minimize the need for daily physical activity have led to the current obesogenic culture that promotes weight gain and the array of chronic conditions caused by excessive weight.

The number of people who are obese and overweight in the United States has increased dramatically during the past 25 years, a direct result of a lack of physical activity and poor dietary habits by the American people. The average weight of American adults between the ages of 20 and 74 has increased 25 pounds or more since 1965, most of the weight gain (15 pounds) coming since 1990. Nearly half of all adults in the United States do not achieve the minimum recommended amount of physical activity (see Figure 1.8, page 12). According to the U.S. Department of Agriculture, in 2008, the average American was consuming an additional 505 calories as compared to 1970.

Data indicate that 68.5 percent of U.S. adults age 20 and older are overweight (have a BMI greater than 25), and 34.9 percent are obese (Figure 5.1).[1] About 41 million women and 37 million men aged 20 and over are obese. Between 1960 and 2012, the overall (men and women combined) prevalence of adult obesity increased from about 13 percent to 35 percent. Most of this increase occurred in the 1990s.

FIGURE 5.1 Percentage of the adult population (≥20 years) that is normal weight (BMI <25), overweight (BMI 25–29.99), or obese (BMI >30) in the United States.

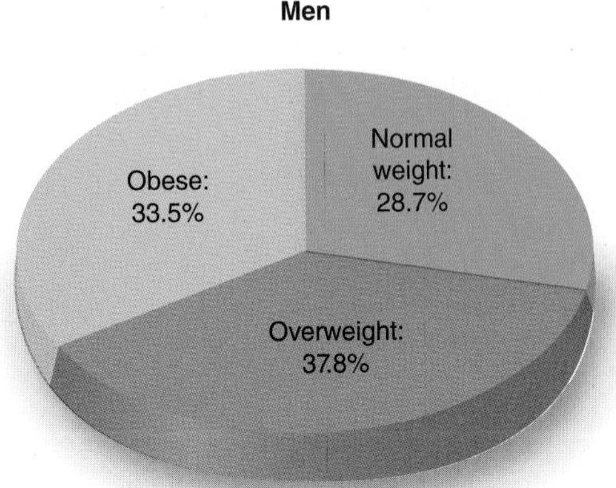

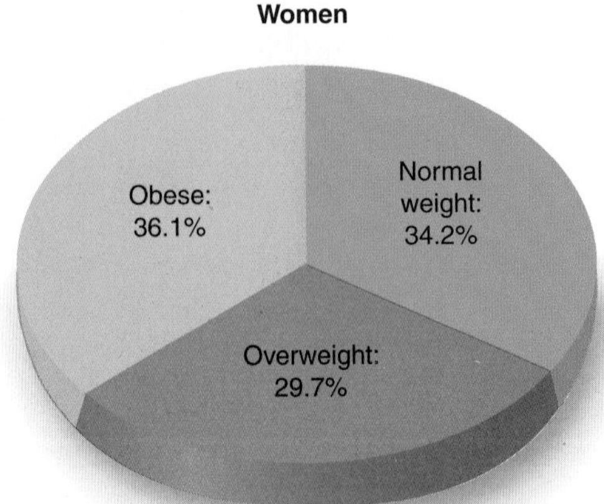

Source: Centers for Disease Control and Prevention, 2011.

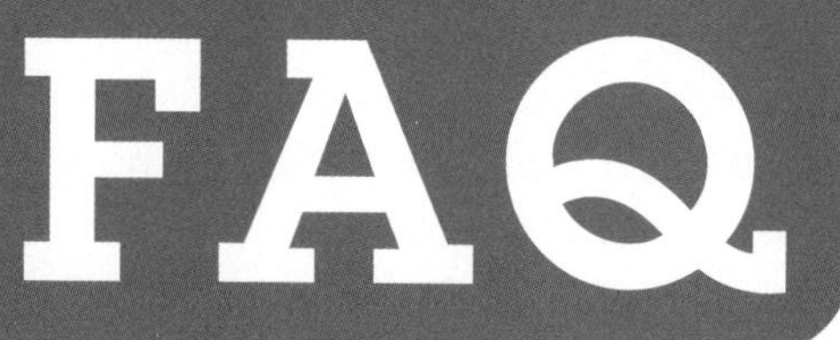

Why can't I lose weight with exercise?

During the past few years, there has been a fair amount of media distortion stating "exercise makes a person fat," "why most of us believe that exercise makes us thinner—and why we are wrong," and "the myth about exercise: of course it's good for you, but it won't make you lose weight." There is ample scientific evidence that exercise is an important component of a successful weight loss program. The problem is that following exercise, many people eat more (particularly more junk food). They feel justified in doing so because they exercised. It is clear that weight loss is more effective when you cut back on calories (dieting), as opposed to only increasing physical activity or exercise.

When attempting to lose weight, initial lengthy exercise sessions (longer than 60 minutes) by unfit people may not be the best approach to weight loss—unless they carefully monitor daily caloric intake and avoid caloric compensation for the energy expended during exercise. In active or fit individuals, lengthy exercise sessions are not counterproductive.

Body composition changes are also more effective when dieting and exercise are combined while attempting to lose body weight. Most weight loss when dieting with exercise comes in the form of body fat and not lean body tissue, a desirable outcome. Weight loss maintenance, however, in most cases is possible only with 60 to 90 minutes of sustained daily physical activity and exercise.

If you are still not convinced that exercise is the best approach to weight management, take a look around the gym or the jogging trail. If this were the case, wouldn't those who regularly exercise be the fattest? Additional information on this subject is provided throughout this chapter, in particular in the section "The Roles of Exercise Intensity and Duration in Weight Management" on page 185.

Are we making any progress in the fight against obesity?

For the first time in three decades, the U.S. obesity rate did not rise in 2013. According to the U.S. Department of Agriculture, Americans have slimmed down total caloric intake by an average of 118 calories per day. Although not a precise science (see discussion on page 178), 118 calories per day represents about 12 pounds of body fat per year (118 calories $\times$ 365 days per year $\div$ 3,500 calories per pound of fat). The trend is attributed to five factors. People are: (1) preparing more meals at home, (2) eating fewer restaurant and fast-food meals, (3) paying more attention to nutrition labels, (4) limiting spending because of the lengthy most recent recession, and (5) becoming more physically active. The fight against excessive body weight, however, still has a long way to go—68.5 percent of all adults ($\geq$20 years) are overweight, and 34.9 percent are obese.

Are some diet plans more effective than others?

The term "diet" implies a negative caloric balance. A negative caloric balance means that you are consuming fewer calories than those required to maintain your current weight. When energy output surpasses energy intake, weight loss occurs. Popular diets differ widely in the food choices that you are allowed to have, but regardless of which diet you follow, as long as there is a negative caloric balance, you will lose weight. The more limited the choices, the lower the chances to overeat and thus the lower the caloric intake. And the fewer calories you consume, the greater the weight loss. For health reasons, to obtain the variety of nutrients the body needs, even during weight loss periods, you should not consume less than 1,500 calories per day (unless you are a very small individual). These calories should be distributed over a range of foods, emphasizing grains, fruits, vegetables, and small amounts of low-fat animal products or fish.

Why is it so difficult to change dietary habits?

In most developed countries, there is an overabundance of food and practically an unlimited number of food choices. With unlimited supply and choices, most people do not have the willpower, stemming from their core values, to avoid overconsumption.

Our bodies were not created to go hungry or to overeat. We are uncomfortable overeating, and we feel even worse when we have to go hungry. Our health values, however, are not strong enough to prevent overconsumption. The end result: weight gain. Next, we restrict calories (go on a diet), we feel hungry, and we have a difficult time adhering to the diet. Stated quite simply, going hungry is an uncomfortable and unpleasant experience.

To avoid this vicious cycle, our dietary habits (and most likely physical activity habits) must change. A question you need to ask yourself is, do I value health and quality of life more than food overindulgence? If you do not, then the achievement and maintenance of recommended body weight and good health is a moot point. If you desire to avoid disease and increase quality of life, you have to value health more than food overconsumption. If you have spent the past 20 years tasting and "devouring" every food item in sight, it is time to make healthy choices and consume only moderate amounts of food at a time (portion control). You do not have to taste and eat everything that is placed before your eyes. If you can make such a change in your eating habits, you may not have to worry about another diet for the rest of your life.

MyProfile: Personal Weight Management Program

To the best of your ability, answer the following questions. If you do not know the answer(s), this chapter will guide you through them.

I. Do you understand the concept of recommended body weight? ___ Yes ___ No Do you consider yourself to be at this weight? ___ Yes ___ No Explain your answer.

II. What type of exercise program do you consider most effective for weight management (mark one): ___ aerobic exercise or ___ strength training? Indicate why you feel this way.

III. Have you gained weight since you started college? ___ Yes ___ No If yes, what do you attribute this weight gain to?

IV. What can you learn from David's experience, and what strategies can you use to help properly manage your body weight?

V. Do you understand the concept of long-term gratification derived through a lifetime exercise program and the required process to do so? ___ Yes ___ No

Obesity rates in the U.S. have drastically increased since 1985. Based on data from 1985, no single state reported an obesity rate above 15 percent of the state's total population (which includes both adults and children). By 2012 (see Figure 5.2), no state had a prevalence of obesity less than 20 percent. Nine states and the District of Columbia had prevalence between 20 and 25 percent. Thirteen had a prevalence equal to or greater than 30 percent.

As of the end of 2012, the average man now weighs in at 196 pounds and the average woman at 156 pounds. As pointed out in Chapter 2, the human mind has a tremendous capability to adapt and accept change, even if such is detrimental to one's health. And so it is with body weight. According to a Gallup poll conducted in November 2012, men indicate their "ideal" body weight is 185 pounds, the highest ever, and 14 pounds above the 1990 weight as determined by this same poll. Women indicate their "ideal" weight to be 11 pounds heavier than in 1990, at 140 pounds.

The prevalence of obesity is even higher in certain ethnic groups, especially African Americans and Hispanic Americans. Furthermore, as the nation continues to evolve into a more mechanized and automated society (relying on escalators, elevators, remote controls, computers, e-mail, cell phones, and automatic-sensor doors), the amount of required daily physical activity continues to decrease. People are being lulled into a high-risk sedentary lifestyle.

The data in Figure 5.3 illustrate that the current obesity epidemic is not due to a change in the genetic code, as it doesn't change from one generation to the next. The data compare the obesity rates in the United States from 1988 to 1994 and with those from 2005 to 2008 and quite clearly illustrate that lifestyle changes over the past 15 to 20 years are

FIGURE 5.2 Obesity trends in the United States based on BMI 30 or 30 pounds overweight, 2012.

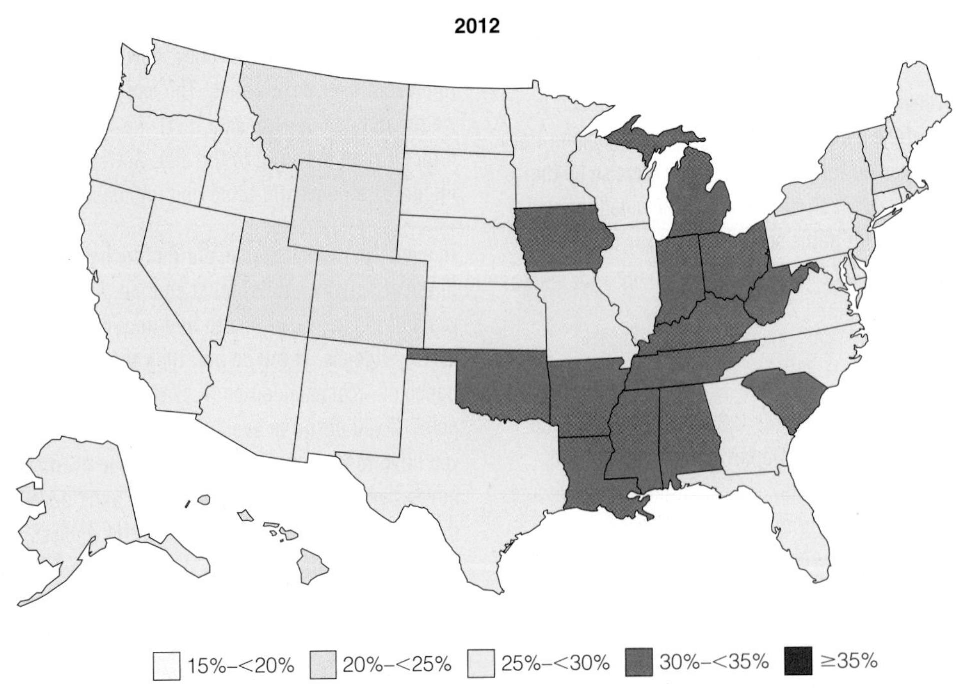

Source: Obesity Trends Among U.S. Adults Between 1985-2010. (Atlanta: Centers for Disease Control and Prevention, 2012).

Health Consequences of Excessive Body Weight

Being overweight or obese increases the risk for

- high blood pressure
- elevated blood lipids (high blood cholesterol and triglycerides)
- type 2 (non-insulin-dependent) diabetes
- insulin resistance
- glucose intolerance
- coronary heart disease
- angina pectoris
- congestive heart failure
- stroke
- gallbladder disease
- gout
- osteoarthritis
- orthopedic problems
- back pain
- gastroesophageal reflux disease (GERD or acid reflux)
- obstructive sleep apnea and respiratory problems
- some types of cancer (endometrial, breast, prostate, and colon)
- complications of pregnancy (gestational diabetes, gestational hypertension, preeclampsia, and complications during C-sections)
- poor female reproductive health (menstrual irregularities, infertility, and irregular ovulation)
- bladder control problems (stress incontinence)
- skin infections
- psychological disorders (depression, eating disorders, distorted body image, discrimination, and low self-esteem)
- cognitive decline
- shortened life expectancy
- decreased quality of life

Sources: Centers for Disease Control and Prevention, downloaded March 17, 2014 and J. O. Hill and H. R. Wyatt, "The Myth of Healthy Obesity," *Annals of Internal Medicine* 159 (2013): 789-790.

responsible for the drastic increase in the escalating obesity rate. Furthermore, the prevalence of obesity is significantly lower among college graduates compared to those with only a high school degree or less.

More than a third of the population is on a diet at any given moment. People spend about $40 billion yearly attempting to lose weight, with more than $10 billion going to memberships in weight reduction centers and another $30 billion to diet food sales. Furthermore, the total cost attributable to treating obesity-related diseases is estimated at $117 billion per year.[2]

FIGURE 5.3 **Prevalence of obesity among U.S. adults (≥20 years) by gender and education, 1988–1994 and 2005–2008.**

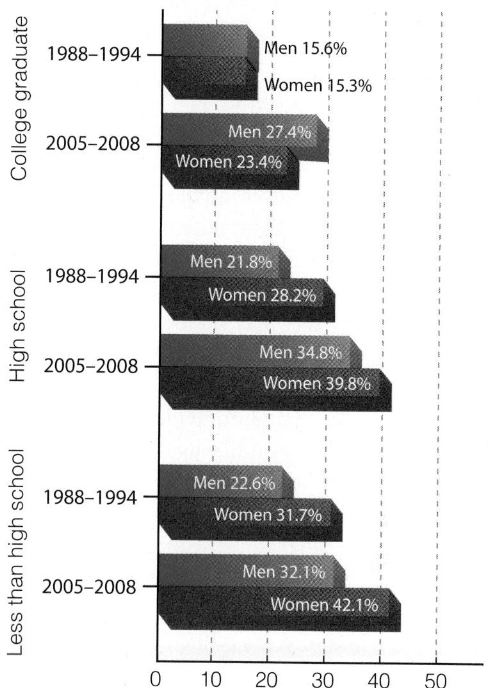

Source: Centers for Disease Control and Prevention, 2010.

Excessive body weight combined with physical inactivity is the second-leading cause of preventable death in the United States, resulting in more than 112,000 deaths each year.[3] Furthermore, obesity is more prevalent than smoking (19 percent), poverty (14 percent), or problem drinking (6 percent).[4] Obesity and unhealthy lifestyle habits are the most critical public health problems in the 21st century.

Excessive body weight and obesity are associated with poor health status and are risk factors for many physical ailments, including cardiovascular disease, type 2 diabetes, and some types of cancer. Evidence indicates that health risks associated with increased body weight start at a BMI greater than 25 and are enhanced greatly at a BMI greater than 30.

The American Heart Association has identified obesity as one of the six major risk factors for coronary heart disease. Estimates also indicate that 14 percent of all cancer deaths among men and 20 percent among women are related to current overweight and obesity patterns in the United States.[5] Excessive body weight also is implicated in psychological maladjustment and a higher accidental death rate. Extremely obese people have a lower mental health-related quality of life.

Overweight versus Obese

Overweight and obese are not the same thing. Many overweight people (who weigh about 10 to 20 pounds over the recommended weight) are not obese. Although a few pounds of excess weight may not be harmful to most people, this is not always the case. People with excessive body fat who have type 2 diabetes and other cardiovascular risk factors (elevated blood lipids, high blood pressure, physical inactivity, and poor eating habits) benefit from losing weight. People who have a few extra pounds of weight but are otherwise healthy and physically active, exercise regularly, and eat a healthy diet may not be at higher risk for early death. Such is not the case, however, with obese individuals.

Research indicates that an individual who is 30 or more pounds overweight during middle age (30 to 49 years of age) loses about 7 years of life, whereas being 10 to 30 pounds overweight decreases the lifespan by about 3 years.[6] These decreases are similar to those seen with tobacco use. Nonetheless, severe obesity (BMI greater than 45) at a young age may cut up to 20 years off a person's life.[7]

Although the loss of years of life is significant, the decreased life expectancy doesn't even begin to address the loss in quality of life, considerably compromised by obesity, and increase in illness and disability throughout the years. Even a modest reduction of 2 to 3 percent can reduce the risk for chronic diseases, including heart disease, high blood pressure, high cholesterol, and diabetes.[8]

A primary objective to achieve overall physical fitness and enhanced quality of life is to attain recommended body composition. Individuals at their recommended body weight are able to participate in a variety of moderate-to-vigorous activities without functional limitations. These people have the freedom to enjoy most of life's recreational activities to their fullest potential. Excessive body weight does not afford people the fitness level to enjoy many lifetime activities, such as basketball, soccer, racquetball, surfing, mountain cycling, or mountain climbing. Maintaining high fitness and recommended body weight gives a degree of independence throughout life that most people in developed nations no longer enjoy.

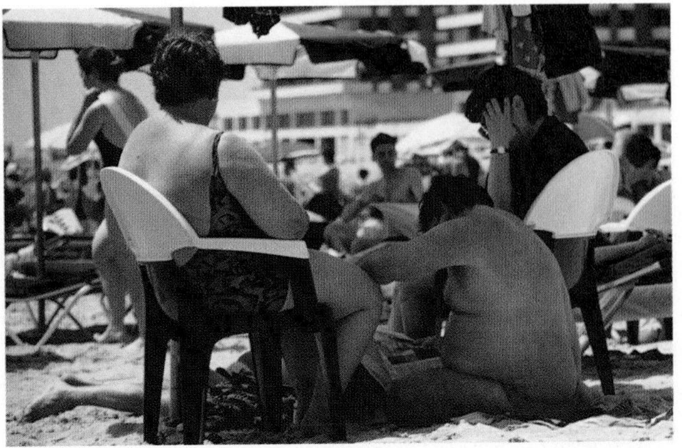

Obesity is a health hazard of epidemic proportions in industrialized nations.

Scientific evidence also recognizes problems with being underweight. Although the social pressure to be thin has declined slightly in recent years, the pressure to attain model-like thinness is still with us and contributes to the gradual increase in the number of people who develop eating disorders (anorexia nervosa and bulimia, discussed under "Eating Disorders" on pages 174–177).

Extreme weight loss can lead to medical conditions such as heart damage, gastrointestinal problems, shrinkage of internal organs, abnormalities of the immune system, disorders of the reproductive system, loss of muscle tissue, damage to the nervous system, and even death. About 14 percent of people in the United States are underweight.

Tolerable Weight

Many people want to lose weight so that they will look better. That's a worthy goal. The problem, however, is that they have a distorted image of what they would look like if they were to reduce to what they think is their ideal weight. Hereditary factors play a big role, and only a small fraction of the population has the genes for a "perfect body."

> **CRITICAL THINKING**
>
> Do you consider yourself overweight? If so, how long have you had a weight problem, what attempts have you made to lose weight, and what has worked best for you?

The media have the greatest influence on people's perception of what constitutes "ideal" body weight. Most people consult fashion, fitness, and beauty magazines to determine what they should look like. The "ideal" body shapes, physiques, and proportions illustrated in these magazines are rare and are achieved mainly through airbrushing and medical reconstruction.[9] Many individuals, primarily young women, go to extremes in attempts to achieve these unrealistic figures. Failure to attain a "perfect body" may lead to eating disorders in some individuals.

When people set their target weight, they should be realistic. Attaining the "excellent" percent of body fat shown in Table 4.11 (page 153) is extremely difficult for some people. It is even more difficult to maintain over time without a commitment to a vigorous lifetime exercise program and permanent dietary changes. Few people are willing to do that. The moderate category for percentage of body fat may be more realistic for many people.

The question you should ask yourself is, am I happy with my weight? Part of enjoying a higher quality of life is being happy with yourself. If you are not, you need to either do something about it or learn to live with it.

If your percentage of body fat is higher than the relevant percentage in the moderate category of Table 4.11 in Chapter 4, you should try to reduce it and stay in this category for health reasons. This is the category that seems to pose no detriment to health.

If you are in the moderate category but would like to reduce your percentage of body fat further, you need to ask yourself additional questions: How badly do I want it? Do I want it badly enough to implement lifetime exercise and dietary changes? If you are not willing to change, you should stop worrying about your weight and deem the moderate category "tolerable" for you.

The Weight Loss Dilemma

Yo-yo dieting carries as great a health risk as being overweight and remaining overweight. Epidemiological data show that frequent fluctuations in weight (up or down) markedly increase the risk for dying from cardiovascular disease. Experts theorize that the constant shrinking and growing with yo-yo dieting causes micro tears in the blood vessels that increase their susceptibility to atherosclerosis (obstruction of the arteries-see Chapter 11). Based on the findings that constant losses and regains can be hazardous to health, quick-fix diets should be replaced by a slow but permanent weight loss program (as described under "Losing Weight the Sound and Sensible Way," page 188). Individuals reap the benefits of recommended body weight when they get to that weight and stay there throughout life.

Unfortunately, only about 10 percent of all people who begin a traditional weight loss program without exercise are able to lose the desired weight. Worse, only 5 in 100 people are able to keep the weight off. The body is highly resistant to permanent weight changes through caloric restrictions alone.

Traditional diets have failed because few of them incorporate permanent behavioral changes in food selection and an overall increase in physical activity and exercise as fundamental to successful weight loss and weight maintenance. When the diet stops, weight gain begins. The $40 billion diet industry tries to capitalize on the false idea that a person can lose weight quickly without considering the consequences of fast weight loss or the importance of lifetime behavioral changes to ensure proper weight loss and maintenance.

In addition, research indicates that most people, especially obese people, underestimate their energy intake. Those who try to lose weight but apparently fail to do so are often described as "diet resistant." A benchmark study found that while on a "diet," a group of obese individuals with a self-reported history of diet resistance underreported their average daily caloric intake by almost 50 percent (1,028 self-reported versus 2,081 actual calories).[10] These individuals also overestimated their amount of daily physical activity by about 25 percent (1,022 self-reported versus 771 actual calories). These differences represent an additional 1,304 calories of energy per day unaccounted for by the subjects in the study. The findings indicate that failing to lose weight often is related to misreports of actual food intake and level of physical activity.

DIVERSITY CONSIDERATIONS: Racial and Ethnic Disparities in Obesity Rates

Significant racial and ethnic disparities in overweight and obesity prevalence exist in the United States.

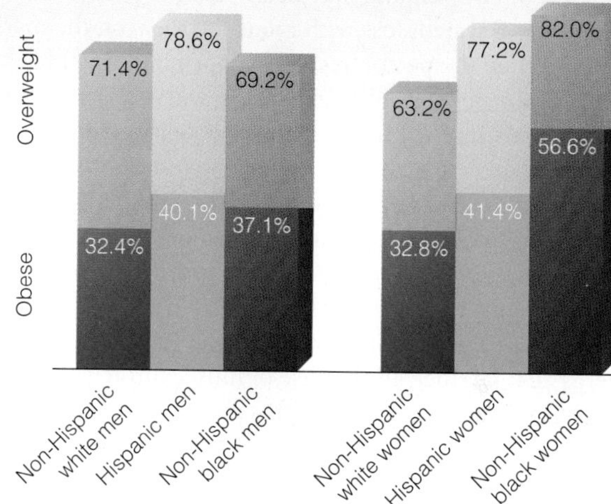

Source: Centers for Disease Control and Prevention, 2014.

Although limited research is available, data also indicate that African American women exhibit fewer lost pounds than African American men and non-Hispanic white men and women on medication therapy for the treatment of diabetes. More research is necessary to understand the complex sociocultural and lifestyle-related issues associated with weight management and the obesity problem among groups of varied ethnic backgrounds.

Diet Crazes

Capitalizing on hopes that the latest diet to hit the market will work, fad diets continue to appeal to people of all shapes and sizes. These diets may work for a while, but their success is usually short lived. Regarding the effectiveness of these diets, Kelly Brownell, one of the foremost researchers in the field of weight management, has stated: "When I get the latest diet fad, I imagine a trick birthday cake candle that keeps lighting up and we have to keep blowing it out."

Fad diets deceive people and claim that dieters will lose weight by following all instructions. Many fad diets are very low in calories. Under these conditions, a lot of the weight lost is in the form of water and protein, not fat.

On average, a 150-pound person stores about 1.3 pounds of glycogen (carbohydrate or glucose storage) in the body. This amount of glycogen is higher in aerobically trained individuals, because intense training (i.e., by elite athletes) can more than double the body's capacity to store glycogen. About 80 percent of the glycogen is stored in muscles, and the remaining 20 percent is in the liver. Water, however, is required to store glycogen. A 2.6-to-1 water-to-glycogen ratio is necessary to store **glycogen.**[11] Thus, this 150-pound person stores about 3.4 pounds of water (1.3 × 2.6), along with the 1.3 pounds of glycogen, accounting for a total of 4.7 pounds of the individual's normal body weight.

When someone is fasting or on a crash diet (typically defined as less than 800 calories per day), glycogen storage can be depleted in just a few days. This loss of weight is not in the form of body fat and is typically used to promote and guarantee rapid weight loss with many fad diets on the market today. When the person resumes a normal eating plan, the body again stores its glycogen, along with the water required to do so, and the individual subsequently gains weight.

Furthermore, on a crash diet, close to half the weight loss is in lean (protein) tissue. When the body uses protein instead of a combination of fats and carbohydrates as a source of energy, weight is lost as much as 10 times faster. This is because a gram of protein produces half the amount of energy that fat does. In the case of muscle protein, one-fifth protein is mixed with four-fifths water. Therefore, each pound of muscle yields only one-tenth the amount of energy of a pound of fat. As a result, most weight lost is in the form of water, which looks good on the scale.

Long-term or frequent crash dieting also increases the risk of heart attacks, because low caloric intake eventually leads to heart muscle (protein) loss. Limiting potassium, magnesium, and copper intake as a result of very low-calorie diets may induce fatal cardiac arrhythmias. Furthermore, sodium depletion may cause a dangerous drop in blood pressure. Very low-calorie diets should always be followed under a physician's supervision. Unfortunately, most crash dieters simply consult a friend rather than seeking a physician's advice.

Diet books are frequently found on best-seller lists. The market is flooded with these books. Examples include *The DASH Diet,* the *Volumetrics Eating Plan,* the *Ornish Diet,* the *Atkins Diet,* the *Zone Diet,* the *South Beach Diet,* the *Best Life Diet,* the *Abs Diet,* and *The Biggest Loser Diet.* Some of these popular diets have sound dietary principles, while others are becoming more nutritionally balanced and encourage consumption of fruits and vegetables, whole grains, some lean meat and fish, and low-fat milk and dairy products. Such plans reduce the risk for chronic diseases, including cardiovascular diseases and cancer.

While it is clear that some diets are healthier than others, strictly from a weight loss point of view, it doesn't matter what diet plan you follow: If caloric intake is lower than caloric output, weight will come off. Dropout rates for many popular diets, however, are high because of the difficulty in long-term adherence to limited dietary plans.

Low-Carb Diets Among the most popular diets on the market in recent years were the low-carbohydrate/high-protein (LCHP) diet plans. Although they vary slightly, low-carb diets, in general, limit the intake of carbohydrate-rich foods—bread, potatoes, rice, pasta, cereals, crackers, juices, sodas, sweets (candy, cake, cookies, etc.), and even fruits and vegetables. Dieters are allowed to eat all the protein-rich foods they desire, including steak, ham, chicken, fish, bacon, eggs, nuts, cheese, tofu, high-fat salad dressings, butter, and small amounts of a few fruits and vegetables. Typically, these diets also are high in fat content. Examples of these diets are the Atkins Diet, the Zone Diet, Protein Power, the Scarsdale Diet, the Carb Addict's Diet, the South Beach Diet, and Sugar Busters.

During digestion, carbohydrates are converted into glucose, a basic fuel used by every cell in the body. As blood glucose rises, the pancreas releases insulin. Insulin is a hormone that facilitates the entry of glucose into the cells, thereby lowering the glucose level in the bloodstream. A rapid rise in glucose also causes a rapid spike in insulin, which is followed by a rapid removal and drop in blood glucose that leaves you hungry again. A slower rise in blood glucose is desirable because the level is kept constant longer, delaying the onset of hunger. If the cells don't need the glucose for normal cell functions or to fuel physical activity, and if cellular glucose stores are already full, glucose is converted to, and stored as, body fat.

Not all carbohydrates cause a similar rise in blood glucose. The rise in glucose is based on the speed of digestion, which depends on a number of factors, including the size of the food particles. Small-particle carbohydrates break down rapidly and cause a quick, sharp rise in blood glucose. Thus, to gauge a food's effect on blood glucose, carbohydrates are classified by their **glycemic index.**

A high glycemic index signifies a food that causes a quick rise in blood glucose. At the top of the 100-point scale is glucose itself. This index is not directly related to simple and complex carbohydrates, and the glycemic values are not always what you might expect. Rather, the index is based on the actual laboratory-measured speed of absorption. Processed foods generally have a high glycemic index, whereas high-fiber foods tend to have a lower index (Table 5.1). Other factors that affect the index are the amount of carbohydrate, fat, and protein in the food; how refined the ingredients are; and whether the food was cooked.

The body functions best when blood sugar remains at a constant level. Although this is best accomplished by consuming foods with a low glycemic index (nuts, apples, oranges, low-fat yogurt, etc.), a person does not have to eliminate all high–glycemic index foods (sugar, potatoes, bread, white rice, soda drinks, etc.) from the diet. Foods with a high glycemic index along with some protein are useful to replenish depleted glycogen stores

Glycogen Manner in which carbohydrates (glucose molecules) are stored in the human body, predominantly in the muscles and liver.

Glycemic index A measure used to rate the plasma glucose response of carbohydrate-containing foods, comparing it with the response produced by the same amount of carbohydrates from a standard source, usually glucose or white bread.

Popular Diets

The DASH Diet

The Dietary Approaches to Stop Hypertension (DASH) diet was originally designed as a heart-healthy diet to help lower high blood pressure. The diet plan is rich in fruits, vegetables, fat-free or low-fat milk and milk products, whole grains, fish, poultry, beans, seeds, and nuts. It also contains less sodium, fats, red meats, sweets, added sugars, and sugar-containing beverages than the typical American diet. Because it is such a healthy diet, the plan has been embraced by people seeking to lose weight. For weight loss purposes, the recommended daily caloric intake ranges from about 1,600 to 2,200 calories. The macronutrient composition of the diet includes 50 to 60 percent carbohydrates, less than 30 percent fat, and 15 to 20 percent protein.

The Volumetrics Eating Plan

The Volumetrics diet plan focuses on maximizing the volume of food and limiting calories by emphasizing high-water content or low-fat foods (lower energy density), low-fat cooking techniques, and extensive use of vegetables. The average daily caloric intake is reduced by 500 to 1,000 calories, with a macronutrient composition of approximately 55 percent carbohydrates, less than 30 percent fat, and more than 20 percent protein.

The Best Life Diet

The initial phase of the Best Life Diet plan encourages exercise and a recommended eating schedule. The second phase requires a reduction in caloric intake through consumption of healthful foods to satisfy hunger. The plan deals extensively with emotional eating. Caloric intake averages about 1,700 calories, with maintenance of daily moderate physical activity. The diet composition is about 50 percent carbohydrates, 30 percent fat, and 20 percent protein.

The Weight Watchers Diet

Dieters are given a daily point allowance in which calorie-dense foods with a higher fat content, simple carbohydrate content, or both are given more points. The points are determined using the patented Weight Watchers Point Calculator formula that looks to create an approximate 1,000-calorie per day deficit. The program encourages dieters to use points wisely by eating filling foods that keep hunger at bay, primarily foods rich in protein and fiber. The diet contains approximately 50 percent carbohydrates, 30 percent fat, and 20 percent protein.

The Ornish Diet

Ornish is a very low-fat, vegetarian-type diet. Dieters are not allowed to drink alcohol or eat meat, fish, oils, sugar, or white flour. Data indicate that strict adherence to the Ornish Diet can prevent and reverse heart disease. An average daily caloric intake is about 1,500 calories, composed of approximately 75 percent carbohydrates, less than 10 percent fat, and 15 percent protein.

The Zone Diet

The Zone Diet proposes that proper macronutrient (carbohydrate/fat/protein) distribution is critical to keep blood sugar and hormones in balance and thus prevent weight gain and disease. Daily caloric allowance is about 1,100 calories for women and 1,400 for men. All meals need to provide 40 percent carbohydrate calories, 30 percent fat calories, and 30 percent protein calories.

The Atkins Diet

In the LCHP Atkins Diet, practically all carbohydrates are eliminated during the first 2 weeks. Thereafter, very small amounts of carbohydrates are allowed, primarily in the form of limited fruits, vegetables, and wine. No caloric guidelines are given, but a typical daily diet plan is about 1,500 calories and is extremely high in fat (about 60 percent of calories), followed by protein (about 30 percent of calories), and limited carbohydrates (about 10 percent of calories). Dieters may not be as hungry on the Atkins Diet but may find it too restrictive for long-term adherence.

The South Beach Diet

Also an LCHP diet, the South Beach Diet is not as restrictive as the Atkins Diet. It emphasizes low-glycemic foods thought to decrease cravings for sugar and refined carbohydrates. Sugar, fruits, and grains are initially eliminated. In phase two, some high-fiber grains, fruit, and dark chocolate are permitted. No caloric guidelines are given, but a typical dietary plan provides about 1,400 calories per day, composed of 40 percent carbohydrate, 40 percent fat, and 20 percent protein calories.

The Glycemic Index Diet

The Glycemic Index Diet is based on the system of ranking carbohydrate foods according to how much each food raises the person's blood sugar level. This diet is also the basis for the Zone and South Beach diets. Dieters are encouraged to choose carbohydrate foods with a low glycemic index, such as whole fruits, vegetables, and beans. The hypothesis behind the diet is that low–glycemic index foods are absorbed more slowly, delaying hunger and making you less likely to overeat. Caloric intake ranges between 1,000 and 1,500 calories per day, and the diet composition is around 40 to 50 percent carbohydrates, 30 percent fat, and 30 percent protein.

The Biggest Loser Diet

Based on the popular TV show, The Biggest Loser Diet encourages small, frequent meals that emphasize filling calories from

Continued

fruits, vegetables, lean protein sources, and whole grains; portion control; a food journal to monitor food intake; and an increase in daily physical activity and exercise. Caloric intake ranges from about 1,200 to 1,800 calories. The macronutrient composition of the diet is approximately 45 percent carbohydrate, 25 percent fat, and 30 percent protein calories.

The Mediterranean Diet

Although not specifically a dietary plan for weight reduction, the Mediterranean Diet (different cultures around the Mediterranean have slightly different patterns) emphasizes daily fruits, vegetables, whole grains, beans, nuts, legumes, olive oil, and flavorful herbs and spices; seafood at least twice a week; and poultry, eggs, cheese, yogurt, and red wine in moderation. Sweets and red meat are reserved for special occasions only, and physically activity is a part of the daily pattern. A calorie-restricted plan of the dietary pattern has been used to promote weight loss. Typically, the diet includes 40 to 50 percent carbohydrates, 25 to 40 percent fat, and 10 to 20 percent protein.

following prolonged or exhaustive aerobic exercise. Combining high– with low–glycemic index items or with some fat and protein brings down the average index.

Regular consumption of high-glycemic foods by themselves may increase the risk for cardiovascular disease, especially in people at risk for diabetes. A person does not need to plan the diet around the index, as many popular diet programs indicate. The glycemic index deals with single foods eaten alone. Most people eat high–glycemic index foods with other foods as part of a meal. In combination, these foods have a lower effect on blood sugar. People who follow a healthy diet; that is, consume more fruits, vegetables, whole grains, beans, fiber, fish, and lean meats, and cut back on sugar and highly processed foods; will most likely have a diet in the low to moderate glycemic index category. Even people at risk for diabetes or who have the disease can eat high-glycemic foods, but in moderation.

Low-glycemic foods may also aid in weight loss and weight maintenance. As blood sugar levels drop between snacks and meals, hunger increases. Keeping blood sugar levels constant by including low-glycemic foods in the diet helps stave off hunger, appetite, and overeating (Figure 5.4).

Proponents of LCHP diets claim that if a person eats fewer carbohydrates and more protein, the pancreas will produce less insulin; then, as insulin drops, the body will turn to its own fat deposits for energy. There is no scientific proof, however, that high levels of insulin lead to weight gain. None of the authors of these diets published studies validating their claims. Yet, these authors base their diets on the faulty premise that high insulin leads to obesity. We know the opposite to be true: Excessive body fat causes insulin levels to rise, thereby increasing the risk for developing diabetes.

The reason for rapid weight loss in LCHP dieting is that a low carbohydrate intake forces the liver to produce glucose. The source for most of this glucose is body proteins—lean body mass, including muscle. As indicated earlier, protein contains a lot of water; thus, weight is lost rapidly. When a person terminates the diet, the body rebuilds some protein tissue and quickly regains some weight.

Research studies indicated that individuals on an LCHP (Atkins) diet lost slightly more weight in the first few months than those on a low-fat diet.[12] The effectiveness of the diet, however, seemed to dwindle over time. In one of

TABLE 5.1 Glycemic Index of Selected Foods

Item	Index	Item	Index	Item	Index	Item	Index
All-Bran cereal	38	Carrots, raw	47	Honey	58	Peas	50
Apples	40	Cherries	20	Milk, chocolate, low fat	34	Pizza, cheese	60
Bagel, white	72	Colas	65	Milk, skim	32	Potato, baked	56–100
Banana	56	Corn, sweet	60	Milk, whole	40	Potato, French fries	75
Bread, French	95	Corn Flakes	92	Jelly beans	80	Potato, sweet	51
Bread, wheat	73	Doughnut	76	Oatmeal	75	Rice, white	56
Bread, white	70	Frosted Flakes	55	Oranges	48	Sugar, table	65
Carrots, boiled (Australia)	41	Fruit cocktail	55	Pasta, white	50	Watermelon	72
Carrots, boiled (Canada)	92	Gatorade	78	Pasta, wheat	32	Yogurt, low-fat	32
		Glucose	100	Peanuts	20		

the studies, at 12 months into the diet, participants in the LCHP diet had regained more weight than those on the low-fat diet plan.

Years of research are required to determine the extent to which adhering over the long term to LCHP diets increases the risk for heart disease, cancer, and kidney or bone damage. Low-carb diets are contrary to the nutrition advice of most leading national health organizations (which recommend a diet lower in saturated fat and trans fats and high in complex carbohydrates). Without fruits, vegetables, and whole grains, high-protein diets lack many vitamins, minerals, antioxidants, phytonutrients, and fiber—all dietary factors that protect against an array of ailments and diseases.

The major risk associated with long-term adherence to LCHP diets could be the increased risk for heart disease, because high-protein foods are also high in fat content (see Chapter 10). Short-term (a few weeks or months) adherence to LCHP diets does not appear to increase heart disease risk. The long-term (years) effects of these types of diet, nonetheless, have not been evaluated by scientific research (few people would be willing to adhere to such a diet for several years). A possible long-term adverse effect of adherence to an LCHP diet is a potential increase in cancer risk. Phytonutrients found in fruits, vegetables, and whole grains protect against certain types of cancer. A low carbohydrate intake also produces a loss of vitamin B, calcium, and potassium. Potential bone loss can accentuate the risk for osteoporosis.

Side effects commonly associated with LCHP diets include weakness, nausea, bad breath, constipation, irritability, lightheadedness, and fatigue. If you choose to go on an LCHP diet for longer than a few weeks, let your physician know so that he or she may monitor your blood lipids, bone density, and kidney function.

The benefit of adding extra protein to a weight loss program may be related to the hunger-suppressing effect of protein. Data suggest that protein curbs hunger more effectively than carbohydrates or fat. Dieters feel less hungry when caloric intake from protein is increased to about 30 percent of

How to Recognize Fad Diets

Fad diets have characteristics in common. These diets typically

- are nutritionally unbalanced.
- rely primarily on a single food (e.g., grapefruit).
- are based on testimonials.
- were developed according to "confidential research."
- are based on a "scientific breakthrough."
- promote rapid and "painless" weight loss.
- promise miraculous results.
- restrict food selection.
- are based on pseudoclaims that excessive weight is related to a specific condition, such as insulin resistance, combinations or timing of nutrient intake, food allergies, hormone imbalances, and certain foods (e.g., fruits).
- require the use of selected products.
- use liquid formulas instead of foods.
- misrepresent salespeople as individuals qualified to provide nutrition counseling.
- fail to provide information on risks associated with weight loss and of the diet use.
- do not involve physical activity.
- do not encourage healthy behavioral changes.
- are not supported by the scientific community or national health organizations.
- fail to provide information for weight maintenance upon completion of the diet phase.

FIGURE 5.4 Effects of high- and low-glycemic carbohydrate intake on blood glucose levels.

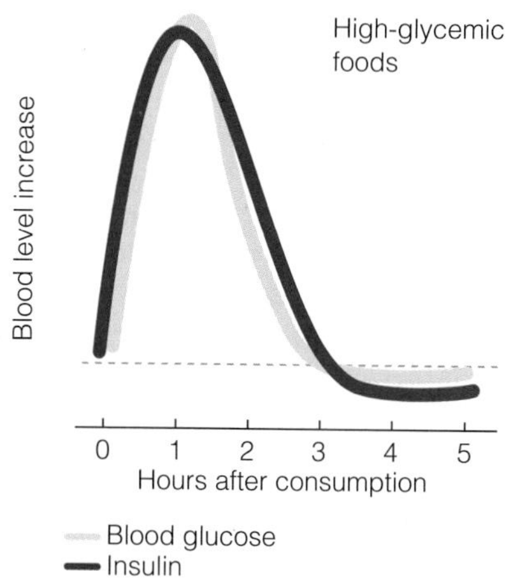

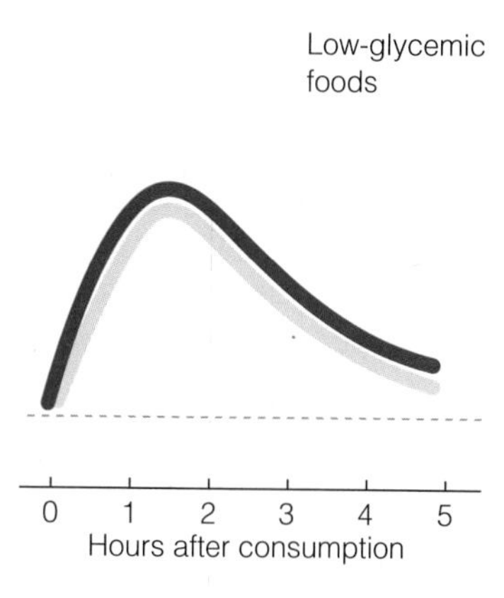

total calories and fat intake is cut to about 20 percent (while carbohydrate intake is kept constant at 50 percent of total calories). Thus, if you struggle with frequent hunger pangs, try to include some lean protein with each meal. This amount of protein is the equivalent of 1.5 ounces of lean meat (beef, fowl, or fish), two tablespoons of natural peanut butter, or 8 ounces of plain low-fat yogurt.

Many of these diets succeed because they restrict a large number of foods. Thus, people tend to eat less food overall. With the extraordinary variety of foods available to us, it is unrealistic to think that people will adhere to these diets for long. People eventually tire of eating the same thing day in and day out and start eating less, leading to weight loss. If they happen to achieve the lower weight but do not make permanent dietary changes, they regain the weight quickly once they go back to their previous eating habits.

A few diets recommend exercise along with caloric restrictions—the best method for weight reduction. People who adhere to these programs succeed, so the diet has achieved its purpose. Unfortunately, if the people do not change their food selection and activity level permanently, they gain back the weight once they discontinue dieting and exercise.

If people would only accept that no magic foods provide all necessary nutrients and that they have to eat a variety of foods to be well nourished, dieters would be more successful and the diet industry would go broke. Also, people eat for pleasure and for health. Two of the most essential components of a wellness lifestyle are healthy eating and regular physical activity, and they provide the best weight management program available today.

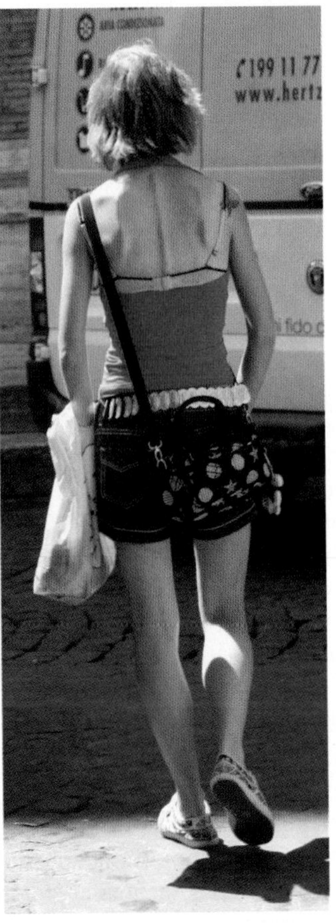

Society's unrealistic view of what constitutes recommended weight and "ideal" body image contributes to the development of eating disorders.

Eating Disorders

Eating disorders are medical illnesses that involve crucial disturbances in eating behaviors thought to stem from some combination of environmental pressures. These disorders are characterized by an intense fear of becoming fat, which does not disappear even when the person is losing weight in extreme amounts. The three most common types of eating disorders are anorexia nervosa, bulimia nervosa, and binge-eating disorder. A fourth disorder, emotional eating, can also be listed under disordered eating.

Most people who have eating disorders are afflicted by significant family and social problems. They may lack fulfillment in many areas of their lives. The eating disorder then becomes the coping mechanism to avoid dealing with these problems. Taking control of their body weight helps them believe that they are restoring some sense of control over their lives.

Anorexia nervosa and bulimia nervosa are common in industrialized nations whose society encourages low-calorie diets and thinness. The female role in society has changed rapidly, which makes women more susceptible to eating disorders. Although frequently seen in young women, eating disorders are most prevalent among individuals between the ages of 25 and 50. Surveys, nonetheless, indicate that as many as 40 percent of college-age women are struggling with an eating disorder.

Eating disorders are not limited to women. Every 1 in 10 cases occurs in men. But because men's role and body image are viewed differently in most societies, these cases often go unreported.

Although genetics may play a role in the development of eating disorders, most cases are environmentally related. Individuals who have clinical depression and obsessive-compulsive behavior are more susceptible. About half of all people with eating disorders have some sort of chemical dependency (alcohol and drugs), and most of them come from families with alcohol- and drug-related problems. Of reported cases of eating disorders, a large number are individuals who are, or have been, victims of sexual molestation.

Eating disorders develop in stages. Typically, individuals who are already dealing with significant issues in life start a diet. At first, they feel in control and are happy about the weight loss, even if they are not overweight. Encouraged by the prospect of weight loss and the control they can exert over their weight, the dieting becomes extreme and often is combined with exhaustive exercise and overuse of laxatives and diuretics.

The syndrome typically emerges following emotional issues or a stressful life event and uncertainty about the ability to cope efficiently. Life experiences that can trigger the syndrome might be gaining weight, starting the menstrual period, beginning college, losing a boyfriend, having poor self-esteem, being socially rejected, starting a professional career, or becoming a wife or a mother.

The eating disorder then takes on a life of its own and becomes the primary focus of attention for the individual afflicted with it. Self-worth revolves around what the scale reads every day, the individual's relationship with food, and that person's perception of how he or she looks each day.

Anorexia Nervosa An estimated 1 percent of the population in the United States has the eating disorder **anorexia nervosa**. Anorexic individuals seem to fear weight gain more than death from starvation. Furthermore, they have a distorted image of their bodies and think of themselves as being fat even when they are emaciated.

Anorexic patients commonly develop obsessive and compulsive behaviors and emphatically deny their condition. They are preoccupied with food, meal planning, and grocery shopping, and they have unusual eating habits. As they lose weight and their health begins to deteriorate, they feel weak and tired. They might realize they have a problem, but they will not stop the starvation and refuse to consider the behavior abnormal.

Once they have lost a lot of weight and malnutrition sets in, the physical changes become more visible. Typical changes are amenorrhea (absence of menstruation), digestive problems, extreme sensitivity to cold, hair problems, fluid and electrolyte abnormalities (which may lead to an irregular heartbeat and sudden stopping of the heart), injuries to nerves and tendons, abnormalities of immune function, anemia, growth of fine body hair, mental confusion, inability to concentrate, lethargy, depression, dry skin, lower skin and body temperature, and osteoporosis.

The following diagnostic criteria are for anorexia nervosa[13]:

- Refusal to maintain body weight over a minimal normal weight for age and height (weight loss leading to maintenance of body weight less than 85 percent of that expected or failure to make expected weight gain during periods of growth, leading to body weight less than 85 percent of that expected).
- Intense fear of gaining weight or becoming fat, even though underweight.
- Disturbance in the way in which the individual's body weight, size, or shape is perceived; undue influences of body weight or shape on self-evaluation; or denial of the seriousness of current low body weight.
- In postmenarcheal females, amenorrhea (absence of at least three consecutive menstrual cycles; a woman is considered to have amenorrhea if her periods occur only following estrogen therapy).

Many changes induced by anorexia nervosa can be reversed, and individuals with this condition can get better with professional therapy. However, they sometimes turn to bulimia nervosa, or they die from the disorder. Anorexia nervosa has the highest mortality rate of all psychosomatic illnesses today—20 percent of anorexic individuals die as a result of their condition. The disorder is 100 percent curable, but treatment almost always requires professional help. The sooner it is started, the better the chances for reversibility and cure. Therapy consists of a combination of medical and psychological techniques to restore proper nutrition, prevent medical complications, and modify the environment or events that triggered the syndrome.

Seldom can anorexia sufferers overcome the problem by themselves. They strongly deny their condition. They are able to hide it and deceive friends and relatives. Based on their behavior, many of them meet all characteristics of anorexia nervosa, but it goes undetected because both thinness and dieting are socially acceptable. Only a well-trained clinician is able to diagnose anorexia nervosa.

Bulimia Nervosa **Bulimia nervosa** is more prevalent than anorexia nervosa. As many as one in five women on college campuses may be bulimic, according to some estimates. Bulimia nervosa also is more prevalent than anorexia nervosa in males, although bulimia is still more prevalent in females.

People with bulimia usually are healthy looking, well educated, and near recommended body weight. They seem to enjoy food and often socialize around it. In actuality, they are emotionally insecure, rely on others, and lack self-confidence and self-esteem. Recommended weight and food are important to them.

The binge–purge cycle usually occurs in stages. As a result of stressful life events or the simple compulsion to eat, bulimic individuals engage periodically in binge eating that may last an hour or longer. With some apprehension, bulimics anticipate and plan the cycle. Next, they feel an urgency to begin large and uncontrollable food consumption, during which time they may eat several thousand calories (up to 10,000 calories in extreme cases). After a short period of relief and satisfaction, feelings of deep guilt and shame and intense fear of gaining weight emerge. Purging seems to be an easy answer, because the bingeing cycle can continue without fear of gaining weight.

The following diagnostic criteria are for bulimia nervosa[14]:

- Recurrent episodes of binge eating. An episode of binge eating is characterized by both of the following: (1) eating in a discrete period (e.g., within any two-hour period) an amount of food that is more than most

Anorexia nervosa An eating disorder characterized by self-imposed starvation to lose and maintain very low body weight.

Bulimia nervosa An eating disorder characterized by a pattern of binge eating and purging in an attempt to lose weight and maintain low body weight.

people would eat during a similar period and under similar circumstances and (2) a sense of lack of control over eating during the episode (feeling unable to stop eating or control what or how much is being consumed).

- Recurring inappropriate compensatory behaviors to prevent weight gain, such as self-induced vomiting; misuse of laxatives, diuretics, other medications, or emetics; fasting; or excessive exercise.
- Occurrence of the binge eating and inappropriate compensatory behaviors occurring, on average, at least twice a week for 3 months.
- Undue influence of body shape and weight on self-evaluation.

The most typical form of purging is self-induced vomiting. Bulimics also frequently ingest strong laxatives and emetics. Near-fasting diets and strenuous bouts of exercise are common. Medical problems associated with bulimia nervosa include cardiac arrhythmias, amenorrhea, kidney and bladder damage, ulcers, colitis, tearing of the esophagus or stomach, tooth erosion, gum damage, and general muscular weakness.

Unlike anorexics, bulimia sufferers realize that their behavior is abnormal and feel shame about it. Fearing social rejection, they pursue the binge–purge cycle in secrecy and at unusual hours of the day.

Bulimia nervosa can be treated successfully when the person realizes that this destructive behavior is not the solution to life's problems. A change in attitude can prevent permanent damage or death.

Binge-Eating Disorder

Binge-eating disorder is probably the most common of the three main eating disorders. About 2 percent of American adults are afflicted with binge-eating disorder in any six-month period. Although most people overeat occasionally, eating more than appropriate now and then does not mean someone has a binge-eating disorder. The disorder is slightly more common in women than in men; three women for every two men have the disorder.

Binge-eating disorder is characterized by uncontrollable episodes of eating excessive amounts of food within a relatively short time. The causes of binge-eating disorder are unknown, although depression, anger, sadness, boredom, and worry can trigger an episode. Unlike bulimic sufferers, binge eaters do not purge; thus, most people with this disorder are either overweight or obese.

Typical symptoms of binge-eating disorder include the following:

- Eating what most people think is an unusually large amount of food
- Eating until uncomfortably full
- Eating out of control
- Eating faster than usual during binge episodes
- Eating alone because of embarrassment of how much food is consumed
- Feeling disgusted, depressed, or guilty after overeating

Emotional Eating

In addition to physiological purposes, eating fulfills psychological, social, and cultural purposes. We eat to sustain our daily energy requirements, but we also eat at family celebrations, national holidays, social gatherings, and sporting events (as spectators) and even when we become emotional (some people stop eating when emotional). **Emotional eating** involves the consumption of large quantities of food, mostly "comfort" and junk food, to suppress negative emotions. Such emotions include stress, anxiety, uncertainty, guilt, anger, pain, depression, loneliness, sadness, boredom, and foods that have a nostalgic or sentimental appeal. In such circumstances, we eat for comfort when we are at our weakest point emotionally. Comfort foods often include calorie-dense, sweet, salty, and fatty foods. Excessive emotional eating hinders proper weight management.

Some palatable foods, such as chocolate, cause the body to release small amounts of mood-elevating opiates, helping offset negative emotions. A preference for certain foods is also present when people experience specific feelings (loneliness, anxiety, and fear). Eating helps divert the stressor, but the distraction is only temporary. The emotions return and may be compounded by a feeling of guilt from overeating.

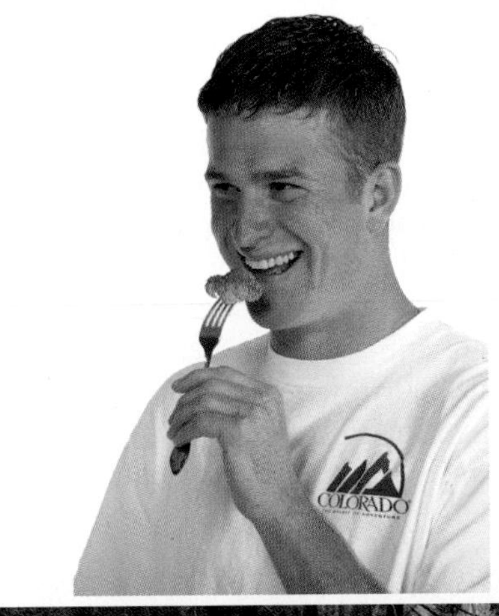

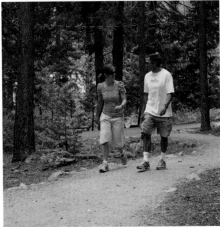

Achieving and maintaining a high physical fitness percent body fat standard requires a lifetime commitment to regular physical activity and proper nutrition.

If you are an emotional overeater, you can always seek help from a therapist at the school's counseling center. The following list of suggestions may help:

1. Learn to differentiate between emotional and physical hunger.
2. Avoid storing and snacking on unhealthy foods.
3. Keep healthy snacks handy.
4. Use countering techniques (going for a walk instead of reaching for the ice cream, or listening to music instead of eating the candy bar).
5. Keep a "trigger log" and get to know what triggers your emotional food consumption.
6. Work it out with exercise instead of food.

Eating Disorder Not Otherwise Specified (EDNOS) The American Psychiatric Association introduced EDNOS, a diagnostic category for individuals who don't fall into the previously discussed categories but still have troubled relationships with food or distorted body images. EDNOS diagnoses outnumber both anorexia and bulimia nervosa cases. These conditions also lead to malnourishment.

Orthoxia

An eating disorder characterized by a fixation with healthy or righteous eating. These individuals attempt to eat organic foods only or anything that isn't "pure in quality," often eliminating entire food groups. They are primarily motivated by fear of bad health and not necessarily thinness.

Pregorexia

Because of the social pressure to look thin during and after child bearing, some women fear gaining the recommended 25 to 35 pounds of weight during pregnancy, resulting in excessive dieting and exercising during this time. Common health risks include anemia, hypertension, depression, and malnourished babies who may be born with birth defects or miscarried.

Drunkorexia

Individuals who decrease caloric intake or skip meals to save those calories for alcohol and binge drinking. One survey found that close to 30 percent of female college students engage in drunkorexic behavior. Such action increases the risk for alcohol poisoning, unplanned sexual relations, and, in the long term, it raises the risk for heart and liver disease.

Anorexia Athletica

People who engage daily in compulsive lengthy and rigorous exercise routines to reach and maintain low body weight. These individuals feel extremely guilty if they miss a workout or are unable to keep up with the exercise regimen. Health risks of this behavior include depression and fatal heart disease.

Treatment Treatment for eating disorders is available on most school campuses through the school's counseling center or health center. Local hospitals also offer treatment for these conditions. Many communities have support groups, frequently led by professional personnel and often free of charge. All information and the individual's identity are kept confidential, so the person need not fear embarrassment or repercussions when seeking professional help.

The Physiology of Weight Loss

Traditional concepts related to weight control have centered on three assumptions:

1. Balancing food intake against output allows a person to achieve recommended weight.
2. All fat people simply eat too much.
3. The human body doesn't care how much (or how little) fat it stores.

Although these statements contain some truth, they are open to much debate and research. We now know that the causes of obesity are complex, involving a combination of genetics, behavior, and lifestyle factors.

Energy-Balancing Equation The principle embodied in the **energy-balancing equation** is simple: As long as caloric input equals caloric output, the person does not gain or lose weight. If caloric intake exceeds output, the person gains weight; when output exceeds input, the person loses weight. If daily energy requirements could be determined accurately, caloric intake could be balanced against output. This is not always the case, though, because genetic and lifestyle-related individual differences determine the number of calories required to maintain or lose body weight.

Table 5.3 (page 191) offers general guidelines to determine the **Estimated Energy Requirement (EER)** in calories per day. This is an estimated figure and (as discussed

Binge-eating disorder An eating disorder characterized by uncontrollable episodes of eating excessive amounts of food within a relatively short time.

Emotional eating The consumption of large quantities of food to suppress negative emotions.

Energy-balancing equation A principle holding that as long as caloric input equals caloric output, the person does not gain or lose weight. If caloric intake exceeds output, the person gains weight; when output exceeds input, the person loses weight.

Estimated Energy Requirement (EER) Average dietary energy (caloric) intake that is predicted to maintain energy balance in a healthy adult of defined age, gender, weight, height, and level of physical activity, consistent with good health.

under "Losing Weight the Sound and Sensible Way," page 188) serves only as a starting point from which individual adjustments have to be made.

The total daily energy requirement has three basic components (Figure 5.5):

1. Resting metabolic rate
2. Thermic effect of food
3. Physical activity

The **resting metabolic rate (RMR)**—the energy requirement to maintain the body's vital processes in the resting state—accounts for approximately 60 to 70 percent of the total daily energy requirement. The thermic effect of food—the energy required to digest, absorb, and store food—accounts for about 5 to 10 percent of the total daily requirement. Physical activity accounts for 15 to 30 percent of the total daily requirement.

One pound of fat is the equivalent of 3,500 calories. If a person's EER is 2,500 calories and that person were to decrease intake by 500 calories per day, it should result in a loss of 1 pound of fat in 7 days (500 × 7 = 3,500). But research has shown—and many people have experienced—that even when dieters carefully balance caloric input against caloric output, weight loss does not always result as predicted. Furthermore, two people with similar measured caloric intake and output seldom lose weight at the same rate.

The rule of thumb is that a person needs a 3,500-calorie deficit to lose a pound of fat. This figure, however, is an oversimplification of what really happens. There are too many individual, behavior, and lifestyle variables that keep weight loss from happening at the same rate among individuals, including gender, body composition, metabolic rate, age, and activity level. As will be discussed in this chapter, most notably are differences in daily physical activity and the drop in basal metabolic rate as a person loses weight (that is, the body burns fewer calories as weight is lost). The 3,500-calorie rule, nonetheless, is a good guideline to work off when writing weight-loss programs.

FIGURE 5.5 **Components of total daily energy requirement.**

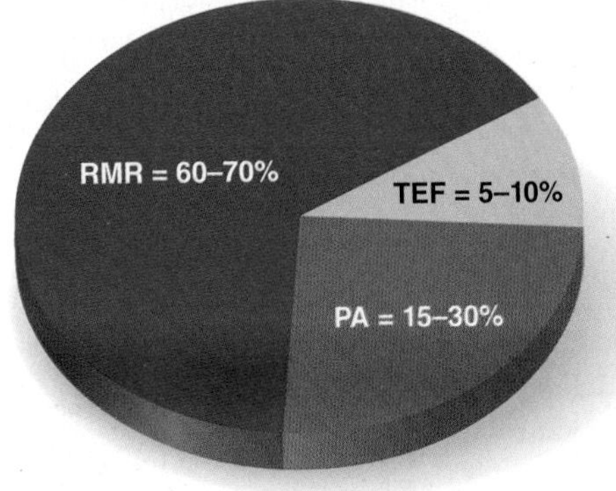

The most common explanation for individual differences in weight loss and weight gain has been variation in human metabolism from one person to another. We are all familiar with people who can eat "all day long" and not gain an ounce of weight and others who cannot even "dream about food" without gaining weight. Because experts did not believe that human metabolism alone could account for such extreme differences, they developed other theories that might better explain these individual variations.

In terms of physical activity, all activity or movement a person does during the course of the day counts. This principle is known as "spontaneous non-exercise activity," or "fidgeting." Such activity can easily account for several hundred calories a day, resulting in significant differences in weight management among people.

Setpoint Theory Results of research studies point toward a **weight-regulating mechanism (WRM)** in the human body that has a **setpoint** for controlling both appetite and amount of fat stored. The setpoint is hypothesized to work like a thermostat for body fat, maintaining fairly constant body weight, because it "knows" at all times the exact amount of adipose tissue stored in the fat cells. Some people have high settings; others have low settings.

If body weight decreases (as in dieting), the setpoint senses this change and triggers the WRM to increase appetite or make the body conserve energy to maintain the "set" weight. The opposite also may be true. Some people have a hard time gaining weight. In this case, the WRM decreases appetite or causes the body to waste energy to maintain the lower weight.

Every person has a certain body fat percentage (as established by the setpoint) that the body attempts to maintain. The genetic instinct to survive tells the body that fat storage is vital; therefore, the body sets an acceptable fat level. This level may remain somewhat constant or may climb gradually because of poor lifestyle habits.

For instance, under strict caloric reduction, the body may make extreme metabolic adjustments in an effort to maintain its setpoint for fat. The **basal metabolic rate (BMR)**, the lowest level of caloric intake necessary to sustain life, may drop dramatically when operating under a consistent negative caloric balance, and that person's weight loss may plateau for days or even weeks. A low BMR compounds a person's problems in maintaining recommended body weight.

These findings were substantiated by research conducted at Rockefeller University in New York.[15] The authors showed that the body resists maintaining altered weight. Obese and lifetime nonobese individuals were used in the investigation. Following a 10 percent weight loss, the body, in an attempt to regain the lost weight, compensated by burning up to 15 percent fewer calories than expected for the new reduced weight (after accounting for the 10 percent loss). The effects were similar in the obese and nonobese participants. These results imply that after a 10 percent weight loss, a person would have to eat even less or exercise even more to compensate for the estimated 15 percent slowdown (a difference of about 200 to 300 calories).

CRITICAL THINKING

Do you see a difference in the amount of food that you are now able to eat compared with the amount that you ate in your mid- to late-teen years? If so, to what do you attribute this difference? What actions are you taking to account for the difference?

In this same study, when the participants were allowed to increase their weight to 10 percent above their "normal" body (before weight loss) weight, the body burned 10 to 15 percent *more* calories than expected—attempting to waste energy and maintain the preset weight. This is another indication that the body is highly resistant to weight changes unless additional lifestyle changes are incorporated to ensure successful weight management. (These methods are discussed under "Losing Weight the Sound and Sensible Way," page 188.)

Dietary restriction alone does not lower the setpoint, even though the person may lose weight and fat. When the dieter goes back to the normal or even below-normal caloric intake (at which the weight may have been stable for a long time), he or she quickly regains the lost fat as the body strives to regain a comfortable fat store.

An Example

Let's use a practical illustration. A person would like to lose some body fat and assumes that his or her current stable body weight has been reached at an average daily caloric intake of 1,800 calories (no weight gain or loss occurs at this daily intake). In an attempt to lose weight rapidly, this person now goes on a **very low-calorie diet** (defined as 800 calories per day or less) or, even worse, a near-fasting diet. This immediately activates the body's survival mechanism and readjusts the metabolism to a lower caloric balance. After a few weeks of dieting at the 800-calories-per-day level, the body now can maintain its normal functions at 1,300 calories per day. This new figure (1,300 calories) represents a drop of 500 calories per day in the BMR. Having lost the desired weight, the person terminates the diet but realizes that the original intake of 1,800 calories per day has to be lower to maintain the new lower weight. To adjust to the new lower body weight, the person restricts intake to about 1,600 calories per day. The individual is surprised to find that even at this lower daily intake (200 fewer calories), the weight comes back at a rate of 1 pound every 1 to 2 weeks. After the diet is over, this new lowered BMR may take several months to kick back up to its normal level.

Based on this explanation, individuals clearly should not go on very low-calorie diets. This slows the BMR and deprives the body of basic daily nutrients required for normal function. Very low-calorie diets should be used only in conjunction with dietary supplements and under proper medical supervision. Furthermore, people who use very low-calorie diets are not as effective in keeping the weight off once the diet is terminated.

Recommendations

A daily caloric intake of approximately 1,500 calories provides the necessary nutrients if a variety of nonprocessed foods are distributed properly over the basic food groups (meeting the daily recommended amounts from each group). Of course, the individual will have to learn to select healthy foods from among 100-percent whole grains, fiber-rich fruits and vegetables, beans, lean proteins, modest amounts of healthy oils (olive and canola), and nuts while on a calorie-restricted plan.

Under no circumstances should petite women go on a diet that calls for a level of 1,200 or fewer calories or should most men and women eat 1,500 or fewer calories. Weight (fat) is gained over months and years, not overnight. Likewise, weight loss should be gradual, not abrupt. At 1,200 calories per day, you may require a multivitamin supplement. Your health care professional should be consulted regarding such a supplement.

A second way in which the setpoint may work is by keeping track of the nutrients and calories consumed daily. It is thought that the body, like a cash register, records the daily food intake and that the brain does not feel satisfied until the calories and nutrients have been "registered."

This setpoint for calories and nutrients seems to operate even when people participate in moderately intense exercise. Some evidence suggests that people do not become hungrier with moderate physical activity. Therefore, people can choose to lose weight either by going hungry or by combining a sensible calorie-restricted diet with an increase in daily physical activity.

Lowering the Setpoint

The most common question regarding the setpoint is how to lower it so that the body feels comfortable at a reduced fat percentage. The following factors seem to affect the setpoint directly by lowering the fat thermostat:

- Exercise
- A diet high in complex carbohydrates
- Nicotine
- Amphetamines

Resting metabolic rate (RMR) The energy requirement to maintain the body's vital processes in the resting state.

Weight-regulating mechanism (WRM) A feature of the hypothalamus of the brain that controls how much the body should weigh.

Setpoint Weight control theory that the body has an established weight and strongly attempts to maintain that weight.

Basal metabolic rate (BMR) The lowest level of oxygen consumption (and energy requirement) necessary to sustain life.

Very low-calorie diet A diet that allows an energy intake (consumption) of only 800 calories or less per day.

The last two are more destructive than the extra fat weight, so they are not reasonable alternatives (as far as extra strain on the heart is concerned, smoking one pack of cigarettes per day is said to be the equivalent of carrying 50 to 75 pounds of excess body fat). A diet high in fats and refined carbohydrates, near-fasting diets, and perhaps even artificial sweeteners seem to raise the setpoint. Therefore, the only practical and sensible way to lower the setpoint and lose fat weight is a combination of exercise and a diet high in complex carbohydrates and only moderate amounts of fat.

Because of the effects of proper food management on the body's setpoint, most of the successful dieter's effort should be spent in reforming eating habits, increasing intake of complex carbohydrates and high-fiber foods, and decreasing consumption of processed foods that are high in refined carbohydrates (sugars) and fats. This change in eating habits brings about a decrease in total daily caloric intake. Because one gram of carbohydrates provides only four calories, as opposed to nine calories per gram of fat, the person could eat twice the volume of food (by weight) when substituting carbohydrates for fat. Some fat, however, is recommended in the diet—preferably polyunsaturated and monounsaturated fats. These so-called good fats do more than help protect the heart; they help delay hunger pangs.

A "diet" should not be viewed as a temporary tool to aid in weight loss but instead as a permanent change in eating behaviors to ensure weight management and better health. The role of increased physical activity also must be considered, because successful weight loss, maintenance, and recommended body composition are seldom attained without a moderate reduction in caloric intake combined with a regular exercise program.

Diet and Metabolism

Fat can be lost by selecting the proper foods, exercising, or restricting calories. However, when dieters try to lose weight by dietary restrictions alone, they also lose lean body mass (muscle protein, along with vital organ protein). The amount of lean body mass lost depends on caloric limitation. When people go on a near-fasting diet, up to half of the weight loss is lean body mass and the other half is actual fat loss (Figure 5.6).[16] When diet is combined with exercise, close to 100 percent of the weight loss is in the form of fat; lean tissue actually may increase. Loss of lean body mass is never good, because it weakens organs and muscles and slows metabolism. Large losses in lean tissue can cause disturbances in heart function and damage to other organs.

BEHAVIOR MODIFICATION PLANNING

Eating Right When on the Run

Current lifestyles often require people to be on the run. We don't seem to have time to eat right, but fortunately it doesn't have to be that way. If you are on the run, it is even more critical to make healthy choices to keep up with a challenging schedule. Do you regularly consume the following foods when you are eating on the run?

I PLAN TO	I DID IT	
❑	❑	Water
❑	❑	Whole-grain cereal and skim milk
❑	❑	Whole-grain bread and bagels
❑	❑	Whole-grain bread with peanut butter
❑	❑	Nonfat or low-fat yogurt
❑	❑	Fresh fruits
❑	❑	Frozen fresh fruit (grapes, cherries, banana slices)
❑	❑	Dried fruits
❑	❑	Raw vegetables (carrots, red peppers, cucumbers, radishes, cauliflower, asparagus)
❑	❑	Crackers
❑	❑	Pretzels
❑	❑	Bread sticks
❑	❑	Low-fat cheese sticks
❑	❑	Granola bars
❑	❑	Snack-size cereal boxes
❑	❑	Nuts
❑	❑	Trail mix
❑	❑	Plain popcorn
❑	❑	Vegetable soups

Try It

In your Online Journal or class notebook, plan your fast-meal menus for the upcoming week. It may require extra shopping and some food preparation (for instance, cutting vegetables to place in snack plastic bags). At the end of the week, evaluate how many days you had a "healthy eating on the run day." What did you learn from the experience?

Equally important is not to overindulge (binge) following a very low-calorie diet, because this may cause changes in BMR and electrolyte balance, which could trigger fatal cardiac arrhythmias.

Contrary to some beliefs, aging is not the main reason for the lower BMR. It is not so much that metabolism slows down as that people slow down. As people age, they tend to rely more on the amenities of life (remote controls, cell phones, intercoms, single-level homes, riding lawnmowers, etc.) that lull them into sedentary living.

Basal metabolism also is related to lean body weight. More lean tissue yields a higher BMR. As a consequence of sedentary living and less physical activity, the lean component decreases and fat tissue increases. The human body requires a certain amount of oxygen per pound of lean body mass. Given that fat is considered metabolically inert from the point of view of caloric use, the lean tissue uses most of the oxygen, even at rest. As muscle and organ mass (lean body mass) decrease, so do the energy requirements at rest.

Diets with caloric intakes below 1,500 calories cannot guarantee the retention of lean body mass. Even at this intake level, some loss is inevitable unless the diet is combined with exercise. Despite the claims of many diets that they do not alter the lean component, the simple truth is that regardless of what nutrients may be added to the diet, severe caloric restrictions always prompt the loss of lean tissue. Sadly, many people go on very low-calorie diets constantly. Every time they do, their BMR slows as more lean tissue is lost.

People in their 40s and older who weigh the same as they did when they were 20 tend to think they are at recommended body weight. During this span of 20 years or more, though, they may have dieted many times without participating in an exercise program. After they terminate each diet, they regain the weight, and much of that gain is additional body fat. Maybe at age 20 they weighed 150 pounds, of which only 15 percent was fat. Now at age 40, even though they still weigh 150 pounds, they might be 30 percent fat (Figure 5.7). At "recommended" body weight, they wonder why they are eating little and still having trouble staying at that weight.

FIGURE 5.7 **Body composition changes as a result of frequent dieting without exercise.**

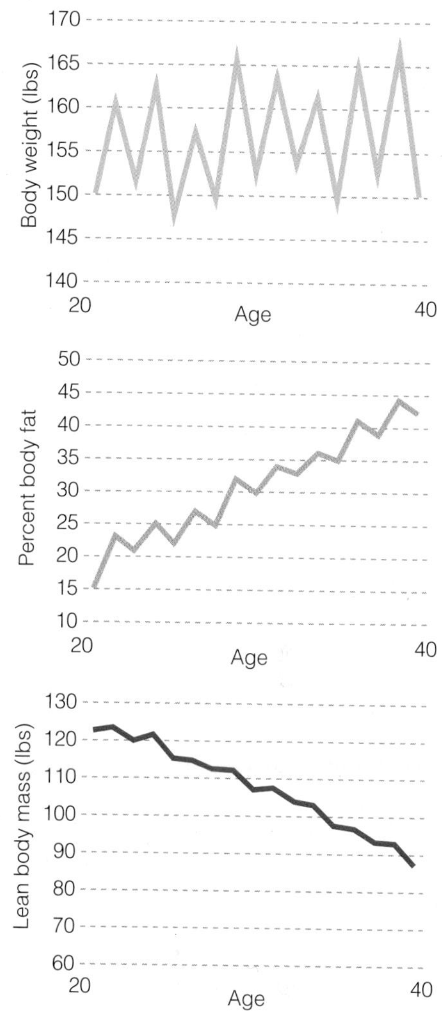

FIGURE 5.6 **Outcome of three forms of diet on fat loss.**

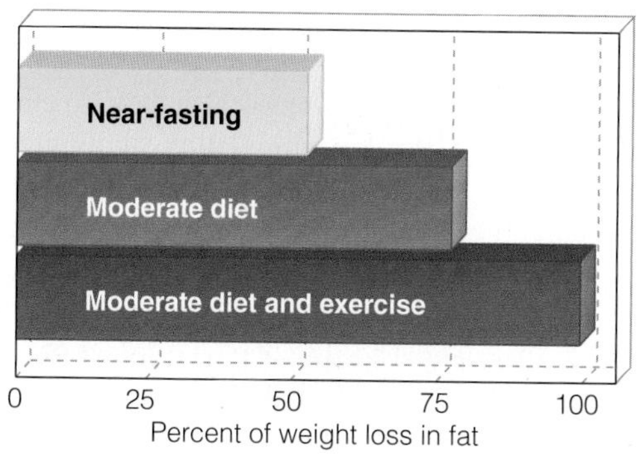

Source: Adapted from R. J. Shephard, Alive Man: The Physiology of Physical Activity (Springfield, IL: Charles C. Thomas, 1975): pp. 484–488.

Hormonal Regulation of Appetite

Ghrelin and leptin are two hormones currently being extensively researched because they appear to play a role in appetite. Ghrelin, produced primarily in the stomach, stimulates appetite: that is, the more ghrelin the body produces, the more you want to eat. However, leptin, produced by fat cells, lets the brain know when you are full; the more leptin you produce, the less you want to eat. Similar to insulin resistance (leading to type 2 diabetes), research is beginning to show that a lack of physical activity leads to leptin resistance, setting up a vicious cycle that in turn leads to excessive eating. Scientists are now looking into the role these hormones play in weight gain and weight loss, as well as the effects of sleep deprivation and exercise on these hormones and subsequent appetite regulation.

Sleep and Weight Management

As presented under the Healthy Lifestyle Habits box in Chapter 1 (see page 28), adequate sleep is 1 of the 12 key components that enhance health and extend life. New evidence shows that sleep is also important to adequate weight management. Sleep deprivation appears to be conducive to weight gain and may interfere with the body's capability to lose weight.

Current obesity and sleep deprivation data point toward a possible correlation between excessive body weight and sleep deprivation. About 68 percent of the U.S. population is overweight or obese, and according to the National Sleep Foundation, 63 percent of Americans report that they do not get 8 hours of sleep per night. The question must be raised, is there a connection? Let's examine some data.

One of the most recent studies examining this issue showed that individuals who get less than 6 hours of sleep per night have a higher average BMI (28.3) compared with those who average 8 hours per night (24.5).[17] Another study on more than 68,000 women between the ages of 30 and 55 found that those who got 5 hours or less of sleep per night were 30 percent more likely to gain 30 or more pounds compared with women who got 8 hours per night.[18]

Researchers think that lack of sleep disrupts normal body hormonal balances. Sleep deprivation has now been shown to elevate ghrelin levels and decrease leptin levels, potentially leading to weight gain or keeping you from losing weight.[19] Data comparing these hormone levels in five-hour versus eight-hour sleepers found that the short sleepers had a 14.9 percent increase in ghrelin levels and a 15.5 percent decrease in leptin levels. The short sleepers also had a 3.6 percent higher BMI than the regular sleepers.[20]

Based on all these studies, the data appear to indicate that sleep deprivation has a negative impact on weight loss or maintenance. Thus, an important component to a well-designed weight management program should include a good night's rest (8 hours of sleep).

Monitoring Body Weight

A most critical component to lifetime weight management is to regularly monitor your body weight. Get into the habit of weighing yourself, preferably at the same time of day and under the same conditions—for instance, in the morning just as you get out of bed. Data indicate that daily weigh-ins are associated with better weight maintenance and enhanced weight loss, while infrequent weighing leads to weight gain.

Depending on your body size, activity patterns, rehydration level, and dietary intake on any given day, your weight will fluctuate by a pound or more from one day to the next. You do not want to be obsessed with body weight that can potentially lead to an eating disorder, but monitoring *"healthy" recommended body weight* regularly allows you to make immediate adjustments in food intake and physical activity if your weight increases and stays there for several days. Do not adapt and accept the higher weight as your new stable weight. Understand that it is easier to make sensible short-term dietary and activity changes to lose 1 or 2 pounds of weight than to make drastic long-term changes to lose 10, 20, 50, or more pounds that you allowed yourself to gain over the course of several months or years. Whenever feasible, you also want to do periodic assessments of body composition using experienced technicians and valid techniques.

Exercise and Weight Management

To tilt the energy-balancing equation in your favor, you need to burn more calories through physical activity. Research indicates that exercise accentuates weight loss while on a negative caloric balance (diet) as long as you do not replenish the calories expended during exercise. The debate, however, centers on what amount of exercise is best for individuals who are trying to lose weight and those who are trying to maintain weight. Nonetheless, the data are clear that exercise is the best predictor of long-term maintenance of weight loss.[21]

Regular exercise seems to exert control over how much a person weighs. On average, the typical adult American gradually becomes overweight by gaining one to two pounds of weight per year. A one-pound weight gain represents a simple energy surplus of fewer than 10 calories per day (10×365 days $= 3{,}650$ calories, and one pound of fat represents 3,500 calories). This simple surplus of fewer than 10 calories per day is the equivalent of less than one teaspoon of sugar. Weight gain is clearly related to a decrease in physical activity and an increase in caloric intake. Physical inactivity, however, might well be the primary cause, leading to excessive weight and obesity. The human body was meant to be physically active, and a minimal level of activity appears to be necessary to accurately balance caloric intake to caloric expenditure. In sedentary individuals, the body seems to lose control over this fine energy balance.

Most people understand that exercise enhances the rate of weight loss, enhances body composition, and is vital in maintaining the lost weight. Not only does exercise maintain lean tissue, but advocates of the setpoint theory also say that exercise resets the fat thermostat to a new, lower level.

Most people who struggle with weight management need 60 to 90 minutes of daily physical activity to effectively manage body weight. While accumulating 30 minutes of moderate-intensity activity per day provides substantial health benefits (the minimum daily recommended amount of activity), from a weight management point of view, the Institute of Medicine of the National Academy of Sciences recommends that people accumulate 60 minutes of moderate-intensity physical activity most days of the week.[22] The evidence shows that people who maintain recommended weight typically accumulate an hour or more of daily physical activity.

According to the American College of Sports Medicine "Position Stand on Strategies for Weight Loss and Prevention of Weight Regain for Adults" (Figure 5.8), greater weight loss is achieved by increasing the amount of weekly physical activity. Of even greater significance, physical activity is required for weight maintenance following weight loss. People who exercise regain less weight than those who do not. And those who exercise the most regain the least amount of weight. Individuals who remain physically active for 60 minutes or longer per day are able to keep the weight off.

Furthermore, data from the National Weight Control Registry (www.nwcr.ws) on more than 6,000 individuals who have lost at least 30 pounds and have kept them off for a minimum of 5 years indicate that they typically expend about 300 calories through daily moderate-intensity exercise.[23] Three hundred calories represents about three miles jogging in 30 minutes or walking briskly the same distance in 60 minutes. Individuals who stop physical activity regain almost 100 percent of the weight within 18 months of discontinuing the weight loss program. Most successful "weight maintainers" also show greater dietary restraint and follow a low-fat diet, consuming less than 30 percent of the total daily calories from fat.

Most experts and leading organizations now recognize that if weight management is not a consideration, 30 minutes of daily activity 5 days per week provides substantial health benefits. Nonetheless, to prevent weight gain, 60 minutes of daily activity is recommended; to maintain substantial weight loss, 90 minutes may be required.

The most important reason physical activity and exercise are vital for weight loss maintenance is that sedentary living expends no additional energy (calories) over the RMR. With limited physical activity throughout the day, sedentary people cannot afford to eat many calories; perhaps only 1,000 to 1,200 calories per day. Such a low level of energy intake is not sufficient to keep people from constantly feeling hungry. The only choice they then have is to go hungry every day, an impossible task to sustain. After terminating the diet, energy intake climbs in just a few days, with an end result of weight regain. Thus, the only logical way to increase caloric intake and maintain weight loss is by burning more calories through exercise and incorporating physical activity throughout daily living.

For people trying to lose weight, a combination of aerobic and strength-training exercises works best. Aerobic exercise is the best exercise modality to offset the setpoint, and the continuity and duration of these types of activities cause many calories to be burned in the process. The role of aerobic exercise in successful lifetime weight management cannot be overestimated.

FIGURE 5.8 Approximate decrease in body weight based on total weekly minutes of physical activity (PA) without caloric restrictions.

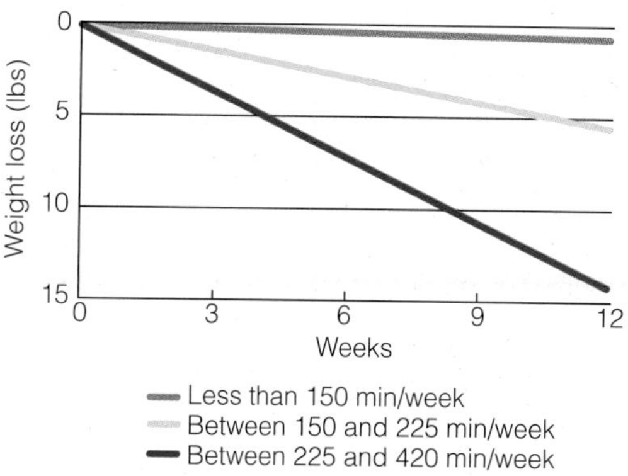

Source: Adapted from American College of Sports Medicine, "Position Stand: Appropriate Physical Activity Intervention Strategies for Weight Loss and Prevention of Weight Regain for Adults," *Medicine and Science in Sports and Exercise* 41 (2009): 459–471.

BEHAVIOR MODIFICATION PLANNING

Physical Activity Guidelines for Weight Management

The following physical activity guidelines are recommended to effectively manage body weight:

- 30 minutes of physical activity on most days of the week if you do not have difficulty maintaining body weight (more minutes and/or higher intensity if you choose to reach a high level of physical fitness).
- Between 30 and 60 minutes of light-to-moderate exercise on most days of the week if you are trying to lose weight. Incorporate as many light ambulatory activities as possible during the course of each day.
- 60 minutes of daily activity if you want to prevent weight gain.
- Between 60 and 90 minutes of physical activity each day if you want to keep weight off following extensive weight loss (30 pounds of weight loss or more). Be sure to include some high-intensity/low-impact activities at least twice a week in your program.

Try It

In your Behavior Change Planner Progress Tracker, online journal, or class notebook, record how many minutes of daily physical activity you accumulate on a regular basis and record your thoughts on how effectively your activity has helped you manage your body weight. Is there one thing you could do today to increase your physical activity?

Strength training is critical in helping maintain and increase lean body mass. Fewer calories are burned during a typical hour-long strength-training session than during an hour of aerobic exercise. Because of the high intensity of strength training, the person needs frequent rest intervals to recover from each set of exercises. In the long run, however, the person enjoys the benefits of gains in lean tissue. Guidelines for developing aerobic and strength-training programs are given in Chapters 6 and 7.

Although the increase in BMR through increased muscle mass is being debated in the literature and merits further research, data indicate that each additional pound of muscle tissue raises the BMR in the range of 6 to 35 calories per day.[24] The latter figure is based on calculations that an increase of 3 to 3.5 pounds of lean tissue through strength training increased BMR by about 105 to 120 calories per day.[25]

Most likely, the benefit of strength training goes beyond the new muscle tissue. Maybe a pound of muscle tissue requires only 6 calories per day to sustain itself, but as all muscles undergo strength training, they undergo increased protein synthesis to build and repair themselves, resulting in increased energy expenditure of 1 to 1.5 calories per pound in all trained muscle tissue. Such an increase would explain the 105- to 120-calorie BMR increase in this research study.

To examine the effects of a small increase in BMR on long-term body weight, let's use a conservative estimate of an additional 50 calories per day as a result of a regular strength-training program. An increase of 50 calories represents an additional 18,250 calories per year (50 × 365), or the equivalent of 5.2 pounds of fat (18,250 ÷ 3,500). This increase in BMR would more than offset the typical adult weight gain of 1 to 2 pounds per year.

This figure of 18,250 calories per year does not include the actual energy cost of the strength-training workout. If you use an energy expenditure of only 150 calories per strength-training session, done twice per week, over a year's time it would represent 15,600 calories (150 × 2 × 52), or the equivalent of another 4.5 pounds of fat (15,600 ÷ 3,500).

In addition, although the amounts seem small, the previous calculations do not account for the increase in BMR following the strength-training workout (the number of hours it takes the body to return to its preworkout resting rate, according to the intensity and duration of training). Depending on the training volume (see Chapter 7, page 270), this recovery energy expenditure ranges from 20 to 100 calories following each strength-training workout. All these "apparently small" changes make a big difference in the long run.

Although size (inches) and percent body fat both decrease when sedentary individuals begin an exercise program, body weight often remains the same or may even increase during the first couple of weeks of the program. Exercise helps increase muscle tissue, connective tissue, blood volume (as much as 500 milliliters, or the equivalent of one pound, following the first week of aerobic exercise), enzymes and other structures within the cell, and glycogen (which binds water). All of these changes lead to a higher functional capacity of the human body. With exercise, most weight loss becomes apparent after a few weeks of training, when the lean component has stabilized.

We know that a negative caloric balance of 3,500 calories does not always result in a loss of one pound of fat, but the role of exercise in achieving a negative balance by burning additional calories is significant in weight reduction and maintenance programs. Sadly, some individuals claim that the number of calories burned during exercise is hardly worth the effort. They think that cutting their daily intake by 300 calories is easier than participating in some sort of exercise that would burn the same number of calories. The

BEHAVIOR MODIFICATION PLANNING

Weight-Maintenance Benefits of Lifetime Aerobic Exercise

The authors of this book have been jogging together a minimum of 15 miles per week (3 miles, 5 times per week) for the past 38 years. Without considering the additional energy expenditure from their regular strength-training program and their many other sport and recreational activities, the energy cost of this regular jogging program over 38 years has been approximately 2,964,000 calories (15 miles × 100 calories/mile × 52 weeks × 38 years), or the equivalent of 847 pounds of fat (2,964,000 ÷ 3,500). In essence, without this 30-minute workout 5 times per week, the authors would weigh 989 and 963 pounds respectively! Such is the long-term gratification (reward) of a lifetime exercise program—not to mention the myriad health benefits, joy, and quality of life derived through this program.

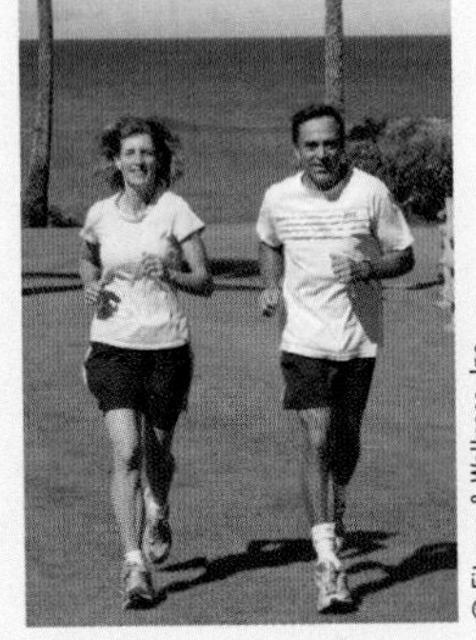

Try It!

Ask yourself whether a regular aerobic exercise program is part of your long-term gratification and health enhancement program. If the answer is no, are you ready to change your behavior? Use the Behavior Change Planner to help you answer the question.

confidentconsumer

Federal Trade Commission's Weight-Loss Gimmick "7 Gut Check Claims"

To make it easier to spot false weight-loss representations—the "gut check" claims—the Federal Trade Commission (FTC—the nation's consumer protection agency) has compiled a list of seven statements in ads that experts say simply can't be true. If you spot one of these claims in an ad a marketer wants to run in your media outlet, it's likely to be a tip-off to deception.

By the way, several of the "gut check" claims refer to "substantial weight loss." This means "a lot of weight" and includes weight loss of a pound a week for more than four weeks or a total weight loss of more than 15 pounds in any time period. But as the examples illustrate, advertisers can convey that "substantial weight loss" message without using specific numbers. Substantial weight loss can be suggested by reference to dress size, inches, or body fat.

If one of these seven claims crosses your desk, do a "gut check." Consult the appropriate person in your company, and think twice before running any ad that says a product:

1. causes weight loss of two pounds or more a week for a month or more without dieting or exercise;
2. causes substantial weight loss no matter what or how much the consumer eats;
3. causes permanent weight loss even after the consumer stops using product;
4. blocks the absorption of fat or calories to enable consumers to lose substantial weight;
5. safely enables consumers to lose more than three pounds per week for more than four weeks;
6. causes substantial weight loss for all users; or
7. causes substantial weight loss by wearing a product on the body or rubbing it into the skin.

Some gutsy con artists may repeat a "gut check" claim verbatim. That's a sure sign that false advertising is afoot. But "gut check" claims can be conveyed in more subtle ways, too. Knowing you'll be on the look-out for specific false claims, some advertisers are careful not to use the exact wording of "gut check" claims. Others may try to work in limiting phrases that consumers may not catch. For example, they may claim a product "*helps* consumers lose substantial weight without diet or exercise" or that people can take off "*up to* three pounds a week for a month or more."

You can outfox the fraudsters by understanding what makes each of those claims bogus. Fine-tuning your falsity detector will make it easier for you to spot deception when marketers try to slip a false claim past you by paraphrasing or using synonyms.

Source: http://www.business.ftc.gov/documents/0492-gut-check-reference-guide-media-spotting-false-weight-loss-claims. Released January 7, 2014.

problem is that the willpower to cut those 300 calories lasts only a few weeks, and then people go back to the old eating patterns.

If a person gets into the habit of exercising regularly, say three times a week, jogging three miles per exercise session (about 300 calories burned), this represents 900 calories in one week, about 3,600 calories in one month, or 46,800 calories per year. This minimal amount of exercise represents as many as 13.5 extra pounds of fat in one year, 27 pounds in 2 years, and so on.

Does this seem hardly worth the effort? We tend to forget that our weight creeps up gradually over the years, not overnight. And we have not even taken into consideration the increase in lean tissue, possible resetting of the setpoint, benefits to the cardiorespiratory system, and most important, the improved quality of life. Fundamental reasons for excessive weight and obesity, few could argue, are sedentary living and lack of a regular exercise program.

In terms of preventing disease, many health benefits that people seek by losing weight are reaped through exercise alone, even without weight loss. Exercise offers protection against premature morbidity and mortality for people who are overweight or already have risk factors for disease.

One additional benefit of exercise and physical activity is that it attenuates a person's predisposition to obesity. Genetic epidemiological studies have established that genetic factors play a role in obesity development in our 21st century obesogenic environment abundant in energy-dense foods and labor-saving devices. The data indicate that even in the most genetically predisposed individuals, regular physical activity, exercise, and an active lifestyle significantly reduce the predisposition to obesity.[26]

The Roles of Exercise Intensity and Duration in Weight Management

A hotly debated and controversial topic is the exercise volume required for adequate weight management. Depending on the degree of the initial weight problem and the person's fitness level, there appears to be a difference in the volume of exercise that is most conducive toward adequate weight loss, weight loss maintenance, and weight management.

We have known for years that compared with vigorous exercise, a greater proportion of calories burned during light-intensity exercise is derived from fat. The lower the intensity of exercise, the higher the percentage of fat utilization as an energy source. During light-intensity exercise, up to 50 percent of the calories burned may be derived from fat (the other 50 percent from glucose, which is converted from carbohydrates). With vigorous exercise, only 30 to 40 percent of the caloric expenditure comes from fat.

However, you can burn twice as many calories overall—and subsequently more fat—during vigorous exercise. Let's look at a practical illustration (also see Table 5.2). If you exercised for 30 to 40 minutes at a light intensity level and burned 200 calories, about 100 of those calories (50 percent) would come from fat. If you exercised with vigorous intensity during those same 30 to 40 minutes, you could burn 400 calories, with 120 to 160 of the calories (30 to 40 percent) coming from fat. Thus, even though it is true that the percentage of fat used is greater during light-intensity exercise, the overall amount of fat used is still less during light-intensity exercise. Plus, if you were to exercise at a light intensity level, you would have to do so twice as long to burn the same number of total calories.

Another benefit is that the metabolic rate remains at a slightly higher level longer after vigorous-intensity exercise, so you continue to burn a few extra calories following exercise. Very few calories are burned during recovery following a 45-minute moderate-intensity (50 percent or less of maximal capacity) exercise session, whereas when exercising at or above 70 percent of the maximal capacity for the same 45 minutes, nearly 40 percent of the total energy expenditure of the exercise bout is achieved during the recovery phase as the body returns to its pre-exercise baseline. A 500-calorie 45-minute vigorous exercise session will bring about another 200-calorie energy expenditure during the post-exercise recovery session.[27] Researchers believe that the extra caloric expenditure following vigorous exercise is because (a) the body uses more fat and less carbohydrates following a hard exercise session, (b) additional energy is required to replenish glycogen stores used during intense exercise, and (c) hormones released during vigorous exercise remain high, maintaining an elevated metabolism for several hours thereafter.

This example does not mean that light-intensity exercise is ineffective. Light-intensity exercise provides substantial health benefits, including a decrease in premature morbidity among overweight individuals. In addition, beginners are more willing to participate and stay with light-intensity programs. The risk of injury when starting out is quite low with this type of program. Light-intensity exercise does promote weight loss.

In terms of overall weight loss, there is additional controversy regarding the optimal duration of exercise. Research conducted in the 1990s at Laval University in Quebec, Canada, using both men and women participants, showed that subjects who performed a high-intensity intermittent training (HIIT) program lost more body fat than participants in a light- to moderate-intensity continuous aerobic endurance group.[28] Even more surprisingly, this finding occurred despite the fact that the vigorous-intensity group burned fewer total calories per exercise session. The researchers concluded that the "results reinforce the notion that for a given level of energy expenditure, vigorous exercise favors negative energy and lipid balance to a greater extent than exercise of light to moderate intensity. Moreover, the metabolic adaptations taking place in the skeletal muscle in response to the HIIT program appear to favor the process of lipid oxidation." If time constraints do not allow extensive exercise, to increase energy expenditure, a vigorous 20- to 30-minute exercise program is recommended.

In addition, it has been suggested that with attempts to lose weight, particularly by women, lengthy exercise sessions may not be helpful because they trigger greater food consumption following exercise, whereas shorter exercise sessions do not lead to greater caloric intake. Thus, some people think that the potential weight reduction effect of lengthy exercise sessions may be attenuated, because people end up eating more food when they exercise.

A 2009 study had postmenopausal women exercise at 50 percent of their maximal aerobic capacity for about 20, 40, and 60 minutes three to four times per week.[29] On average, the groups lost 3, 4.6, and 3.3 pounds of weight, respectively. The data indicated that the 20- and 40-minute groups lost weight close to the amounts that had been predicted, whereas the 60-minute group lost significantly less than predicted. The researchers concluded that 60 minutes of exercise led this group of women to compensate with greater food intake, possibly triggered by an increase in ghrelin levels. Nonetheless, all three groups exhibited a significant decrease in waist circumference, independent of total weight lost. Researchers theorize that the biological mechanism to maintain fat stores in women is stronger than the one in men.

Over the years, moderate-intensity exercise is still beneficial for weight maintenance. A 2010 study of more than 34,000 women who were followed for 13 years, starting at an average age of 54, found that on average the women gained six pounds of weight. However, a small group of them who reported 60 minutes of almost daily exercise at a moderate intensity level closely maintained their body weight.[30] The routine of this group was not new but rather exercise that they had been doing for years.

Thus, while the best exercise dose for optimal weight loss may not be a precise science, the research is quite clear that regular exercise is the best predictor of long-term weight maintenance. The data also indicate that even as little as 80 weekly minutes of aerobic or strength-training exercise prevents regain of the harmful visceral fat (also see pages 150–152 in Chapter 4).

The take-home message from these studies is that when trying to lose weight, initial lengthy exercise sessions (longer than 60 minutes) may not be the best approach to weight loss, *unless* you track daily caloric intake and avoid caloric compensation. The data show that people who carefully monitor caloric intake, instead of "guesstimating" energy intake, are by far more successful with weight loss.

Caloric compensation in response to extensive exercise in overweight individuals may be related to a low initial fit-

TABLE 5.2 **Comparison of Approximate Energy Expenditure between 30–40 Minutes of Exercise at Three Intensity Levels**

Exercise Intensity	Total Energy Expenditure (Calories)	Percent Calories from Fat	Total Fat Calories	Percent Calories from CHO*	Total CHO* Calories	Calories Burned per Minute	Calories per Pound per Minute
Light Intensity	200	50%	100	50%	100	6.67	0.045
Moderate Intensity	280	40%	112	60%	168	9.45	0.063
Vigorous Intensity	400	30%	120	70%	280	13.50	0.090

*CHO = Carbohydrates

FTO: The Obesity-Associated Gene

Researchers recently discovered a variant of the fat mass and obesity-associated (FTO) gene that appears to have a strong link to BMI and increases the risk that carriers will be overweight or obese. The strength of the genetic association depends on whether the individual has inherited one or two copies of the FTO gene variant. Having one copy of the variant has a corresponding modest effect on body weight. On average, such a person weighs an extra 2.5 pounds compared to those who do not have the variant. Someone with two copies of the variant typically weighs an extra 6.5 pounds. Nonetheless, obesity is only partially driven by genes, and the genetic code does not substantially change in just a few generations. In contrast, people's lifestyles and their environment have changed significantly over the past 100 years.

People with one or two variants of the gene are not destined to be obese. The gene variant does not cause a sluggish metabolism but rather causes them to eat more, in particular calorie-dense foods. And lifestyle plays a crucial role in enabling or minimizing susceptibility to weight gain. Physical activity is effective in controlling weight in people with this genetic predisposition toward obesity. Shortly after the discovery of FTO in 2007, researchers found that physical activity and exercise attenuate the effect of the gene on weight gain. As little as 60 minutes of moderate- to vigorous-intensity activity per week thwarts the genetic inheritance and reduces the effects of the FTO variant. Thus, the benefits of physical activity and exercise are strong enough to keep at recommended body weight people who could otherwise become seriously overweight.

ness level and an already-low caloric intake. Overall, inactive people tend to eat fewer calories, and a lengthy exercise session may well trigger a greater appetite due to the large negative caloric balance. Research confirms that energy deficit, and not exercise, is the most significant regulator of the hormonal responses seen in previously inactive individuals who begin an exercise program.[31] In active or fit individuals, lengthy exercise sessions are not counterproductive. If such was the case, health clubs and jogging trails would be full of overweight and obese people.

New research is beginning to look into the role of increasing light-intensity ambulation (walking) and standing activities (doing some work on your feet instead of sitting the entire time) on weight loss. In essence, people increase light-intensity physical activity throughout the day. Light-intensity activities do not seem to trigger the increase in ghrelin levels seen in previously inactive individuals who undertake long moderate-intensity or vigorous exercise sessions. The difference in energy expenditure by increasing light-intensity activities throughout the day can represent several hundred calories. As people achieve a higher fitness level, they can combine light-intensity activities performed throughout the day with moderate-intensity or vigorous exercise—or both. A graphic illustration of such lifestyle patterns and their effects on the metabolic rate and overall energy expenditure is provided in Figure 5.9.

If you wish to engage in vigorous-intensity exercise to either maintain lost weight or for adequate weight management, a word of caution is in order: Be sure that it is medically safe for you to participate in such activities and that you build up gradually to that level. If you are cleared to participate in vigorous exercise, do not attempt to do too much too quickly, because you may incur injuries and become discouraged. You must allow your body a proper conditioning period of 8 to 12 weeks, and perhaps even longer.

In addition, keep in mind that vigorous intensity does not mean high impact. High-impact activities are the most common cause of exercise-related injuries. More information on proper exercise prescription is presented in Chapter 6. And remember, when on a weight loss program, always carefully monitor your daily caloric intake to avoid food overconsumption.

Overweight and Fit Debate

A hotly debated topic in the exercise and medical community is the topic most commonly referred to as "fit and fat." Can a person possibly be overweight/obese and still be fit?

Initially, the debate started with research indicating that the higher the aerobic fitness level, as measured by total treadmill-walking time, the lower the mortality rate, regardless of body weight. Most recently, fitness has been defined as "accumulating 30 minutes of moderate intensity activity on most days of the week." Overweight people who reach this goal are not predisposed to premature death. In fact, data indicate that death rates for thin but unfit individuals is twice as high as that of obese and "fit" people. Furthermore, looking at every category of body composition, "unfit" people have a higher rate of premature death than "fit" individuals. Thus, at least partially, lack of physical activity (fitness), and not the weight problem itself, may be the cause of premature death in most overweight people. However, it's not simply a matter of fitness or fatness. Research has shown that both obesity and physical inactivity are independent risk factors for heart disease, type 2 diabetes, and other chronic ailments.

Fitness does offer substantial benefits, but regular physical activity in itself does not completely reverse chronic disease risks associated with excess body fat. Studies are encouraging because they show that overweight/obese people who focus on healthy eating and become physically active decrease the risk of premature mortality, regardless of whether they lose weight or not. Few obese people, however, eat healthy and exercise regularly for 30 minutes on most days of the week. Most obese people either chose not to exercise or are unable to do so because of functional limitations as a result of the excessive body weight.

The answer to the question as to whether a person can be fit and fat depends on the definition of fitness. If cardiorespiratory fitness is determined by "accumulating 30 minutes of moderate-intensity activity on most days of the week," then the answer is a definite "yes." If you measure fitness based on maximal oxygen uptake (VO_{2max}—see chapter 6, page 231), the answer is a clear "no." Many fitness experts do not agree with the concept of fit and fat. And according to Dr. JoAnn Manson of Harvard Medical School, "it's a rare bird" to find someone who is truly overweight and yet truly fit from a cardiorespiratory standpoint. Additionally, just because an obese individual is considered "metabolically healthy" at one point does not indicate that the person will stay that way in the future.

Most nutritionists and exercise scientists agree that healthy eating and healthy exercise contribute to healthy body weight. There are more than 50 medical conditions—from type 2 diabetes, acid reflux, arthritis, sleep apnea, and some types of cancers, that are directly related to excessive body weight. At this point, most fitness leaders do not support the notion that people can enjoy vibrant health and good quality of life while being overweight or obese.

Healthy Weight Gain

"Skinny" people should realize that the only healthy way to gain weight is also through exercise (mainly strength training) and a slight increase in caloric intake. Attempting to gain weight by overeating alone raises the fat component and not the lean component—which is not the path to better health. Exercise is the best solution to weight (fat) reduction and weight (lean) gain alike.

A strength-training program, such as the one explained in Chapter 7, is the best approach to add body weight. The training program should include at least two exercises of one to three sets for each major body part. Each set should consist of about 8 to 12 repetitions maximum.

Even though the metabolic cost of synthesizing a pound of muscle tissue is still unclear, consuming an estimated 500 additional calories per day is recommended to gain lean tissue. Your diet should include a daily total intake of about 1.5 grams of protein per kilogram of body weight. If your daily protein intake already exceeds 1.5 grams per day, the extra 500 calories should be primarily in the form of complex carbohydrates. The higher caloric intake must be accompanied by a strength-training program; otherwise, the increase in body weight will be in the form of fat, not muscle tissue (Lab 5D can be used to monitor your caloric intake for healthy weight gain). Additional information on nutrition to optimize muscle growth and strength development is provided in Chapter 7 in the section "Dietary Guidelines for Muscular and Strength Development," pages 277–278.

Weight Loss Myths

Cellulite and spot reducing are mythical concepts. **Cellulite** is caused by the herniation of subcutaneous fat within fibrous connective tissue, giving the tissue a padded appearance.

Spot reducing, or exercising a body part to reduce fat in that specific area, is also impossible. Doing several sets of daily sit-ups will not get rid of fat in the midsection of the body. When fat comes off, it does so throughout the entire body, not just the exercised area. The greatest proportion of fat may come off the biggest fat deposits, but the caloric output of a few sets of sit-ups has practically no effect on reducing total body fat. You have to exercise longer to see results.

Other touted means toward quick weight loss, such as steam baths, rubberized sweat suits, and mechanical vibrators, are misleading. When you step into a sauna, the weight lost is not fat but merely a significant amount of water. It looks nice when you step on the scale immediately afterward, but this represents a false loss of weight. As soon as you replace body fluids, you gain the weight back quickly.

Wearing rubberized sweat suits hastens the rate of body fluid that is lost—fluid that is vital during prolonged exercise—and raises core temperature at the same time. This combination puts a person in danger of dehydration, which impairs cellular function and, in extreme cases, can even cause death.

Similarly, mechanical vibrators are worthless in a weight control program. Vibrating belts and turning rollers may feel good, but they require no effort. Fat cannot be shaken off. It is lost primarily by burning it in muscle tissue.

Losing Weight the Sound and Sensible Way

Dieting never has been fun and never will be. People who are overweight and are serious about losing weight, however, have to include regular physical activity and exercise in their

FIGURE 5.9 Effects of lifestyle patterns on overall daily expenditure.

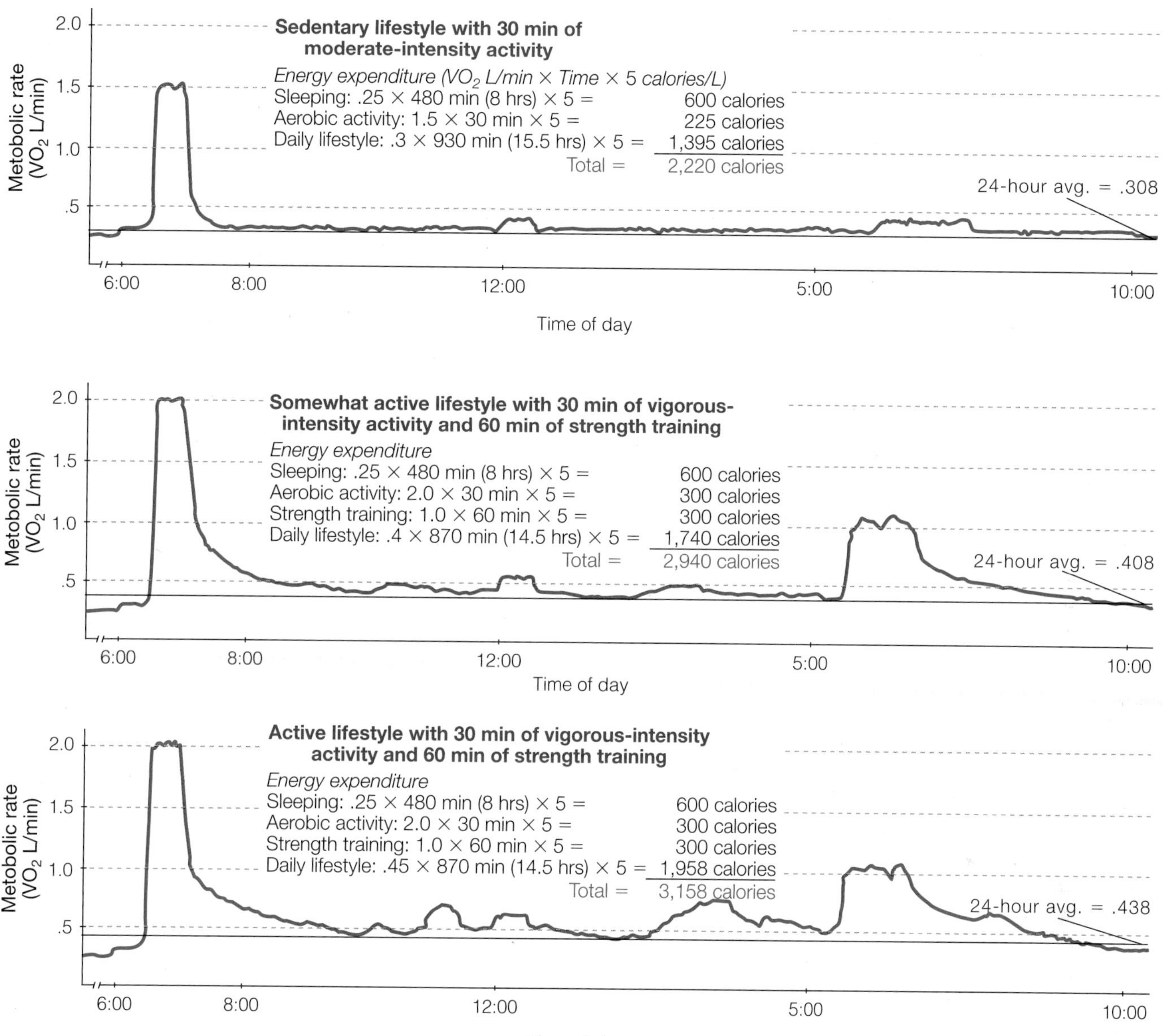

lives, along with proper food management and a sensible reduction in caloric intake.

Because excessive body fat is a risk factor for cardiovascular disease, some precautions are in order. Depending on the extent of the weight problem, a medical examination is a good idea before undertaking the exercise program. Consult a physician in this regard.

Significantly overweight individuals need to choose activities in which they do not have to support their body weight but that still are effective in burning calories. Injuries to joints and muscles are common in excessively overweight individuals who participate in weight-bearing exercises such as walking, jogging, and aerobics.

Swimming may not be a good weight loss exercise modality. Additional body fat makes a person more buoyant, and many people are not at the skill level required to swim fast enough to get a good training effect, thus limiting the number of calories burned as well as the benefits to the cardiorespiratory system. Additionally, swimmers often conduct "land training" to more effectively manage body weight. Research indicates that swimming has minimal effect on weight loss.[32] The data further shows that swimming in cold water stimulates appetite, so people tend to eat more following

Cellulite Term frequently used in reference to fat deposits that "bulge out," caused by the herniation of subcutaneous fat within fibrous connective tissue and giving the tissue a padded appearance.

Spot reducing Fallacious theory proposing that exercising a specific body part results in significant fat reduction in that area.

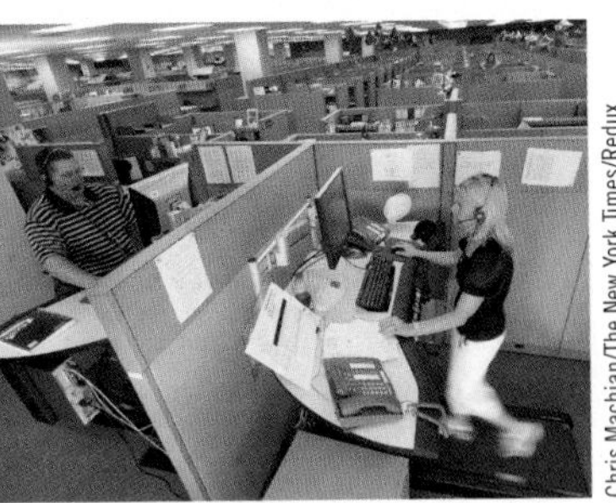

Chris Machian/The New York Times/Redux

Increasing ambulatory activities throughout the day enhances fitness and is an excellent weight management strategy.

their exercise session.[33] If your preferred mode of exercise is swimming, guard against eating more after you swim. During the initial stages of exercise, better alternatives include walking, riding a bicycle (either road or stationary), elliptical training, low-impact aerobics/zumba, or walking in a warm shallow pool. These forms of exercise aid with weight loss without fear of injuries.

How long should each exercise session last? The amount of exercise needed to lose weight and maintain weight loss is different from the amount of exercise needed to improve fitness. For health fitness, accumulating 30 minutes of physical activity a minimum of 5 days per week is recommended. To develop and maintain cardiorespiratory fitness, 20 to 60 minutes of vigorous exercise, three to five times per week, is suggested (see Chapter 6). For successful weight loss, however, 30 to 60 minutes of light to vigorous exercise on most days of the week is recommended. Additional light-intensity ambulation and standing throughout the day are also strongly encouraged. To maintain substantial weight loss, 60 to 90 minutes of physical activity nearly daily is recommended.

People should not try to do too much too fast. Unconditioned beginners should start with about 15 minutes of aerobic exercise three times a week, and during the next 3 to 4 weeks gradually increase the duration by approximately 5 minutes per week and the frequency by one day per week.

In addition to exercise and food management, a sensible reduction in caloric intake and careful monitoring of this intake are recommended. Research indicates that a negative caloric balance is required to lose weight for the following reasons:

1. People tend to underestimate their caloric intake and are eating more than they should be eating.
2. Developing new behaviors takes time, and most people have trouble changing and adjusting to new eating habits.
3. Many individuals are in such poor physical condition that they take a long time to increase their activity level enough to offset the setpoint and burn enough calories to aid in losing body fat.
4. Most successful dieters carefully monitor their daily caloric intake.
5. A few people simply will not alter their food selection (high unhealthy fat foods). For those who will not (which increases their risk for chronic diseases), the only solution to lose weight successfully is a large increase in physical activity, a negative caloric balance, or a combination of the two.

Perhaps the only exception to a decrease in caloric intake for weight loss purposes is in people who already are eating too few calories. A nutrient analysis (see Chapter 3) often reveals that long-term dieters are not consuming enough calories. These people actually need to increase their daily caloric intake and combine it with an exercise program to get their metabolism to kick back up to a normal level.

You also must learn to make wise food choices. Think in terms of long-term benefits (weight management) instead of instant gratification (unhealthy eating and subsequent weight gain). Making healthful choices allows you to eat more food, eat more nutritious food, and ingest fewer calories. For example, instead of eating a high-fat, 700-calorie scone, you could eat as much as one orange, one cup of grapes, a hardboiled egg, two slices of whole-wheat toast, two teaspoons of jam, one-half cup of honey-sweetened oatmeal, and one glass of skim milk (for other meal alternatives, see Figure 5.10).

You can estimate your daily energy (caloric) requirement by consulting Tables 5.3 and 5.4 and completing Lab 5A. Given that this is only an estimated value, individual adjustments related to many of the factors discussed in this chapter may be necessary to establish a more precise value. Nevertheless, the estimated value offers beginning guidelines for weight control or reduction.

The EER without additional planned activity and exercise is based on age, total body weight, height, and gender. Individuals who hold jobs that require a lot of walking or heavy manual labor burn more calories during the day than those who have sedentary jobs (e.g., working behind a desk). To estimate your EER, refer to Table 5.3. For example, the EER computation for a 20-year-old man who is 71 inches tall and weighs 160 pounds would be as follows:

1. Body weight (BW) in kilograms = 72.6 kg (160 lb ÷ 2.2046)

   Height (HT) in meters = 1.8 m (71 inches × .0254)
2. EER = 662 − (9.53 × Age) + (15.91 × BW) + (539 × HT)

   EER = 662 − (9.53 × 20) + (15.91 × 72.6) + (539 × 1.8)

   EER = 662 − 190.6 + 1155 + 970

   EER = 2,596 calories/day

Thus, the EER to maintain body weight for this individual would be 2,596 calories per day.

To determine the average number of calories you burn daily as a result of exercise, figure out the total number of minutes you exercise weekly, and then figure the daily average exercise time. For instance, the man in the prior example cycling at 10 miles per hour five times a week, 60 minutes

FIGURE 5.10 Making wise food choices.

These illustrations provide a comparison of how much more food you can eat when you make healthy choices. You also get more vitamins, minerals, antioxidants, phytonutrients, and fiber by making healthy choices.

Breakfast

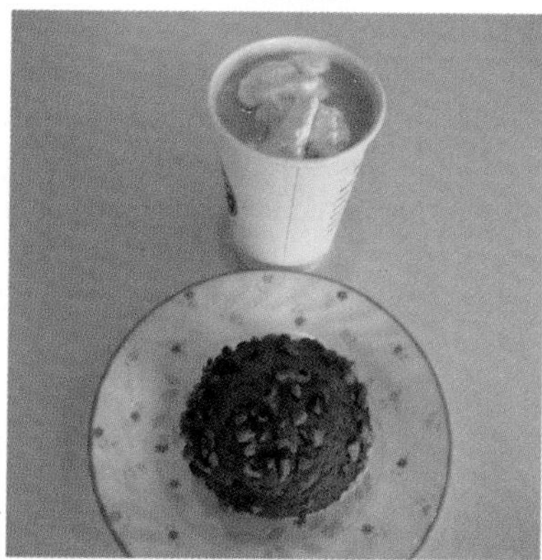

1 banana nut muffin, 1 cafe mocha

Calories: 940

Percent fat calories: 48%

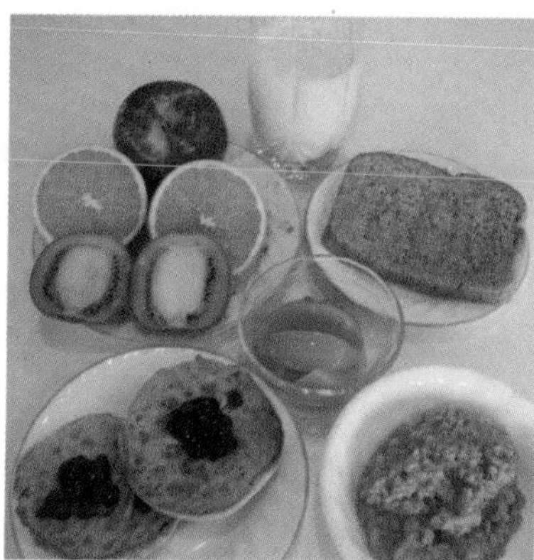

1 cup oatmeal, 1 English muffin with jelly, 1 slice whole wheat bread with honey, ½ cup peaches, 1 kiwi fruit, 1 orange, 1 apple, 1 cup skim milk

Calories: 900

Percent fat calories: 5%

Lunch

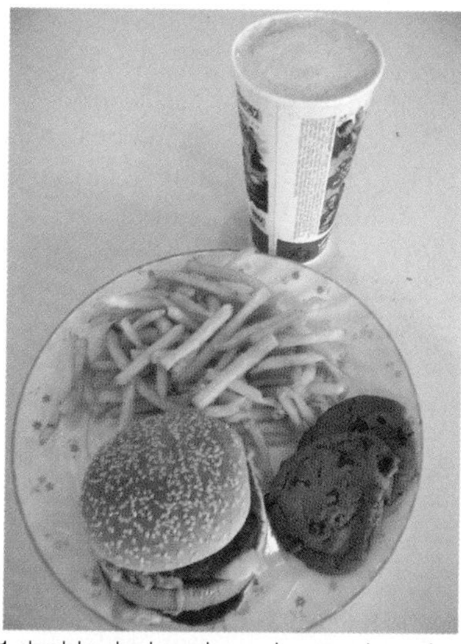

1 double-decker cheeseburger, 1 serving medium French fries, 2 chocolate chip cookies, 1 medium strawberry milkshake

Calories: 1790

Percent fat calories: 37%

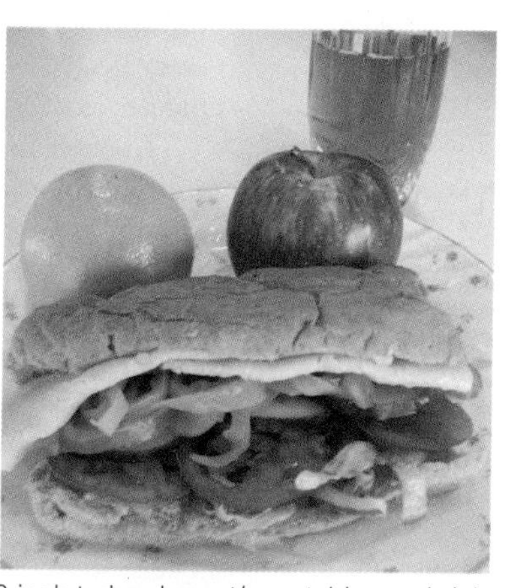

6-inch turkey breast/vegetable sandwich, 1 apple, 1 orange, 1 cup sweetened green tea

Calories: 500

Percent fat calories: 10%

Dinner

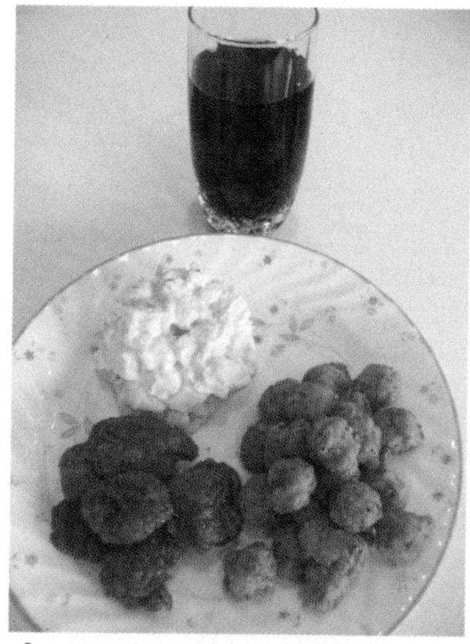

6 oz. popcorn chicken, 3 oz. barbecue chicken wings, 1 cup potato salad, 1 12-oz. cola drink

Calories: 1250

Percent fat calories: 42%

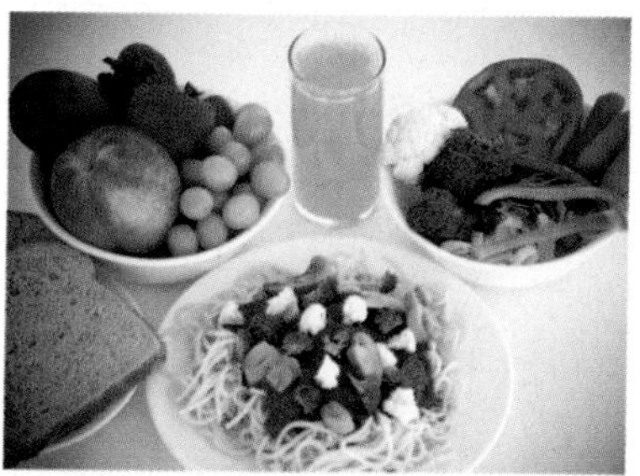

2 cups spaghetti with tomato sauce and vegetables, a 2-cup salad bowl with two tablespoons Italian dressing, 2 slices whole wheat bread, 1 cup grapes, 3 large strawberries, 1 kiwi fruit, 1 peach, 1 12-oz. fruit juice drink

Calories: 1240

Percent fat calories: 14%

TABLE 5.3 Estimated Energy Requirement (EER) Based on Age, Body Weight, and Height

Men	EER = 662 − (9.53 × Age) + (15.91 × BW) + (539 × HT)
Women	EER = 354 − (6.91 × Age) + (9.36 × BW) + (726 × HT)

Note: Includes activities of independent living only and no moderate physical activity or exercise.
BW = body weight in kilograms (divide BW in pounds by 2.2046),
HT = height in meters (multiply HT in inches by .0254).

Table 5.4 Caloric Expenditure of Selected Physical Activities

Activity*	Cal/lb/min	Activity*	Cal/lb/min
Aerobics		Jogging/running (on a level surface)	
Moderate	0.065	11.0 min/mile	0.070
Vigorous	0.095	8.5 min/mile	0.090
Step aerobics	0.070	7.0 min/mile	0.102
Archery	0.030	6.0 min/mile	0.114
Badminton		Deep water**	0.100
Recreation	0.038	Racquetball	0.065
Competition	0.065	Rope jumping	0.060
Baseball	0.031	Rowing (vigorous)	0.090
Basketball		Skating (moderate)	0.038
Moderate	0.046	Skiing	
Competition	0.063	Downhill	0.060
Bowling	0.030	Level (5 mph)	0.078
Calisthenics	0.033	Soccer	0.059
Circuit training		Stationary cycling	
Moderate	0.070	Moderate	0.055
Vigorous	0.100	Vigorous	0.070
Cross-country skiing		Strength training	0.050
Moderate	0.090	Swimming (crawl)	
Vigorous	0.120	20 yds/min	0.031
Cycling (on a level surface)		25 yds/min	0.040
5.5 mph	0.033	45 yds/min	0.057
10.0 mph	0.050	50 yds/min	0.070
13.0 mph	0.071	Table tennis	0.030
Dance		Tennis	
Moderate	0.030	Moderate	0.045
Vigorous	0.055	Competition	0.064
Elliptical training		Volleyball	0.030
Moderate	0.070	Walking	
Vigorous	0.090	4.5 mph	0.045
Golf	0.030	Shallow pool	0.090
Gymnastics		Water aerobics	
Light	0.030	Moderate	0.050
Heavy	0.056	Vigorous	0.070
Handball	0.064	Wrestling	0.085
High-intensity interval training	0.120	Zumba	
		Moderate	0.065
Hiking	0.040	Vigorous	0.095
Judo/karate	0.086		

*Values are for actual time engaged in the activity.
** Treading water
Adapted from: P. E. Allsen, J. M. Harrison, and B. Vance, *Fitness for Life: An Individualized Approach* (Dubuque, IA: Wm. C. Brown, 1989). C. A. Bucher and W. E. Prentice, *Fitness for College and Life* (St. Louis: Times Mirror/Mosby College Publishing, 1989). C. F. Consolazio, R. E. Johnson, and L. J. Pecora, *Physiological Measurements of Metabolic Functions in Man* (New York: McGraw-Hill, 1963). R. V. Hockey, *Physical Fitness: The Pathway to Healthy Living* (St. Louis: Times Mirror/Mosby College Publishing, 1989). W. W. K. Hoeger et al., Research conducted at Boise State University, 1986–2009.

each time, exercises 300 minutes per week (5 × 60). The average daily exercise time, therefore, is 42 minutes (300 ÷ 7, rounded off to the lowest unit).

Next, from Table 5.4, find the energy expenditure for the activity (or activities) chosen for the exercise program. In the case of cycling (10 miles per hour), the expenditure is .05 calories per pound of body weight per minute of activity (cal/lb/min). With a body weight of 160 pounds, this man would burn 8 calories each minute (body weight × .05, or 160 × .05). In 42 minutes, he would burn approximately 336 calories (42 × 8).

Now obtain the daily energy requirement, with exercise, needed to maintain body weight. To do this, add the EER obtained from Table 5.3 and the average calories burned through exercise. In our example, it is 2,932 calories (2,596 + 336).

If a negative caloric balance is recommended to lose weight, this person has to consume less than 2,932 calories daily to achieve the objective. Because of the many factors that play a role in weight control, this 2,932-calorie value is only an estimated daily requirement. Furthermore, we cannot predict that the man in the example will lose exactly one pound of fat in one week if he cuts his daily intake by 500 calories (500 × 7 = 3,500 calories, or the equivalent of one pound of fat).

The daily energy requirement figure is only a target guideline for weight control. Periodic readjustments are necessary because individuals differ, and the daily requirement changes as they lose weight and modify their exercise habits.

To determine your target caloric intake to lose weight, multiply your current weight by 5 and subtract this amount from the total daily energy requirement with exercise. For our example, this would mean 2,132 calories per day to lose weight (160 × 5 = 800 and 2,932 − 800 = 2,132 calories).

This final caloric intake to lose weight should not be below 1,500 daily calories for most people. If distributed properly over the various food groups, 1,500 calories provide the necessary nutrients the body needs. In terms of percentages of total calories, the daily distribution should be approximately 50 to 60 percent carbohydrates (mostly complex carbohydrates), less than 30 percent fat, and about 20 percent protein.

Many experts believe that a person can take off weight more efficiently by reducing daily fat intake to about 20 percent of total daily caloric intake. Because one gram of fat supplies more than twice the number of calories that carbohydrates and protein do, the tendency when someone eats less fat is to consume fewer calories. With fat intake at 20 percent of total calories, the individual has sufficient fat in the diet to feel satisfied and avoid frequent hunger pangs.

Furthermore, it takes only 3 to 5 percent of ingested calories to store fat as fat, whereas it takes approximately 25 percent of ingested calories to convert carbohydrates to fat. Some evidence indicates that if people eat the same number of calories as carbohydrate or as fat, those on the fat diet store more fat. Long-term successful weight loss and weight management programs are low in fat content.

Many people have trouble adhering to a low-fat-calorie diet. During times of weight loss, however, you are strongly encouraged to do so. Refer to Table 5.5 to aid you in determining the grams of fat at 20 percent of the total calories for selected energy intakes. Also, use the form provided in Lab 3A to monitor your daily fat intake. For weight maintenance, individuals who have been successful in maintaining an average weight loss of 30 pounds for more than 5 years are consuming about 24 percent of calories from fat, 56 percent from carbohydrates, and 20 percent from protein.[34]

Breakfast is a critical meal while on a weight loss program. Many people skip breakfast because it's the easiest meal to skip. For years, a common recommendation when attempting to lose weight has been that intake should consist of a minimum of 25 percent of the total daily calories for breakfast, 50 percent for lunch, and no more than 25 percent for dinner. Evidence indicates that people who skip breakfast are hungrier later in the day and end up consuming more total daily calories than those who eat breakfast. Furthermore, regular breakfast eaters have less of a weight problem, lose weight more effectively, and have less difficulty maintaining the weight loss.

This concept was most recently substantiated by researchers who found that people who eat a larger meal at breakfast are more likely to lose weight and waist line circumference than those who eat a larger meal for dinner.[35] In the 12-week study, participants were divided into two 1,400-calorie diet groups. Group one distributed the daily intake so that 700, 500, and 200 calories were consumed respectively at breakfast, lunch, and dinner; whereas group two consumed 200, 500, and 700 calories respectively over breakfast, lunch, and dinner. The participants in the larger breakfast group lost almost 18 pounds and three inches off their waist line as compared to only 7.3 pound and a 1.4-inch loss for those in the larger dinner group. The larger breakfast group was also found to have lower levels of the appetite-increasing hormone ghrelin, indicating that they were more satiated and exhibited a lower desire for snacking

TABLE 5.5 Grams of Fat at 20 and 30 Percent of Total Calories for Selected Energy Intakes

	Grams of fat			Grams of fat	
Caloric Intake	20%	30%	Caloric Intake	20%	30%
1,200	27	40	2,200	49	73
1,300	29	43	2,300	51	77
1,400	31	47	2,400	53	80
1,500	33	50	2,500	56	83
1,600	36	53	2,600	58	87
1,700	38	57	2,700	60	90
1,800	40	60	2,800	62	93
1,900	42	63	2,900	64	97
2,000	44	67	3,000	67	100
2,100	47	70			

BEHAVIOR MODIFICATION PLANNING

Healthy Breakfast Choices

Breakfast is the most important meal of the day. Skipping breakfast makes you hungrier later in the day and leads to overconsumption and greater caloric intake throughout the rest of the day. Regular breakfast eaters have less of a weight problem, lose weight more effectively, have less difficulty maintaining lost weight, and live longer. Skipping breakfast also temporarily raises LDL (bad) cholesterol and lowers insulin sensitivity, changes that may increase the risk for heart disease and diabetes. Below are some healthy breakfast food choices. Have you tried these options for breakfast?

I PLAN TO	I DID IT	
❑	❑	Fresh fruit
❑	❑	Low-fat or skim milk
❑	❑	Low-fat yogurt with berries
❑	❑	Whole-grain cereal
❑	❑	Whole-grain bread or bagel with fat-free cream cheese and slices of red or green pepper
❑	❑	Hummus over a whole-grain bagel
❑	❑	Peanut butter with whole-grain bread or bagel
❑	❑	Low-fat cottage cheese with fruit
❑	❑	Oatmeal
❑	❑	Reduced-fat cheese
❑	❑	Egg Beaters with salsa
❑	❑	A scrambled egg with veggies (limit oil or butter use)

Try It

Select a healthy breakfast choice each day for the next 7 days. Evaluate how you feel the rest of the morning. What effect did eating breakfast have on your activities of daily living and daily caloric intake? Be sure to record your food choices, how you felt, and what activities you engaged in.

throughout the day. Another benefit was a significant decrease in insulin, glucose, and triglyceride levels in the larger breakfast group, and they did not experience the large spike in blood glucose level that occurs after a meal and is believed to increase cardiovascular disease risk.

Thus it can be concluded that eating most of your calories earlier in the day aids with weight loss. Furthermore, be sure to include protein and fiber with breakfast (whole-wheat toast with eggs or peanut butter or oatmeal with nuts) to further keep yourself fueled and full for hours. Eating only carbohydrates for breakfast (or with any meal) substantially increases food cravings within a relative short time of that particular meal.

If most daily calories are consumed during one meal (as in the typical evening meal), the body may perceive that something is wrong and slow the metabolism so that it can store more calories in the form of fat. Also, eating most daily calories during one meal causes a person to go hungry the rest of the day, making it more difficult to adhere to the diet. Also, try not to eat within 3 hours of going to bed. At this time of day, your metabolism is slowest; your caloric intake is less likely to be used for energy and more likely to be stored as fat.

Consuming most of the calories earlier in the day seems helpful in losing weight and in managing **atherosclerosis**. The time of day when most of the fats and cholesterol are consumed can influence blood lipids and coronary heart disease. Peak digestion time following a heavy meal is about 7 hours after that meal. If most lipids, or fats, are consumed during the evening meal, digestion peaks while the person is sound asleep and the metabolism is at its lowest rate. Consequently, the body may not metabolize fats and cholesterol as well, leading to a higher blood lipid count and increasing the risk for atherosclerosis and coronary heart disease.

Before you proceed to develop a thorough weight loss program, take a moment to identify, in Lab 5B, your current stage of change as it pertains to your recommended body weight. If applicable—that is, if you are not at recommended weight—list also the processes and techniques for change that you will use to accomplish your goal. In Lab 5B, also outline your exercise program for weight management.

Monitoring Your Diet with Daily Food Logs

To help you monitor and adhere to a weight loss program, use the daily food logs provided in Lab 5C. If the goal is to maintain or increase body weight, use Lab 5D.

Evidence indicates that people who monitor daily caloric intake are more successful at weight loss than those who don't self-monitor. "If you eat it, record it." Most people underestimate what they eat and wonder why they aren't losing weight. Before using the forms in Lab 5C, make a master copy for your files so that you can make future copies as needed. Guidelines are provided for 1,200-, 1,500-, 1,800-, and 2,000-calorie diet plans. These plans have been developed based on the MyPlate and the *Dietary Guidelines for Americans* to meet the Recommended Dietary Allowances.[36] The objective is to meet (not exceed) the number of servings allowed for each diet plan. Each time you eat a serving of a certain food, record it in the appropriate box.

To lose weight, you should use the diet plan that most closely approximates your target caloric intake. The plan is based on the following caloric allowances for these food groups:

- Grains: 80 calories per serving
- Fruits: 60 calories per serving
- Vegetables: 25 calories per serving
- Dairy (use low-fat products): 120 calories per serving
- Protein: Use low-fat (300 calories per serving) frozen entrees or an equivalent amount if you prepare your own main dish (see the following discussion)

As you start your diet plan, pay particular attention to food serving sizes. Take care with cup and glass sizes. A standard cup is 8 ounces, but most glasses nowadays contain between 12 and 16 ounces. If you drink 12 ounces of fruit juice, in essence you are getting two servings of fruit because a standard serving is three-fourths cup of juice.

Read food labels carefully to compare the caloric value of the serving listed on the label with the caloric guidelines provided previously. Here are some examples:

- One slice of standard whole-wheat bread has about 80 calories. A plain bagel may have 200 to 350 calories. Although it is low in fat, a 350-calorie bagel is equivalent to almost four servings in the grains group.
- The standard serving size listed on the food label for most cereals is one cup. As you read the nutrition information, however, you will find that for the same cup of cereal, one type of cereal has 120 calories and another cereal has 200 calories. Because a standard serving in the grains group is 80 calories, the first cereal would be 1.5 servings and the second would be 2.5 servings.
- A medium-size fruit is usually considered one serving. A large fruit provides more than one serving.
- In the dairy group, one serving represents 120 calories. A cup of whole milk has about 160 calories, compared with a cup of skim milk, which contains 88 calories. A cup of whole milk, therefore, would provide 1.33 servings in this food group.

Low-Fat Entrees To be more accurate with caloric intake and to simplify meal preparation, use commercially prepared low-fat frozen entrees as the main dish for lunch and dinner meals (only one entree per meal for the 1,200-calorie diet plan; see Lab 5C). Look for entrees that provide about 300 calories and no more than six grams of fat per entree. This entree can be used as a selection for the protein group and will provide most of your daily requirement. Along with each entree, supplement the meal with some of your servings from the other food groups. This diet plan has been used successfully in weight loss research programs.[37] If you choose not to use low-fat frozen entrees, prepare a similar meal using three ounces (cooked) of lean meat, poultry, or fish with additional vegetables, rice, or pasta that will provide 300 calories with less than six grams of fat per dish.

In your daily logs, be sure to record the precise amount in each serving. You also can run a computerized nutrient analysis to verify your caloric intake and food distribution pattern (percent of total calories from carbohydrate, fat, and protein).

Protein Intake To minimize the loss of lean body mass and hunger pangs while dieting, it is extremely important that you consume sufficient protein with each meal. You need to insure that you are consuming between 1.0 grams and 1.2 grams of protein per kilogram of body weight per day (more if you are doing vigorous aerobic exercise and strength-training). As explained in Chapter 3, Table 3.4 (page 90), if you weigh 141 pounds (64 kg), your total daily protein intake would be between 96 and 128 grams per day (64 × 1.5 and 64 × 2.0) or the equivalent of 384 to 512 calories from protein every day (96 × 4 and 128 × 4), distributed in 32 to 43 grams of protein for each of your daily three meals. High protein/low-calorie foods include fat-free or low-fat dairy products (milk, plain Greek yogurt, and cheese), eggs, lean meats and poultry, fish, soybeans and soy milk, tofu, quinoa, and beans. To help monitor your daily protein intake, you can calculate and record your daily intake in Lab 5C as well.

Effect of Food Choices on Long-Term Weight Gain

Although still in its infancy, research published in 2011 on more than 120,000 people, who were evaluated every 4 years over a 20-year period, showed that food choices have a significant effect on weight gain.[38] On average, study participants gained 17 pounds over the course of 20 years. Regardless of other lifestyle habits, individuals who consumed unhealthy foods gained the most weight, whereas those who made healthy food choices gained the least amount of weight. Although more research is needed, in this study, 4-year weight change was most strongly associated with consumption of potato chips, potatoes, sugar-sweetened beverages, and unprocessed and processed red meats and inversely associated with consumption of vegetables, whole grains, fruits, nuts, and yogurt. The take-home message: Consume more fruits, vegetables, whole grains, low-fat dairy products, and nuts (the latter in moderation because of their high caloric content).

Behavior Modification and Adherence to a Weight Management Program

Achieving and maintaining recommended body composition is possible, but it requires desire and commitment. If weight management is to become a priority, people must realize that they have to transform their behavior to some extent.

Modifying old habits and developing new, positive behaviors takes time. Individuals who apply the management techniques provided in the Behavior Modification Planning box on pages 196–198 are more successful at changing detrimental behavior and adhering to a positive lifetime weight control program. In developing a retraining program, you are not expected to incorporate all of the strategies given but should note the ones that apply to you. The form provided

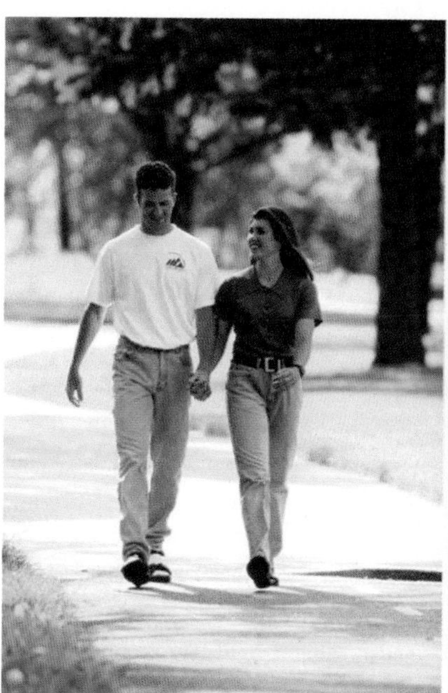
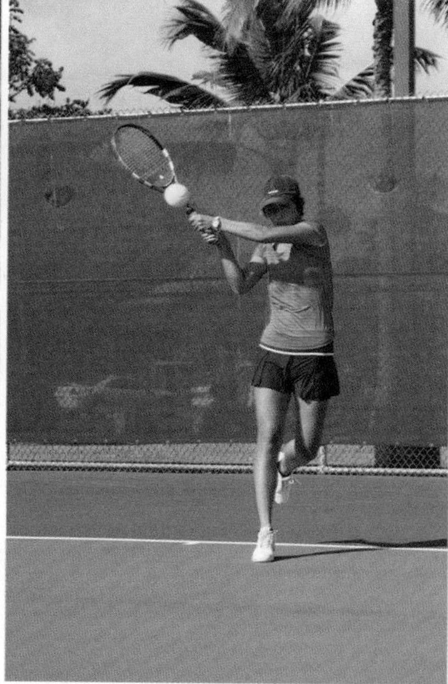
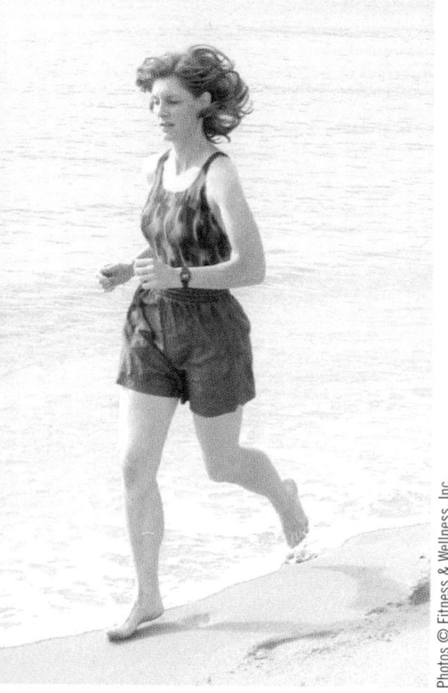

Exercising with other people and in different places helps people maintain exercise regularity.

in Lab 5E will allow you to evaluate and monitor your own weight management behaviors.

CRITICAL THINKING

What behavioral strategies have you used to properly manage your body weight? How do you think those strategies would work for others?

During the weight loss process, surround yourself with people who have the same goal that you have (weight loss). Data released in 2007 showed that obesity can spread through "social networks."[39] That is, if your friends, siblings, or spouse gain weight, you are more likely to gain weight as well. People tend to accept a higher weight standard if someone they are close to or care about gains weight.

In the study, the social ties of more than 12,000 people were examined over 32 years. The findings revealed that if a close friend becomes obese, a person's risk of becoming obese during the next 2 to 4 years increases 171 percent. In addition, the risk increases 57 percent for casual friends, 40 percent for siblings, and 37 percent for the person's spouse. The reverse was also found to be true: When a person loses weight, the likelihood of friends, siblings, or spouse to lose weight is also enhanced.

Furthermore, the research found that gender plays a role in social networks. A male's weight has a greater effect on the weight of male friends and brothers than on female friends or sisters. Similarly, a woman's weight has a far greater influence on sisters and girlfriends than on brothers or male friends. Thus, if you are trying to lose weight, choose your friendships carefully: Do not surround yourself with people who either have a weight problem or are still gaining weight.

The Simple Truth

There is no quick and easy way to take off excess body fat and keep it off for good. Weight management is accomplished by making a lifetime commitment to physical activity and proper food selection. When taking part in a weight (fat) reduction program, people also have to decrease their caloric intake moderately, use portion control, be physically active, and implement strategies to modify unhealthy eating behaviors.

During the process, relapses into past negative behaviors are almost inevitable. The three most common reasons for relapse are as follows:

1. Stress-related factors (e.g., major life changes, depression, job changes, or illness)
2. Social reasons (e.g., entertaining, eating out, or business travel)
3. Self-enticing behaviors (placing yourself in a situation to see how much you can get away with: "One small taste won't hurt" leads to "I'll eat just one slice" and finally to "I haven't done well, so I might as well eat some more")

Making mistakes is human and does not necessarily mean failure. Failure comes to those who give up and do not build on previous experiences and thereby develop skills that will prevent self-defeating behaviors in the future. Where there's a will, there's a way, and those who persist will reap the rewards.

BEHAVIOR MODIFICATION PLANNING

Weight Loss Strategies

I PLAN TO	I DID IT	
❑	❑	1. Make a commitment to change. The first necessary ingredient is the desire to modify your behavior. You have to stop precontemplating or contemplating change and get going! You must accept that you have a problem and decide by yourself whether you really want to change. Sincere commitment increases your chances for success.
❑	❑	2. Set realistic goals. The weight problem developed over several years. Similarly, new lifetime eating and exercise habits take time to develop. A realistic long-term goal also will include short-term objectives that allow for regular evaluation and help maintain motivation and renewed commitment to attain the long-term goal.
❑	❑	3. Monitor caloric intake. Keep an accurate daily record of food consumption. "If you eat it, record it." People who keep accurate food logs are more successful at weight loss.
❑	❑	4. Plan on three small meals and possibly one to two snacks each day. Eating less but more often helps keep your blood sugar levels steady and avoid hunger pangs. Include adequate protein intake with each meal and use primarily high-volume, low-calorie foods. Space your meals and snacks so that you eat every three to four hours. Snacks need to be nutrient-rich, including fruits, vegetables, low-fat/plain yogurt, or a small amount of nuts.

BEHAVIOR MODIFICATION PLANNING

❑ ❑ 5. Weigh yourself regularly, preferably at the same time of day and under the same conditions. Do not adapt and accept a higher body weight as a new stable weight. Make dietary and physical activity adjustments accordingly.

❑ ❑ 6. Incorporate exercise into the program. Choosing enjoyable activities, places, times, equipment, and people to work out with will help you adhere to an exercise program (see Chapters 6–9). If time is a factor, you can easily create extra time in your day by recording your favorite TV programs and watching them later. You can then skip the commercials and end with extra time to fit in exercise.

❑ ❑ 7. Differentiate between hunger and appetite. Hunger is the actual physical need for food. Appetite is a desire for food, usually triggered by factors such as stress, habit, boredom, depression, availability of food, or just the thought of food. Developing and sticking to a regular meal pattern will help control hunger.

❑ ❑ 8. Eat less fat. Small amounts of healthy fats are encouraged with your meals to curb appetite and help delay hunger. However, each gram of fat provides 9 calories, and protein and carbohydrates provide only 4. In essence, you can eat more food on a low-fat diet because you consume fewer calories with each meal. Most of your fat intake should come from healthy unsaturated sources.

❑ ❑ 9. Pay attention to calories. Just because food is labeled "low-fat" does not mean you can eat as much as you want. When reading food labels—and when eating—don't just look at the fat content. Pay attention to calories as well. Many low-fat foods are high in calories.

❑ ❑ 10. Cut unnecessary items from your diet. Substituting water for a daily can of soda would cut 51,100 (140 × 365) calories yearly from the diet—the equivalent of 14.6 (51,000 ÷ 3,500) pounds of fat. If you always drink water when thirsty and with your meals, instead of sugar-sweetened beverages, you can do even better and decrease caloric intake by an average of 300 daily calories. Studies also indicate that liquid calories do little to suppress hunger.

❑ ❑ 11. Maintain a daily intake of calcium-rich foods, especially low-fat or nonfat dairy products.

❑ ❑ 12. Add foods to your diet that reduce cravings, such as eggs; small amounts of red meat, fish, poultry, tofu, oils, and fats; and nonstarchy vegetables such as lettuce, green beans, peppers, asparagus, broccoli, mushrooms, and brussels sprouts. Also, increasing the intake of low-glycemic carbohydrates with your meals helps you go longer before you feel hungry again.

❑ ❑ 13. Avoid morning snacks. Dieters who skip morning snacks (which are usually calorie-dense, refined-carbohydrate, or high-fat snacks) lose more weight than morning snackers. The time between breakfast and lunch is not that long, and most people aren't hungry but eat because food is available at work or at home. The opposite is true for afternoon snacks. The time frame may be between 5 and 6 hours, and being too hungry at dinnertime may cause you to devour supersized meal portions. Research indicates that an afternoon snack that fills you with nutrients, not calories (e.g., a fruit, vegetable, or a small amount of nuts), aids weight loss.

❑ ❑ 14. Avoid automatic eating. Many people associate certain daily activities with eating, for example, cooking, watching television, or reading. Most foods consumed in these situations lack nutritional value or are high in sugar and fat.

❑ ❑ 15. Stay busy. People tend to eat more when they sit around and do nothing. Occupying the mind and body with activities not associated with eating helps take away the desire to eat. Some options are walking; cycling; playing sports; gardening; sewing; or visiting a library, a museum, or a park. You also might develop other skills and interests not associated with food.

❑ ❑ 16. Plan meals and shop sensibly. Always shop on a full stomach, because hungry shoppers tend to buy unhealthy foods impulsively—and then snack on the way home. Always use a shopping list, which should include 100 percent whole-grains (breads and cereals), fruits and vegetables, low-fat milk and dairy products, lean meats, fish, and poultry.

(Continued)

BEHAVIOR MODIFICATION PLANNING

❑ ❑ 17. Cook wisely:

- ❑ Use less fat and fewer refined and processed foods in food preparation.
- ❑ Trim all visible fat from meats and remove skin from poultry before cooking.
- ❑ Skim the fat off gravies and soups.
- ❑ Bake, broil, boil, or steam instead of frying.
- ❑ Sparingly use butter, cream, mayonnaise, and salad dressings.
- ❑ Avoid coconut oil, palm oil, and cocoa butter.
- ❑ Prepare plenty of foods that contain fiber.
- ❑ Include whole-grain breads and cereals, vegetables, and legumes in most meals.
- ❑ Eat fruits for dessert.
- ❑ Stay away from soda, fruit juices, fruit-flavored drinks, and sports and energy drinks.
- ❑ Use less sugar, and cut down on other refined carbohydrates, such as corn syrup, malt sugar, dextrose, and fructose.
- ❑ Drink plenty of water throughout the day.

❑ ❑ 18. Do not serve more food than you should eat. Measure the food in portions and keep serving dishes away from the table. Do not force yourself or anyone else to "clean the plate" after they are satisfied (including children after they already have had a healthy, nutritious serving).

❑ ❑ 19. Try "junior size" instead of "super size." People who are served larger portions eat more, whether they are hungry or not. Use smaller plates, bowls, cups, and glasses. Try eating half as much food as you commonly eat. Watch for portion sizes at restaurants as well: Supersized foods create supersized people.

❑ ❑ 20. Eat out infrequently. The more often people eat out, the more body fat they have. People who eat out six or more times per week consume about 300 extra calories per day and 30 percent more fat than those who eat out less often.

❑ ❑ 21. Eat slowly and at the table only. Eating on the run promotes overeating because the body doesn't have enough time to "register" consumption and people overeat before the body perceives the fullness signal. Eating at the table encourages people to take time out to eat and deters snacking between meals. After eating, do not sit around the table but, rather, clean up and put away the food to avoid snacking.

❑ ❑ 22. Avoid social binges. Social gatherings tend to entice self-defeating behavior. Use visual imagery to plan ahead. Do not feel pressured to eat or drink and rationalize in these situations. Choose low-calorie foods and entertain yourself with other activities, such as dancing and talking.

❑ ❑ 23. Do not place unhealthy foods within easy reach. Ideally, avoid bringing high-calorie, high-sugar, or high-fat foods into the house. If they are there already, store them where they are hard to get to or see—perhaps the garage or basement.

❑ ❑ 24. Avoid evening food raids. Most people do really well during the day but then "lose it" at night. Take control. Stop and think. To avoid excessive nighttime snacking, stay busy after your evening meal. Go for a short walk, floss and brush your teeth, and get to bed earlier. Even better, close the kitchen after dinner and try not to eat anything 3 hours prior to going to sleep.

❑ ❑ 25. Practice stress management techniques (discussed in Chapter 10). Many people snack and increase their food consumption in stressful situations.

❑ ❑ 26. Get support. People who receive support from friends, relatives, and formal support groups are much more likely to lose and maintain weight loss than those without such support. The more support you receive, the better off you will be.

❑ ❑ 27. Monitor changes and reward accomplishments. Being able to exercise without interruption for 15, 20, 30, or 60 minutes; swimming a certain distance; running a mile—all these accomplishments deserve recognition. Create rewards that are not related to eating: new clothing, a tennis racquet, a bicycle, exercise shoes, or something else that is special and you would not have acquired otherwise.

❑ ❑ 28. Prepare for slipups. Most people will slip and occasionally splurge. Do not despair and give up. Reevaluate and continue with your efforts. An occasional slip won't make much difference in the long run.

BEHAVIOR MODIFICATION PLANNING

❑ ❑ 29. Think positive. Avoid negative thoughts about how difficult changing past behaviors might be. Instead, think of the benefits you will reap, such as feeling, looking, and functioning better, plus enjoying better health and improving the quality of life. Avoid negative environments and unsupportive people.

Try It

In your Online Journal or class notebook, answer the following questions: How many of the above strategies do you use to help you maintain recommended body weight? Do you feel that any of these strategies specifically help you manage body weight more effectively? If so, explain why.

ASSESS YOUR BEHAVIOR

CENGAGE brain.com To access course materials, including companion resources, please visit **www.cengagebrain.com**.

1. Are you satisfied with your current body composition (including body weight) and quality of life? If not, are you willing to do something about it to properly resolve the problem?
2. Are physical activity, aerobic exercise, and strength training a regular part of your lifetime weight management program?
3. Do you weigh yourself regularly and make adjustments in energy intake and physical activity habits if your weight starts to shift upward?
4. Do you exercise portion control, watch your overall fat intake, and plan ahead before you eat out or attend social functions that entice overeating?

ASSESS YOUR KNOWLEDGE

1. During the past five decades, the rate of obesity in the United States has
   a. been on the decline.
   b. increased at an alarming rate.
   c. increased slightly.
   d. remained steady.
   e. increased in men and decreased in women.
2. Obesity is defined as a BMI equal to or above
   a. 10.
   b. 25.
   c. 30.
   d. 45.
   e. 50.
3. Obesity increases the risk for
   a. hypertension.
   b. congestive heart failure.
   c. atherosclerosis.
   d. type 2 diabetes.
   e. All of the choices are correct.
4. Tolerable weight is a body weight
   a. that is not ideal but one that you can live with.
   b. that tolerates the increased risk for chronic diseases.
   c. with a BMI range between 25 and 30.
   d. that meets both ideal values for percent body weight and BMI.
   e. All of the choices are correct.
5. When the body uses protein instead of a combination of fats and carbohydrates as a source of energy,
   a. weight loss is very slow.
   b. a large amount of weight loss is in the form of water.
   c. muscle turns into fat.
   d. fat is lost rapidly.
   e. fat cannot be lost.
6. Eating disorders
   a. are characterized by an intense fear of becoming fat.
   b. are physical and emotional conditions.
   c. almost always require professional help for successful treatment of the disease.
   d. are common in societies that encourage thinness.
   e. All of the choices are correct.
7. The mechanism that seems to regulate how much a person weighs is known as the
   a. setpoint.
   b. weight factor.
   c. BMR.
   d. metabolism.
   e. energy-balancing equation.

8. The key to maintaining weight loss successfully is
a. frequent dieting.
b. very low-calorie diets when "normal" dieting doesn't work.
c. a lifetime physical activity program.
d. regular LCHP meals.
e. All of the choices are correct.

9. The daily duration of physical activity recommended for weight loss purposes is
a. 15 to 20 minutes.
b. 20 to 30 minutes.
c. 30 to 60 minutes.
d. 60 to 90 minutes.
e. Any duration is sufficient as long as physical activity is done daily.

10. A daily energy expenditure of 300 calories through physical activity is the equivalent of approximately ___ pounds of fat per year.
a. 12
b. 15
c. 22
d. 27
e. 31

Correct answers can be found at the back of the book.

NOTES

1. C. L. Ogden, M. D. Carroll, B. K. Kit, and K. M. Flegal. "Prevalence of Childhood and Adult Obesity in the United States, 2011-2012," *Journal of the American Medical Association* 311(2014): 806–814.
2. J. Stein, "The Epidemic of Obesity," *Journal of Clinical Endocrinology & Metabolism* 89 (2004): 2522–2525.
3. A. H. Mokdad, J. S. Marks, D. F. Stroup, and J. L. Gerberding, "Actual Causes of Death in the United States, 2000," *Journal of the American Medical Association* 291 (2004): 1238–1241.
4. R. Sturm and K. B. Wells, "Does Obesity Contribute as Much to Morbidity as Poverty or Smoking?" *Public Health* 115 (2001): 229–235.
5. E. E. Calle et al., "Overweight, Obesity, and Mortality from Cancer in a Prospectively Studied Cohort of U.S. Adults," *New England Journal of Medicine* 348 (2003): 1625–1638.
6. A. Peeters et al., "Obesity in Adulthood and Its Consequences for Life Expectancy: A Life-Table Analysis," *Annals of Internal Medicine* 138 (2003): 2432.
7. K. R. Fontaine et al., "Years of Life Lost Due to Obesity," *Journal of the American Medical Association* 289 (2003): 187–193.
8. American College of Sports Medicine, "Position Stand: Appropriate Physical Activity Intervention Strategies for Weight Loss and Prevention of Weight Regain for Adults," *Medicine & Science in Sports & Exercise* 41 (2009): 459–471.
9. S. Thomsen, "A Steady Diet of Images," *BYU Magazine* 57, no. 3 (2003): 20–21.
10. S. Lichtman et al., "Discrepancy Between Self-Reported and Actual Caloric Intake and Exercise in Obese Subjects," *New England Journal of Medicine* 327 (1992): 1893–1898.
11. J. H. Wilmore, D. L. Costill, and W. L. Kenney, *Physiology of Sport and Exercise* (Champaign, IL: Human Kinetics, 2008).
12. C. D. Gardner et al., "Comparison of the Atkins, Zone, Ornish, and LEARN Diets for Change in Weight and Related Risk Factors among Overweight Premenopausal Women," *Journal of the American Medical Association* 297 (2007): 969–977; G. D. Foster et al., "A Randomized Trial of a Low-Carbohydrate Diet for Obesity," *New England Journal of Medicine* 348 (2003): 2082–2090.
13. American Psychiatric Association, *Diagnostic and Statistical Manual of Mental Disorders* (Washington, DC: APA, 1994).
14. See note 13.
15. R. L. Leibel, M. Rosenbaum, and J. Hirsh, "Changes in Energy Expenditure Resulting from Altered Body Weight," *New England Journal of Medicine* 332 (1995): 621–628.
16. R. J. Shepard, *Alive Man: The Physiology of Physical Activity* (Springfield, IL: Charles C. Thomas, 1975), pp. 484–488.
17. A. Eliasson et al., "Sleep Is a Critical Factor in the Maintenance of Healthy Weight," paper presented at the American Thoracic Society International Conference (2009).
18. S. Pattel et al., "Sleep Your Way to Weight Loss?" paper presented at the American Thoracic Society International Conference (2006).
19. K. Knutson, "Impact of Sleep and Sleep Loss on Glucose Homeostasis and Appetite Regulation," *Sleep Medicine Clinic* 2 (2007): 187–197.
20. S. Taheri et al., "Short Sleep Duration Is Associated with Reduced Leptin, Elevated Ghrelin, and Increased Body Mass Index," *PLoS Medicine* 1 (2004): e62, doi:10.1371/journal.pmed.0010062.
21. W. C. Miller, D. M. Koceja, and E. J. Hamilton, "A Meta-Analysis of the Past 25 Years of Weight Loss Research Using Diet, Exercise, or Diet Plus Exercise Intervention," *International Journal of Obesity* 21 (1997): 941–947.
22. National Academy of Sciences, Institute of Medicine, *Dietary Reference Intakes for Energy, Carbohydrates, Fiber, Fat, Protein and Amino Acids (Macronutrients)* (Washington, DC: National Academy Press, 2002).
23. J. G. Thomas et al., "The National Weight Control Registry: A Study of Successful Losers," *ACSM's Health & Fitness Journal* 15, no. 2 (2011): 8–12.
24. E. T. Poehlman et al., "Effects of Endurance and Resistance Training on Total Daily Energy Expenditure in Young Women: A Controlled Randomized Trial," *Journal of Clinical Endocrinology and Metabolism* 87 (2002): 1004–1009; L. M. Van Etten et al., "Effect of an 18-Wk Weight-Training Program on Energy Expenditure and Physical Activity," *Journal of Applied Physiology* 82 (1997): 298–304; W. W. Campbell, M. C. Crim, V. R. Young, and W. J. Evans, "Increased Energy Requirements and Changes in Body Composition with Resistance Training in Older Adults," *American Journal of Clinical Nutrition* 60 (1994): 167–175; Z. Wang et al., "Resting Energy Expenditure: Systematic Organization and Critique of Prediction Methods," *Obesity Research* 9 (2001): 331–336.

25. J. R. Karp and W. L. Wescott, "The Resting Metabolic Rate Debate," *Fitness Management* 23, no. 1 (2007): 44–47.

26. L. Shengxu, et al., "Physical Activity Attenuates the Genetic Predisposition to Obesity in 20,000 Men and Women from EPIC-Norfolk Prospective Population Study," *PLOS Medicine* 7 (2010): 10.1371/e1000332.

27. A. M. Knab, et al., "A 45-Minute Vigorous Exercise Bout Increases Metabolic rate for 14 Hours," *Medicine and Science in Sports and Exercise* 43 (2011): 1643–1648.

28. A. Tremblay, J. A. Simoneau, and C. Bouchard, "Impact of Exercise Intensity on Body Fatness and Skeletal Muscle Metabolism," *Metabolism* 43 (1994): 814–818.

29. T. S. Church et al., "Changes in Weight, Waist Circumference and Compensatory Responses with Different Doses of Exercise Among Sedentary, Overweight Postmenopausal Women," *PLoS ONE* 4, no. 2 (2009): e4515, doi:10.1371/journal.pone.0004515.

30. I. Lee et al., "Physical Activity and Weight Gain Prevention," *Journal of the American Medical Association* 303 (2010): 1173–1179.

31. T. A. Hagobian and B. Braun, "Physical Activity and Hormonal Regulation of Appetite: Sex Differences and Weight Control," *Exercise and Sport Sciences Reviews* 38 (2010): 25–30.

32. G. Gwinup, "Weight Loss Without Dietary restriction: Efficacy of Different Forms of Aerobic Exercise," *American Journal of Sports Medicine,* 15 (1987): 275–279

33. L. J. White, et al., "Increased Caloric Intake Soon After Exercise in Cold water," *International Journal of Sport Nutrition and Exercise Metabolism* 15 (2005): 38–47.

34. M. L. Klem, R. R. Wing, M. T. McGuire, H. M. Seagle, and J. O. Hill, "A Descriptive Study of Individuals Successful at Long-Term Maintenance of Substantial Weight Loss," *American Journal of Clinical Nutrition* 66 (1997): 239–246.

35. D. Jakubowicz, M. Barnea, J. Waistein, and O. Froy, "High Caloric Intake at Breakfast vs. Dinner Differentially Influences Weight Loss of Overweight and Obese Women," *Obesity, A Research Journal* (2013): 10.1002/oby.20460.

36. See note 23; U.S. Department of Health and Human Services and U.S. Department of Agriculture, *Dietary Guidelines for Americans 2005* (Washington, DC: DHHS, 2005).

37. W. W. K. Hoeger, C. Harris, E. M. Long, and D. R. Hopkins, "Four-Week Supplementation with a Natural Compound Produces Favorable Changes in Body Composition," *Advances in Therapy* 15, no. 5 (1998): 305–313; W. W. K. Hoeger et al., "Dietary Supplementation with Chromium Picolinate/L-Carnitine Complex in Combination with Diet and Exercise Enhances Body Composition," *Journal of the American Nutraceutical Association* 2, no. 2 (1999): 40–45.

38. D. Mozaffarian et al., "Changes in Diet and Lifestyle and Long-Term Weight Gain in Women and Men," *New England Journal of Medicine* 364 (2011): 2392–2404.

39. N. A. Christakis and J. H. Fowler, "The Spread of Obesity in a Large Social Network over 32 Years," *New England Journal of Medicine* 357 (2007): 370–379.

SUGGESTED READINGS

American College of Sports Medicine. "Position Stand: Appropriate Physical Activity Intervention Strategies for Weight Loss and Prevention of Weight Regain for Adults," *Medicine & Science in Sports & Exercise* 41 (2009): 459-471.

American Diabetes Association and American Dietetic Association. *Exchange Lists for Meal Planning.* Chicago, IL: American Dietetic Association and American Diabetes Association, 2008.

National Academy of Sciences, Institute of Medicine. *Dietary Reference Intakes for Energy, Carbohydrates, Fiber, Fat, Protein and Amino Acids (Macronutrients).* Washington, DC: National Academy Press, 2002.

Lab 5A: Computing Your Daily Caloric Requirement

Name ______________________ Date ____________ Grade ____________

Instructor ______________________ Course ____________ Section ____________

NECESSARY LAB EQUIPMENT

Tables 5.3 and 5.4 (page 191–192).

OBJECTIVE

To estimate your daily caloric requirement for weight maintenance or reduction and to select fitness activities for your exercise program.

INSTRUCTIONS

Complete all of the sections provided in this lab.

A. Current body weight (BW) in kilograms (body weight in pounds ÷ 2.2046) .... [ ]

B. Current height (HT) in meters (HT in inches × .0254) .... [ ]

C. Estimated energy requirement (EER) (Table 5.3, page 191)

Men: $EER = 663 - (9.53 \times Age) + (15.91 \times BW) + (539.6 \times HT)$

Women: $EER = 354 - (6.91 \times Age) + (9.36 \times BW) + (726 \times HT)$

EER = [ ] – ([ ] × [ ]) + ([ ] × [ ]) + ([ ] × [ ])

EER = [ ] – [ ] + [ ] + [ ] = [ ] calories

D. Selected physical activity (e.g., jogging)[a] .... [ ]

E. Number of exercise sessions per week .... [ ]

F. Duration of exercise session (in minutes) .... [ ]

G. Total weekly exercise time in minutes (E × F) .... [ ]

H. Average daily exercise time in minutes (G ÷ 7) .... [ ]

I. Caloric expenditure per pound per minute (cal/lb/min) of physical activity (use Table 5.4, page 192) .... [ ]

J. Body weight in pounds .... [ ]

K. Total calories burned per minute of physical activity (I × J) .... [ ]

L. Average daily calories burned as a result of the exercise program (H × K) .... [ ]

M. Total daily energy requirement with exercise to maintain body weight (C + L) .... [ ]

Stop here if no weight loss is required, otherwise proceed to items N and O.

N. Number of calories to subtract from daily requirement to achieve a negative caloric balance (J × 5) .... [ ]

O. Target caloric intake to lose weight (M – N)[b] .... [ ]

[a] *If more than one physical activity is selected, you will need to estimate the average daily calories burned as a result of each additional activity (steps D through K) and add all of these figures to L above.*

[b] *This figure should never be below 1,200 calories for small women or 1,500 for everyone else. See Lab 5C for the 1,200-, 1,500-, and 2,000-calorie diet plans.*

Lab 5B: Weight-Loss Behavior Modification Plan

Name ______________________ Date ____________ Grade ____________

Instructor ______________________ Course ____________ Section ____________

NECESSARY LAB EQUIPMENT

Tables 5.3 and 5.4 (page 179).

OBJECTIVE

To estimate your daily caloric requirement for weight management and to select fitness activities for your exercise program.

INSTRUCTIONS

Complete all of the sections provided in this lab.

1. Using Figure 2.6 (page 66) and Table 2.3 (page 65), identify your current stage of change regarding **recommended body weight:** [ ]
2. How much weight do you want to lose? [ ] Is it a realistic goal? [ ]
3. Target caloric intake to lose weight (diet plan—see Lab 5A, item O) [ ].
4. Based on the processes and techniques of change discussed in Chapter 2, indicate what you can do to help yourself implement a weight management program.

   ____

   ____

5. How much effort are you willing to put into reaching your weight loss goal? ______________________

   Indicate your feelings about participating in an exercise program.

   ____

6. Will you commit to participate in a combined aerobic and strength-training program?* Yes [ ] No [ ]

   If your answer is "Yes," proceed to the next question; if you answered "No," please read Chapters 3–9.

7. Select one or two aerobic activities in which you will participate regularly: [ ]

   List facilities available to you where you can carry out the aerobic and strength-training programs.

   ____

8. Indicate days and times you will set aside for your aerobic and strength-training program (5 or 6 days per week should be devoted to aerobic exercise and 1 to 3 nonconsecutive days per week to strength training).

   Monday: [ ]

   Tuesday: [ ]

   Wednesday: [ ]

   Thursday: [ ]

   Friday: [ ]

   Saturday: [ ]

   Sunday: A complete day of rest once a week is recommended to allow your body to fully recover from exercise.

Behavior Modification

Briefly describe whether you think you can meet the goals of your aerobic and strength-training program. What obstacles will you have to overcome, and how will you overcome them?

____

____

Flexibility programs are necessary for adequate fitness, possible injury prevention, and good health but do not help with weight loss. Stretching exercises can be conducted regularly during the cool-down phase of your aerobic and strength-training programs (see Chapter 8).

Lab 5C: Calorie-Restricted Diet Plans

Name ______________________ Date __________ Grade __________

Instructor ______________________ Course __________ Section __________

NECESSARY LAB EQUIPMENT

None required.

OBJECTIVE

To help you implement a calorie-restricted diet plan according to your target caloric intake obtained in Lab 5A.

INSTRUCTIONS

Read Chapter 5 prior to this lab and make additional copies (as needed) of your selected diet plan.

1,200 CALORIE DIET PLAN

The objective of the diet plan is to meet (not exceed) the number of servings allowed for the food groups listed. Each time that you eat a particular food, record it in the space provided for each group along with the amount you ate. Refer to the number of calories below to find out what counts as one serving for each group listed. Instead of the meat, poultry, fish, dry beans, eggs, and nuts group, you are allowed to have a commercially available low-fat frozen entree for your main meal (this entree should provide no more than 300 calories and less than 6 grams of fat). You can make additional copies of this form as needed.

Bread, Cereal, Rice, Pasta Group (80 calories/serving): 6 servings

1 ______________________

2 ______________________

3 ______________________

4 ______________________

5 ______________________

6 ______________________

Vegetable Group (25 calories/serving): 3 servings

1 ______________________

2 ______________________

3 ______________________

Fruit Group (60 calories/serving): 2 servings

1 ______________________

2 ______________________

Milk Group (120 calories/serving, use low-fat milk and milk products): 2 servings

1 ______________________

2 ______________________

Low-fat Frozen Entree (300 calories and less than 6 grams of fat): 1 serving

1 ______________________

Today's physical activity: ______ Intensity: ______ Duration: ______ min Number of steps: ______

Grams of protein consumed with each meal: Breakfast: _______ g, Lunch: _______ g, Dinner: _______ g

1,500-CALORIE DIET PLAN

Instructions:

The objective of the diet plan is to meet (not exceed) the number of servings allowed for the food groups listed. Each time that you eat a particular food, record it in the space provided for each group along with the amount you ate. Refer to the number of calories below to find out what counts as one serving for each group listed. Instead of the meat, poultry, fish, dry beans, eggs, and nuts group, you are allowed to have two commercially available low-fat frozen entrees for your main meal (these entrees should provide no more than 300 calories and less than 6 grams of fat). You can make additional copies of this form as needed.

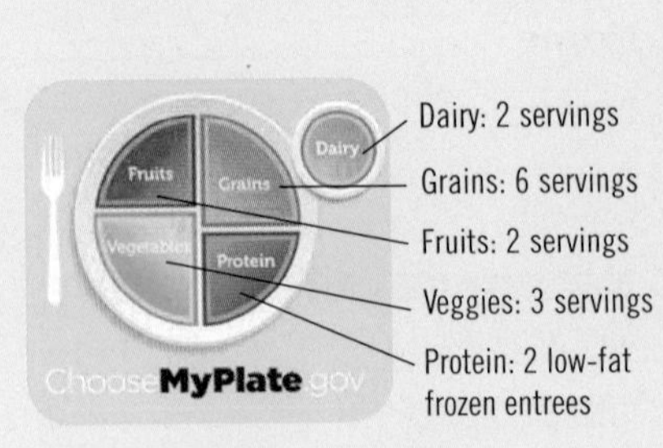

Bread, Cereal, Rice, Pasta Group (80 calories/serving): 6 servings

1	
2	
3	
4	
5	
6	

Vegetable Group (25 calories/serving): 3 servings

1	
2	
3	

Fruit Group (60 calories/serving): 2 servings

1	
2	

Milk Group (120 calories/serving, use low-fat milk and milk products): 2 servings

1	
2	

Two Low-fat Frozen Entrees (300 calories and less than 6 grams of fat): 2 servings

1	
2	

Today's physical activity: ______ Intensity: ______ Duration: ______ min Number of steps: ______

Grams of protein consumed with each meal: Breakfast: _______ g, Lunch: _______ g, Dinner: _______ g

1,800-CALORIE DIET PLAN

Instructions:

The objective of the diet plan is to meet (not exceed) the number of servings allowed for the food groups listed. Each time that you eat a particular food, record it in the space provided for each group along with the amount you ate. Refer to the number of calories below to find out what counts as one serving for each group listed. Instead of the meat, poultry, fish, dry beans, eggs, and nuts group, you are allowed to have two commercially available low-fat frozen entrees for your main meal (these entrees should provide no more than 300 calories and less than 6 grams of fat). You can make additional copies of this form as needed.

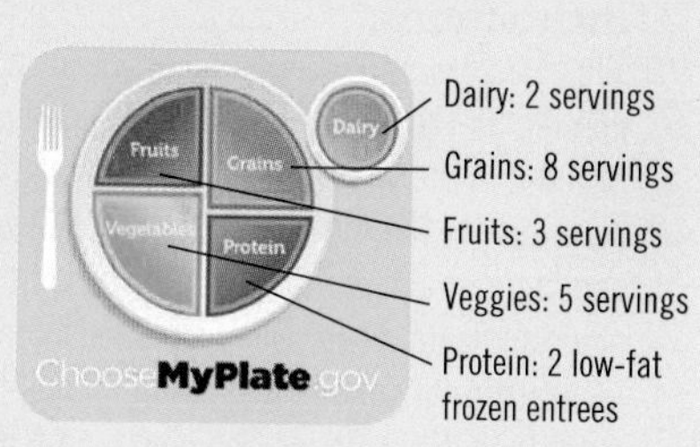

Bread, Cereal, Rice, Pasta Group (80 calories/serving): 8 servings

1
2
3
4
5
6
7
8

Vegetable Group (25 calories/serving): 5 servings

1
2
3
4
5

Fruit Group (60 calories/serving): 3 servings

1
2
3

Milk Group (120 calories/serving, use low-fat milk and milk products): 2 servings

1
2

Two Low-fat Frozen Entrees (300 calories and less than 6 grams of fat): 2 servings

1
2

Today's physical activity: ______ Intensity: ______ Duration: ______ min Number of steps: ______

Grams of protein consumed with each meal: Breakfast: _______ g, Lunch: _______ g, Dinner: _______ g

2,000-CALORIE DIET PLAN

Instructions:

The objective of the diet plan is to meet (not exceed) the number of servings allowed for the food groups listed. Each time that you eat a particular food, record it in the space provided for each group along with the amount you ate. Refer to the number of calories below to find out what counts as one serving for each group listed. Instead of the meat, poultry, fish, dry beans, eggs, and nuts group, you are allowed to have two commercially available low-fat frozen entrees for your main meal (these entrees should provide no more than 300 calories and less than 6 grams of fat). You can make additional copies of this form as needed.

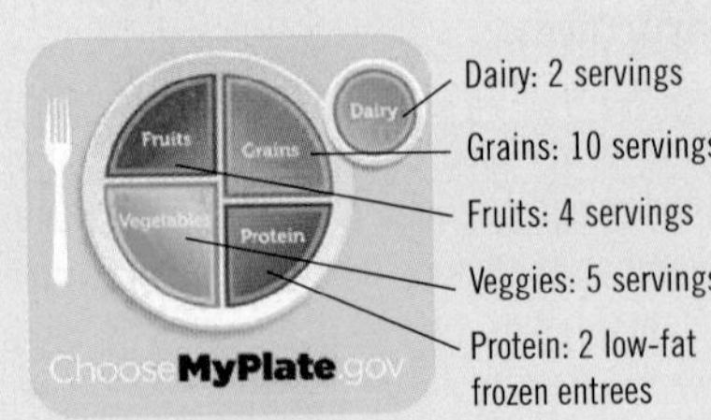

Bread, Cereal, Rice, Pasta Group (80 calories/serving): 10 servings

#	
1	
2	
3	
4	
5	
6	
7	
8	
9	
10	

Vegetable Group (25 calories/serving): 5 servings

#	
1	
2	
3	
4	
5	

Fruit Group (60 calories/serving): 4 servings

#	
1	
2	
3	
4	

Milk Group (120 calories/serving, use low-fat milk and milk products): 2 servings

#	
1	
2	

Two Low-fat Frozen Entrees (300 calories and less than 6 grams of fat): 2 servings

#	
1	
2	

Today's physical activity: ______ Intensity: ______ Duration: ______ min Number of steps: ______

Grams of protein consumed with each meal: Breakfast: ______ g, Lunch: ______ g, Dinner: ______ g

Lab 5D: Healthy Plan for Weight Maintenance or Gain

Name ______________________ Date ____________ Grade ____________

Instructor ______________________ Course ____________ Section ____________

NECESSARY LAB EQUIPMENT
None.

OBJECTIVE
To design a sample daily healthy diet plan to maintain current body weight or increase body weight.

LAB PREPARATION
Read Chapters 3, 4, and 5 prior to this lab.

I. Daily Caloric Requirement

A. Current body weight in pounds........ ☐

B. Current percent body fat........ ☐

C. Current body composition classification (Table 4.11, page 153)........ ☐

D. Total daily energy requirement with exercise to maintain body weight (use item L from Lab 5A). Use this figure and stop further computations if the goal is to maintain body weight........ ☐

E. Target body weight to (if your goal is to increase body weight)........ ☐

F. Number of additional daily calories to increase body weight (500 calories are recommended—combine this increased caloric intake with a strength-training program, see Chapter 7)........ ☐

G. Total daily energy (caloric) requirement with exercise to increase body weight (D + F) ☐

II. Strength-Training Program

For weight gain purposes, indicate three days during the week and the time when you will engage in a strength-training program.

____

____

III. Healthy Diet Plan

Design a sample healthy daily diet plan according to the total daily energy requirement computed in D (maintenance) or G (weight gain) above. Using Appendix A, list all individual food items that you can consume on that day, along with their caloric, carbohydrate, fat, and protein content. Be sure that the diet meets the recommended number of servings from the five food groups.

Breakfast

	Food item	Serving size	Calories	Carbohydrates (g)	Fat (g)	Protein (g)
1.						
2.						
3.						
4.						
5.						

Breakfast

	Food item	Serving size	Calories	Carbohydrates (g)	Fat (g)	Protein (g)
6.						
7.						
8.						
Lunch						
1.						
2.						
3.						
4.						
5.						
6.						
7.						
8.						
Snack						
1.						
Dinner						
1.						
2.						
3.						
4.						
5.						
6.						
7.						
8.						
		Totals:				

IV. Percent of Macronutrients

Determine the percent of total calories that are derived from carbohydrates, fat, and protein.

A. Total calories = ______

B. Grams of carbohydrates ______ × 4 ÷ ______ (total calories) = ______ %

C. Grams of fat ______ × 9 ÷ ______ (total calories) = ______ %

D. Grams of protein ______ × 4 ÷ ______ (total calories) = ______ %

E. Body weight (BW) in kilograms (BW in pounds divided by 2.2046) = ______ kg

F. Grams of protein per kilogram of body weight ______ (grams of protein) ÷ ______ (BW in kg) = ______ gr/kg

G. Please summarize your diet and protein intake to either maintain or gain weight.

____

____

Lab 5E: Weight Management: Measuring Progress

Name ______________________ Date ____________ Grade ____________
Instructor ______________________ Course ____________ Section ____________

NECESSARY LAB EQUIPMENT
None.

OBJECTIVE
To prepare and monitor behavioral changes for weight management.

LAB PREPARATION
Read Chapters 2, 3, 4, and 5 prior to this lab.

I. Please answer all of the following:

1. State your own feelings regarding your current body weight, your target body composition, and a completion date for this goal.

Completion date: ____________

2. Do you have an eating disorder? If so, express your feelings about it. Can your instructor help you find professional advice so that you can work toward resolving this problem?

3. Is your present diet adequate according to the nutrient analysis? Yes ________ No ________

4. State dietary changes necessary to achieve a balanced diet and/or to lose weight (increase or decrease caloric intake, decrease fat intake, increase intake of complex carbohydrates, etc.). List specific foods that will help you improve in areas where you may have deficiencies and food items to avoid or consume in moderation to help you achieve better nutrition.

Changes to make: ____________

Foods that will help: ____________

Foods to avoid: ____________

II. Behavior Modification Progress Form

Instructions: Read the section on *Behavior Modification and Adherence to a Weight Management Program* (pages 195–199). On a weekly or biweekly basis, go through the list of strategies and provide a "Yes" or "No" answer to each statement. If you are able to answer "Yes" to most questions, you have been successful in implementing positive weight management behaviors. (Make additional copies of this page as needed.)

Strategy Date						
1. I have made a commitment to change.						
2. I set realistic goals.						
3. I exercise regularly.						
4. I have healthy eating patterns.						
5. I exercise control over my appetite.						
6. I am consuming less fat in my diet.						
7. I pay attention to the number of calories in food.						
8. I have eliminated unnecessary food items from my diet.						
9. I use craving-reducing foods in my diet.						
10. I avoid automatic eating.						
11. I stay busy.						
12. I plan meals ahead of time.						
13. I cook wisely.						
14. I do not serve more food than I should eat.						
15. I use portion control in my diet.						
16. I eat slowly and at the table only.						
17. I avoid social binges.						
18. I avoid food raids.						
19. I do not eat out more than once per week. When I do, I eat low-fat meals.						
20. I practice stress management.						
21. I have a strong support group.						
22. I monitor behavior changes.						
23. I prepare for lapses/relapses.						
24. I reward my accomplishments.						
25. I think positive.						

6

Cardiorespiratory Endurance

Physical activity is the miracle medication that people are looking for. It makes you look and feel younger, boosts energy, provides lifetime weight management, improves self-confidence and self-esteem, and enhances independent living, health, and quality of life. It further allows you to enjoy a longer life by decreasing the risk of many chronic conditions, including heart disease, high blood pressure, stroke, diabetes, some cancers, and osteoporosis. Your attitude should be: I do not fear nor will I avoid physical activity: Bring it on!

OBJECTIVES

- Define cardiorespiratory (CR) endurance and describe the benefits of CR endurance training in maintaining health and well-being.
- Define and give examples of aerobic and anaerobic exercise.
- Be able to assess CR fitness through five test protocols: 1.5-Mile Run Test, 1.0-Mile Walk Test, Step Test, Astrand-Ryhming Test, and 12-Minute Swim Test.
- Be able to interpret the results of CR endurance assessments according to health fitness and physical fitness standards.
- Determine your readiness to start an exercise program.
- Explain the principles that govern CR exercise prescription: intensity, mode, duration, frequency, volume, and rate of progression.
- Learn ways to foster adherence to exercise.

CENGAGE brain.com

Visit **www.cengagebrain.com** to access course materials and companion resources for this text, including digital labs, quiz questions designed to check your understanding of the chapter contents, and more! See the preface on page xii for more information.

REAL LIFE STORY | Karen's Experience

I've never been very active. Just about the only activity I did in high school was going to dances once in a while. I didn't participate in many activities that required physical exertion. I enjoyed being home and during my spare time I would read a book or watch TV or a movie. At 5 feet 10 inches, I was careful with my diet and I was able to keep my weight pretty consistent at 150 pounds. When I got to college, I had to take a required wellness course. What a drag! I knew I wasn't very active, but I felt I was okay fitness wise. That notion was reinforced when I learned that my BMI was 22. The following week, however, I found out that I was in "fair" cardiovascular shape and my body fat was 26.2 percent. Even though it met the health fitness standard, I didn't feel good about being in the "moderate" body composition category. I knew my caloric intake was within recommended guidelines but I needed to step up my fitness. I joined a zumba class and started to lift weights. It was hard at the beginning and I even gained a couple of pounds the first 2 weeks. The zumba class was intense, but what a blast it was. It took me a while, but eventually I was able to participate for the full 45 minutes. As I became more fit, I added 30 minutes of walking/jogging three times per week the second half of the semester. I started to eat healthier foods and snacked mainly on fruits and vegetables. I lost 6 pounds in 4 months and my body fat went down to 21 percent! Also, my maximal oxygen uptake came up to 38.2 mL/kg/min, meeting the health fitness standard, which was okay for me at that point. I was also more energetic, did better in school, and I even started joining people in activities that I had never considered in the past. Little did I know all that I was missing. My whole outlook on life changed and now my goal is to never stop exercising.

Cardiorespiratory (CR) endurance is the most important component of health-related physical fitness. The exception occurs among older adults, for whom muscular strength is particularly important. In any case, people can get by without high levels of strength and flexibility, but they cannot do without a good CR system, facilitated by aerobic exercise.

Aerobic exercise is especially important in preventing cardiovascular disease. A poorly conditioned heart, which has to pump more often just to keep a person alive, is subject to more wear and tear than a well-conditioned heart. In situations that place strenuous demands on the heart, such as doing yard work, lifting heavy objects or weights, or running to catch a bus, the unconditioned heart may not be able to sustain the strain. Regular participation in CR endurance activities also helps a person achieve and maintain recommended body weight—the fourth component of health-related physical fitness.

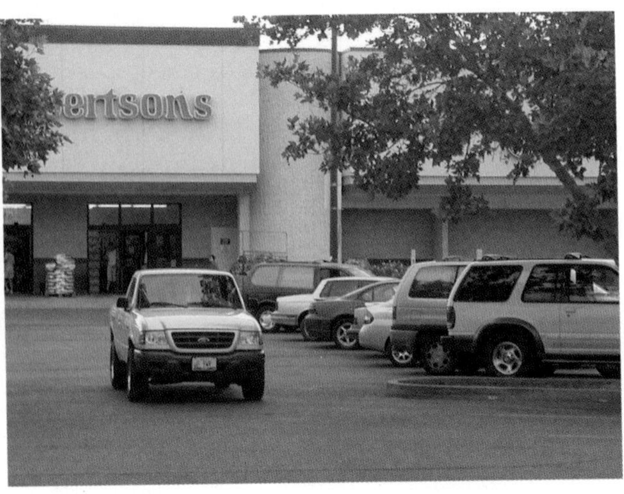

The epitome of physical inactivity: driving around a parking lot for several minutes in search of a parking spot 20 yards closer to the store's entrance.

Physical activity, unfortunately, is no longer a natural part of human existence. Technological developments have driven most people in developed countries into sedentary lifestyles. For instance, when many people go to a store only a couple of blocks away, they drive their automobiles and then spend a couple of minutes driving around the parking lot to find a spot 20 yards closer to the store's entrance. At times, they don't even have to carry the groceries to the car, because an employee working at the store offers to do this for them.

Similarly, during a visit to a multilevel shopping mall, almost everyone chooses to take the escalator instead of the stairs (which tend to be inaccessible). Automobiles, elevators, escalators, telephones, intercoms, remote controls, electric garage door openers—all are modern-day conveniences that minimize the amount of movement and effort required of the human body.

One of the most harmful effects of modern-day technology is an increase in chronic conditions related to a lack of physical activity. These

Cardiorespiratory (CR) endurance Ability of the lungs, heart, and blood vessels to deliver adequate amounts of oxygen to the cells to meet the demands of prolonged physical activity.

FAQ

Does aerobic exercise make people immune to heart and blood vessel disease?

Although aerobically fit individuals as a whole have a lower incidence of cardiovascular disease, a regular aerobic exercise program by itself does not guarantee against cardiovascular disease. The best way to minimize the risk for cardiovascular disease is to manage the risk factors. Many factors, including a genetic predisposition, can increase the risk. Research data, however, indicate that a regular aerobic exercise program delays the onset of cardiovascular problems and improves the chances of surviving a heart attack. Even moderate increases in aerobic fitness significantly lower the incidence of premature cardiovascular deaths. Data from a research study on death rates by physical fitness groups (illustrated in Figure 1.11, page 19) indicate that the decrease in cardiovascular mortality is greatest between the unfit and the moderately fit groups. A further decrease in cardiovascular mortality is observed between the moderately fit and the highly fit groups.

Is light-intensity aerobic exercise more effective in burning fat?

During light- and moderate-intensity exercise, a greater percentage of the energy is derived from fat. It is also true, however, that an even greater percentage of the energy comes from fat when doing nothing (resting or sleeping). And when someone does nothing, as in a sedentary lifestyle, that person doesn't burn many calories.

Let's examine this issue. During resting conditions, the human body is an efficient "fat-burning machine." That is, most energy, approximately 70 percent, is derived from fat, and only 30 percent comes from carbohydrates. But we burn few calories per minute at rest, about 1.5 calories compared with 3 to 4 calories during light-intensity exercise, 5 to 7 calories during moderate-intensity exercise, and 8 to 10 (or more) calories during vigorous exercise. As we begin to exercise and subsequently increase exercise intensity, we progressively rely more on carbohydrates and less on fat for energy until we reach maximal intensity, when 100 percent of the energy is derived from carbohydrates. Even though a lower percentage of the energy is derived from fat during vigorous exercise, the total caloric expenditure is so much greater (twice as high or more) that the total fat burned overall is still higher than it is during activities of moderate intensity.

A word of caution, nonetheless: Do not start vigorous, intense exercise without several weeks of proper and gradual conditioning. Effects can be even worse is if such exercise is a weight-bearing activity. If you do such exercise from the outset, you increase the risk of injury and may have to stop exercising. Also, people with an initial low level of fitness often compensate with greater caloric intake following vigorous exercise, thus defeating the added energy expenditure obtained through exercise (additional information on this subject is provided on pages 185–187).

Do energy drinks enhance performance?

People associate energy with work. If an energy drink can enhance work capacity, the benefits of such drinks would surpass plain thirst-quenching drinks. Energy drinks typically contain sugar (discussed in Chapter 3), herbal extracts, large amounts of caffeine, and water-soluble vitamins. Consumers are led to believe that these ingredients increase energy metabolism, provide an energy boost, improve endurance, and aid in weight loss. These purported benefits are yet to be proven through scientific research.

The energy content of many of these drinks is around 60 grams of sugar and 240 calories in a 16-ounce drink, with little additional nutritive value. If you are going to participate in an intense and lengthy workout, the carbohydrate content can boost performance and help you get through the workout. If, however, you are concerned with weight management, 240 calories is an extraordinarily large amount of calories in a two-cup drink. Weight gain may be the end result if you drink a few of these throughout the day to give you a boost while studying or while at work. Sugar-free energy drinks provide little or no energy (calories), although they are packed with nervous system stimulants.

The high caffeine content in energy drinks can cause adverse health effects. Caffeine intake above 400 mg can precipitate adverse health effects. Many of the popular energy drinks (Red Bull, Sobe Adrenaline Rush, Full Throttle, Rip It Energy Fuel) contain about 80 mg of caffeine per 8-ounce cup. If you drink two 16-ounce cans, you'll end up with upward of 300 mg of caffeine through these drinks alone. You may also have to consider additional caffeine intake from other beverages that you routinely consume during the day (coffee, tea, sodas).

Consumption of energy drinks has been linked with a rapid heart rate, (palpitations and tachycardia), ischemia (lack of blood flow to the heart muscle), chest pain, increased blood pressure, tremors, jitters, convulsions, agitation, restlessness, gastrointestinal disturbance, increased urination, nausea, dizziness, irritability, nervousness, syncope (loss of consciousness), paraesthesia (tingling or numbing of the skin), insomnia, respiratory distress, headaches, and, most seriously, based on circumstantial evidence, myocardial infarctions and sudden cardiac deaths. At least one sudden cardiac death has been reported in a 28-year-old man who consumed eight cans of an energy drink containing 80 mg of caffeine each over a 7-hour span of time. Between 2008 and 2012, the Food and Drug Administration (FDA) received reports of 13 deaths possibly linked to the highly caffeinated drink 5-Hour Energy (215 mg of caffeine per drink—about two cups of coffee) and more than 90 filings of adverse effects, including more than 30 citing life-threatening complications.

Energy drinks manufacturers' state that the products are safe when used as directed. The potential for excessive use or abuse, however, is real because the products are not regulated by the FDA. As with most addictive substances, invariably a sugar and caffeine rush is likely to end up in a physiological crash, requiring a subsequent larger intake to obtain a similar "physical high," thus augmenting the risk for adverse and life-threatening effects.

MyProfile: Cardiorespiratory Fitness—A Personal Survey

To the best of your ability, answer the following questions. If you do not know the answer(s), this chapter will guide you through them.

I. Have you ever experienced the feeling of being aerobically fit? ___ Yes ___ No If yes, can you describe that feeling?

____

____

____

II. Do you understand the concept of oxygen uptake and the difference between absolute and relative oxygen uptake? ___ Yes ___ No What are the applications of the latter two? ______________________________

____

III. At 70 percent training intensity, your exercise prescription requires a heart rate of 156 beats per minute. Is there a difference between jogging and doing zumba when exercising at this same heart rate? ___ Yes ___ No Expound on your response.

____

____

____

IV. Can you identify and relate to the factors that motivated Karen to become aerobically fit and what helped her stay with the exercise program? ___ Yes ___ No ___ What factors do you think can help you start or stay with aerobic exercise?

____

____

V. Your cardiorespiratory fitness test indicates that your maximal oxygen uptake (VO_{2max}) is 48 mL/kg/min. If you chose to exercise at 50 percent of your VO_{2max} (moderate intensity, as most people like to do during aerobic exercise), can you compute how many calories you burn per minute at this intensity level and the total minutes that you'd have to exercise to burn the equivalent of one pound of fat? Yes ___ No ___ If yes, show your computations on a separate sheet of paper.

hypokinetic diseases include hypertension, heart disease, chronic low back pain, and obesity. ("Hypo" means low or little, and "kinetic" implies motion.) Lack of adequate physical activity is a fact of modern life that most people can no longer avoid. To enjoy modern-day conveniences and still expect to live life to its fullest, people have to make a personalized lifetime exercise program a part of daily living.

Basic Cardiorespiratory Physiology: A Quick Survey

Before people begin to overhaul their bodies with an exercise program, they should understand the mechanisms they propose to alter and survey the ways in which they can measure how well they perform these mechanisms. CR endurance is a measure of how the pulmonary (lungs), cardiovascular (heart and blood vessels), and muscular systems work together during aerobic activities. As people breathe, part of the oxygen in the air is taken up by the **alveoli** in the lungs. As blood passes through the alveoli, oxygen is picked up by **hemoglobin** and transported in the blood to the heart. The heart then is responsible for pumping the oxygenated blood through the circulatory system to all organs and tissues of the body.

At the cellular level, oxygen is used to convert food substrates (primarily carbohydrates and fats) through aerobic metabolism into **adenosine triphosphate (ATP)**. This compound provides the energy for physical activity, body functions, and maintenance of a constant internal equilibrium. During physical exertion, more ATP is needed to perform the activity. As a result, the lungs, heart, and blood vessels have to deliver more oxygen to the muscle cells to supply the required energy.

During prolonged exercise, an individual with a high level of CR endurance is able to deliver the required amount

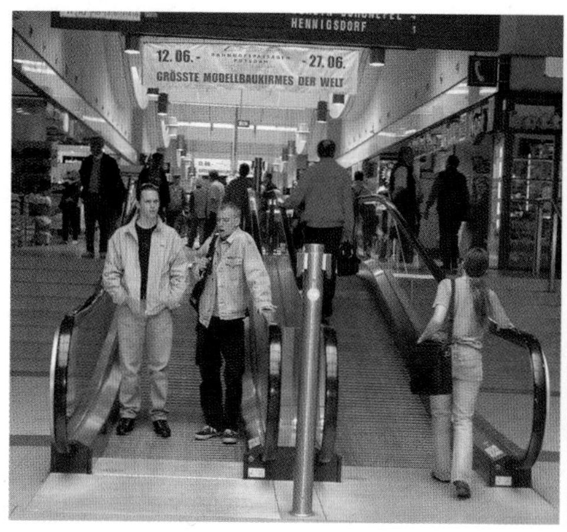

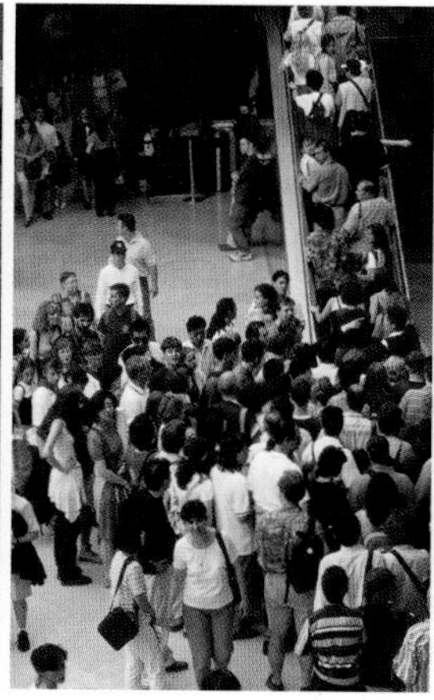

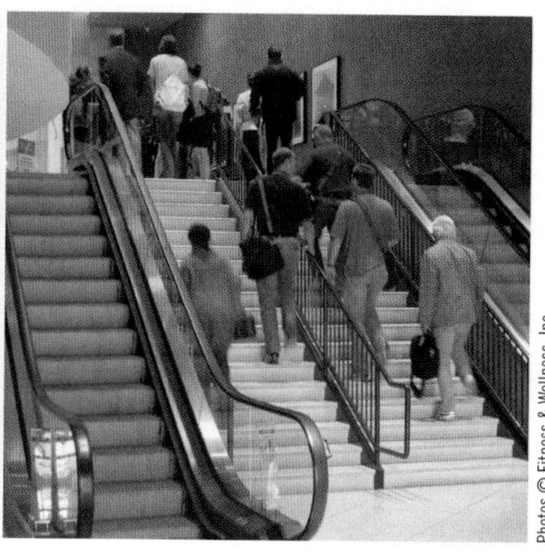

Photos © Fitness & Wellness, Inc.

Advances in modem technology have almost completely eliminated the need for physical activity, but you can choose to be physically active and greatly decrease the risk for premature mortality.

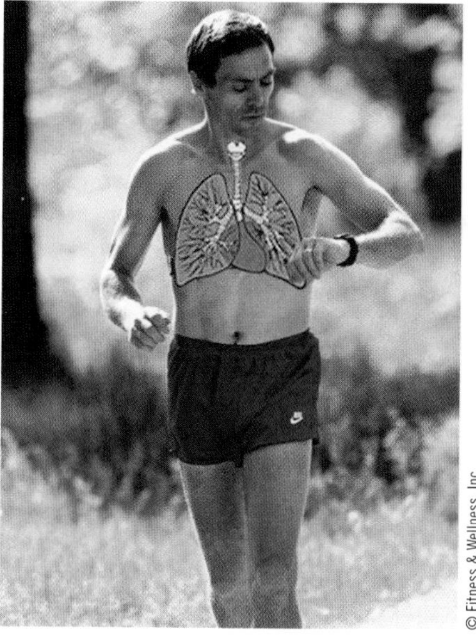

© Fitness & Wellness, Inc.

CR endurance refers to the ability of the lungs, heart, and blood vessels to deliver adequate amounts of oxygen to the cells to meet the demands of prolonged physical activity.

of oxygen to the tissues with relative ease. In contrast, the CR system of a person with a low level of endurance has to work harder, the heart has to work at a higher rate, less oxygen is delivered to the tissues, and consequently, the individual fatigues faster. Hence, a higher capacity to deliver and utilize oxygen—called **oxygen uptake**, or **VO_2**—indicates a more efficient CR system. Therefore, measuring VO_2 is an important way to evaluate CR health.

Aerobic and Anaerobic Exercise

CR endurance activities often are called **aerobic** exercises. Examples are walking, jogging, swimming, cycling, cross-country skiing, aerobics (including water aerobics), and rope skipping. By contrast, the intensity of **anaerobic** exercise is so high that oxygen cannot be delivered and utilized to produce energy. Because energy production is limited in the absence of oxygen, anaerobic activities can be carried out for only short periods—2 to 3 minutes. The higher the intensity of the activity, the shorter the duration.

CRITICAL THINKING

Your friend Joe is not physically active and doesn't exercise. He manages to keep his weight down by dieting and tells you that because he feels and looks good, he doesn't need to exercise. How do you respond to your friend?

Good examples of anaerobic activities are races of 100, 200, and 400 meters in track and field, a 100-meter race in swimming, gymnastics routines, and strength training. Anaerobic activities do not contribute much to developing the CR system. Only aerobic activities increase CR endurance. The basic guidelines for CR exercise prescription are set forth later in this chapter.

Hypokinetic diseases Hypo denotes "lack of"; therefore, chronic ailments that result from a lack of physical activity.

Alveoli Air sacs in the lungs where oxygen is taken up and carbon dioxide (produced by the body) is released from the blood.

Hemoglobin Protein–iron compound in red blood cells that transports oxygen in the blood.

Adenosine triphosphate (ATP) High-energy chemical compound that the body uses for immediate energy.

Oxygen uptake (VO2) The amount of oxygen the human body uses.

Aerobic Exercise that requires oxygen to produce the necessary energy (ATP) to carry out the activity.

Anaerobic Exercise that does not require oxygen to produce the necessary energy (ATP) to carry out the activity.

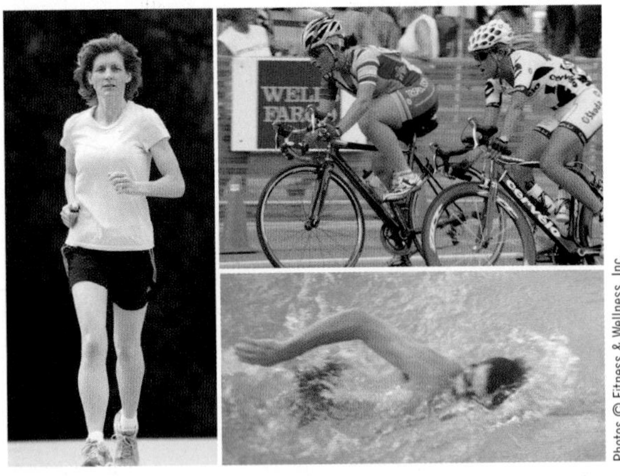

Aerobic activities

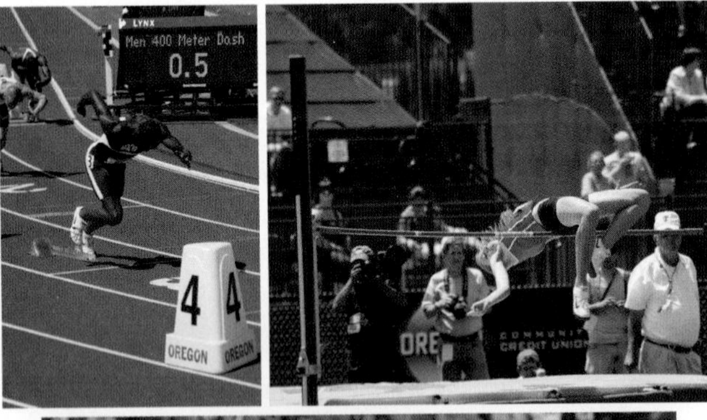

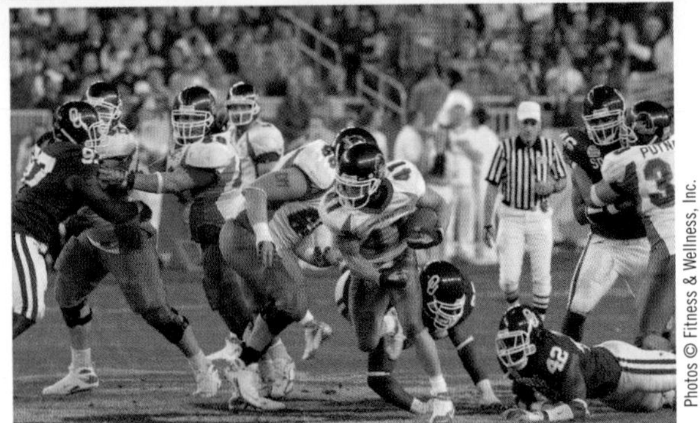

Anaerobic activities

Benefits of Aerobic Training

Everyone who participates in a CR or aerobic exercise program can expect a number of beneficial physiological adaptations from training (Figure 6.1). Among them are the following:

1. A higher **maximal oxygen uptake (VO_{2max})**. The amount of oxygen that the body is able to use during exercise increases significantly. This allows the individual to exercise longer and more intensely before becoming fatigued. Depending on the initial fitness level, the increases in VO_{2max} average 15 to 20 percent, although increases greater than 50 percent have been reported in people who have very low initial levels of fitness or who were significantly overweight prior to starting the aerobic exercise program.
2. An increase in the oxygen-carrying capacity of the blood. As a result of training, the red blood cell count goes up. Red blood cells contain hemoglobin, which transports oxygen in the blood.
3. A decrease in **resting heart rate (RHR)** and an increase in cardiac muscle strength. During resting conditions, the heart ejects between 5 and 6 liters of blood per minute (a liter is slightly larger than a quart). This amount of blood, also referred to as **cardiac output**, meets the body's energy demands in the resting state. Like any other muscle, the heart responds to training by increasing in strength and size. As the heart gets stronger, the muscle can produce a more forceful contraction, which helps the heart to eject more blood with each beat. This **stroke volume** yields a lower heart rate. The lower heart rate also allows the heart to rest longer between beats. Average resting and maximal cardiac outputs, stroke volumes, and heart rates for sedentary, trained, and highly trained (elite) males are shown in Table 6.1. RHRs frequently decrease by 10 to 20 beats per minute (bpm) after only 6 to 8 weeks of training. A reduction of 20 bpm saves the heart about 10,483,200 beats per year. The average heart beats between 70 and 80 bpm. As seen in Table 6.1, RHRs in highly trained athletes are often around 45 bpm.
4. A lower heart rate at given workloads. When compared with untrained individuals, trained people have a lower heart rate response to a given task because of greater efficiency of the CR system. Individuals are surprised to find that following several weeks of training, a given **workload** (let's say a 10-minute mile) elicits a lower heart rate response than their response when they first started training.
5. An increase in the number, size, and capacity of mitochondria. All energy necessary for cell function is produced in the **mitochondria**. As their size and numbers increase, so does their potential to produce energy for muscular work.
6. An increase in the number of functional capillaries. **Capillaries** allow exchange of oxygen and carbon dioxide between the blood and the cells. As more vessels open up, more gas exchange can take place, delaying the onset of fatigue during prolonged exercise. This increase in capillaries also speeds the rate at which waste products of cell metabolism can be removed. This increased capillarization occurs in the heart as well, which enhances the oxygen delivery capacity to the heart muscle.
7. Ability to recover rapidly. Trained individuals have a faster **recovery time** after exercising. A fit body system is able to more quickly restore any internal equilibrium disrupted during exercise.
8. Lower blood pressure and blood lipid levels. A regular aerobic exercise program leads to lower blood pressure

TABLE 6.1 **Average Resting and Maximal Cardiac Output, Stroke Volume, and Heart Rate for Sedentary, Trained, and Highly Trained Males***

	Resting			Maximal		
	Cardiac Output (L/min)	Stroke Volume (mL)	Heart Rate (bpm)	Cardiac Output (L/min)	Stroke Volume (mL)	Heart Rate (bpm)
Sedentary	5–6	68	74	20	100	200
Trained	5–6	90	56	30	150	200
Highly trained	5–6	110	45	35	175	200

* Cardiac output and stroke volume in women are about 25 percent lower than in men.

FIGURE 6.1 **Selected benefits of cardiorespiratory (aerobic) fitness.**

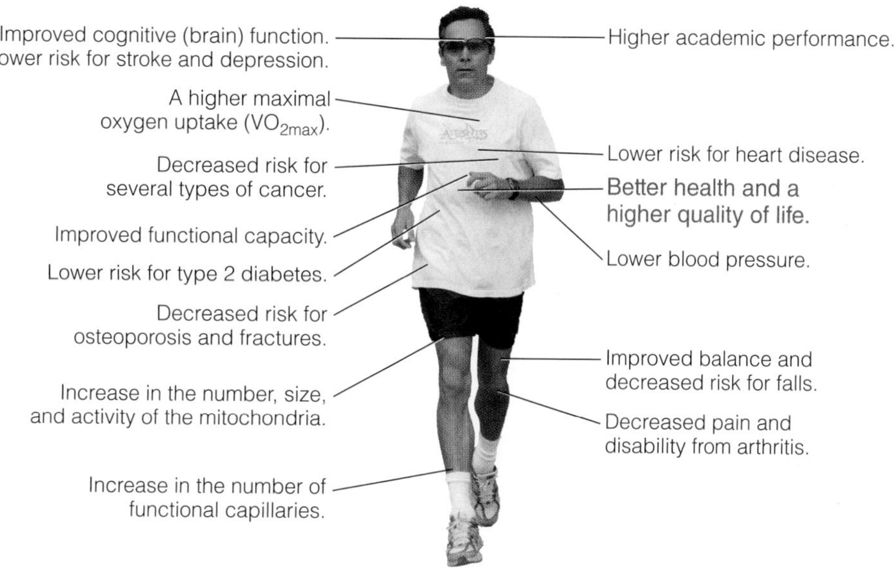
Improved cognitive (brain) function.
Lower risk for stroke and depression.
A higher maximal oxygen uptake (VO_{2max}).
Decreased risk for several types of cancer.
Improved functional capacity.
Lower risk for type 2 diabetes.
Decreased risk for osteoporosis and fractures.
Increase in the number, size, and activity of the mitochondria.
Increase in the number of functional capillaries.
Higher academic performance.
Lower risk for heart disease.
Better health and a higher quality of life.
Lower blood pressure.
Improved balance and decreased risk for falls.
Decreased pain and disability from arthritis.

(thereby reducing a major risk factor for stroke) and lower levels of fats (e.g., cholesterol and triglycerides), which have been linked to the formation of atherosclerotic plaque that obstructs the arteries (see Chapter 11). A decrease in "bad" low-density lipoprotein (LDL) cholesterol and an increase in "good" high-density lipoprotein (HDL) cholesterol, commonly seen in people who reduce dietary intake of saturated fat, are seen primarily when exercise is combined with weight loss. These beneficial changes lower the risk for coronary heart disease (see Chapter 11).

9. An increase in fat-burning enzymes. These enzymes are significant because fat is lost primarily by burning it in muscle. As the concentration of the enzymes increases (along with the number and size of mitochondria), so does the ability to burn fat (triglycerides) as opposed to carbohydrates (glucose or glycogen) during submaximal workloads (below a pace that you can comfortably sustain for at least 20 minutes).

Maximal oxygen uptake (VO_{2max}) Maximum amount of oxygen the body is able to utilize per minute of physical activity, commonly expressed in milliliters per kilogram per minute (mL/kg/min); the best indicator of CR or aerobic fitness.

Resting heart rate (RHR) Heart rate after a person has been sitting quietly for 15 to 20 minutes.

Cardiac output Amount of blood pumped by the heart in one minute.

Stroke volume Amount of blood pumped by the heart in one beat.

Workload Load (or intensity) placed on the body during physical activity.

Mitochondria Structures within the cells where energy transformations take place.

Capillaries Smallest blood vessels carrying oxygenated blood to the tissues in the body.

Recovery time Amount of time that the body takes to return to resting levels after exercise.

BEHAVIOR MODIFICATION PLANNING

Tips to Increase Daily Physical Activity

Adults need recess, too! There are 1,440 minutes in every day. Schedule a minimum of 30 of these minutes for physical activity. With a little creativity and planning, even the person with the busiest schedule can make room for physical activity. For many folks, before or after work or meals is often an available time to cycle, walk, or play. Think about your weekly or daily schedule and look for or make opportunities to be more active. Every little bit helps. Consider the following suggestions:

I PLAN TO	I DID IT	
❑	❑	Walk, cycle, jog, skate, etc., to school, work, the store, or place of worship.
❑	❑	Use a pedometer to count your daily steps.
❑	❑	Walk while doing errands.
❑	❑	Get on or off the bus several blocks away.
❑	❑	Park the car farther away from your destination.
❑	❑	At work, walk to nearby offices instead of sending e-mails or using the phone.
❑	❑	Walk or stretch a few minutes every hour that you are at your desk.
❑	❑	Take fitness breaks—walking or doing desk exercises—instead of taking cigarette breaks or coffee breaks.
❑	❑	Incorporate activity into your lunch break (walk to the restaurant).
❑	❑	Take the stairs instead of the elevator or escalator.
❑	❑	Play with children, grandchildren, or pets. Everybody wins. If you find it too difficult to be active after work, try it before work.
❑	❑	Do household tasks.
❑	❑	Work in the yard or garden.
❑	❑	Avoid labor-saving devices. Turn off the self-propelled option on your lawnmower or vacuum cleaner.
❑	❑	Use leg power. Take small trips on foot to get your body moving.
❑	❑	Exercise while watching TV (e.g., use hand weights or stationary bicycle/treadmill, elliptical training, or stretch).
❑	❑	Spend more time playing sports than sitting in front of the TV or the computer.
❑	❑	Dance to music.
❑	❑	Keep a pair of comfortable walking or running shoes in your car and office. You'll be ready for activity wherever you go!
❑	❑	Make a Saturday morning walk a group habit.
❑	❑	Learn a new sport or join a sports team.
❑	❑	Avoid carts when golfing.
❑	❑	When out of town, stay in hotels with fitness centers.

Try It

Keep a 3-day log of all your activities. List the activities performed, time of day, and how long you were engaged in these activities. You may be surprised by your findings.

Source: Adapted from Centers for Disease Control and Prevention, Atlanta, 2014.

Physical Fitness Assessment

The assessment of physical fitness serves several purposes:

- To educate participants regarding their present fitness levels and compare them with health fitness and physical fitness standards
- To motivate individuals to participate in exercise programs
- To provide a starting point for an individualized exercise prescription and establish realistic goals
- To evaluate improvements in fitness achieved through exercise programs and adjust exercise prescription and fitness goals accordingly
- To monitor changes in fitness throughout the years

Responders versus Nonresponders

Individuals who follow similar training programs show wide variation in physiological responses. Heredity plays a crucial role in how each person responds to and improves after beginning an exercise program. Several studies have documented that following exercise training, most individuals, called **responders**, readily show improvements but a few, the **nonresponders**, exhibit small or no improvements. This concept is referred to as the **principle of individuality**.

After several months of aerobic training, increases in VO_{2max} are between 15 and 20 percent on the average, although individual responses can range from 0 percent (in a few cases) to more than 50 percent improvement, even when all participants follow the same training program. Nonfitness and low-fitness participants, however, should not label themselves as nonresponders based on the previous discussion. Nonresponders constitute less than 5 percent of exercise participants. Although additional research is necessary, lack of improvement in CR endurance among nonresponders might be related to low levels of leg strength. A lower-body strength-training program has been shown to help these individuals improve VO_{2max} through aerobic exercise.[1]

If through your self-assessment of CR fitness you find your fitness level is less than adequate, do not let that discourage you; rather, set a priority to be physically active every day. In addition to regular exercise, lifestyle behaviors—walking, taking stairs, cycling to work, parking farther from the office, doing household tasks, gardening and doing yard work, for example—provide substantial benefits. In this regard, daily **physical activity** and **exercise** habits should be monitored, in conjunction with fitness testing, to evaluate adherence among nonresponders. After all, it is through increased daily activity that you will reap the health benefits that improve your quality of life.

Assessment of Cardiorespiratory Endurance

CR endurance, CR fitness, or aerobic capacity is determined by the maximal amount of oxygen the human body is able to utilize (the oxygen uptake) per minute of physical activity (VO_{2max}). This value can be expressed in liters per minute (L/min) or milliliters per kilogram per minute (mL/kg/min). The relative value in mL/kg/min is used most often for VO_{2max}, because it considers total body mass (weight) in kilograms. When comparing two individuals with the same absolute value, the one with the lesser body mass will have a higher relative value, indicating that more oxygen is available to each kilogram (2.2 pounds) of body weight. Because all tissues and organs of the body need oxygen to function, higher oxygen consumption indicates a more efficient CR system.

VO_2 expressed in liters per minute is valuable in determining the caloric expenditure of physical activity. The human body burns about five calories for each liter of oxygen consumed. A complete discussion of this principle is given under the section "Predicting Oxygen Uptake and Caloric Expenditure from Walking and Jogging" in this same chapter (pages 230–232).

Components of VO_2

The amount of oxygen the body uses at rest or during submaximal (VO_2) or maximal (VO_{2max}) exercise is determined by heart rate, stroke volume, and the amount of oxygen removed from the vascular system (for use by all organs and tissues of the body, including the muscular system).

Heart Rate

Normal heart rate ranges from about 45 bpm or lower during resting conditions in trained athletes to 200 bpm or higher during maximal exercise. The **maximal heart rate (MHR)** that a person can achieve starts to drop by about one beat per year beginning around 12 years of age. The MHR in trained endurance athletes is sometimes slightly lower than in an untrained individual. This adaptation to training is thought to allow the heart more time to effectively fill with blood so as to produce a greater stroke volume.

Stroke Volume

Stroke volume can range from 50 milliliters (mL) per beat (stroke) during resting conditions in highly sedentary people to as high as 200 mL per beat at maximum in elite endurance-trained athletes (Table 6.1). Following endurance training, stroke volume increases significantly. Some of the increase is the result of a stronger heart muscle, but it also is related to an increase in total blood volume and a greater filling capacity of the ventricles during the resting phase (diastole) of the cardiac cycle. As more blood enters the heart, more blood can be ejected with each heartbeat (systole). The increase in stroke volume is primarily responsible for the increase in VO_{2max} with endurance training.

Amount of Oxygen Removed from Blood

The amount of oxygen removed from the vascular system is known as the **arterial–venous oxygen difference** **($a\text{-}\bar{v}O_{2diff}$)**. The

Responders Individuals who exhibit improvements in fitness as a result of exercise training.

Nonresponders Individuals who exhibit small or no improvements in fitness compared to others who undergo the same training program.

Principle of individuality Training concept holding that genetics plays a major role in individual responses to exercise training and these differences must be considered when designing exercise programs for different people.

Physical activity Bodily movement produced by skeletal muscles, which requires expenditure of energy and produces progressive health benefits. Examples include walking, taking the stairs, dancing, gardening, working in the yard, cleaning the house, shoveling snow, washing the car, and all forms of structured exercise.

Exercise Type of physical activity that requires planned, structured, and repetitive bodily movement with the intent of improving or maintaining one or more components of physical fitness.

Maximal heart rate (MHR) Highest heart rate for a person, related primarily to age.

Arterial–venous oxygen difference ($a\text{-}\bar{v}O_{2diff}$) Amount of oxygen removed from the blood as determined by the difference in oxygen content between arterial and venous blood.

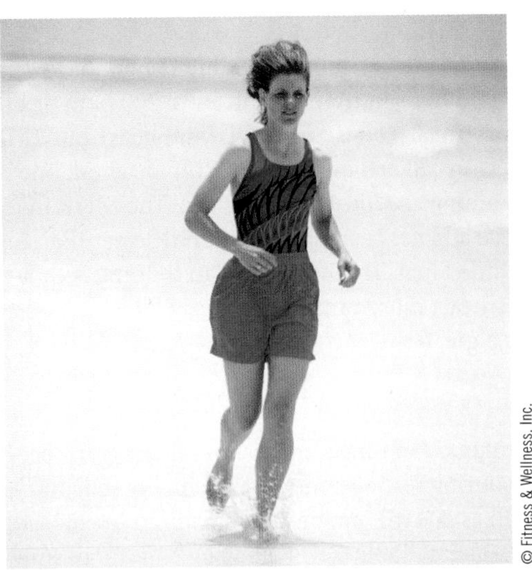
© Fitness & Wellness, Inc.

Aerobic fitness leads to better health and a higher quality of life.

oxygen content in the arteries at sea level is typically 20 mL of oxygen per 100 mL of blood. (This value decreases at higher altitudes because of the drop in barometric pressure, which affects the amount of oxygen picked up by hemoglobin.) The oxygen content in the veins during a resting state is about 15 mL per 100 mL. Thus, the $a\text{-}\bar{v}O_{2diff}$—the amount of oxygen in the arteries minus the amount in the veins—at rest is 5 mL per 100 mL. The arterial value remains constant during both resting and exercise conditions. Because of the additional oxygen removed during maximal exercise, the venous oxygen content drops to about 5 mL per 100 mL, yielding an $a\text{-}\bar{v}O_{2diff}$ of 15 mL per 100 mL. The latter value may be slightly higher in endurance athletes.

These three factors are used to compute VO_2 using the following equation:

$$VO_2 \text{ in L/min} = (HR \times SV \times a\text{-}\bar{v}O_{2diff}) \div 100{,}000,$$

where HR is the heart rate and SV is the stroke volume. For example, the resting VO_2 (also known as the resting metabolic rate) of an individual with an RHR of 76 bpm and a stroke volume of 79 mL would be

$$VO_2 \text{ in L/min} = (76 \times 79 \times 5) \div 100{,}000 = .3 \text{ L/min}.$$

Likewise, the VO_{2max} of a person exercising maximally who achieves a heart rate of 190 bpm and a maximal stroke volume of 120 mL would be

$$VO_{2max} \text{ in L/min} = (190 \times 120 \times 15) \div 100{,}000 = 3.42 \text{ L/min}.$$

To convert L/min to mL/kg/min, multiply the L/min value by 1,000 and divide by body weight in kilograms. In the preceding example, if the person weighs 70 kilograms, the VO_{2max} would be 48.9 mL/kg/min (3.42 × 1000 ÷ 70).

Because the actual measurement of the stroke volume and the $a\text{-}\bar{v}O_{2diff}$ is impractical in the fitness setting, VO_2 also is determined through gas (air) analysis. To do so, the air exhaled by a person being tested is analyzed by a metabolic cart that measures the difference in oxygen content between the person's exhaled air and the atmosphere. The air we breathe contains 21 percent oxygen; thus, VO_2 can be assessed by establishing the difference between 21 percent and the percentage of oxygen left in the air the person exhales, according to the total volume of air taken into the lungs. This type of equipment, however, is expensive. Consequently, several alternative methods of estimating VO_{2max} using limited equipment have been developed. These methods are discussed next.

VO_{2max} is affected by genetics, training, gender, age, and body composition. Although aerobic training can help people attain good or excellent CR fitness, only those with a strong genetic component are able to reach an "elite" level of aerobic capacity (60 to 80 mL/kg/min). Furthermore, VO_{2max} is 15 to 30 percent higher in men. This is related to a greater hemoglobin content, lower body fat (see "Essential and Storage Fat" in Chapter 4, page 138), and larger heart size in men (a larger heart pumps more blood and thus produces a greater stroke volume). VO_{2max} also decreases by about 1 percent per year starting at age 25. This decrease, however, is only .5 percent per year in physically active individuals.

Tests to Estimate VO_{2max}

Even though most CR endurance tests probably are safe to administer to apparently healthy individuals (those with no major coronary risk factors or symptoms), a health history questionnaire (including the PAR-Q), such as found in Activity 1.3 in Chapter 1, should be used as a minimum screening tool prior to exercise testing or participation. The American College of Sports Medicine (ACSM) also recommends that individuals at risk, or diagnosed with cardiovascular disease, undergo a medical examination prior to exercise testing or exercise participation.[2]

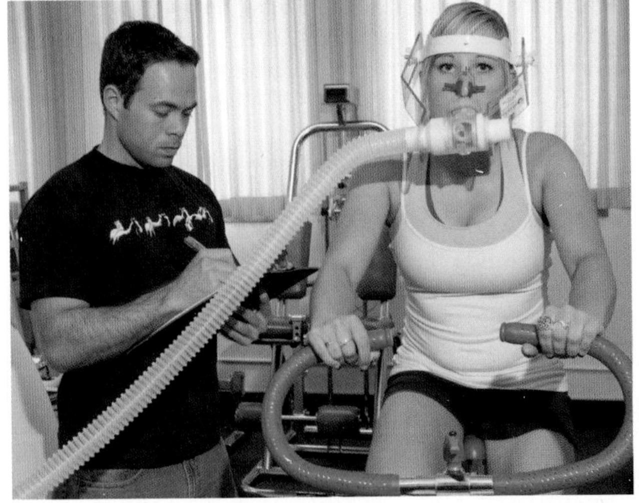
© Fitness & Wellness, Inc.

Oxygen uptake (VO_2), as determined through direct gas analysis.

FIGURE 6.2 Procedure for the 1.5-Mile Run Test.

1. Make sure you qualify for this test. This test is contraindicated for unconditioned beginners, individuals with symptoms of heart disease, and those with known heart disease or risk factors.
2. Select the testing site. Find a school track (each lap is one-fourth of a mile) or a premeasured 1.5-mile course.
3. Have a stopwatch available to determine your time.
4. Conduct a few warm-up exercises prior to the test. Do some stretching exercises, some walking, and slow jogging.
5. Initiate the test and try to cover the distance in the fastest time possible (walking or jogging). Time yourself during the run to see how fast you have covered the distance. If any unusual symptoms arise during the test, do not continue. Stop immediately and retake the test after another 6 weeks of aerobic training.
6. At the end of the test, cool down by walking or jogging slowly for another 3 to 5 minutes. Do not sit or lie down after the test.
7. According to your performance time, look up your estimated maximal oxygen uptake (VO_{2max}) in Table 6.2.

Example: A 20-year-old female runs the 1.5-mile course in 12 minutes and 40 seconds. Table 6.2 shows a VO_{2max} of 39.8 mL/kg/min for a time of 12:40. According to Table 6.8, this VO_{2max} would place her in the "good" cardiorespiratory fitness category.

Five exercise tests used to assess CR fitness are introduced in this chapter: the 1.5-Mile Run Test, the 1.0-Mile Walk Test, the Step Test, the Astrand-Ryhming Test, and the 12-Minute Swim Test. The procedures for each test are explained in detail in Figures 6.2, 6.3, 6.4, 6.5, and 6.6, respectively. The 1.5-Mile Run Test and the Swim Test are considered maximal tests, as they require an all-out or nearly all-out effort on the part of the participant. Submaximal exercise tests do not require all-out efforts.

You may choose one or more of these tests depending on time, equipment, and individual physical limitations. For example, people who can't jog or walk can take the Astrand-Ryhming (bicycle) Test or 12-Minute Swim Test. However, because these tests are different and only estimate VO_{2max}, they may not yield the same results. Therefore, to make valid comparisons, you should take the same test when doing pre- and postassessments. You can record the results of your test or tests in Lab 6A.

1.5-Mile Run Test

The 1.5-Mile Run Test is used most frequently to predict VO_{2max}, according to the time the person takes to run or walk a 1.5-mile course (Figure 6.2). VO_{2max} is estimated based on the time the person takes to cover the distance (Table 6.2).

The only equipment necessary to conduct this test is a stopwatch and a track or premeasured 1.5-mile course. This perhaps is the easiest test to administer, but a note of caution is in order when conducting the test: Given that the objective is to cover the distance in the shortest time, it is considered a maximal exercise test. The 1.5-Mile Run Test should be limited to conditioned individuals who have been cleared for exercise. The test is not recommended for unconditioned beginners, men over age 45 and women over age 55 without proper medical clearance, symptomatic individuals, or those with known disease or risk factors for heart disease. A program of at least 6 weeks of aerobic training is recommended before unconditioned individuals take this test.

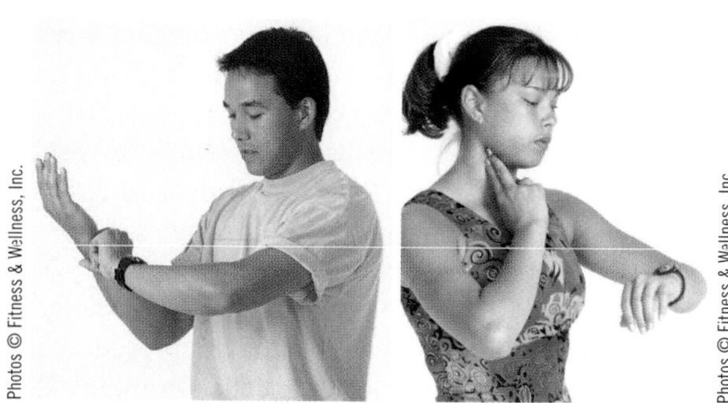

Photos © Fitness & Wellness, Inc.

Pulse taken at the radial artery. Pulse taken at the carotid artery.

1.0-Mile Walk Test

The 1.0-Mile Walk Test can be used by individuals who are unable to run because of low fitness levels or injuries. All that is required is a brisk 1.0-mile walk that elicits an exercise heart rate of at least 120 bpm at the end of the test.

You need to know how to take your heart rate by counting your pulse. You can do this by gently placing the middle and index fingers over the radial artery on the inside of the wrist on the side of the thumb or over the carotid artery in the neck just below the jaw next to the voice box. You should not use the thumb to check the pulse because it has a strong pulse of its own, which can make you miscount. When checking the carotid pulse, do not press too hard, because it may cause a reflex action that slows the heart. For checking the pulse over the carotid artery, some exercise experts recommend that the hand on the same side of the neck (right hand over right carotid artery) be used to avoid excessive pressure on the artery. With minimum experience, however, you can be accurate using either hand as long as you apply only gentle pressure. If available, heart rate monitors can be used to increase the accuracy of heart rate assessment.

VO_{2max} is estimated according to a prediction equation that requires the following data: 1.0-mile walk time, exercise heart rate at the end of the walk, gender, and body weight in pounds. The procedure for this test and the equation are given in Figure 6.3.

Step Test

The Step Test requires little time and equipment and can be administered to almost anyone, because a submaximal

TABLE 6.2 Estimated Maximal Oxygen Uptake (VO_{2max}) for the 1.5-Mile Run Test

Time	VO_{2max} (mL/kg/min)	Time	VO_{2max} (mL/kg/min)
6:10	80.0	12:40	39.8
6:20	79.0	12:50	39.2
6:30	77.9	13:00	38.6
6:40	76.7	13:10	38.1
6:50	75.5	13:20	37.8
7:00	74.0	13:30	37.2
7:10	72.6	13:40	36.8
7:20	71.3	13:50	36.3
7:30	69.9	14:00	35.9
7:40	68.3	14:10	35.5
7:50	66.8	14:20	35.1
8:00	65.2	14:30	34.7
8:10	63.9	14:40	34.3
8:20	62.5	14:50	34.0
8:30	61.2	15:00	33.6
8:40	60.2	15:10	33.1
8:50	59.1	15:20	32.7
9:00	58.1	15:30	32.2
9:10	56.9	15:40	31.8
9:20	55.9	15:50	31.4
9:30	54.7	16:00	30.9
9:40	53.5	16:10	30.5
9:50	52.3	16:20	30.2
10:00	51.1	16:30	29.8
10:10	50.4	16:40	29.5
10:20	49.5	16:50	29.1
10:30	48.6	17:00	28.9
10:40	48.0	17:10	28.5
10:50	47.4	17:20	28.3
11:00	46.6	17:30	28.0
11:10	45.8	17:40	27.7
11:20	45.1	17:50	27.4
11:30	44.4	18:00	27.1
11:40	43.7	18:10	26.8
11:50	43.2	18:20	26.6
12:00	42.3	18:30	26.3
12:10	41.7	18:40	26.0
12:20	41.0	18:50	25.7
12:30	40.4	19:00	25.4

Source: Adapted from K. H. Cooper, "A Means of Assessing Maximal Oxygen Intake," *Journal of the American Medical Association,* 203 (1968): 201–204; M. L. Pollock, J. H. Wilmore, and S. M. Fox III, *Health and Fitness Through Physical Activity,* (New York: John Wiley & Sons, 1978); and J. H. Wilmore and D. L. Costill, *Training for Sport and Activity* (Dubuque, IA: Wm. C. Brown Publishers, 1988).

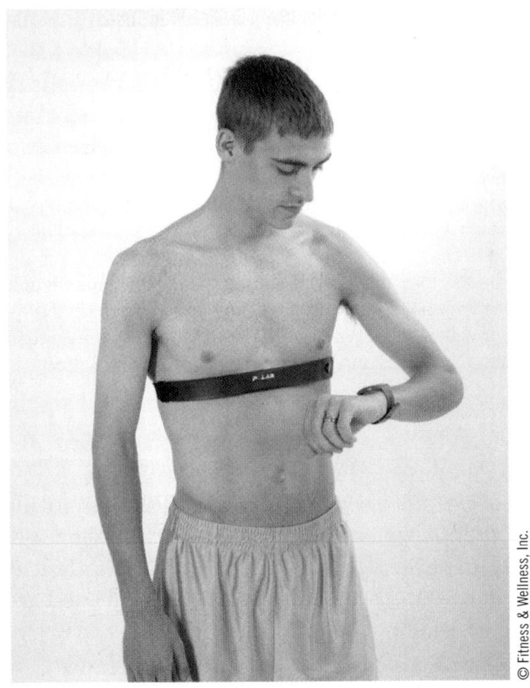

Heart rate monitors increase the accuracy of heart rate assessment.

workload is used to estimate VO_{2max}. Symptomatic and diseased individuals should not take this test. Significantly overweight individuals and those with joint problems in the lower extremities may have difficulty performing the test.

The actual test takes only 3 minutes. A 15-second recovery heart rate is taken between 5 and 20 seconds following the test (Figure 6.4 and Table 6.3). The required equipment consists of a bench or gymnasium bleacher $16^1/_4$ inches high, a stopwatch, and a metronome.

People taking this test also need to know how to take their heart rate by counting their pulse, as just discussed for the 1.0-Mile Walk Test. Once people learn to take their own heart rate, a large group of people can be tested at once, using gymnasium bleachers for the steps.

Astrand-Ryhming Test

Because of its simplicity and practicality, the Astrand-Ryhming Test is one of the most popular tests used to estimate VO_{2max} in a laboratory setting. The test is conducted on a bicycle ergometer and, similar to the Step Test, requires only submaximal workloads and little time to administer.

The cautions given for the Step Test also apply to the Astrand-Ryhming Test. Nevertheless, because the participant does not have to support his or her own body weight while riding the bicycle, overweight individuals and those with limited joint problems in the lower extremities can take this test.

The bicycle ergometer to be used for this test should allow the regulation of workloads (see the test procedure in Figure 6.5). Besides the bicycle ergometer, a stopwatch and an additional technician to monitor the participant's heart rate are needed to conduct the test.

FIGURE 6.3 **Procedure for the 1.0-Mile Walk Test.**

1. Select the testing site. Use a 440-yard track (4 laps to a mile) or a premeasured 1.0-mile course.
2. Determine your body weight in pounds prior to the test.
3. Have a stopwatch available to determine total walking time and exercise heart rate.
4. Walk the 1.0-mile course at a brisk but even pace throughout (the exercise heart rate at the end of the test should be above 120 beats per minute).
5. At the end of the 1.0-mile walk, check your walking time and immediately count your pulse for 10 seconds. Multiply the 10-second pulse count by 6 to obtain the exercise heart rate in beats per minute.
6. Convert the walking time from minutes and seconds to minute units. Because each minute has 60 seconds, divide the seconds by 60 to obtain the fraction of a minute. For instance, a walking time of 12 minutes and 15 seconds would equal 12 + (15 ÷ 60), or 12.25 minutes.
7. To obtain the estimated maximal oxygen uptake (VO_{2max}) in mL/kg/min, plug your values in the following equation: $VO_{2max} = 88.768 - (0.0957 \times W) + (8.892 \times G) - (1.4537 \times T) - (0.1194 \times HR)$

Where:

W = Weight in pounds
G = Gender (use 0 for women and 1 for men)
T = Total time for the one-mile walk in minutes (see item 6)
HR = Exercise heart rate in beats per minute at the end of the 1.0-mile walk

Example: A 19-year-old female who weighs 140 pounds completed the 1.0-mile walk in 14 minutes 39 seconds with an exercise heart rate of 148 beats per minute. Her estimated VO_{2max} would be:

W = 140 lbs
G = 0 (female gender = 0)
T = 14:39 = 14 + (39 ÷ 60) = 14.65 min
HR = 148 bpm
$VO_{2max} = 88.768 - (0.0957 \times 140) + (8.892 \times 0) - (1.4537 \times 14.65) - (0.1194 \times 148)$
$VO_{2max} = 36.4$ mL/kg/min

Source: F. A. Dolgener, L. D. Hensley, J. J. Marsh, and J. K. Fjelstul, "Validation of the Rockport Fitness Walking Test in College Males and Females," *Research Quarterly for Exercise and Sport* 65 (1994): 152–158.

TABLE 6.3 **Predicted Maximal Oxygen Uptake for the Step Test**

15-Sec Heart Rate	Heart Rate (bpm)	VO_{2max} (mL/kg/min) Men	Women
30	120	60.9	43.6
31	124	59.3	42.9
32	128	57.6	42.2
33	132	55.9	41.4
34	136	54.2	40.7
35	140	52.5	40.0
36	144	50.9	39.2
37	148	49.2	38.5
38	152	47.5	37.7
39	156	45.8	37.0
40	160	44.1	36.3
41	164	42.5	35.5
42	168	40.8	34.8
43	172	39.1	34.0
44	176	37.4	33.3
45	180	35.7	32.6
46	184	34.1	31.8
47	188	32.4	31.1
48	192	30.7	30.3
49	196	29.0	29.6
50	200	27.3	28.9

FIGURE 6.4 **Procedure for the Step Test.**

1. Conduct the test with a bench or gymnasium bleacher 16¼ inches high.
2. Perform the stepping cycle to a four-step cadence (up-up-down-down). Men should perform 24 complete step-ups per minute, regulated with a metronome set at 96 beats per minute. Women perform 22 step-ups per minute, or 88 beats per minute on the metronome.
3. Allow a brief practice period of 5 to 10 seconds to familiarize yourself with the stepping cadence.
4. Begin the test and perform the step-ups for exactly 3 minutes.
5. Upon completing the 3 minutes, remain standing and take your heart rate for a 15-second interval from 5 to 20 seconds into recovery. Convert recovery heart rate to beats per minute (multiply 15-second heart rate by 4).
6. Maximal oxygen uptake (VO_{2max}) in mL/kg/min is estimated according to the following equations:

Men:
$VO_{2max} = 111.33 - (0.42 \times \text{recovery heart rate in bpm})$
Women:
$VO_{2max} = 65.81 - (0.1847 \times \text{recovery heart rate in bpm})$

Example: The recovery 15-second heart rate for a male following the 3-minute step test is found to be 39 beats. His VO_{2max} is estimated as follows:

15-second heart rate = 39 beats
Minute heart rate = 39 × 4 = 156 bpm
$VO_{2max} = 111.33 - (0.42 \times 156) = 45.81$ mL/kg/min
VO_{2max} also can be obtained according to recovery heart rates in Table 6.3.

The heart rate is taken every minute for 6 minutes. At the end of the test, the heart rate should be in the range given for each workload in Table 6.5 (generally between 120 and 170 bpm).

When administering the test to older people, good judgment is essential. Low workloads should be used, because if the higher heart rates (around 150 to 170 bpm) are reached, these individuals could be working near or at their maximal capacity, making this an unsafe test without adequate medical supervision. When testing older people, choose workloads so that the final exercise heart rates do not exceed 130 to 140 bpm.

12-Minute Swim Test

Similar to the 1.5-Mile Run Test, the 12-Minute Swim Test is considered a maximal exercise test, and the same precautions apply. The objective is to swim as far as possible during the 12-Minute Swim Test (Figure 6.6).

Unlike land-based tests, predicting VO_{2max} through a swimming test is difficult. A swimming test is practical only for those who are planning to take part in a swimming program or who cannot perform any of the other tests. Differences in skill level, swimming conditioning, and body composition greatly affect the energy requirements (VO_2) of swimming. A skilled swimmer is able to swim more efficiently and expend less energy than an unskilled swimmer. Unskilled and unconditioned swimmers can expect lower CR fitness ratings than can be obtained with a land-based test. In addition, improper breathing patterns cause premature fatigue. Overweight individuals are more buoyant in the water, and the larger surface area (body size) produces more friction against movement in the water medium.

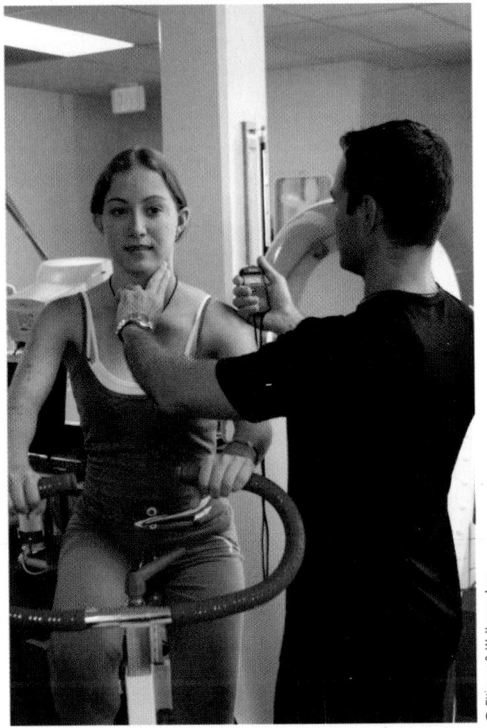

Monitoring heart rate on the carotid artery during the Astrand-Ryhming Test.

Lack of conditioning affects swimming test results as well. An unconditioned yet skilled swimmer who is in good CR shape because of a regular jogging program will not perform as effectively in a swimming test.

FIGURE 6.5 Procedure for the Astrand-Ryhming Test.

1. Adjust the bike seat so the knees are almost completely extended as the foot goes through the bottom of the pedaling cycle.
2. During the test, keep the speed constant at 50 revolutions per minute. Test duration is 6 minutes.
3. Select the appropriate workload for the bike based on gender, age, weight, health, and estimated fitness level. For unconditioned individuals: women, use 300 kpm (kilopounds per meter) or 450 kpm; men, 300 kpm or 600 kpm. Conditioned adults: women, 450 kpm or 600 kpm; men, 600 kpm or 900 kpm.*
4. Ride the bike for 6 minutes and check the heart rate every minute, during the last 15 seconds of each minute. Determine heart rate by recording the time it takes to count 30 pulse beats and then converting to beats per minute using Table 6.4.
5. Average the final two heart rates (5th and 6th minutes). If these two heart rates are not within 5 beats per minute of each other, continue the test for another few minutes until this is accomplished. If the heart rate continues to climb significantly after the 6th minute, stop the test and rest for 15 to 20 minutes. You may then retest, preferably at a lower workload. The final average heart rate should also fall between the ranges given for each workload in Table 6.5 (men: 300 kpm = 120 to 140 beats per minute; 600 kpm = 120 to 170 beats per minute).
6. Based on the average heart rate of the final 2 minutes and your workload, look up the maximal oxygen uptake (VO_{2max}) in Table 6.5 (for example: men: 600 kpm and average heart rate = 145, VO_{2max} = 2.4 L/min).
7. Correct VO_{2max} using the correction factors found in Table 6.6 (if VO_{2max} = 2.4 and age 35, correction factor = .870. Multiply 2.4 × .870 and final corrected VO_{2max} = 2.09 L/min).
8. To obtain VO_{2max} in mL/kg/min, multiply the VO_{2max} by 1,000 (to convert liters to milliliters) and divide by body weight in kilograms (to obtain kilograms, divide your body weight in pounds by 2.2046).

Example: Corrected VO_{2max} = 2.09 L/min
Body weight = 132 pounds ÷ 2.2046 = 60 kilograms

$$VO_{2max} \text{ in mL/kg/min} = \frac{2.09 \times 1{,}000}{60} = 34.8 \text{ mL/kg/min}$$

*On the Monark bicycle ergometer, at a speed of 50 revolutions per minutes a load of 1 kp = 300kpm, 1.5 kp = 450 kpm, 2 kp = 600 kpm, and so forth with increases of 150 kpm to each half kp.

TABLE 6.4 Conversion of the Time for 30 Pulse Beats to Pulse Rate per Minute

Sec	bpm	Sec	bpm	Sec	bpm	Sec	bpm	Sec	bpm	Sec	bpm
22.0	82	19.6	92	17.2	105	14.8	122	12.4	145	10.0	180
21.9	82	19.5	92	17.1	105	14.7	122	12.3	146	9.9	182
21.8	83	19.4	93	17.0	106	14.6	123	12.2	148	9.8	184
21.7	83	19.3	93	16.9	107	14.5	124	12.1	149	9.7	186
21.6	83	19.2	94	16.8	107	14.4	125	12.0	150	9.6	188
21.5	84	19.1	94	16.7	108	14.3	126	11.9	151	9.5	189
21.4	84	19.0	95	16.6	108	14.2	127	11.8	153	9.4	191
21.3	85	18.9	95	16.5	109	14.1	128	11.7	154	9.3	194
21.2	85	18.8	96	16.4	110	14.0	129	11.6	155	9.2	196
21.1	85	18.7	96	16.3	110	13.9	129	11.5	157	9.1	198
21.0	86	18.6	97	16.2	111	13.8	130	11.4	158	9.0	200
20.9	86	18.5	97	16.1	112	13.7	131	11.3	159	8.9	202
20.8	87	18.4	98	16.0	113	13.6	132	11.2	161	8.8	205
20.7	87	18.3	98	15.9	113	13.5	133	11.1	162	8.7	207
20.6	87	18.2	99	15.8	114	13.4	134	11.0	164	8.6	209
20.5	88	18.1	99	15.7	115	13.3	135	10.9	165	8.5	212
		18.0	100	15.6	115	13.2	136	10.8	167	8.4	214
		17.9	101	15.5	116	13.1	137	10.7	168	8.3	217
		17.8	101	15.4	117	13.0	138	10.6	170	8.2	220
		17.7	102	15.3	118	12.9	140	10.5	171	8.1	222
		17.6	102	15.2	118	12.8	141	10.4	173	8.0	225
		17.5	103	15.1	119	12.7	142	10.3	175		
		17.4	103	15.0	120	12.6	143	10.2	176		
		17.3	104	14.9	121	12.5	144	10.1	178		

FIGURE 6.6 Procedure for the 12-Minute Swim Test.

1. Enlist a friend to time the test. The only other requisites are a stopwatch and a swimming pool. Do not attempt to do this test in an unsupervised pool.
2. Warm up by swimming slowly and doing a few stretching exercises before taking the test.
3. Start the test and swim as many laps as possible in 12 minutes. Pace yourself throughout the test and do not swim to the point of complete exhaustion.
4. After completing the test, cool down by swimming another 2 or 3 minutes at a slower pace.
5. Determine the total distance you swam during the test and look up your fitness category in Table 6.7.

CRITICAL THINKING

Should fitness testing be a part of a fitness program? Why or why not? Does preparticipation fitness testing have benefits, or should fitness testing be done at a later date?

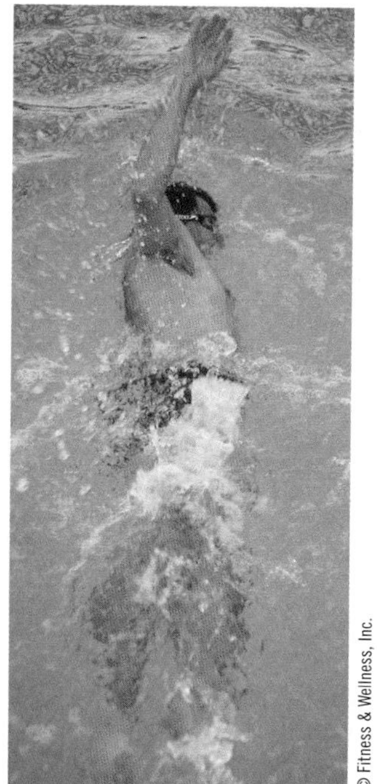

Only those with swimming skill and proper conditioning should take the 12-Minute Swim Test.

TABLE 6.5 **Maximal Oxygen Uptake (VO_{2max}) Estimates in L/min for the Astrand-Ryhming Test**

	Men					Women				
	Workload (kpm)					Workload (kpm)				
Heart Rate	300	600	900	1,200	1,500	300	450	600	750	900
120	2.2	3.4	4.8			2.6	3.4	4.1	4.8	
121	2.2	3.4	4.7			2.5	3.3	4.0	4.8	
122	2.2	3.4	4.6			2.5	3.2	3.9	4.7	
123	2.1	3.4	4.6			2.4	3.1	3.9	4.6	
124	2.1	3.3	4.5	6.0		2.4	3.1	3.8	4.5	
125	2.0	3.2	4.4	5.9		2.3	3.0	3.7	4.4	
126	2.0	3.2	4.4	5.8		2.3	3.0	3.6	4.3	
127	2.0	3.1	4.3	5.7		2.2	2.9	3.5	4.2	
128	2.0	3.1	4.2	5.6		2.2	2.8	3.5	4.2	4.8
129	1.9	3.0	4.2	5.6		2.2	2.8	3.4	4.1	4.8
130	1.9	3.0	4.1	5.5		2.1	2.7	3.4	4.0	4.7
131	1.9	2.9	4.0	5.4		2.1	2.7	3.4	4.0	4.6
132	1.8	2.9	4.0	5.3		2.0	2.7	3.3	3.9	4.5
133	1.8	2.8	3.9	5.3		2.0	2.6	3.2	3.8	4.4
134	1.8	2.8	3.9	5.2		2.0	2.6	3.2	3.8	4.4
135	1.7	2.8	3.8	5.1		2.0	2.6	3.1	3.7	4.3
136	1.7	2.7	3.8	5.0		1.9	2.5	3.1	3.6	4.2
137	1.7	2.7	3.7	5.0		1.9	2.5	3.0	3.6	4.2
138	1.6	2.7	3.7	4.9		1.8	2.4	3.0	3.5	4.1
139	1.6	2.6	3.6	4.8		1.8	2.4	2.9	3.5	4.0
140	1.6	2.6	3.6	4.8	6.0	1.8	2.4	2.8	3.4	4.0
141		2.6	3.5	4.7	5.9	1.8	2.3	2.8	3.4	3.9
142		2.5	3.5	4.6	5.8	1.7	2.3	2.8	3.3	3.9
143		2.5	3.4	4.6	5.7	1.7	2.2	2.7	3.3	3.8
144		2.5	3.4	4.5	5.7	1.7	2.2	2.7	3.2	3.8
145		2.4	3.4	4.5	5.6	1.6	2.2	2.7	3.2	3.7
146		2.4	3.3	4.4	5.6	1.6	2.2	2.6	3.2	3.7
147		2.4	3.3	4.4	5.5	1.6	2.1	2.6	3.1	3.6
148		2.4	3.2	4.3	5.4	1.6	2.1	2.6	3.1	3.6
149		2.3	3.2	4.3	5.4		2.1	2.6	3.0	3.5
150		2.3	3.2	4.2	5.3		2.0	2.5	3.0	3.5
151		2.3	3.1	4.2	5.2		2.0	2.5	3.0	3.4
152		2.3	3.1	4.1	5.2		2.0	2.5	2.9	3.4
153		2.2	3.0	4.1	5.1		2.0	2.4	2.9	3.3
154		2.2	3.0	4.0	5.1		2.0	2.4	2.8	3.3
155		2.2	3.0	4.0	5.0		1.9	2.4	2.8	3.2
156		2.2	2.9	4.0	5.0		1.9	2.3	2.8	3.2
157		2.1	2.9	3.9	4.9		1.9	2.3	2.7	3.2
158		2.1	2.9	3.9	4.9		1.8	2.3	2.7	3.1
159		2.1	2.8	3.8	4.8		1.8	2.2	2.7	3.1
160		2.1	2.8	3.8	4.8		1.8	2.2	2.6	3.0
161		2.0	2.8	3.7	4.7		1.8	2.2	2.6	3.0
162		2.0	2.8	3.7	4.6		1.8	2.2	2.6	3.0
163		2.0	2.8	3.7	4.6		1.7	2.2	2.6	2.9
164		2.0	2.7	3.6	4.5		1.7	2.1	2.5	2.9
165		2.0	2.7	3.6	4.5		1.7	2.1	2.5	2.9
166		1.9	2.7	3.6	4.5		1.7	2.1	2.5	2.8
167		1.9	2.6	3.5	4.4		1.6	2.1	2.4	2.8
168		1.9	2.6	3.5	4.4		1.6	2.0	2.4	2.8
169		1.9	2.6	3.5	4.3		1.6	2.0	2.4	2.8
170		1.8	2.6	3.4	4.3		1.6	2.0	2.4	2.7

Source: I. Astrand, "Aerobic Work Capacity in Men and Women with Special Reference to Age," *Acta Physiologica Scandinavica Supplementum* 49, no. 169 (1960): 45–60.

Because of these limitations, VO_{2max} cannot be estimated for a swimming test, and the fitness categories given in Table 6.7 are only estimated ratings.

Interpreting the Results of Your VO_{2max}

After obtaining your VO_{2max}, you can determine your current level of CR fitness by consulting Table 6.8. Locate the VO_{2max} in your age category; then, on the top row, find your present level of CR fitness. For example, a 19-year-old male with a VO_{2max} of 35 mL/kg/min would be classified in the average CR fitness category. After you initiate your personal CR exercise program (Lab 6D), you may wish to retest yourself periodically to evaluate your progress.

Predicting VO_2 and Caloric Expenditure from Walking and Jogging

As indicated earlier in the chapter, VO_{2max} can be expressed in liters per minute or milliliters per kilogram per minute. The latter is used to classify individuals into the various CR fitness categories (Table 6.8).

TABLE 6.6 Age-Based Correction Factors for Maximal Oxygen Uptake

Age	Correction Factor	Age	Correction Factor	Age	Correction Factor	Age	Correction Factor	Age	Correction Factor	Age	Correction Factor
14	1.11	23	1.02	32	.909	41	.820	50	.750	59	.686
15	1.10	24	1.01	33	.896	42	.810	51	.742	60	.680
16	1.09	25	1.00	34	.883	43	.800	52	.734	61	.674
17	1.08	26	.987	35	.870	44	.790	53	.726	62	.668
18	1.07	27	.974	36	.862	45	.780	54	.718	63	.662
19	1.06	28	.961	37	.854	46	.774	55	.710	64	.656
20	1.05	29	.948	38	.846	47	.768	56	.704	65	.650
21	1.04	30	.935	39	.838	48	.762	57	.698		
22	1.03	31	.922	40	.830	49	.756	58	.692		

Source: I. Astrand, "Aerobic Work Capacity in Men and Women with Special Reference to Age," *Acta Physiologica Scandinavica Supplementum* 49, no. 169 (1960): 45–60.

TABLE 6.7 12-Minute Swim Test Fitness Categories

Distance (yd)	Fitness Category
≥700	Excellent
500–700	Good
400–500	Average
200–400	Fair
≤200	Poor

Source: Adapted from K. H. Cooper, *The Aerobics Program for Total Well-Being* (New York: Bantam Books, 1982).

VO_2 expressed in liters per minute is valuable in determining the caloric expenditure of physical activity. The human body burns about five calories for each liter of oxygen consumed. During aerobic exercise, the average person trains around 50 percent of VO_{2max}.

A person with a VO_{2max} of 3.5 L/min who trains at 60 percent of maximum uses 2.1 liters of oxygen per minute of physical activity (3.5 × .60). This indicates that 10.5 calories are burned each minute of exercise (2.1 × 5). If the activity is carried out for 30 minutes, 315 calories have been burned (10.5 × 30).

For individuals concerned about weight management, these computations are valuable in determining energy

TABLE 6.8 Cardiorespiratory Fitness Classification According to Maximal Oxygen Uptake (VO_{2max})

		Fitness Category (based on VO_{2max} in mL/kg/min)				
Gender	Age	Poor	Fair	Average	Good	Excellent
Men	<29	<24.9	25–33.9	34–43.9	44–52.9	>53
	30–39	<22.9	23–30.9	31–41.9	42–49.9	>50
	40–49	<19.9	20–26.9	27–38.9	39–44.9	>45
	50–59	<17.9	18–24.9	25–37.9	38–42.9	>43
	60–69	<15.9	16–22.9	23–35.9	36–40.9	>41
	≥70	≤12.9	13–20.9	21–32.9	33–37.9	≥38
Women	<29	<23.9	24–30.9	31–38.9	39–48.9	>49
	30–39	<19.9	20–27.9	28–36.9	37–44.9	>45
	40–49	<16.9	17–24.9	25–34.9	35–41.9	>42
	50–59	<14.9	15–21.9	22–33.9	34–39.9	>40
	60–69	<12.9	13–20.9	21–32.9	33–36.9	>37
	≥70	≤11.9	12–19.9	20–30.9	31–34.9	≥35

Health fitness standard   High physical fitness standard

See the Chapter 1 discussion on health fitness versus physical fitness.

expenditure. Because a pound of body fat represents 3,500 calories, this individual would have to exercise for a total of 333 minutes to burn the equivalent of a pound of body fat (3,500 ÷ 10.5). At 30 minutes per exercise session, approximately 11 sessions would be required to expend the 3,500 calories.

Applying the principle of 5 calories burned per liter of oxygen consumed, you can determine with reasonable accuracy your own caloric output for walking and jogging. Table 6.9 contains the oxygen requirement (VO_2 uptake) for walking speeds between 50 and 100 meters per minute and for jogging speeds in excess of 80 meters per minute.

There is a transition period from walking to jogging for speeds in the range of 80 to 134 meters per minute. Consequently, you must be truly jogging at these lower speeds to use the estimated VO_2 for jogging in Table 6.9. Because these uptakes are expressed in mL/kg/min, you need to convert this figure to L/min to predict caloric output. This is done by multiplying the VO_2 in mL/kg/min by your body weight in kilograms (kg) and then dividing by 1,000.

For example, let's estimate the caloric cost for an individual who weighs 145.5 pounds and runs 3 miles in 21 minutes. Each mile is about 1,600 meters, or four laps around a 400-meter (440-yard) track. Three miles then would be 4,800 meters (1,600 × 3). Therefore, 3 miles (4,800 meters) in 21 minutes represents a pace of 228.6 meters per minute (4,800 ÷ 21), which we can round up to 230 meters per minute.

Table 6.9 indicates an oxygen requirement (VO_2) of 49.5 mL/kg/min for a speed of 230 meters per minute. A weight of 145.5 pounds equals 66 kilograms (145.5 ÷ 2.2046). The VO_2 in L/min now can be calculated by multiplying the value in mL/kg/min by body weight in kg and dividing by 1,000. In our example, it is (49.5 × 66) ÷ 1,000 = 3.3 L/min. This VO_2 in 21 minutes represents a total of 347 calories (3.3 × 5 × 21).

In Lab 6B, you have an opportunity to determine your VO_2 and caloric expenditure for walking and jogging. Using your VO_2 information in conjunction with exercise heart rates allows you to estimate your caloric expenditure for almost any activity, as long as the heart rate ranges from 110 to 180 bpm.

To make an accurate estimate, you have to be skilled in assessing exercise heart rate. Also, as your level of fitness improves, you need to reassess your exercise heart rate, because it will drop (given the same workload) with improved physical condition.

TABLE 6.9 Oxygen Requirement Estimates for Selected Walking and Jogging Speeds

Walking		Jogging			
Speed (m/min)	VO_2 (mL/kg/min)	Speed (m/min)	VO_2 (mL/kg/min)	Speed (m/min)	VO_2 (mL/kg/min)
50	8.5	96	13.1	180	39.5
52	8.7	98	13.3	185	40.5
54	8.9	100	13.5	190	41.5
56	9.1	80	19.5	195	42.5
58	9.3	85	20.5	200	43.5
60	9.5	90	21.5	205	44.5
62	9.7	95	22.5	210	45.5
64	9.9	100	23.5	215	46.5
66	10.1	105	24.5	220	47.5
68	10.3	110	25.5	225	48.5
70	10.5	115	26.5	230	49.5
72	10.7	120	27.5	235	50.5
74	10.9	125	28.5	240	51.5
76	11.1	130	29.5	245	52.5
78	11.3	135	30.5	250	53.5
80	11.5	140	31.5	255	54.5
82	11.7	145	32.5	260	55.5
84	11.9	150	33.5	265	56.5
86	12.1	155	34.5	270	57.5
88	12.3	160	35.5	275	58.5
90	12.5	165	36.5	280	59.5
92	12.7	170	37.5		
94	12.9	175	38.5		

m/min = meters per minute
mL/kg/min = milliliters per kilogram per minute

Source: Table developed using the metabolic calculations contained in *Guidelines for Exercise Testing and Exercise Prescription*, by the American College of Sports Medicine (Baltimore: Williams & Wilkins, 2014).

Principles of CR Exercise Prescription

Before proceeding with the principles of exercise prescription, you should ask yourself if you are willing to give exercise a try. A low percentage of the U.S. population is truly committed to exercise. The first 6 weeks of the program are most critical. Adherence to exercise is greatly enhanced if you are able to make it through 4 to 6 weeks of training. The benefits of exercise cannot help unless you commit and participate in a lifetime program of physical activity.

Readiness for Exercise

The first step is to ask yourself, am I ready to start an exercise program? The information provided in Lab 6C can help you answer this question. You are evaluated in four categories: mastery (self-control), attitude, health, and commitment. The higher you score in any category—mastery, for example—the more important that reason for exercising is to you.

Scores can vary from 4 to 16. A score of 12 or above is a strong indicator that the factor is important to you, whereas 8 or below is low. If you score 12 or more points in each category, your chances of initiating and sticking to an exercise program are good. If you do not score at least 12 points in each of any three categories, your chances of succeeding at exercise may be slim. You need to be better informed about the benefits of exercise, and a retraining process might be helpful to change core values regarding exercise. More tips on how you can become committed to exercise are provided in the section "Getting Started and Adhering to a Lifetime Exercise Program" (page 242).

Next you have to decide positively that you will try. Using Lab 6C, you can list the advantages and disadvantages of incorporating exercise into your lifestyle. Your list might include the following advantages:

- It will make me feel better.
- I will lose weight.
- I will have more energy.
- It will lower my risk for chronic diseases.

Your list of disadvantages might include the following:

- I don't want to take the time.
- I'm too out of shape.
- There's no good place to exercise.
- I don't have the willpower to do it.

When your reasons for exercising outweigh your reasons for not exercising, you will find it easier to try. In Lab 6C, you can also determine your stage of change for aerobic exercise. Using the information learned in Chapter 2, you can outline specific processes and techniques for change (also see the example in Chapter 9, page 370).

Guidelines for CR Exercise Prescription

As far back as 380 BC, Plato, the renowned Greek philosopher stated: "Lack of activity destroys the good condition of every human being, while movement and methodical physical exercise save it and preserve it." In the 20th century, Dr. Calvin Wells, a scholar in the study of ancient disease indicates in his book *Bones, Bodies, and Disease:* "The pattern of disease or injury that affects any group of people is never a matter of chance. It is invariably the expression of stresses and strains to which they were exposed, a response to everything in their environment and behaviour...It is influenced by their daily occupations, their habits of diet...Man is a whole with his environment." These statements are more applicable than ever in our modern-day technologically driven culture.

In spite of the release of the U.S. Surgeon General's statement on physical activity and health in 1996 indicating that regular moderate physical activity provides substantial health benefits,[3] and the overwhelming evidence validating the benefits of exercise on health, longevity, and quality of life, the majority of adults in the United States still do not meet the minimum recommendations for the improvement and maintenance of CR fitness. According to a survey by the Centers for Disease Control and Prevention (CDC), overall, only 46.1 percent of adults (50.4 percent of men and 42.1 percent of women) in the United States met the 2008 federal guidelines for aerobic physical activity. Furthermore, almost 34 percent did not engage in leisure-time physical activities.

To develop the CR system, the heart muscle has to be overloaded like any other muscle in the human body. Just as the biceps muscle in the upper arm is developed through strength-training exercises, the heart muscle has to be exercised to increase in size, strength, and efficiency. To better understand how the CR system can be developed, you have to be familiar with the different variables that govern exercise prescription.[4]

First, however, you should be aware that the ACSM recommends that individuals with two or more risk factors for cardiovascular disease (men 45 or older and women 55 or older, family history, cigarette smoking, sedentary lifestyle, obesity, high blood pressure, high LDL cholesterol, low HDL cholesterol [see Chapter 11], or prediabetes) get a medical exam prior to **vigorous exercise.**[5] They may, however, initiate a light-to-moderate intensity exercise program without medical clearance. The ACSM has defined vigorous exercise as an exercise intensity above 60 percent of maximal capacity. For individuals initiating an exercise program, this intensity is the equivalent of exercise that "substantially increases heart rate and breathing." Anyone at high risk, symptomatic, or diagnosed with disease should undergo a medical examination prior to initiating even a **moderate exercise** program (one that noticeably increases heart rate and breathing or between 40 percent and 60 percent of maximal capacity).

For exercise prescription purposes, the ACSM uses the **FITT-VP** principle. This acronym stands for Frequency, Intensity, Time (duration), Type (mode), Volume, and Progression. A discussion of each of these principles follows. For practicability and ease of understanding, these principles are discussed in a different order.

Intensity of Exercise

When trying to develop the CR system, many people ignore **intensity** of exercise. For muscles to develop, they have to be overloaded to a given point. The training stimulus to develop the biceps muscle, for example, can be accomplished with arm curl exercises with increasing weights. Likewise, the CR system is stimulated by making the heart pump faster for a specified period.

Health and CR fitness benefits result when the person is working between 30 and 90 percent of heart rate reserve (HRR) combined with an appropriate duration and

FITT-VP Acronym used to describe the four CR exercise prescription variables: frequency, intensity, type (mode), time (duration), volume, and progression.

Vigorous exercise CR exercise that requires an intensity level of approximately 70 percent of capacity.

Heart rate reserve (HRR) The difference between the MHR and the RHR.

Moderate-intensity exercise CR exercise that noticeably increases heart rate and breathing, one that requires an intensity level of approximately 50 percent of capacity.

Intensity In CR exercise, how hard a person has to exercise to improve or maintain fitness.

frequency of training (discussed next).[6] Health benefits are achieved when training at a lower exercise intensity, that is, between 30 and 60 percent of the person's HRR. Even greater health and cardioprotective benefits, as well as higher and faster improvements in CR fitness (VO_{2max}), are achieved primarily through vigorous programs.[7]

Most people who initiate exercise programs have a difficult time adhering to vigorous exercise. Thus, unconditioned individuals (those in the poor CR fitness category of Table 6.8) and older adults should start at a 30 to 40 percent training intensity (TI). For people in the fair fitness category, training is recommended between 40 and 50 percent TI. For those in the average category, a 50 to 60 percent TI is recommended. Active and fit people in the good category should exercise between 60 and 70 percent TI, while active people in the excellent fitness category can exercise at the higher TIs between 70 and 90 percent.

Following 4 to 8 weeks of progressive training (depending on your starting TI) at light to moderate (30 to 60 percent) intensities, exercise can be performed between 60 and 90 percent TI. Increases in VO_{2max} are accelerated when the heart is working closer to 90 percent of HRR. Exercise training above 90 percent is recommended only for healthy, performance-oriented individuals and competitive athletes. For most people, training above 90 percent is discouraged to avoid potential cardiovascular problems associated with very high-intensity exercise. As intensity increases, exercise adherence decreases and the risk of orthopedic injuries increases.

Intensity of exercise can be calculated easily, and training can be monitored by checking your pulse. To determine the intensity of exercise or **cardiorespiratory (CR) training zone** according to HRR, follow these steps (also refer to Lab 6D):

1. Estimate your MHR* according to the following formula[8]:

$$MHR = 207 - (.7 \times age)$$

2. Check your RHR for a full minute in the evening, after you have been sitting quietly for about 30 minutes reading or watching a relaxing TV show. As explained on page 225, you can check your pulse on the wrist by placing two fingers over the radial artery or in the neck, using the carotid artery.
3. Determine the HRR by subtracting the RHR from the MHR:

$$HRR = MHR - RHR$$

4. Calculate the TIs at 30, 40, 50, 60, 70, and 90 percent. Multiply the HRR by the respective .30, .40, .50, .60, .70, and .90, and then add the RHR to all four of these figures (e.g., 60% TI = HRR × .60 + RHR).

   Example. The 30, 40, 50, 60, 70, and 90 percent TIs for a 20-year-old with an RHR of 68 bpm would be as follows:

   MHR = 207 − (.70 × 20) = 193 bpm

   RHR = 68 bpm

   HRR = 193 − 68 = 125 beats

   30% TI = (125 × .30) + 68 = 106 bpm

   40% TI = (125 × .40) + 68 = 118 bpm

   50% TI = (125 × .50) + 68 = 131 bpm

   60% TI = (125 × .60) + 68 = 143 bpm

   70% TI = (125 × .70) + 68 = 155 bpm

   90% TI = (125 × .90) + 68 = 181 bpm

   Light-intensity CR training zone: 106 to 118 bpm

   Moderate-intensity CR training zone: 118 to 143 bpm

   Vigorous CR training zone: 143 to 181 bpm

Once you reach the vigorous-intensity CR training zone, continue to exercise between the 60 and 90 percent TIs to further improve or maintain your CR fitness (Figure 6.7).

Following a few weeks of training, you may have a considerably lower RHR (10 to 20 beats fewer in 8 to 12 weeks). Therefore, you should recompute your target zone periodically. You can compute your CR training zone using Lab 6D. Once you have reached an ideal level of CR endurance, frequent training in the 60 to 90 percent range allows you to maintain your fitness level.

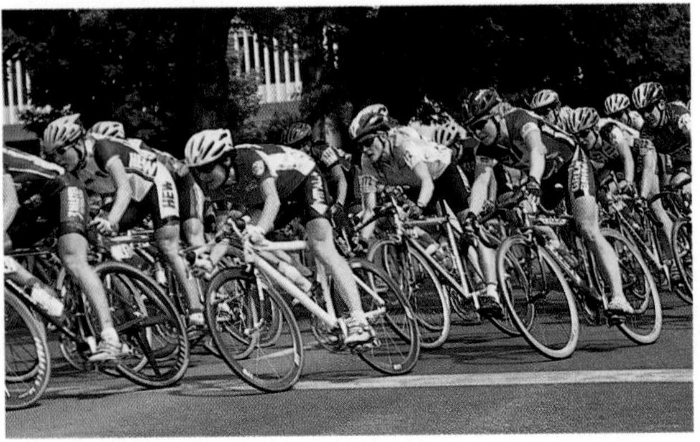

High-intensity exercise is required to achieve the high physical fitness standard (good or excellent category) for CR endurance.

Moderate- versus Vigorous-Intensity Exercise

As fitness programs became popular in the 1970s, vigorous exercise (about 70 percent TI) was routinely prescribed for all fitness participants. Following extensive research in the late 1980s and 1990s, we learned that moderate-intensity physical activity (about 50 percent TI) provided many health benefits, including decreased risk for cardiovascular mortality—a statement endorsed by the U.S. Surgeon General in 1996.[9] Thus, the emphasis switched from vigorous to moderate-intensity training in the late 1990s. In the 1996 report, the Surgeon General also stated that vigorous exercise would provide even greater benefits. Limited attention, however, was paid to this recommendation.

Vigorous-intensity programs yield higher improvements in VO_{2max} than do moderate-intensity programs, especially in people with higher fitness levels.[10] Furthermore, a comprehensive review of research articles looking at the protective benefits of physical fitness versus the weekly amount of physical activity found that higher levels of aerobic fitness are asso-

FIGURE 6.7 **Recommended cardiorespiratory or aerobic training pattern.**

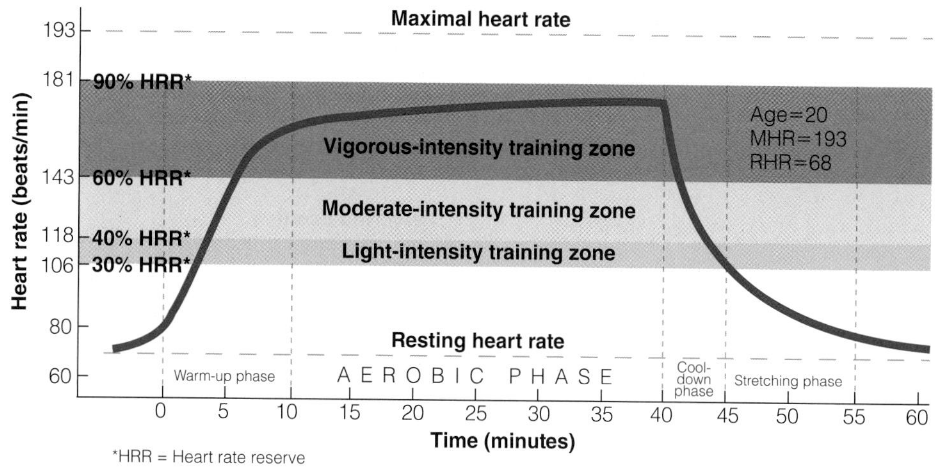

ciated with a lower incidence of cardiovascular disease (Figure 6.8), even when the duration of moderate-intensity activity is prolonged to match the energy expenditure performed during a shorter vigorous effort.[11] The results showed that people who accumulate the greatest amount of weekly physical activity (the 100th percentile rank in Figure 6.8), have a 28 percent reduction in the risk of cardiovascular disease; whereas the individuals with the highest level of aerobic fitness (also the 100th percentile rank in Figure 6.8) reduce their risk by 64 percent, more than twice the level of risk reduction in the most active group.

Another review of several clinical studies substantiated that vigorous, compared with moderate-intensity, exercise leads to better improvements in coronary heart disease risk factors, including aerobic endurance, blood pressure, and blood glucose control.[12] As a result, the pendulum is again swinging toward vigorous intensity because of the added aerobic benefits, greater protection against disease, and larger energy expenditure that helps with weight management.

Monitoring Exercise Heart Rate

During the first few weeks of an exercise program, you should monitor your exercise heart rate regularly to make sure you are training in the proper zone. Wait until you are about 5 minutes into the aerobic phase of your exercise session before taking your first reading. When you check your heart rate, count your pulse for 10 seconds, and then multiply by 6 to get the per minute pulse rate. The exercise heart rate will remain at the same level for about 15 seconds following aerobic exercise but then drop rapidly. Do not hesitate to stop during your exercise bout to check your pulse. If the rate is too low, increase the intensity of exercise. If the rate is too high, slow down.

When determining the TI for

Cardiorespiratory (CR) training zone Recommended TI range, in terms of exercise heart rate, to obtain adequate CR endurance development.

Health and Fitness Apps

An app is a software application designed to help the user perform a specific task related to accounting, graphics, office suites, education, media, music and entertainment, or health and fitness, among others. Be careful when selecting apps. Many people are designing apps with limited or no knowledge in the related field. When it comes to fitness, one size doesn't fit all, because fitness levels and needs vary widely among participants. An instructor or personal trainer may be a better option when getting started. If you are looking for apps, search for those designed by health and fitness experts who hold degrees and certifications in the related field. A good place to start is the government's app store (apps.usa.gov) that lists apps designed by experts.

Apps are now a part of our ever-changing world. As you search for a personal health/fitness app, take into consideration your desired activities and outcome, current fitness level, personal budget, and whether you wish to use a device other than your smart phone (wrist band, chest strap, clip on, arm band). Apps provide motivation, training guidance, activity tracking, nutrition recommendations, and health advice. Some apps involve a cost, while others are free. An Internet search can help identify apps in your area of need and interest. Among popular apps are MyFitnessPal, Hot5, Endomondo, GymPact, and RunKeeper.

As a consumer, you are strongly encouraged to research available apps and search for the best that fit your interests but still follow recommended exercise guidelines by leading national health, fitness, and sportsmedicine organizations.

FIGURE 6.8 Relative risk of cardiovascular disease (CVD) based on weekly volume of physical activity and aerobic fitness.

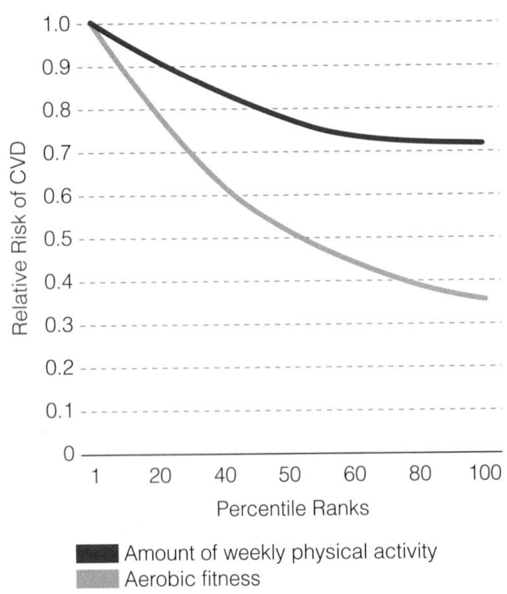

FIGURE 6.9 Physical activity perceived exertion scale.

The H-PAPE (Hoeger-Physical Activity Perceived Exertion) Scale provides a subjective rating of the perceived exertion or difficulty of physical activity and exercise when training at a given intensity level. The intensity level is associated with the corresponding perceived exertion phrase provided. These phases are based on common terminology used in physical activity and exercise prescription guidelines.

Perceived Exertion	Training Intensity
Light	40%
Moderate	50%
Somewhat hard	60%
Vigorous	70%
Hard	80%
Very hard	90%
All-out effort	100%

Source: Adapted from Werner W. K. Hoeger, "Training for a Walkathon," Diabetes Self-Management 24, no. 4 (2007):56–68.

your program, you need to consider your personal fitness goals and possible cardiovascular risk factors. Individuals who exercise around 50 percent TI still reap significant health benefits—in particular, improvements in the metabolic profile (see "Health Fitness Standards" in Chapter 1, page 20). Training at this lower percentage, however, may place you in only the "average" (moderate fitness) category (Table 6.8). Exercising at this lower intensity will not allow you to achieve a good or excellent CR endurance fitness rating (the physical fitness standard). The latter ratings, and even greater health benefits, are obtained by exercising closer to the 90 percent threshold.

Rate of Perceived Exertion

Because many people do not check their heart rate during exercise, an alternative method of prescribing intensity of exercise has been devised using the **physical activity perceived exertion (or H-PAPE) scale** (Figure 6.9). This scale uses phrases based on terminology common in physical activity and exercise prescription guidelines. Using the scale, a person subjectively rates the perceived exertion or difficulty of exercise when training at different intensity levels. The exercise heart rate then is associated with the corresponding perceived exertion phrase provided.

For example, if someone is training between 143 bpm (60 percent TI) and 155 bpm (70 percent TI), the person may associate this with training between "somewhat hard" and "vigorous." Some individuals perceive less exertion than others when training at a certain intensity level. Therefore, people have to associate their inner perception of the task with the phrases given on the scale. They then may proceed to exercise at that rate of perceived exertion.

Be sure to cross-check your target zone with your perceived exertion during the first weeks of your exercise program. To help you develop this association, you should regularly keep a record of your activities, using the form provided in Figure 6.12 (page 243). After several weeks of training, you should be able to predict your exercise heart rate just by your perceived exertion of the intensity of exercise.

Whether you monitor the intensity of exercise by checking your pulse or using the H-PAPE scale, you should be aware that changes in normal exercise conditions affect the TI. For example, exercising on a hot, humid day or at a high altitude increases the heart rate response to a given task, requiring adjustments in the intensity of your exercise.

Mode (type) of Exercise

The **mode**, or type, of exercise that develops the CR system has to be aerobic in nature. Once you have established your CR training zone, any activity or combination of activities that get your heart rate up to that zone and keep it there for as long as you exercise gives you adequate development. Examples of these activities are walking, jogging, elliptical activity, aerobics, water aerobics, road cycling, spinning, elliptical training, and stationary jogging or cycling. The latter activities require little skill to perform and can be enjoyed by most adults to improve health and fitness. Other aerobic activities, such as swimming, cross-country skiing, mountain cycling, rope skipping, racquetball, basketball, and soccer, can also be used and are recommended for individuals who already possess the skills to perform these activities or have adequate fitness to learn the necessary skills to safely perform them.

To be aerobic, exercise has to involve the major muscle groups of the body, and it has to be rhythmic and continuous. As the amount of muscle mass involved during exercise increases, so do the demands on the CR system. The activity you choose should be pleasant—based on your personal preferences, what you most enjoy doing, and your physical limita-

confidentconsumer

getting fit fast

A popular myth that is often pitched through mass media (TV infomercials, radio advertisements, the Internet, magazines, and newspapers) is the "get fit fast" gimmick. This myth has been built into mass marketing to deceive consumers into buying products that purportedly provide fast and miraculous results. Statements such as: the 10-minute fitness program, lose 16 pounds in a month, tone up in just 5 minutes a day, and fit into your bikini in just 30 days are often used to catch consumers' attention.

It is time to get over this quick-fix mentality. There are no shortcuts to fitness. If it sounds too good to be true, it is! Getting fit is a process that takes commitment and perseverance, to be done according to exercise guidelines. The American College of Sports Medicine guidelines for exercise prescription are quoted extensively throughout this book. They are quite clear as to the mode, intensity, duration, and frequency of exercise required to achieve optimal results. Thus, if you are looking to get in shape overnight or in just a few days, you are only setting yourself up for failure. Furthermore, 5 to 10 minutes of daily physical activity will not make a dent in the current obesity epidemic afflicting most developed countries throughout the world.

tions. Low-impact activities greatly reduce the risk for injuries. Most injuries to beginners result from high-impact activities. Also, general strength conditioning (see Chapter 7) is recommended prior to initiating an aerobic exercise program for individuals who have been inactive. Strength conditioning can significantly reduce the incidence of injuries.

The amount of strength or flexibility you develop through various activities differs. In terms of CR development, though, the heart doesn't know whether you are walking, swimming, or cycling. All the heart knows is that it has to pump at a certain rate, and as long as that rate is in the desired range, your CR fitness will improve. From a health fitness point of view, training in the lower end of the CR zone yields substantial health benefits. The closer the heart rate is to the higher end of the CR training zone, however, the greater the health benefits and improvements in VO_{2max} (high physical fitness).

Because of the specificity of training, to ascertain changes in fitness, it is recommended that you use the same mode of exercise for training and testing. If your primary mode of training is cycling, it is best to assess your VO_{2max} using a bicycle test. For joggers, a field or treadmill running test is ideal. Swimmers should use a swim test.

Duration (time) of Exercise The general recommendation is that a person exercise between 20 and 60 minutes per session. For vigorous-intensity exercise, a minimum of 75 total minutes per week are recommended, while those in a moderate-intensity program should accumulate at least 150 minutes per week.

The duration of exercise is based on how intensely a person trains. The variables are inversely related. If the training intensity is around 90 percent, a session of 20 to 30 minutes is sufficient. With intensity around 50 percent, the person should train close to 60 minutes. As mentioned in the section "Intensity of Exercise," an unconditioned person or older adult should train at a lower percentage; therefore, the activity should be carried out over a longer period.

Although the recommended guideline is 20 to 60 minutes of aerobic exercise per session, in the early stages of conditioning and for individuals who are pressed for time, accumulating 30 minutes or more of moderate-intensity physical activity throughout the day still provides health benefits. Three 10-minute exercise sessions per day, separated by at least 4 hours, and at approximately 70 percent of MHR, have been shown to produce training benefits.[13] Although the increases in VO_{2max} with the latter program were not as large (57 percent) as those found in a group performing a continuous 30-minute bout of exercise per day, the researchers concluded that the accumulation of 30 minutes of moderate-intensity physical activity, conducted for at least 10 minutes three times per day, benefits the CR system significantly. Activity bouts of less than 10 minutes in duration do not count toward the 30-minute daily guideline.

Results of this and other similar studies are meaningful because people often mention lack of time as the reason they do not take part in an exercise program. Many think they have to exercise at least 20 continuous minutes to get any benefits at all. Even though a duration of 20 to 30 minutes of continuous vigorous-intensity activity is ideal, short, intermittent physical activity bouts, of at least 10 minutes long each, are beneficial to the CR system.

The 2008 *Federal Guidelines for Physical Activity* measure duration of exercise in terms of the total quantity of physical activity performed on a weekly basis. Two hours and 30 minutes (150 minutes) of moderate-intensity aerobic activity or 1 hour and 15 minutes (75 minutes) of vigorous-intensity aerobic activity per week, or an equivalent combination of the two are recommended (30 minutes of moderate-intensity twice per week combined with 20 minutes of vigorous-intensity another two times per week).

Two hours and 30 minutes per week represents the accumulation of 30 minutes of moderate-intensity aerobic activity (done in bouts of at least 10 minutes each) per daily session performed 5 days per week, whereas 1 hour and 15 minutes is approximately 25 minutes of vigorous aerobic activity done three times per week.

Physical activity perceived exertion (or H-PAPE) scale A perception scale to monitor or interpret the intensity of aerobic exercise.

Mode Form or type of exercise.

The federal guidelines indicate that 5 hours of moderate-intensity activity, or 2 hours and 30 minutes of vigorous activity, per week provide additional benefits. Thus, when possible, people are encouraged to go beyond the minimum recommendation.

From a weight management point of view, the recommendation to prevent weight gain is for people to accumulate 60 minutes of moderate-intensity physical activity most days of the week,[14] whereas 60 to 90 minutes of daily moderate-intensity activity is necessary to prevent weight regain.[15] These recommendations are based on evidence that people who maintain healthy weight typically accumulate this amount of physical activity at least five times per week. The duration of exercise should be increased gradually to avoid undue fatigue and exercise-related injuries.

If lack of time is a concern, you should exercise at a vigorous intensity for about 30 minutes, which can burn as many calories as 60 minutes of moderate-intensity exercise (also see "The Role of Exercise Intensity and Duration in Weight Management," Chapter 5, page 185). Unfortunately, only 19 per cent of adults in the United States typically exercise at a vigorous intensity level. Novice and overweight exercisers also need proper conditioning prior to vigorous exercise to avoid injuries or cardiovascular-related problems.

Exercise sessions always should be preceded by a 5- to 10-minute **warm-up** and be followed by a 10-minute **cooldown** period (Figure 6.7). The purpose of the warm-up is to aid in the transition from rest to exercise. A good warm-up increases extensibility of the muscles and connective tissue, extends joint range of motion, and enhances muscular activity. A warm-up consists of general calisthenics, mild stretching exercises, and walking, jogging, or cycling for a few minutes at a lower intensity than the actual target zone. The concluding phase of the warm-up is a gradual increase in exercise intensity to the lower end of the target training zone.

In the cooldown, the intensity of exercise is decreased gradually to help the body return to near-resting levels, followed by stretching and relaxation activities. Stopping abruptly causes blood to pool in the exercised body parts, diminishing the return of blood to the heart. Less blood return can cause a sudden drop in blood pressure, dizziness and faintness, or cardiac abnormalities. The cooldown phase also helps dissipate body heat and remove the lactic acid produced during high-intensity exercise.

In its latest guidelines, the ACSM recommends at least 10 minutes of stretching exercises performed immediately following the warm-up phase (prior to exercising in the appropriate target zone) or after the cool-down phase. The purpose of stretching following either the warm-up or the cool-down phase is because warm muscles achieve a greater range of motion, thus helping enhance the flexibility program (discussed in Chapter 8). While two to three stretching sessions per week are recommended, near daily stretching is most effective.

Frequency of Exercise The recommended exercise **frequency** for aerobic exercise is 3 to 5 days per week. When performing vigorous-intensity exercise, three 20- to 30-minute exercise sessions per week, on nonconsecutive days, are sufficient to improve or maintain VO_{2max}. When exercising at a moderate intensity, 30 to 60 minutes 5 days per week are required. A combination of moderate- and vigorous-intensity may also be used 3 to 5 days per week. Research indicates that when vigorous training is conducted more than 5 days a week, further improvements in VO_{2max} are minimal. Although endurance athletes often train 6 or 7 days per week (often twice per day), their training programs are designed to increase training mileage to endure

BEHAVIOR MODIFICATION PLANNING

Tips for People Who Have Been Physically Inactive

I PLAN TO	I DID IT	
❏	❏	Take the sensible approach by starting slowly.
❏	❏	Begin by choosing moderate-intensity activities you enjoy the most. By choosing activities you enjoy, you'll be more likely to stick with them.
❏	❏	Gradually build up the time spent exercising by adding a few minutes every few days or so until you can comfortably perform a minimum recommended amount of exercise (30 minutes per day).
❏	❏	As the minimum amount becomes easier, gradually increase either the length of time exercising or increase the intensity of the activity, or both.
❏	❏	Vary your activities, both for interest and to broaden the range of benefits.
❏	❏	Explore new physical activities.
❏	❏	Reward and acknowledge your efforts.

Try It

Fill out the cardiorespiratory exercise prescription in Lab 6D either in your text or online. In your Online Journal or class notebook, describe how well you implement the above suggestions.

long-distance races (6 to 100 miles) at a high percentage of VO_{2max}, frequently at or above the **anaerobic threshold**.

Although three vigorous exercise sessions per week maintain CR fitness, when exercising at a moderate intensity, 30 to 60 minutes 5 days per week are recommended. The importance of almost daily physical activity in preventing disease and enhancing quality of life has been stated clearly by the ACSM, the U.S. Centers for Disease Control and Prevention, and the President's Council on Fitness, Sports & Nutrition. These organizations, along with the U.S. Surgeon General, advocate at least 30 minutes of moderate-intensity physical activity on most (defined as 5 days) or preferably all days of the week. This routine has been promoted as an effective way to improve health and quality of life. Furthermore, the Surgeon General states that no one, including older adults, is too old to enjoy the benefits of regular physical activity. Also, be aware that most benefits of exercise and activity diminish within 2 weeks of substantially decreased physical activity and the benefits are lost within a few months of inactivity.

"Physical Stillness:" A Deadly Proposition

As introduced in Chapters 1 and 2 under "Sitting Disease" (page 13) and "Environmental Influences on Physical Activity" (pages 46–48), if you meet the guidelines and you are physically active five times per week, but spend most of your day sitting, your sedentary lifestyle may be voiding the health benefits of exercise. The nature of our society nowadays is such that physical activity is not required in our environment. Even people with excellent exercise habits tend to spend most of the remainder of their day in a sedentary environment: commuting to and from work, riding escalators and elevators, sitting behind a desk, sitting at a computer, reading, watching TV, and lying down. In essence, people spend most of their non-exercise time not moving.

If you are physically active or exercise seven times per week for 30 minutes a day, you will accumulate 210 weekly minutes of intentional activity. Even though you perceive yourself as being physically active because of the daily 30 minutes of activity, the issue at hand is the physical stillness the rest of the day. Two hundred and ten minutes translates into just 2 percent of the total 10,080 minutes available to you on a weekly basis. Thus, the difference between a regular exerciser and a sedentary individual is 30 minutes of activity per day. The other 98 percent of the time, most exercisers and sedentary people spend their time in very similar non-moving activities. Research indicates that people who spend most of their day sitting have a greater risk of dying prematurely from all causes and an even greater risk of dying from cardiovascular disease.[16] The data further indicate that death rates are still high for people who spend most of their day sitting, even though they meet the current minimum moderate-physical activity recommendations (30 minutes, at least five times per week).[17]

Hypokinetic diseases are the result of a sedentary lifestyle. Thirty daily minutes of activity per day are certainly a good step toward decreasing absolute sedentarism, but it's only a small step. Your challenge is not only to exercise for a minimum of 30 minutes on most days of the week, but to consciously incorporate as much physical activity throughout the day as possible—at least 10 minutes every waking hour of the day. To meet this challenge, a change in attitude is required on your part. Your frame of mind should be: *"I do not fear nor will I avoid physical activity: Bring it on!"* Learn to move as much as possible all through the day for health, quality of life, wellness, and a long life.

Exercise Volume A relatively new concept, volume of exercise is the product of frequency, intensity, and duration. The recommended absolute minimum volume is an energy expenditure of 1,000 calories per week or the equivalent of 150 minutes of moderate-intensity exercise each week. Volume can also be measured using a pedometer and achieving 10,000 or more steps each day. This minimal amount of volume is essential to achieve health benefits and adequate body composition. A minimum of 75 minutes of vigorous-intensity activity, along with at least 2 days of 30 minutes of moderate intensity is required for substantial fitness benefits. Training volume is also used as an indicator of excessive exercise. Too much exercise and physical activity leads to overtraining, muscle soreness, undue fatigue, shortness of breath, and increase risk for injury. Should you experience any adverse effects as a result of your physical activity/exercise program, downward adjustments are recommended to the exercise prescription, including the rate of exercise progression (discussed next).

Rate of Progression How quickly an individual progresses through an exercise program depends on the person's health status, fitness status, exercise tolerance, training responses, and exercise program goals. Initially, only three weekly training sessions of 15 to 20 minutes are recommended to avoid excessive muscle soreness and musculoskeletal injuries. You may then increase the duration by 5 to 10 minutes per week and the frequency so that by the fourth or fifth week you are exercising five times per week (see Lab 6D). Thereafter, you can adjust frequency, duration, and intensity of exercise until you reach your fitness and maintenance goals. All increases in FITT-VP variables should be gradual to minimize the risk of overtraining and injuries.

To sum up: Ideally, a person should engage in physical activity six or seven times per week. Based

Warm-up Starting a workout slowly.

Cooldown Tapering off an exercise session slowly.

Frequency Number of times per week a person engages in exercise.

Anaerobic threshold The highest percentage of VO_{2max} at which an individual can exercise (maximal steady state) for an extended time without accumulating significant amounts of lactic acid, which forces an individual to reduce exercise intensity or stop exercising.

FIGURE 6.10 **The physical activity pyramid.**

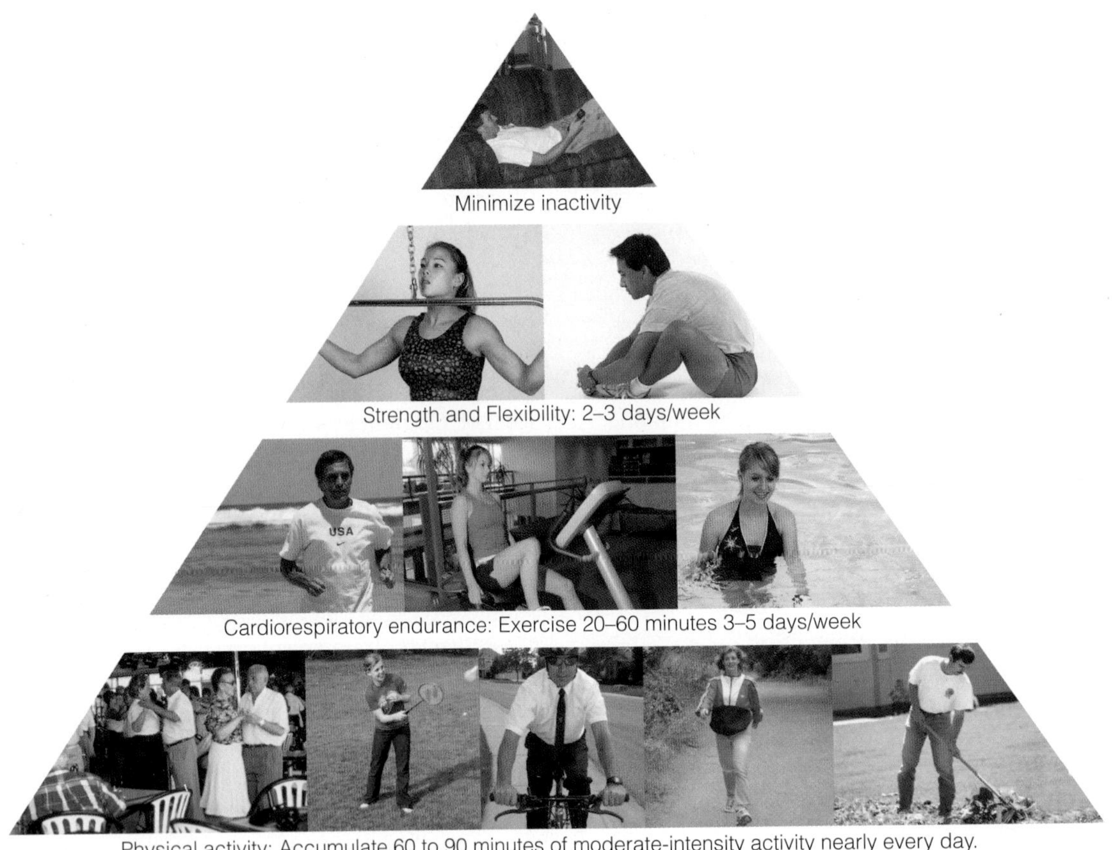
Minimize inactivity
Strength and Flexibility: 2–3 days/week
Cardiorespiratory endurance: Exercise 20–60 minutes 3–5 days/week
Physical activity: Accumulate 60 to 90 minutes of moderate-intensity activity nearly every day.

on the previous discussion, to reap both the high physical fitness and the health fitness benefits of exercise, a person should do vigorous exercise three times per week for high physical fitness maintenance and two to four additional times per week in moderate-intensity activities (Figure 6.10) to maintain good health. Depending on the intensity of the activity and the health and fitness goals, all exercise sessions should last between 20 and 60 minutes. For adequate weight-management purposes, additional daily physical activity, up to 90 minutes, may be necessary. A summary of the CR exercise prescription guidelines according to the ACSM is provided in Figure 6.11.

Fitness Benefits of Aerobic Activities

The contributions of different aerobic activities to the health-related components of fitness vary. Although an accurate assessment of the contributions to each fitness component is difficult to establish, a summary of likely benefits of several activities is provided in Table 6.10. Instead of a single rating or number, ranges are given for some categories. The benefits derived are based on the person's effort while participating in the activity.

FIGURE 6.11 **Cardiorespiratory exercise prescription guidelines.**

Mode: Moderate- or vigorous-intensity aerobic activity (examples: walking, jogging, stair climbing, elliptical activity, aerobics, water aerobics, cycling, stair climbing, swimming, cross-country skiing, racquetball, basketball, and soccer)

Intensity: 30% to 90% of heart rate reserve (the training intensity is based on age, health status, initial fitness level, exercise tolerance, and exercise program goals)

Duration: Be active 20 to 90 minutes. At least 20 minutes of continuous vigorous-intensity or 30 minutes of moderate-intensity aerobic activity (the latter may be accumulated in segments of at least 10 minutes in duration each over the course of the day)

Frequency: 3 to 5 days per week for vigorous-intensity aerobic activity to accumulate at least 75 minutes per week, or 5 days per week of moderate-intensity aerobic activity for a minimum total of 150 minutes weekly

Rate of progression:

- Start with three training sessions per week of 15 to 20 minutes
- Increase the duration by 5 to 10 minutes per week and the frequency so that by the fourth or fifth week you are exercising five times per week
- Progressively increase frequency, duration, and intensity of exercise until you reach your fitness goal prior to exercise maintenance

Source: Adapted from American College of Sports Medicine, *ACSM's Guidelines for Exercise Testing and Prescription* (Philadelphia: Wolters Kluwer/Lippincott Williams & Wilkins, 2014).

Table 6.10 **Ratings of Selected Aerobic Activities**

Activity	Recommended Starting Fitness Level[1]	Injury Risk[2]	Potential Cardiorespiratory Endurance Development (VO_{2MAX})[3,4]	Upper Body Strength Development[3]	Lower Body Strength Development[3]	Upper Body Flexibility Development[3]	Lower Body Flexibility Development[3]	Weight Management[3]	MET Level[4,5,6]	Caloric Expenditure (cal/hour)[4,6]
Aerobics										
High-Impact Aerobics	A	H	3–4	2	4	3	2	4	6–12	450–900
Moderate-Impact Aerobics	I	M	2–4	2	3	3	2	3	6–12	450–900
Low-Impact Aerobics	B	L	2–4	2	3	3	2	3	5–10	375–750
Step Aerobics	I	M	2–4	2	3–4	3	2	3–4	5–12	375–900
Circuit Training	B	M	2-3	3-4	3-4	2	2-3	3-4	5-12	375-900
Cross-Country Skiing	B	M	4–5	4	4	2	2	4–5	8–16	600–1,200
Cross-Training	I	M	3–5	2–3	3–4	2–3	1–2	3–5	6–15	450–1,125
Cycling										
Road	I	M	2–5	1	4	1	1	3	6–12	450–900
Stationary	B	L	2–4	1	4	1	1	3	6–10	450–750
Elliptical training/Stair Climbing	B	L	3–5	1	4	1	1	4–5	8–15	600–1,125
Functional Fitness	B	L	2-3	2-3	2-3	2-3	2-3	2-3	5-10	375-750
High-Intensity Interval Training	I	M	4-5	2	3-4	1	1	4-5	8-16	600-1,200
Jogging	I	M	3–5	1	3	1	1	5	6–15	450–1,125
Jogging, Deep Water	I	L	3–5	2	2	1	1	5	5–12	375–900
Racquet Sports	I	M	2–4	3	3	3	2	3	6–10	450–750
Rowing	B	L	3–5	4	2	3	1	4	8–14	600–1,050
Strength Training	B	L	1	4-5	4-5	2-3	2-3	3-4	4-8	300-600
Swimming (front crawl)	B	L	3–5	4	2	3	1	3	6–12	450–900
Walking	B	L	1–2	1	2	1	1	3	4–6	300–450
Walking, Water, Chest-Deep	I	L	2–4	2	3	1	1	3	5–10	375–750
Water Aerobics	B	L	2–4	3	3	3	2	3	6–10	450–750
Yoga	B	L	1	1-2	1-2	3-5	3-5	1-3	4-8	300-600
Zumba	B	M	3-4	2	3	3	2	3-4	6-12	450-900

[1]B = Beginner, I = Intermediate, A = Advanced
[2]L = Low, M = Moderate, H = High
[3]1 = Low, 2 = Fair, 3 = Average, 4 = Good, 5 = Excellent
[4]Varies according to the person's effort (intensity) during exercise.
[5]1 MET represents the rate of energy expenditure at rest (3.5 mL/kg/min). Each additional MET is a multiple of the resting value. For example, 5 METs represents an energy expenditure equivalent to five times the resting value, or about 17.5 mL/kg/min.
[6]Varies according to body weight.

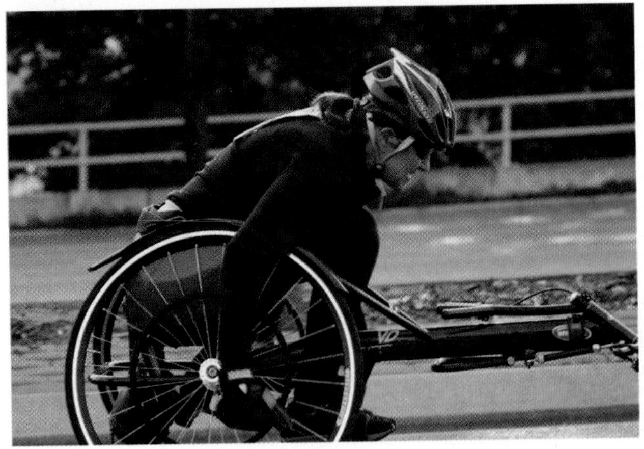

© Fitness & Wellness, Inc.

Physically challenged people can participate in and derive health and fitness benefits through a vigorous-intensity exercise program.

The nature of the activity often dictates the potential aerobic development. For example, jogging is more strenuous than walking. The effort during exercise also affects the amount of physiological development. For example, during a low-impact aerobics routine, accentuating all movements (instead of just going through the motions) increases training benefits by orders of magnitude.

Table 6.10 indicates a starting fitness level for each aerobic activity. Attempting to participate in vigorous activities without proper conditioning often leads to injuries, not to mention discouragement. Beginners should start with light-intensity activities that carry a minimum risk for injuries.

In some cases, such as high-impact aerobics and rope skipping, the risk for orthopedic injuries remains high even if the participants are adequately conditioned. These activities should be supplemental only and are not recommended as the sole mode of exercise. Most exercise-related injuries occur as a result of high-impact activities, not high intensity of exercise.

An alternative method of prescribing exercise intensity is through **metabolic equivalents (METs)**. One MET represents the rate of energy expenditure at rest, that is, 3.5 mL/kg/min. METs are used to measure the intensity of physical activity and exercise in multiples of the resting metabolic rate. At an intensity level of 10 METs, the activity requires a 10-fold increase in the resting energy requirement (or approximately 35 mL/kg/min). MET levels for a given activity vary according to the effort expended. The MET range for various activities is included in Table 6.10. The harder a person exercises, the higher the MET level.

The effectiveness of various aerobic activities in weight management is also charted in Table 6.10. As a rule, the greater the muscle mass involved in exercise, the better the results. Rhythmic and continuous activities that involve large amounts of muscle mass are most effective in burning calories.

CRITICAL THINKING

Mary started an exercise program last year as a means to lose weight and enhance her body image. She now runs about six miles every day, strength-trains daily, participates in step aerobics twice per week, and plays tennis or racquetball twice a week. Evaluate her program and make suggestions for improvements.

Vigorous activities increase caloric expenditure as well. Exercising longer, however, compensates for lower intensities. If carried out long enough (45 to 60 minutes five or six times per week), even walking can be a good exercise mode for weight management. Additional information on a comprehensive weight management program was given in Chapter 5.

Getting Started and Adhering to a Lifetime Exercise Program

Following the guidelines provided in Lab 6D, you may proceed to initiate your own CR endurance program. If you have not been exercising regularly, you might begin by attempting to train five or six times a week for 30 minutes at a time. You might find this discouraging and be tempted to drop out before getting too far, because you will probably develop some muscle soreness and stiffness and possibly incur minor injuries. However, muscle soreness and stiffness and the risk for injuries can be lessened or eliminated by increasing the intensity, duration, and frequency of exercise progressively, as outlined in Lab 6D.

Once you have determined your exercise prescription, the difficult part begins: starting and sticking to a lifetime exercise program. Although you may be motivated after reading about the benefits to be gained from physical activity, lifelong dedication and perseverance are necessary to reap and maintain good fitness. Just reading and thinking about fitness will not provide benefits; you need active participation to derive benefits.

The first few weeks probably will be the most difficult for you, but where there's a will, there's a way. Once you begin to see positive changes, it won't be as hard. Soon you will develop a habit of exercising that will be deeply satisfying and will bring about a sense of self-accomplishment. The suggestions provided in the accompanying Behavior Modification Planning box (see page 244) have been used successfully to help people change behavior and adhere to a lifetime exercise program.

Metabolic equivalent (MET) Rate of energy expenditure at rest; 1 MET is the equivalent of a VO_2 of 3.5 mL/kg/min.

FIGURE 6.12 Cardiorespiratory Exercise Record Form.

Name: ______________ Date: __________ Course: __________ Section: __________ Gender: ________ Age: ________

Month ____________

Date	Body Weight	Exercise Heart Rate	Type of Activity	Distance in Miles	Time Minutes	H-PAPE*	Daily Steps
1							
2							
3							
4							
5							
6							
7							
8							
9							
10							
11							
12							
13							
14							
15							
16							
17							
18							
19							
20							
21							
22							
23							
24							
25							
26							
27							
28							
29							
30							
31							
			Total				

*Physical activity perceived exertion.

Month ____________

Date	Body Weight	Exercise Heart Rate	Type of Activity	Distance in Miles	Time Minutes	H-PAPE*	Daily Steps
1							
2							
3							
4							
5							
6							
7							
8							
9							
10							
11							
12							
13							
14							
15							
16							
17							
18							
19							
20							
21							
22							
23							
24							
25							
26							
27							
28							
29							
30							
31							
			Total				

*Physical activity perceived exertion.

BEHAVIOR MODIFICATION PLANNING

Tips to Enhance Exercise Compliance

I PLAN TO | I DID IT

❑ ❑ 1. Set aside a regular time for exercise. If you don't plan ahead, it is a lot easier to skip. On a weekly basis, using red ink, schedule your exercise time into your day planner. Next, hold your exercise hour "sacred." Give exercise priority equal to the most important school or business activity of the day.

If you are too busy, attempt to accumulate 30 to 60 minutes of daily activity by doing separate 10-minute sessions throughout the day. Try reading the mail while you walk, taking stairs instead of elevators, walking the dog, or riding the stationary bike as you watch the evening news.

❑ ❑ 2. Exercise early in the day, when you will be less tired and the chances of something interfering with your workout are minimal; thus, you will be less likely to skip your exercise session.

❑ ❑ 3. Select aerobic activities you enjoy. Exercise should be as much fun as your favorite hobby. If you pick an activity you don't enjoy, you will be unmotivated and less likely to keep exercising. Don't be afraid to try out a new activity, even if that means learning new skills.

❑ ❑ 4. Combine different activities. You can train by doing two or three different activities the same week. This cross-training may reduce the monotony of repeating the same activity every day. Try lifetime sports. Many endurance sports, such as racquetball, basketball, soccer, badminton, roller skating, cross-country skiing, and body surfing (paddling the board), provide a nice break from regular workouts.

❑ ❑ 5. Use the proper clothing and equipment for exercise. A poor pair of shoes, for example, can make you more prone to injury, discouraging you from the beginning.

❑ ❑ 6. Find a friend or group of friends to exercise with. Social interaction will make exercise more fulfilling. Besides, exercise is harder to skip if someone is waiting to go with you.

❑ ❑ 7. Set goals and share them with others. Quitting is tougher when someone else knows what you are trying to accomplish. When you reach a targeted goal, reward yourself with a new pair of shoes or a jogging suit.

❑ ❑ 8. Purchase a pedometer (step counter) and build up to 10,000 steps per day. These 10,000 steps may include all forms of daily physical activity combined. Pedometers motivate people toward activity because they track daily activity, provide feedback on activity level, and remind the participant to enhance daily activity.

❑ ❑ 9. Don't become a chronic exerciser. Overexercising can lead to chronic fatigue and injuries. Exercise should be enjoyable, and in the process you should stop and smell the roses.

❑ ❑ 10. Exercise in different places and facilities. This will add variety to your workouts.

❑ ❑ 11. Exercise to music. People who listen to fast-tempo music tend to exercise more vigorously and longer. Using headphones when exercising outdoors, however, can be dangerous. Even indoors, it is preferable not to use headphones so that you are still aware of your surroundings.

❑ ❑ 12. Keep a regular record of your activities. Keeping a record allows you to monitor your progress and compare it against previous months and years (see Figure 6.12, page 243).

❑ ❑ 13. Conduct periodic assessments. Improving to a higher fitness category is often a reward in itself, and creating your own rewards is even more motivating.

❑ ❑ 14. Listen to your body. If you experience pain or unusual discomfort, stop exercising. Pain and aches are an indication of potential injury. If you do suffer an injury, don't return to your regular workouts until you are fully recovered. You may cross-train using activities that don't aggravate your injury (e.g., swimming instead of jogging).

❑ ❑ 15. If a health problem arises, see a physician. When in doubt, it's better to be safe than sorry.

Try It

The most difficult challenge about exercise is to keep going once you start. The above behavioral change tips will enhance your chances for exercise adherence. In your Online Journal or class notebook, describe which suggestions were most useful.

A Lifetime Commitment to Fitness

The benefits of fitness can be maintained only through a regular lifetime program. Exercise is not like putting money in the bank. It doesn't help much to exercise 4 or 5 hours on Saturday and not do anything else the rest of the week. If anything, exercising only once a week is not safe for unconditioned adults.

The time involved in losing the benefits of exercise varies among the components of physical fitness and depends on the person's condition before the interruption. In regard to CR endurance, it has been estimated that 4 weeks of aerobic training are reversed in 2 consecutive weeks of physical inactivity. But if someone has been exercising regularly for months or years, 2 weeks of inactivity won't hurt that person as much as it will someone who has exercised only a few weeks. As a rule, after 48 to 72 hours of aerobic inactivity, the CR system starts to lose some of its capacity.

To maintain fitness, you should keep up a regular exercise program, even during vacations. If you have to interrupt your program for reasons beyond your control, you should not attempt to resume training at the same level you left off; rather, build up gradually again.

Even the greatest athletes, if they were to stop exercising, would be around the same risk for disease after just a few years as someone who has never done any physical activity. Staying with a physical fitness program long enough brings about positive physiological and psychological changes. Once you are there, you will not want to have it any other way.

ASSESS YOUR BEHAVIOR

1. Do you consciously attempt to incorporate as much physical activity as possible in your daily living (walk, take stairs, cycle, participate in sports and recreational activities)?
2. Are you accumulating at least 30 minutes of moderate intensity physical activity over a minimum of five days per week?
3. Is aerobic exercise in the appropriate target zone a priority in your life a minimum of three times per week for at least 20 minutes per exercise session?
4. Do you own a pedometer and do you accumulate 10,000 or more steps on most days of the week?
5. Have you evaluated your aerobic fitness, and do you meet at least the health fitness category?

ASSESS YOUR KNOWLEDGE

1. CR endurance is determined by
   a. the amount of oxygen the body is able to utilize per minute of physical activity.
   b. the length of time it takes the heart rate to return to 120 bpm following the 1.5-Mile Run Test.
   c. the difference between the MHR and the RHR.
   d. the product of heart rate and blood pressure at rest versus exercise.
   e. the time it takes a person to reach a heart rate between 120 and 170 bpm during the Astrand-Ryhming Test.
2. Which of the following is not a benefit of aerobic training?
   a. higher VO_{2max}
   b. increase in red blood cell count
   c. decrease in RHR
   d. increase in heart rate at a given workload
   e. increase in functional capillaries
3. The VO_2 for a person with an exercise heart rate of 130 bpm, a stroke volume of 100 mL, and an $a\text{-}\bar{v}O_{2diff}$ of 10 mL per 100 mL is
   a. 130,000 mL/kg/min.
   b. 1,300 L/min.
   c. 1.3 L/min.
   d. 130 mL/kg/min.
   e. 13 mL/kg/min.
4. The VO_2 in mL/kg/min for a person with a VO_2 of 2.0 L/min who weighs 60 kilograms is
   a. 120 mL/kg/min.
   b. 26.5 mL/kg/min.
   c. 33.3 mL/kg/min.
   d. 30 mL/kg/min.
   e. 120,000 mL/kg/min.
5. The Step Test estimates VO_{2max} according to
   a. how long a person is able to sustain the proper Step Test cadence.
   b. the lowest heart rate achieved during the test.
   c. the recovery heart rate following the test.
   d. the difference between the MHR achieved and the RHR.
   e. the exercise heart rate and the total stepping time.
6. An "excellent" CR fitness rating for young male adults is about
   a. 10 mL/kg/min.
   b. 20 mL/kg/min.
   c. 30 mL/kg/min.
   d. 40 mL/kg/min.
   e. 50 mL/kg/min.

7. How many minutes would a person training at 2.0 L/min have to exercise to burn the equivalent of one pound of fat?
   a. 700 minutes
   b. 350 minutes
   c. 120 minutes
   d. 60 minutes
   e. 20 minutes
8. The vigorous CR training zone for a 22-year-old individual with an RHR of 68 bpm is
   a. 120 to 148 bpm.
   b. 132 to 156 bpm.
   c. 138 to 164 bpm.
   d. 142 to 180 bpm.
   e. 154 to 188 bpm.
9. Which of the following activities does not contribute to the development of CR endurance?
   a. light-impact aerobics
   b. jogging
   c. 400-yard dash
   d. racquetball
   e. All of these activities contribute to its development.
10. The recommended duration for each CR training session is
   a. 10 to 20 minutes.
   b. 15 to 30 minutes.
   c. 20 to 60 minutes.
   d. 45 to 70 minutes.
   e. 60 to 120 minutes.

Correct answers can be found at the back of the book.

NOTES

1. R. B. O'Hara et al., "Increased Volume Resistance Training: Effects upon Predicted Aerobic Fitness in a Select Group of Air Force Men," *ACSM's Health & Fitness Journal* 8, no. 4 (2004): 16–25.
2. American College of Sports Medicine, *ACSM's Guidelines for Exercise Testing and Prescription* (Philadelphia: Wolters Kluwer/ Lippincott Williams & Wilkins, 2014).
3. U.S. Department of Health and Human Services, *Physical Activity and Health: A Report of the Surgeon General* (Atlanta, GA: Centers for Disease Control and Prevention, National Center for Chronic Disease Prevention and Health Promotion, 1996).
4. American College of Sports Medicine, "Quantity and Quality of Exercise for Developing and Maintaining Cardiorespiratory, Musculoskeletal, and Neuromotor Fitness in Apparently Healthy Adults: Guidance for Prescribing Exercise," *Medicine & Science in Sports & Exercise* 43 (2011): 1334–1359.
5. See note 2.
6. See note 2.
7. S. E. Gormley et al., "Effect of Intensity of Aerobic Training on VO_{2max}," *Medicine & Science in Sports & Exercise* 40 (2008): 1336–1343.
8. R. L. Gellish et al., "Longitudinal Modeling of the Relationship between Age and Maximal Heart Rate," *Medicine & Science in Sports & Exercise* 39 (2007): 822–829.
9. See note 3.
10. D. P. Swain, "Moderate or Vigorous Intensity Exercise: Which Is Better for Improving Aerobic Fitness?" *Preventive Cardiology* 8, no. 1 (2005): 55–58.
11. P. T. Williams, "Physical Fitness and Activity as Separate Heart Disease Risk Factors: A Meta-analysis," *Medicine & Science in Sports & Exercise* 33 (2001): 754–761.
12. D. P. Swain and B. A. Franklin, "Comparative Cardioprotective Benefits of Vigorous vs. Moderate Intensity Aerobic Exercise," *American Journal of Cardiology* 97, no. 1 (2006): 141–147.
13. R. F. DeBusk, U. Stenestrand, M. Sheehan, and W. L. Haskell, "Training Effects of Long Versus Short Bouts of Exercise in Healthy Subjects," *American Journal of Cardiology* 65 (1990): 1010–1013.
14. National Academy of Sciences, Institute of Medicine, *Dietary Reference Intakes for Energy, Carbohydrates, Fiber, Fat, Protein and Amino Acids (Macronutrients)* (Washington, DC: National Academy Press, 2002).
15. U.S. Department of Health and Human Services and U.S. Department of Agriculture, *Dietary Guidelines for Americans 2005* (Washington, DC: DHHS, 2005).
16. W. Dunstan et al., "Television Viewing Time and Mortality: The Australian Diabetes, Obesity, and Lifestyle Study (AusDiab)," *Circulation* 121 (2010): 384–391.
17. P. T. Katzmarzyk et al., "Sitting Time and Mortality from All Causes, Cardiovascular Disease, and Cancer," *Medicine & Science in Sports & Exercise* 41 (2009): 998–1005.
18. See note 2.

SUGGESTED READINGS

American College of Sports Medicine. *ACSM's Guidelines for Exercise Testing and Prescription*. Philadelphia: Wolters Kluwer/Lippincott Williams & Wilkins, 2014.

American College of Sports Medicine. *ACSM's Resource Manual for Guidelines for Exercise Testing and Prescription*. Philadelphia: Wolters Kluwer/ Lippincott Williams & Wilkins, 2014.

Hoeger, W. W. K., and S. A. Hoeger. *Fitness and Wellness*. Belmont, CA: Wadsworth/Cengage Learning, 2015.

Hoeger, W. W. K., and S. A. Hoeger. *Lifetime Physical Fitness & Wellness*. Belmont, CA: Wadsworth/ Cengage Learning, 2015.

Karvonen, M. J., E. Kentala, and O. Mustala. "The Effects of Training on the Heart Rate: A Longitudinal Study," *Annales Medicinae Experimetalis et Biologiae Fenniae* 35 (1957): 307-315.

McArdle, W. D., F. I. Katch, and V. L. Katch. *Exercise Physiology: Energy, Nutrition, and Human Performance*, 5th ed. Philadelphia: Wolters Kluwer/Lippincott Williams & Wilkins, 2014.

Nieman, D. C. *Exercise Testing and Prescription: A Health-Related Approach*. Boston: McGraw-Hill, 2011.

Wilmore, J. H., and D. L. Costill. *Physiology of Sport and Exercise*. Champaign, IL: Human Kinetics, 2012.

Lab 6A: Cardiorespiratory Endurance Assessment

Name ______________________ Date ____________ Grade ____________

Instructor ______________________ Course ____________ Section ____________

NECESSARY LAB EQUIPMENT

1.5-Mile Run: School track or premeasured course and a stopwatch.

1.0-Mile Walk Test: School track or premeasured course and a stopwatch.

STEP TEST: A bench or gymnasium bleachers 16¼ inches high, a metronome, and a stopwatch.

ASTRAND-RYHMING TEST: A bicycle ergometer that allows for regulation of workloads in kilopounds per meter (or watts) and a stopwatch.

12-MINUTE SWIM TEST: Swimming pool and a stopwatch.

OBJECTIVE

To estimate maximal oxygen uptake (VO_{2max}) and cardiorespiratory endurance classification.

LAB PREPARATION

Wear appropriate exercise clothing including jogging shoes and a swimsuit if required. Be prepared to take the 1.0-Mile Walk Test, the Step Test, the Astrand–Ryhming Test, the 1.5-Mile Run Test, and/or the 12-Minute Swim Test. If more than one test will be conducted, perform them in the order just listed and allow at least 15 minutes between tests. Avoid vigorous physical activity 24 hours prior to this lab.

I. 1.5-Mile Run Test

1.5-Mile Run Time: ________ min and ________ sec VO_{2max} (see Table 6.2, page 226): ________ mL/kg/min

Cardiorespiratory Fitness Category (Table 6.8, page 231): ______________________

II. 1.0-Mile Walk Test

Weight (W) = ________ lbs Gender (G) = _____ (female = 0, male = 1) Time = _____ min and _____ sec

Heart Rate (HR) = ________ bpm

Time in minutes (T) = min + (sec ÷ 60) or T = ________ + (________ ÷ 60) = ________ min

VO_{2max} = 88.768 – (0.0957 × W) + (8.892 × G) – (1.4537 × T) – (0.1194 × HR)

VO_{2max} = 88.768 – (0.0957 × _____) + (8.892 × _____) – (1.4537 × ________) – (0.1194 × ________)

VO_{2max} = 88.768 – (________) + (________) – (________) – (________) = ________ mL/kg/min

Cardiorespiratory Fitness Category (Table 6.8, page 231): ______________________

III. Step Test

15-second recovery heart rate: ________ beats VO_{2max} (Table 6.3, page 227): ________ mL/kg/min

Cardiorespiratory Fitness Category (Table 6.8, page 231): ______________________

IV. Astrand–Ryhming Test

Weight (W) = ________ lbs   Weight (BW) in kilograms = (W ÷ 2.2046) = ________ kg   Workload = ________ kpm

Excercise Heart Rates	Time to count 30 beats	Heart Rate (bpm) (from Table 6.4, page 229)		Time to count 30 beats	Heart Rate (bpm) (from Table 6.4, page 229)
First minute:			Fourth minute:		
Second minute:			Fifth minute:		
Third minute:			Sixth minute:		

Average heart rate for the fifth and sixth minutes = ________ bpm

VO_{2max} in L/min (Table 6.5, page 230) = ________ L min   Correction factor (from Table 6.6, page 231) = ________

Corrected VO_{2max} = VO_{2max} in L/min × correction factor = ________ × ________ = ________ L/min

VO_{2max} in mL/kg/min = corrected VO_{2max} in L/min × 1000 ÷ BW in kg = ______ × 1000 ÷ ______ = ______ mL/kg/min

Cardiorespiratory Fitness Category (Table 6.8, page 231): ____________________

V. 12-Minute Swim Test

Distance swum in 12 minutes: ________ yards

Cardiorespiratory Fitness Category (Table 6.7, page 231): ____________________

VI. What I Learned and Where I Go from Here:

1. Interpret the results of your cardiorespiratory endurance test(s). Indicate the cardiorespiratory fitness classification you would like to achieve by the end of the term and explain how you are planning to achieve this goal.

____

____

____

____

____

____

____

2. Briefly discuss the advantages and disadvantages of the cardiorespiratory endurance tests used in this lab.

____

____

____

____

____

____

____

Lab 6B: Caloric Expenditure and Exercise Heart Rate

Name ______________________ Date __________ Grade __________

Instructor ______________________ Course __________ Section __________

NECESSARY LAB EQUIPMENT

A school track (or premeasured course) and a stopwatch. Each student also should bring a watch with a second hand.

OBJECTIVE

To monitor exercise heart rate and determine the caloric cost of physical activity based on exercise heart rate.

LAB PREPARATION

Wear exercise clothing, including jogging shoes. Do not engage in vigorous physical activity prior to this lab. Read the information on predicting oxygen uptake and caloric expenditure in this chapter, pages 230–232.

Procedure

1. **Cardiorespiratory Training Zone.** Look up your cardiovascular training zone at 60 percent and 85 percent of heart rate reserve in Lab 6D. Record this information in beats per minute (bpm) and in 10-second pulse counts in the blank spaces provided below.

		Beats/minute	10-sec count
60% intensity	=		
85% intensity	=		

2. **Resting Heart Rate (HR) and Body Weight (BW).** Determine your resting HR prior to exercise and your body weight in kilograms (divide pounds by 2.2046).

Resting HR: ______ bpm

BW: ______ lbs ÷ 2.2046 = ______ kg

3. **Walking HR, Oxygen Uptake (VO_2), and Caloric Expenditure.** Walk two laps around a 400-meter (440-yard) track at an average speed of 75 to 100 meters per minute. Try to maintain a constant speed around the track. You can monitor your speed by starting the walk at the beginning of the 100-meter straightway and making sure you have walked at least 75 meters and no more than 100 meters in one minute. As soon as you complete the two laps (800 meters), notice the time required to walk this distance and immediately check your exercise HR by taking a 10-second pulse count. Record this information in the spaces provided below. Do not record the time until after you have checked your pulse. Exercise HR will remain at the same rate for about 15 seconds following cessation of exercise. Therefore, you need to check your pulse as soon as you finish the walk, after noticing the 800-meter walk time.

10-sec. pulse count: ________ beats (from question 1 above)

800-meter time: ________ min ________ sec

HR in bpm = 10-sec pulse count × 6

HR in bpm = ________ × 6 = ________ bpm

800-meter time in minutes = min + (sec ÷ 60)

800-meter time in minutes = ________ + (________ ÷ 60) = ________ min

Speed in meters per minute (mts/min) = 800 ÷ 800-meter time in min

Speed in mts/min = 800 ÷ ________ = ________ mts/min

VO_2 in mL/kg/min at this walking speed (Use Table 6.9, page 232) = ________ mL/kg/min

VO_2 in L/min = VO_2 in mL/kg/min × BW in kg ÷ 1,000

VO_2 in L/min = ________ × ________ ÷ 1,000 = ________ L/min

Caloric expenditure for 800-meter walk = VO_2 in L/min × 5 × 800-meter time in min

Caloric expenditure for 800-meter walk = ________ × 5 × ________ = ________ calories

4. **Slow-Jogging HR, VO_2, and Caloric Expenditure.** Slowly jog 800 meters (two laps) around the track. Try to maintain the same slow-jogging pace throughout the two laps. Do NOT jog fast or sprint. This is not a speed test and is intended to be a slow jog only. As soon as you complete the 800 meters, notice the time required to complete the distance and check your exercise HR immediately by taking another 10-second pulse count. Record this information below.

   10-sec pulse count: ________ beats

   800-meter time: ________ min ________ sec

   HR in bpm = 10-sec pulse count × 6

   HR in bpm = ________ × 6 = ________ bpm

   800-meter time in minutes = min + (sec ÷ 60)

   800-meter time in minutes = ________ + (________ ÷ 60) = ________ min

   Speed in mts/min = 800 ÷ 800-meter time in min

   Speed in mts/min = 800 ÷ ________ = ________ mts/min

   VO_2 in mL/kg/min at this slow-jogging speed (Use Table 6.9, page 232) = ________ mL/kg/min

   VO_2 in L/min = VO_2 in mL/kg/min × BW in kg ÷ 1,000

   VO_2 in L/min = ________ × ________ ÷ 1,000 = ________ L/min

   Caloric expenditure for 800-meter slow jog = VO_2 in L/min × 5 × 800-meter time in min

   Caloric expenditure for 800-meter slow jog = ________ × 5 × ________ = ________ calories

5. **Fast-Jogging HR, VO_2, Caloric Expenditure, and Recovery HR.** Jog another 800 meters at a faster speed around the track. Again try to maintain the same jogging pace throughout the two laps. Do NOT sprint. Your HR should not exceed 180 bpm on this test. As soon as you complete the 800 meters, notice your time for the two laps and check your 10-second pulse count. Record this information below. You also should check your 2- and 5-minute recovery HRs after the run and record these rates below.

   10-sec pulse count: ________ beats

   800-meter time: ________ min ________ sec

   HR in bpm = 10-sec pulse count × 6

   HR in bpm = ________ × 6 = ________ bpm

   800-meter time in minutes = min + (sec ÷ 60)

   800-meter time in minutes = ________ + (________ ÷ 60) = ________ min

   Speed in mts/min = 800 ÷ 800-meter time in min

   Speed in mts/min = 800 ÷ ________ = ________ mts/min

   VO_2 in mL/kg/min at this fast-jogging speed (Use Table 6.9, page 232) = ________ mL/kg/min

   VO_2 in L/min = VO_2 in mL/kg/min × BW in kg ÷ 1,000

VO_2 in L/min = ________ × ________ ÷ 1,000 = ________ L/min

Caloric expenditure for 800-meter fast jog = VO_2 in L/min × 5 × 800-meter time in min

Caloric expenditure for 800-meter fast jog = ________ × 5 × ________ = ________ calories

Recovery HRs

	10-sec count	bpm
2 minutes		
5 minutes*		

6. **Resting, Exercise, and Recovery HRs.** Plot your resting, exercise, and recovery HRs on the graph provided below.

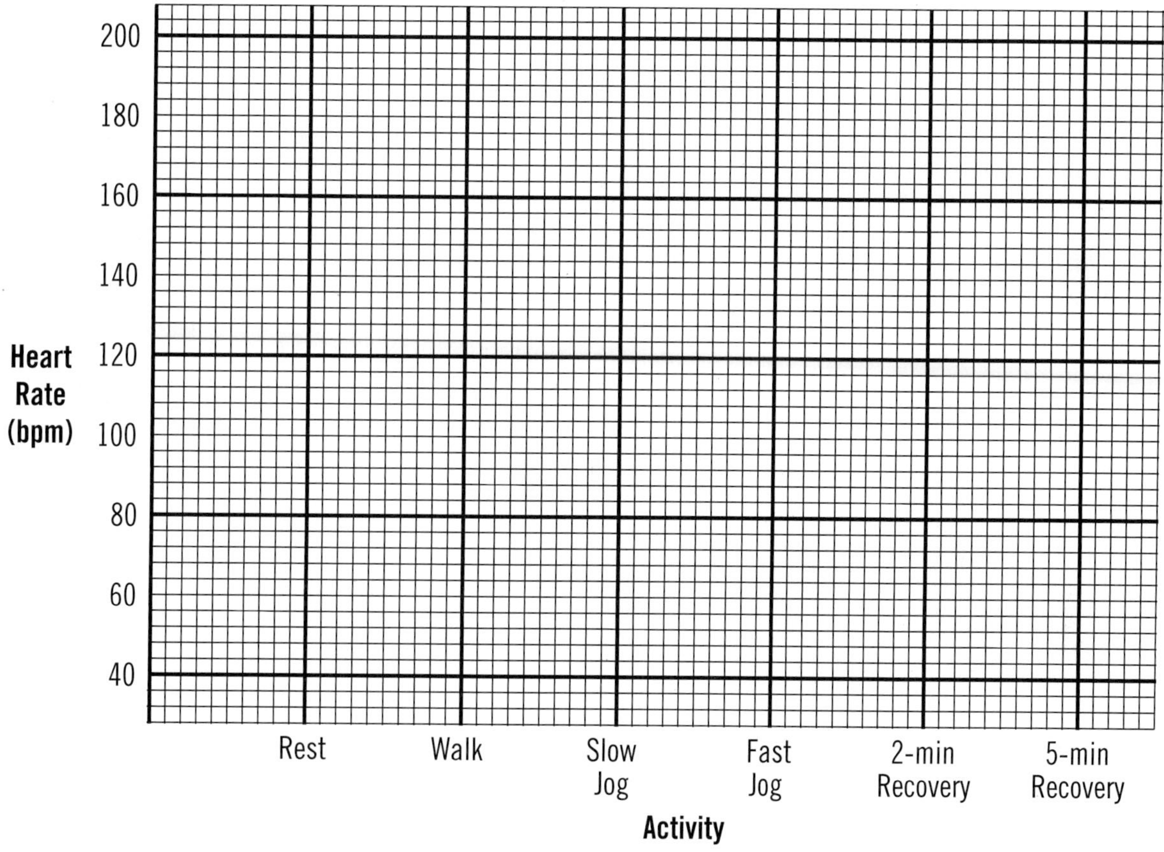

7. **Training Exercise HR and Equivalent Caloric Expenditure.** This part of the lab should be completed outside your regular lab time, during the next 2 or 3 days prior to turning in the assignment. According to the previous exercise HRs (items 3, 4, and 5), try to select a walking or jogging speed that will allow you to maintain your exercise HR in the appropriate cardiorespiratory training zone. Using a 400-meter track, walk or jog for 20 minutes at the selected speed and again try to maintain a constant speed throughout the exercise time. At the end of the 20 minutes, check your 10-second pulse count and estimate the distance covered in meters. Record this information below and estimate the VO_2 and caloric expenditure.

10-sec pulse count: ________ beats

HR in bpm = 10-sec pulse count × 6

HR in bpm = ________ × 6 = ________ bpm

Approximate distance covered in 20 minutes: ________ meters

---

*Your 5-minute recovery HR should be below 120 bpm. If it is above 120, you most likely have overexerted yourself and, therefore, need to decrease the intensity of exercise (and/or duration when exercising for long periods of time). If your 5-minute recovery HR is still above 120 after decreasing the intensity of exercise, you should consult a physician regarding this condition.

Speed in mts/min = distance in meters ÷ 20 minutes

Speed in mts/min = ________ ÷ 20 = ________ mts/min

VO_2 at this speed (see Table 6.9, page 232) = ________ mL/kg/min

VO_2 in L/min = VO_2 in mL/kg/min × BW in kg ÷ 1,000

VO_2 in L/min = ________ × ________ ÷ 1,000 = ________ L/min

Caloric expenditure for 20-min walk/jog = VO_2 in L/min × 5 × 20 min

Caloric expenditure for 20-min walk/jog = ________ × 5 × 20 = ________ calories

Using the previous information, how many calories would you have burned if you had maintained this pace for:

10 minutes (VO_2 in L/min × 5 × 10) = ________ × 5 × 10 = ________ calories

30 minutes (VO_2 in L/min × 5 × 30) = ________ × 5 × 30 = ________ calories

60 minutes (VO_2 in L/min × 5 × 60) = ________ × 5 × 60 = ________ calories

Predicting Caloric Expenditure According to Exercise HR

Research indicates that there is a linear relationship between HR and VO_2, as long as the HR ranges from about 110 to 180 bpm. If you obtain two exercise HRs in this range and the equivalent oxygen uptakes (in L/min), you can easily predict your VO_2 and caloric expenditure for any given HR in the specified range. Plot your two exercise HRs and the corresponding VO_2 values on the graph provided below. Next, draw a line between these two points on the graph and extend the line to 110 and 180 bpm. You now may look up the VO_2 for any HR by finding the desired HR on the Y axis, then going across to the reference line and straight down to the X axis, where you will find the corresponding VO_2 in L/min. To obtain the caloric expenditure in calories per minute, simply multiply the VO_2 by 5. You also may predict your maximal VO_2 (in L/min) by extending the line up to your estimated maximal HR. The maximal HR is estimated by subtracting your age from 220. To convert the maximal VO_2 to mL/kg/min, multiply the L/min value by 1,000 and divide by body weight in kilograms.

Using the results from your lab and the graph below, indicate the VO_2 in L/min and the caloric expenditure at the following HRs:

	VO_2 (L/min)	Caloric Expenditure (calories per minute)
120 bpm		
150 bpm		
170 bpm		

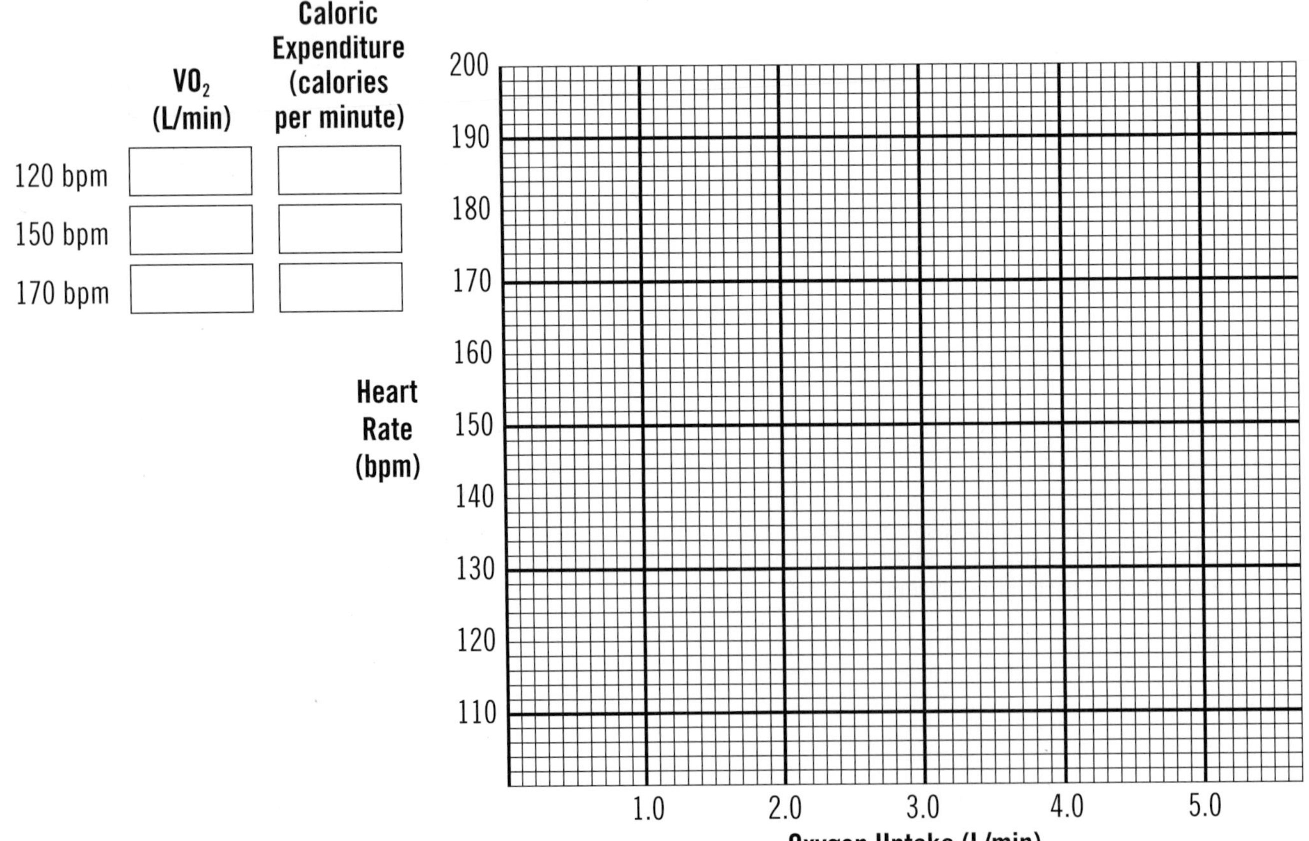

Lab 6C: Exercise Readiness Questionnaire

Name ______________________ Date ____________ Grade ____________

Instructor ______________________ Course ____________ Section ____________

NECESSARY LAB EQUIPMENT
None required.

OBJECTIVE
To determine your preparedness to start an exercise program.

INSTRUCTIONS
Read each statement carefully and circle the number that best describes your feelings in each statement. Please be completely honest with your answers. Interpret the results of this questionnaire using the guidelines provided on the next page.

I.	Strongly Agree	Mildly Agree	Mildly Disagree	Strongly Disagree
1. I can walk, ride a bike (or use a wheelchair), swim, or walk in a shallow pool.	4	3	2	1
2. I enjoy exercise.	4	3	2	1
3. I believe exercise can help decrease the risk for disease and premature mortality.	4	3	2	1
4. I believe exercise contributes to better health.	4	3	2	1
5. I have previously participated in an exercise program.	4	3	2	1
6. I have experienced the feeling of being physically fit.	4	3	2	1
7. I can envision myself exercising.	4	3	2	1
8. I am contemplating an exercise program.	4	3	2	1
9. I am willing to stop contemplating and give exercise a try for a few weeks.	4	3	2	1
10. I am willing to set aside time at least three times a week for exercise.	4	3	2	1
11. I can find a place to exercise (the streets, a park, a YMCA, a health club).	4	3	2	1
12. I can find other people who would like to exercise with me.	4	3	2	1
13. I will exercise when I am moody, fatigued, and even when the weather is bad.	4	3	2	1
14. I am willing to spend a small amount of money for adequate exercise clothing (shoes, shorts, leotards, swimsuit).	4	3	2	1
15. If I have any doubts about my present state of health, I will see a physician before beginning an exercise program.	4	3	2	1
16. Exercise will make me feel better and improve my quality of life.	4	3	2	1

Scoring Your Test:

This questionnaire allows you to examine your readiness for exercise. You have been evaluated in four categories: mastery (self-control), attitude, health, and commitment. Mastery indicates that you can be in control of your exercise program. Attitude examines your mental disposition toward exercise. Health measures the strength of your convictions about the wellness benefits of exercise. Commitment shows dedication and resolution to carry out the exercise program. Write the number you circled after each statement in the corresponding spaces below. Add the scores on each line to get your totals. Scores can vary from 4 to 16. A score of 12 and above is a strong indicator that that factor is important to you, and 8 and below is low. If you score 12 or more points in each category, your chances of initiating and adhering to an exercise program are good. If you fail to score at least 12 points in three categories, your chances of succeeding at exercise may be slim. You need to be better informed about the benefits of exercise, and a retraining process may be required.

Mastery:	1.		+	5.		+	6.		+	9.		=	
Attitude:	2.		+	7.		+	8.		+	13.		=	
Health:	3.		+	4.		+	15.		+	16.		=	
Commitment:	10.		+	11.		+	12.		+	14.		=	

II. Stage of Change for Cardiorespiratory Endurance Exercise

Using Figure 2.6 (page 66) and Table 2.3 (page 65), identify your current stage of change in regard to participation in a cardiorespiratory endurance exercise program:

III. Advantages and Disadvantages for Adding Aerobic Exercise to Your Lifestyle

Advantages: ______________________________

____

____

____

____

____

____

____

Disadvantages: ______________________________

____

____

____

____

____

____

____

Lab 6D: Cardiorespiratory Exercise Prescription

Name ______________________ Date ____________ Grade ____________

Instructor ______________________ Course ____________ Section ____________

NECESSARY LAB EQUIPMENT
None required.

OBJECTIVE
To write your own cardiorespiratory exercise prescription.

I. Intensity of Exercise

1. Estimate your own maximal heart rate (MHR)

   MHR = 207 – (.70 × age)

   MHR = 207 – (.70 × [ ]) = [ ] bpm

2. Resting Heart Rate (RHR). Determine your RHR by counting your pulse for a full minute in the evening after you have been sitting quietly, reading, or watching a relaxing TV show.

   RHR = [ ] bpm

3. Heart Rate Reserve (HRR) = MHR – RHR

   HRR = [ ] – [ ] = [ ] beats

4. Training Intensities (TI) = HRR × TI + RHR

   30 Percent TI = [ ] × .30 + [ ] = [ ] bpm

   40 Percent TI = [ ] × .40 + [ ] = [ ] bpm

   50 Percent TI = [ ] × .50 + [ ] = [ ] bpm

   60 percent TI = [ ] × .60 + [ ] = [ ] bpm

   70 percent TI = [ ] × .70 + [ ] = [ ] bpm

   85 Percent TI = [ ] × .85 + [ ] = [ ] bpm

5. Current cardiorespiratory fitness category (see Lab 6A): [ ]

   Cardiorespiratory Training Zone: unconditioned individuals, persons in the poor cardiorespiratory fitness category, and older adults starting an exercise program should use a 30 to 40 percent TI. Individuals in fair and average fitness are encouraged to exercise between 40 and 60 percent TI. Active individuals in the good or excellent categories should exercise between 60 and 85 percent TI.

   Light-intensity cardiorespiratory training zone (30% to 40% TI): [ ] to [ ] bpm

   Moderate-intensity cardiorespiratory training zone (40% to 60% TI): [ ] to [ ] bpm

   Vigorous-intensity cardiorespiratory training zone (60% to 85% TI): [ ] to [ ] bpm

II. Mode of Exercise

Select any activity or combination of activities that you enjoy doing. The activity has to be continuous in nature and must get your heart rate up to the cardiorespiratory training zone and keep it there for as long as you exercise. Indicate your preferred mode(s) of exercise:

1. ________ 2. ________ 3. ________

4. ________ 5. ________ 6. ________

III. Cardiorespiratory Exercise Program

The following is your weekly program for development of cardiorespiratory endurance. If you are in the poor or fair cardiorespiratory fitness category, start with week 1. If you are in the average category, you may start at week 5. If you are already active and in the good or excellent category, you may start at week 9 (otherwise start at week 5). After completing the goal for week 12, you can maintain fitness by training between a 70 and 85 percent TI for about 20 to 30 minutes, a minimum of three times per week, on nonconsecutive days. You should also recompute your TIs periodically because you will experience a significant reduction in resting heart rate with aerobic training (approximately 10 to 20 beats in 8 to 12 weeks).

Week	Duration (min)	Frequency	Training Intensity	Heart Rate (bpm)	Perceived Exertion*
1	15	3	Between 30% and 40%	____ to ____	____ to ____ beats
2	15	4	Between 30% and 40%		
3	20	4	Between 30% and 40%		
4	20	5	Between 30% and 40%		
5	20	4	Between 40% and 60%	____ to ____	____ to ____ beats
6	20	5	Between 40% and 60%		
7	30	4	Between 40% and 60%		
8	30	5	Between 40% and 60%		
9	30	4	Between 60% and 90%	____ to ____	____ to ____ beats
10	30	5	Between 60% and 90%		
11	30–40	5	Between 60% and 90%		
12	30–40	5	Between 60% and 90%		

*See Figure 6.9, page 236.

Maintenance cardiorespiratory training zone (60% to 90% TI): ________ to ________ bpm

IV. Briefly State Your Experiences and Feelings Regarding Aerobic Exercise:

V. Monitoring Daily Physical Activity

What is your average total number of daily steps (use a 7-day average): ________

What is your current activity category (use Table 1.2, page 12): ________

Do you accumulate 10,000 steps on most days of the week (at least five days)? ☐ Yes ☐ No

7

Muscular Fitness: Strength and Endurance

Progressive resistance strength training enhances fitness, health, self-esteem and self-confidence, functional capacity, and overall well-being.

OBJECTIVES

- Explain the importance of adequate muscular fitness levels in maintaining good health and well-being.
- Clarify misconceptions about strength fitness.
- Define muscular fitness, muscular strength, and muscular endurance.
- Be able to assess muscular strength and endurance, and learn to interpret test results according to health fitness and physical fitness standards.
- Identify the factors that affect strength.
- Understand the principles of overload and specificity of training for strength development.
- Learn dietary guidelines for optimum strength development.
- Become familiar with core strength training and realize its importance for overall quality of life.
- Become acquainted with two distinct strength-training programs—with weights and without weights.

REAL LIFE STORY | Demetrio's Experience

© Jason Stitt/Shutterstock.com

My fitness class in high school emphasized aerobic endurance. Our teacher would ask that we run/walk laps around the track. We never did any strength training and not much stretching. I can't say I really enjoyed the class, and I never really felt I was getting fit. Our fitness and wellness college course required a balanced approach to fitness. We used a circuit aerobic/strength-training approach followed by stretching the last 10 minutes of class. The fitness center was set up so that we had treadmills, bikes, elliptical trainers, jump ropes, and weight machines. I had never lifted weights before. Our work-to-rest ratio was 60-to-15 seconds, and we had a total of 20 stations (10 each aerobic and strength). During the 15-second rest period, we would switch between aerobic and strength units. It was quite a workout. Once we started, we were locked into the circuit and just kept going till all 20 stations were completed. A "traffic stoplight" on the one end of the gym was our guide. Green (55 seconds) meant work. The yellow light (5 seconds) meant we had to get ready to change. The red light (15 seconds) was an indication that we had a total of 15 seconds to switch units and set up the next station (treadmill speed or resistance on other aerobic and weight machines). I truly loved the class and developed fitness like never before. Strength training has really improved my confidence and daily functional capacity. I also started to eat better and really paid attention to pre- and postexercise snacks and meals. It has made a world of difference in my body composition. Because of how I feel, my approach to lifetime fitness has changed. I now do the aerobics and strength-training workouts separately, and I always stretch after I lift. I don't ever want to lose this feeling of "fitness," independence, and my newly found quality of life.

MyProfile: Personal Understanding of Muscular Fitness Concepts

To the best of your ability, answer the following questions. If you do not know the answer(s), this chapter will guide you through them.

I. In terms of health and wellness, is muscular fitness or aerobic fitness more important? Explain your answer. ______

____

____

____

II. Body weight may not drop or even increase as a result of a progressive resistance strength-training program; nonetheless, circumference measurements and percent body fat may decrease. Can you describe the reason for these changes? ___ Yes ___ No ______________

____

____

III. Performing at least one set of each strength-training exercise within the repetition maximum zone produces substantial strength development. Is this a program you could follow? ___ Yes ___ No How does it differ from traditional programs? ______________

____

____

IV. A periodized strength-training program is frequently used to maximize muscular strength and endurance gains. Have you ever used such an approach? ___ Yes ___ No How did it contribute to your muscular fitness? ________

____

____

V. In your training, have single-joint exercises been more effective than multiple-joint exercises in developing strength? ___ Yes ___ No Share your experience.

____

____

____

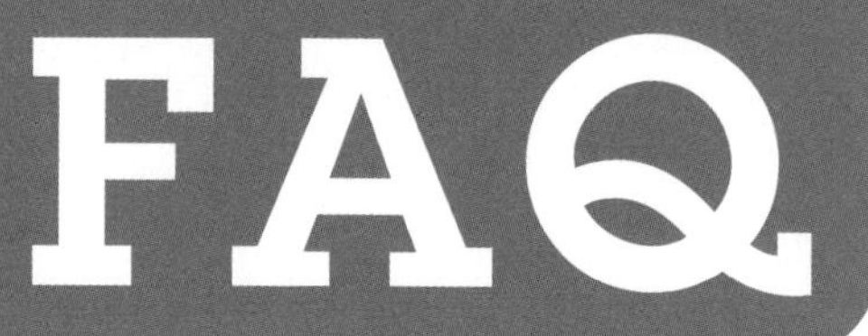

Which is more important for good health: aerobic fitness or muscular fitness (muscular strength and muscular endurance)?

They are both important. During the initial fitness boom in the 1970s and 1980s, the emphasis was almost exclusively on aerobic fitness. We now know that a comprehensive training routine that combines aerobic fitness and muscular strength (along with regular flexibility training) contribute to health, fitness, work capacity, independent living, and overall quality of life. Among many health benefits, aerobic fitness is important in the prevention of cardiovascular diseases and some types of cancer, whereas muscular fitness builds strong muscles and bones, prevents sarcopenia (age-related muscle loss), increases functional capacity, helps prevent osteoporosis and type 2 diabetes, and decreases the risk for low back pain and other musculoskeletal injuries.

Should I do aerobic exercise or strength training first?

Ideally, allow some recovery hours between the two types of training. If you can't afford the time, the training order should be based on your fitness goals and preferences. Unless extremely exhausting, aerobics provides a good lead into strength training. Excessive fatigue from vigorous aerobic exercise leads to bad form while lifting and may result in injury. Vigorous-intensity aerobic exercise prior to strength training also decreases strength, power, and muscle hypertrophy development. If your primary goal is strength development, lift first, because you'll be less fatigued and will end up with a more productive workout. On the other hand, if you are trying to develop the cardiorespiratory system or enhance caloric expenditure for weight loss purposes, heavy lower body lifting makes it difficult to sustain a good cardio workout thereafter. Thus, evaluate your goals, and select the training order accordingly. In adults over the age of 65, strength training first seems more effective in enhancing aerobic power because in older adults VO_{2max} is somewhat limited to age-related loss of muscle and strength.

Do big muscles turn into fat when you stop training?

Muscle and fat tissue are two different types of tissue. Just as an apple will not turn into an orange, muscle tissue cannot turn into fat, or vice versa. Muscle cells increase and decrease in size according to your training program. If you train quite hard, muscle cells increase in size. This increase is limited in women compared with men due to hormonal differences. When you stop training, muscle cells again decrease in size. If you maintain a high caloric intake without physical training, however, fat cells will increase in size as weight (fat) is gained.

What strength-training exercises are best to get an abdominal "six-pack"?

Most men tend to store body fat around the waist, while women do so around the hips. There are, however, no "miracle" exercises to spot reduce. Multiple sets of abdominal curl-ups, crunches, reverse crunches, or sit-ups performed three to five times per week strengthen the abdominal musculature but are not sufficient to allow the muscles to appear through the layer of fat between the skin and the muscles. The total energy (caloric) expenditure of a few sets of abdominal exercises is not sufficient to lose a significant amount of weight (fat). If you want to get a "washboard stomach" (or, for women, achieve shapely hips), you need to engage in a moderate to vigorous aerobic and strength-training program combined with a moderate reduction in daily caloric intake (diet).

The benefits of **muscular fitness**, achieved through **strength training** or **resistance training**, on health and well-being are well documented. Muscular fitness, achieved through **progressive resistance training**, involves both muscular strength and muscular endurance, with the corresponding improvements in muscle tone and power.

The need for muscular fitness is not confined to highly trained athletes, fitness enthusiasts, or individuals who have jobs that require heavy muscular work. All people need adequate muscular fitness for good health, improved functional capacity, and a better quality of life. Unfortunately, according to the 2013 survey released by the Centers for Disease Control and Prevention (CDC), only 27 percent of men and 19 percent of women met the 2008 Federal Physical Activity

Muscular fitness A term used in reference to the general health, strength, and endurance of a person's muscular system.

Strength training A program designed to improve muscular strength and/or endurance through a series of progressive resistance (weight) training exercises that overload the muscular system and cause physiological development.

Resistance training See **strength training** (resistance training).

Progressive resistance training A gradual increase of resistance used during strength training over a period of time.

Guidelines for muscular fitness. Worse yet, almost 74 percent or nearly 3 out of every 4 American adults, did not participate in any type of muscular fitness activity; that is, they did not strength train or take a class that required some sort of muscular strength activity such as cardio/strength training, Pilates, boot camp, PX90, CrossFit, or even a single push-up during their available leisure time.

Strength Training Benefits

A well-planned strength-training program leads to increased muscle strength and endurance, power, muscle tone, and tendon and ligament strength—all of which help improve and maintain everyday functional physical capacity. Muscular fitness is a basic health-related fitness component and is an important wellness component for optimal performance in daily activities such as sitting, walking, running, lifting and carrying objects, doing housework, and enjoying recreational activities. Strength also is of great value in improving posture, personal appearance, and self-image; in developing sports skills; in promoting stability of joints; and in meeting certain emergencies in life.

From a health standpoint, increasing strength helps increase or maintain muscle and a higher resting metabolic rate; encourages weight loss and maintenance; prevents obesity; lessens the risk for injury; reduces chronic low back pain; reduces pressure on the joints alleviating arthritic pain; aids in childbearing; improves bone density; prevents osteoporosis; improves cholesterol levels, decreases triglyceride levels, and reduces high blood pressure, thus reducing the risk for cardiovascular disease and premature mortality; and promotes psychological well-being. Furthermore, it decreases the risk of developing physical function limitations and the overall risk of nonfatal disease.[1]

Regular strength training also helps control blood sugar. Much of the blood glucose from food consumption goes to the muscles, where it is stored as glycogen. When muscles are not used, muscle cells may become insulin resistant, and glucose cannot enter the cells, thereby increasing the risk for type 2 diabetes. Research indicates that even a single strength-training exercise session enhances insulin sensitivity for the next 24 hours. Additionally, following 16 weeks of strength training, a group of diabetic men and women improved their blood sugar control, gained strength, increased lean body mass, lost body fat, and lowered blood pressure.[2] Across all ages, the greater the amount of muscle mass, relative to body size, the better the insulin sensitivity and the lower the risk for diabetes.

Furthermore, with time, the heart rate and blood pressure response to lifting a heavy resistance (a weight) decreases. This adaptation reduces the demands on the cardiovascular system when you perform activities such as carrying a child, the groceries, or a suitcase.

Because of the many health benefits provided by a regular muscular fitness training program, the American Medical Association (AMA), the American Heart Association (AHA), the American College of Sports Medicine, the American Diabetic Association (ADA), and the CDC have offered strong support of strength training as an exercise modality to promote health and prevent disease.

Muscular Fitness and Aging

In the older adult population (65 and older), muscular fitness may be the most important health-related component of physical fitness. Although proper cardiorespiratory endurance is necessary to help maintain a healthy heart, good strength contributes more to independent living than any other fitness component. Studies indicate that, on average, a 30-year-old loses 25 percent of muscle strength by age 70 and about half by age 90. Once in the 50s, older adults who strength train can successfully perform most **activities of daily living**. Those who don't become weaker and less functional.

A common occurrence as people age is **sarcopenia** (loss of muscle mass), strength, and function. How much of this loss of muscle mass is related to the aging process itself or to actual physical inactivity and faulty nutrition is unknown. Sarcopenia leads to mobility disability and loss of independence. Muscle mass loss is also related to a lower metabolic rate, high prevalence of obesity, insulin resistance, type 2 diabetes, abnormal blood lipids, and high blood pressure. Muscular strength has also been shown to be inversely associated with all-cause mortality; the lower the strength level, the higher the risk for early mortality.[3] Estimates indicate that half of all adults 65 and older in the United States currently suffer from age-related muscle loss. Early muscle loss doesn't appear to bother them or hold them back. They think they are fine until they lose functional independence, at that point they realize the serious mistake made and subsequent loss of quality of life.

Studies[4] further indicate that adults who do not strength train lose between 4 and 6 pounds of muscle tissue per decade of life. As a result, a person who has maintained body weight but did not strength train between the ages of 40 and 60 can remain at the same body mass index (BMI), but percent body fat can easily go up 7 to 10 percentage points (i.e., 20 percent to 27 to 30 percent). And a summary of 49 research studies also indicates that older adults gain an average of 2.42 pounds of lean body mass following 20 weeks of strength training.[5] The findings are significant because so many older adults are affected by sarcopenia and strength training can prevent much of this loss and allow these older adults to preserve independent living throughout the aging process.

Currently, according to a CDC report in 2013, less than 20 percent of older adults engage in strength-training exercises. And whereas thinning of the bones from osteoporosis renders them prone to fractures, the gradual loss of muscle mass and ensuing frailty are what lead to falls and subsequent loss of function in older adults. Strength training helps to slow the age-related loss of muscle function. Protein deficiency, seen in some older adults, also contributes to loss of lean tissue.

More than anything else, older adults want to enjoy good health and to function independently. Many of them, however, are confined to nursing homes because they lack sufficient strength to move about. They cannot walk very far, and many have to be helped in and out of beds, chairs, and bathtubs.

A strength-training program can enhance quality of life tremendously, and nearly everyone can benefit from it. Only people with advanced heart disease are advised to refrain from strength training. Inactive adults between the ages of 56 and 86 who participated in a 12-week strength-training program increased their lean body mass by about 3 pounds, lost about 4 pounds of fat, and increased their resting metabolic rate by almost 7 percent.[6] Research data have also confirmed significant drops in unhealthy visceral fat (intra-abdominal fat) through strength training, despite little or no change in total body weight (the loss of fat is compensated by an increase in muscle mass). Furthermore, when strength-training is accompanied by a calorie-restricted diet, visceral fat losses are greater than total whole-body subcutaneous fat.

In other research, leg strength improved by as much as 200 percent in previously inactive adults older than 90 years.[7] As strength improves, so does the ability to move about, the capacity for independent living, and enjoyment of life during the "golden years." More specifically, good strength enhances quality of life in that it

- improves balance and restores mobility
- makes lifting and reaching easier
- decreases the risk for injuries and falls
- stresses the bones and preserves bone mineral density, thereby decreasing the risk for osteoporosis

Another benefit of maintaining a good strength level is its relationship to human **metabolism**. A primary outcome of a strength-training program is an increase in muscle mass or size (lean body mass), known as muscle **hypertrophy**.

Muscle tissue uses more energy than does fatty tissue. That is, your body expends more calories to maintain muscle than to maintain fat. All other factors being equal, if two individuals both weigh 150 pounds but have different amounts of muscle mass, the one with more muscle mass will have a higher **resting metabolism**. Even small increases in muscle mass have a long-term positive effect on metabolism.

Loss of lean tissue also is thought to be a primary reason for the decrease in metabolism as people grow older. Contrary to some beliefs, metabolism does not have to slow down significantly with aging. It is not so much that metabolism slows down, it's that we slow down. Lean body mass decreases with sedentary living, which in turn slows down the resting metabolic rate. Thus, if people continue eating at the same rate as they age, body fat increases.

Daily energy requirements decrease an average of 360 calories between age 26 and age 60.[8] Participating in a strength-training program can offset much of the decline and prevent and reduce excess body fat. One research study found an increase in resting metabolic rate of 35 calories per pound of muscle mass in older adults who participated in a strength-training program.[9]

Gender Differences A common misconception about physical fitness concerns women in strength training. Because of the increase in muscle mass typically seen in men, some women still think that a strength-training program will result in the development of large musculature.

Even though the quality of muscle in men and women is the same, endocrinological differences do not allow women to achieve the same amount of muscle hypertrophy (size) as men. Men also have more muscle fibers, and because of the sex-specific male hormones, each individual fiber has more potential for hypertrophy. On the average, following 6 months of training, women can achieve up to a 50 percent increase in strength but only a 10 percent increase in muscle size.

The idea that strength training allows women to develop muscle hypertrophy to the same extent as men is as false as the notion that playing basketball turns women into giants. Masculinity and femininity are established by genetic inheritance, not by amount of physical activity. Variations in the extent of masculinity and femininity are determined by individual differences in hormonal secretions of androgen, testosterone, estrogen, and progesterone. Women with a bigger-than-average build often are inclined to participate in sports because of their natural physical advantage. As a result, many people have associated women's participation in sports and strength training with large muscle size.

As the number of females who participate in sports has increased steadily, the myth of strength training in women leading to large increases in muscle size has abated somewhat. For example, per pound of body weight, female gymnasts are among the strongest athletes in the world. These athletes engage regularly in vigorous strength-training programs. Yet, female gymnasts have some of the most well-toned and graceful figures of all women.

Improved body appearance has become the rule rather than the exception for women who participate in strength-training programs. Some

Activities of daily living Everyday behaviors that people normally do to function in life (cross the street, carry groceries, lift objects, do laundry, sweep floors, etc.).

Sarcopenia Age-related loss of lean body mass, strength, and function.

Metabolism All energy and material transformations that occur within living cells and are necessary to sustain life.

Hypertrophy An increase in the size of the cell, as in muscle hypertrophy.

Resting metabolism Amount of energy (expressed in milliliters of oxygen per minute or total calories per day) an individual requires during resting conditions to sustain proper body function.

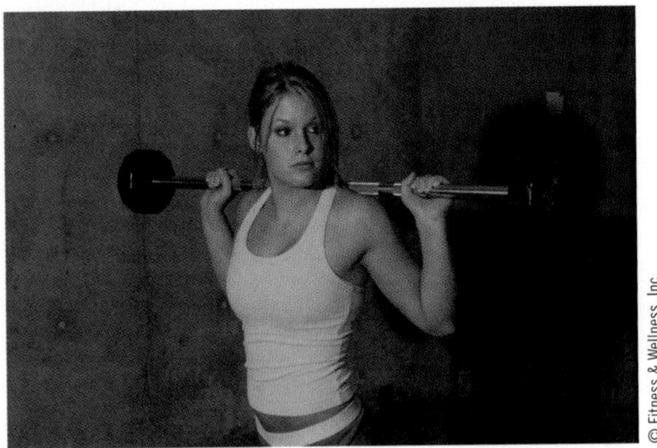

Improved body appearance has become the rule rather than the exception for women who participate in strength-training exercises.

of the most attractive female movie stars also train with weights to further improve their personal image.

Nonetheless, you may ask if weight training does not masculinize women, why do so many women body builders develop such heavy musculature? In the sport of body building, the athletes follow intense training routines consisting of 2 or more hours of constant weight lifting with short rest intervals between sets. Many body-building training routines call for back-to-back exercises using the same muscle groups. The objective of this type of training is to cause sarcoplasmic hypertrophy (see page 268) and to pump extra blood into the muscles. This additional fluid makes the muscles appear much bigger than they do in a resting condition. Based on the intensity and the length of the training session, the muscles can remain filled with blood, appearing measurably larger for an hour or longer after completing the training session. Performing such routines is a common practice before competitions. Therefore, in real life, these women are not as muscular as they seem to be when they are participating in a contest.

CRITICAL THINKING

What role should strength training have in a fitness program? Should people be motivated for the health fitness benefits, or should they participate to enhance their body image? What are your feelings about individuals (male or female) with large body musculature?

In the sport of body building (among others), a big point of controversy is the use of **anabolic steroids** and human growth hormones. These hormones produce detrimental and undesirable side effects, even more so in women (e.g., hypertension, fluid retention, decreased breast size, deepening of the voice, and whiskers and other atypical body hair growth), which some women deem tolerable. Anabolic steroid use in general—except for medical reasons and when carefully monitored by a physician—can lead to serious health consequences.

Selected Detrimental Effects from Using Anabolic Steroids

- Liver tumors
- Hepatitis
- Hypertension
- Reduction of high-density lipoprotein (HDL) cholesterol
- Elevation of low-density lipoprotein (LDL) cholesterol
- Hyperinsulinism
- Impaired pituitary function
- Impaired thyroid function
- Mood swings
- Aggressive behavior
- Increased irritability
- Acne
- Fluid retention
- Decreased libido
- HIV infection (via injectable steroids)
- Prostate problems (men)
- Testicular atrophy (men)
- Reduced sperm count (men)
- Clitoral enlargement (women)
- Decreased breast size (women)
- Increased body and facial hair (nonreversible in women)
- Deepening of the voice (nonreversible in women)

Use of anabolic steroids by female body builders and female track-and-field athletes is not uncommon. Athletes use anabolic steroids to remain competitive at the highest level. During the 2012 Olympic Games in London, the woman shot put gold medal winner was expelled from the games and stripped of her medal for using steroids. Women who take steroids undoubtedly will build heavy musculature, and if they take them long enough, the steroids will produce masculinizing effects.

To prevent steroid use, the International Federation of Body Building and Fitness instituted a mandatory steroid-testing program for women participating in the Ms. Olympia contest. When drugs are not used to promote development, improved body image is the rule rather than the exception among women who participate in body building, strength training, and sports in general.

Changes in Body Composition A benefit of strength training, accentuated even more when combined with aerobic exercise, is a decrease in adipose or fatty tissue

FIGURE 7.1 **Changes in body composition as a result of a combined aerobic and strength-training program.**

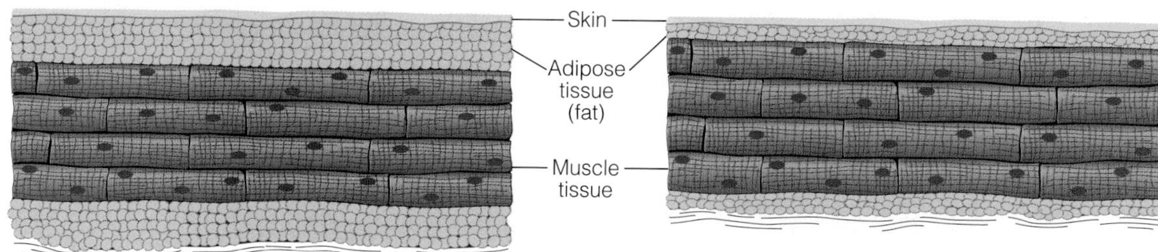

around muscle fibers. This decrease is often greater than the amount of muscle hypertrophy (Figure 7.1). Therefore, losing inches but not body weight is common.

Because muscle tissue is denser than fatty tissue (and even though inches are lost during a combined strength-training and aerobic program), people, especially women, often become discouraged because they cannot see the results readily on the scale. They can offset this discouragement by determining body composition regularly to monitor their changes in percent body fat rather than simply measuring changes in total body weight (see Chapter 4).

Assessment of Muscular Strength and Endurance

Although muscular strength and endurance are interrelated, they do differ. **Muscular strength** is the ability to exert maximum force against resistance. **Muscular endurance** is the ability of a muscle to exert submaximal force repeatedly over time.

Muscular endurance (also referred to as localized muscular endurance) largely depends on muscular strength. Weak muscles cannot repeat an action several times or sustain it. Based on these principles, strength tests and training programs have been designed to measure and develop absolute muscular strength, muscular endurance, or a combination of the two.

Muscular strength is usually determined by the maximal amount of resistance (weight)—**one repetition maximum**, or **1 RM**—that an individual is able to lift in a single effort. Although this assessment yields a good measure of absolute strength, it requires considerable time, because the 1 RM is determined through trial and error. For example, strength of the chest muscles is frequently measured through the bench press exercise. If a man has not trained with weights, he may try 100 pounds and lift this resistance easily. After adding 50 pounds, he may fail to lift the resistance. Then he decreases resistance by 20 or 30 pounds. Finally, after several trials, the 1 RM is established.

Using this method, a true 1 RM might be difficult to obtain the first time an individual is tested, because fatigue becomes a factor. By the time the 1 RM is established, the person already has made several maximal or near-maximal attempts.

In contrast, muscular endurance typically is established by the number of repetitions an individual can perform against a submaximal resistance or by the length of time a given contraction can be sustained. For example: How many push-ups can an individual do? Or how many times can a 30-pound resistance be lifted? Or how long can a person hold a chin-up?

If time is a factor and only one test item can be done, the Hand Grip Strength Test, described in Figure 7.2, is commonly used to assess strength. This test, though, provides only a weak correlation with overall body strength. Two additional strength tests are provided in Figures 7.3 and 7.4. Lab 7A also offers you the opportunity to assess your level of muscular strength or endurance with all three tests. You may take one or more of these tests, according to your time and the facilities available.

In strength testing, several body sites should be assessed, because muscular strength and muscular endurance are both highly specific. A high degree of strength or endurance in one body part does not necessarily indicate similarity in other parts, so no single strength test provides a good assessment of overall body strength. Accordingly, exercises for the strength tests were selected to include the upper body, lower body, and abdominal regions.

Before strength testing, you should become familiar with the procedures for the respective tests. For safety reasons, always take at least one friend with you whenever you train with weights or undertake any type of strength assessment. Also, these are different tests, so to make valid comparisons, you should use the same test

Anabolic steroids Synthetic versions of the male sex hormone testosterone, which promotes muscle development and hypertrophy.

Muscular strength The ability of a muscle to exert maximum force against resistance (e.g., 1 repetition maximum [or 1 RM] on the bench press exercise).

Muscular endurance The ability of a muscle to exert submaximal force repeatedly over time.

One repetition maximum (1 RM) The maximum amount of resistance an individual is able to lift in a single effort.

FIGURE 7.2 Procedure for the Hand Grip Strength Test.

1. Adjust the width of the dynamometer* so the middle bones of your fingers rest on the distant end of the dynamometer grip.
2. Use your dominant hand for this test. Place your elbow at a 90° angle and about 2 inches away from the body.

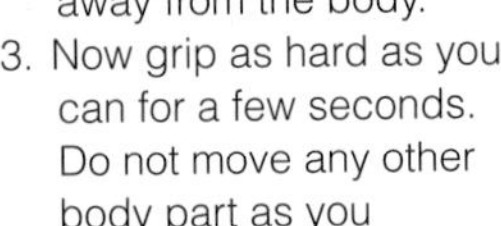

3. Now grip as hard as you can for a few seconds. Do not move any other body part as you perform the test (do not flex or extend the elbow, do not move the elbow away or toward the body, and do not lean forward or backward during the test).
4. Record the dynamometer reading in pounds (if reading is in kilograms, multiply by 2.2046).
5. Three trials are allowed for this test. Use the highest reading for your final test score. Look up your percentile rank for this test in Table 7.1.
6. Based on your percentile rank, obtain the hand grip strength fitness category according to the following guidelines:

Percentile Rank	Fitness Category
≥90	Excellent
70–80	Good
50–60	Average
30–40	Fair
≤20	Poor

*A Lafayette 78010 dynamometer is recommended for this test (Lafayette Instruments Co., Sagamore and North 9th Street, Lafayette, IN 47903).

for pre- and postassessments. The following are your options.

Muscular Strength: Hand Grip Strength Test As indicated previously, when time is a factor, the Hand Grip Strength Test can be used to provide a rough estimate of strength. Unlike the next two tests, this one is isometric (involving static contraction, discussed later in the chapter). If the proper grip is used, no finger motion or body movement is visible during the test. The test procedure is given in Figure 7.2, and percentile ranks based on results are provided in Table 7.1. You can record your results of this test in Lab 7A.

TABLE 7.1 Scoring Table for Hand Grip Strength Test

Percentile Rank	Men	Women
99	153	101
95	145	94
90	141	91
80	139	86
70	132	80
60	124	78
50	122	74
40	114	71
30	110	66
20	100	64
10	91	60
5	76	58

Changes in strength are more difficult to evaluate with the Hand Grip Strength Test than with other muscular strength tests. Most strength-training programs are dynamic (body segments are moved through a range of motion), whereas this test provides an isometric assessment. Furthermore, grip strength exercises are seldom used in strength training, and increases in strength are specific to the body parts exercised. This test, however, can be used to supplement the following strength tests.

Muscular Endurance Test Three exercises were selected to assess the endurance of the upper body, lower body, and midbody muscle groups (Figure 7.3). The advantage of the Muscular Endurance Test is that it does not require strength-training equipment—only a stopwatch, a metronome, a bench or gymnasium bleacher $16^1/_4$ inches high, a cardboard strip $3^1/_2$ inches wide by 30 inches long, and a partner. A percentile rank is given for each exercise according to the number of repetitions performed (Table 7.2). An overall endurance rating can be obtained by totaling the number of points obtained on each exercise. Record your results of this test in Lab 7A and Appendix A.

Muscular Strength and Endurance Test In the Muscular Strength and Endurance Test,

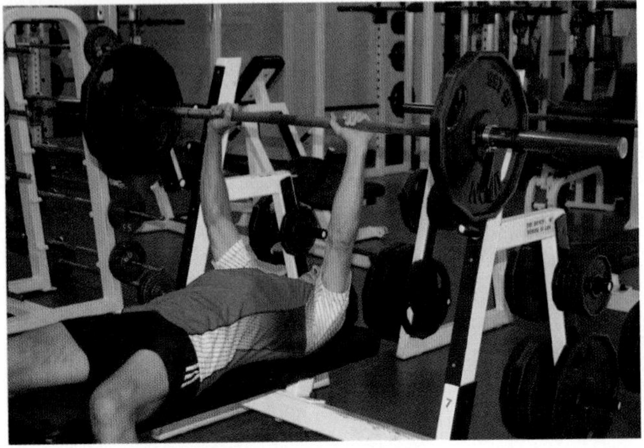

The maximal amount of resistance that an individual is able to lift in one single effort (1 RM) is a measure of absolute strength.

The Hand Grip Strength Test

FIGURE 7.3 **Muscular Endurance Test.**

Three exercises are conducted on this test: bench jumps, modified dips (men) or modified push-ups (women), and bent-leg curl-ups or abdominal crunches. All exercises should be conducted with the aid of a partner. The correct procedure for performing each exercise is as follows:

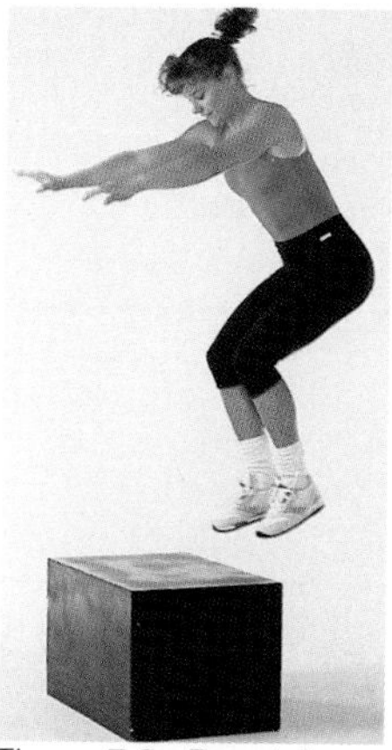

Bench-jump. Using a bench or gymnasium bleacher 16¼" high, attempt to jump up onto and down off of the bench as many times as possible in 1 minute. If you cannot jump the full minute, you may step up and down. A repetition is counted each time both feet return to the floor.

Figure 7.3a Bench jump

Modified dip. Men only: Using a bench or gymnasium bleacher, place the hands on the bench with the fingers pointing forward. Have a partner hold your feet in front of you. Bend the hips at approximately 90° (you also may use three sturdy chairs: Put your hands on two chairs placed by the sides of your body and place your feet on the third chair in front of you). Lower your body by flexing the elbows until they reach a 90° angle, then return to the starting position (also see Exercise 6, page 287). Perform the repetitions to a two-step cadence (down-up) regulated with a metronome set at 56 beats per minute. Perform as many continuous repetitions as possible. Do not count any more repetitions if you fail to follow the metronome cadence.

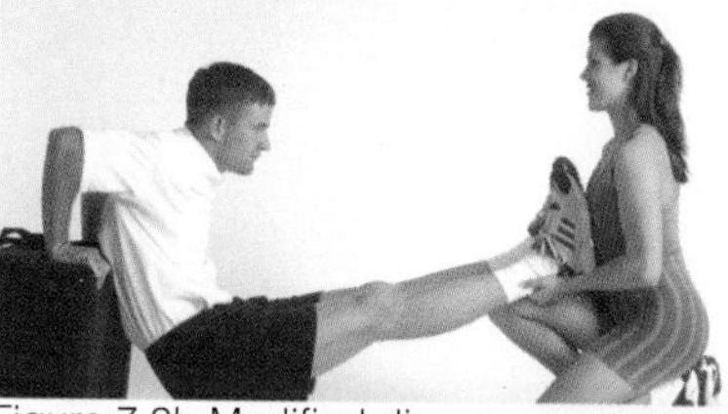

Figure 7.3b Modified dip

Modified push-up. Women: Lie down on the floor (face down), bend the knees (feet up in the air), and place the hands on the floor by the shoulders with the fingers pointing forward. The lower body will be supported at the knees (as opposed to the feet) throughout the test (see Figure 7.3c). The chest must touch the floor on each repetition. As with the modified-dip exercise (above), perform the repetitions to a two-step cadence (up-down) regulated with a metronome set at 56 beats per minute. Perform as many continuous repetitions as possible. Do not count any more repetitions if you fail to follow the metro-nome cadence.

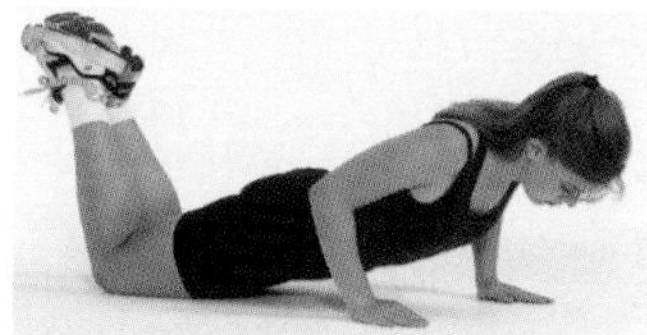

Figure 7.3c Modified push-up

Bent-leg curl-up. Lie down on the floor (face up) and bend both legs at the knees at approximately 100°. The feet should be on the floor, and you must hold them in place yourself throughout the test. Cross the arms in front of the chest, each hand on the opposite shoulder. Now raise the head off the floor, placing the chin against the chest. This is the starting and finishing position for each curl-up (see Figure 7.3d). **The back of the head may not come in contact with the floor, the hands cannot be removed from the shoulders, nor may the feet or hips be raised off the floor at any time during the test. The test is terminated if any of these four conditions occur.** When you curl up, the upper body must come to an upright position before going back down (see Figure 7.3e). The repetitions are performed to a two-step cadence (up-down) regulated with the metronome set at 40 beats per minute. For this exercise, you should allow a brief practice period of 5 to 10 seconds to familiarize yourself with the cadence (the *up* movement is initiated with the first beat, then you must wait for the next beat to initiate the *down* movement; one repetition is accomplished every two beats of the metronome). Count as many repetitions as you are able to perform following the proper cadence. The test is also terminated if you fail to maintain the appropriate cadence or if you accomplish 100 repetitions. Have your partner check the angle at the knees throughout the test to make sure to maintain the 100° angle as close as possible.

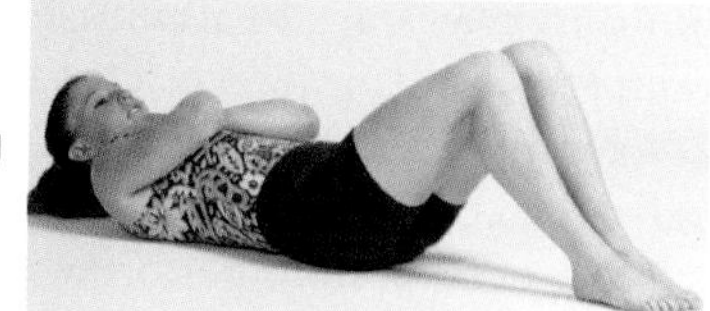

Figure 7.3d Bent-leg curl-up

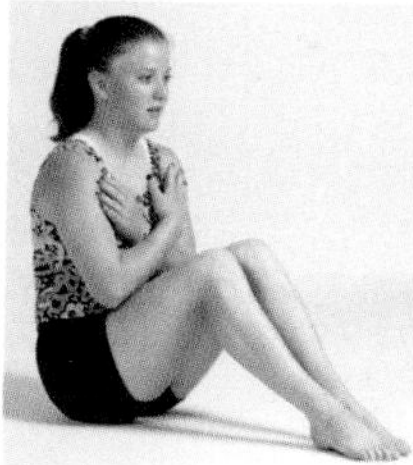

Figure 7.3e Bent-leg curl-up

Abdominal crunch. This test is recommended only for individuals who are unable to perform the bent-leg curl-up test because of susceptibility to low-back injury. Exercise form must be carefully monitored during the test. Several authors and researchers have indicated that proper form during this test is extremely difficult to control. Subjects often slide their bodies, bend their elbows, or shrug their shoulders during the test. Such actions facilitate the performance of the test and misrepresent the actual test results. Biomechanical factors also limit the ability to perform this test. Further, lack of spinal flexibility keeps some individuals from being able to move the full 3½" range of motion. Others are unable to keep their heels on the floor during the test. The validity of this test as an effective measure of abdominal strength or abdominal endurance has also been questioned through research.

Tape a 3½" × 30" strip of cardboard onto the floor. Lie down on the floor in a supine position (face up) with the knees bent at approximately 100° and the legs slightly apart. The feet should be on the floor, and you must hold them in place yourself throughout the test. Straighten out your arms and place them on the floor alongside the trunk with the palms down and the fingers fully extended. The fingertips of both hands should barely touch the closest edge of the cardboard (see Figure 7.3f). Bring the head off the floor until the chin is 1" to 2" away from your chest. Keep the head in this position during the entire test (do not move the head by flexing or extending the neck). You are now ready to begin the test.

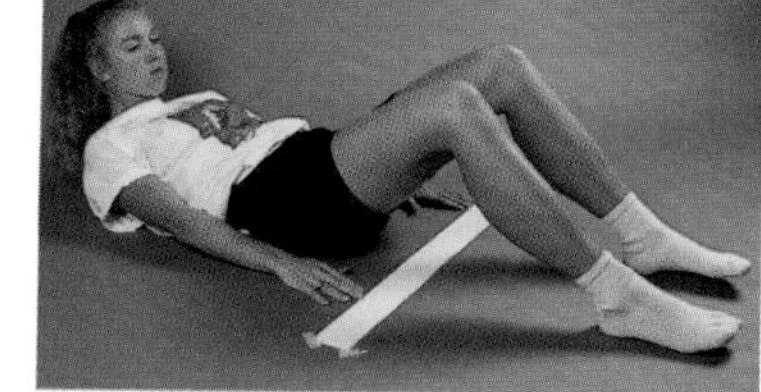

Figure 7.3f Abdominal crunch test

Perform the repetitions to a two-step cadence (up-down) regulated with a metronome set at 60 beats per minute. As you curl up, slide the fingers over the cardboard until the fingertips reach the far edge (3½") of the board (see Figure 7.3g), then return to the starting position.

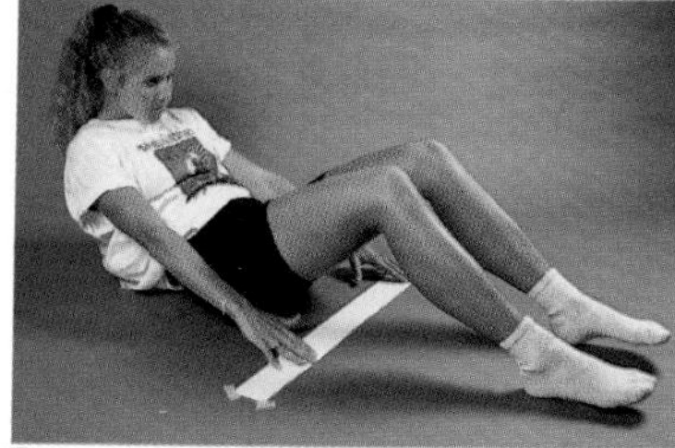

Figure 7.3g Abdominal crunch test

Allow a brief practice period of 5 to 10 seconds to familiarize yourself with the cadence. Initiate the *up* movement with the first beat and the *down* movement with the next beat. Accomplish one repetition every two beats of the metronome. Count as many repetitions as you are able to perform following the proper cadence. You may not count a repetition if the fingertips fail to reach the distant edge of the cardboard.

Terminate the test if you (a) fail to maintain the appropriate cadence, (b) bend the elbows, (c) shrug the shoulders, (d) slide

FIGURE 7.3 Muscular Endurance Test. (continued)

the body, (e) lift heels off the floor, (f) raise the chin off the chest, (g) accomplish 100 repetitions, or (h) no longer can perform the test. Have your partner check the angle at the knees throughout the test to make sure that the 100° angle is maintained as closely as possible.

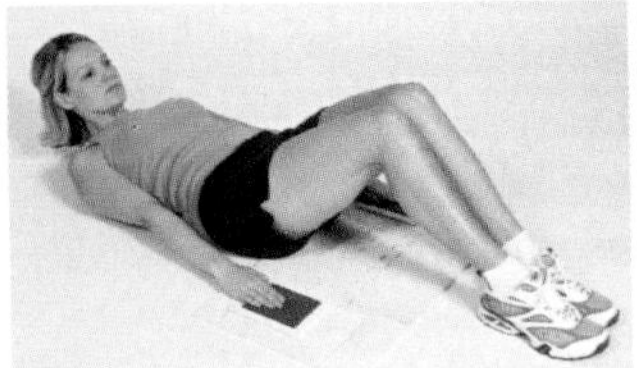
Figure 7.3h

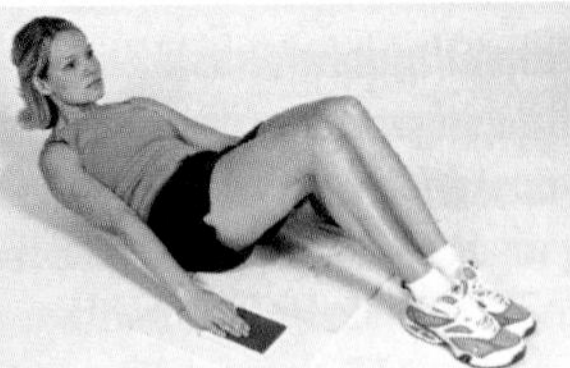
Figure 7.3i

Abdominal crunch test performed with a Crunch-Ster Curl-Up Tester.

For this test you may also use a Crunch-Ster Curl-Up Tester, available from Novel Products.* An illustration of the test performed with this equipment is provided in Figures 7.3h and 7.3i.

According to the results, look up your percentile rank for each exercise in the far left column of Table 7.2 and determine your muscular endurance fitness category according to the following classification:

Average Score	Fitness Category	Points
≥90	Excellent	5
70–80	Good	4
50–60	Average	3
30–40	Fair	2
≤20	Poor	1

Look up the number of points assigned for each fitness category above. Total the number of points and determine your overall strength endurance fitness category according to the following ratings:

Total Points	Strength Endurance Category
≥13	Excellent
10–12	Good
7–9	Average
4–6	Fair
≤3	Poor

TABLE 7.2 Muscular Endurance Scoring Table

	Men				Women			
Percentile Rank	Bench Jumps	Modified Dips	Bent-Leg Curl-Ups	Abdominal Crunches	Bench Jumps	Modified Push-Ups	Bent-Leg Curl-Ups	Abdominal Crunches
99	66	54	100	100	58	95	100	100
95	63	50	81	100	54	70	100	100
90	62	38	65	100	52	50	97	69
80	58	32	51	66	48	41	77	49
70	57	30	44	45	44	38	57	37
60	56	27	31	38	42	33	45	34
50	54	26	28	33	39	30	37	31
40	51	23	25	29	38	28	28	27
30	48	20	22	26	36	25	22	24
20	47	17	17	22	32	21	17	21
10	40	11	10	18	28	18	9	15
5	34	7	3	16	26	15	4	0

you lift a submaximal resistance as many times as possible using the six strength-training exercises listed in Figure 7.4. The resistance for each lift is determined according to selected percentages of body weight shown in Figure 7.4 and Lab 7A.

With this test, if an individual does only a few repetitions, primarily absolute strength is measured. For those who are able to do a lot of repetitions, the test is an indicator of muscular endurance. If you are not familiar with the different lifts, see the illustrations provided at the end of this chapter.

A strength/endurance rating is determined according to the maximum number of repetitions you are able to perform on each exercise. Fixed-resistance strength units are necessary to administer all but the abdominal exercises in this test (see "Dynamic Training" on page 272 for an explanation of fixed-resistance equipment).

A percentile rank for each exercise is given based on the number of repetitions performed (Table 7.3). As with the Muscular Endurance Test, an overall muscular strength/

FIGURE 7.4 Muscular Strength and Endurance Test.

1. Familiarize yourself with the six lifts used for this test: lat pull-down, leg extension, bench press, bent-leg curl-up or abdominal crunch,* leg curl, and arm curl. Graphic illustrations for each lift are given on pages 294, 296, 291, 287, 292, and 295, respectively. For the leg curl exercise, the knees should be flexed to 90°. A description and illustration of the bent-leg curl-up and the abdominal crunch exercises are provided in Figure 7.3. On the leg extension lift, maintain the trunk in an upright position.
2. Determine your body weight in pounds.
3. Determine the amount of resistance to be used on each lift. To obtain this number, multiply your body weight by the percent given below for each lift.

Lift	Percent of Body Weight	
	Men	Women
Lat Pull-Down	.70	.45
Leg Extension	.65	.50
Bench Press	.75	.45
Bent-Leg Curl-Up or Abdominal Crunch*	NA**	NA**
Leg Curl	.32	.25
Arm Curl	.35	.18

*The abdominal crunch exercise should be used only by individuals who suffer or are susceptible to low-back pain.
**NA = not applicable—see Figure 7.3.

4. Perform the maximum continuous number of repetitions possible.
5. Based on the number of repetitions performed, look up the percentile rank for each lift in the left column of Table 7.3.
6. The individual strength fitness category is determined according to the following classification:

Percentile Rank	Fitness Category	Points
≥90	Excellent	5
70–80	Good	4
50–60	Average	3
30–40	Fair	2
≤20	Poor	1

7. Look up the number of points assigned for each fitness category under item 6 above. Total the number of points and determine your overall strength fitness category according to the following ratings:

Total Points	Strength Category
≥25	Excellent
19–24	Good
13–18	Average
7–12	Fair
≤6	Poor

8. Record your results in Lab 7A.

endurance rating is obtained by totaling the number of points obtained on each exercise.

If no fixed-resistance equipment is available, you can still perform the test using different equipment. In that case, though, the percentile rankings and strength fitness categories may not be accurate, because a certain resistance (e.g., 50 pounds) is seldom the same on two different strength-training machines (e.g., Universal Gym versus Nautilus). The industry has no standard calibration procedure for strength equipment. Consequently, if you lift a certain resis-

TABLE 7.3 Muscular Strength and Endurance Scoring Table

Percentile Rank	Men							Women						
	Lat Pull-Down	Leg Extension	Bench Press	Bent-Leg Curl-Up	Abdominal Crunch	Leg Curl	Arm Curl	Lat Pull-Down	Leg Extension	Bench Press	Bent-Leg Curl-Up	Abdominal Crunch	Leg Curl	Arm Curl
>99	30	25	26	100	100	24	25	30	25	27	100	100	20	25
95	25	20	21	81	100	20	21	25	20	21	100	100	17	21
90	19	19	19	65	100	19	19	21	18	20	97	69	12	20
80	16	15	16	51	66	15	15	16	13	16	77	49	10	16
70	13	14	13	44	45	13	12	13	11	13	57	37	9	14
60	11	13	11	31	38	11	10	11	10	11	45	34	7	12
50	10	12	10	28	33	10	9	10	9	10	37	31	6	10
40	9	10	7	25	29	8	8	9	8	5	28	27	5	8
30	7	9	5	22	26	6	7	7	7	3	22	24	4	7
20	6	7	3	17	22	4	5	6	5	1	17	21	3	6
10	4	5	1	10	18	3	3	3	3	0	9	15	1	3
5	3	3	0	3	16	1	2	2	1	0	4	0	0	2

tance for a specific exercise (e.g., bench press) on one machine, you may or may not be able to lift the same amount for this exercise on a different machine.

Even though the percentile ranks may not be valid across different equipment, test results can be used to evaluate changes in fitness. For example, you may be able to do 7 repetitions during the initial test, but if you can perform 14 repetitions after 12 weeks of training, that's a measure of improvement. Results of the Muscular Strength and Endurance Test can be recorded in Lab 7A.

Strength-Training Prescription

The capacity of muscle cells to exert force increases and decreases according to the demands placed upon the muscular system. If muscle cells are overloaded beyond their normal use, such as in strength-training programs, the cells increase in size (hypertrophy) and strength. If the demands placed on the muscle cells decrease, such as in sedentary living or required rest because of illness or injury, the cells **atrophy** and lose strength. A good level of muscular fitness is important to develop and maintain fitness, health, and total well-being.

Two types of muscular hypertrophy are known: **myofibrillar hypertrophy** and **sarcoplasmic hypertrophy**. Myofibrils are composed of the myosin and actin filaments (see Figure 7.5), the contractile portion of the muscle. Several hundred myofibrils make up a single muscle fiber. A bundle of muscle fibers (about 10 to 100) make up a fasciculus. In turn, many of these bundles together (fasciculi) make up an entire muscle. The **sarcoplasm** in muscle is comparable to the cytoplasm in other cells. This semifluid substance in muscle contains primarily myosin and actin myofibrils, but also large amounts of glycosomes (organelles that store glycogen and enzymes) and myoglobin (the oxygen-binding protein in muscle).

Myofibrillar hypertrophy is the result of increased synthesis of the protein filaments myosin and actin that slide past one another to produce muscle contraction. With this type of hypertrophy, the area density (size) of the myofibrils increases and results in a greater ability of the muscle to generate tension (exert muscle strength). This type of hypertrophy is achieved by training with heavy resistances and low repetitions (1 to 6). Strength and power athletes use this training method because it results in greater strength increases.

Sarcoplasmic hypertrophy is achieved primarily through an increase in sarcoplasm as a result of training conducted with lower resistances but performing a larger number of repetitions (8 to 15). The latter training results in greater muscle size than observed in myofibrillar hypertrophy but lower increases in strength. Muscular strength is primarily dependent on the amount and the density of the muscle fibers. Adding more muscle fluid (sarcoplasm) does

FIGURE 7.5 Basic Muscle Structure

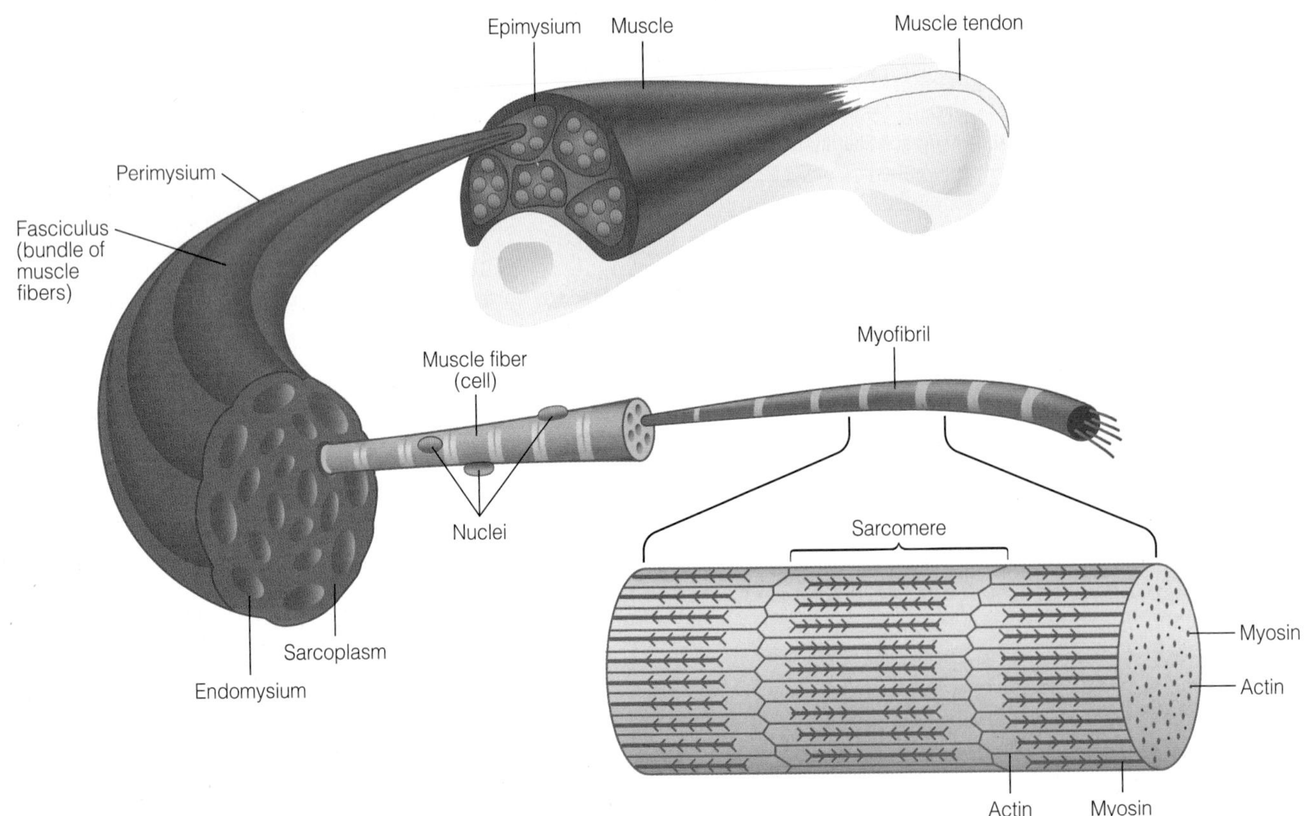

not increase strength to the same extent. Bodybuilders typically rely on training that leads to sarcoplasmic hypertrophy as they are judged by appearance and not by the amount of resistance lifted.

Factors That Affect Muscular Fitness

Several physiological factors combine to create muscle contraction and subsequent strength gains: neural stimulation, type of muscle fiber, overload, specificity of training, training volume, and periodization. Basic knowledge of these concepts is important for understanding the principles involved in strength development.

Neural Function

Within the neuromuscular system, single **motor neurons** branch and attach to multiple muscle fibers. The motor neuron and the fibers it innervates (supplies with nerves) form a **motor unit**. The number of fibers that a motor neuron can innervate varies from just a few in muscles that require precise control (e.g., eye muscles) to as many as 1,000 or more in large muscles that do not perform refined or precise movements.

Stimulation of a motor neuron causes the muscle fibers to contract maximally or not at all. Variations in the number of fibers innervated and the frequency of their stimulation determine the strength of the muscle contraction. As the number of fibers innervated and frequency of stimulation increase, so does the strength of the muscular contraction.

Neural adaptations are prominent in the early stages of strength training. In novice participants, significant strength increases seen during the first 2 to 3 weeks of training are largely related to enhanced neural function by increasing motor neuron stimulation and muscle fiber recruitment (skill acquisition). Long-term strength development is primarily related to increased physiological adaptation within the muscle(s) and to a lesser extent to continued neural adaptations.

Types of Muscle Fiber

The human body has two basic types of muscle fibers: (1) slow-twitch or red fibers and (2) fast-twitch or white fibers. **Slow-twitch fibers** have a greater capacity for aerobic work. **Fast-twitch fibers** have a greater capacity for anaerobic work and produce more overall force. The latter are important for quick and powerful movements commonly used in strength-training activities.

The proportion of slow- and fast-twitch fibers is determined genetically and consequently varies from one person to another. Nevertheless, training increases the functional capacity of both types of fiber, and more specifically, strength training increases their ability to exert force.

During muscular contraction, slow-twitch fibers always are recruited first. As the force and speed of muscle contraction increase, the relative importance of the fast-twitch fibers increases. To activate the fast-twitch fibers, an activity must be intense and powerful.

Overload

Strength gains are achieved in two ways:

1. Through increased ability of individual muscle fibers to generate a stronger contraction
2. By recruiting a greater proportion of the total available fibers for each contraction

These two factors combine in the **overload principle**. The demands placed on the muscle must be increased systematically and progressively over time, and the resistance must be of a magnitude significant enough to cause physiological adaptation. In simpler terms, just like all other organs and systems of the human body, to increase in physical capacity, muscles have to be taxed repeatedly beyond their accustomed loads. Because of this principle, strength training also is called progressive resistance training.

Several procedures can be used to overload in strength training[10]:

1. Increasing the intensity (the resistance or the amount of weight used)
2. Increasing the number of repetitions at the current intensity
3. Increasing or decreasing the speed at which the repetitions are performed
4. Decreasing the rest interval for endurance improvements (with lighter resistances) or lengthening the rest interval for strength and power development (with higher resistances)
5. Increasing the volume (the sum of the repetitions performed multiplied by the resistance used)
6. Using any combination of the preceding procedures

Atrophy Decrease in the size of a cell.

Myofibrillar hypertrophy Muscle hypertrophy as a result of increased protein synthesis in the myosin and actin myofibrils.

Sarcoplasmic hypertrophy Muscle hypertrophy as a result of an increase in sarcoplasm.

Sarcoplasm The equivalent of the cytoplasm in other cells—a semifluid substance that contains myosin and actin filaments, as well other muscle cell organelles.

Motor neurons Nerves connecting the central nervous system to the muscle.

Motor unit The combination of a motor neuron and the muscle fibers that neuron innervates.

Slow-twitch fibers Muscle fibers with greater aerobic potential and slow speed of contraction.

Fast-twitch fibers Muscle fibers with greater anaerobic potential and fast speed of contraction.

Overload principle Training concept that the demands placed on a system (cardiorespiratory or muscular) must be increased systematically and progressively over time to cause physiological adaptation (development or improvement).

Specificity of Training

Training adaptations are specific to the impetus applied. In strength training, the principle of **specificity of training** holds that for a muscle to increase in strength or endurance, the training program must be specific to obtain the desired effects (see also the discussion on resistance on page 274).

The principle of specificity also applies to activity- or sport-specific development and is commonly referred to as **specific adaptation to imposed demand (SAID) training**. The SAID principle implies that if an individual is attempting to improve specific activity or sport skills, the strength-training exercises performed should resemble as closely as possible the movement patterns encountered in that particular activity or sport.

For example, a soccer player who wishes to become stronger and faster emphasizes exercises that develop leg strength and power. In contrast, an individual recovering from a lower-limb fracture initially exercises to increase strength and stability and subsequently to improve muscle endurance.

Training Volume **Volume** is the sum of all repetitions performed multiplied by the resistances used during a strength-training session. Volume frequently is used to quantify the amount of work performed in a given training session. For example, an individual who does three sets of six repetitions with 150 pounds has performed a training volume of 2,700 ($3 \times 6 \times 150$) for this exercise. The total training volume can be obtained by totaling the volume of all exercises performed.

The volume of training done in a strength-training session can be modified by changing the total number of exercises performed, the number of sets done per exercise, or the number of repetitions performed per set. Athletes typically use high training volumes and low intensities to achieve muscle hypertrophy and low volumes and high intensities to increase strength and power.

Periodization The concept of **periodization** (variation) entails systematically altering training variables over time to keep the program challenging and lead to greater strength development. Periodization means cycling training objectives (hypertrophy, strength, and endurance), with each phase of the program, which lasts anywhere from 2 to 12 weeks. Training variables that can be altered include resistance (weight lifted), number of repetitions, number of sets, and number of exercises performed.

The periodized training approach is popular among athletes and is frequently used to prevent **overtraining**. Training volume should not increase by more than 5 percent from one phase to the next. Periodization is now popular among fitness participants who wish to achieve maximal strength gains. Over the long run, for intermediate and advanced participants, the periodized approach has been shown to be superior to nonperiodized training (using the same exercises, sets, and repetitions repeatedly).

Three types of periodized training, based on program design and objectives, are commonly used:

- **Classical periodization**, used by individuals seeking maximal strength development. It starts with an initial high volume of training using low resistances. In subsequent cycles, the program gradually switches to a lower volume and higher resistances.
- **Reverse periodization**, used primarily by individuals seeking greater muscular endurance. Also a linear model, it is opposite of the classical model: The resistances are highest at the beginning of training, with a low volume, and subsequently followed by progressive decreases in resistances and increases in training volume.
- **Undulating periodization**, using a combination of volumes and resistances within a cycle by alternating now (randomly or systematically) among the muscular fitness components: strength, hypertrophy, power, and endurance. The undulating model compares favorably, and in some cases is superior to, the classical and reverse models.

Understanding all five training concepts that affect strength (neural stimulation, muscle fiber types, overload, specificity, and periodization) discussed thus far is required to design an effective strength-training program.

Principles Involved in Strength Training

Because muscular strength and endurance are important in developing and maintaining overall fitness and well-being, the principles necessary to develop a strength-training program have to be understood, just as in the prescription for cardiorespiratory endurance (see Chapter 6). These principles are mode, resistance, sets, and frequency, in addition to volume of training, as described previously. The key factor in successful muscular fitness development, however, is the individualization of the program according to these principles and the person's goals, as well as the magnitude of the individual's effort during training.

Mode of Training Two types of training methods are used to improve strength: isometric (static) and dynamic (previously called "isotonic"). In **isometric training**, muscle contractions produce little or no movement, such as pushing or pulling against an immovable object or holding a given position against resistance for a given period. In **dynamic training**, the muscle contractions produce movement, such as extending the knees with resistance on the ankles (leg extension). The specificity of training principle applies here too. To increase isometric versus dynamic strength, an individual must use static instead of dynamic training to achieve the desired results.

Isometric Training

Isometric training does not require much equipment. Because strength gains with isometric training are specific to

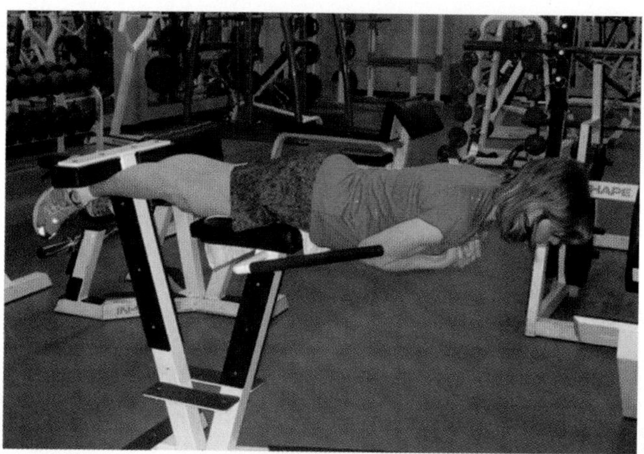
© Fitness & Wellness, Inc.

In isometric (static) training, muscle contraction produces little or no movement.

the angle of muscle contraction, this type of training is beneficial in a sport such as gymnastics, which requires regular static contractions during routines. As presented in Chapter 8, however, isometric training is a critical component of health conditioning programs for the low back (see "Preventing and Rehabilitating Low Back Pain," page 321–326) and for spinal-stabilization musculature and healthy posture. Selected exercises, in particular core exercises, are recommended as a part of a comprehensive strength-training program.

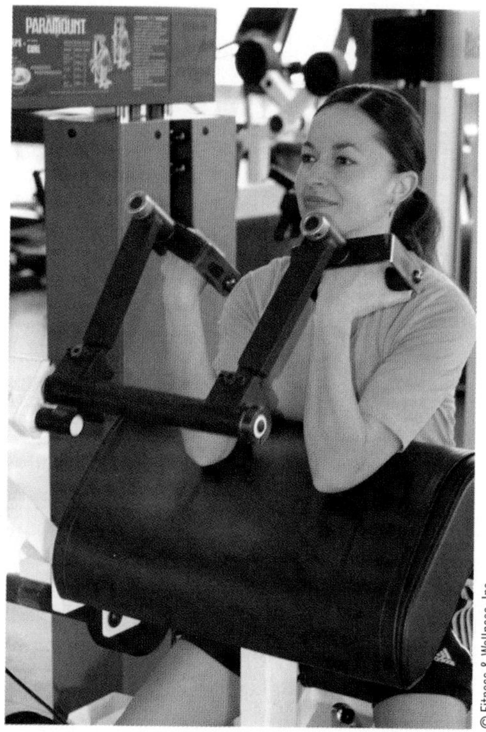
© Fitness & Wellness, Inc.

In dynamic training, muscle contraction produces movement in the respective joint.

Dynamic Training

Dynamic training is the most common mode for strength training. The primary advantage is that strength is gained through the full **range of motion.** Most daily activities are dynamic. We are constantly lifting, pushing, and pulling objects, and strength is needed through a complete range of motion. Another advantage is that improvements are measured easily by the amount lifted.

Dynamic training consists of two action phases when an exercise is performed: (1) **concentric** or **positive resistance** and (2) **eccentric** or **negative resistance.** In the concentric phase, the muscle shortens as it contracts to overcome the resistance. In the eccentric phase, the muscle lengthens to overcome the resistance. For example, during a bench press exercise, when the person lifts the resistance from the chest to full-arm extension, the triceps muscle on the back of the upper arm shortens to extend

Specificity of training Principle that training must be done with the specific muscle(s) the person is attempting to improve.

Specific adaptation to imposed demand (SAID) training Training principle stating that, for improvements to occur in a specific activity, the exercises performed during a strength-training program should resemble as closely as possible the movement patterns encountered in that particular activity.

Volume (in strength training) The sum of all repetitions performed multiplied by resistances used during a strength-training session.

Periodization A training approach that divides the season into three cycles (macrocycles, mesocycles, and microcycles) using systematic variation in intensity and volume of training to enhance fitness and performance.

Overtraining An emotional, behavioral, and physical condition marked by increased fatigue, decreased performance, persistent muscle soreness, mood disturbances, and feelings of "staleness" or "burnout" as a result of excessive physical training.

Isometric training Strength-training method referring to a muscle contraction that produces little or no movement, such as pushing or pulling against an immovable object.

Dynamic training Strength-training method referring to a muscle contraction with movement.

Range of motion Entire arc of movement of a given joint.

Concentric Shortening of a muscle during muscle contraction.

Positive resistance The lifting, pushing, or concentric phase of a repetition during a strength-training exercise.

Eccentric Lengthening of a muscle during muscle contraction.

Negative resistance The lowering or eccentric phase of a repetition during a strength-training exercise.

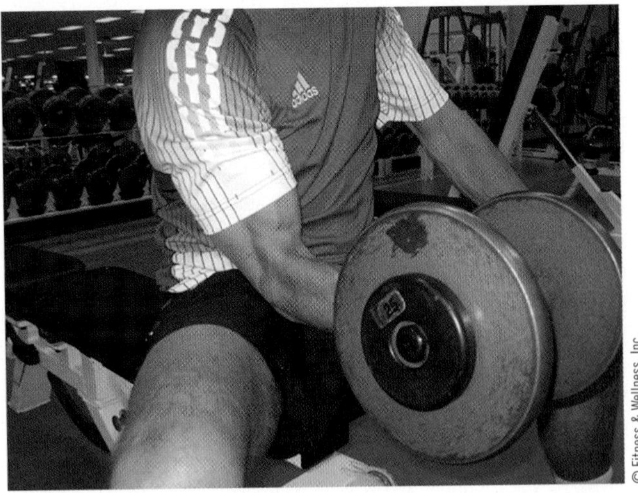

Strength training can be done using free weights.

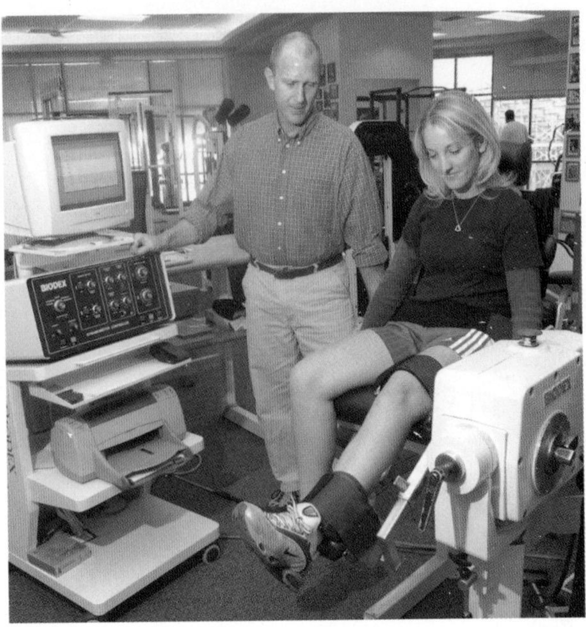

In isokinetic training, the speed of muscle contraction is constant.

(straighten) the elbow. During the eccentric phase, the same triceps muscle is used to lower the weight during elbow flexion, but the muscle lengthens slowly to avoid dropping the resistance. Both motions work the same muscle against the same amount of resistance.

Eccentric muscle contractions allow you to lower weights in a smooth, gradual, and controlled manner. Without eccentric contractions, weights would be suddenly dropped on the way down. Because the same muscles work when you lift and lower a resistance, always be sure to execute both actions in a controlled manner. Failure to do so diminishes the benefits of the training program and increases the risk for injuries. Eccentric contractions seem to be more effective in producing muscle hypertrophy but result in greater muscle soreness.[11]

Dynamic training programs can be conducted without weights; using exercise bands; and with **free weights**, **fixed-resistance** machines, **variable-resistance** machines, or isokinetic equipment. When you perform dynamic exercises without weights (e.g., pull-ups and push-ups), with free weights, or with fixed-resistance machines, you move a constant resistance through a joint's full range of motion. The greatest resistance that can be lifted equals the maximum weight that can be moved at the weakest angle of the joint. This is because of changes in length of muscle and angle of pull as the joint moves through its range of motion. This type of training is also referred to as **dynamic constant external resistance** or DCER.

As strength training became more popular, new strength-training machines were developed. This technology brought about **isokinetic training** and variable-resistance training programs, which require special machines equipped with mechanical devices that provide differing amounts of resistance, with the intent of overloading the muscle group maximally through the entire range of motion. A distinction of isokinetic training is that the speed of the muscle contraction is kept constant because the machine provides resistance to match the user's force through the range of motion. The mode of training that an individual selects depends mainly on the type of equipment available and the specific objective the training program is attempting to accomplish.

The benefits of isokinetic and variable-resistance training are similar to those of the other dynamic training methods. Theoretically, strength gains should be better because maximum resistance is applied at all angles. Research, however, has not shown this type of training to be more effective than other modes of dynamic training.

Free Weights versus Machines in Dynamic Training

The most popular weight-training devices available during the first half of the 20th century were plate-loaded barbells (free weights). Strength-training machines were developed in the middle of the century but did not become popular until the 1970s. With subsequent technological improvements to these machines, a debate arose over which of the two training modalities was better.

Free weights require that the individual balance the resistance through the entire lifting motion. Free weights may provide greater strength development because additional muscles are needed to balance the resistance as it is moved through the range of motion. Strength-training machines, nonetheless, are an excellent training modality for individuals who are either starting strength training for the first time, those who are primarily attempting to maintain strength levels, and for older adults concerned with safety and ease of use. Let's examine the advantages of each system.

Advantages of Free Weights

Following are the advantages of using free weights instead of machines in a strength-training program:

- Cost. Free weights are less expensive than most exercise machines. On a limited budget, free weights are a better option.
- Variety. A bar and a few plates can be used to perform many exercises to strengthen most muscles in the body.
- Portability. Free weights can be easily moved from one area or station to another.
- Coordination. Free weights require greater muscular coordination to mimic movement requirements of specific tasks.
- Balance: Free weights require that a person balance the weight through the entire range of motion. This feature involves additional support and stabilizing muscles to keep the weight moving properly.
- One size fits all. People of almost all ages can use free weights. A drawback of machines is that individuals who are at the extremes in terms of height or limb length often do not fit into the machines. In particular, small women and adolescents are at a disadvantage.

Advantages of Machines

Strength-training machines have the following advantages over free weights:

- Safety: Machines are safer because spotters are rarely needed to monitor lifting
- Ease of use: Only a minimal amount of skill is required because the machines guide and control the movement through the entire range of motion
- Selection. A few exercises—such as hip flexion, hip abduction, leg curls, lat pull-downs, and neck exercises—can be performed only with machines.
- Variable resistance. Most machines provide variable resistance. Free weights provide only fixed resistance.
- Isolation. Individual muscles are better isolated with machines, because stabilizing muscles are not used to balance the weight during the exercise.
- Time. Exercising with machines requires less time, because you can set the resistance quickly by using a selector pin instead of having to manually change dumbbells or weight plates on both sides of a barbell.
- Flexibility. Most machines can provide resistance over a greater range of movement during the exercise, thereby contributing to more flexibility in the joints. For example, a barbell pullover exercise provides resistance over a range of 100 degrees, whereas a weight machine may allow for as much as 260 degrees.
- Rehabilitation. Machines are more useful during injury rehabilitation. A knee injury, for instance, is practically impossible to rehab using free weights, whereas with a weight machine, small loads can be easily selected through a limited range of motion.
- Skill acquisition. Learning a new exercise movement—and performing it correctly—is faster, because the machine controls the direction of the movement.

confidentconsumer

I have been told that certain types of equipment are better for strength development. Which one is best?

Free weights, as opposed to strength-training machines, require that the individual balance the resistance through the entire lifting motion. We could logically assume that free weights are a better training modality, because additional stabilizing muscles are needed to balance the resistance as it is moved through the range of motion. Research, however, has not shown any differences in strength development among different exercise modalities. Proper technique and degree of effort are more important than the specific type of equipment used. Muscles do not know whether the source of a resistance is a barbell, a dumbbell, a weight machine, or a simple cinder block. What determines the extent of a person's strength development is the quality of the program (number of exercises, sets, reps, frequency, and progression), the individual's effort during the training program—not the type of equipment used, and proper nutrition. Selection comes down to personal preference, equipment availability, and a program that fits personal lifestyle.

An ideal training program actually incorporates both free weights and machines. You can chose free weights for some exercises and machines for others. Although each modality has pros and cons, muscles do not know whether the source of a resistance is a barbell, a dumbbell, a Universal Gym machine, a Nautilus machine, or a simple cinder block. The most important component that determines the extent of a person's strength development is the quality of the program and the individual's effort during the training program itself—not the type of equipment used, thus, the general recommendation that machines be

Free weights Barbells and dumbbells.

Fixed resistance Type of exercise in which a constant resistance is moved through a joint's full range of motion (dumbbells, barbells, and machines using a constant resistance).

Variable resistance Training using special machines equipped with mechanical devices that provide differing amounts of resistance through the range of motion.

Dynamic constant external resistance (DCER) See **fixed resistance**.

Isokinetic training Strength-training method in which the speed of the muscle contraction is kept constant because the equipment (machine) provides an accommodating resistance to match the user's force (maximal) through the range of motion.

used early on. Subsequently, both machines and free weights can be used by intermediate and advanced participants.

Resistance **Resistance** in strength training is the equivalent of intensity in cardiorespiratory exercise prescription. To stimulate strength development, the general recommendation has been to use a resistance of approximately 80 percent of the maximum capacity (the 1 RM). For example, a person with a 1 RM of 150 pounds should work with about 120 pounds (150 × .80).

The number of repetitions that someone can perform at 80 percent of the 1 RM, however, varies among exercises (i.e., bench press, lat pull-down, and leg curl; Table 7.4). Data indicate that the total number of repetitions performed at a certain percentage of the 1 RM depends on the amount of muscle mass involved (bench press versus triceps extension) and whether it is a single or multi-joint exercise (leg press versus leg curl). In trained and untrained subjects alike, the number of repetitions is greater with larger muscle mass involvement and multi joint exercises.[12]

Because of the time factor involved in constantly determining the 1 RM on each lift to ensure that the person is indeed working around 80 percent, the accepted rule for many years has been that individuals perform between 8 and 12 repetitions maximum (or in the 8 to 12 RM zone) for adequate strength gains. For example, if a person is training with a resistance of 120 pounds and cannot lift it more than 12 times—that is, the person reaches volitional fatigue at or before 12 repetitions—the training stimulus (weight used) is adequate for strength development. It is important to note that volitional fatigue means to the point of muscle fatigue but not muscle failure. Exerting muscles to failure substantially increases the risk of excessive soreness and injury among beginner lifters and older adults. Once the person can lift the resistance more than 12 times, the resistance is increased by 5 to 10 pounds and the person again should build up to 12 repetitions. This is referred to as **progressive resistance training**.

TABLE 7.4 Number of Repetitions Performed at 80 Percent of the One Repetition Maximum (1 RM)

	Trained		Untrained	
Exercise	**Men**	**Women**	**Men**	**Women**
Leg press	19	22	15	12
Lat pull-down	12	10	10	10
Bench press	12	14	10	10
Leg extension	12	10	9	8
Sit-up*	12	12	8	7
Arm curl	11	7	8	6
Leg curl	7	5	6	6

*Sit-up exercise performed with weighted plates on the chest and feet held in place with an ankle strap.

Source: W. W. K. Hoeger, D. R. Hopkins, S. L. Barette, and D. F. Hale, "Relationship Between Repetitions and Selected Percentages of One Repetition Maximum: A Comparison Between Untrained and Trained Males and Females," *Journal of Applied Sport Science Research* 4, no. 2 (1990): 47–51.

Strength development, however, also can occur when working with less than 80 percent of the 1 RM (60 percent to 80 percent). Although the 8 to 12 RM zone is the most commonly prescribed resistance training zone, benefits still accrue when working with less than 8 RM or above 12 RM. Older adults and individuals susceptible to musculoskeletal injuries are encouraged to work with 10 to 15 repetitions using moderate resistances (about 50 percent to 60 percent of the 1 RM).If the main objective of the training program is muscular endurance, 15 to 25 repetitions per set are recommended.

In both young and older individuals, all repetitions should be performed at a moderate velocity (about 1 second concentric and 1 second eccentric), which yields the greatest strength gains. For advanced training, varying training velocity among sets, from very slow to fast, is recommended.

Elite strength and power athletes typically work between 1 and 6 RM, but they often shuffle training (periodized training) with a different number of repetitions and sets for selected periods (weeks). Body builders tend to work with moderate resistance levels (60 to 85 percent of the 1 RM) and perform 8 to 15 repetitions to near fatigue. A foremost objective of body building is to increase muscle size. Moderate resistance promotes blood flow to the muscles, "pumping up the muscles" (also known as "the pump"), which makes them look larger than they do in a resting state.

From a general fitness point of view, a moderate resistance of only about 50 percent should be used initially while learning proper form and lifting technique. Following the first 2 weeks of training, working near a 10-repetition threshold seems to improve overall performance most effectively. We live in a dynamic world in which muscular strength and endurance are both required to lead an enjoyable life. Working around 10 RM produces good balanced results between strength, endurance, and hypertrophy. To maximize training development, advanced participants are encouraged to cycle between 1 and 12 RM.

Sets In strength training, a **set** is the number of repetitions performed for a given exercise. For example, a person lifting 120 pounds eight times has performed one set of 8 repetitions (1 × 8 × 120) with 2 to 3 minutes rest interval between sets. For general fitness, muscular strength, and muscular hypertrophy, the recommendation is two to four sets per exercise (advanced participants often train with up to six sets per exercise). For a person looking to improve muscular endurance, no more than two sets (of 15 to 25 repetitions each) per exercise are recommended.

When performing multiple sets using the RM zone with the same resistance, if the person truly performs 12 RM to muscle fatigue (or close to it), in subsequent sets fewer RM will be performed (perhaps 10, 9, and 7 RM). Because of the characteristics of muscle fiber, the number of sets the exerciser can do is limited. As the number of sets increases, so does the amount of muscle fatigue and subsequent recovery time.

When time is a factor, and although multiple-set training is most beneficial, single-set programs are still effective, as long as the single set is performed within the RM zone to muscular fatigue. You may also choose to do two sets for multi-joint exercises (bench press, leg press, lat pull-down, etc.) and a single RM-zone set for single-joint exercises (arm curl, triceps extension, knee extension, etc.).

A recommended program for beginners in their first year of training is one or two light warm-up sets per exercise, using about 50 percent of the 1 RM (no warm-up sets are necessary for subsequent exercises that use the same muscle group), followed by one to four sets to near fatigue per exercise. Maintaining resistance and effort that temporarily fatigue the muscle (volitional exhaustion) from the number of repetitions selected in at least one of the sets is crucial to achieve optimal progress. Because of the lower resistances used in body building, four to eight sets can be done for each exercise.

To avoid muscle soreness and stiffness, new participants should build up gradually to the three to four sets of maximal repetitions. They can do this by performing only one set of each exercise with a lighter resistance on the first day of training and two sets of each exercise on the second day—the first light and the second with the required resistance to volitional exhaustion. They then could choose to increase to three sets on the third day—one light and two heavy. After that, they should be able to perform anywhere from two to four sets as planned.

The time necessary to recover between sets depends mainly on the resistance used during each set. In strength training, the energy to lift heavy weights is derived primarily from the system involving adenosine triphosphate (ATP) and creatine phosphate (CP) or phosphagen (see "Energy (ATP) Production," Chapter 3, page 117).Ten seconds of maximal exercise nearly depletes the CP stores in the exercised muscle(s). These stores are replenished in about 3 to 5 minutes of recovery.

Based on this principle, rest intervals between sets vary in length depending on the program goals and are dictated by the amount of resistance used in training. Short rest intervals of less than 2 minutes are commonly used when people are trying to develop local muscular endurance. Moderate rest intervals of 2 to 4 minutes are used for strength development. Long intervals of more than 4 minutes are used when people are training for power development.[13] Using these guidelines, individuals training for health fitness purposes might allow 2 minutes of rest between sets. Body builders, who use lower resistances, should rest no more than 1 minute to maximize the "pumping" effect.

For someone trying to maximize strength gains, the exercise program is more time effective if two or three exercises are alternated that require different muscle groups, called **circuit training**. In this way, an individual does not have to wait 2 to 3 minutes before proceeding to a new set on a different exercise. For example, the bench press, leg extension, and abdominal curl-up exercises may be combined so that the person can go almost directly from one exercise set to the next.

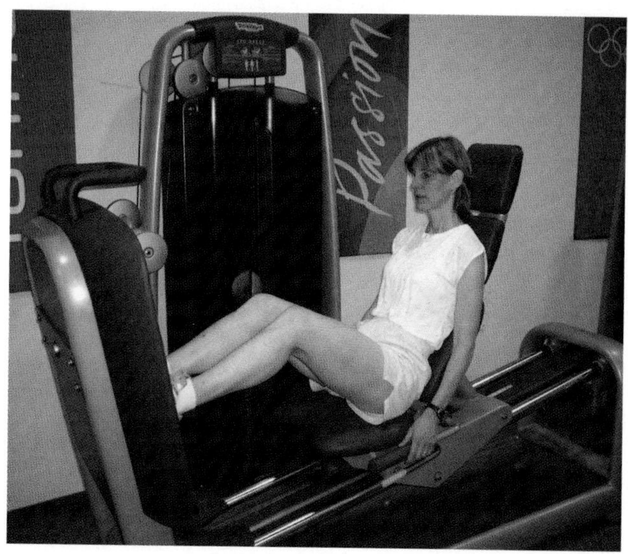

From a health-fitness standpoint, one to two strength-training sessions per week are sufficient to maintain strength.

Men and women alike should observe the guidelines given previously. However, many women do not follow them. They erroneously believe that training with low resistances and many repetitions is best to enhance body composition and maximize energy expenditure. Unless people are seeking to increase muscular endurance for a specific sport-related activity, the use of low resistances and high repetitions is not recommended to achieve optimal strength fitness goals and maximize long-term energy expenditure.

Frequency Strength training should be done through a total body workout two to three times a week. Strength training two times per week produces about 80 percent of the strength gains seen in a traditional three times per week program. Training can be performed more frequently if using a split-body routine, that is, upper body one day and lower body the next. After a maximum strength workout, a rest interval of 48 to 72 hours between sessions is recommended to promote the adaptations required for optimal muscle hypertrophy and the respective strength gains. If not recovered in 2 to 3 days, the person most likely is overtraining and therefore not reaping the full benefits of the program. In that case, the person should do fewer sets of exercises than in the previous workout. A summary of strength-training guidelines for health fitness purposes is provided in Figure 7.6.

To achieve significant strength gains, a minimum of 8 weeks of consecutive training is recommended. After an individual has achieved an adequate strength level, from a health fitness standpoint, one to two train-

Resistance Amount of weight lifted.

Set A fixed number of repetitions; one set of bench presses might be 10 repetitions.

Circuit training Alternating exercises by performing them in a sequence of three to six or more.

ing session per week are sufficient to maintain it. Highly trained athletes have to train twice a week to maintain their strength levels.

Frequency of strength training for body builders varies from person to person. Because body builders use moderate resistance, daily or even two-a-day workouts are common. The frequency depends on the amount of resistance, number of sets performed per session, and the person's ability to recover from the previous exercise bout (Table 7.5). The latter often is dictated by level of conditioning.

Exercise Variations Multiple- and single-joint exercises are used in strength training. Multiple-joint exercises, such as the squat, bench press, and lat pull-down, require more skill and complex neural responses than single-joint exercises. Multiple-joint exercises also allow you to lift more weight and develop more strength. Single-joint exercises, such as the arm curl or knee extension, are used to target specific muscles for further development. Both are recommended for a comprehensive training program.

Many strength-training exercises can be performed bilaterally and unilaterally. Muscle activation differs between the two modes. Unilateral training can enhance selected sport skills, such as single-leg jumping, high jumping, and single-arm throwing. Unilateral training is also used extensively in rehab programs. For example, bilateral concentric knee extension followed by unilateral eccentric knee flexion is strongly recommended for individuals with weak knees and to prevent potential knee problems (see Exercise 28B). Both modes of training are recommended to maximize strength gains.

Plyometrics Strength, speed, and explosiveness are all crucial for success in athletics. All three of these factors are enhanced with a progressive resistance training program, but greater increases in speed and explosiveness are thought to be possible with **plyometric exercise**. The objective is to generate the greatest amount of force in the shortest time. A solid strength base is necessary before attempting plyometric exercises.

TABLE 7.5 **Guidelines for Various Strength-Training Programs**

Strength-Training Program	Resistance	Sets	Rest Between Sets*	Frequency (workouts per week)**
General fitness	8–12 reps max	2–4	2–3 min	2–3
Muscular endurance	15–25 reps	1–2	1–2 min	2–3
Maximal strength	1–6 reps max	2–5	3 min	2–3
Body building	8–15 reps near max	3–8	up to 1 min	4–12

*Recovery between sets can be decreased by alternating exercises that use different muscle groups.
**Weekly training sessions can be increased by using a split-body routine.

FIGURE 7.6 **Strength-training guidelines.**

Mode: Select 8 to 10 dynamic strength-training exercises that involve the body's major muscle groups and include opposing muscle groups (chest and upper back, abdomen and lower back, front and back of the legs).

Resistance: Sufficient resistance to perform 8 to 12 repetitions maximum for muscular strength and 15 to 25 repetitions to near fatigue for muscular edurance. Older adults and injury prone individuals should use 10 to 15 repetitions with moderate resistance (50% to 60% of their 1 RM).

Sets: 2 to 4 sets per exercise with 2 to 3 minutes recovery between sets for optimal strength development. Less than 2 minutes per set if exercises are alternated that require different muscle groups (chest and upper back) or between muscular endurance sets.

Frequency: 2 to 3 days per week on nonconsecutive days. More frequent training can be done if different muscle groups are exercised on different days. (Allow at least 48 hours between strength-training sessions of the same muscle group.)

Source: Adapted from American College of Sports Medicine, *ACSM's Guidelines for Exercise Testing and Prescription* (Philadelphia: Wolters Kluwer/Lippincott Williams & Wilkins, 2014).

Plyometric training is popular in sports that require powerful movements, such as basketball, volleyball, sprinting, jumping, and gymnastics. A typical plyometric exercise involves jumping off and back onto a box, attempting to rebound as quickly as possible on each jump. Box heights are increased progressively from about 12 to 22 inches.

The bounding action attempts to take advantage of the stretch–recoil and stretch reflex characteristics of muscle. The rapid stretch applied to the muscle during contact with the ground is thought to augment muscle contraction, leading to more explosiveness. Plyometrics also can be used for strengthening upper body muscles. An example is doing push-ups so that the extension of the arms is forceful enough to drive the hands (and body) off the floor during each repetition.

A drawback of plyometric training is its higher risk for injuries compared with conventional modes of progressive resistance training. For instance, the potential for injury in rebound exercise escalates with the increase in box height or the number of repetitions.

Strength Gains A common question by many strength-training participants is, how quickly can strength gains be observed? Strength-training studies have revealed that most strength gains are seen in the first 8 weeks of training. The amount of improvement, however, is related to previous training status. Increases of 40 percent are seen in individuals with no previous strength-training experience, 16 percent in previously strength-trained people, and 10 percent in advanced individuals.[14] Using a periodized strength-training program can yield further improvements (see "Periodization," Chapter 9, page 369).

Strength-Training Exercises

The strength-training programs introduced on pages 286–303 provide a complete body workout. The major muscles of the human body referred to in the exercises are pointed out in Figure 7.7 and within the exercises themselves at the end of the chapter.

Only a minimum of equipment is required for the first program, Strength-Training Exercises without Weights (Bodyweight Training—see exercises 1 through 14). You can conduct this program at home. Your body weight is used as the primary resistance for most exercises. A few exercises call for a friend's help or some basic implements from around your house to provide greater resistance.

CRITICAL THINKING

A friend started a strength-training program last year and has seen good results. He is now strength training nearly daily and taking performance-enhancing supplements hoping to accelerate results. What are your feelings about his program? What would you say (and not say) to him?

Strength-Training Exercises with Weights (Exercises 15 through 37) require machines, as shown in the accompanying photographs. These exercises can be conducted on either fixed- or variable-resistance equipment. Many of these exercises also can be performed with free weights. The first 13 of these exercises (15 to 27) are recommended to get a complete workout. You can do these exercises as circuit training. If time is a factor, as a minimum perform the first nine (15 through 23) exercises. Exercises 28 to 37 are supplemental or can replace some of the basic 13 (e.g., substitute Exercise 29 or 30 for 15; 31 for 16; 33 for 19; 34 for 24; 35 for 26; 32 for 27). Exercises 38 to 46 are stability ball exercises that can be used to complement your workout. Some of these exercises can also take the place of others that you use to strengthen similar muscle groups.

Selecting different exercises for a given muscle group is recommended between training sessions (e.g., chest press for bench press). No evidence indicates that a given exercise is best for a given muscle group. Changing exercises works the specific muscle group through a different range of motion and may change the difficulty of the exercise. Alternating exercises is also beneficial to avoid the monotony of repeating the same training program each training session.

Dietary Guidelines for Muscular and Strength Development

Individuals who wish to enhance muscle growth and strength during periods of intense strength training should increase protein to 1.2 to 2.0 grams per kilogram of body weight per day. The selected amount should be based on the volume of the undertaken strength-training program. An additional 500 daily calories are also recommended to optimize muscle mass gain. If protein intake is already in the range of 1.2 to 2.0 grams per kilogram of body weight, the additional 500 calories should come primarily from complex carbohydrates to provide extra nutrients to the body and glucose for the working muscles.

The timing, dose, and type of protein are all important in promoting muscle growth. Studies suggest that consuming a pre-exercise snack consisting of a combination of carbohydrates and protein leads to greater amino acid (the building blocks of protein) uptake by the muscle cells. The carbohydrates supply energy for training, and the availability of amino acids in the blood during training enhances muscle building. A peanut butter, turkey, or tuna sandwich; milk or yogurt and fruit; or nuts and fruit consumed 20 to 60 minutes before training are excellent choices for a pre-workout snack. As an added benefit, research showed that a whey protein (18 grams) supplement ingested 20 minutes prior to strength training resulted in a greater increase in resting energy expenditure during the 24 hours following the exercise session as compared to a carbohydrate-only (19 grams) supplement.[15]

Consuming a carbohydrate/protein snack immediately following strength training and a meal or second snack an hour thereafter further promotes muscle growth and strength development. Postexercise carbohydrates help restore muscle glycogen depleted during training and, in combination with protein, induce an increase in blood insulin and growth hormone levels. These hormones are essential to the muscle-building process. The higher level of circulating amino acids in the bloodstream immediately following training is believed to increase protein synthesis to a greater extent than amino acids made available later in the day. People who consume a carbohydrate/protein preexercise/postexercise supplement gain significantly more muscle mass than those who consume a similar supplement morning and evening.[16] A ratio of 4 to 1 grams of carbohydrates to protein is recommended—such as a snack containing 40 grams of carbohydrates (160 calories) and 10 grams of protein (40 calories).

The type of protein you consume is also important for optimal development. Whey protein, found in milk, has been shown to be the most effective type of protein for strength development and myofibrillar hypertrophy. Milk contains two major types of proteins: whey and casein. Whey can be separated from the casein or formed as a by-product of cheese production. Whey protein has been reported to be superior to casein, soy, or egg proteins for muscular development.

The relatively immediate preexercise/

Plyometric exercise Explosive jump training, incorporating speed and strength training to enhance explosiveness.

FIGURE 7.7 **Major muscles of the human body.**

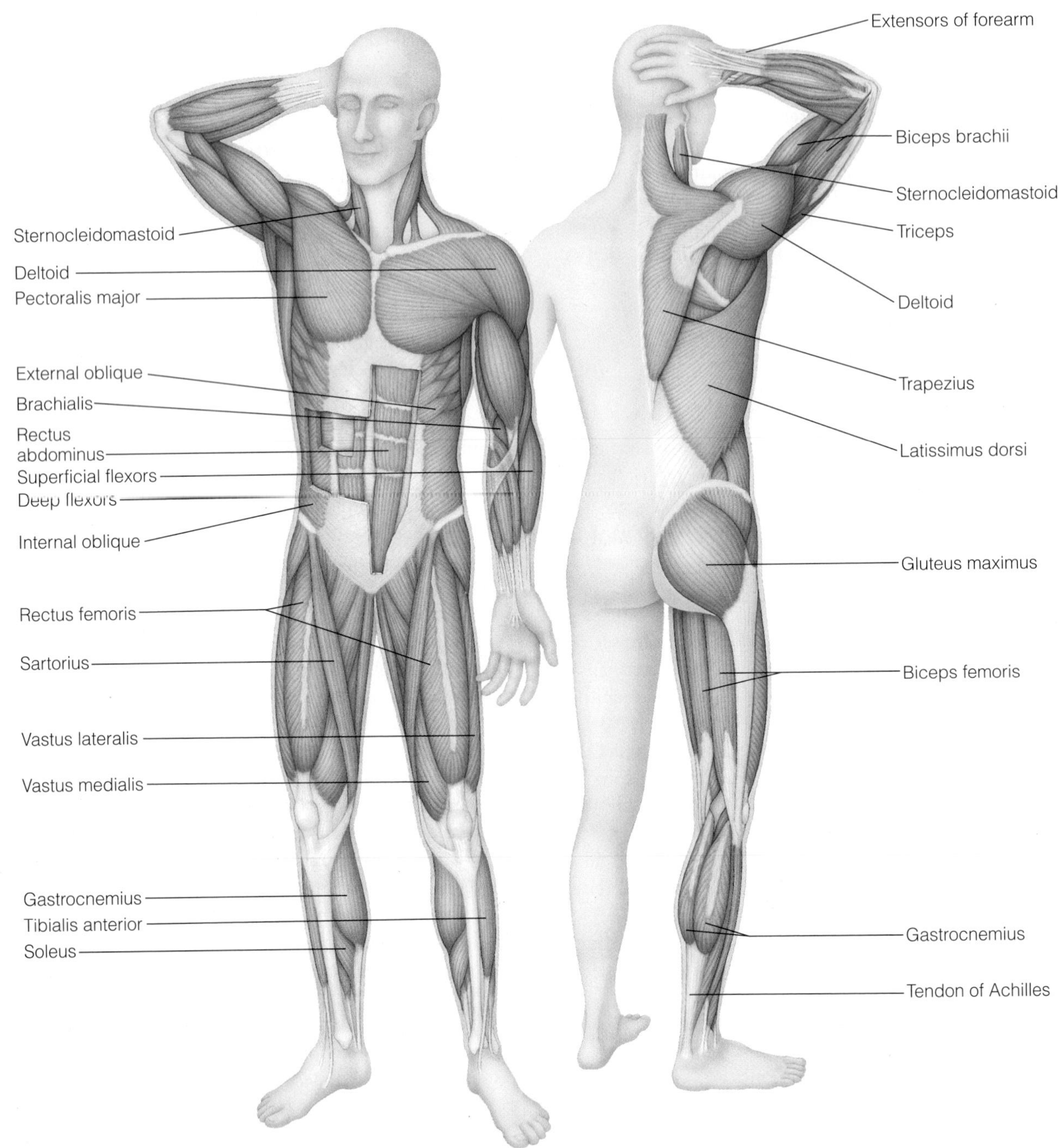

postexercise carbohydrate/protein consumption is critical, but muscle fibers do continue to absorb a greater amount of amino acids up to 48 hours following strength training. Thus, while attempting to increase muscular strength and size, proper distribution of protein intake at regular intervals throughout the day is important.Research indicates that further myofibrillar protein synthesis and muscle development are best accomplished with a 20-gram dose of whey protein taken every 3 hours throughout the day.[17] The latter has proven to be more effective than taking a similar total amount of protein with morning and evening meals.

Once you have reached your strength and hypertrophy goals, do not neglect your daily protein intake. Spreading the intake over three meals (about 20 to 40 grams of high-quality protein per meal based on your body size and level of activity) is most effective in keeping you satisfied, maintaining your muscle tissue, and helping reduce your caloric intake the rest of the day.

BEHAVIOR MODIFICATION PLANNING

Healthy Strength Training

I PLAN TO | I DID IT

❑ ❑ Make a progressive resistance strength-training program a priority in your weekly schedule.

❑ ❑ Strength-train at least once a week; even better, 2 to 3 times per week.

❑ ❑ Find a facility where you feel comfortable training and where you can get good professional guidance.

❑ ❑ Learn the proper technique for each exercise.

❑ ❑ Train with a friend or group of friends.

❑ ❑ Consume a pre-exercise snack consisting of a combination of carbohydrates and some protein about 20 to 60 minutes before each strength-training session.

❑ ❑ Use a minimum of 8 to 10 exercises that involve all major muscle groups of your body.

❑ ❑ Perform at least one set of each exercise to near muscular fatigue.

❑ ❑ To enhance protein synthesis, consume one post-exercise snack with a 4-to-l gram ratio of carbohydrates to protein (preferably whey protein) immediately following strength training; a second snack or meal with some whey protein 1 hour thereafter; and then continue to consume 20 grams of whey protein every 3 hours throughout the day.

❑ ❑ Allow at least 48 hours between strength-training sessions that involve the same muscle groups.

Try It

Attend the school's fitness or recreation center and have an instructor or fitness trainer help you design a progressive resistance strength-training program. Train twice a week for the next 4 weeks. Thereafter, evaluate the results and write down your feelings about the program.

Core Strength Training

The trunk (spine) and pelvis are referred to as the "core" of the body. Core muscles include the abdominal muscles (rectus, transversus, and internal and external obliques), hip muscles (front and back), and spinal muscles (lower and upper back muscles). These muscle groups are responsible for maintaining the stability of the spine and pelvis.

Many major muscle groups of the legs, shoulders, and arms attach to the core. A strong core allows a person to perform activities of daily living with greater ease, improve sports performance through a more effective energy transfer from large to small body parts, and decrease the incidence of low back pain. **Core strength training** also contributes to better posture and balance.

A major objective of core training is to exercise the abdominal and lower back muscles in unison. Furthermore, individuals should spend as much time training the back muscles as they do the abdominal muscles. Besides enhancing stability, core training improves dynamic balance, which is often required during physical activity and participation in sports.

Key core training exercises include the abdominal crunch and bent-leg curl-up, reverse crunch, pelvic tilt, side plank, plank, leg press, seated back, lat pull-down, back extension, lateral trunk flexion, supine bridge, and pelvic clock (Exercises 4, 11, 12, 13, 14, 16, 20, 24, 36, and 37 in this chapter and Exercises 26 and 27 in Chapter 8, respectively). Stability ball exercises 38 through 46 are also used to strengthen the core.

When core training is used in athletic conditioning programs, athletes attempt to mimic the dynamic skills they use in their sport. To do so, they use special equipment such as balance boards, stability balls, and foam pads. Using this equipment allows the athletes to train the core while seeking balance and stability in a sport-specific manner.

Pilates Exercise System

Previously, Pilates training was used primarily by dancers, but now this exercise modality is embraced by a large number of fitness participants, rehab patients, models, actors, and even professional athletes. Pilates studios, college courses, and classes at health clubs are available nationwide.

The **Pilates** training system was originally developed in the 1920s by German physical therapist Joseph Pilates. He designed the

Core strength training A program designed to strengthen the abdominal, hip, and spinal muscles (the core of the body).

Pilates A training program that uses exercises designed to help strengthen the body's core by developing pelvic stability and abdominal control; exercises are coupled with focused breathing patterns.

exercises to help strengthen the body's core by developing pelvic stability and abdominal control, coupled with focused breathing patterns.

Pilates exercises are performed either on a mat (floor) or with specialized equipment to help increase strength and flexibility of deep postural muscles. The intent is to improve muscle tone and length (a limber body), instead of increasing muscle size (hypertrophy). Pilates mat classes focus on body stability and proper body mechanics. The exercises are performed in a slow, controlled, precise manner. When performed properly, these exercises require intense concentration. Initially, Pilates training should be conducted under the supervision of certified instructors with extensive Pilates teaching experience.

Fitness goals of Pilates programs include better flexibility, muscle tone, posture, spinal support, body balance, low back health, sports performance, and mind–body awareness. Individuals with loose or unstable joints benefit from Pilates, because the exercises are designed to enhance joint stability. The Pilates program is also used to help lose weight, increase lean tissue, and manage stress. Although Pilates programs are quite popular, more research is required to corroborate the benefits attributed to this training system.

Stability Exercise Balls

A stability exercise ball is a large, flexible, inflatable ball used for exercises that combine the principles of Pilates with core strength training. Stability exercises are specifically designed to develop abdominal, hip, chest, and spinal muscles by addressing core stabilization while the exerciser maintains a balanced position over the ball. Emphasis is placed on correct movement and maintenance of proper body alignment to involve as much of the core as possible. Although the primary objective is core strength and stability, many stability exercises can be performed to strengthen other body areas as well.

Stability exercises are thought to be more effective than similar exercises on the ground. For example, just sitting on the ball requires the use of stabilizing core muscles (including the rectus abdominis and the external and internal obliques) to keep the body from falling off the ball. Traditional strength-training exercises are primarily for strength and power development and do not contribute as much to body balance.

When performing stability exercises, choose a ball size based on your height. Your thighs should be parallel to the floor when you sit on the ball. A slightly larger ball may be used if you suffer from back problems. Several stability ball exercises are provided on pages 300–303. For best results, have a trained specialist teach you the proper technique and watch your form while you learn the exercises. Individuals who have a weak muscular system or poor balance or who are over the age of 65 should perform stability exercises under the supervision of a qualified trainer.

Elastic-Band Resistive Exercise

Elastic bands and tubing can also be used for strength training. This type of constant-resistance training has increased in popularity and can be used to supplement traditional strength training, because it has shown to help increase strength, mobility, and functional ability (particularly in older adults) and to aid in the rehab of many types of injuries. Some advantages to using this type of training include low cost, versatility (you can create resistance in almost all angles and directions of the range of motion), use of a large number of exercises to work all joints of the body, and accessibility to a workout while traveling (exercise bands and tubes can be easily packed in a suitcase). This type of resistance training can also add variety to your routine workout.

Elastic-band resistive exercise workouts can be just as challenging as with free weights or machines. Due to the constant resistance provided by the bands or tubing, the training may appear more difficult to some individuals, because the resistance is used during both the eccentric and the concentric phases of the repetition. In addition, the bands can be used by beginners and strength-trained individuals. This is because several tension cords (up to eight bands) are available and all participants can progress through various resistance levels.

At the beginning, it may be a little confusing to determine how to use the bands and create the proper loops to grip the bands. The assistance of a training video, an instructor, or a personal trainer is helpful. The bands can be wrapped around a post or a doorknob, or you can stand on them for some exercises. A few sample elastic-band resistive exercises are provided in Figure 7.8. Instructional booklets are available for purchase with elastic bands or tubing.

Exercise Safety Guidelines

As you prepare to design your strength-training program, keep the following guidelines in mind:

- Safety is the most important component in strength training. If you are new to strength training or if you are lifting alone, strength-training machines are the best option for you. Experienced lifters like to use a combination of both free weights and strength-training machines.
- Select exercises that will involve all major muscle groups: chest, shoulders, back, legs, arms, hip, and trunk.
- Select exercises that will strengthen the core. Use controlled movements and start with light-to-moderate resistances. (Later, athletes may use explosive movements with heavier resistances.)
- Never lift weights alone. Always have someone work out with you in case you need a spotter or help with an injury. When you use free weights, one to two spotters are rec-

FIGURE 7.8 Sample elastic-band resistive exercises

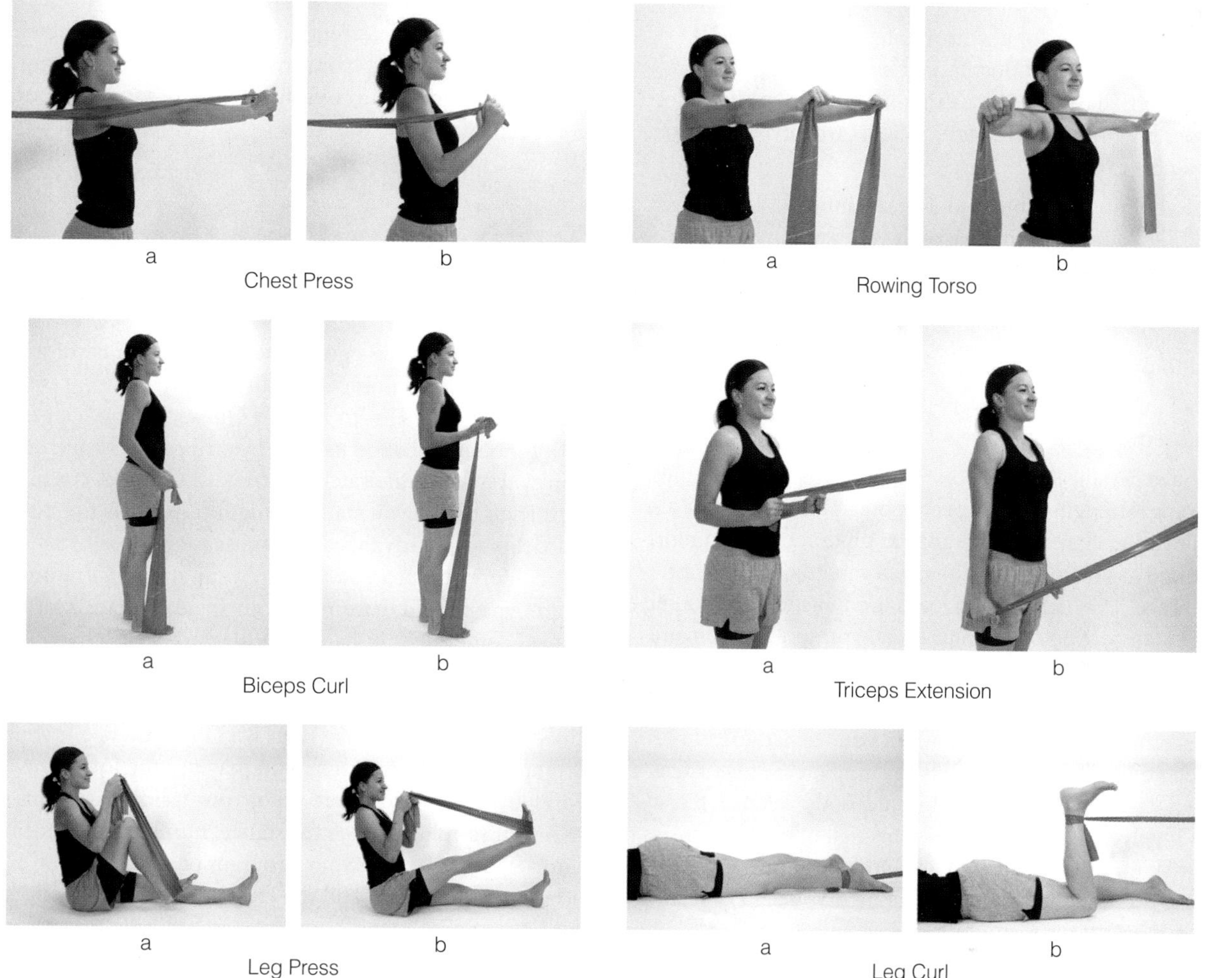

ommended for certain exercises (e.g., bench press, squats, and overhead press).

- Prior to lifting weights, warm up properly by performing a light- to moderate-intensity aerobic activity (5 to 7 minutes) and some gentle stretches for a few minutes.
- Use proper lifting technique for each exercise. The correct lifting technique will involve only those muscles and joints intended for a specific exercise. Involving other muscles and joints to "cheat" during the exercise to complete a repetition or to be able to lift a greater resistance decreases the long-term effectiveness of the exercise and can lead to injury (such as arching the back during the push-up, squat, or bench press exercises). Proper lifting technique also implies performing the exercises in a controlled manner and throughout the entire range of motion. Perform each repetition in a rhythmic manner and at a moderate speed. Avoid fast and jerky movements, and do not throw the entire body into the lifting motion. Do not arch the back when lifting a weight.
- Don't lock your elbows and knee joints while lifting. See that you always leave a slight bend in the elbows and knees when straightening out the legs and arms.
- Maintain proper body balance while lifting. Proper balance involves good posture, a stable body position, and correct seat and arm/leg settings on exercise machines. Loss of balance places undue strain on smaller muscles and leads to injuries because of the heavy resistances suddenly placed on them. In the early stages of a program, first-time lifters often struggle with bar control and balance when using free weights. This problem is overcome quickly with practice following a few training sessions.
- Exercise larger muscle groups (such as those in the chest, back, and legs) before exercising smaller muscle groups (arms, abdominals, ankles, and neck). For example, the bench press exercise works the chest, shoulders, and back of the upper arms (triceps), whereas the triceps extension works the back of the upper arms only.
- Exercise opposing muscle groups for a balanced workout. When you work the chest (bench press), also work the

back (rowing torso). If you work the biceps (arm curl), also work the triceps (triceps extension).

- Breathe naturally. Inhale during the eccentric phase (bringing the weight down), and exhale during the concentric phase (lifting or pushing the weight up). Practice proper breathing with lighter weights when you are learning a new exercise.
- Avoid holding your breath while straining to lift a weight. Holding your breath increases the pressure inside the chest and abdominal cavity greatly, making it nearly impossible for the blood in the veins to return to the heart. Although rare, a sudden high intrathoracic pressure may lead to dizziness, blackout, stroke, heart attack, or hernia.
- Based on the program selected, allow adequate recovery time between sets of exercises (see Table 7.5).
- If you experience unusual discomfort or pain, discontinue training. Strength-training exercises should not cause pain while lifting. Stay within a range of motion that is comfortable and as you progress along, you can gradually extend the range. The high tension loads used in strength training can exacerbate potential injuries. Discomfort and pain are signals to stop and determine what's wrong. Be sure to evaluate your condition properly before you continue training.
- Use common sense on days when you feel fatigued or when you are performing sets to complete fatigue. Excessive fatigue affects lifting technique, body balance, muscles involved, and range of motion—all of which increase the risk for injury. Learn to listen to your body and decrease exercise intensity and volume if you are not feeling right. A spotter is recommended when sets are performed to complete fatigue. The spotter's help through the most difficult part of the repetition will relieve undue stress on muscles, ligaments, and tendons—and help ensure that you perform the exercise correctly.
- At the end of each strength-training workout, stretch for a few minutes to help your muscles return to their normal resting length and to minimize muscle soreness and risk for injury.

Setting Up Your Own Strength-Training Program

The same pre-exercise guidelines outlined for cardiorespiratory endurance training apply to strength training (see Lab 1C, "PAR-Q and Health History Questionnaire," pages 39–40). If you have concerns about your present health status or ability to participate safely in strength training, consult a physician before you start. Strength training is not advised for people with advanced heart disease.

Before you proceed to write your strength-training program, you should determine your stage of change for this fitness component in Lab 7B at the end of the chapter. Next, if you are prepared to do so, and depending on the facilities available, you can choose one of the training programs outlined in this chapter (use Lab 7B). Once you begin your strength-training program, you may use the form provided in Figure 7.9 to keep a record of your training sessions.

You should base the resistance, number of repetitions, and sets you use with your program on your current strength-fitness level and the amount of time that you have for your strength workout. If you are training for reasons other than general health fitness, review Table 7.5 for a summary of the guidelines.

FIGURE 7.9 Strength-training record form.

Name ____________________

Date										
Exercise	St/Reps/Res*	St/Reps/Res*	St/Reps/Res*	St/Reps/Res*	St/Reps/Res*	St/Reps/Res*	St/Reps/Res*	St/Reps/Res*	St/Reps/Res*	St/Reps/Res*

*Sets, Repetitions, and Resistance (e.g., 1/6/125 = 1 set of 6 repetitions with 125 pounds)

ASSESS YOUR BEHAVIOR

CENGAGE brain.com To access course materials, including companion resources, please visit **www.cengagebrain.com**.

1. Are your strength levels sufficient to perform tasks of daily living (climbing stairs, carrying a backpack, opening jars, doing housework, mowing the yard, etc.) without requiring additional assistance or feeling unusually fatigued?
2. Do you regularly participate in a strength-training program that includes all major muscle groups of the body, and do you perform at least one set of each exercise to near fatigue?

ASSESS YOUR KNOWLEDGE

1. The ability of a muscle to exert submaximal force repeatedly over time is known as
   a. muscular strength.
   b. plyometric training.
   c. muscular endurance.
   d. isokinetic training.
   e. isometric training.
2. Muscle hypertrophy as a result of a similar strength-training program is greater in men than in women
   a. due to endocrinological differences.
   b. because the former have more muscle fibers.
   c. due to differences in muscle quality between both genders.
   d. Choices a and b are correct.
   e. Choices a through c are correct.
3. The Hand Grip Strength Test is an example of
   a. an isometric test.
   b. an isotonic test.
   c. a dynamic test.
   d. an isokinetic test.
   e. a plyometric test.
4. A 70th percentile rank places an individual in the ___ fitness category.
   a. excellent
   b. good
   c. average
   d. fair
   e. poor
5. During an eccentric muscle contraction,
   a. the muscle shortens as it overcomes the resistance.
   b. there is little or no movement during the contraction.
   c. a joint has to move through the entire range of motion.
   d. the muscle lengthens as it contracts.
   e. the speed is kept constant throughout the range of motion.
6. The training concept stating that the demands placed on a system must be increased systematically and progressively over time to cause physiological adaptation is referred to as
   a. the overload principle.
   b. positive-resistance training.
   c. specificity of training.
   d. variable-resistance training.
   e. progressive resistance.
7. A set in strength training refers to
   a. the starting position for an exercise.
   b. the recovery time required between exercises.
   c. a given number of repetitions.
   d. the starting resistance used in an exercise.
   e. the sequence in which exercises are performed.
8. For health fitness, the recommendation of the American College of Sports Medicine is that a person should perform a maximum of between
   a. 1 and 6 reps.
   b. 4 and 10 reps.
   c. 8 and 12 reps.
   d. 10 and 25 reps.
   e. 20 and 30 reps.
9. Nutrition guidelines for optimum myofibrillar hypertrophy indicate that
   a. the timing, dose, and type of protein following strength training are all important.
   b. you consume a carbohydrate/protein snack immediately following strength training.
   c. you consume between 1.2 and 2.0 grams of protein per kilogram of body weight per day.
   d. whey protein is superior to other types of protein.
   e. All of the choices are correct.
10. The posterior deltoid, rhomboids, and trapezius muscles can be developed with the
   a. bench press.
   b. lat pull-down.
   c. rotary torso.
   d. squat.
   e. rowing torso.

Correct answers can be found at the back of the book.

NOTES

1. American College of Sports Medicine, *ACSM's Guidelines for Exercise Testing and Prescription* (Baltimore: Wolters Kluwer/ Lippincott Williams & Wilkins, 2014).
2. C. Castaneda et al., "A Randomized Controlled Trial of Resistance Exercise Training to Improve Glycemic Control in Older Adults with Type 2 Diabetes," *Diabetes Care* 25 (2002): 2335–2341.
3. S. J. Fitzgerald, et al., "Muscular Fitness and All-cause Mortality: Prospective Observations," *Journal of Physical Activity and Health 1* (2004): 7–18.
4. G. B. Forbes, "The Adult Decline in Lean Body Mass," *Human Biology* 48 (1976): 161–173; W. R. Frontera et al., "A Cross-sectional Study of Muscle Strength and Mass in 45 to 78 Yr-Old Men and Women," *Journal of Applied Physiology* 71 (1991): 644–650; W. R. Frontera et al., "Aging of Skeletal Muscle: A 12-Yr Longitudinal Study," *Journal of Applied Physiology* 88 (2000): 1321–1326.
5. M. D. Peterson, A. Sen, and P. M. Gordon, "Influence of Resistance Exercise on Lean Body Mass in Aging Adults: A Meta-Analysis," *Medicine and Science in Sports and Exercise* 43 (2011): 249–258.
6. W. W. Campbell, M. C. Crim, V. R. Young, and W. J. Evans, "Increased Energy Requirements and Changes in Body Composition with Resistance Training in Older Adults," *American Journal of Clinical Nutrition* 60 (1994): 167–175.
7. W. J. Evans, "Exercise, Nutrition and Aging," *Journal of Nutrition* 122 (1992): 796–801.
8. P. E. Allsen, *Strength Training: Beginners, Body Builders and Athletes* (Dubuque, IA: Kendall/Hunt, 2009).
9. See note 6.
10. American College of Sports Medicine, "Progression Models in Resistance Training for Healthy Adults," *Medicine & Science in Sports & Exercise* 41 (2009): 687–708.
11. B. M. Hather, P. A. Tesch, P. Buchanan, and G. A. Dudley, "Influence of Eccentric Actions on Skeletal Muscle Adaptations to Resistance Training," *Acta Physiologica Scandinavica* 143 (1991): 177–185; C. B. Ebbeling and P. M. Clarkson, "Exercise-Induced Muscle Damage and Adaptation," *Sports Medicine* 7 (1989): 207–234.
12. W. W. K. Hoeger, D. R. Hopkins, S. L. Barette, and D. F. Hale, "Relationship Between Repetitions and Selected Percentages of One Repetition Maximum: A Comparison Between Untrained and Trained Males and Females," *Journal of Applied Sport Science Research* 4, no. 2 (1990): 47–51.
13. W. J. Kraemer and M. S. Fragala, "Personalize It: Program Design in Resistance Training," *ACSM's Health and Fitness Journal* 10, no. 4 (2006): 7–17.
14. See note 10.
15. K. J. Hartman, A. J. Bruenger, and J. T. Lemmer, "Timing Protein Intake Increases Energy Expenditure 24 h After Resistance Training," *Medicine & Science in Sports & Exercise* 42 (2010): 998–1003.
16. P. Cribb and A. Hayes, "Effect of Supplement Timing on Skeletal Muscle Hypertrophy," *Medicine & Science in Sports & Exercise* 38 (2006): 1918–1925.
17. J. L. Areta, et al., "Timing and Distribution of Protein Ingestion During Prolonged Recovery from Resistance Exercise Alters Myofibrillar Protein Synthesis," *Journal of Physiology* (2013): 1–13, DOI: 10.1113/ jphysiol.2012.244897; D. R. Moore, et al., "Daytime Pattern of Post-exercise Protein Intake Affects Whole-Body Protein Turnover in Resistance-Trained Males," *Nutrition & Metabolism* 9, no. 1 (2012): 91. DOI:10.1186/1743-7075-9-91

SUGGESTED READINGS

American College of Sports Medicine. "Progression Models in Resistance Training for Healthy Adults," *Medicine & Science in Sports & Exercise* 41 (2009): 687-708.

Hesson, J. L. *Weight Training for Life.* Belmont, CA: Wadsworth/Cengage Learning, 2012.

Heyward, V. H. *Advanced Fitness Assessment and Exercise Prescription.* Champaign, IL: Human Kinetic Press, 2010.

Hoeger, W. W. K., and S. A. Hoeger. *Lifetime Physical Fitness and Wellness: A Personalized Program.* Belmont, CA: Wadsworth/Cengage Learning, 2015.

Kraemer, J. K., and N. A. Ratamess. "Fundamentals of Resistance Training: Progression and Exercise Prescription," *Medicine & Science in Sports & Exercise* 36 (2004): 674-688.

Kraemer, W. J., and S. J. Fleck. *Optimizing Strength Training.* Champaign, IL: Human Kinetic Press, 2007.

Volpe, S. L. "How to Increase Muscle Mass: What Science Tells Us?" *ACSM's Health & Fitness Journal* 17, no. 5 (2013): 37-38.

Strength-Training Exercises without Weights

EXERCISE 1 Step Up

ACTION Step up and down using a box or chair approximately 12 to 15 inches high (a). Conduct one set using the same leg each time you step up, and then conduct a second set using the other leg. You also could alternate legs on each step-up cycle. You may increase the resistance by holding an object in your arms (b). Hold the object close to the body to avoid increased strain in the lower back.

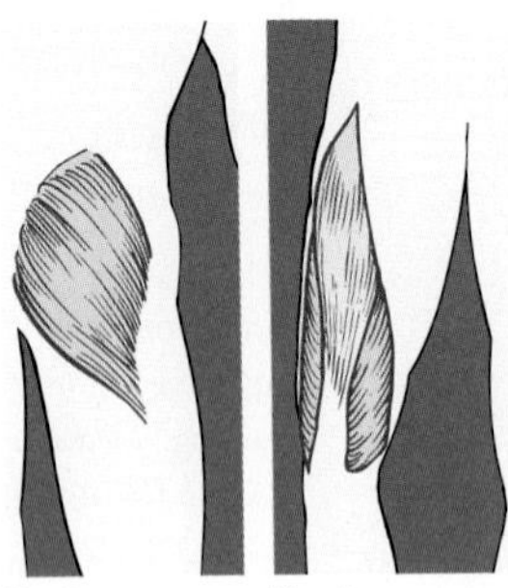

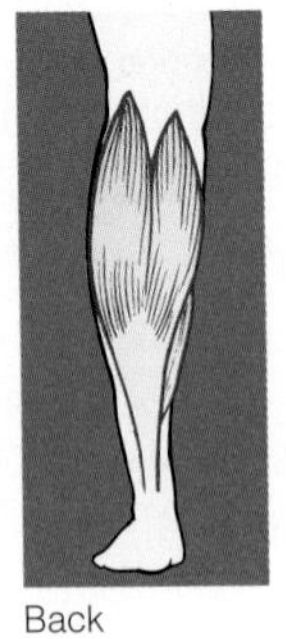

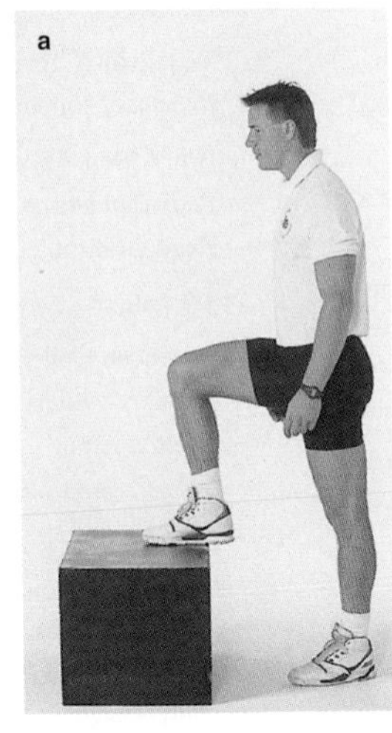

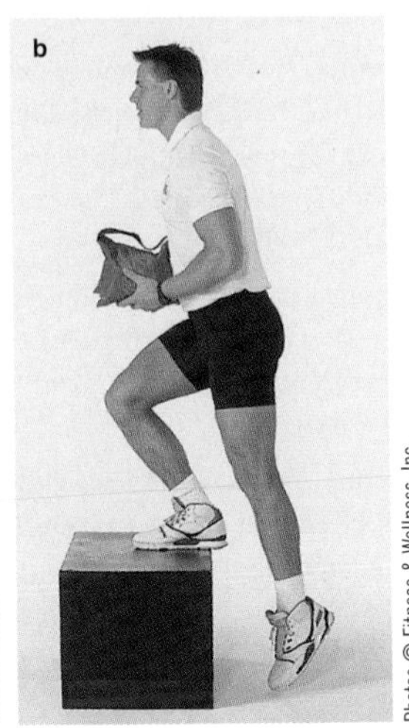

Photos © Fitness & Wellness, Inc.

MUSCLES DEVELOPED Gluteal muscles, quadriceps, gastrocnemius, and soleus

EXERCISE 2 Rowing Torso

ACTION Raise your arms laterally (abduction) to a horizontal position and bend your elbows to 90°. Have a partner apply enough pressure on your elbows to gradually force your arms forward (horizontal flexion) while you try to resist the pressure. Next, reverse the ACTION, horizontally forcing the arms backward as your partner applies sufficient forward pressure to create resistance.

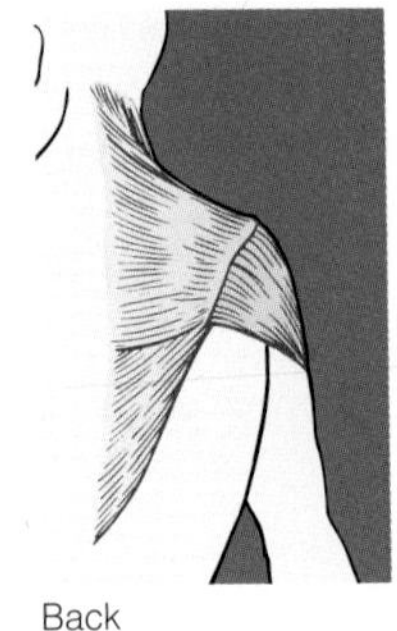

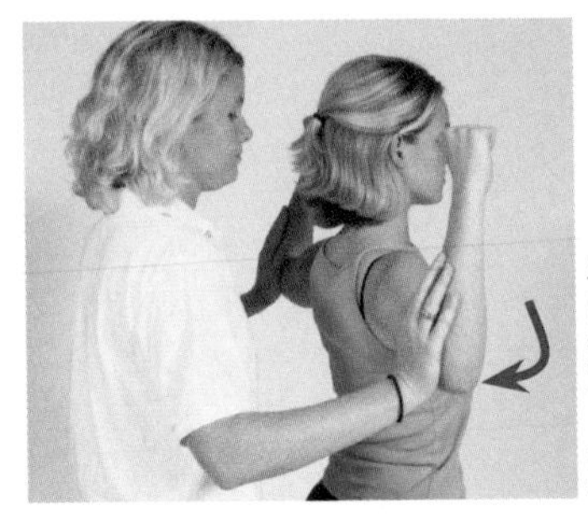

© Fitness & Wellness, Inc.

MUSCLES DEVELOPED Posterior deltoid, rhomboids, and trapezius

EXERCISE 3 Push-Up

ACTION Maintaining your body as straight as possible (a), flex the elbows, lowering the body until you almost touch the floor (b), then raise yourself back up to the starting position. If you are unable to perform the push-up as indicated, decrease the resistance by supporting the lower body with the knees rather than the feet (c).

MUSCLES DEVELOPED Triceps, deltoid, pectoralis major, abdominals, and erector spinae

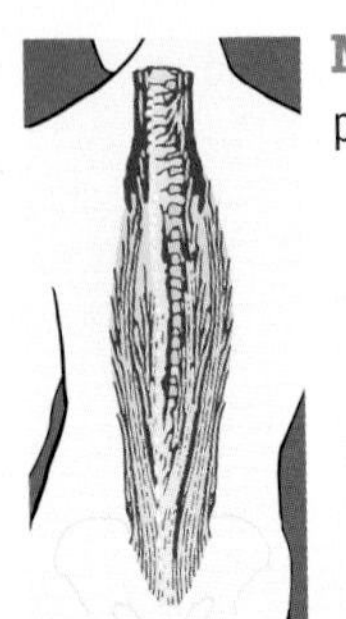

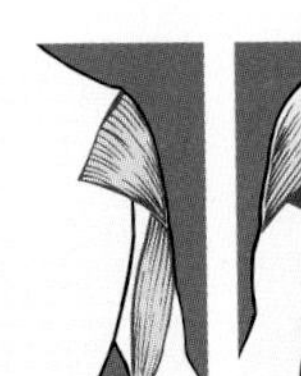

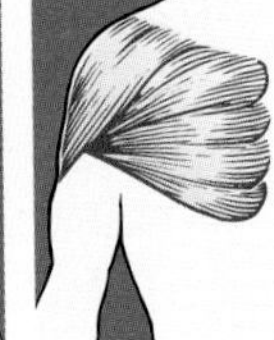

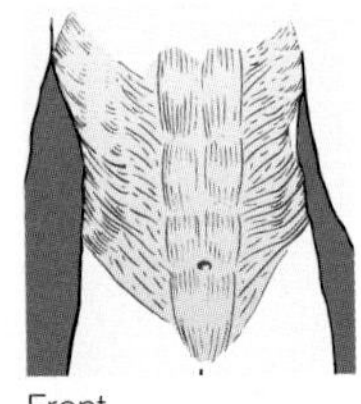

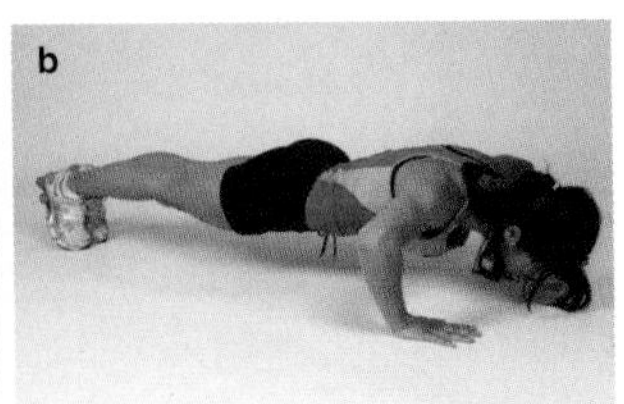

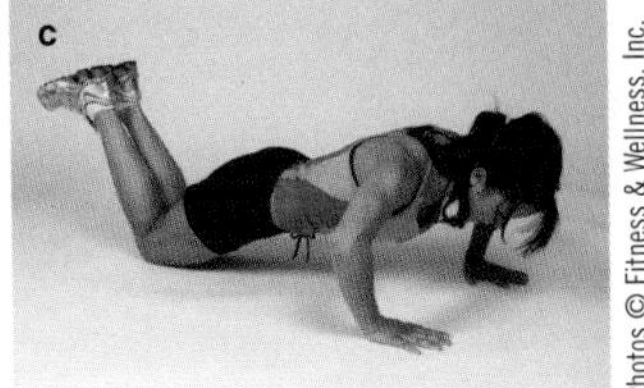

Photos © Fitness & Wellness, Inc.

EXERCISE 4 **Abdominal Crunch and Bent-Leg Curl-Up**

ACTION Start with your head and shoulders off the floor, arms crossed on your chest, and knees slightly bent (a). The greater the flexion of the knee, the more difficult the curl-up. Now curl up to about 30° (abdominal crunch—illustration b) or curl up all the way (abdominal curl-up—illustration c), then return to the starting position without letting the head or shoulders touch the floor or allowing the hips to come off the floor. If you allow the hips to raise off the floor and the head and shoulders to touch the floor, you most likely will "swing up" on the next crunch or curl-up, which minimizes the work of the abdominal muscles. If you cannot curl up with the arms on the chest, place the hands by the side of the hips or even help yourself up by holding on to your thighs (d and e). Do not perform the sit-up exercise with your legs completely extended, because this will strain the lower back.

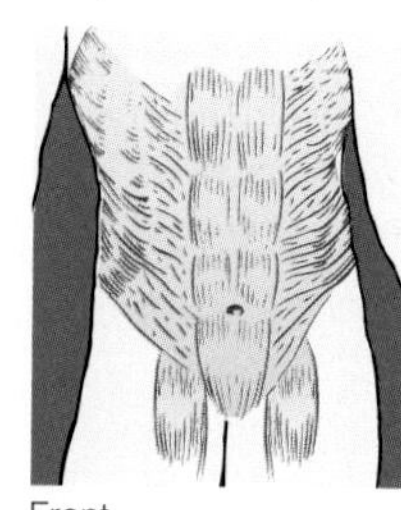
Front

MUSCLES DEVELOPED Abdominal muscles and hip flexors

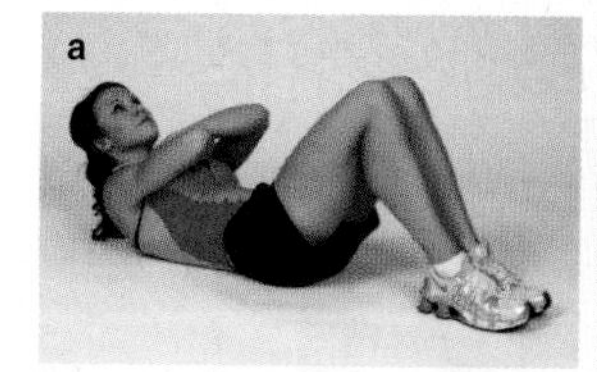
a

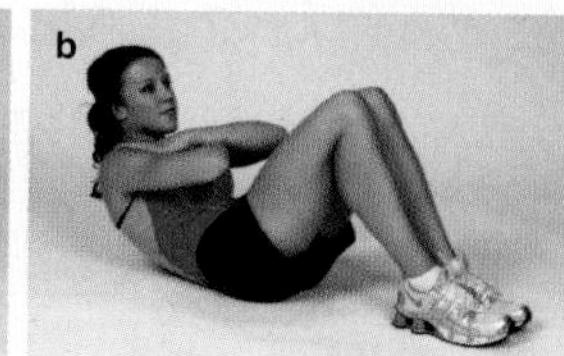
b

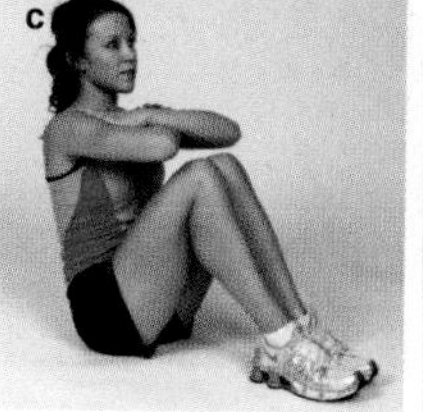
c

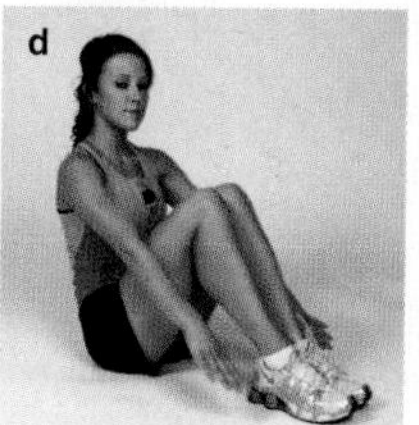
d

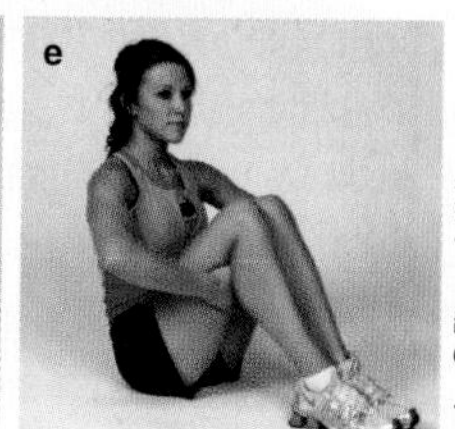
e

EXERCISE 5 **Leg Curl**

ACTION Lie on the floor face down. Cross the right ankle over the left heel (a). Apply resistance with your right foot while you bring the left foot up to 90° at the knee joint (b). Apply enough resistance so the left foot can only be brought up slowly. Repeat the exercise, crossing the left ankle over the right heel.

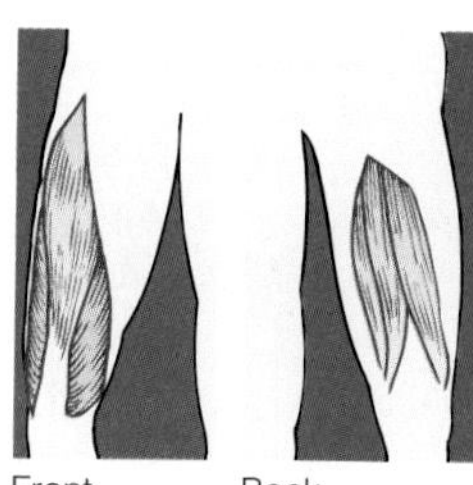
Front Back

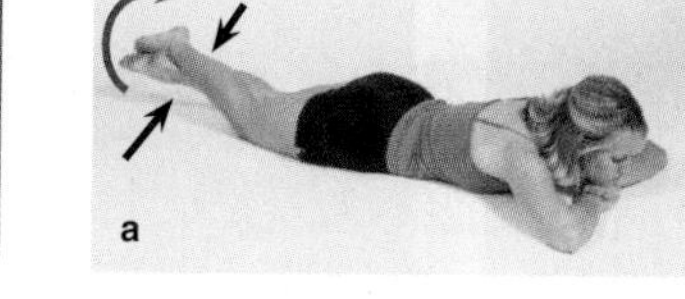
a

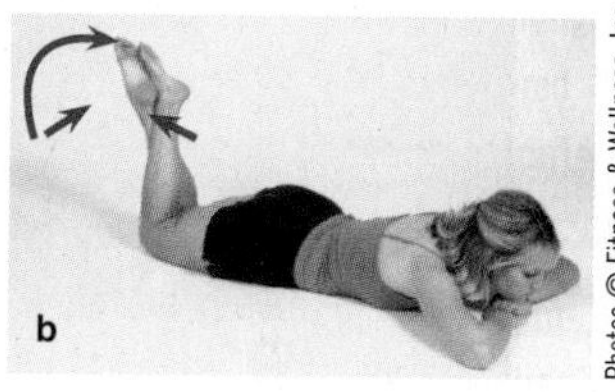
b

MUSCLES DEVELOPED Hamstrings (and quadriceps)

EXERCISE 6 **Modified Dip**

ACTION Using a gymnasium bleacher or box and with the help of a partner, dip down at least to a 90° angle at the elbow joint and then return to the initial position.

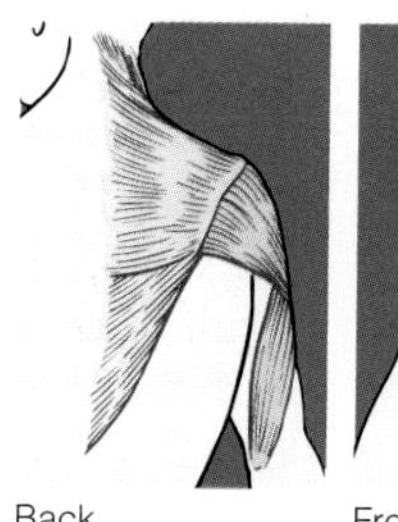
Back

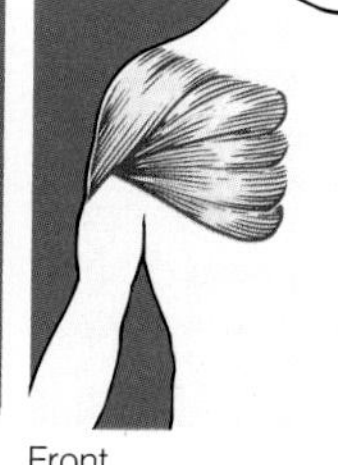
Front

MUSCLES DEVELOPED Triceps, deltoid, and pectoralis major

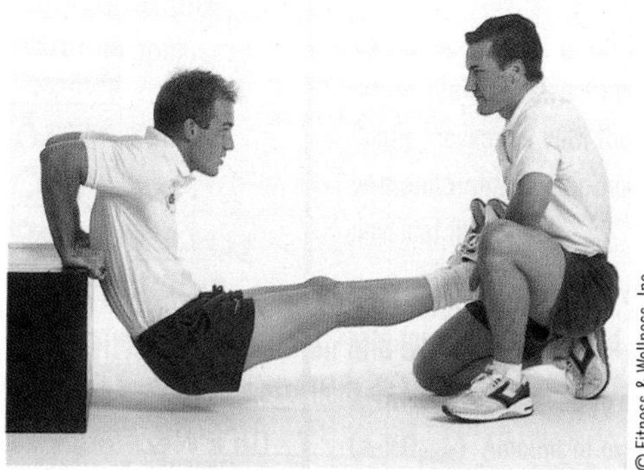

EXERCISE 7 **Pull-Up**

ACTION Suspend yourself from a bar with a pronated (thumbs-in) grip (a). Pull your body up until your chin is above the bar (b), then lower the body slowly to the starting position. If you are unable to perform the pull-up as described, have a partner hold your feet to push off and facilitate the movement upward (c and d).

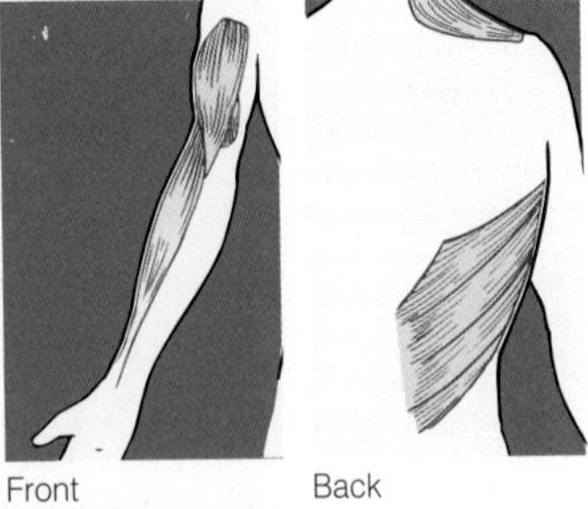

MUSCLES DEVELOPED Biceps, brachioradialis, brachialis, trapezius, and latissimus dorsi

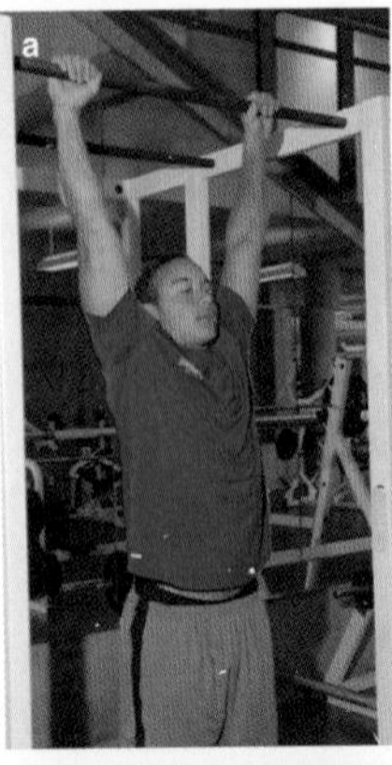

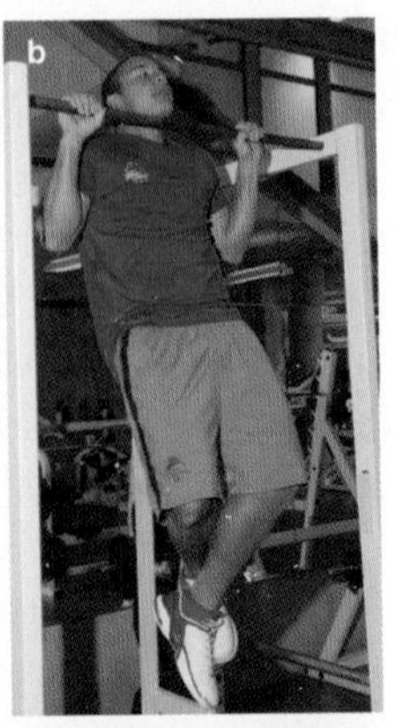

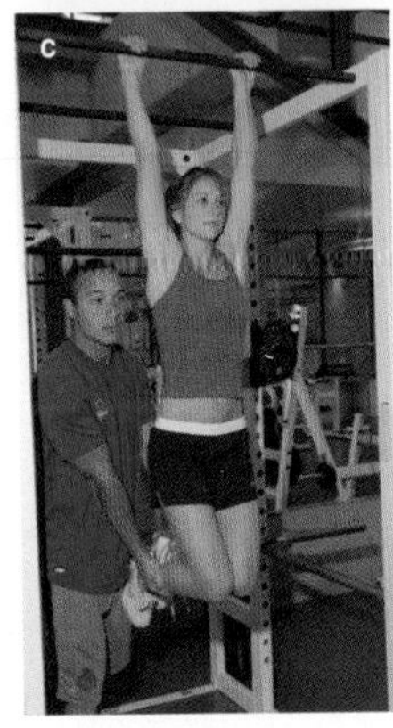

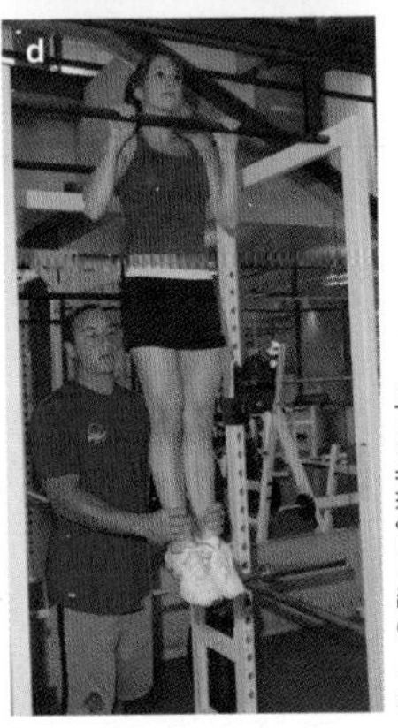

EXERCISE 8 **Arm Curl**

ACTION Using a palms-up grip, start with the arm completely extended and, with the aid of a sandbag or bucket filled (as needed) with sand or rocks (a), curl up as far as possible (b), then return to the initial position. Repeat the exercise with the other arm.

MUSCLES DEVELOPED Biceps, brachioradialis, and brachialis

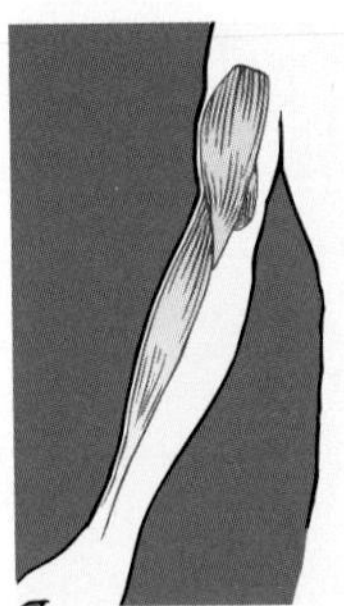

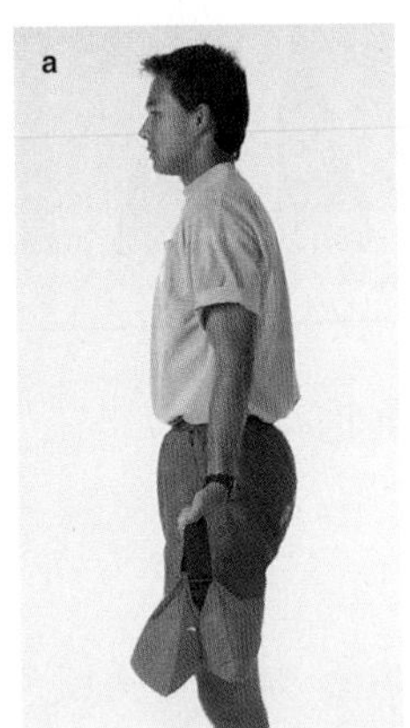

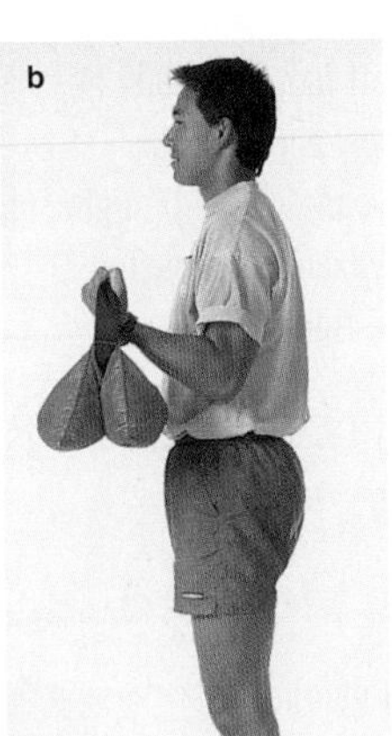

EXERCISE 9 **Heel Raise**

ACTION From a standing position with feet flat on the floor or at the edge of a step (a), raise and lower your body weight by moving at the ankle joint only (b). For added resistance, have someone else hold your shoulders down as you perform the exercise.

MUSCLES DEVELOPED Gastrocnemius and soleus

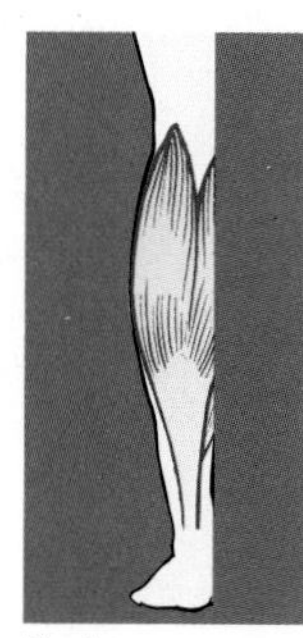
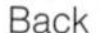
Back

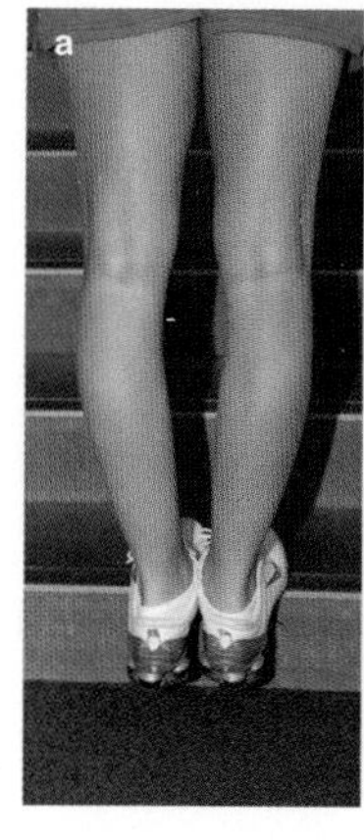

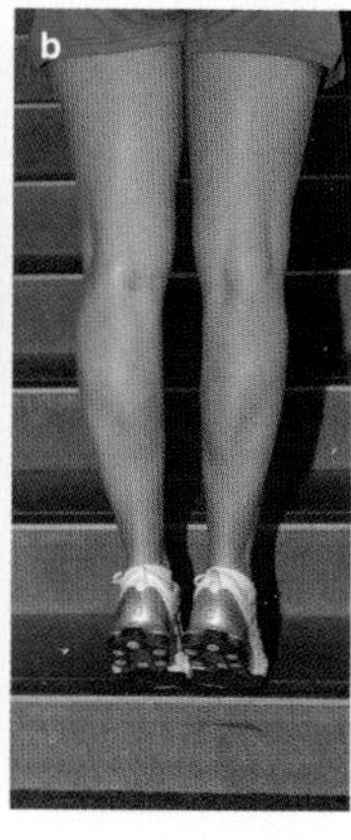

EXERCISE 10 **Leg Abduction and Adduction**

ACTION Both participants sit on the floor. The person on the left places the feet on the inside of the other person's feet. Simultaneously, the person on the left presses the legs laterally (to the outside—abduction), while the person on the right presses the legs medially (adduction). Hold the contraction for 5 to 10 seconds. Repeat the exercise at all three angles, and then reverse the pressing sequence: The person on the left places the feet on the outside and presses inward while the person on the right presses outward.

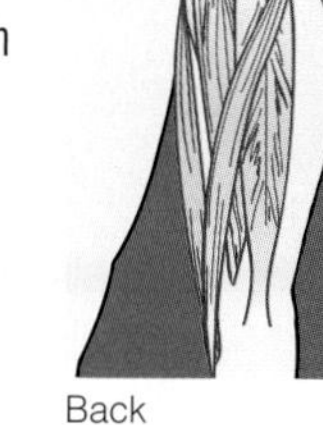
Back

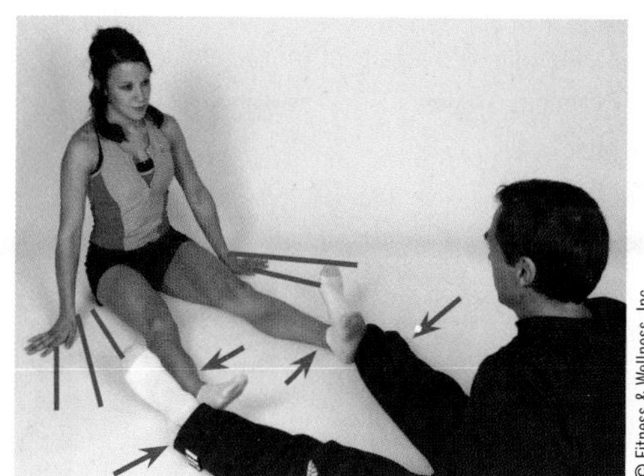

MUSCLES DEVELOPED Hip abductors (rectus femoris, sartori, gluteus medius and minimus) and adductors (pectineus, gracilis, adductor magnus, adductor longus, and adductor brevis)

EXERCISE 11 **Reverse Crunch**

ACTION Lie on your back with arms to the sides and knees and hips flexed at 90° (a). Now attempt to raise the pelvis off the floor by lifting vertically from the knees and lower legs (b). This is a challenging exercise that may be difficult for beginners to perform.

MUSCLES DEVELOPED Abdominals

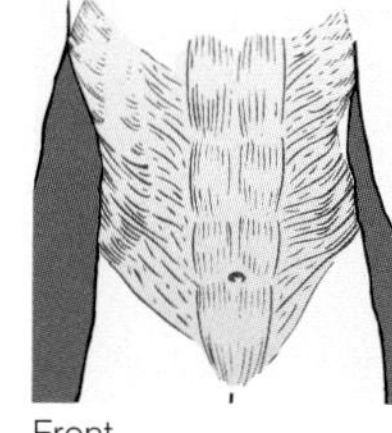
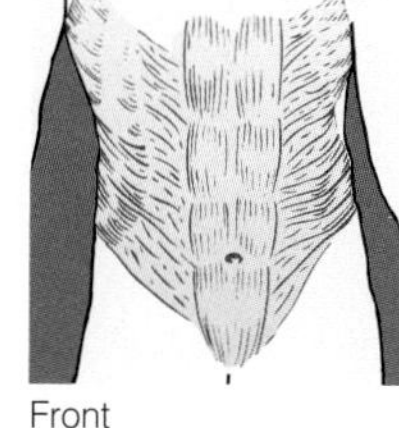
Front

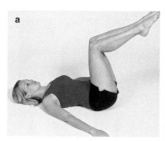

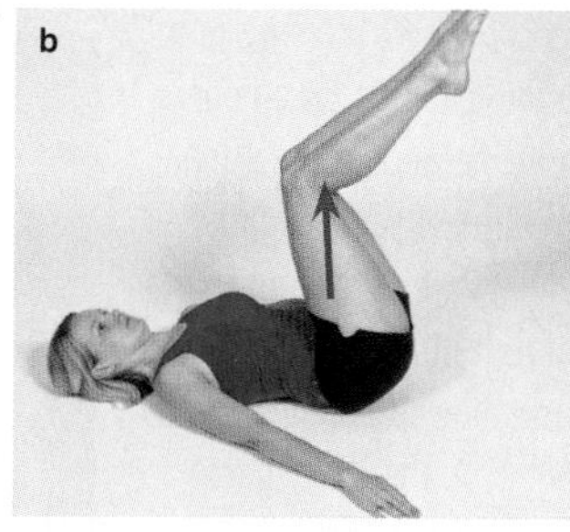

EXERCISE 12 **Pelvic Tilt**

ACTION Lie flat on the floor with the knees bent at about a 90° angle (a). Tilt the pelvis by tightening the abdominal muscles, flattening your back against the floor, and raising the lower gluteal area ever so slightly off the floor (b). Hold the final position for several seconds.

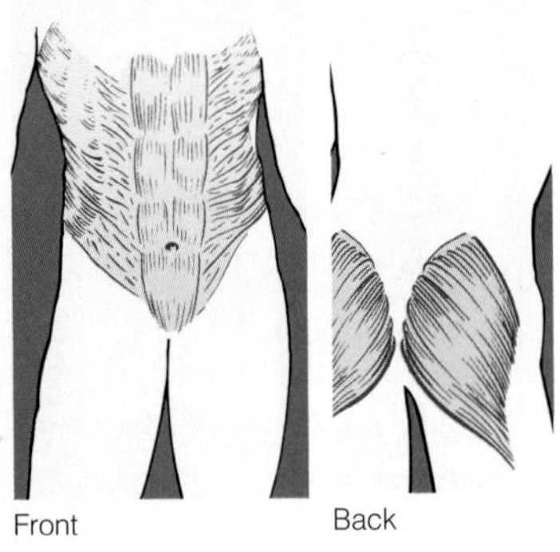

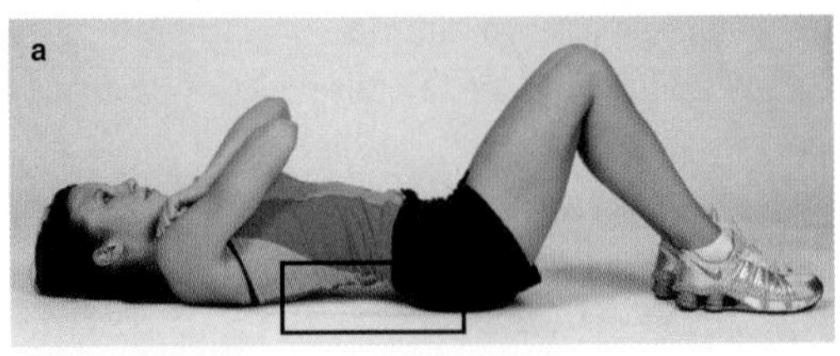

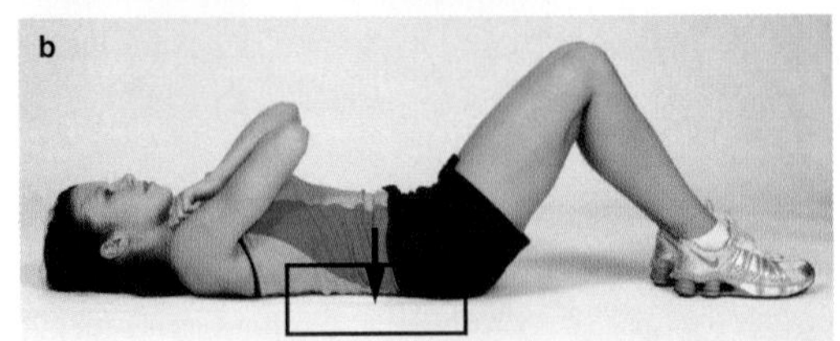

Photos © Fitness & Wellness, Inc.

AREAS STRETCHED Low back muscles and ligaments

AREAS STRENGTHENED Abdominal and gluteal muscles

EXERCISE 13 **Side Plank**

ACTION Lie on your side with legs bent (a: easier version) or straight (b: harder version) and support the upper body with your arm. Straighten your body by raising the hip off the floor and hold the position for several seconds. Repeat the exercise with the other side of the body.

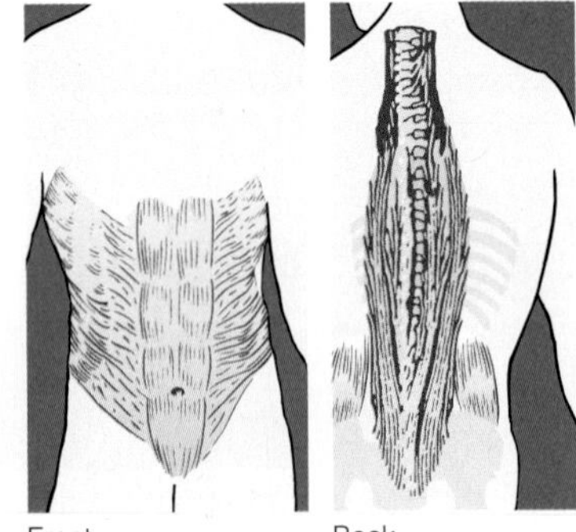

MUSCLES DEVELOPED Abdominals (obliques and transversus abdominus) and quadratus lumborum (lower back)

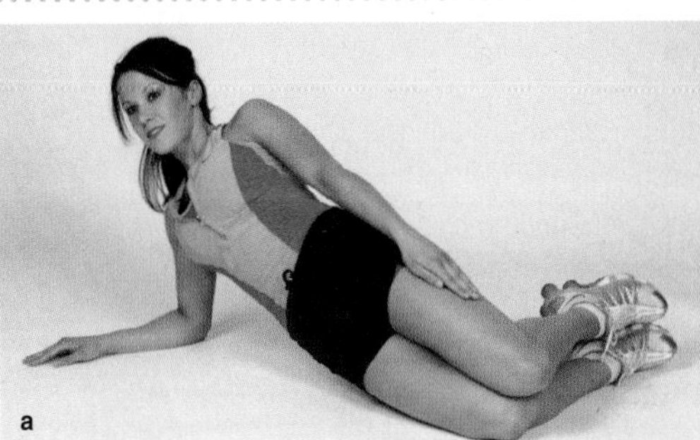

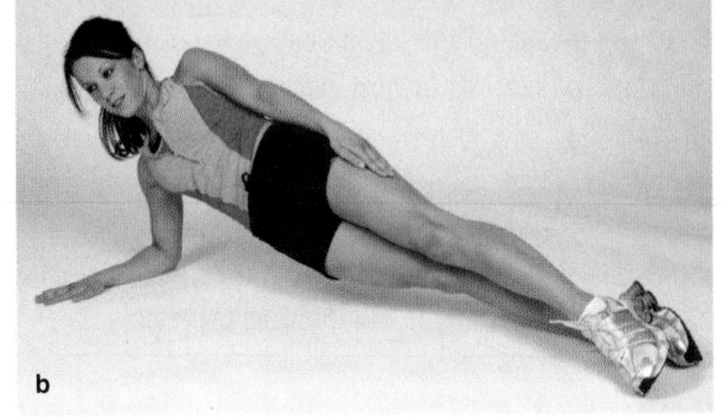

Photos © Fitness & Wellness, Inc.

EXERCISE 14 **Plank**

ACTION Starting in a prone position on a floor mat, balance yourself on the tips of your toes and elbows while attempting to maintain a straight body from heels to shoulders (do not arch the lower back) (a). You can increase the difficulty of this exercise by placing your hands in front of you and straightening the arms (elbows off the floor) (b).

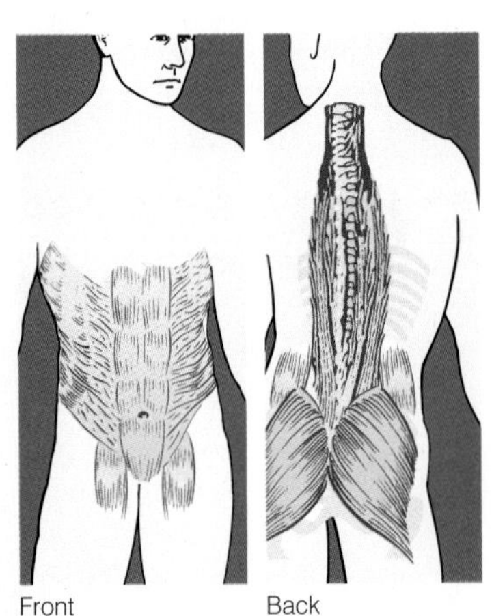

MUSCLES DEVELOPED Anterior and posterior muscle groups of the trunk and pelvis

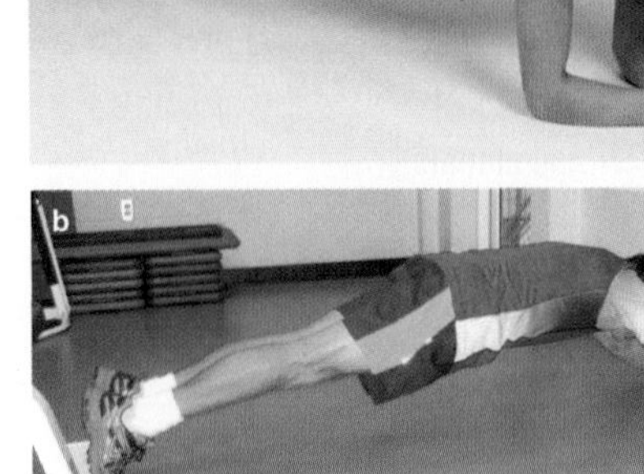

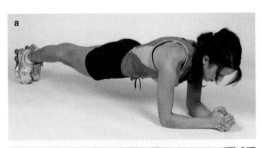

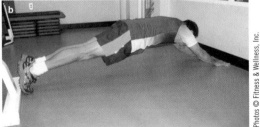

Photos © Fitness & Wellness, Inc.

Strength-Training Exercises with Weights

EXERCISE 15 Chest/Bench Press

MACHINE From a seated position, grasp the bar handles (a) and press forward until the arms are completely extended (b), then return to the original position. Do not arch the back during this exercise.

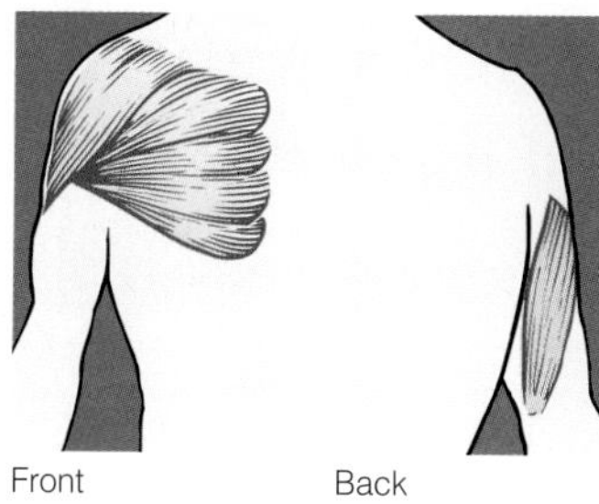

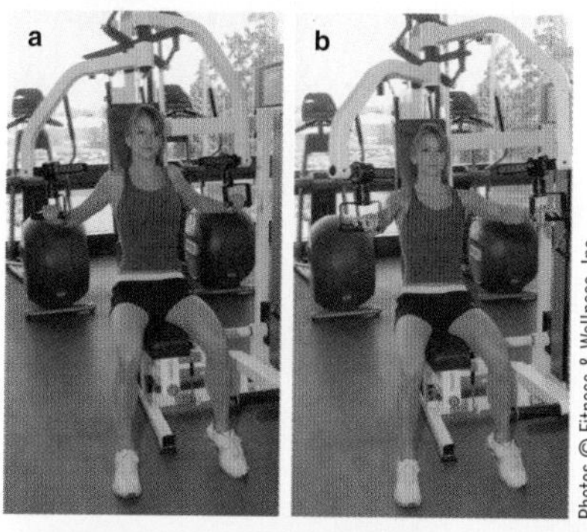

Photos © Fitness & Wellness, Inc.

FREE WEIGHTS Lie on the bench with arms extended and have one or two spotters help you place the barbell directly over your shoulders (a). Lower the weight to your chest (b) and then push it back up until you achieve full extension of the arms. Do not arch the back during this exercise.

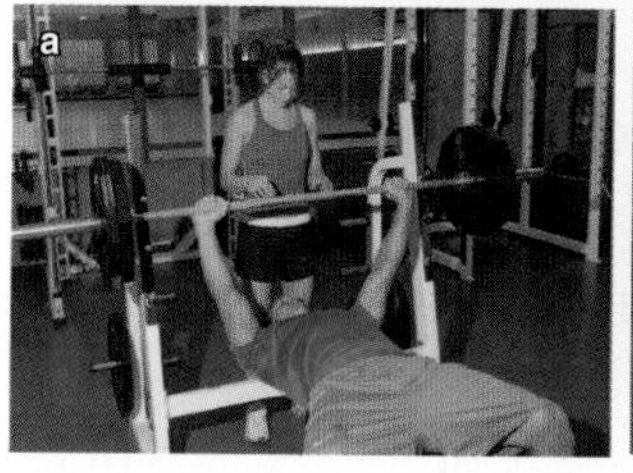

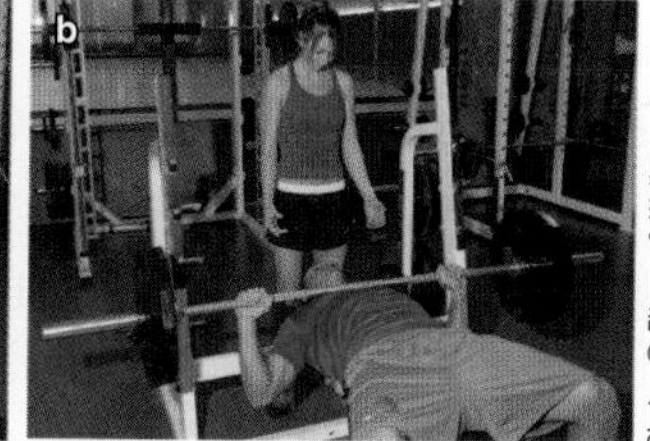

Photos © Fitness & Wellness, Inc.

MUSCLES DEVELOPED Pectoralis major, triceps, and deltoid

EXERCISE 16 Leg Press

ACTION From a sitting position with the knees flexed at about 90° and both feet on the footrest (a), extend the legs fully (b), then return slowly to the starting position.

MUSCLES DEVELOPED Quadriceps and gluteal muscles

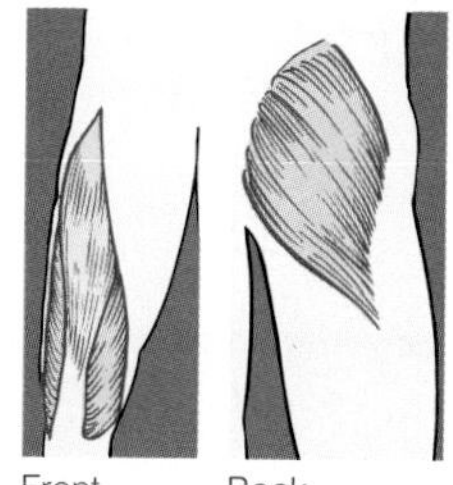

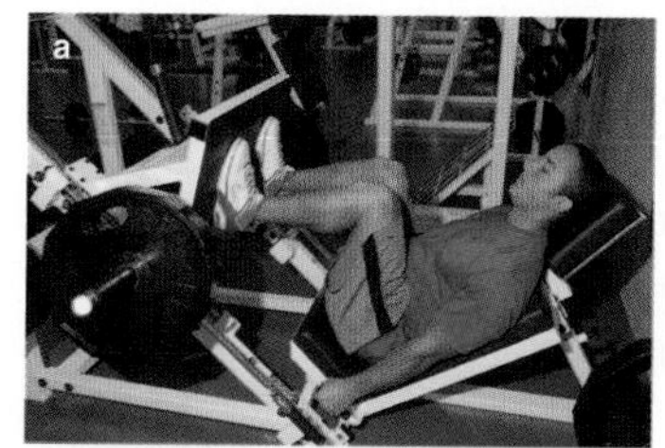

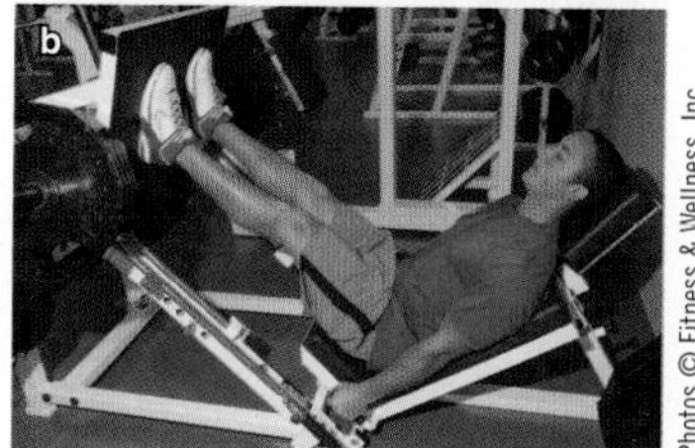

Photos © Fitness & Wellness, Inc.

EXERCISE 17 Abdominal Crunch

ACTION Sit in an upright position. Grasp the handles in front of you and crunch forward. Return slowly to the original position.

MUSCLES DEVELOPED Abdominals

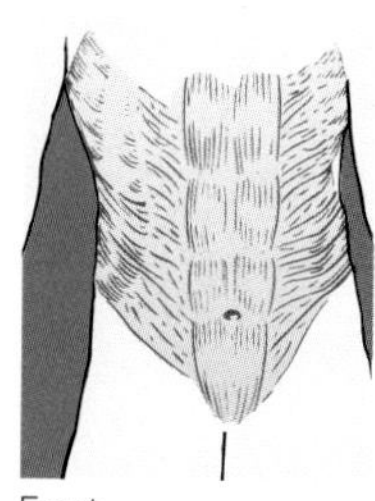

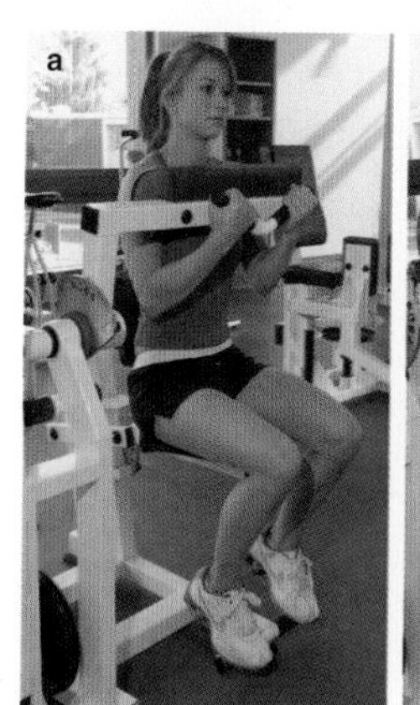

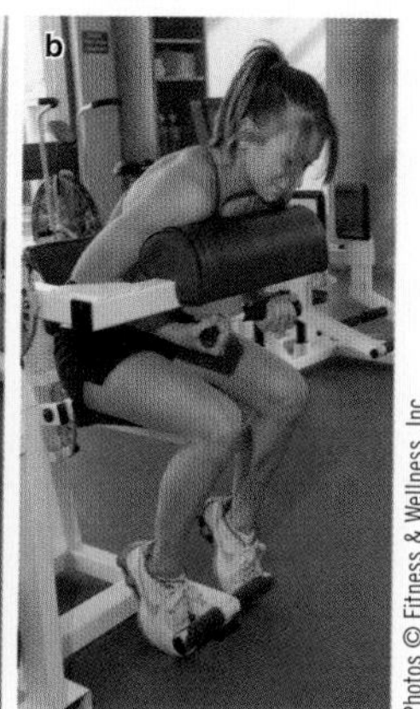

Photos © Fitness & Wellness, Inc.

EXERCISE 18A **Rowing Torso**

ACTION Sit in the machine and grasp the handles in front of you (a). Press back as far as possible, drawing the shoulder blades together (b). Return to the original position.

MUSCLES DEVELOPED Posterior deltoid, rhomboids, and trapezius

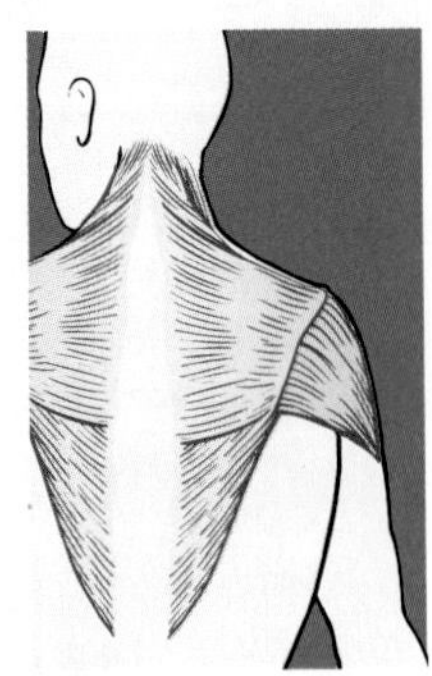

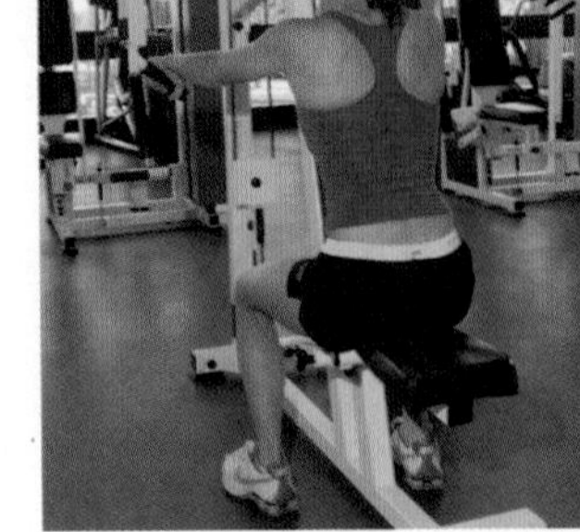

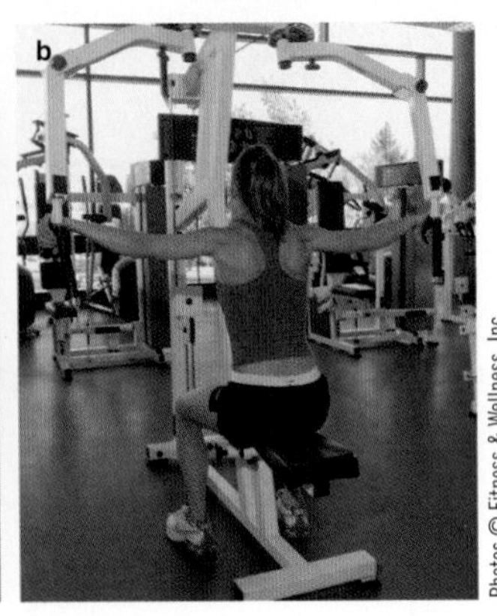

Photos © Fitness & Wellness, Inc.

EXERCISE 18B **Bent-over Lateral Raise**

ACTION Bend over with your back straight and knees bent at about 5 to 10° (a). Hold one dumbbell in each hand. Raise the dumbbells laterally to about shoulder level (b) and then slowly return them to the starting position.

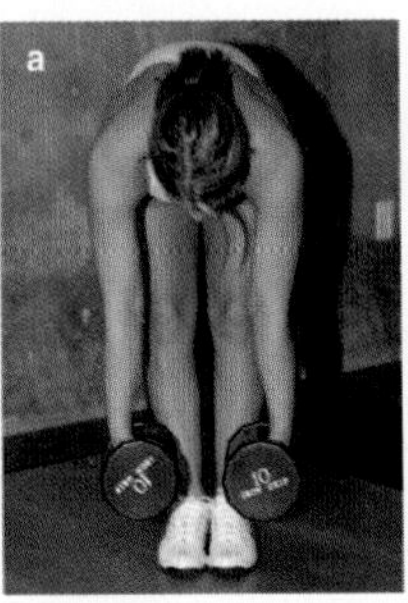

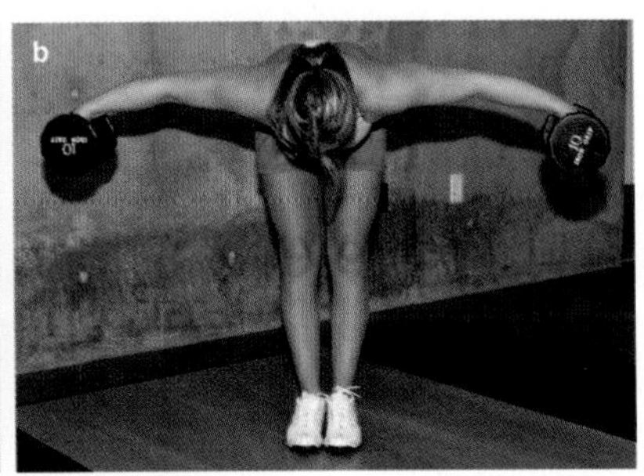

Photos © Fitness & Wellness, Inc.

EXERCISE 19 **Leg Curl**

ACTION Lie face down on the bench, legs straight, and place the back of the feet under the padded bar (a). Curl up to at least 90° (b), and return to the original position.

MUSCLES DEVELOPED Hamstrings

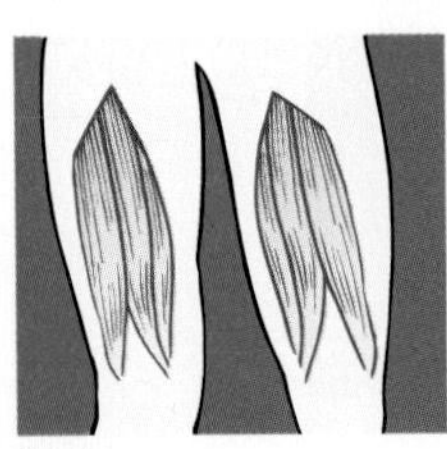

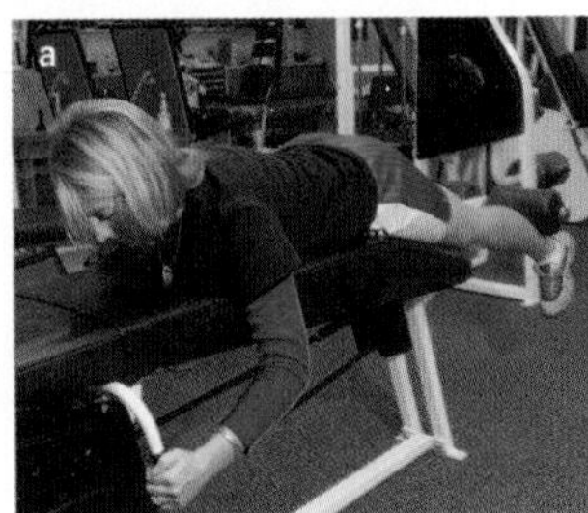

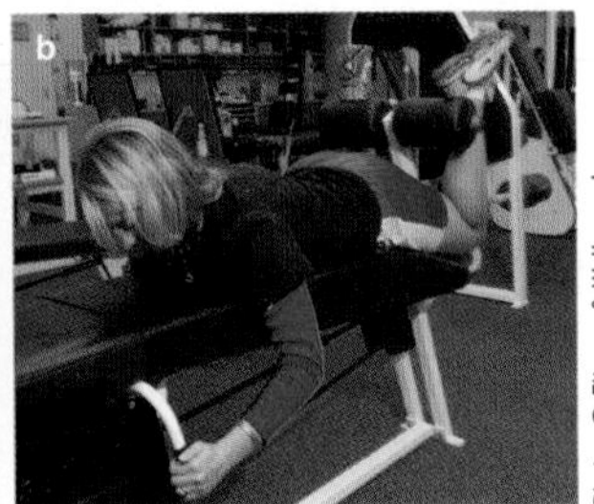

Photos © Fitness & Wellness, Inc.

EXERCISE 20 Seated Back

ACTION Sit in the machine with your trunk flexed and the upper back against the shoulder pad. Place the feet under the padded bar and hold on with your hands to the bars on the sides (a). Start the exercise by pressing backward, simultaneously extending the trunk and hip joints (b). Slowly return to the original position.

MUSCLES DEVELOPED Erector spinae and gluteus maximus

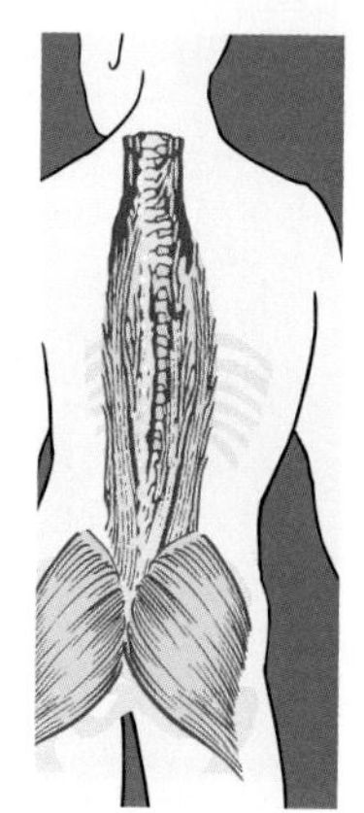

Back

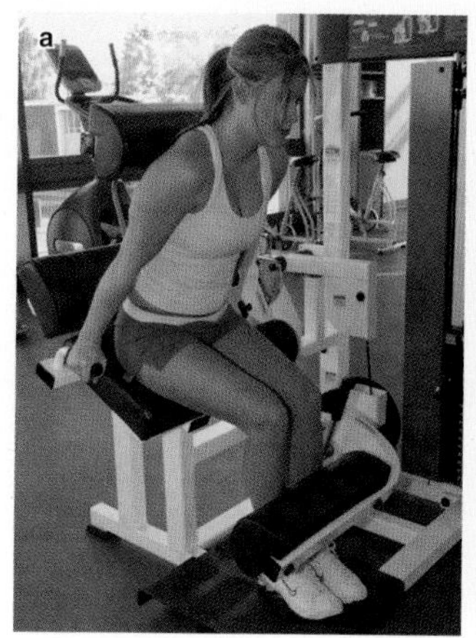

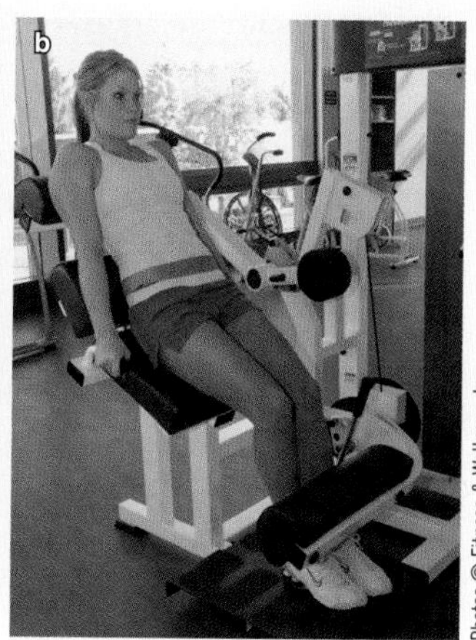

Photos © Fitness & Wellness, Inc.

EXERCISE 21 Calf Press

FREE WEIGHTS In a standing position, place a barbell across the shoulders and upper back. Grip the bar by the shoulders (a). Raise your heels off the floor or step box as far as possible (b) and then slowly return them to the starting position.

MACHINE Start with your feet flat on the plate (a). Now extend the ankles by pressing on the plate with the balls of your feet (b).

MUSCLES DEVELOPED Gastrocnemius, soleus

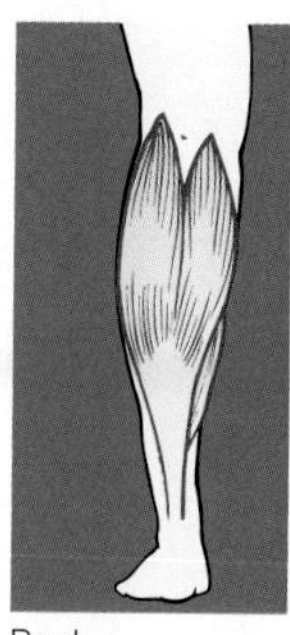
Back

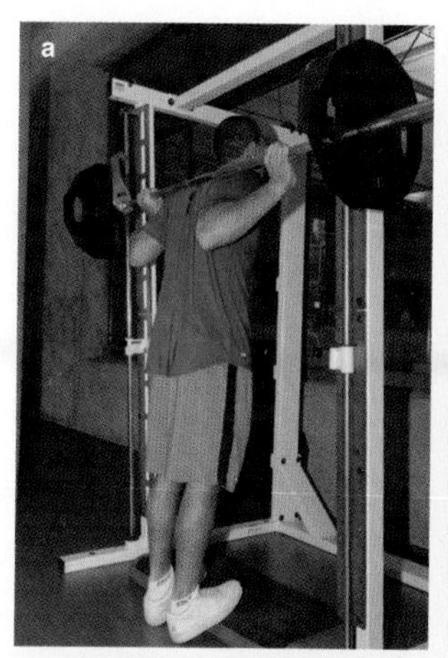

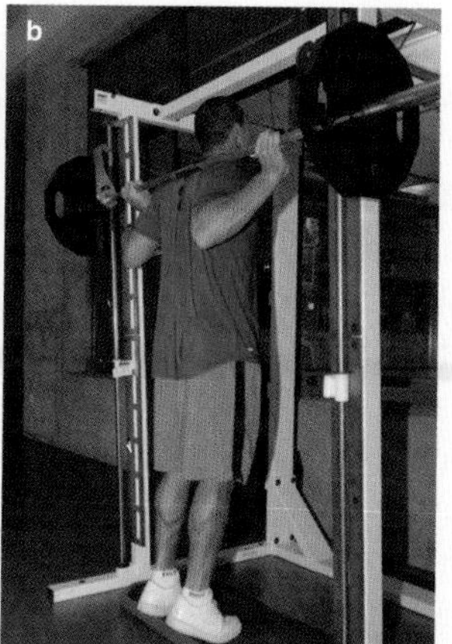

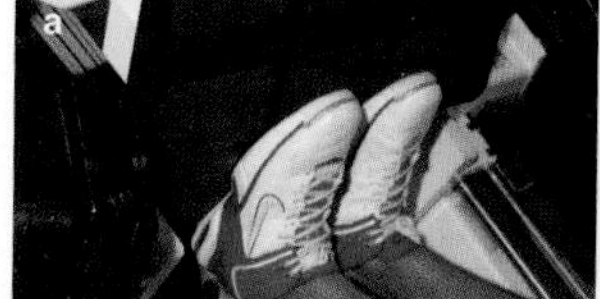

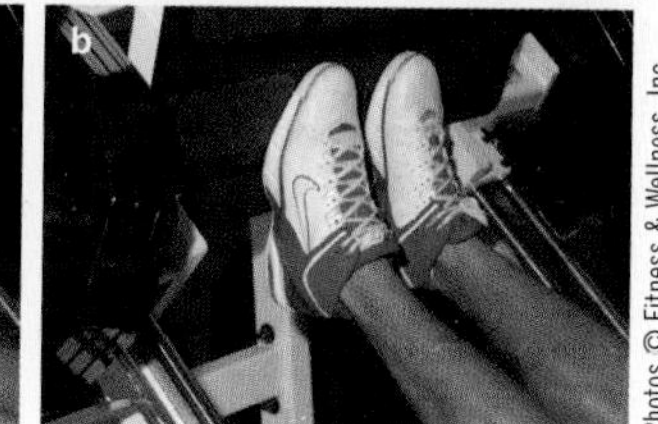

Photos © Fitness & Wellness, Inc.

EXERCISE 22 Leg (Hip) Adduction

ACTION Adjust the pads on the inside of the thighs as far out as the desired range of motion to be accomplished during the exercise (a). Press the legs together until both pads meet at the center (b). Slowly return to the starting position.

MUSCLES DEVELOPED Hip adductors (pectineus, gracilis, adductor magnus, adductor longus, and adductor brevis)

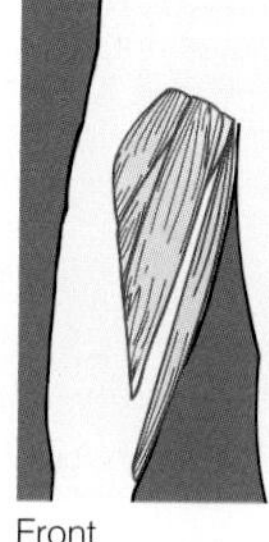
Front

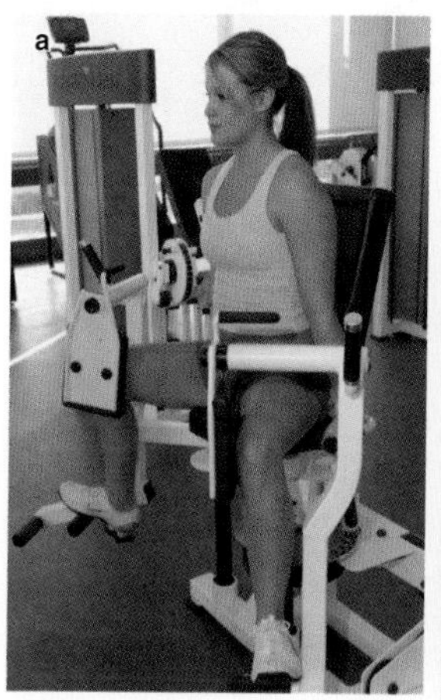

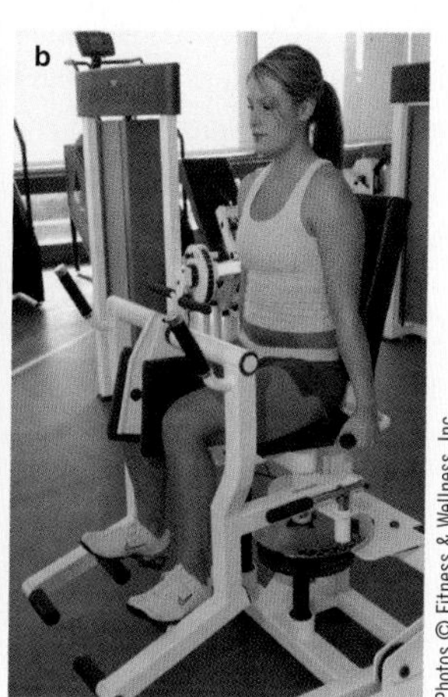

Photos © Fitness & Wellness, Inc.

EXERCISE 23 **Leg (Hip) Abduction**

ACTION Place your knees together with the pads directly outside the knees (a). Press the legs laterally out as far as possible (b). Slowly return to the starting position.

MUSCLES DEVELOPED Hip abductors (rectus femoris, sartori, gluteus medius and minimus)

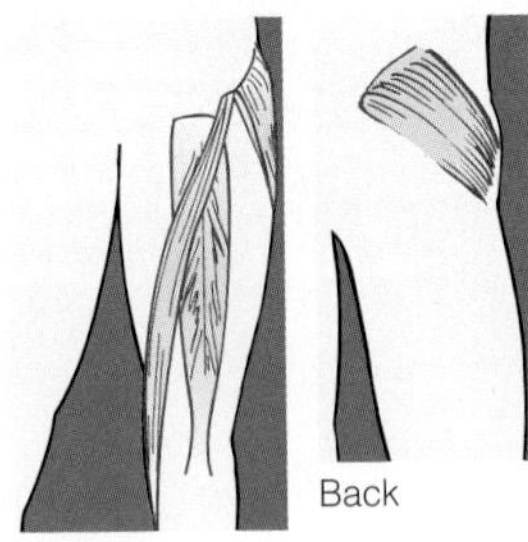

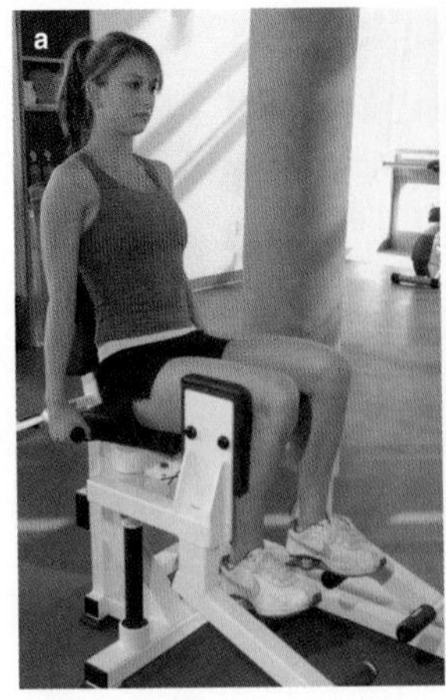

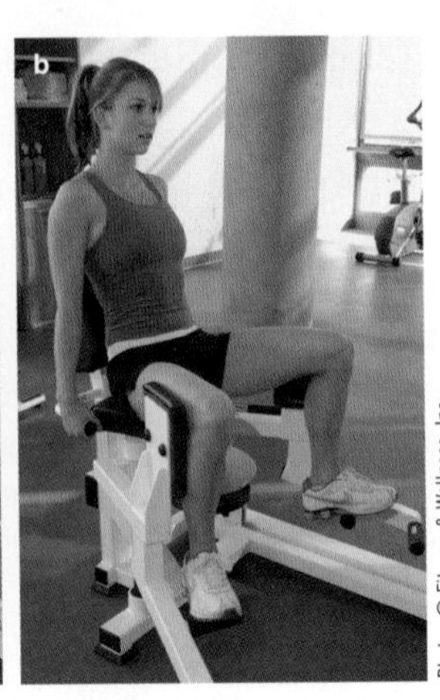

Photos © Fitness & Wellness, Inc.

EXERCISE 24 **Lat Pull-Down**

ACTION Starting from a sitting position, hold the exercise bar with a wide grip (a). Pull the bar down in front of you until it reaches the upper chest (b), then return to the starting position.

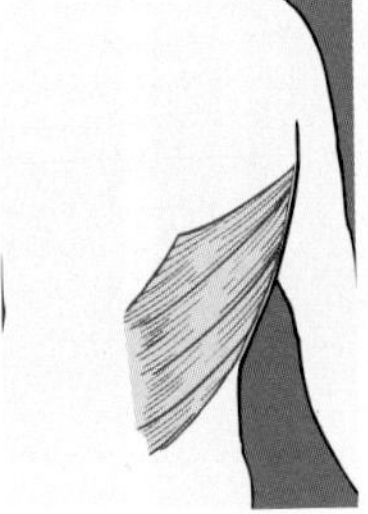

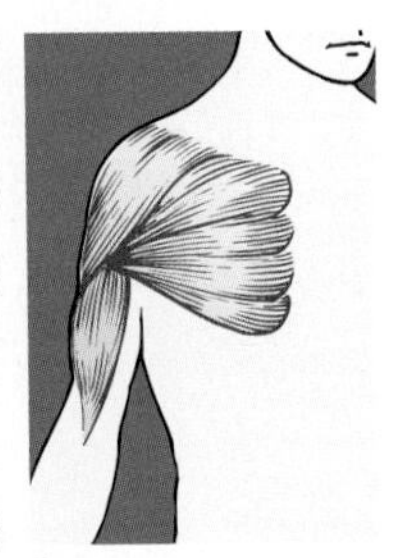

MUSCLES DEVELOPED Latissimus dorsi, pectoralis major, and biceps

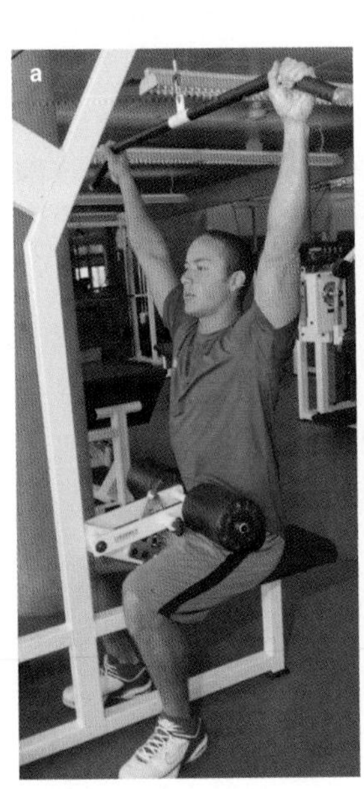

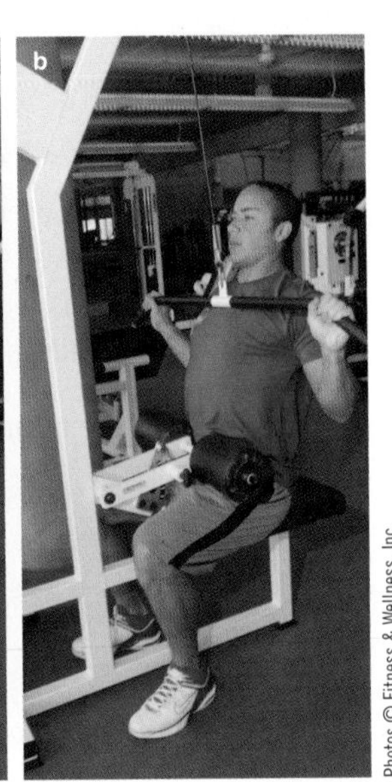

Photos © Fitness & Wellness, Inc.

EXERCISE 25 **Rotary Torso**

FREE WEIGHTS Stand with your feet slightly apart. Place a barbell across your shoulders and upper back, holding on to the sides of the barbell. Now gently, and in a controlled manner, twist your torso to one side as far as possible and then do so in the opposite direction.

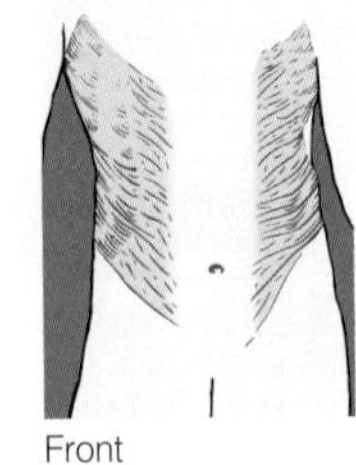

MUSCLES DEVELOPED Internal and external obliques (abdominal muscles)

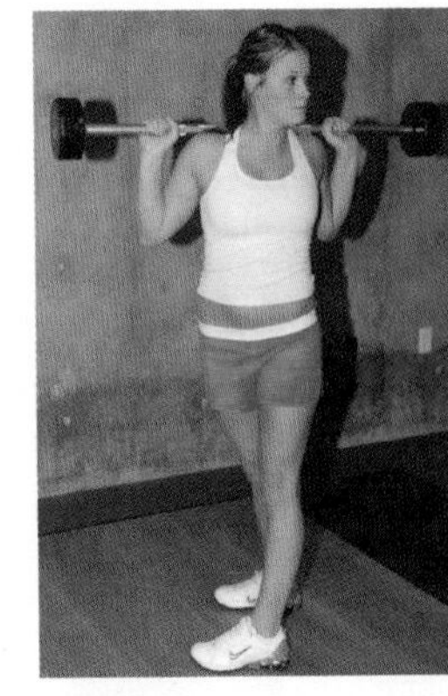

© Fitness & Wellness, Inc.

EXERCISE 26 Triceps Extension

MACHINE Sit in an upright position and grasp the bar behind the shoulders (a). Fully extend the arms (b) and then return to the original position.

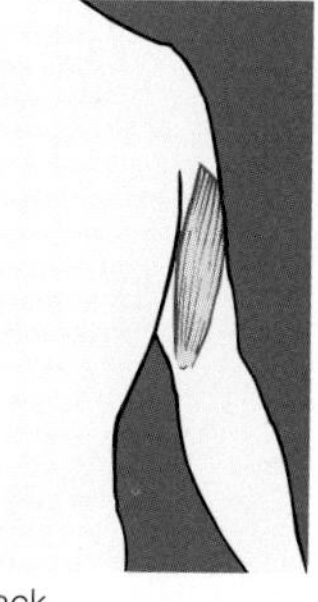
Back

MACHINE Using a palms-down grip, grasp the bar slightly closer than shoulder-width and start with the elbows almost completely bent (a). Extend the arms fully (b), then return to starting position.

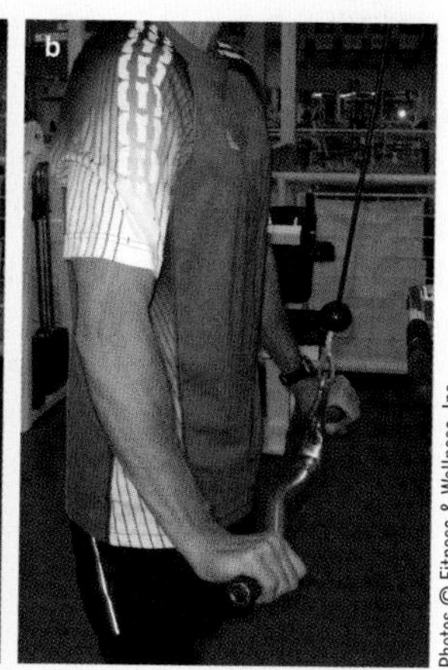
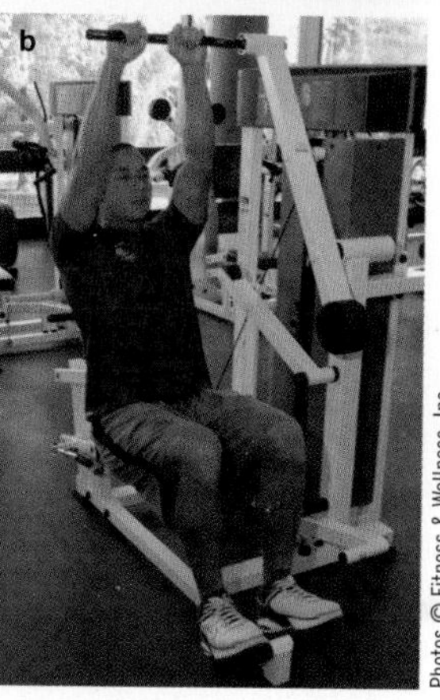
Photos © Fitness & Wellness, Inc.

FREE WEIGHTS In a standing position, hold a barbell with both hands overhead and with the arms in full extension (a). Slowly lower the barbell behind your head (b) and then return it to the starting position.

MUSCLES DEVELOPED Triceps

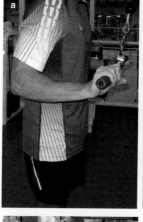

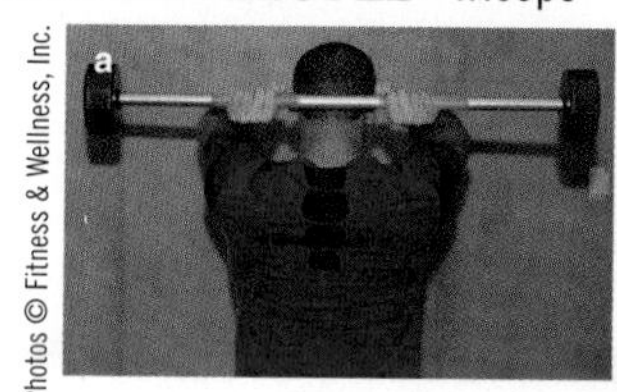
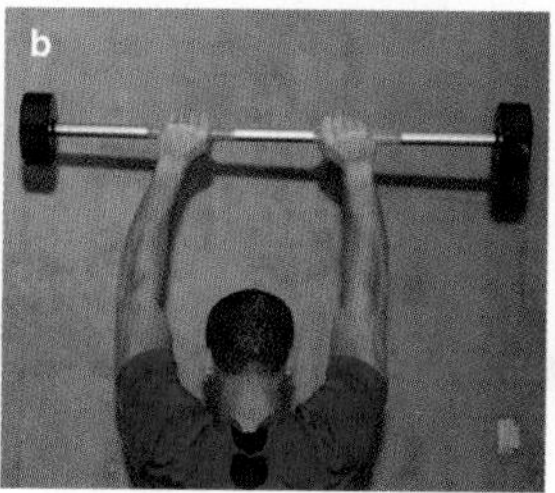
Photos © Fitness & Wellness, Inc.

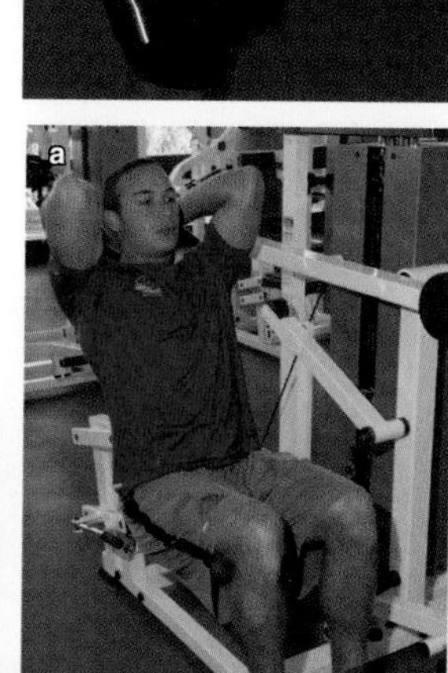
Photos © Fitness & Wellness, Inc.

EXERCISE 27 Arm Curl

MACHINE Using a supinated (palms-up) grip, start with the arms almost completely extended (a). Curl up as far as possible (b), then return to the starting position.

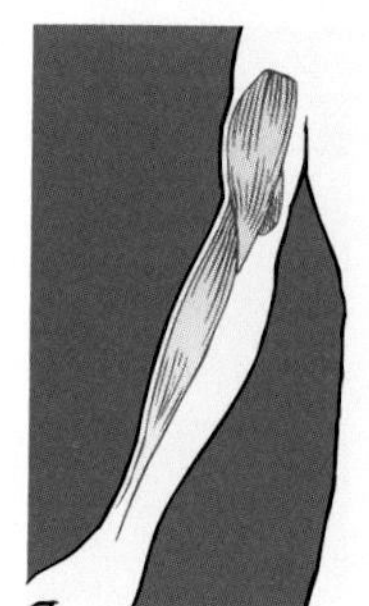
Front

FREE WEIGHTS Standing upright, hold a barbell in front of you at about shoulder width with arms extended and the hands in a thumbs-out position (supinated grip) (a). Raise the barbell to your shoulders (b) and slowly return it to the starting position.

MUSCLES DEVELOPED Biceps, brachioradialis, and brachialis

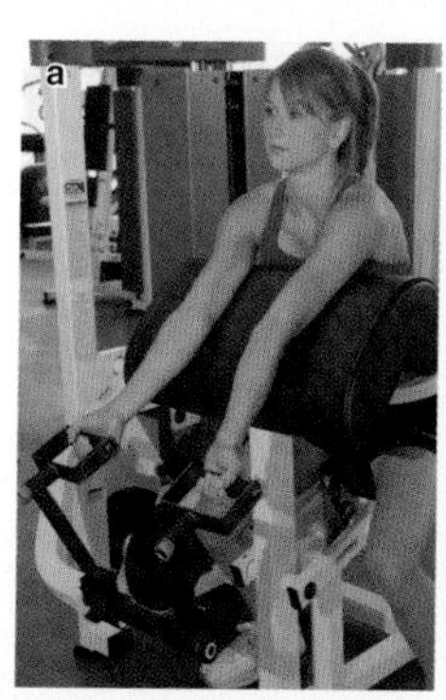
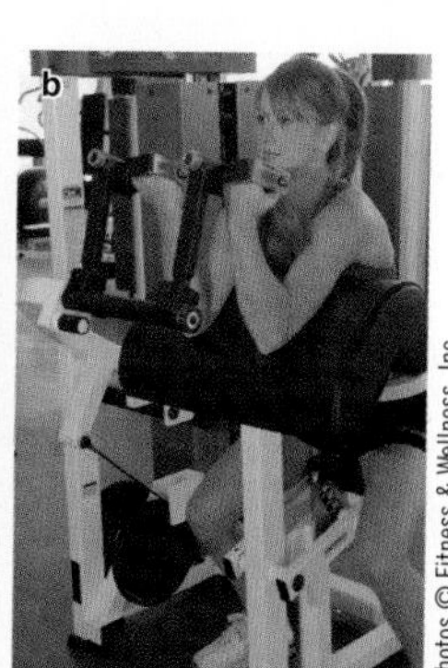
Photos © Fitness & Wellness, Inc.

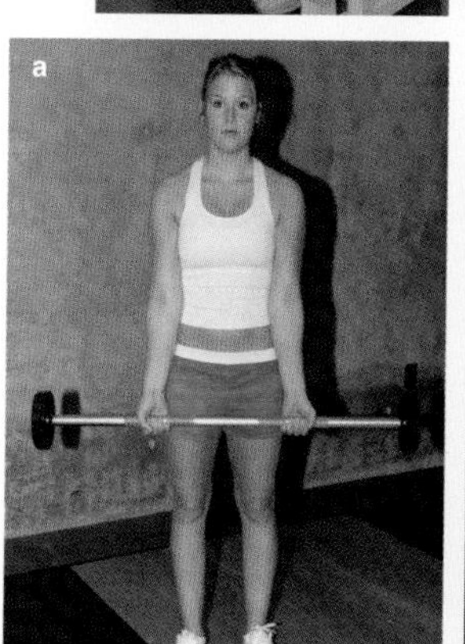
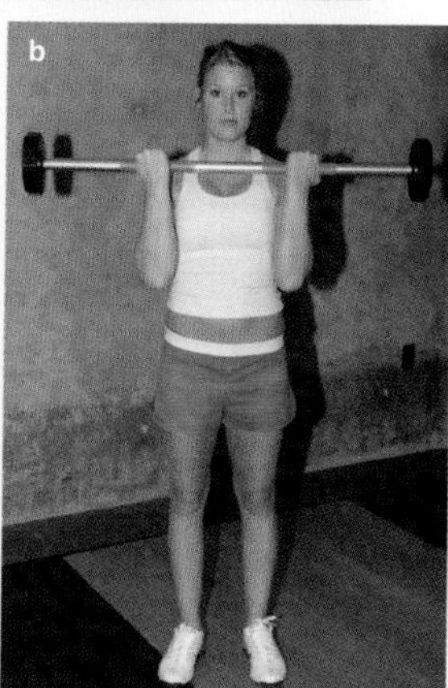
Photos © Fitness & Wellness, Inc.

EXERCISE 28A **Leg Extension**

ACTION Sit in an upright position with the feet under the padded bar and grasp the handles at the sides (a). Extend the legs until they are completely straight (b), then return to the starting position.

MUSCLES DEVELOPED Quadriceps

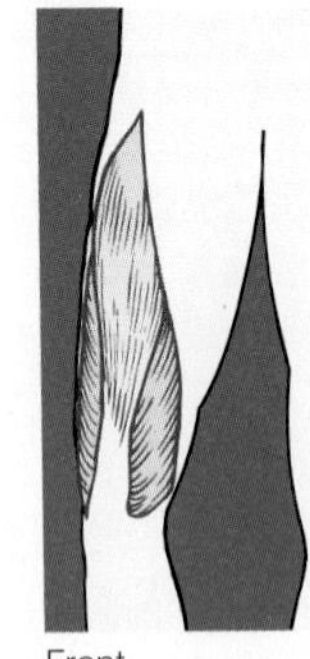

Front

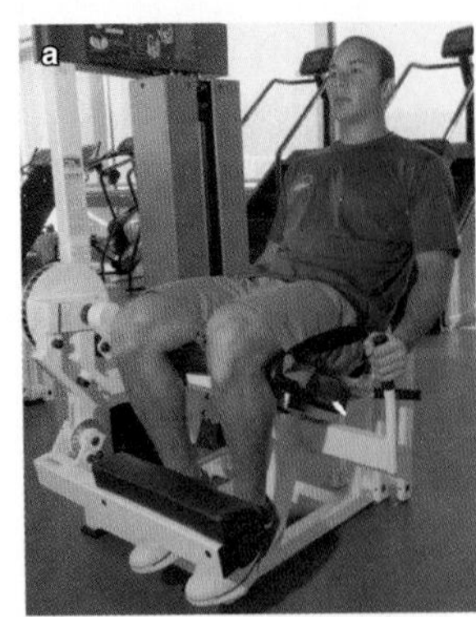

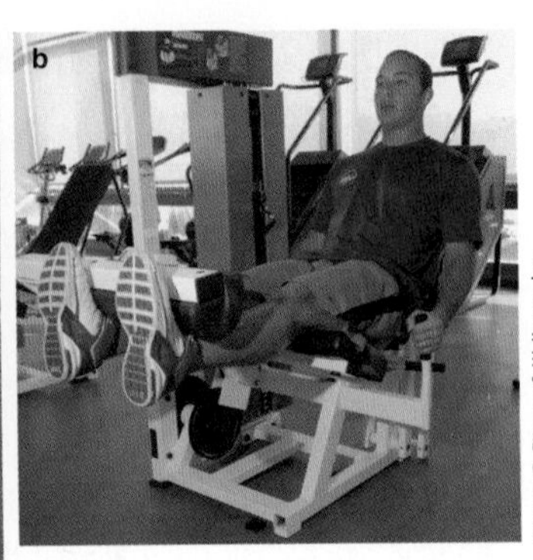

EXERCISE 28B **Unilateral Eccentric Knee Flexion**

ACTION Using a *moderate resistance*, raise the padded bar by extending both knees (see exercise 28A, a and b). Next, remove the left foot from the padded bar while holding the bar in place with the right leg (c). Now slowly lower the resistance (padded bar) to about 45 degrees (d). Return the left foot to the padded bar and once again press the bar up to full knee extension. Alternate legs by releasing the right foot next and lower the resistance with the left foot. Repeat the exercise about 10 times with each leg. **THIS EXERCISE IS *QUITE HELPFUL* TO STRENGTHEN WEAK KNEES AND PREVENT POTENTIAL FUTURE KNEE PROBLEMS.**

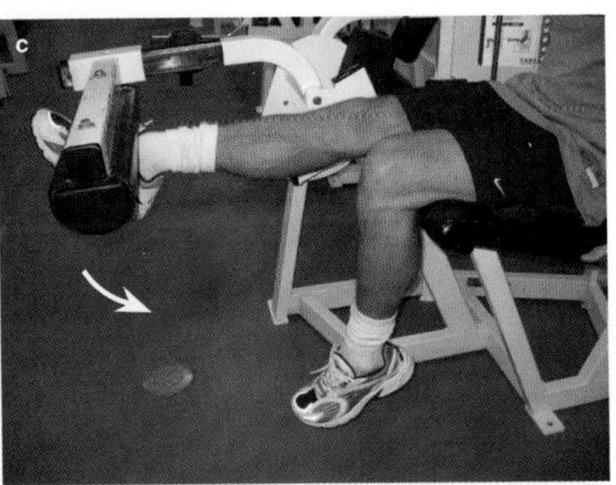

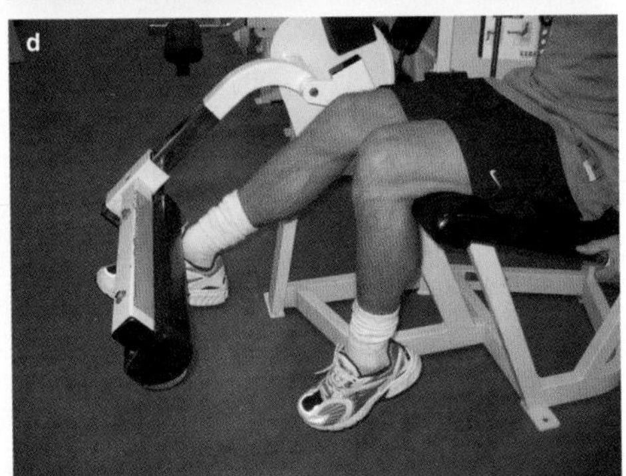

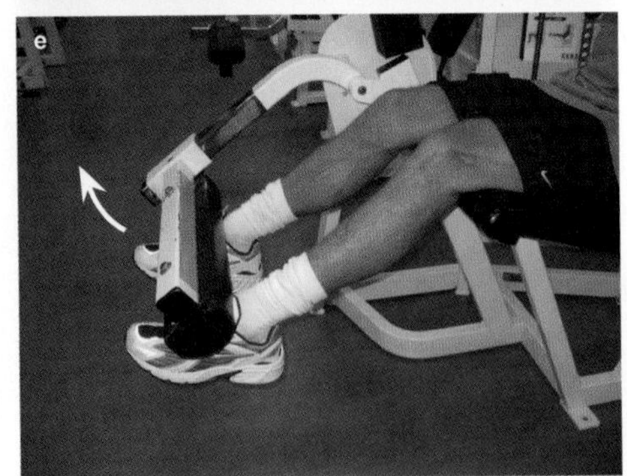

EXERCISE 29 Shoulder Press

MACHINE Sit in an upright position and grasp the bar wider than shoulder width (a). Press the bar all the way up until the arms are fully extended (b), then return to the initial position.

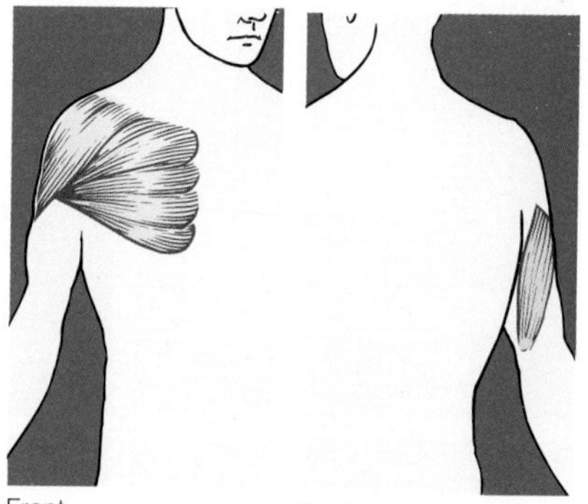

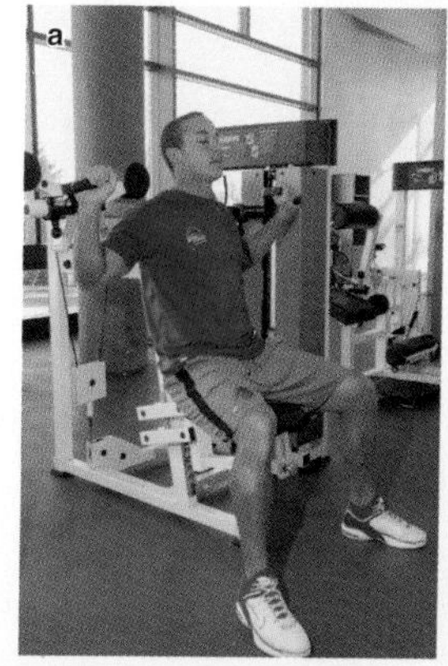

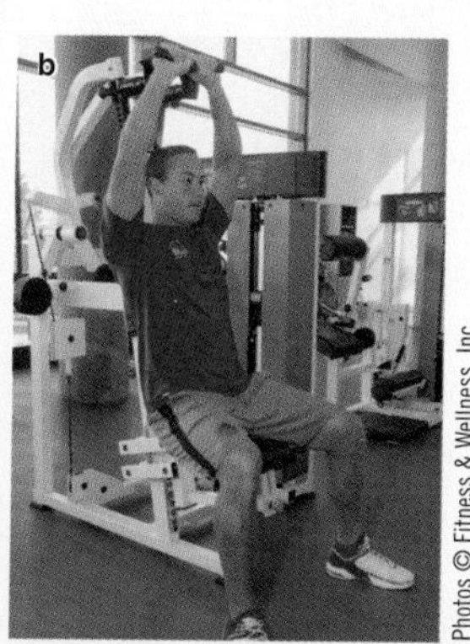

Photos © Fitness & Wellness, Inc.

FREE WEIGHTS Place a barbell on your shoulders in front of the body (a) and press the weight overhead until complete extension of the arms is achieved (b). Return the weight to the original position. Be sure not to arch the back or lean back during this exercise.

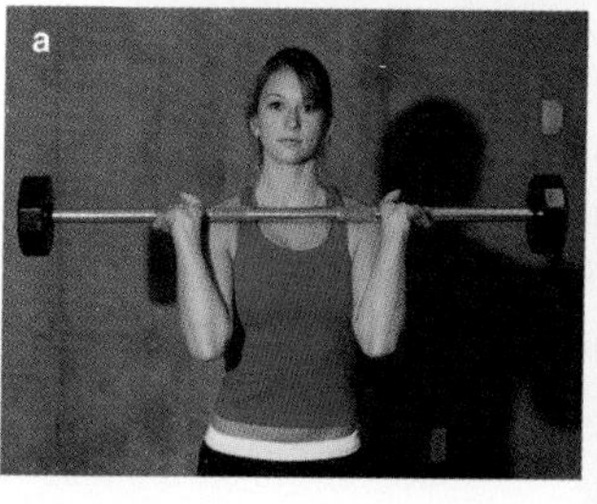

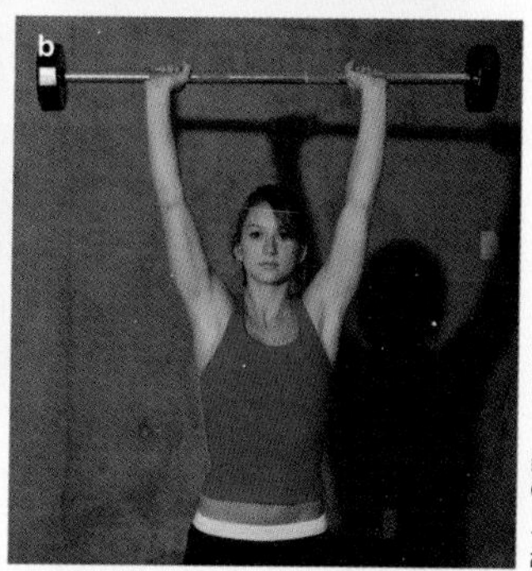

Photos © Fitness & Wellness, Inc.

MUSCLES DEVELOPED Triceps, deltoid, and pectoralis major

EXERCISE 30 Chest Fly

ACTION Start with the arms out to the side, and grasp the handle bars with the arms straight (a). Press the movement arms forward until they are completely in front of you (b). Slowly return to the starting position.

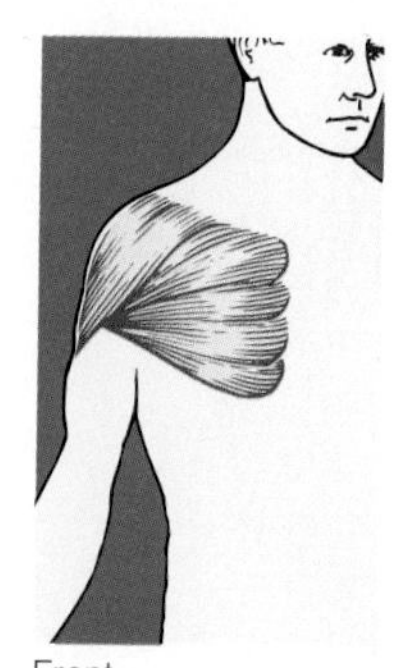

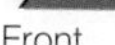

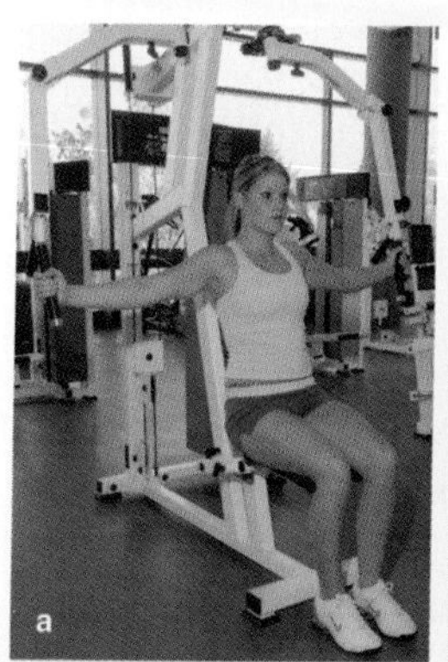

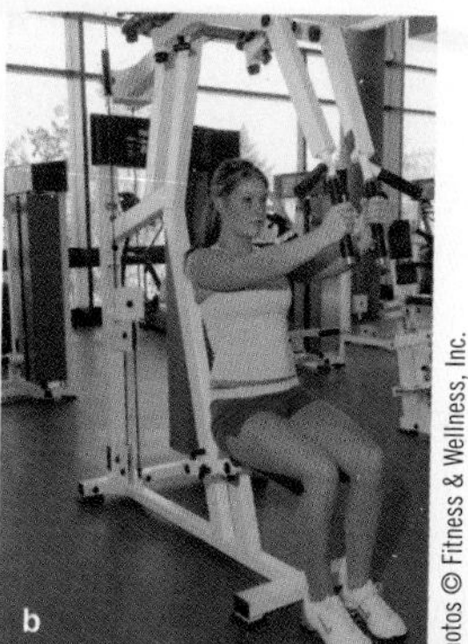

Photos © Fitness & Wellness, Inc.

FREE WEIGHTS Bent Arm Fly
Lie down on your back on a bench and hold a dumbbell in each hand directly overhead (a). Keeping your elbows slightly bent, lower the weights laterally to a horizontal position (b) and then bring them back up to the starting position.

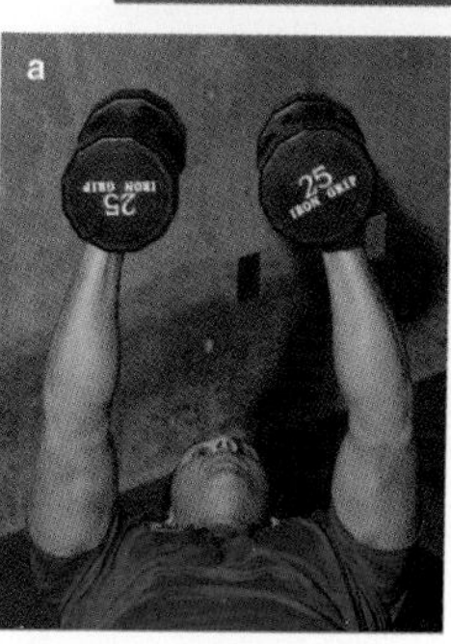

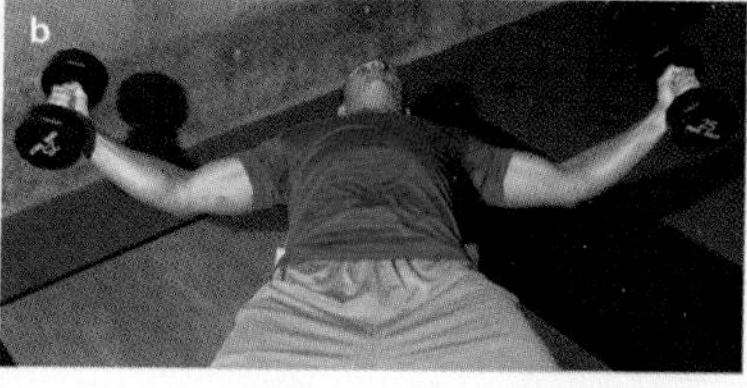

Photos © Fitness & Wellness, Inc.

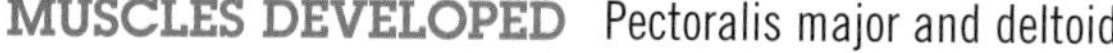

MUSCLES DEVELOPED Pectoralis major and deltoid

EXERCISE 31 Squat

MACHINE Place the shoulders under the pads and grasp the bars by the sides of the shoulders (a). Slowly bend the knees to between 90° and 120° (b). Return to the starting position.

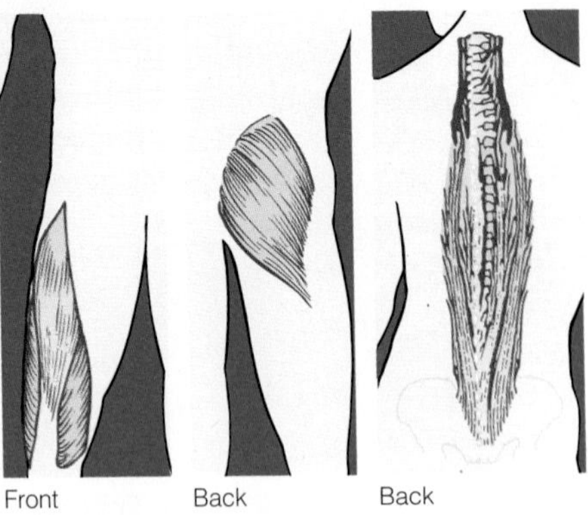

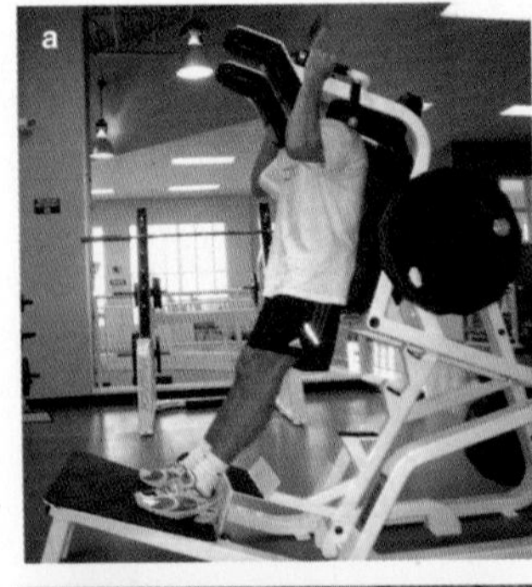

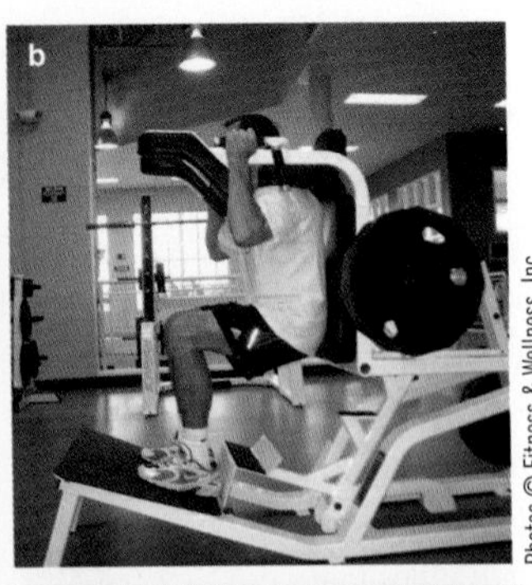

Photos © Fitness & Wellness, Inc.

FREE WEIGHTS From a standing position, and with a spotter to each side, support a barbell over your shoulders and upper back (a). Keeping your head up and back straight, bend at the knees and the hips until you achieve an approximate 120° angle at the knees (b). Return to the starting position. *Do not perform this exercise alone.* If no spotters are available, use a squat rack to ensure that you will not get trapped under a heavy weight.

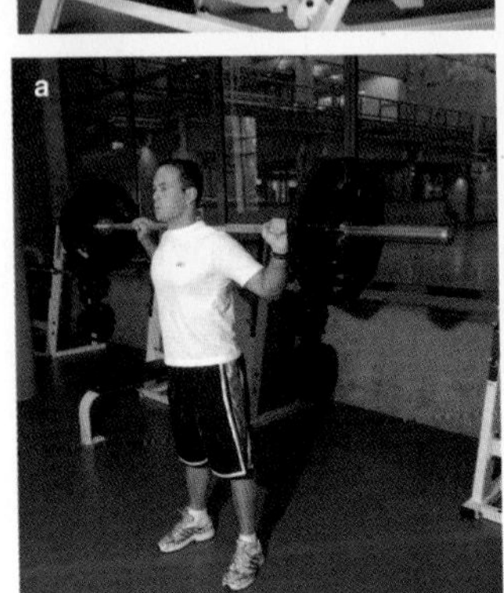

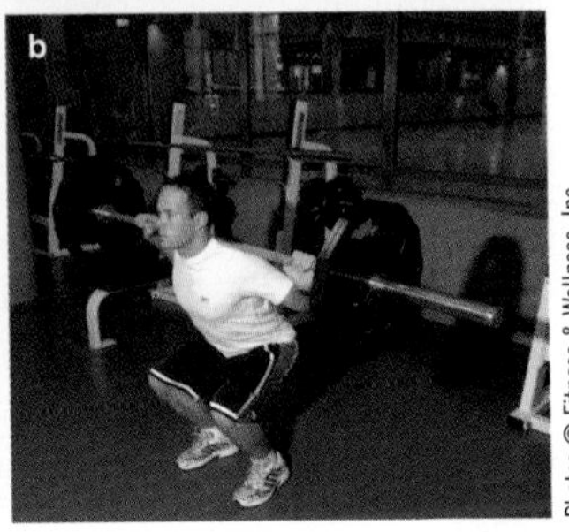

Photos © Fitness & Wellness, Inc.

MUSCLES DEVELOPED Quadriceps, gluteus maximus, erector spinae

EXERCISE 32 Upright Rowing

MACHINE Start with the arms extended and grip the handles with the palms down (a). Pull all the way up to the chin (b), then return to the starting position.

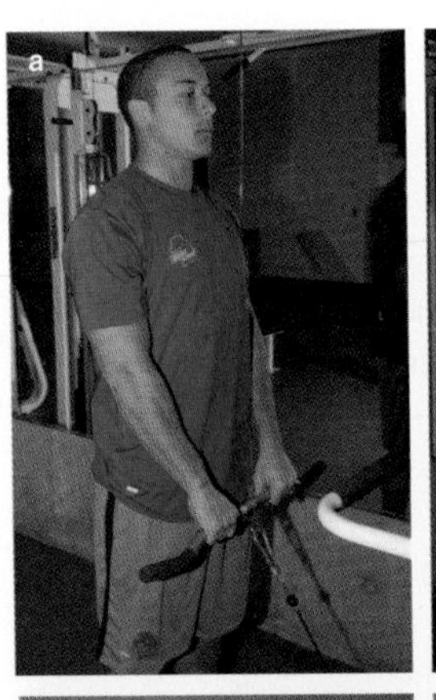

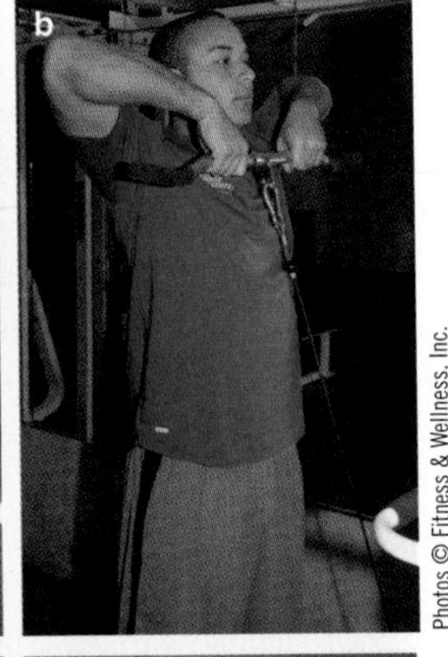

Photos © Fitness & Wellness, Inc.

FREE WEIGHTS Hold a barbell in front of you, with the arms fully extended and hands in a thumbs-in (pronated) grip less than shoulder-width apart (a). Pull the barbell up until it reaches shoulder level (b) and then slowly return it to the starting position.

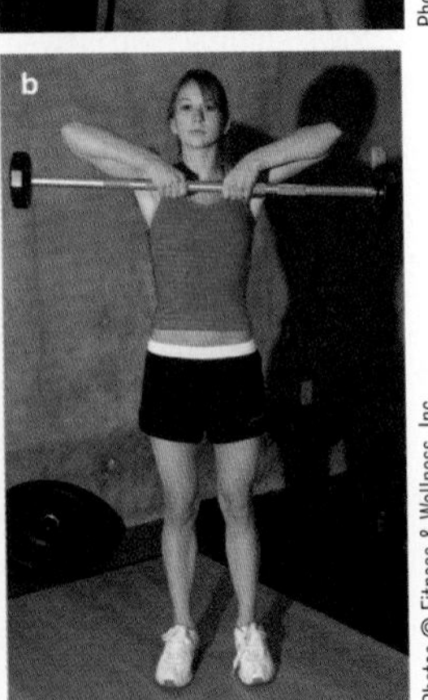

Photos © Fitness & Wellness, Inc.

MUSCLES DEVELOPED Biceps, brachioradialis, brachialis, deltoid, and trapezius

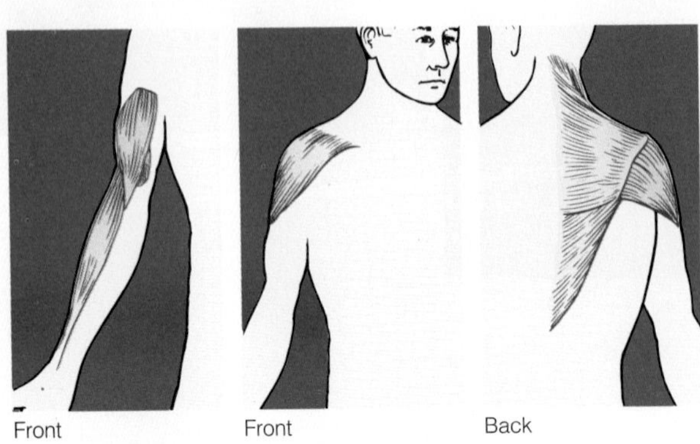

EXERCISE 33 **Seated Leg Curl**

ACTION Sit in the unit and place the strap over the upper thighs. With legs extended, place the back of the feet over the padded rollers (a). Flex the knees until you reach a 90° to 100° angle (b). Slowly return to the starting position.

MUSCLES DEVELOPED Hamstrings

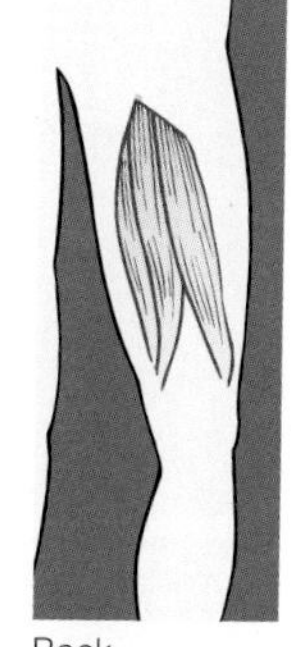
Back

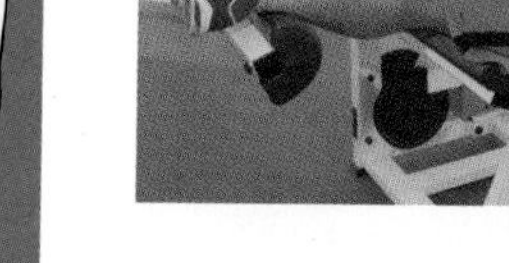

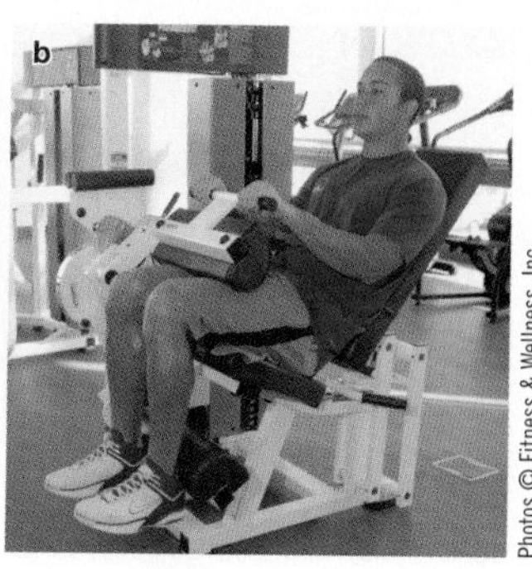

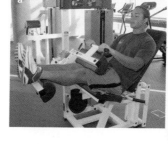

Photos © Fitness & Wellness, Inc.

EXERCISE 34 **Bent-Arm Pullover**

MACHINE Sit back into the chair and grasp the bar behind your head (a). Pull the bar over your head all the way down to your abdomen (b) and slowly return to the original position.

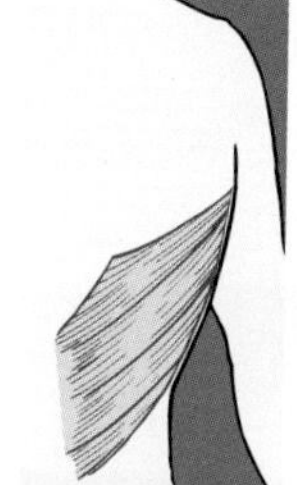
Back

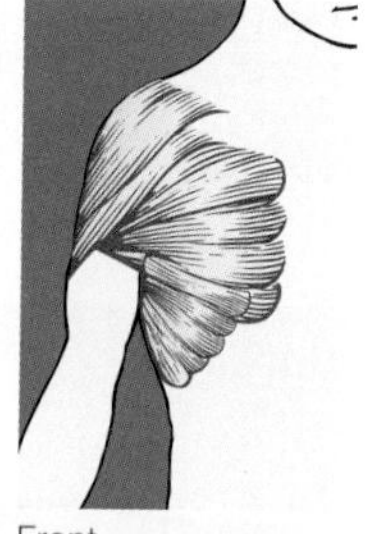
Front

FREE WEIGHTS Lie on your back on an exercise bench with your head over the edge of the bench. Hold a barbell over your chest with the hands less than shoulder-width apart (a). Keeping the elbows shoulder-width apart, lower the weight over your head until your shoulders are completely extended (b). Slowly return the weight to the starting position.

MUSCLES DEVELOPED Latissimus dorsi, pectoral muscles, deltoid, and serratus anterior

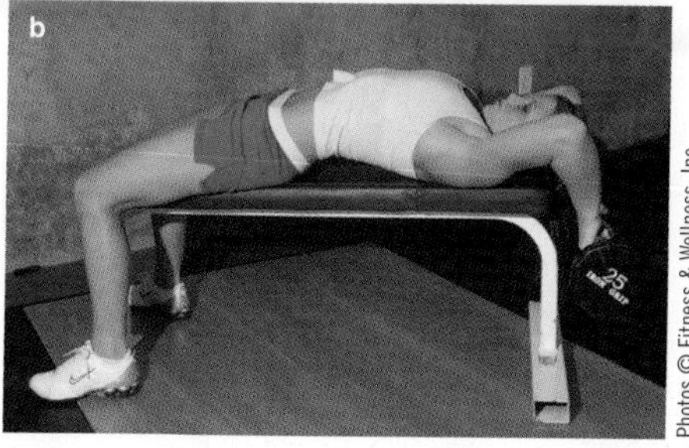

Photos © Fitness & Wellness, Inc.

EXERCISE 35 **Dip**

ACTION Start with the elbows flexed (a), then extend the arms fully (b), and return slowly to the initial position.

MUSCLES DEVELOPED Triceps, deltoid, and pectoralis major

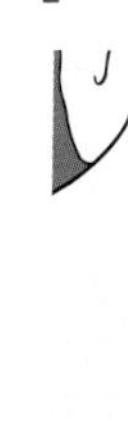

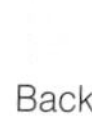
Back

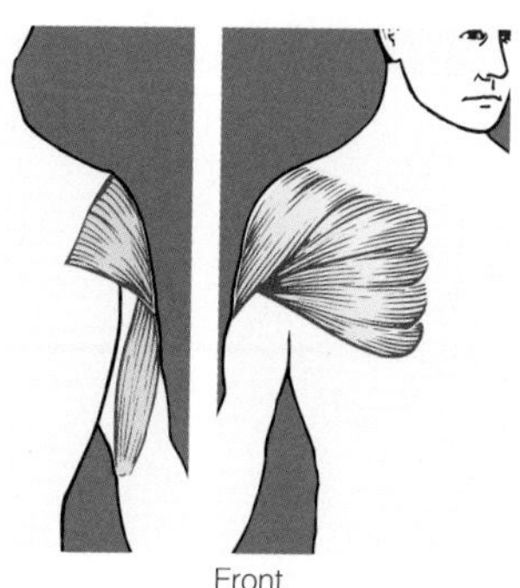
Front

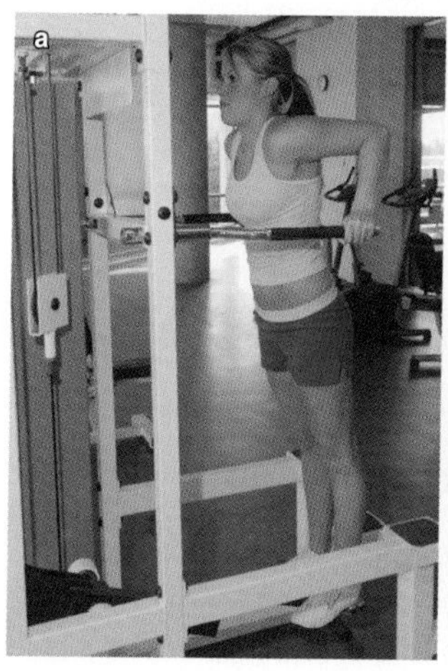

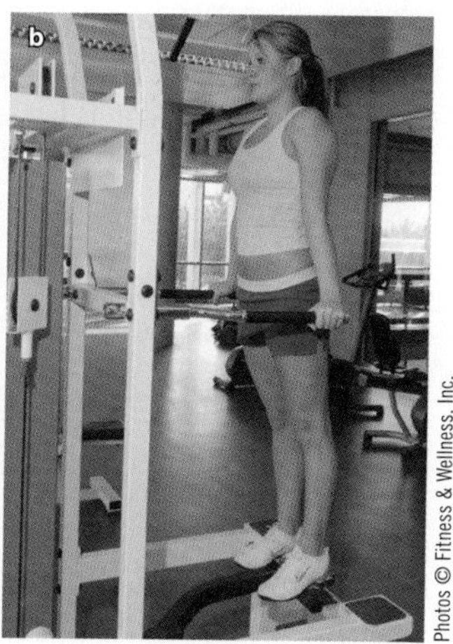

Photos © Fitness & Wellness, Inc.

EXERCISE 36 Back Extension

ACTION Place your feet under the ankle rollers and the hips over the padded seat. Start with the trunk in a flexed position and the arms crossed over the chest (a). Slowly extend the trunk to a horizontal position (b), hold the extension for 2 to 5 seconds, then slowly flex (lower) the trunk to the original position.

MUSCLES DEVELOPED Erector spinae, gluteus maximus, and quadratus lumborum (lower back)

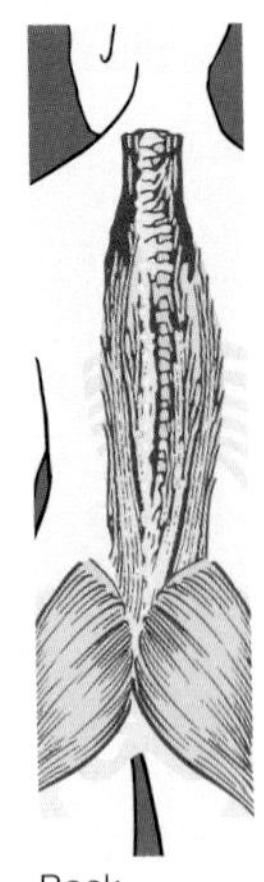

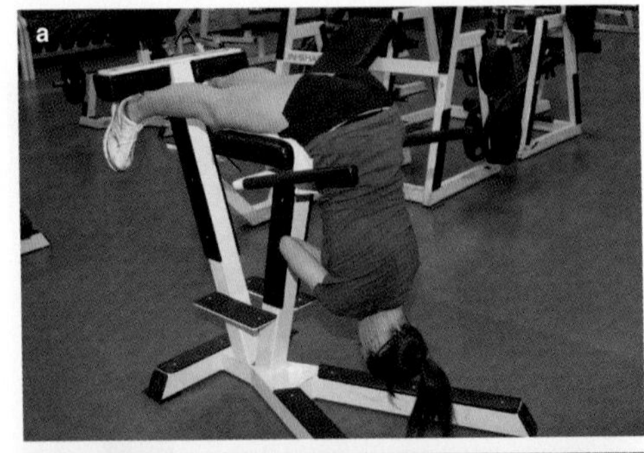

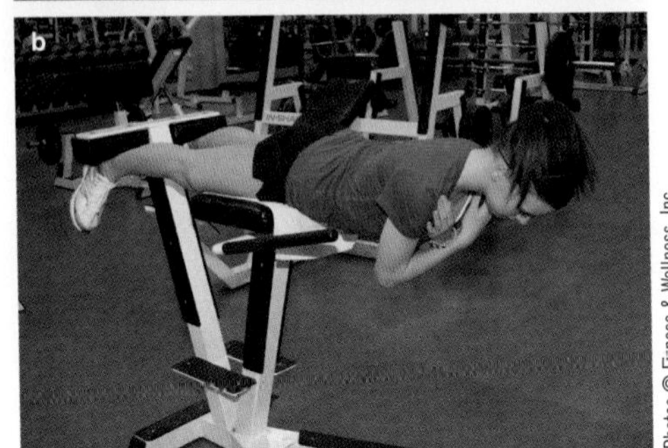

EXERCISE 37 Lateral Trunk Flexion

ACTION Lie sideways on the padded seat with the right foot under the right side of the padded ankle pad (right knee slightly bent) and the left foot stabilized on the vertical bar. Cross the arms over the abdomen or chest and start with the body in a straight line. Raise (flex) your upper body about 30 to 40° and then slowly return to the starting position.

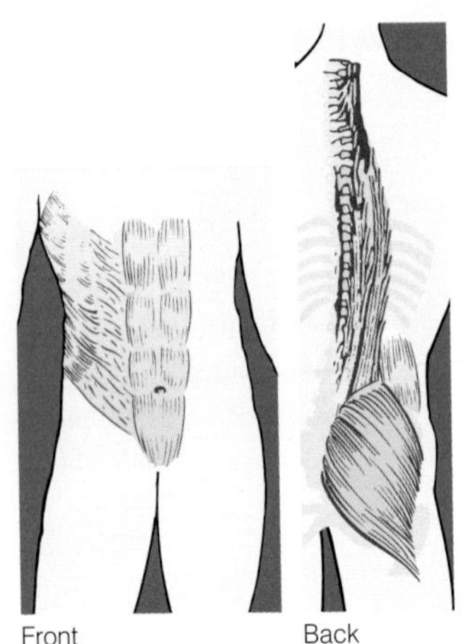

MUSCLES DEVELOPED Erector spinae, rectus abdominus, internal and external abdominal obliques, quadratus lumborum, gluteal muscles

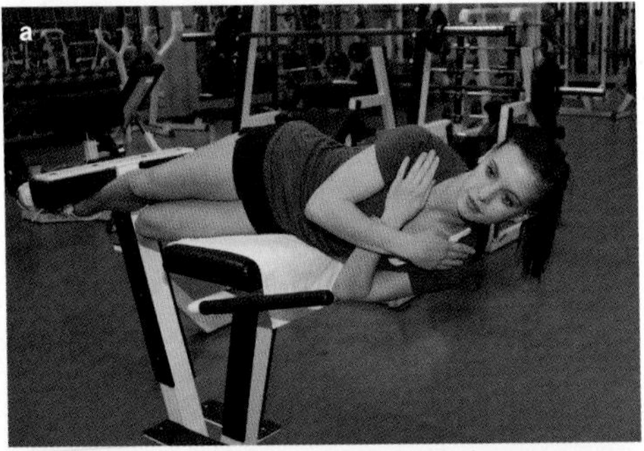

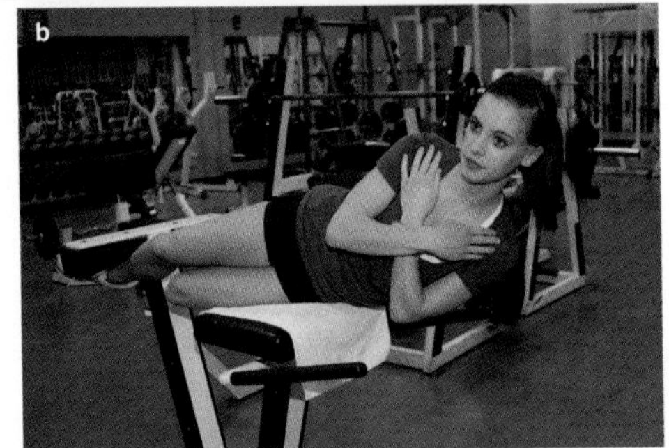

Stability Ball Exercises

EXERCISE 38 The Plank

ACTION Place your knees or feet (increased difficulty) on the ball and raise your body off the floor to a horizontal position. Pull the abdominal muscles in and hold the body in a straight line for 5 to 10 seconds. Repeat the exercise 3 to 5 times.

MUSCLES INVOLVED Abdominals, erector spinae, lower back, hip flexors, gluteal, quadriceps, hamstrings, chest, shoulder, and triceps

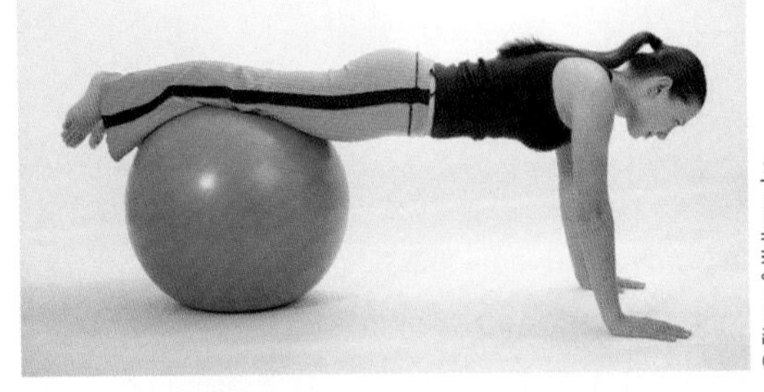

EXERCISE 39 **Abdominal Crunches**

ACTION On your back and with the feet slightly separated, lie with the ball under your back and shoulder blades. Cross the arms over your chest (a). Press your lower back into the ball and crunch up 20 to 30°. Keep your neck and shoulders in line with your trunk (b). Repeat the exercise 10 to 20 times (you may also do an oblique crunch by rotating the ribcage to the opposite hip at the end of the crunch [c]).

MUSCLES INVOLVED Rectus abdominus, internal and external abdominal obliques

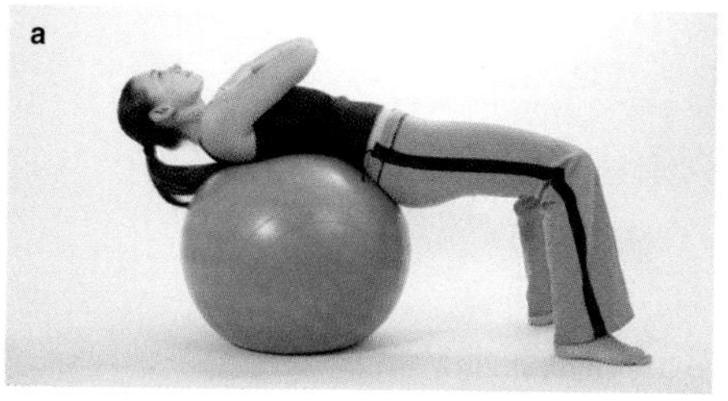
a

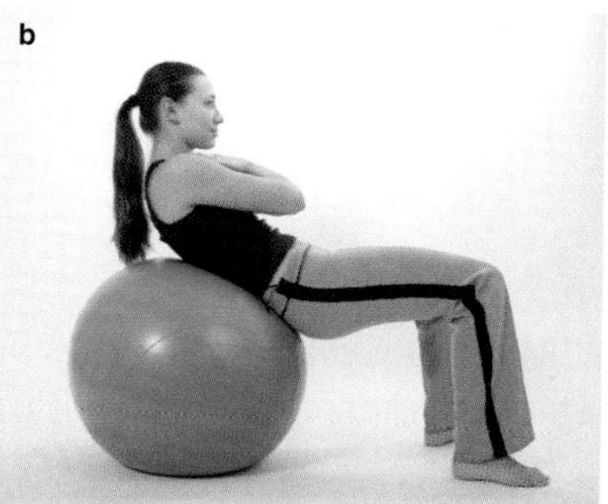
b

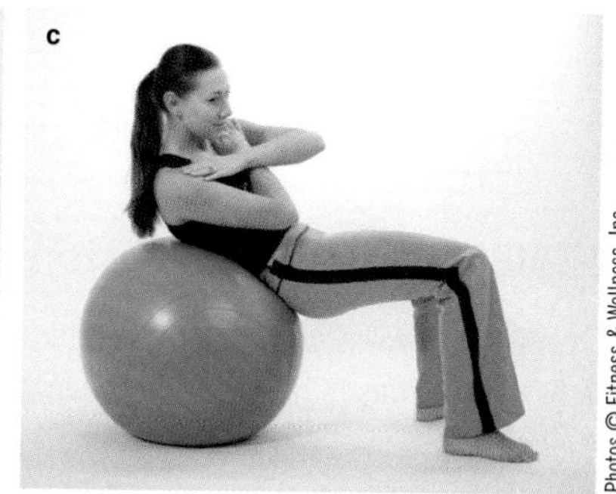
c

EXERCISE 40 **Supine Bridge**

ACTION With the feet slightly separated and knees bent, lie with your neck and upper back on the ball; hands placed on the abdomen. Gently squeeze the gluteal muscles while raising your hips off the floor until the upper legs and trunk reach a straight line. Hold this position for 5 to 10 seconds. Repeat the exercise 3 to 5 times.

MUSCLES INVOLVED Gluteal, abdominals, lower back, hip flexors, quadriceps, and hamstrings

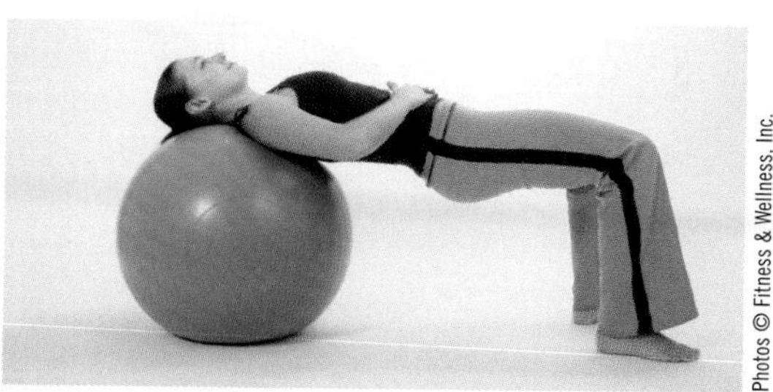

EXERCISE 41 **Reverse Supine Bridge**

ACTION Lie face up on the floor with the heels on the ball. Keeping the abdominal muscles tight, slowly lift the hips off the floor and squeeze the gluteal muscles until the body reaches a straight line. Hold the position for 5 to 10 seconds. Repeat the exercise 3 to 5 times.

MUSCLES INVOLVED Gluteal, abdominals, lower back, erector spinae, hip flexors, quadriceps, and hamstring

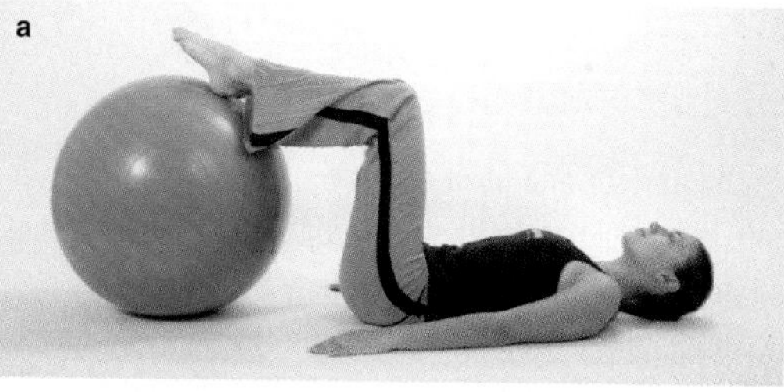
a

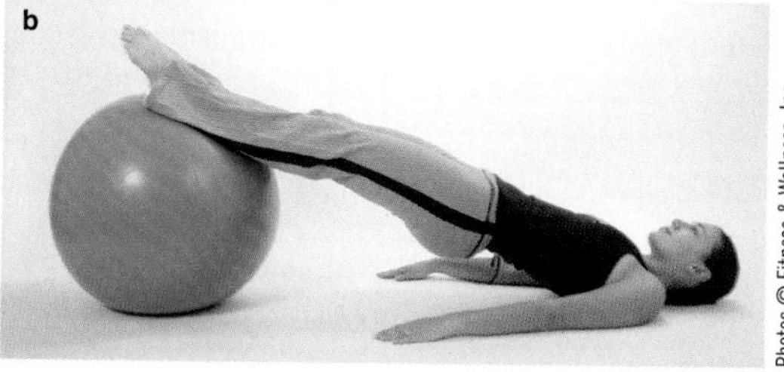
b

EXERCISE 42 **Push-Ups**

ACTION Place the front of your thighs (knees or feet—more difficult) over the ball with the body straight, the arms extended, and the hands under your shoulders. Now bend the elbows and lower the upper body as far as possible. Return to the original position. Repeat the exercise 10 times.

MUSCLES INVOLVED Triceps, chest, shoulder, abdominals, erector spinae, lower back, hip flexors, quadriceps, and hamstring

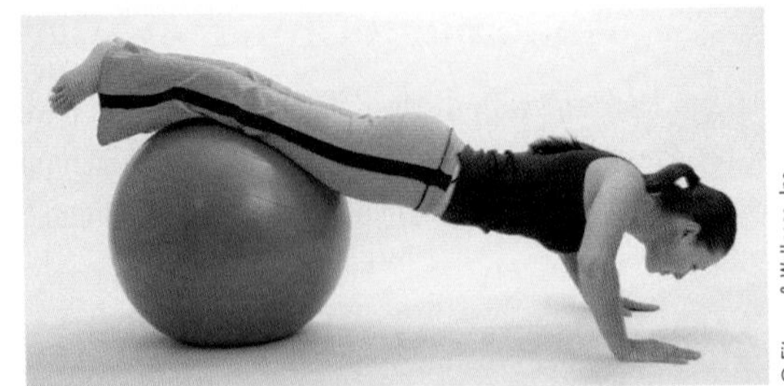

EXERCISE 43 **Back Extension**

ACTION Lie face down with the hips over the ball. Keep the legs straight with the toes on the floor and slightly separated (a). Keep your arms to the sides and extend the trunk until the body reaches a straight position (b). Repeat the exercise 10 times.

MUSCLES INVOLVED Erector spinae, abdominals, and lower back

a

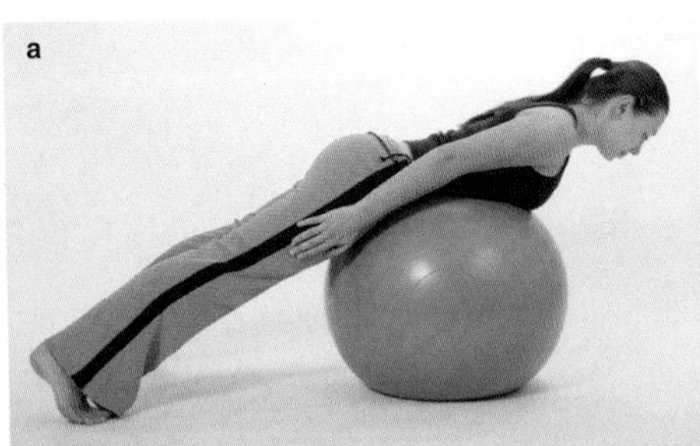

b

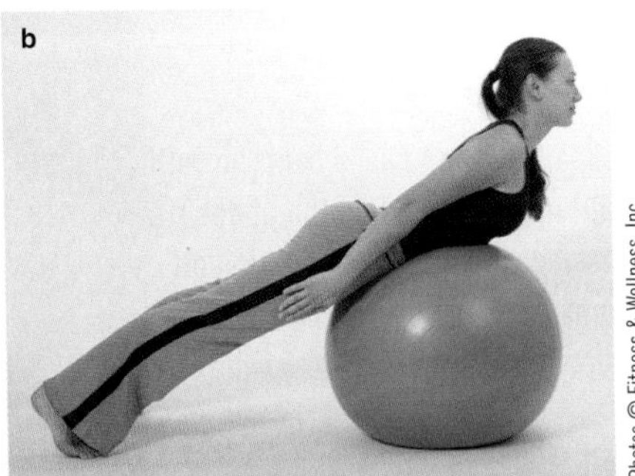

EXERCISE 44 **Wall Squat**

ACTION Stand upright and position the ball between your lower back and a wall. Place your feet slightly in front of you, about a foot apart (a). Lean into the ball and lower your body by bending the knees until the thighs are parallel to the ground (b) (to avoid excessive strain on the knees, it is not recommended that you go beyond this point). Return to the starting position. Repeat the exercise 10 to 20 times.

MUSCLES INVOLVED Quadriceps, hip flexors, hamstrings, abdominals, erector spinae, lower back, gastrocnemius, and soleus

a

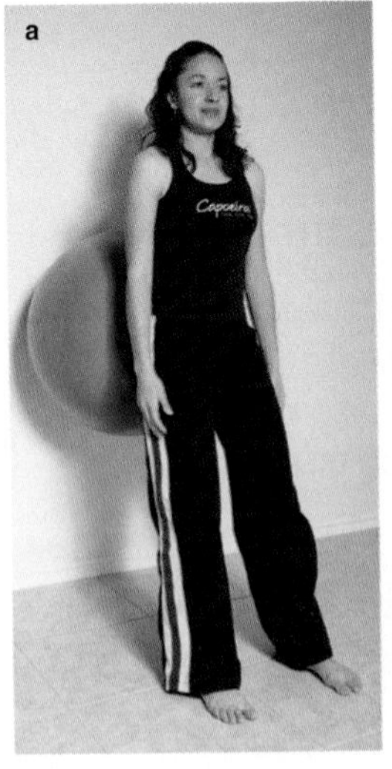

b

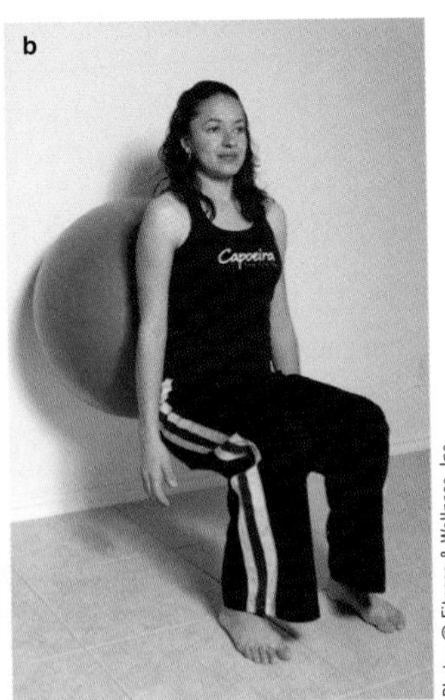

EXERCISE 45 **Jackknives**

ACTION Lie face down with the hips on the ball and walk forward with your hands until the thighs are over the ball. Keep the arms fully extended, hands on floor, and the body straight (a). Now, pull the ball forward with your legs by bending at the knees and raising your hips while keeping the abdominal muscles tight (b). Repeat the exercise 10 times.

MUSCLES INVOLVED Hip flexors, abdominals, erector spinae, lower back, quadriceps, hamstrings, chest, and shoulder

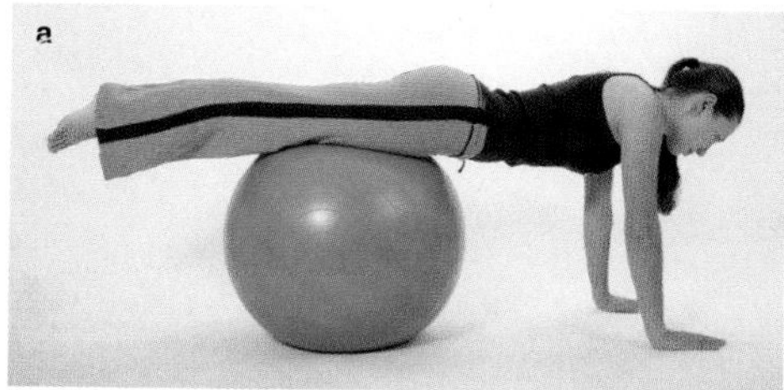
a

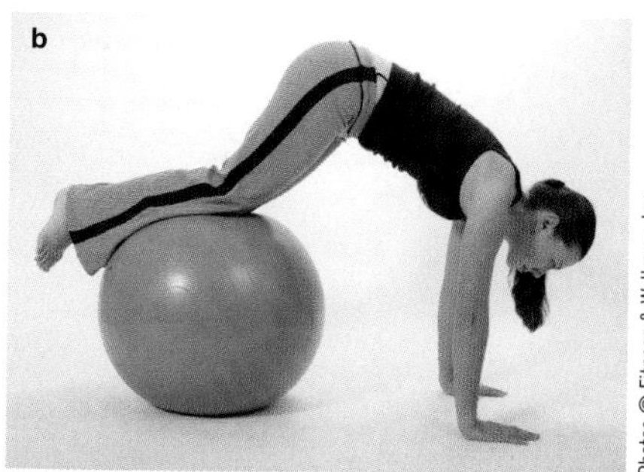
b

Photos © Fitness & Wellness, Inc.

EXERCISE 46 **Hamstring Roll**

ACTION Lie on your back with your knees bent and the heels on the ball. Raise your hips off the floor, while keeping the knees bent (a). Tighten the abdominal muscles and roll the ball out with your feet to extend the legs (b). Now roll the ball back into the original position. Repeat the exercise 10 times.

MUSCLES INVOLVED Hamstrings, abdominals, erector spinae, lower back, hip flexors, quadriceps, and chest

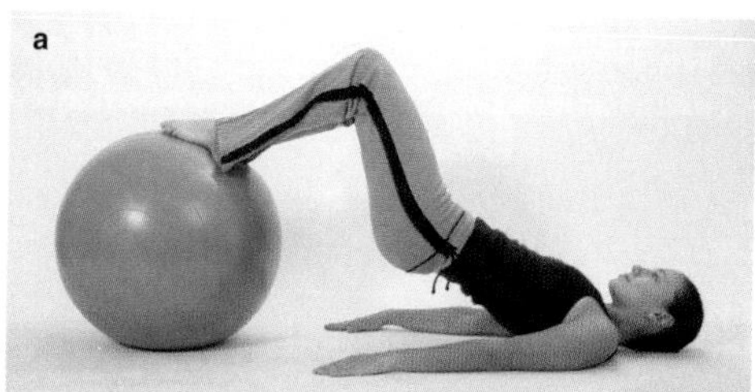
a

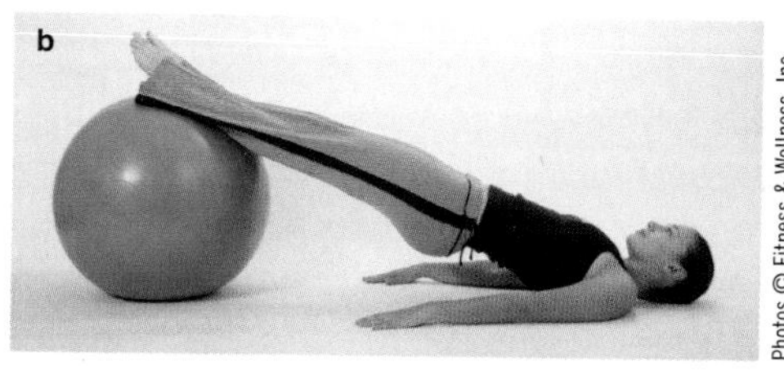
b

Photos © Fitness & Wellness, Inc.

Lab 7A: Muscular Strength and Endurance Assessment

Name ______________________ Date ____________ Grade ____________

Instructor ______________________ Course ____________ Section ____________

NECESSARY LAB EQUIPMENT

A Lafayette hand grip dynamometer model 78010 is recommended for the Hand Grip Test. A metronome, gymnasium bleachers, and a stopwatch are needed for the Muscular Endurance Test. A metronome is also needed for the Muscular Strength and Endurance Test.

OBJECTIVE

To determine muscular strength and/or endurance and the respective fitness classification.

LAB PREPARATION

Wear exercise clothing and avoid strenuous strength training 48 hours prior to this lab.

I. Hand Grip Strength Test

The instructions for the Hand Grip Strength Test are provided in Figure 7.2, page 264. Perform the test according to the instructions and look up your results in Table 7.1, page 264.

Hand used: ____________ Right ____________ Left

Reading: ____________ lbs.

Fitness category (see Figure 7.2, page 264): ______________________

II. Muscular Endurance Test

Conduct this test using the guidelines provided in Figure 7.3, page 266, and Table 7.2, page 266. Record your repetitions, fitness category, and points in the spaces provided below.

Exercise	Metronome Cadence	Repetitions	Fitness Category	Points
Bench jumps	none			
Modified dips — men only	56 bpm			
Modified push-ups — women only	56 bpm			
Bent-leg curl-ups	40 bpm			
Abdominal crunches	60 bpm			
			Total Points:	

Overall muscular endurance fitness category (see Figure 7.3, page 266): ______________________

III. Muscular Strength and Endurance Test

Perform the Muscular Strength and Endurance Test according to the procedure outlined in Figure 7.4, page 267. Record the results, fitness category, and points in the appropriate blanks provided below.

Body weight: ___________ lbs.

Lift	Percent of Body Weight (pounds)		Resistance	Repetitions
	Men	Women		
Lat pull-down	.70	.45		
Leg extension	.65	.50		
Bench press	.75	.45		
Bent-leg curl-up or abdominal crunch	NA*	NA*		
Leg curl	.32	.25		
Arm curl	.35	.18		

*Not applicable—no resistance required. Use test described in Figure 7.3, page 265.

IV. Muscular Strength and Endurance Goals

Indicate the muscular strength/endurance category that you would like to achieve by the end of the term:

Briefly state your feelings about your current strength level and indicate how you are planning to achieve your strength objective:

Lab 7B: Strength-Training Program

Name ______________________ Date __________ Grade __________

Instructor ______________________ Course __________ Section __________

NECESSARY LAB EQUIPMENT

Free weights, strength-training machines, or no equipment if the "Strength-Training Exercises without Weights" program is selected.

OBJECTIVE

To develop your personal strength-training exercise program.

LAB PREPARATION

Wear exercise clothing and prepare to participate in a sample strength-training exercise session. All of the strength-training exercises are illustrated on pages 286–303.

I. Stage of Change for Muscular Strength or Endurance

Using Figure 2.6 (page 66) and Table 2.3 (page 65), identify your current stage of change for participation in a muscular strength or muscular endurance program:

[ ]

II. Instructions

Select one of the two strength-training exercise programs. Perform all of the recommended exercises and, with the exception of the abdominal curl-up exercises, determine the resistance required to do approximately 10 repetitions maximum. For "Strength-Training Exercises without Weights," simply indicate the total number of repetitions performed. For the abdominal crunches or curl-up exercises, perform or build up to about 20 repetitions.

1. Strength-Training Exercises without Weights

Exercise	Repetitions
Step-up	
Rowing torso	
Push-up	
Abdominal curl-up or abdominal crunch	
Leg curl	
Modified dip	
Pull-up or arm curl	
Heel raise	
Leg abduction and adduction	
Reverse crunch	
Pelvic tilt	
Lateral bridge	
Prone bridge	

2. Strength-Training Exercises with Weights

Exercise	Repetitions	Resistance
Bench press, shoulder press, or chest press (select and circle one)		
Leg press or squat (select one)		
Abdominal curl-up or abdominal crunch (select one)		N/A
Rowing torso		
Arm curl or upright rowing (select one)		
Leg curl or seated leg curl (select one)		
Seated back or back extension (select one)		
Calf press		
Hip adduction		
Hip abduction		
Lat pull-down or bent-arm pullover (select one)		
Rotary torso		
Triceps extension or dip (select one)		
Leg extension		
Lateral trunk flexion		

3. Stability Ball Exercises

Exercise	Length of hold (if applicable)	Repetitions
The plank		
Abdominal crunches		
Supine bridge or reverse supine bridge		N/A
Push-ups		
Back extension		
Wall squats		
Jackknives		
Hamstring roll		
Lateral trunk flexion		

III. Your Personalized Strength-Training Program

Once you have performed the strength-training exercises in this lab, and depending on your personal preference (strength versus endurance), design your strength-training program selecting a minimum of 8 to 10 exercises. Indicate the number of sets, repetitions, and approximate resistance that you will use. Also state the days of the week, time, and facility that will be used for this program.

Strength-training days: M ☐ T ☐ W ☐ Th ☐ F ☐ Sa ☐ Su ☐ Time of day: ______ Facility: ______

	Exercise	Sets / Reps / Resistance		Exercise	Sets / Reps / Resistance
1.			9.		
2.			10.		
3.			11.		
4.			12.		
5.			13.		
6.			14.		
7.			15.		
8.			16.		

8

Muscular Flexibility

"Regrettably, most people neglect flexibility training, limiting freedom of movement, physical and mental relaxation, release of muscle tension and soreness, and injury prevention."
—*American Council on Exercise (ACE)*

OBJECTIVES

- Explain the importance of muscular flexibility to adequate fitness.
- Identify the factors that affect muscular flexibility.
- Explain the health-fitness benefits of stretching.
- Become familiar with a battery of tests to assess overall body flexibility (Modified Sit-and-Reach Test, Total Body Rotation Test, and Shoulder Rotation Test).
- Be able to interpret flexibility test results according to health-fitness and physical-fitness standards.
- Learn the principles that govern development of muscular flexibility.
- List some exercises that may cause injury.
- Become familiar with a program for preventing and rehabilitating low back pain.
- Create your own personal flexibility program.

REAL LIFE STORY | Gina's Experience

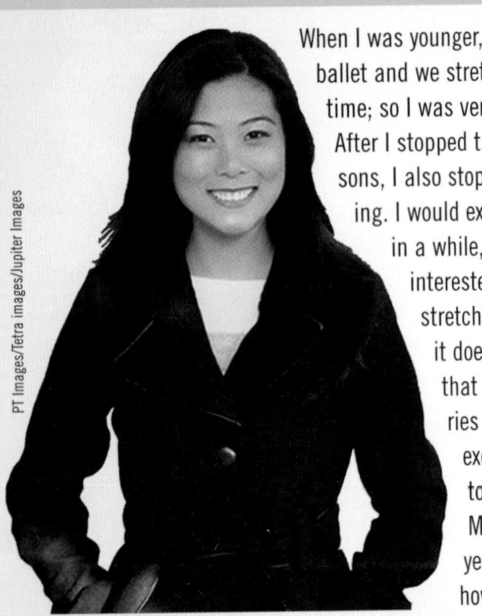
PT Images/Tetra images/Jupiter Images

When I was younger, I was in ballet and we stretched all the time; so I was very flexible. After I stopped taking lessons, I also stopped stretching. I would exercise once in a while, but I wasn't interested in stretching because it doesn't burn that many calories and I was exercising just to lose weight. My second year of college, however, I was really stressed out. I was working a ton of hours, going to classes, keeping up with homework, and on top of that, I had back pain that I had to deal with. Sometimes I would be sitting and trying to do the reading for class, but my back would hurt and I could feel my heart speeding and my breathing rate accelerating really fast because I couldn't stop worrying about all the things that were going on in my life. My back pain was sometimes so bad that I considered taking medication, but I didn't really want to do that. Then my friend got me to go to a yoga class with her. I didn't think I would like it, but I was shocked by how much it helped me. My back pain improved that same day and after each class my body felt great and I was calm and relaxed! In time, my flexibility improved, my back pain disappeared, my usual anxiety was gone, and I was sleeping great at night. I now attend yoga classes two to three times a week. If I can't get to a class, I do a few poses in my room or even some of my old ballet stretches. I am so happy to have found something that has helped my back and also really helps calm me down when I am stressed. For me, stretching is the painkiller and antianxiety medication that has no side effects!

Very few people who exercise take the time to stretch, and only a few of those who stretch do so properly. When joints are not regularly moved through their entire range of motion, muscles and ligaments shorten in time and flexibility decreases. Repetitive movement through regular or structured exercise, such as with running, cycling, or aerobics, without proper stretching also causes muscles and ligaments to tighten. Most fitness participants underestimate and overlook the contribution of good muscular flexibility to overall fitness.

Flexibility refers to the achievable range of motion at a joint or group of joints without causing injury. Some muscular and skeletal problems and injuries are thought to be related to a lack of flexibility. In daily life, we often have to make rapid or strenuous movements that we are not accustomed to making. Abruptly forcing a tight muscle beyond its achievable range of motion may lead to injury.

A decline in flexibility can cause poor posture and subsequent aches and pains that lead to limited and painful joint movement. Inordinate tightness is uncomfortable and debilitating. Approximately 80 percent of all low back problems in the United States stem from improper alignment of the vertebral column and pelvic girdle, a direct result of inflexible and weak muscles. Nationally, low back pain is the most common cause of work-related disability and the second most common neurological condition (disorder of the nervous system). This backache syndrome costs U.S. industries billions of dollars each year in lost productivity, health services, and worker compensation.

Benefits of Good Flexibility

Improving and maintaining good range of motion in the joints enhances the quality of life. Good flexibility promotes healthy muscles and joints. Improving elasticity of muscles and connective tissue around joints enables greater freedom of movement and the individual's ability to participate in many types of sports and recreational activities. Adequate flexibility also makes activities of daily living such as turning, lifting, and bending much easier to perform. A person must take care, however, not to overstretch joints. Too much flexibility leads to unstable and loose joints, which may increase injury rate, including joint **subluxation** and dislocation.

Taking part in a regular **stretching** program increases circulation to the muscle(s) being stretched, prevents low back and other spinal column problems, improves and maintains good postural alignment, promotes proper and graceful body movement, improves personal appearance and self-image, and helps development and maintenance of motor skills throughout life.

Flexibility exercises have been prescribed successfully to treat

Flexibility The achievable range of motion at a joint or group of joints without causing injury.

Subluxation Partial dislocation of a joint.

Stretching Moving the joints beyond the accustomed range of motion.

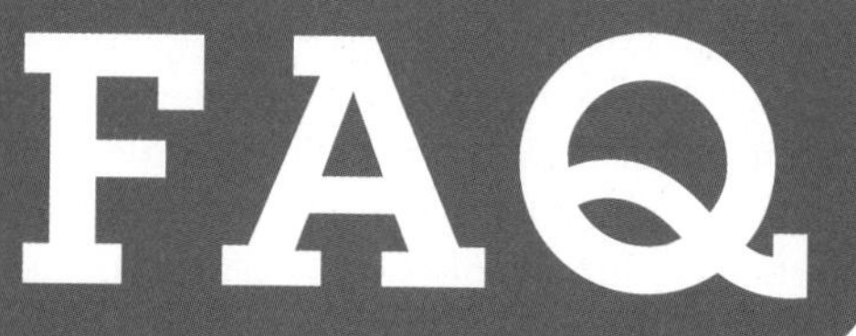

Will stretching before exercise prevent injuries?

The research on this subject is controversial. Some data suggest that intense stretching prior to physical activity modestly increases the risk for injuries and leads to a temporary decrease in muscle contraction velocity, strength, and power. Other studies, however, show no changes and even some improvement with intense pre-exercise stretching. The most important factor prior to vigorous exercise is to gradually increase the exercise intensity through mild calisthenics and light- to moderate-intensity aerobic exercise.

To prevent injuries while participating in activities that require flexibility, the American College of Sports Medicine recommends stretching following an appropriate warm-up phase. For activities that do not require much flexibility, you can perform the flexibility program following the aerobic and/or strength-training phase of your training.

Does strength training limit flexibility?

A popular myth is that individuals with large musculature, frequently referred to as "muscle-bound," are inflexible. Data show that strength-training exercises, when performed through a full range of motion, do not limit flexibility. With few exceptions, most strength-training exercises can be performed from complete extension to complete flexion. Body builders and gymnasts, who train heavily with weights, have better-than-average flexibility.

How much should stretching "hurt" to gain flexibility?

Proper stretching should not cause undue pain. Pain is an indication that you are stretching too aggressively. Stretching exercises should be performed to the point of "mild tension" or "limits of discomfort." It is best to decrease the degree of stretch to mild tension and hold the final position for a longer period of time (10 to 30 seconds).

MyProfile: Personal Flexibility Health

The following questions will allow you to analyze your knowledge and commitment to flexibility fitness. If you can't answer all of the questions, the chapter contents will provide the needed information.

I. Have you ever been able to touch your toes without bending your knees while sitting on the floor? ___ Yes ___ No
Can you elaborate on how your flexibility has changed the last few years? ___ Yes ___ No ________________
____
____

II. Do you feel that the most important factor affecting your degree of flexibility is your current level of physical activity? ___ Yes ___ No Can you expound on your answer? ____
____
____
____

III. What are your feelings about vigorous stretching prior to participating in athletic events that rely on force and power for peak performance? ________________
____
____

IV. Can you explain the role of aerobic, strength, and flexibility training on back health? ___ Yes ___ No __________
____
____

V. Have you ever experienced back pain episodes similar to Gina's? ___ Yes ___ No Can you explain the probable cause of Gina's pain? ___ Yes ___ No ____________
____
____

dysmenorrhea[1] (painful menstruation), general neuromuscular tension (stress), and knots (trigger points) in muscles and fascia. Regular stretching helps decrease the aches and pains caused by psychological stress and contributes to a decrease in anxiety, blood pressure, and breathing rate.[2] Stretching also helps relieve muscle cramps encountered at rest or during participation in exercise.

Mild stretching exercises in conjunction with calisthenics are helpful in warm-up routines to prepare for more vigorous aerobic or strength-training exercises and in cool-down routines following exercise to facilitate the return to a normal

Dysmenorrhea Painful menstruation.

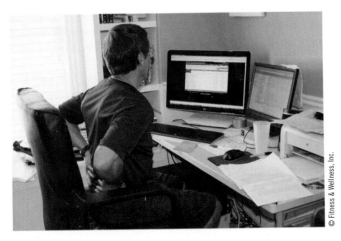

© Fitness & Wellness, Inc.

Excessive sitting and lack of physical activity lead to chronic back pain.

resting state. Fatigued muscles tend to contract to a shorter-than-average resting length, and stretching exercises help fatigued muscles reestablish their normal resting length.

Flexibility in Older Adults

Similar to muscular strength, good range of motion is critical in older life (see "Exercise and Aging" in Chapter 9). Muscle elasticity and bone strength tend to decline as people age. Because of decreased flexibility, older adults lose mobility and may be unable to perform simple daily tasks such as bending forward or turning. Many older adults cannot turn their head or rotate their trunk to look over their shoulder; rather, they must step around 90 to 180 degrees to see behind them. Adequate flexibility is also important in driving. Individuals who lose range of motion with age are unable to look over their shoulder to switch lanes or to parallel park, which increases the risk for automobile accidents.

Physical activity and exercise can be hampered severely by lack of good range of motion. Because of the pain during activity, older people who have tight hip flexors (muscles) cannot jog or walk very far. A vicious circle ensues, because the condition usually worsens with further inactivity. Lack of flexibility also may be a cause of falls and subsequent injury in older adults. A simple stretching program can alleviate or prevent this problem and help people return to an exercise program.

Factors Affecting Flexibility

The total range of motion around a joint is highly specific and varies from one joint to another (hip, trunk, shoulder, etc.), as well as from one individual to the next. Muscular flexibility relates primarily to genetic factors. A regular stretching program helps maintain range of motion around a joint and can help improve it as well. Joint structure (the shape of the bones), joint cartilage, ligaments, tendons, muscles, skin, tissue injury, and adipose tissue (fat) all influence range of motion around a joint. Body temperature, age, and gender also affect flexibility.

The range of motion around a given joint depends mostly on the structure of that joint. Greater range of motion, however, can be attained through plastic and elastic elongation. **Plastic elongation** is the permanent lengthening of soft tissue. Even though joint capsules, ligaments, and tendons are basically nonelastic, they can undergo plastic elongation. This permanent lengthening, accompanied by increased range of motion, is best attained through proper stretching exercises.

Elastic elongation is the temporary lengthening of soft tissue. Muscle tissue has elastic properties and responds to stretching exercises by undergoing elastic or temporary lengthening. Elastic elongation increases extensibility, the ability to stretch the muscles.

Changes in muscle temperature can increase or decrease flexibility. Individuals who warm up properly have better flexibility than people who do not. Cool temperatures have the opposite effect, impeding range of motion. Because of the effects of temperature on muscular flexibility, many people prefer to do their stretching exercises after the aerobic phase of their workout. Aerobic activities raise body temperature, facilitating elastic elongation.

Another factor that influences flexibility is the amount of adipose (fat) tissue in and around joints and muscle tissue. Excess adipose tissue increases resistance to movement, and the added bulk also hampers joint mobility because of the contact between body surfaces.

On average, women have better flexibility than men, and they seem to retain this advantage throughout life. Aging decreases the extensibility of soft tissue, though, resulting in less flexibility in both sexes.

The most significant contributor to lower flexibility is sedentary living. With less physical activity, muscles lose their elasticity and tendons and ligaments tighten and shorten. Inactivity also tends to be accompanied by an increase in adipose tissue, which further decreases the range of motion around a joint. Finally, injury to muscle tissue and tight skin from excessive scar tissue negatively affect range of motion.

Assessment of Flexibility

Because of the lack of practical flexibility tests, most health and fitness centers rely strictly on the Sit-and-Reach Test as an indicator of flexibility. This test measures flexibility of the hamstring muscles (back of the thigh) and, to a lesser extent, the lower back muscles.

Flexibility is joint specific. This means that a lot of flexibility in one joint does not necessarily indicate that other joints are just as flexible. Therefore, the Total Body Rotation Test and the Shoulder Rotation Test—indicators of the ability to perform everyday movements such as reaching, bending, and turning—are included to determine your flexibility profile.

The Sit-and-Reach Test has been modified from the traditional test to take length of arms and legs into consideration

FIGURE 8.1 Procedure for the Modified Sit-and-Reach Test.

To perform this test, you will need the Acuflex I* Sit-and-Reach Flexibility Tester, or you may simply place a yardstick on top of a box 12" high.

1. Warm up properly before the first trial.
2. Remove your shoes for the test. Sit on the floor with the hips, back, and head against a wall, the legs fully extended, and the bottom of the feet against the Acuflex I or sit-and-reach box.
3. Place the hands one on top of the other and reach forward as far as possible without letting the head and back come off the wall (the shoulders may be rounded as much as possible, but neither the head nor the back should come off the wall at this time). The technician then can slide the reach indicator on the Acuflex I (or yardstick) along the top of the box until the end of the indicator touches the participant's fingers. The indicator then must be held firmly in place throughout the rest of the test.

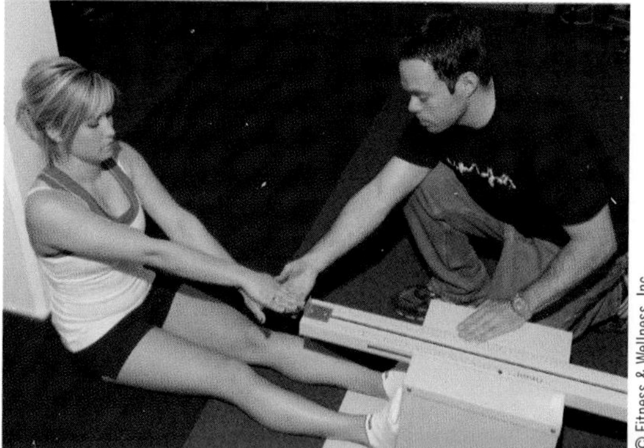

© Fitness & Wellness, Inc.

Determining the starting position for the Modified Sit-and-Reach Test.

4. Now your head and back can come off the wall. Gradually reach forward three times, the third time stretching forward as far as possible on the indicator (or yardstick) and holding the final position for at least 2 seconds. Be sure that during the test you keep the backs of the knees flat against the floor.
5. Record the final number of inches reached to the nearest ½".

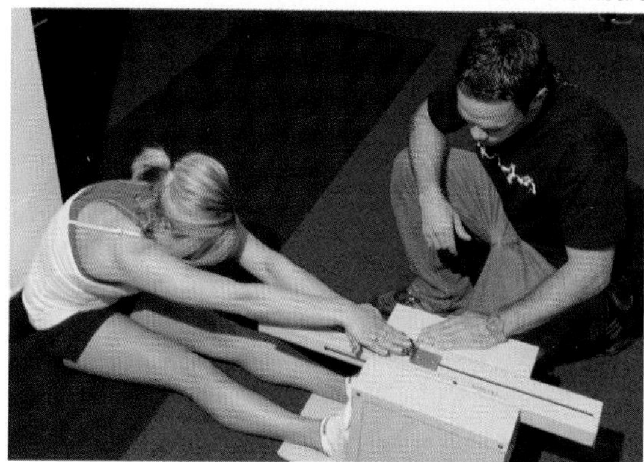

© Fitness & Wellness, Inc.

Modified Sit-and-Reach Test.

You are allowed two trials, and an average of the two scores is used as the final test score. The respective percentile ranks and fitness categories for this test are given in Tables 8.1 and 8.4.

*The Acuflex I Flexibility Tester for the Modified Sit-and-Reach Test can be obtained from Figure Finder Collection, Novel Products, P. O. Box 408, Rockton, IL 61072-0408. Phone: 800-323-5143, Fax 815-624-4866.

in determining the score (Figure 8.1). In the original Sit-and-Reach Test, the 15-inch mark of the yardstick used to measure flexibility is always set at the edge of the box where the feet are placed. This does not take into consideration an individual with long arms, short legs, or both or one with short arms, long legs, or both.[3] All other factors being equal, an individual with longer arms, shorter legs, or both receives a better rating because of the structural advantage.

The procedures and norms for the flexibility tests are described in Figures 8.1, 8.2, and 8.3 and Tables 8.1, 8.2, and 8.3. The flexibility test results in these three tables are provided in both inches and centimeters (cm). Be sure to use the proper column to read your percentile score based on your test results. For the flexibility profile, you should take all three tests. You will be able to assess your flexibility profile in Lab 8A. Because of the specificity of flexibility, pinpointing an "ideal" level of flexibility is difficult. Nevertheless, flexibility is important to health and fitness and independent living, so an assessment gives an indication of your current level of flexibility.

Interpreting Flexibility Test Results

After obtaining your scores and fitness ratings for each test, you can determine the fitness category for each flexibility test using the guidelines given in Table 8.4. You should also look up the number of points assigned for each fitness category in this table. The overall flexibility fitness category is obtained by totaling the number of points from all three tests and using the ratings given in Table 8.5. Record your results in Lab 8A.

Evaluating Body Posture Good posture enhances personal appearance, self-image, and confidence; improves balance and endurance; protects against misalignment-related pains and aches; prevents falls; and enhances your overall sense of well-being.[4] The relationships among different body parts are the essence of posture.

Poor posture is a risk factor for musculoskeletal problems of the neck, shoulders, and lower back. Incorrect posture also strains hips and knees. Faulty posture and weak and inelastic muscles are also leading causes of chronic low back problems. Evaluating these areas is crucial to preventing and rehabilitating low back pain. The results of these tests can be used to prescribe corrective exercises.

Adequate body mechanics also aid in reducing chronic low back pain. Proper body mechanics means using correct positions in

Plastic elongation Permanent lengthening of soft tissue.

Elastic elongation Temporary lengthening of soft tissue.

FIGURE 8.2 Procedure for the Total Body Rotation Test.

An Acuflex II* Total Body Rotation Flexibility Tester or a measuring scale with a sliding panel is needed to administer this test. The Acuflex II or scale is placed on the wall at shoulder height and should be adjustable to accommodate individual differences in height. If you need to build your own scale, use two measuring tapes and glue them above and below the sliding panel centered at the 15" mark. Each tape should be at least 30" long. If no sliding panel is available, simply tape the measuring tapes onto a wall oriented in opposite directions as shown below. A line also must be drawn on the floor and centered with the 15" mark.

1. Warm up properly before beginning this test.
2. Stand with one side toward the wall, an arm's length away from the wall, with the feet straight ahead, slightly separated, and the toes touching the center line drawn on the floor. Hold out the arm away from the wall horizontally from the body, making a fist with the hand. The Acuflex II measuring scale (or tapes) should be shoulder height at this time.
3. Rotate the trunk, the extended arm going backward (always maintaining a horizontal plane) and making contact with the panel, gradually sliding it forward as far as possible. If no panel is available, slide the fist alongside the tapes as far as possible. Hold the final position at least 2 seconds. Position the hand with the little finger side forward during the entire sliding movement. **Proper hand position is crucial. Many people attempt to open the hand, or push with extended fingers, or slide the panel with the knuckles—none of which is acceptable.** During the test the knees can be bent slightly, but **the feet cannot be moved or rotated**—they must point forward. The body must be kept as straight (vertical) as possible.
4. Conduct the test on either the right or the left side of the body. Perform two trials on the selected side. Record the farthest point reached, measured to the nearest half inch and held for at least 2 seconds. Use the average of the two trials as the final test score. Refer to Tables 8.2 and 8.4 to determine the percentile rank and flexibility fitness category for this test.

*The Acuflex II Flexibility Tester for the Total Body Rotation Test can be obtained from Figure Finder Collection, Novel Products, P.O. Box 408, Rockton, IL 61072-0408. Phone: 800-323-5143, Fax 815-624-4866.

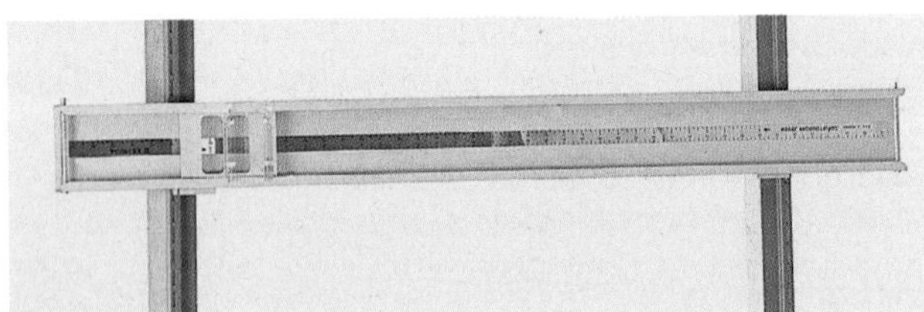
Acuflex II measuring device for the Total Body Rotation Test.

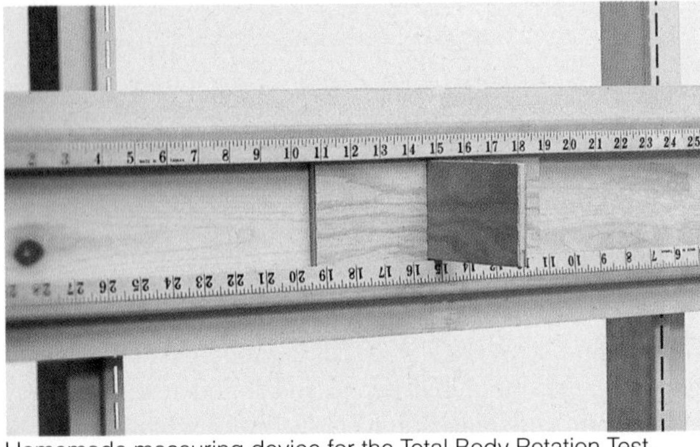
Homemade measuring device for the Total Body Rotation Test.

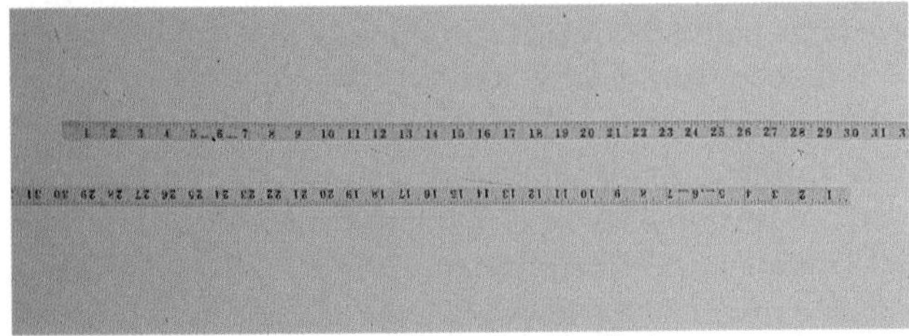
Measuring tapes for the Total Body Rotation Test.

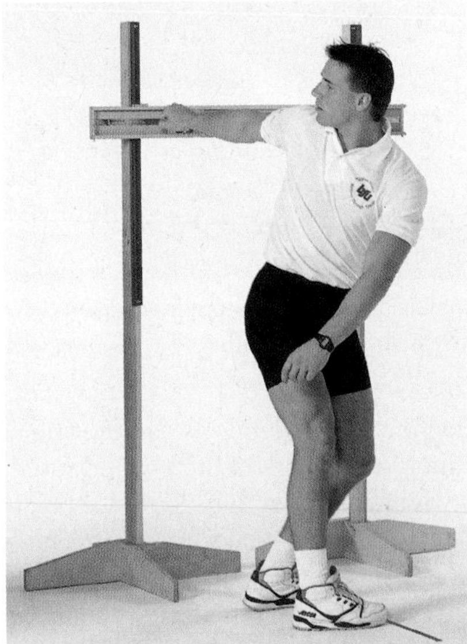
Total Body Rotation Test.

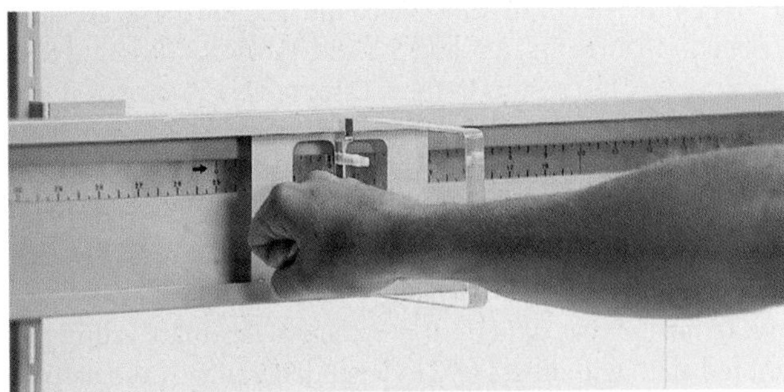
Proper hand position for the Total Body Rotation Test.

FIGURE 8.3 Procedure for the Shoulder Rotation Test.

This test can be done using the Acuflex III* Flexibility Tester, which consists of a shoulder caliper and a measuring device for shoulder rotation. If this equipment is unavailable, you can construct your own device quite easily. The caliper can be built with three regular yardsticks. Nail and glue two of the yardsticks at one end at a 90° angle, and use the third one as the sliding end of the caliper. Construct the rotation device by placing a 60" measuring tape on an aluminum or wood stick, starting at about 6" or 7" from the end of the stick.

1. Warm up before the test.
2. Using the shoulder caliper, measure the biacromial width to the nearest ¼" (use the top scale on the Acuflex III). Measure biacromial width between the lateral edges of the acromion processes of the shoulders.
3. Place the Acuflex III or homemade device behind the back and use a reverse grip (thumbs out) to hold on to the device. Place the index finger of the right hand next to the zero point of the scale or tape (lower scale on the Acuflex III) and hold it firmly in place throughout the test. Place the left hand on the other end of the measuring device wherever comfortable.
4. Standing straight up and extending both arms to full length, with elbows locked, slowly bring the measuring device over the head until it reaches about forehead level. For subsequent trials, depending on the resistance encountered when rotating the shoulders, move the left grip in ½" to 1" at a time, and repeat the task until you no longer can rotate the shoulders without undue strain or starting to bend the elbows. Always keep the right-hand grip against the zero point of the scale. Measure the last successful trial to the nearest ½". Take this measurement at the inner edge of the left hand on the side of the little finger.
5. Determine the final score for this test by subtracting the biacromial width from the best score (shortest distance) between both hands on the rotation test. For example, if the best score is 35" and the biacromial width is 15", the final score is 20" (35 − 15 = 20). Using Tables 8.3 and 8.4, determine the percentile rank and flexibility fitness category for this test.

*The Acuflex III Flexibility Tester for the Shoulder Rotation Test can be obtained from Figure Finder Collection, Novel Products, Inc., P. O. Box 408, Rockton, IL 61072-0408. Phone: (800) 323-5143, Fax 815-624-4866.

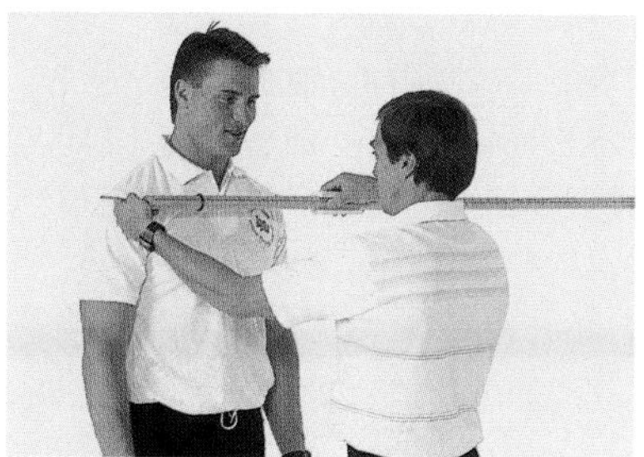
Measuring biacromial width.

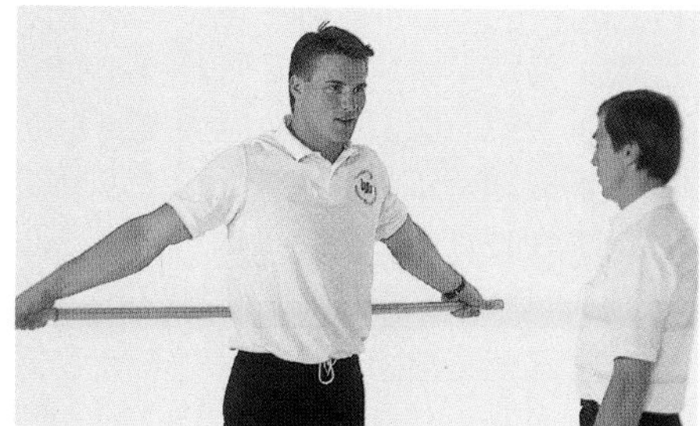
Starting position for the shoulder rotation test (note the reverse grip used for this test).

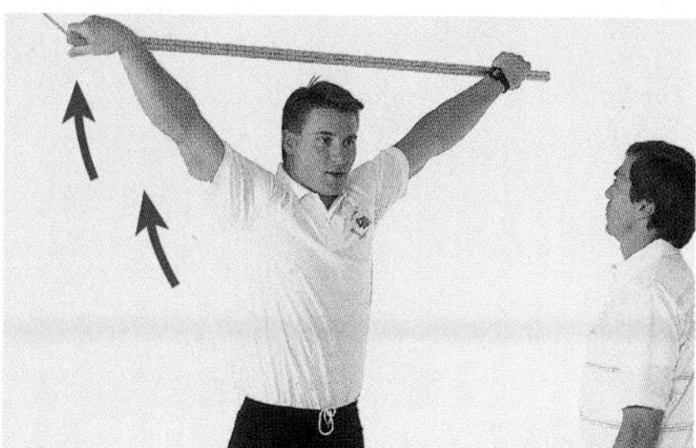
Shoulder rotation test.

TABLE 8.1 Percentile Ranks for the Modified Sit-and-Reach Test

Percentile Rank	Men ≤18 in	Men ≤18 cm	Men 19–35 in	Men 19–35 cm	Men 36–49 in	Men 36–49 cm	Men ≥50 in	Men ≥50 cm	Women ≤18 in	Women ≤18 cm	Women 19–35 in	Women 19–35 cm	Women 36–49 in	Women 36–49 cm	Women ≥50 in	Women ≥50 cm
99	20.8	52.8	20.1	51.1	18.9	48.0	16.2	41.1	22.6	57.4	21.0	53.3	19.8	50.3	17.2	43.7
95	19.6	49.8	18.9	48.0	18.2	46.2	15.8	40.1	19.5	49.5	19.3	49.0	19.2	48.8	15.7	39.9
90	18.2	46.2	17.2	43.7	16.1	40.9	15.0	38.1	18.7	47.5	17.9	45.5	17.4	44.2	15.0	38.1
80	17.8	45.2	17.0	43.2	14.6	37.1	13.3	33.8	17.8	45.2	16.7	42.4	16.2	41.1	14.2	36.1
70	16.0	40.6	15.8	40.1	13.9	35.3	12.3	31.2	16.5	41.9	16.2	41.1	15.2	38.6	13.6	34.5
60	15.2	38.6	15.0	38.1	13.4	34.0	11.5	29.2	16.0	40.6	15.8	40.1	14.5	36.8	12.3	31.2
50	14.5	36.8	14.4	36.6	12.6	32.0	10.2	25.9	15.2	38.6	14.8	37.6	13.5	34.3	11.1	28.2
40	14.0	35.6	13.5	34.3	11.6	29.5	9.7	24.6	14.5	36.8	14.5	36.8	12.8	32.5	10.1	25.7
30	13.4	34.0	13.0	33.0	10.8	27.4	9.3	23.6	13.7	34.8	13.7	34.8	12.2	31.0	9.2	23.4
20	11.8	30.0	11.6	29.5	9.9	25.1	8.8	22.4	12.6	32.0	12.6	32.0	11.0	27.9	8.3	21.1
10	9.5	24.1	9.2	23.4	8.3	21.1	7.8	19.8	11.4	29.0	10.1	25.7	9.7	24.6	7.5	19.0
05	8.4	21.3	7.9	20.1	7.0	17.8	7.2	18.3	9.4	23.9	8.1	20.6	8.5	21.6	3.7	9.4
01	7.2	18.3	7.0	17.8	5.1	13.0	4.0	10.2	6.5	16.5	2.6	6.6	2.0	5.1	1.5	3.8

High physical fitness standard / Health fitness standard

TABLE 8.2 Percentile Ranks for the Total Body Rotation Test

		Age Category—Left Rotation								Age Category—Right Rotation							
	Percentile Rank	≤18		19–35		36–49		≥50		≤18		19–35		36–49		≥50	
		in	cm	in	cm	in	cm	in	cm	in	cm	in	cm	in	cm	in	cm
	99	29.1	73.9	28.0	71.1	26.6	67.6	21.0	53.3	28.2	71.6	27.8	70.6	25.2	64.0	22.2	56.4
	95	26.6	67.6	24.8	63.0	24.5	62.2	20.0	50.8	25.5	64.8	25.6	65.0	23.8	60.5	20.7	52.6
	90	25.0	63.5	23.6	59.9	23.0	58.4	17.7	45.0	24.3	61.7	24.1	61.2	22.5	57.1	19.3	49.0
	80	22.0	55.9	22.0	55.9	21.2	53.8	15.5	39.4	22.7	57.7	22.3	56.6	21.0	53.3	16.3	41.4
	70	20.9	53.1	20.3	51.6	20.4	51.8	14.7	37.3	21.3	54.1	20.7	52.6	18.7	47.5	15.7	39.9
	60	19.9	50.5	19.3	49.0	18.7	47.5	13.9	35.3	19.8	50.3	19.0	48.3	17.3	43.9	14.7	37.3
Men	50	18.6	47.2	18.0	45.7	16.7	42.4	12.7	32.3	19.0	48.3	17.2	43.7	16.3	41.4	12.3	31.2
	40	17.0	43.2	16.8	42.7	15.3	38.9	11.7	29.7	17.3	43.9	16.3	41.4	14.7	37.3	11.5	29.2
	30	14.9	37.8	15.0	38.1	14.8	37.6	10.3	26.2	15.1	38.4	15.0	38.1	13.3	33.8	10.7	27.2
	20	13.8	35.1	13.3	33.8	13.7	34.8	9.5	24.1	12.9	32.8	13.3	33.8	11.2	28.4	8.7	22.1
	10	10.8	27.4	10.5	26.7	10.8	27.4	4.3	10.9	10.8	27.4	11.3	28.7	8.0	20.3	2.7	6.9
	05	8.5	21.6	8.9	22.6	8.8	22.4	0.3	0.8	8.1	20.6	8.3	21.1	5.5	14.0	0.3	0.8
	01	3.4	8.6	1.7	4.3	5.1	13.0	0.0	0.0	6.6	16.8	2.9	7.4	2.0	5.1	0.0	0.0
	99	29.3	74.4	28.6	72.6	27.1	68.8	23.0	58.4	29.6	75.2	29.4	74.7	27.1	68.8	21.7	55.1
	95	26.8	68.1	24.8	63.0	25.3	64.3	21.4	54.4	27.6	70.1	25.3	64.3	25.9	65.8	19.7	50.0
	90	25.5	64.8	23.0	58.4	23.4	59.4	20.5	52.1	25.8	65.5	23.0	58.4	21.3	54.1	19.0	48.3
	80	23.8	60.5	21.5	54.6	20.2	51.3	19.1	48.5	23.7	60.2	20.8	52.8	19.6	49.8	17.9	45.5
	70	21.8	55.4	20.5	52.1	18.6	47.2	17.3	43.9	22.0	55.9	19.3	49.0	17.3	43.9	16.8	42.7
	60	20.5	52.1	19.3	49.0	17.7	45.0	16.0	40.6	20.8	52.8	18.0	45.7	16.5	41.9	15.6	39.6
Women	50	19.5	49.5	18.0	45.7	16.4	41.7	14.8	37.6	19.5	49.5	17.3	43.9	14.6	37.1	14.0	35.6
	40	18.5	47.0	17.2	43.7	14.8	37.6	13.7	34.8	18.3	46.5	16.0	40.6	13.1	33.3	12.8	32.5
	30	17.1	43.4	15.7	39.9	13.6	34.5	10.0	25.4	16.3	41.4	15.2	38.6	11.7	29.7	8.5	21.6
	20	16.0	40.6	15.2	38.6	11.6	29.5	6.3	16.0	14.5	36.8	14.0	35.6	9.8	24.9	3.9	9.9
	10	12.8	32.5	13.6	34.5	8.5	21.6	3.0	7.6	12.4	31.5	11.1	28.2	6.1	15.5	2.2	5.6
	05	11.1	28.2	7.3	18.5	6.8	17.3	0.7	1.8	10.2	25.9	8.8	22.4	4.0	10.2	1.1	2.8
	01	8.9	22.6	5.3	13.5	4.3	10.9	0.0	0.0	8.9	22.6	3.2	8.1	2.8	7.1	0.0	0.0

High physical fitness standard | Health fitness standard

all the activities of daily life, including sleeping, sitting, standing, walking, driving, working, and exercising. Because of the high incidence of low back pain, illustrations of proper body mechanics and a series of corrective and preventive exercises are shown in Figure 8.7 on page 324.

Most people are unaware of how faulty their posture is until they see themselves in a photograph. This can be quite a shock and is often enough to motivate change.

Besides engaging in the recommended exercises to elicit changes in postural alignment, people need to be continually aware of the corrections they are trying to make. As posture improves, you frequently become motivated to change other aspects, such as improving muscular strength and flexibility and decreasing body fat.

Posture tests are used to detect deviations from normal body alignment and prescribe corrective exercises or procedures to improve alignment. These analyses are best conducted early in life, because certain postural deviations are more difficult to correct in an older person. If deviations are allowed to go uncorrected, they usually become more serious as the person grows older. Consequently, corrective exercises or other medical procedures should be used to stop or slow down postural degeneration.

Proper body alignment has been difficult to evaluate because most experts still don't know exactly what constitutes good posture. To objectively analyze a person's posture, an observer either must be adequately trained or must have some guidelines to identify abnormalities and assign ratings according to the amount of deviation from "normal" posture.

A posture rating chart, such as that in Lab 8B, provides simple guidelines for evaluating posture. Assuming the drawings in the left column to be proper alignment and the drawings in the right column to be extreme deviations from normal, an observer is able to rate each body segment on a scale from 1 to 5.

TABLE 8.3 Percentile Ranks for the Shoulder Rotation Test

Percentile Rank	Age Category—Men ≤18 in	≤18 cm	19–35 in	19–35 cm	36–49 in	36–49 cm	≥50 in	≥50 cm
99	2.2	5.6	−1.0	−2.5	18.1	46.0	21.5	54.6
95	15.2	38.6	10.4	26.4	20.4	51.8	27.0	68.6
90	18.5	47.0	15.5	39.4	20.8	52.8	27.9	70.9
80	20.7	52.6	18.4	46.7	23.3	59.2	28.5	72.4
70	23.0	58.4	20.5	52.1	24.7	62.7	29.4	74.7
60	24.2	61.5	22.9	58.2	26.6	67.6	29.9	75.9
50	25.4	64.5	24.4	62.0	28.0	71.1	30.5	77.5
40	26.3	66.8	25.7	65.3	30.0	76.2	31.0	78.7
30	28.2	71.6	27.3	69.3	31.9	81.0	31.7	80.5
20	30.0	76.2	30.1	76.5	33.3	84.6	33.1	84.1
10	33.5	85.1	31.8	80.8	36.1	91.7	37.2	94.5
05	34.7	88.1	33.5	85.1	37.8	96.0	38.7	98.3
01	40.8	103.6	42.6	108.2	43.0	109.2	44.1	112.0

Percentile Rank	Age Category—Women ≤18 in	≤18 cm	19–35 in	19–35 cm	36–49 in	36–49 cm	≥50 in	≥50 cm
99	2.6	6.6	−2.4	−6.1	11.5	29.2	13.1	33.3
95	8.0	20.3	6.2	15.7	15.4	39.1	16.5	41.9
90	10.7	27.2	9.7	24.6	16.8	42.7	20.9	53.1
80	14.5	36.8	14.5	36.8	19.2	48.8	22.5	57.1
70	16.1	40.9	17.2	43.7	21.5	54.6	24.3	61.7
60	19.2	48.8	18.7	47.5	23.1	58.7	25.1	63.8
50	21.0	53.3	20.0	50.8	23.5	59.7	26.2	66.5
40	22.2	56.4	21.4	54.4	24.4	62.0	28.1	71.4
30	23.2	58.9	24.0	61.0	25.9	65.8	29.9	75.9
20	25.0	63.5	25.9	65.8	29.8	75.7	31.5	80.0
10	27.2	69.1	29.1	73.9	31.1	79.0	33.1	84.1
05	28.0	71.1	31.3	79.5	33.4	84.8	34.1	86.6
01	32.5	82.5	37.1	94.2	34.9	88.6	35.4	89.9

High physical fitness standard | Health fitness standard

TABLE 8.4 Flexibility Fitness Categories According to Percentile Ranks

Percentile Rank	Fitness Category	Points
≥90	Excellent	5
70–80	Good	4
50–60	Average	3
30–40	Fair	2
≤20	Poor	1

TABLE 8.5 Overall Flexibility Fitness Category

Total Points	Flexibility Category
≥13	Excellent
10–12	Good
7–9	Average
4–6	Fair
≤3	Poor

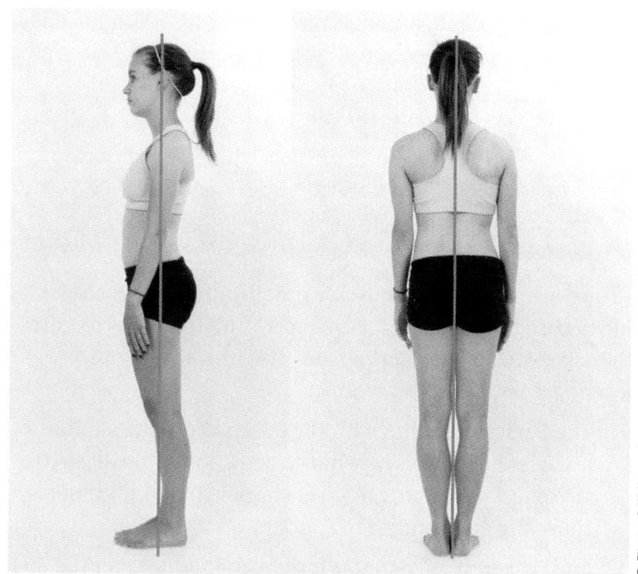

Photographic technique used for posture evaluation.

TABLE 8.6 Posture Evaluation Standards

Total Points	Category
≥45	Excellent
40–44	Good
30–39	Average
20–29	Fair
≤19	Poor

Postural analysis can be done with more precision with the aid of a plumb line and a camera. Two pictures are taken: a lateral and a posterior view. For the lateral view, the plumb line (or a straight line drawn on the photo) is used as a reference to divide the body into front and back halves (try to center the line with the hip joint and the shoulder). For the posterior view, the line divides the body into right and left halves. The two pictures can then be compared to the rating chart given in Lab 8B.

The photographic procedure allows for a better comparison of the different body segment alignments and a more objective analysis. If no plumb line and camera are available, an evaluator can perform a visual assessment of the different body segments.

A final posture score is determined according to the sum of the ratings obtained for each body segment. Table 8.6 contains the various categories as determined by the final posture score.

Principles of Muscular Flexibility Prescription

Even though genetics play a crucial role in body flexibility, the range of joint mobility can be increased and maintained through a regular stretching program. Because range of motion is highly specific to each body part (ankle, trunk, shoulder, etc.), a comprehensive stretching program should include all body parts and follow the basic guidelines for development of flexibility.

The overload and specificity of training principles (discussed in conjunction with strength development in Chapter 7) apply to the development of muscular flexibility. To increase the total range of motion of a joint, the specific muscles surrounding that joint have to be stretched progressively beyond their accustomed length. The principles of mode, intensity, repetitions, and frequency of exercise are also be applied to flexibility programs.

Modes of Training There are several modes of stretching exercises and some modes are safer and more effective in terms of helping to increase flexibility:

1. Static (slow-sustained stretching)
2. Passive stretching
3. Ballistic stretching
4. Dynamic stretching
5. Controlled ballistic stretching
6. Proprioceptive neuromuscular facilitation (PNF) stretching

Static Stretching With **static stretching** or **slow-sustained stretching**, muscles are lengthened gradually through a joint's complete range of motion and the final position is held for a few seconds. A slow-sustained stretch causes the muscles to relax and thereby achieve greater length. This type of stretch causes little pain and has a low risk for injury. In flexibility-development programs, slow-sustained stretching exercises are the most frequently used and recommended.

Passive Stretching Although similar to static stretching, in **passive stretching**, the muscles are relaxed (i.e., they are in a passive state), and an external force, provided by another person or apparatus, is applied to increase the range of motion.

Ballistic Stretching **Ballistic stretching** requires the impetus of a moving body or body part to force a joint or group of joints beyond the normal range of motion. This type of stretching requires a fast and repetitive bouncing motion to achieve a greater degree of stretch. An example would be repeatedly bouncing down and up to touch the toes. Ballistic stretching is the least recommended form of stretching. Fitness professionals feel that it causes muscle soreness and increases the risk of injuries to muscles and nerves. Limited data, however, are available to corroborate such effects. This form of stretching should never be performed without a previous mild aerobic warm-up.

Dynamic Stretching Speed of movement, momentum, and active muscular effort are used in **dynamic stretching** to increase the range of motion around a joint or group of joints. Unlike ballistic stretching, it does not require bouncing motions. Exaggerating a kicking action, walking lunges, and arm circles are all examples of dynamic stretching. Research indicates that dynamic stretches are preferable to static stretches before athletic competition, because dynamic stretching does not seem to have a negative effect on the athlete's strength and power. Dynamic stretching is beneficial for athletes such as gymnasts, dancers, figure skaters, divers, and hurdlers, whose sports activities require ballistic actions.

Precautions must be taken to not overstretch ligaments with ballistic and dynamic stretching. Ligaments undergo plastic or permanent elongation. If the stretching force cannot be controlled—as often occurs with fast, jerky movements—ligaments can easily be overstretched. This, in turn, leads to excessively loose joints, increasing the risk for injuries.

Controlled Ballistic Stretching **Controlled ballistic stretching**—that is, exercises that are performed through slow, gentle, and controlled ballistic movements, instead of jerky, rapid, and bouncy movements—is quite effective in developing flexibility. Properly performed, this type of stretching can be done safely by most individuals.

Proprioceptive Neuromuscular Facilitation

Proprioceptive neuromuscular facilitation (PNF stretching is based on a "contract-and-relax" method and requires the assistance of another person. The procedure is as follows:

1. The person assisting with the exercise provides initial force by pushing slowly in the direction of the desired stretch (assisted stretch). This initial stretch does not cover the entire range of motion.
2. The person being stretched then applies force in the opposite direction of the stretch, against the assistant, who tries to hold the initial degree of stretch as close as pos-

sible. This results in an isometric contraction at the angle of the stretch. The force of the isometric contraction can be anywhere from 20 to 75 percent of the person's maximum contraction.

3. After 3 to 6 seconds of isometric contraction, the person being stretched relaxes the target muscle or muscles completely. The assistant then increases the degree of stretch slowly to a greater angle, and for the PNF technique, the stretch is held for 10 to 30 seconds.
4. If a greater degree of stretch is achievable, the isometric contraction is repeated for another 3 or 6 seconds, after which the degree of stretch is slowly increased again and held for 10 to 30 seconds.

If a progressive degree of stretch is used, steps 1 through 4 can be repeated up to five times. Each isometric contraction is held for 3 to 6 seconds. The progressive stretches are held for about 10 seconds—until the last trial, when the final stretched position is held for up to 30 seconds.

Theoretically, with the PNF technique, the isometric contraction helps relax the muscle being stretched, which results in lengthening of the muscle. Some research indicates that PNF stretching yields greater gains in range of motion than the other forms of stretching.[5] Another benefit of PNF is an increase in strength of the muscle(s) being stretched. Research has shown increases in absolute strength and muscular endurance with PNF stretching. These increases are attributed to the isometric contractions performed during PNF. Disadvantages of PNF are (1) more pain, (2) the need for a second person to assist, and (3) the need for more time to conduct each session.

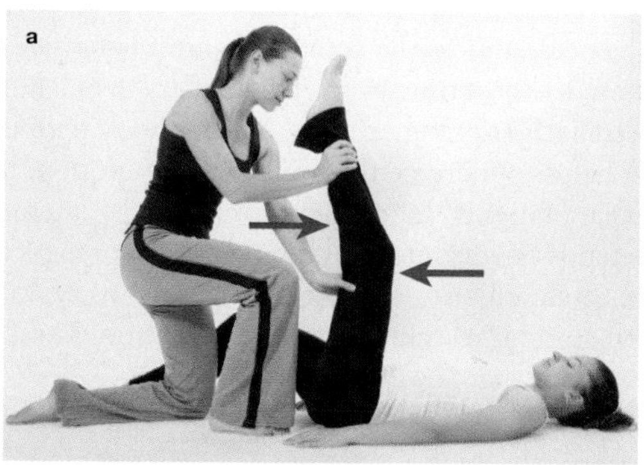

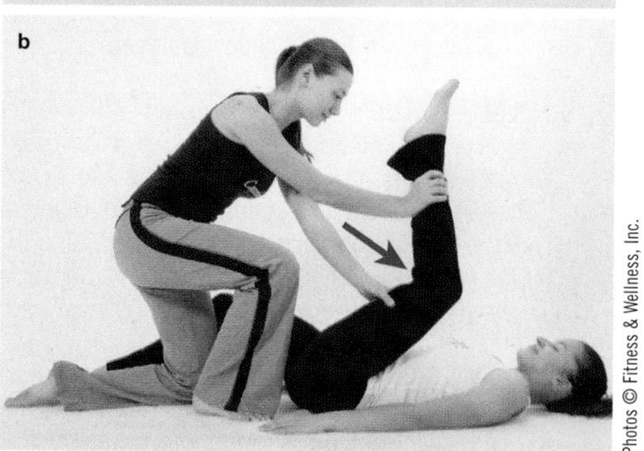

PNF stretching technique: (a) isometric phase, (b) stretching phase.

Physiological Response to Stretching

Located within skeletal muscles are two sensory organs, also known as proprioceptors: the muscle spindle and the Golgi tendon organ. Their function is to protect muscles from injury during stretching.

Muscle spindles are located within the belly of the muscle and their primary function is to detect changes in muscle length. If overstretched or stretched too fast, the spindles send messages to the central nervous system, and through a feedback loop, motor neurons are activated and cause muscle contraction to resist muscle stretch. This mechanism is known as the stretch reflex. Muscle spindle action explains why injury rates are higher with ballistic stretching. Fast stretching speeds trigger the stretch reflex and cause muscles to contract and develop tension that can lead to injury.

Golgi tendon organs are located at the point where muscle fibers attach to the muscle tendon. When excessive force is generated by a muscle, these organs trigger a response opposite to that of the spindles; an inverse stretch reflex action that inhibits the muscle contraction and leads to muscle relaxation. The Golgi tendon organ prevents injury to the muscle by keeping it from generating too much tension while being stretched. This response explains the effectiveness of the PNF technique in increasing joint range of motion. The isometric contraction following the initial stretch triggers the inverse stretch reflex, thus lessening the tension and allowing the muscle to relax. At this point, the muscle tolerates a greater degree of stretch.

Intensity

The **intensity**, or degree of stretch, when doing flexibility exercises should be to only a point of mild discomfort or tightness at the end of the range of motion. Undue pain

Static stretching (slow-sustained stretching) Exercises in which the muscles are lengthened gradually through a joint's complete range of motion.

Passive stretching Stretching exercises performed with the aid of an external force applied by either another individual or an external apparatus.

Ballistic (dynamic) stretching Stretching exercises performed with jerky, rapid, and bouncy movements.

Dynamic stretching Stretching exercises that require speed of movement, momentum, and active muscular effort to help increase the range of motion around a joint or group of joints.

Controlled ballistic stretching Exercises done with slow, short, gentle, and sustained movements.

Proprioceptive neuromuscular facilitation (PNF) A mode of stretching that uses reflexes and neuromuscular principles to relax the muscles being stretched.

Intensity In flexibility exercise, the degree of stretch.

does not have to be part of the stretching routine. All stretching should be done to slightly below the pain threshold. As participants reach this point, they should try to relax the muscle being stretched as much as possible. If they feel pain, the load is too high and may cause injury. After completing the stretch, the body part is gradually brought back to the starting point.

Repetitions

The time required for an exercise session for development of flexibility is based on the number of **repetitions** and the length of time each repetition is held in the final stretched position. As a general recommendation, a minimum of 15 minutes of flexibility exercise, including the major muscle and tendon units of the body, should be performed. Two to four repetitions per exercise should be done, holding the final position each time for 10 to 30 seconds.[6,7] The goal is to achieve 60 seconds of total stretching per exercise by adjusting the duration and repetitions. Older adults may derive greater improvements when the final stretched position is held for 30 to 60 seconds.

Data indicate that stretching for 10 to 60 seconds is better to increase range of motion than stretching for shorter periods of time and is just as effective as stretching for longer durations. Individuals who are susceptible to flexibility injuries should limit each stretch to 20 seconds. Pilates exercises are recommended for these individuals, because they increase joint stability (also see Chapter 7, pages 279–280).

CRITICAL THINKING

Carefully consider the relevance of stretching exercises to your personal fitness program. How much importance do you place on these exercises? Have some conditions improved through your stretching program, or have certain specific exercises contributed to your health and well-being?

Frequency of Exercise

Flexibility exercises should be conducted a minimum of 2 or 3 days per week, but ideally 5 to 7 days per week. After 6 to 8 weeks of almost daily stretching, flexibility can be maintained with 2 or 3 sessions per week, involving the major muscle and tendon groups of the body and doing two to four repetitions for up to a total of 60 seconds for each exercise performed. Figure 8.4 summarizes the guidelines for flexibility development.

Over the years, people who lack adequate flexibility, and those who neglect stretching, can expect to see a decline in functional capacity and to become more susceptible to injuries. Regular stretching increases range of motion not only by increasing muscular elongation but also by enhancing a person's level of stretch tolerance.

When to Stretch?

Many people do not differentiate a warm-up from stretching. Warming up means starting a workout slowly with walking, cycling, or slow jogging, followed by gentle stretching (not through the entire range of motion). Stretching implies movement of joints through their full range of motion and holding the final degree of stretch according to recommended guidelines.

A warm-up that progressively increases muscle temperature and mimics movement that will occur during training enhances performance. For some activities, gentle stretching is recommended in conjunction with warm-up routines. Before steady activities (walking, jogging, cycling, etc.), a warm-up of 3 to 5 minutes is recommended. The recommendation is up to 10 minutes before stop-and-go activities (e.g., racquet sports, basketball, and soccer) and athletic participation in general (e.g., football and gymnastics). Activities that require abrupt changes in direction are more likely to cause muscle strains if they are performed without proper warm-up that includes mild stretching.

Sport-specific or pre-exercise stretching can improve performance in sports that require a greater-than-average range of motion, such as gymnastics, dancing, diving, and figure skating. A few studies indicate that intense stretching during warm-up can lead to a temporary short-term (up to 60 minutes) decrease in strength and power. Thus, intense stretching conducted prior to participating in athletic events that rely on force and power for peak performance is not recommended.[8,9] More recent data show that short-duration static stretching combined with dynamic stretching does not elicit performance impairments.[10]

In general, unless the activity requires extensive range of motion, the best time to stretch appears to be after aerobic or strength-training exercise. Higher body temperature in itself helps to increase the joint range of motion. Muscles also are fatigued following exercise, and a fatigued muscle tends to shorten, which can lead to soreness and spasms. Stretching exercises help fatigued muscles reestablish their normal resting length and prevent unnecessary pain.

FIGURE 8.4 **Guidelines for flexibility development.**

Mode:	Static, dynamic, or proprioceptive neuromuscular facilitation (PNF) stretching to include all major muscle/tendon groups of the body
Intensity:	To the point of mild tension or limits of discomfort
Repetitions:	Repeat each exercise 2 to 4 times, holding the final position between 10 and 30 seconds per repetition, with a cumulative goal of 60 seconds per exercise
Frequency:	At least 2 or 3 days per week Ideally, 5 to 7 days per week
When:	Following cardiorespiratory or strength-training exercises, or as a stand-alone program

Flexibility Exercises

To improve body flexibility, each major muscle group should be subjected to at least one stretching exercise during a stretching session. A complete set of exercises for developing muscular flexibility is presented on pages 329–336.

Although you may not be able to hold a final stretched position with some of these exercises (e.g., lateral head tilts and arm circles), you should still perform the exercise through the joint's full range of motion. Depending on the number and length of repetitions, a complete workout lasts between 15 and 30 minutes.

Contraindicated Exercises Most strength and flexibility exercises are relatively safe to perform, but even safe exercises can be hazardous if they are performed incorrectly. Some exercises may be safe to perform occasionally but, when executed repeatedly, may cause trauma and injury. Pre-existing muscle or joint conditions (old sprains or injuries) can further increase the risk of harm during certain exercises. As you develop your exercise program, you are encouraged to follow the exercise descriptions and guidelines given in this book.

A few exercises, however, are not recommended because of the potential high risk for injury. These exercises are sometimes done in videotaped workouts and some fitness classes. **Contraindicated exercises** may cause harm because of the excessive strain they place on muscles and joints, in particular the spine, lower back, knees, neck, or shoulders.

confidentconsumer

Will stretching exercises help me lose weight?

Good flexibility attained through a regular stretching routine is the most commonly neglected component of fitness. What determines the amount of energy (calories) used by the human body, however, is dictated by the amount of oxygen required by a given activity (sleep, rest, physical activity, exercise, etc.). As described in Chapter 6, each liter of oxygen consumed (VO_2) burns approximately 5 calories. The greater the amount of muscular activity involved, along with the intensity and the duration of the activity, the greater the amount of oxygen required and subsequent energy expenditure. The energy used during stretching exercises is extremely low (100 to 120 calories in 30 minutes) compared to that used during other activities. In 30 minutes of aerobic exercise, you can easily burn an additional 250 to 300 calories as compared to the same amount of time spent stretching. Flexibility exercises are needed for overall fitness and good functional capacity, but they do not contribute much to weight loss or weight maintenance.

Illustrations of contraindicated exercises are presented in Figure 8.5. Safe alternative exercises are listed below each contraindicated exercise and are illustrated in the exercises for strength (pages 286–300) and flexibility (pages 329–336). In isolated instances, a qualified physical therapist may select one or a few of the contraindicated exercises to treat a specific injury or disability in a carefully supervised setting. Unless you are specifically instructed to use one of these exercises, it is best that you select safe exercises from this book.

Preventing and Rehabilitating Low Back Pain

Few people make it through life without having low back pain at some point. An estimated 60 to 80 percent of the population has been afflicted by back pain or injury. Estimates indicate that more than 75 million Americans suffer from chronic back pain. Each year more than $86 billion are spent in the United States to care for back pain, with limited evidence that increased spending really helps people. When it comes to back pain, prevention and treatment through physical exercise are by far the best medicine.

Though low back pain can come as a symptom of chronic illness such as degenerative conditions, bone diseases, or spinal abnormalities, it has been determined that backache syndrome is preventable more than 80 percent of the time and is caused by: (1) physical inactivity, (2) poor postural habits and body mechanics, (3) excessive body weight, and (4) psychological stress. Data also indicate that back injuries are more common among smokers, because smoking reduces blood flow to the spine—increasing back pain susceptibility.

More than 95 percent of all back pain is related to muscle or tendon injury, and only 1 to 5 percent is related to intervertebral disk damage.[11] Usually, back pain is the result of repeated microinjuries that occur over an extended time (sometimes years) until a certain movement, activity, or an excessive overload causes a significant injury to the tissues.[12]

People tend to think of back pain as a problem with the skeleton. Actually, the spine's curvature, alignment, and movement are controlled by surrounding muscles. The most common reason for chronic low back pain is a lack of physical activity. In particular, a major contributor to back pain is excessive sitting, which causes back muscles to shorten, stiffen, and become weaker.

Deterioration or weakening of the abdominal and gluteal muscles, along with tightening of the lower back (erector

Repetitions The number of times a given resistance is performed.

Contraindicated exercises Exercises that are not recommended because they may cause injury to a person.

FIGURE 8.5 **Contraindicated exercises.**

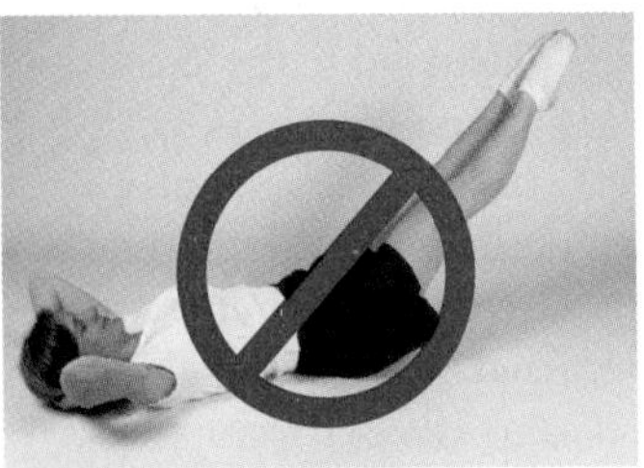

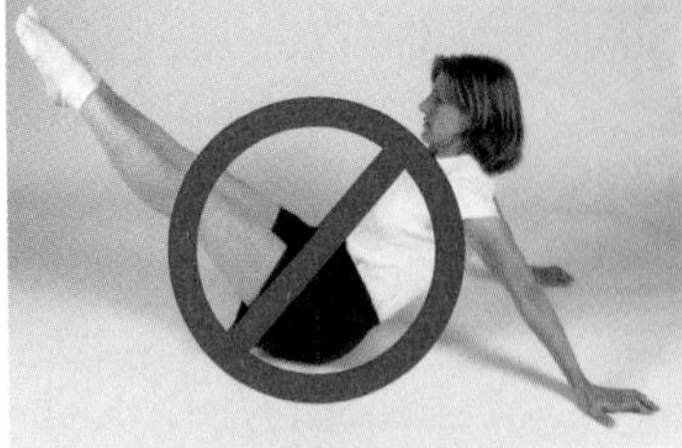

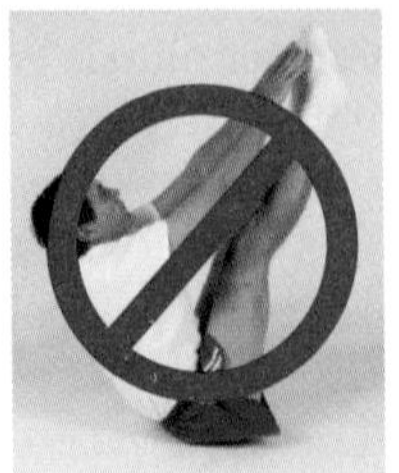

Double-Leg Lift **Upright Double-Leg Lifts** **V-Sits**

All three of these exercises cause excessive strain on the spine and may harm disks.

Alternatives: Strength Exercises 4 and 17, pages 287 and 291

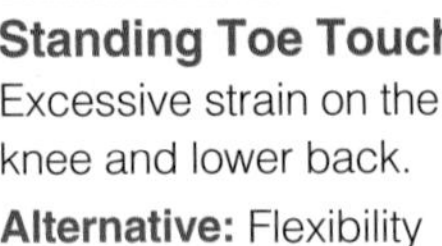

Standing Toe Touch

Excessive strain on the knee and lower back.

Alternative: Flexibility Exercise 12, page 332

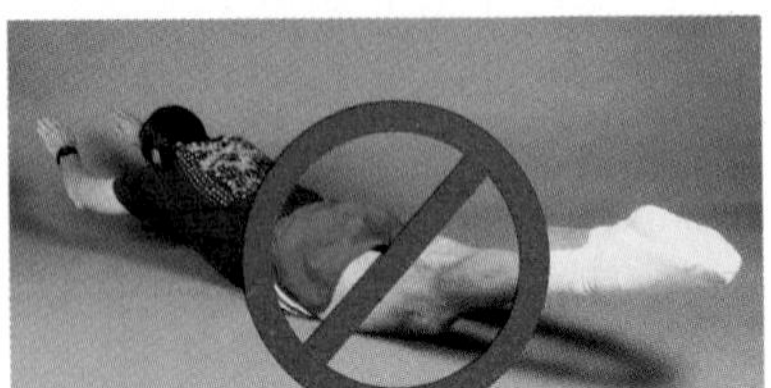

Swan Stretch

Excessive strain on the spine; may harm intervertebral disks.

Alternative: Flexibility Exercise 20, page 334

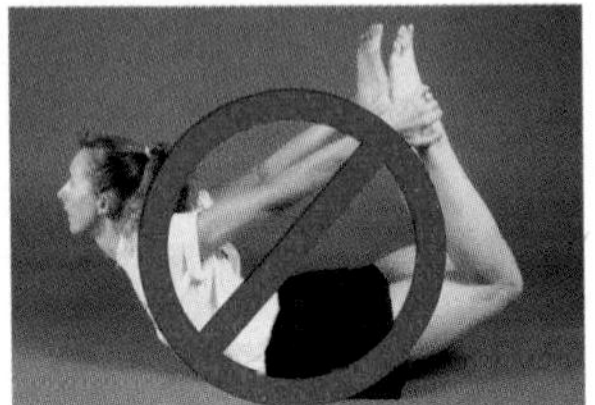

Cradle

Excessive strain on the spine, knees, and shoulders.

Alternatives: Flexibility Exercises 20, 8, and 6, pages 334, 331, and 330

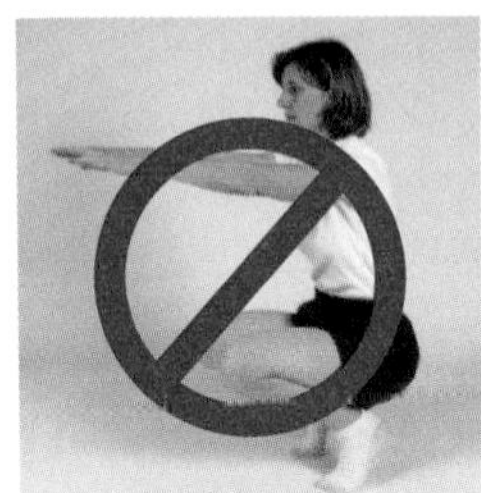

Full Squat

Excessive strain on the knees.

Alternatives: Flexibility Exercise 8, page 331; Strength Exercises 1, 16, 28A, and 28B, pages 286, 291, and 296

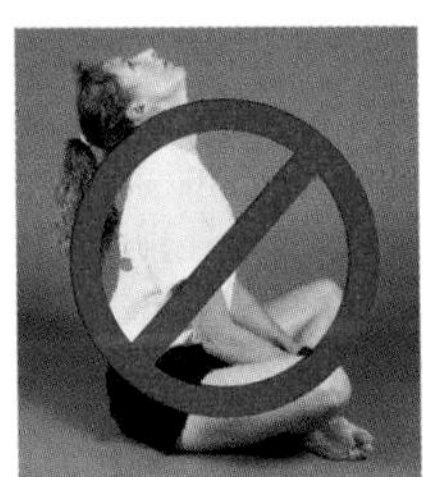

Head Rolls

May injure neck disks.

Alternative: Flexibility Exercise 1, page 329

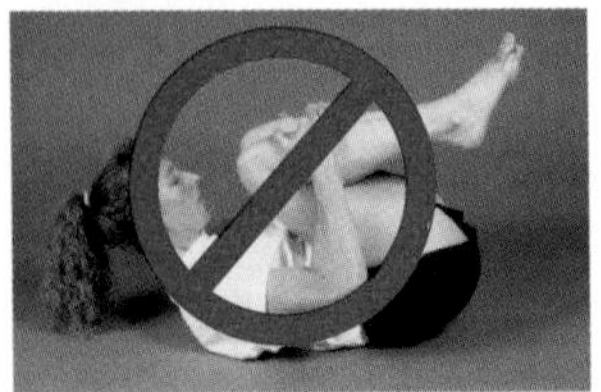

Knee to Chest

(with hands over the shin) Excessive strain on the knee.

Alternative: Flexibility Exercises 15 and 16, page 333

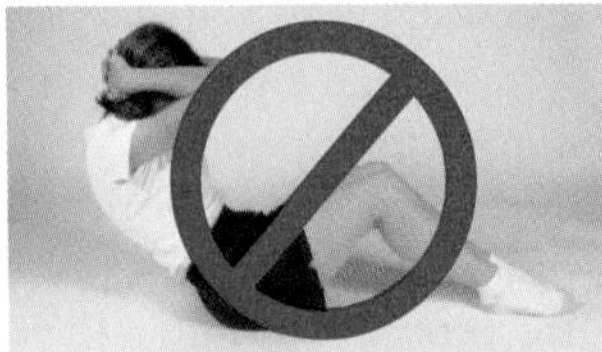

Sit-Ups with Hands Behind the Head

Excessive strain on the neck.

Alternatives: Strength Exercises 4 and 17, pages 287 and 291

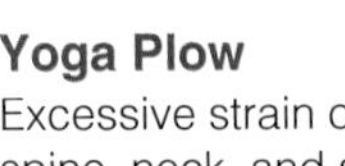

Yoga Plow

Excessive strain on the spine, neck, and shoulders.

Alternatives: Flexibility Exercises 12, 15, 16, 17, and 19, pages 332 and 333

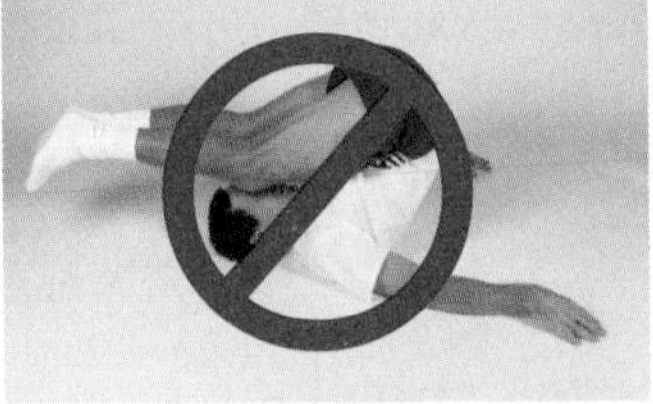

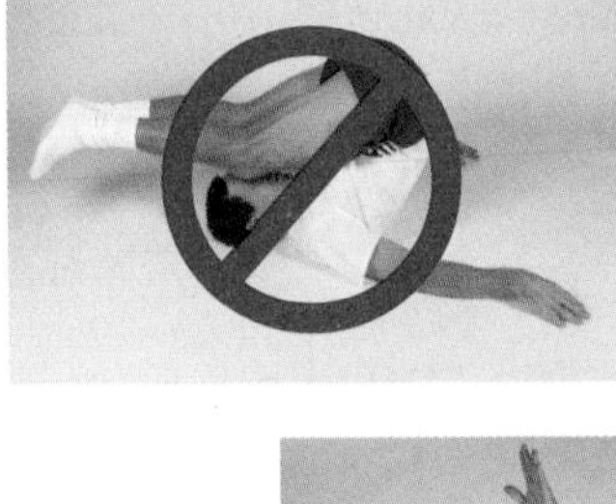

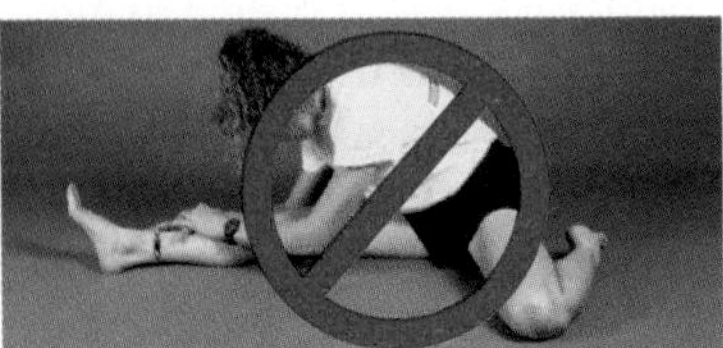

Hurdler Stretch

Excessive strain on the bent knee.

Alternatives: Flexibility Exercises 8 and 12, pages 331 and 332

The Hero

Excessive strain on the knees.

Alternatives: Flexibility Exercises 8 and 14, pages 331 and 332

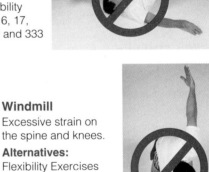

Windmill

Excessive strain on the spine and knees.

Alternatives: Flexibility Exercises 12 and 19, pages 332 and 333

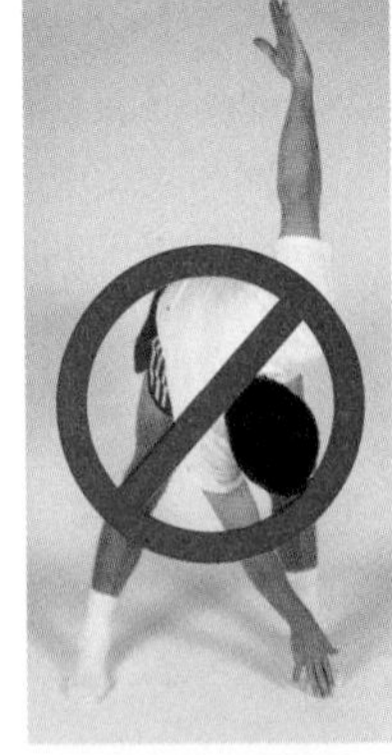

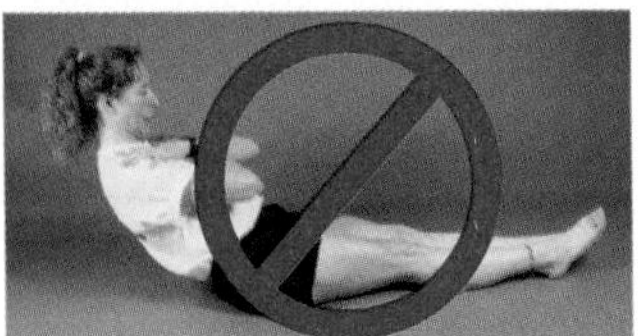

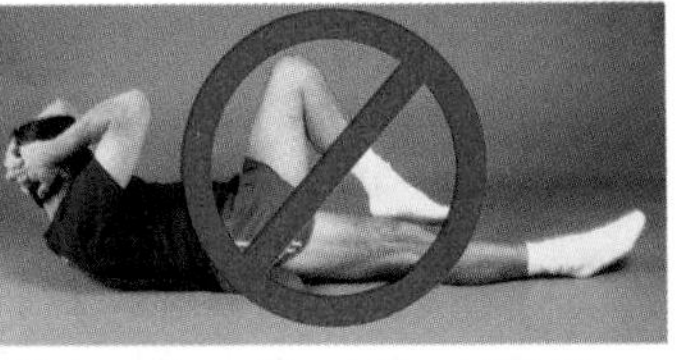

Straight-Leg Sit-Ups **Alternating Bent-Leg Sit-Ups**

These exercises strain the lower back.

Alternatives: Strength Exercises 4 and 17, pages 287 and 291

Donkey Kicks

Excessive strain on the back, shoulders, and neck.

Alternatives: Flexibility Exercises 20, 14, and 1, pages 334, 332, and 329

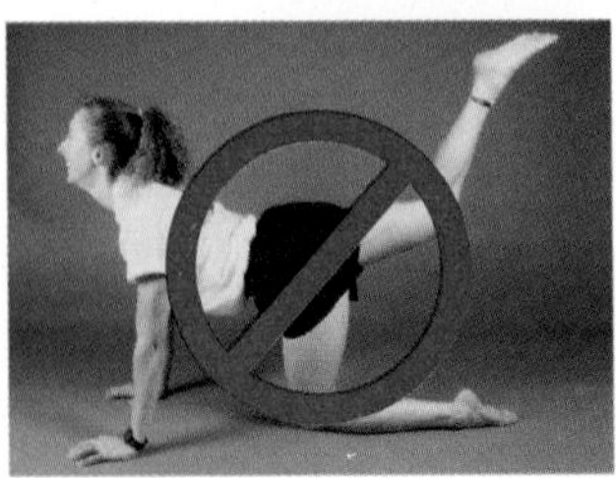

Source: Centers for Disease Control and Prevention.

spinae) muscles, brings about an unnatural forward tilt of the pelvis (Figure 8.6). This tilt puts extra pressure on the spinal vertebrae, causing pain in the lower back. Accumulation of fat around the midsection of the body contributes to the forward tilt of the pelvis, which further aggravates the condition.

Low back pain frequently is associated with faulty posture and improper body mechanics, or body positions. Incorrect posture and poor mechanics, such as prolonged static postures, repetitive bending and pushing, twisting a loaded spine, and prolonged (more than an hour) sitting with little movement increase strain on the lower back and many other bones, joints, muscles, and ligaments. Figure 8.7 provides a summary of proper body mechanics that promote back health.

In the majority of back injuries, pain is present only with movement and physical activity. According to the National Institutes of Health (NIH), most back pain goes away on its own in a few weeks. A physician should be consulted if any of the following conditions are present:

- Numbness in the legs
- Trouble urinating
- Leg weakness
- Fever
- Unintentional weight loss
- Persistent severe pain even at rest

A physician can rule out any disk damage, arthritis, osteoporosis, slipped vertebrae, spinal stenosis (narrowing of the spinal canal), or other serious condition. For common back pain, the physician may prescribe proper bed rest using several pillows under the knees for leg support (Figure 8.7). This position helps relieve muscle spasms by

FIGURE 8.6 Incorrect and correct pelvic alignment.

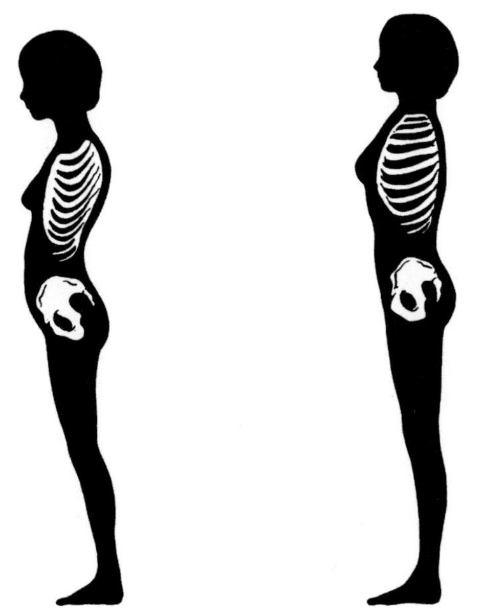

stretching the muscles involved. He or she may also prescribe a muscle relaxant, anti-inflammatory medication, or both, and some type of physical therapy.

In most cases, an x-ray and magnetic resonance imaging are not required unless pain lingers for more than 4 to 6 weeks. In the early stages of back pain, tight muscles and muscle spasms tend to compress the vertebrae, squeezing the intervertebral disks and revealing apparent disk problems on an x-ray. In these cases, the real problem is the tight muscles and subsequent muscle spasms. A daily physical activity and stretching program helps to decompress the spine, stretch tight muscles, strengthen weak muscles, and increase blood flow (promoting healing) to the back muscles.

Time is often the best treatment approach. Even with severe pain, most people feel better within days or weeks without being treated by health care professionals.[13] Up to 90 percent of people heal on their own. To relieve symptoms, you may use over-the-counter pain relievers and hot or cold packs. You should also stay active to avoid further weakening of the back muscles. Low-impact activities such as walking, swimming, water aerobics, and cycling are recommended. Once you are pain free in the resting state, you need to start correcting the muscular imbalance by stretching the tight muscles and strengthening the weak ones. Stretching exercises are always performed first.

If there is no indication of disease or injury (e.g., leg numbness or pain), a herniated disk, or fractures, spinal manipulation by a chiropractor or other health care professional can provide pain relief. Spinal manipulation as a treatment modality for low back pain has been endorsed by the federal Agency for Health Care Policy and Research. The guidelines suggest that spinal manipulation may help alleviate discomfort and pain during the first few weeks of an acute episode of low back pain. Generally, benefits are seen in fewer than 10 treatments. People who have had chronic pain for more than 6 months should avoid spinal manipulation until they have been thoroughly examined by a physician.

Acute or short-term low back pain is most often the result of trauma or injury to the lower back and typically lasts a few days or weeks. Back pain is considered chronic if it persists longer than 3 months. Surgery is seldom the best option, because it often weakens the spine. Scar tissue and surgical alterations also decrease the success rate of a subsequent surgery. Only about 10 percent of people with chronic pain are candidates for surgery. If surgery is recommended, always seek a second opinion. And consider all other options. In many cases, pushing beyond the pain and participating in aggressive physical therapy ("exercise boot camps" for back pain) aimed at strengthening the muscles that support the spine are what's needed to overcome the condition. Data from the Physician's Neck & Back Clinic in Minneapolis showed that only 3 in 38 patients recommended for surgery needed such upon completion of a 10-week aggressive physical therapy program.[14]

Back pain can be reduced greatly through aerobic exercise, muscular flexibility exercise, and muscular strength

FIGURE 8.7 **Your back and how to care for it.**

Low back pain is caused by (a) physical inactivity, (b) poor postural habits and body mechanics, (c) excessive body weight, and/or (d) psychological stress. To protect your back and avoid debilitating low back strain, you need to use proper body mechanics and correct improper body posture. Using appropriate body positions and actions in all daily activities is vital for back health. The following guidelines help avoid unnecessary back strain and protect and support your back.

Correct standing position

To learn the correct standing posture, stand a foot away from a wall and place your upper body completely straight against the wall. You will need to tighten the abdominal and gluteal muscles to do so. Next, walk around for a few minutes holding this same position and at the end return to the wall to evaluate how well you maintained the posture.

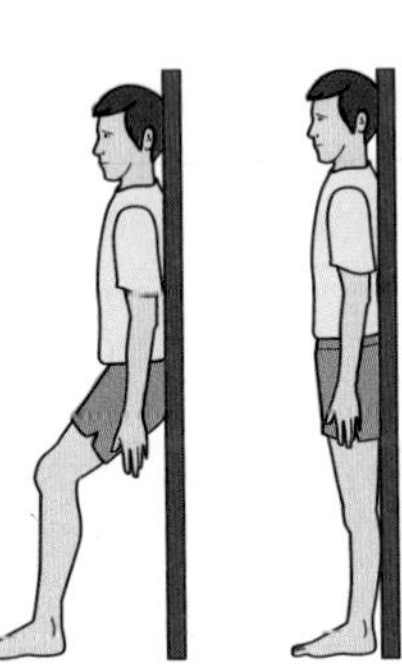

Standing, lifting, and carrying positions

Incorrect: **Correct:**

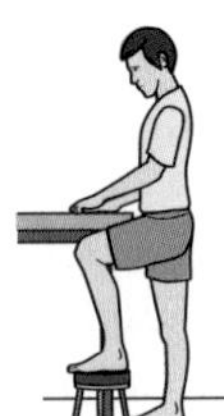

Stand with the aid of a footrest

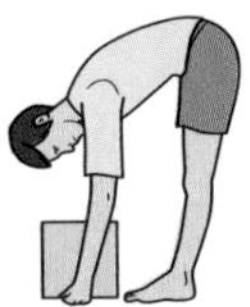

Always bend at the hips and knees

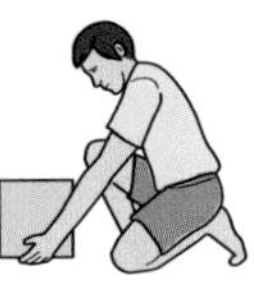

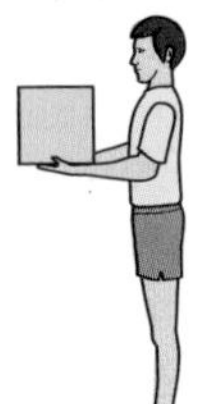

Hold and carry objects close to the body

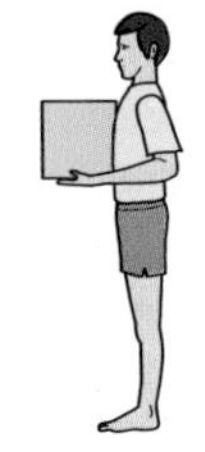

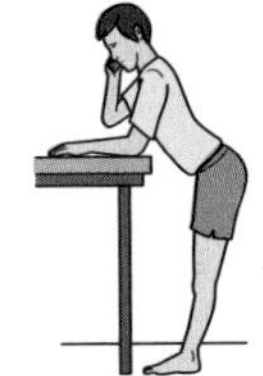

Bend at the knees to lean forward

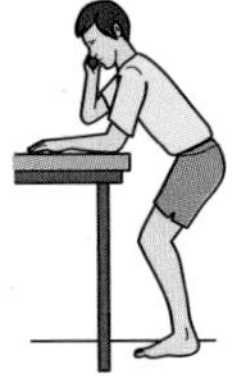

Correct sitting position

Most people spend many daily hours sitting. Proper sitting and preventing a forward slump is essential for back health. To straighten your back (a) put your head back, (b) pull in your chin toward your chest, (c) tighten your abdominal muscles, and (d) raise your chest. You should always sit in this manner. The following guidelines will also help correct improper sitting throughout the day.

Always use a footrest to keep the knees higher than the hips

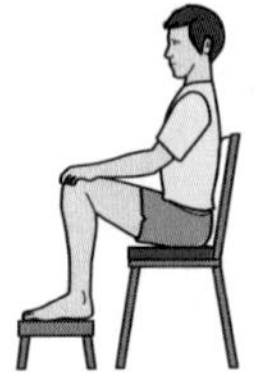

Avoid severe rounding of upper back and neck while seated

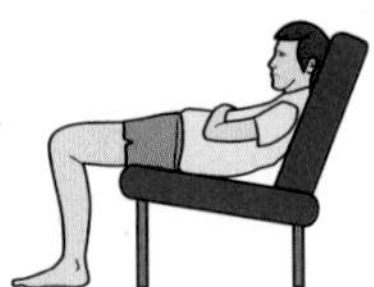

Sit close to the pedals when driving

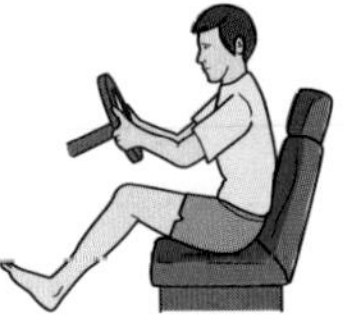

To lean forward, bend at the hips and keep the neck and back as straight as possible

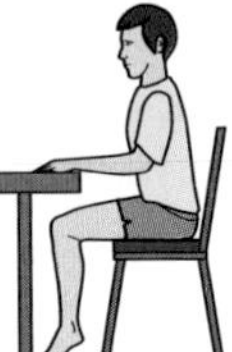

Bed posture

A firm mattress is recommended for proper back support. Avoid sleeping flat on your back or face down with large pillows for head support. Lying sideways in a fetal position with a small pillow for head support and a small pillow between the knees, or on your back with the knees supported by a larger pillow, is best.

Incorrect: **Correct:**

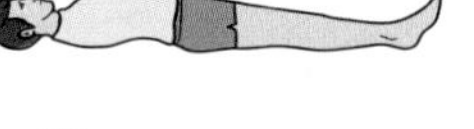

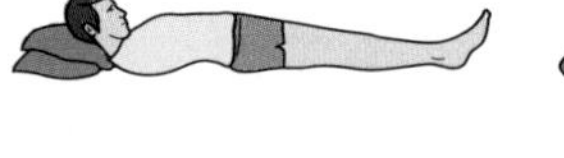

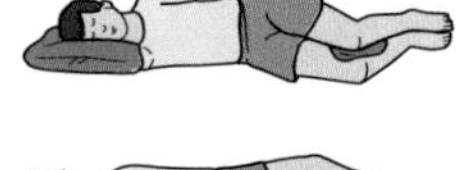

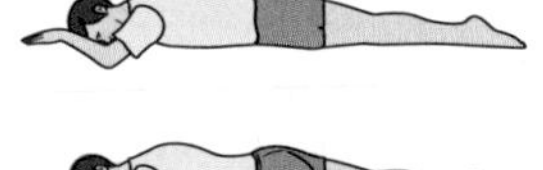

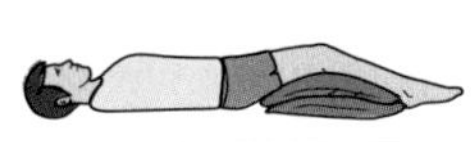

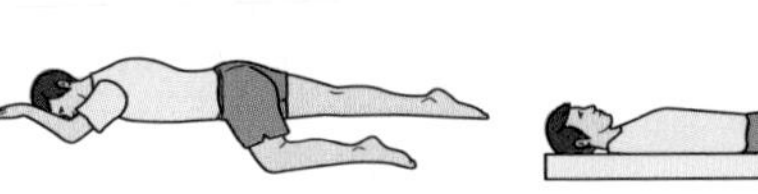

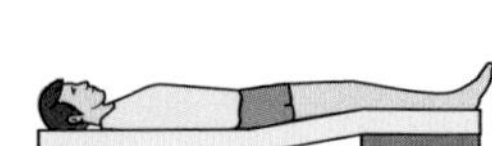

When resting, do it right

When at home resting or relaxing, lie flat on your back with a small pillow under your neck and with pillows under the knees for support. You may also place the lower legs on a chair with your knees bent at 90 degrees. This position is also good to relieve back spasms when suffering from back pain.

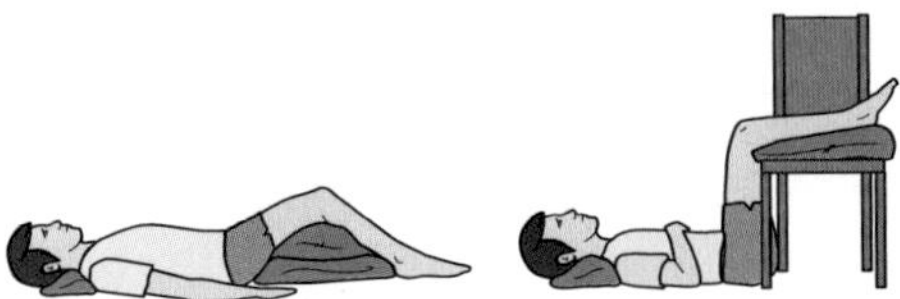

When watching TV or sitting on the floor, do so by lying on a straight-back chair covered with a firm pillow and a second large pillow under the knees.

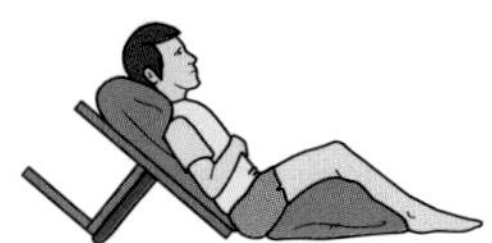

BEHAVIOR MODIFICATION PLANNING

Tips to Prevent Low Back Pain

I PLAN TO | I DID IT

❑ ❑ Be physically active.

❑ ❑ Maintain recommended body weight (excess weight strains the back).

❑ ❑ Stretch often using spinal exercises through a functional range of motion.

❑ ❑ Regularly strengthen the core of the body using sets of 10 to 12 repetitions to near fatigue with isometric contractions when applicable.

❑ ❑ Lift heavy objects by bending at the knees and carry them close to the body. Place one foot forward and keep your knees slightly bent while standing.

❑ ❑ Avoid sitting (over 50 minutes) or standing in one position for lengthy periods of time.

❑ ❑ Maintain correct posture.

❑ ❑ Sleep on your back with a pillow under the knees or on your side with the knees drawn up and a small pillow between the knees.

❑ ❑ Try out different mattresses of firm consistency before selecting a mattress.

❑ ❑ Warm up properly using mild stretches before engaging in physical activity.

❑ ❑ Practice adequate stress management techniques.

❑ ❑ Don't smoke (it reduces blood flow to the spine—increasing back pain risk).

Try It

In your class notebook, record how many of the above actions are a regular part of your healthy low back program. If you are not using all of them, what is necessary to incorporate these behaviors into your lifestyle?

and endurance training that includes specific exercises to strengthen the spine-stabilizing muscles, often referred to as the "core." The core consists of many distinctive muscles running the length of the torso that stabilize the spine. Because having a strong core is the best defense against injury to the spine, a good core-strengthening program can also help reduce back pain or prevent recurring pain. Exercise requires effort by the patient, and it may create discomfort initially, but exercise promotes circulation, healing, muscle size, and muscle strength and endurance. Many patients abstain from aggressive physical therapy, because they are unwilling to commit the time required for the program.

In terms of alleviating back pain, exercise is medicine, but it needs to be the right type of exercise. Aerobic exercise is beneficial because it helps decrease body fat and psychological stress. During an episode of back pain, however, people often avoid activity and cope by getting more rest. In most cases, this restriction on physical activity has been shown in recent studies to be exactly the opposite of what people need to do to reduce low back pain.[15] Patients who continued daily work and physical activity experienced faster recoveries than those treated with bed rest. Rest is recommended if the pain is associated with a herniated disk, but if your physician rules out a serious problem, exercise is a better choice of treatment. Exercise is the most widely used therapy for low back pain, and controlled rehab programs indicate that for chronic low back pain, exercise is more effective at improving long-term function and pain intensity over traditional non-exercise care.[16] Exercise helps restore physical function, and individuals who start and maintain an aerobic exercise program have back pain less frequently. Individuals who exercise also are less likely to require surgery or other invasive treatments.

Regular stretching exercises that help the hip and trunk go through a functional range of motion, rather than increasing the range of motion, are recommended. That is, for proper back care, stretching exercises should not be performed to the extreme range of motion. Individuals with a greater spinal range of motion also have a higher incidence of back injury. Spinal stability, instead of mobility, is desirable for back health.[17]

Yoga exercises are quite beneficial to enhance flexibility and may also help relieve chronic back pain better than conventional medicine. A review of seven studies analyzing the impact of yoga on low back pain and function showed that, overall, yoga was found to significantly reduce pain and increase function in patients suffering from chronic low back pain.[18] **Iyengar yoga** in particular has been shown to relieve chronic low back pain.[19] Following 24 weeks of biweekly classes, yoga participants had greater improvement in functional disability, along with a decrease in pain intensity and low back pain–related depression.

Iyengar yoga A form of yoga that aims to develop flexibility, strength, balance, and stamina using props (belts, blocks, blankets, and chairs) to aid in the correct performance of asanas, or yoga postures.

DESK ERGONOMICS
8 Tips for Improving Your Computer Workspace

1 Center your monitor and keyboard in front of you with the top of the monitor at or below eye level. Be sure your monitor viewing distance is at about an arm's length away to prevent eye strain.

2 Rest your feet flat on the floor and position your knees at or below hip height. Use a footrest if your feet don't comfortably reach the floor or lower the keyboard and chair.

3 Adjust the height of your chair so your elbows are at about keyboard level with your wrists positioned straight and in-line with your forearms. Use a wrist rest if needed to ensure minimal bend at the wrists.

4 Place the mouse next to the keyboard to keep your arms and elbows close to your body as you work. Use a mouse pad to protect your hands and forearms from pressing against the hard surface of the desk.

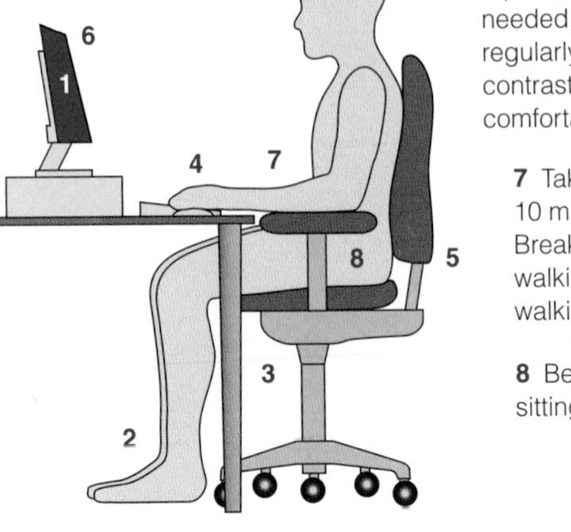

5 Adjust the incline of your chair to provide good support for your lower back. Use a small pillow or lumbar support cushion if needed.

6 Reduce screen glare. Tilt or reposition the monitor as needed, and clean the screen regularly. Set the screen contrast and brightness for comfortable viewing.

7 Take frequent short breaks, 10 minutes per hour of sitting. Breaks can include stretching, walking around, or standing/walking while talking to others.

8 Be mindful to correct your sitting posture often.

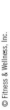

These benefits were still present 6 months after the end of class participation.

A strengthening program for a healthy back should be conducted around the endurance threshold—15 or more repetitions to near fatigue. Muscular endurance of the muscles that support the spine is more important than absolute strength, because these muscles perform their work during the course of an entire day.

Several exercises for preventing and rehabilitating the backache syndrome are given on pages 332–336. These exercises can be done twice or more daily when a person has back pain. Under normal circumstances, doing these exercises three or four times a week is enough to prevent the syndrome. Using some of the additional core exercises listed in Chapter 7 ("Core Strength Training," page 279) further enhances a low back management program. Back pain recurs more often in people who rely solely on medication, compared with people who use both medication and exercise therapy to recover.[20]

Effects of Stress

Psychological stress may lead to back pain.[21] The brain is "hardwired" to the back muscles. Excessive stress causes muscles to contract. Frequent tightening of the back muscles can throw the back out of alignment and constrict blood vessels that supply oxygen and nutrients to the back. Chronic stress also increases the release of hormones that have been linked to muscle and tendon injuries. Furthermore, people under stress tend to forget proper body mechanics, placing themselves at unnecessary risk for injury. If you are undergoing excessive stress and back pain at the same time, proper stress management (see Chapter 10) should be a part of your comprehensive back-care program.

CRITICAL THINKING

Consider your own low back health. Have you ever had episodes of low back pain? If so, how long did it take you to recover, and what helped you recover from this condition?

Personal Flexibility and Low Back Conditioning Program

Lab 8C allows you to develop your own flexibility and low back conditioning programs. Some exercises that help increase spinal stability and muscular strength endurance require isometric contractions. The recommendation calls for these contractions to be held for 2 to 20 seconds. The length of the hold depends on your current fitness level and the difficulty of each exercise. For most exercises, you may start with a 2- to 5-second hold. Over the course of several weeks, you can increase the length of the hold up to 20 seconds.

ASSESS YOUR BEHAVIOR

1. Do you give flexibility exercises the same priority in your fitness program as you do aerobic and strength training?
2. Are stretching exercises a part of your fitness program at least two times per week?
3. Do you include exercises to strengthen and enhance body alignment in your regular strength and flexibility program?

ASSESS YOUR KNOWLEDGE

1. Muscular flexibility is defined as the
   a. capacity of joints and muscles to work in a synchronized manner.
   b. achievable range of motion at a joint or group of joints without causing injury.
   c. capability of muscles to stretch beyond their normal resting length without injury to the muscles.
   d. capacity of muscles to return to their proper length following the application of a stretching force.
   e. limitations placed on muscles as the joints move through their normal planes.
2. Good flexibility
   a. promotes healthy muscles and joints.
   b. decreases the risk of injury.
   c. improves posture.
   d. decreases the risk of chronic back pain.
   e. All of the choices are correct.
3. Plastic elongation is a term used in reference to
   a. permanent lengthening of soft tissue.
   b. increased flexibility achieved through dynamic stretching.
   c. temporary elongation of muscles.
   d. the ability of a muscle to achieve a complete degree of stretch.
   e. lengthening of a muscle against resistance.
4. The most significant contributors to loss of flexibility are
   a. sedentary living and lack of physical activity.
   b. weight and power training.
   c. age and injury.
   d. muscular strength and endurance.
   e. excessive body fat and low lean tissue.
5. Which of the following is not a mode of stretching?
   a. PNF
   b. elastic elongation
   c. ballistic stretching
   d. static stretching
   e. All of the choices are modes of stretching.
6. PNF can help increase
   a. muscular strength.
   b. muscular flexibility.
   c. muscular endurance.
   d. range of motion.
   e. All of the choices are correct.
7. When performing stretching exercises, the degree of stretch should be
   a. through the entire arc of movement.
   b. to about 80 percent of capacity.
   c. to mild tension at the end of the range of motion.
   d. applied until the muscle(s) start shaking.
   e. progressively increased until the desired stretch is attained.
8. The general recommendation when stretching is that the final position reached on each repetition be held for
   a. 1 to 10 seconds.
   b. 10 to 30 seconds.
   c. 30 to 90 seconds.
   d. 1 to 3 minutes.
   e. as long as the person is able to sustain the stretch.
9. Low back pain is associated primarily with
   a. physical inactivity.
   b. faulty posture.
   c. excessive body weight.
   d. improper body mechanics.
   e. All of the choices are correct.
10. The following exercise helps stretch the lower back and hamstring muscles:
    a. adductor stretch.
    b. cat stretch.
    c. back extension stretch.
    d. single-knee-to-chest stretch.
    e. quad stretch.

Correct answers can be found at the back of the book.

NOTES

1. R. Artal, and M. O'Toole, "Guidelines of the American College of Obstetricians and Gynecologists for Exercise During Pregnancy and the Postpartum Period," *British Journal of Sports Medicine* 37 (2003): 6–12.
2. "Stretch Yourself Younger," *Consumer Reports on Health* 11 (August 1999): 6–7.
3. D. R. Hopkins and W. W. K. Hoeger, "A Comparison of the Sit and Reach and the Modified Sit and Reach in the Measurement of Flexibility for Males," *Journal of Applied Sports Science Research* 6 (1992): 7–10; W. W. K. Hoeger and D. R. Hopkins, "A Comparison between the Sit and Reach and the Modified Sit and Reach in the Measurement of Flexibility in Women," *Research Quarterly for Exercise and Sport* 63 (1992): 191–195; W. W. K. Hoeger, D. R. Hopkins, S. Button, and T. A. Palmer, "Comparing the Sit and Reach with the Modified Sit and Reach in Measuring Flexibility in Adolescents," *Pediatric Exercise Science* 2 (1990): 156–162.
4. "Position Yourself to Stay Well," *Consumer Reports on Health* 18 (February 2006): 8–9.
5. American College of Sports Medicine, "Quantity and Quality of Exercise for Developing and Maintaining Cardiorespiratory, Musculoskeletal, and Neuromotor Fitness in Apparently Healthy Adults: Guidance for Prescribing Exercise," *Medicine & Science in Sports & Exercise* 43 (2011): 1334–1359.
6. American College of Sports Medicine, *ACSM's Guidelines for Exercise Testing and Prescription* (Philadelphia: Wolters Kluwer/ Lippincott Williams & Wilkins, 2010).
7. See note 5.
8. K. B. Fields, C. M. Burnworth, and M. Delaney, "Should Athletes Stretch before Exercise?" *Gatorade Sports Science Institute: Sports Science Exchange* 30, no. 1 (2007): 1–5.
9. S. B. Thacker, J. Gilchrist, D. F. Stroup, and C. D. Kimsey Jr., "The Impact of Stretching on Sports Injury Risk: A Systematic Review of the Literature," *Medicine & Science in Sports & Exercise* 36 (2004): 371–378.
10. D. G. Behm et al., "Short Duration of Static Stretching When Combined with Dynamic Stretching Do Not Impair Repeated Sprints and Agility," *Journal of Sport Science and Medicine* 10 (2011): 408–416.
11. D. B. J. Andersson, L. J. Fine, and B. A. Silverstein, "Musculoskeletal Disorders," *Occupational Health: Recognizing and Preventing Work-Related Disease,* edited by B. S. Levy and D. H. Wegman (Boston: Little, Brown, 1995).
12. M. R. Bracko, "Can We Prevent Back Injuries?" *ACSM's Health & Fitness Journal* 8, no. 4 (2004): 5.
13. R. Deyo, "Chiropractic Care for Back Pain: The Physician's Perspective," *HealthNews* 4 (September 10, 1998).
14. B. W. Nelson et al., "Can Spinal Surgery Be Prevented by Aggressive Strengthening Exercise? A Prospective Study of Cervical and Lumbar Patients," *Archives of Physical Medicine and Rehabilitation* 80 (1999): 20–25.
15. B.A. Roy, Greg Vanichkachorn, "Low Back Pain," *ACSM's Health & Fitness Journal* 17, no. 2, (2013): 5.
16. M. van Middelkoop, S.M. Rubinstein, A.P. Verhagen, R.W. Ostelo, B.W. Koes, M.W. van Tulder, "Exercise therapy for chronic nonspecific low back pain," *Best Practice and Research Clinical Rheumatology* 24 (2010): 193–204.
17. See note 12.
18. H. Cramer, R. Lauche, H. Haller, and G. Dobos, "A Systematic Review and Meta-Analysis of Yoga for Low Back Pain," *Clinical Journal of Pain* 29, no. 5 (2013): 450–460.
19. K. Williams et al., "Evaluation of the Effectiveness and Efficacy of Iyegar Yoga Therapy on Chronic Low Back Pain," *Spine* 34 (2009): 2066–2076.
20. J. A. Hides, G. A. Jull, and C. A. Richardson, "Long-Term Effects of Specific Stabilizing Exercises for First-Episode Low Back Pain," *Spine* 26 (2001): E243–E248.
21. A. Brownstein, "Chronic Back Pain Can Be Beaten," *Bottom Line/Health* 13 (October 1999): 3–4.

SUGGESTED READINGS

Alter, M. J. *Science of Flexibility.* Champaign, IL: Human Kinetic Press, 2004.

Bracko, M. R. "Can We Prevent Back Injuries?" *ACSM's Health & Fitness Journal* 8, no. 4 (2004): 5-11.

Hoeger, W. W. K. *The Assessment of Muscular Flexibility: Test Protocols and National Flexibility Norms for the Modified Sit-and-Reach Test, Total Body Rotation Test, and Shoulder Rotation Test.* Rockton, IL: Figure Finder Collection Novel Products, 2010.

Liemohn, W., and G. Pariser. "Core Strength: Implications for Fitness and Low Back Pain," *ACSM's Health & Fitness Journal* 6, no. 5 (2002): 10-16.

McAtee, R. E., and J. Charland. *Facilitated Stretching, Fourth Edition with Online Video.* Champaign, IL: Human Kinetics, 2013.

Nelson, A. G., J. Kokkonen. *Stretching Anatomy.* Champaign, IL: Human Kinetics, 2013.

Flexibility Exercises

EXERCISE 1 Neck Stretches

ACTION Slowly and gently tilt the head laterally (a). You may increase the degree of stretch by gently pulling with one hand (b). You may also turn the head about 30° to one side and stretch the neck by raising your head toward the ceiling (see photo c—do not extend your head backward; look straight forward). Now gradually bring the head forward until you feel an adequate stretch in the muscles on the back of the neck (d). Perform the exercises on both the right and left sides. Repeat each exercise several times, and hold the final stretched position for a few seconds.

AREAS STRETCHED Neck flexors and extensors; ligaments of the cervical spine

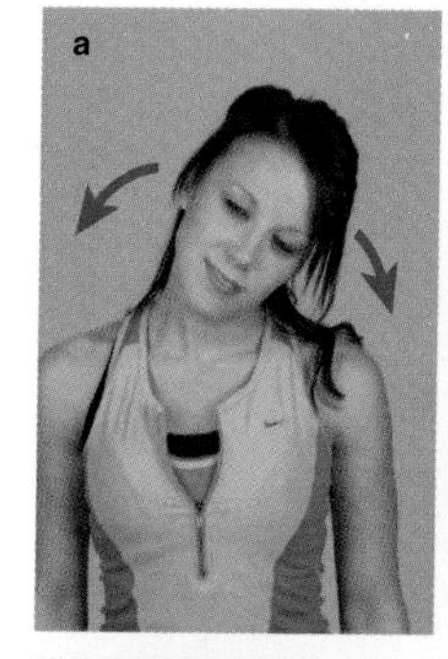

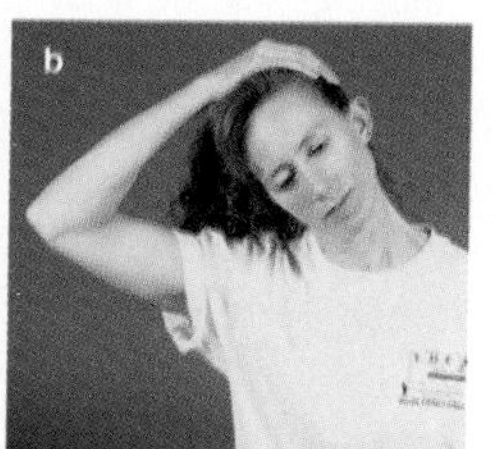

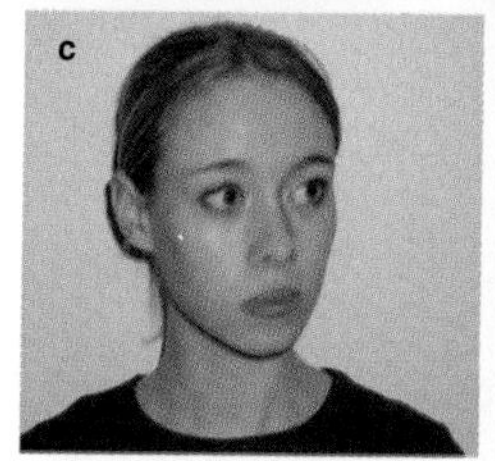

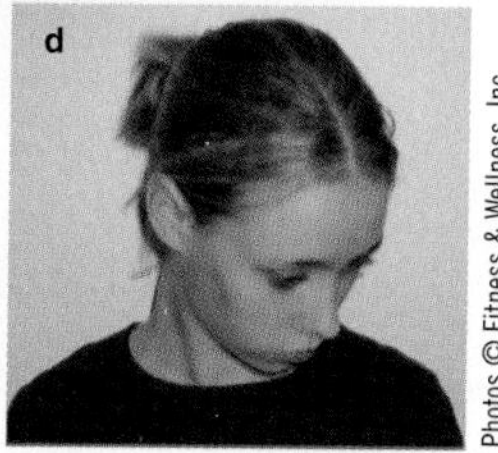

EXERCISE 2 Arm Circles

ACTION Gently circle your arms all the way around. Conduct the exercise in both directions.

AREAS STRETCHED Shoulder muscles and ligaments

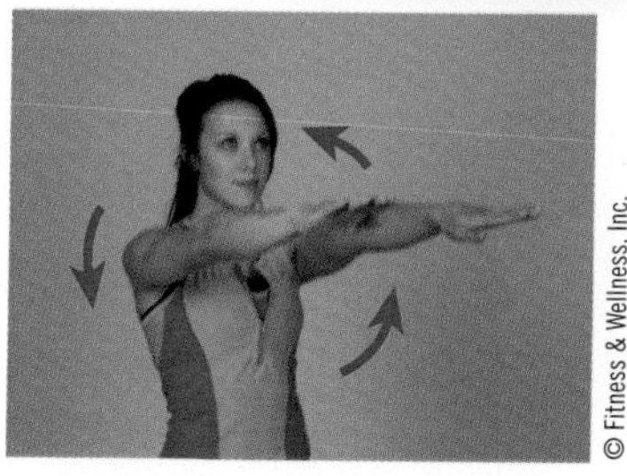

EXERCISE 3 Side Stretch

ACTION Stand straight up, feet separated to shoulder-width, and place your hands on your waist. Now move the upper body to one side and hold the final stretch for a few seconds. Repeat on the other side.

AREAS STRETCHED Muscles and ligaments in the pelvic region

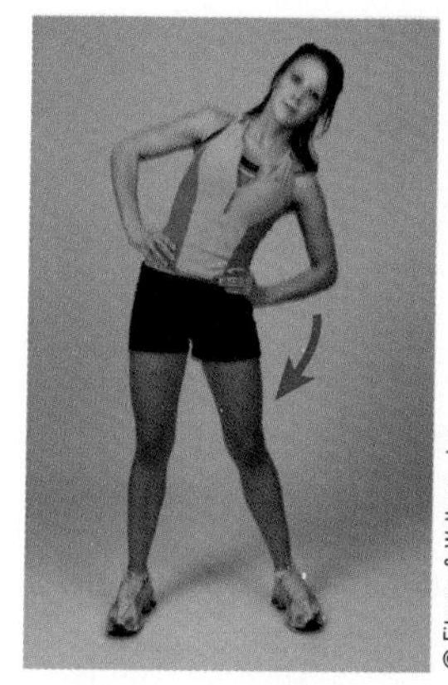

EXERCISE 4 Body Rotation

ACTION Place your arms slightly away from the body and rotate the trunk as far as possible, holding the final position for several seconds. Conduct the exercise for both the right and left sides of the body. You also can perform this exercise by standing about 2 feet away from the wall (back toward the wall) and then rotating the trunk, placing the hands against the wall.

AREAS STRETCHED Hip, abdominal, chest, back, neck, and shoulder muscles; hip and spinal ligaments

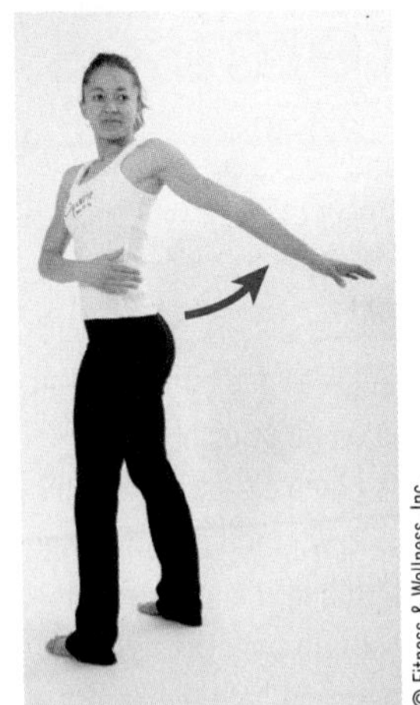

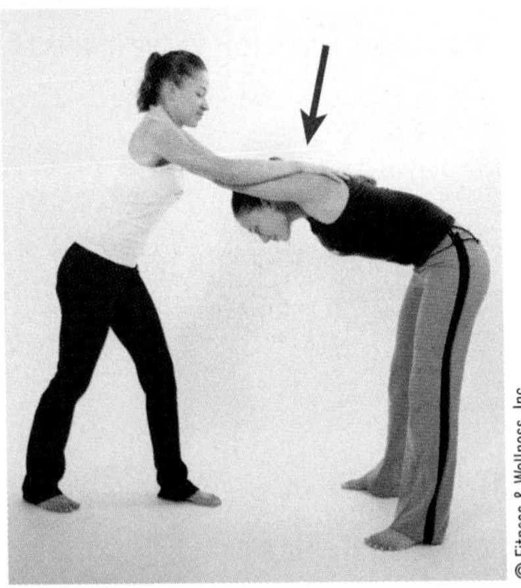

EXERCISE 5 Chest Stretch

ACTION Place your hands on the shoulders of your partner, who in turn will push you down by your shoulders. Hold the final position for a few seconds.

AREAS STRETCHED Chest (pectoral) muscles and shoulder ligaments

EXERCISE 6 Shoulder Hyperextension Stretch

ACTION Have a partner grasp your arms from behind by the wrists and slowly push them upward. Hold the final position for a few seconds.

AREAS STRETCHED Deltoid and pectoral muscles; ligaments of the shoulder joint

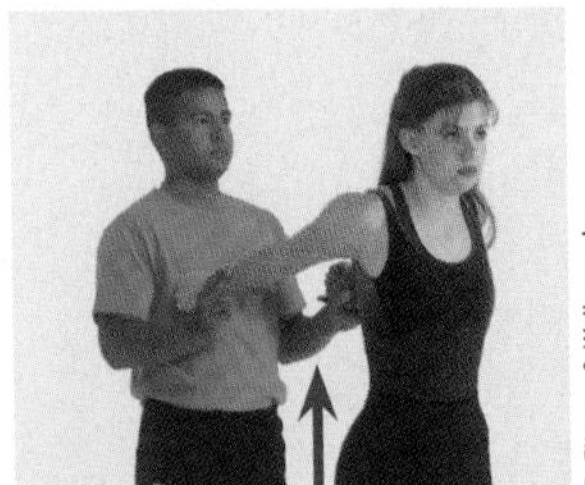

EXERCISE 7 Shoulder Rotation Stretch

ACTION With the aid of surgical tubing or an aluminum or wood stick, place the tubing or stick behind your back and grasp the two ends using a reverse (thumbs-out) grip. Slowly bring the tubing or stick over your head, keeping the elbows straight. Repeat several times (bring the hands closer together for additional stretch).

AREAS STRETCHED Deltoid, latissimus dorsi, and pectoral muscles; shoulder ligaments

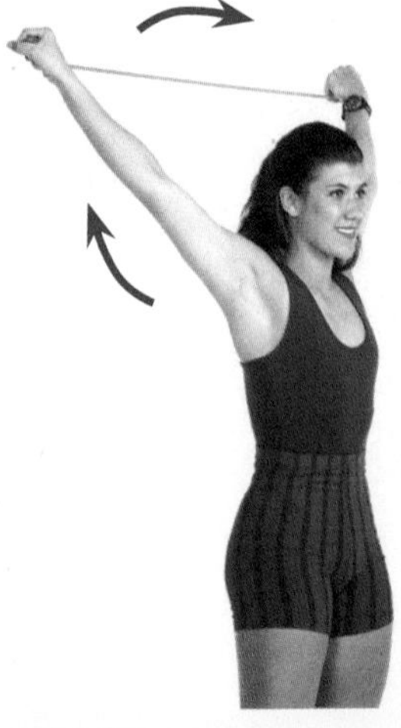

EXERCISE 8 Quad Stretch

ACTION Lie on your side and move one foot back by flexing the knee. Grasp the front of the lower leg and pull the ankle toward the gluteal region. Hold for several seconds. Repeat with the other leg.

AREAS STRETCHED Quadriceps muscle; knee and ankle ligaments

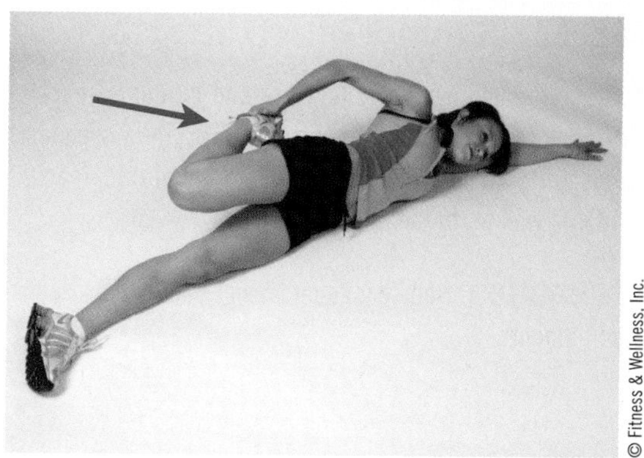

EXERCISE 9 Heel Cord Stretch

ACTION Stand against the wall or at the edge of a step and stretch the heel downward, alternating legs. Hold the stretched position for a few seconds.

AREAS STRETCHED Heel cord (Achilles tendon); gastrocnemius and soleus muscles

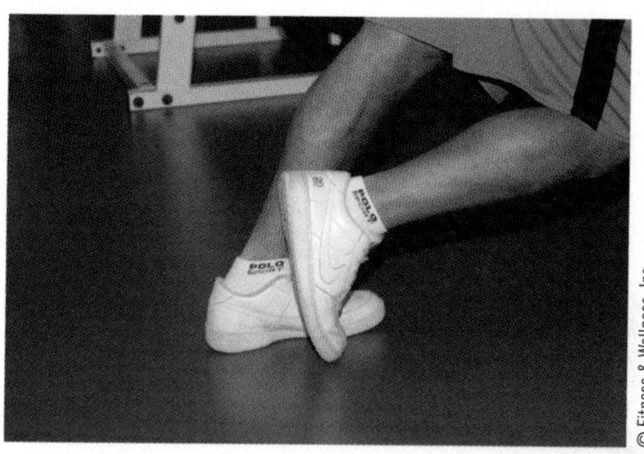

EXERCISE 10 Adductor Stretch

ACTION Stand with your feet about twice shoulder-width apart and place your hands slightly above the knees. Flex one knee and slowly go down as far as possible, holding the final position for a few seconds. Repeat with the other leg.

AREAS STRETCHED Hip adductor muscles

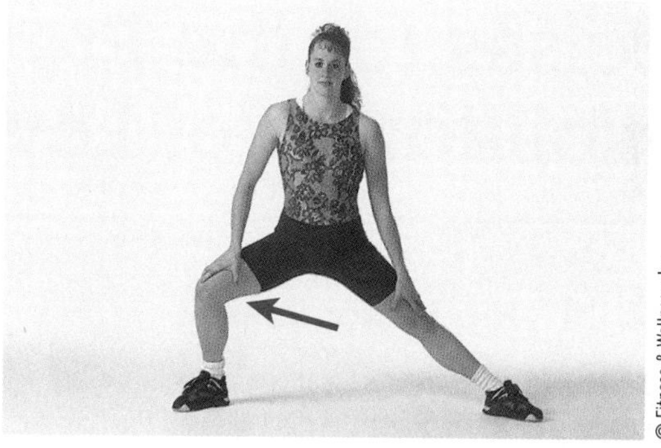

EXERCISE 11 Sitting Adductor Stretch

ACTION Sit on the floor and bring your feet in close to you, allowing the soles of the feet to touch each other. Now place your forearms (or elbows) on the inner part of the thigh and push the legs downward, holding the final stretch for several seconds.

AREAS STRETCHED Hip adductor muscles

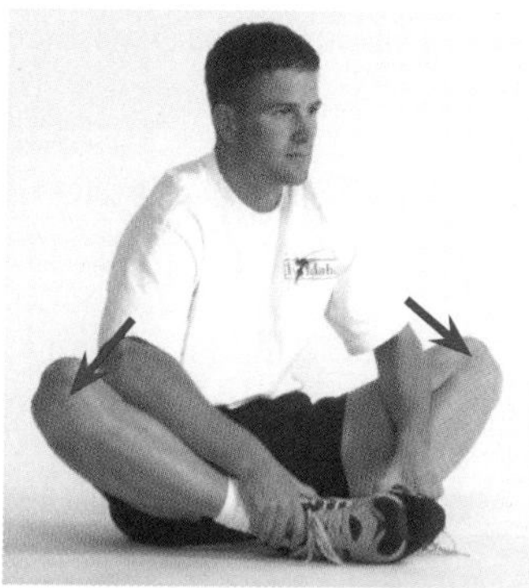

EXERCISE 12 **Sit-and-Reach Stretch**

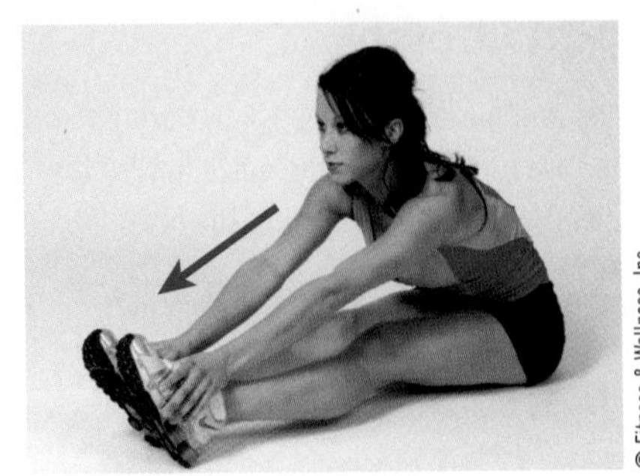
© Fitness & Wellness, Inc.

ACTION Sit on the floor with legs together and gradually reach forward as far as possible. Hold the final position for a few seconds. This exercise also may be performed with the legs separated, reaching to each side as well as to the middle.

AREAS STRETCHED Hamstrings and lower back muscles; lumbar spine ligaments

EXERCISE 13 **Triceps Stretch**

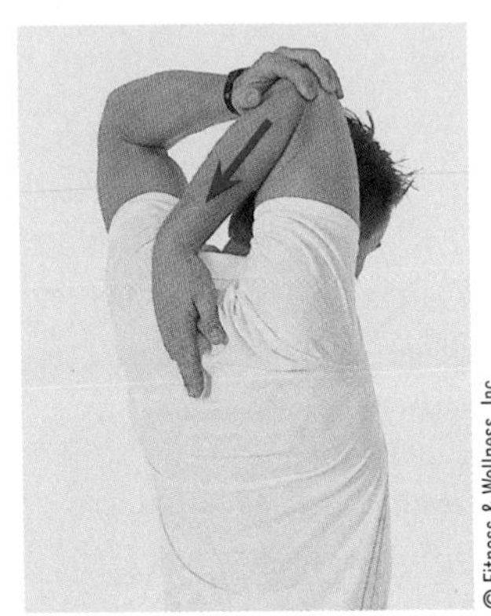
© Fitness & Wellness, Inc.

ACTION Place the right hand behind your neck. Grasp the right arm above the elbow with the left hand. Gently pull the elbow backward. Repeat the exercise with the opposite arm.

AREAS STRETCHED Back of upper arm (triceps muscle); shoulder joint

NOTE Exercises 14 through 21 and 23 are also flexibility exercises and can be added to your stretching program.

Exercises for the Prevention and Rehabilitation of Low Back Pain

EXERCISE 14 **Hip Flexor Stretch**

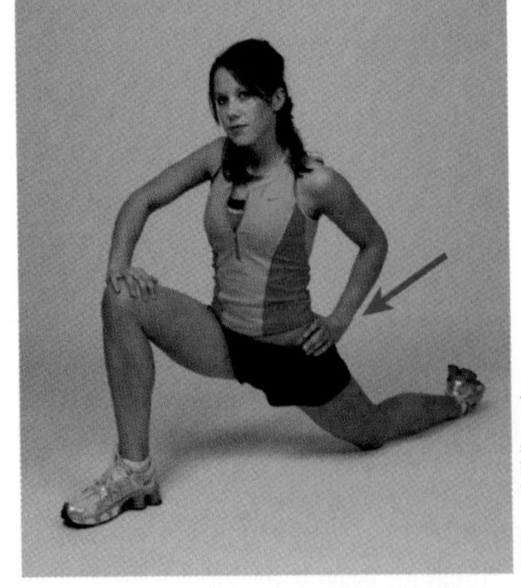
© Fitness & Wellness, Inc.

ACTION Kneel down on an exercise mat or a soft surface, or place a towel under your knees. Raise the right knee off the floor and place the right foot about 3 feet in front of you. Place your right hand over your right knee and the left hand over the back of the left hip. Keeping the lower back flat, slowly move forward and downward as you apply gentle pressure over the left hip. Repeat the exercise with the opposite leg forward.

AREAS STRETCHED Flexor muscles in front of the hip joint

EXERCISE 15 **Single-Knee-to-Chest Stretch**

ACTION Lie down flat on the floor. Bend one leg at approximately 100° and gradually pull the opposite leg toward your chest. Hold the final stretch for a few seconds. Switch legs and repeat the exercise.

AREAS STRETCHED Lower back and hamstring muscles; lumbar spine ligaments

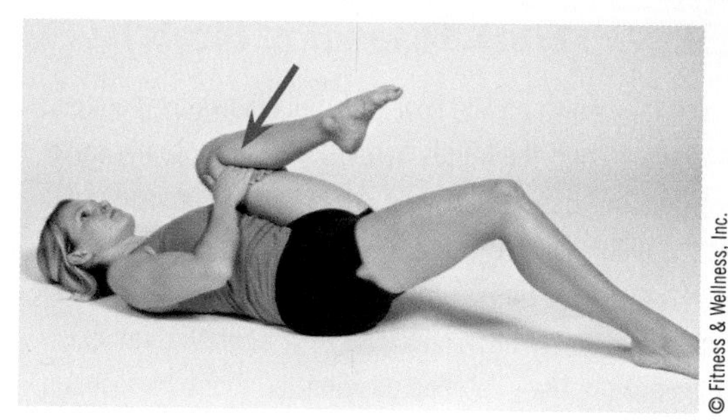

EXERCISE 16 **Double-Knee-to-Chest Stretch**

ACTION Lie flat on the floor and then curl up slowly into a fetal position. Hold for a few seconds.

AREAS STRETCHED Upper and lower back and hamstring muscles; spinal ligaments

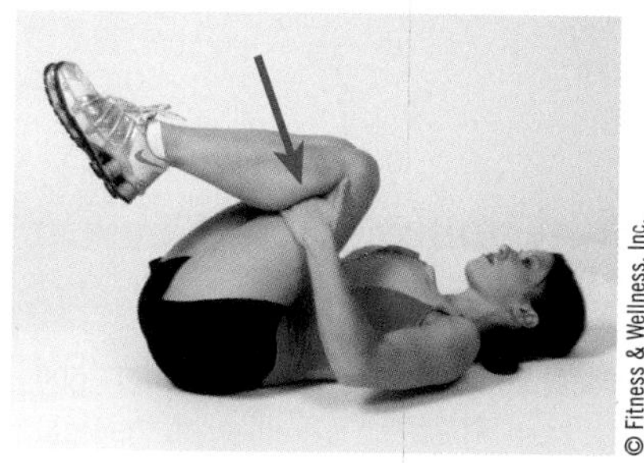

EXERCISE 17 **Upper and Lower Back Stretch**

ACTION Sit on the floor and bring your feet in close to you, allowing the soles of the feet to touch each other. Holding on to your feet, bring your head and upper chest gently toward your feet.

AREAS STRETCHED Upper and lower back muscles and ligaments

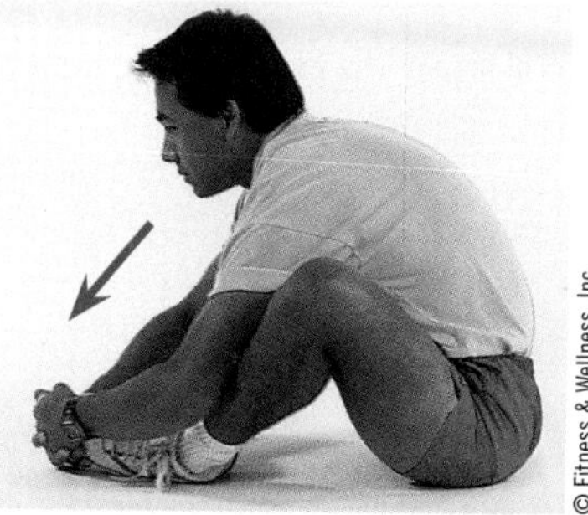

EXERCISE 18 **Sit-and-Reach Stretch**

(See Exercise 12 on page 332)

EXERCISE 19 **Gluteal Stretch**

ACTION Lie on the floor, bend the right leg, and place your right ankle slightly above the left knee. Grasp behind the left thigh with both hands and gently pull the leg toward the chest. Repeat the exercise with the opposite leg.

AREAS STRETCHED Buttock area (gluteal muscles)

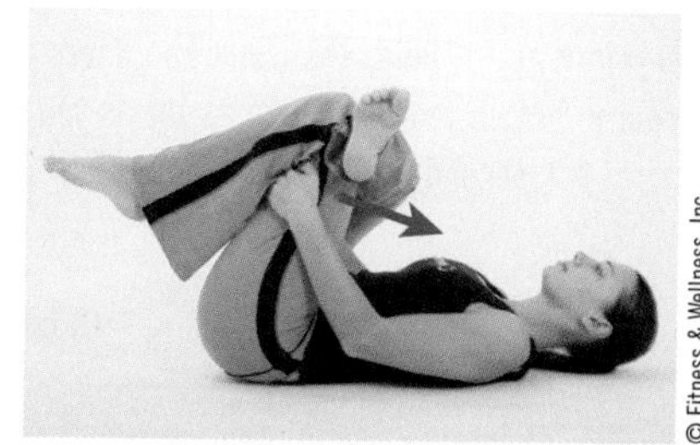

EXERCISE 20 Back Extension Stretch

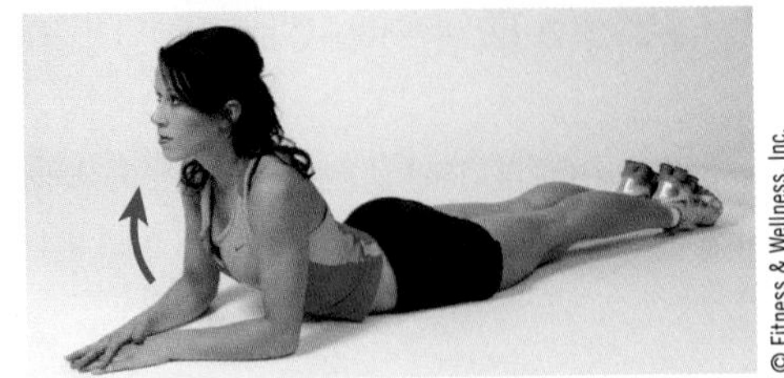

© Fitness & Wellness, Inc.

ACTION Lie face down on the floor with the elbows by the chest, forearms on the floor, and the hands beneath the chin. Gently raise the trunk by extending the elbows until you reach an approximate 90° angle at the elbow joint. Be sure the forearms remain in contact with the floor at all times. Do NOT extend the back beyond this point. Hyperextension of the lower back may lead to or aggravate an existing back problem. Hold the stretched position for about 10 seconds.

AREAS STRETCHED Abdominal region

ADDITIONAL BENEFITS Restore lower back curvature

EXERCISE 21 Trunk Rotation and Lower Back Stretch

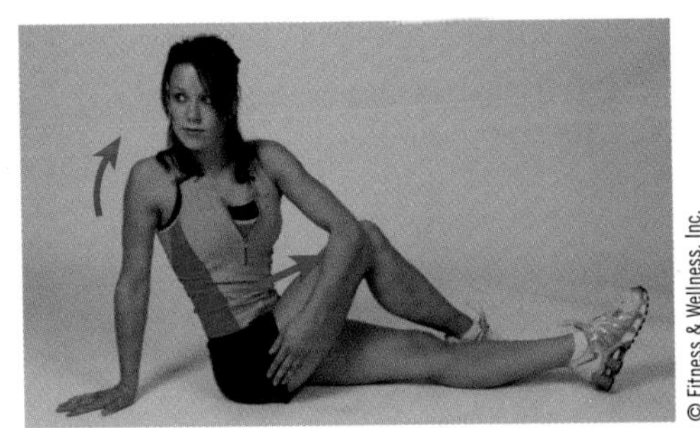

© Fitness & Wellness, Inc.

ACTION Sit on the floor and bend the left leg, placing the right foot on the outside of the left knee. Place the left elbow on the right knee and push against it. At the same time, try to rotate the trunk to the right (clockwise). Hold the final position for a few seconds. Repeat the exercise with the other side.

AREAS STRETCHED Lateral side of the hip and thigh; trunk and lower back

EXERCISE 22 Pelvic Tilt

(See Exercise 12 in Chapter 7, page 290) This is perhaps the most important exercise for the care of the lower back. It should be included as a part of your daily exercise routine and should be performed several times throughout the day when pain in the lower back is present as a result of muscle imbalance.

EXERCISE 23 The Cat

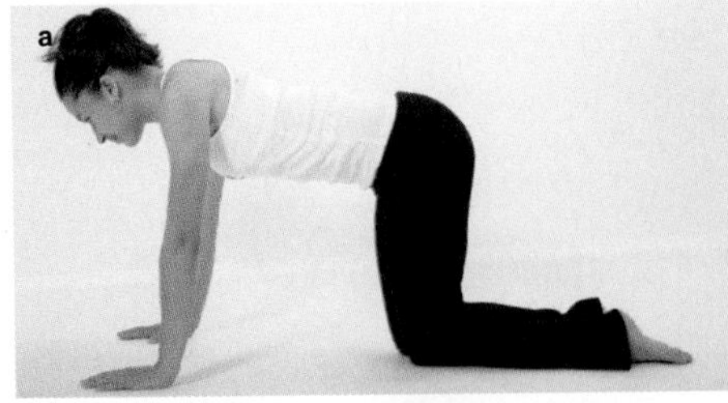

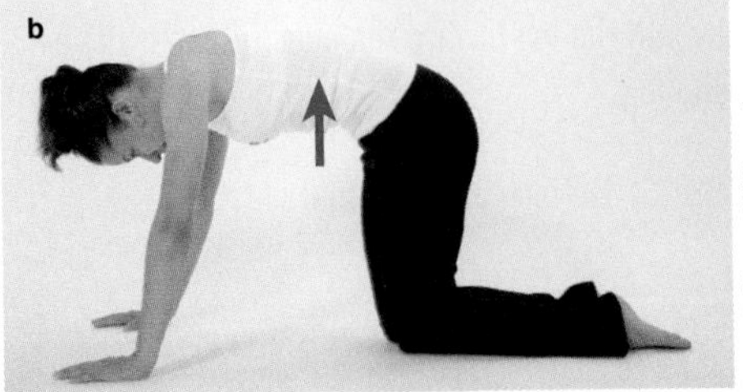

Photos © Fitness & Wellness, Inc.

ACTION Kneel on the floor and place your hands in front of you (on the floor) about shoulder-width apart. Relax the trunk and lower back (a). Now arch the spine and pull in your abdomen as far as you can and hold this position for a few seconds (b). Repeat the exercise 4–5 times.

AREAS STRETCHED Low back muscles and ligaments

AREAS STRENGTHENED Abdominal and gluteal muscles

EXERCISE 24 Abdominal Crunch or Abdominal Curl-Up

(See Exercise 4 in Chapter 7, page 287) It is important that you do not stabilize your feet when performing either of these exercises, because doing so decreases the work of the abdominal muscles. Also, remember not to "swing up" but, rather, to curl up as you perform these exercises.

EXERCISE 25 Reverse Crunch

(See Exercise 11 in Chapter 7, page 289)

EXERCISE 26 Supine Bridge

ACTION Lie face up on the floor with the knees bent at about 120°. Do a pelvic tilt (Exercise 12 in Chapter 7, page 290) and maintain the pelvic tilt while you raise the hips off the floor until the upper body and upper legs are in a straight line. Hold this position for several seconds.

AREAS STRENGTHENED Gluteal and abdominal flexor muscles

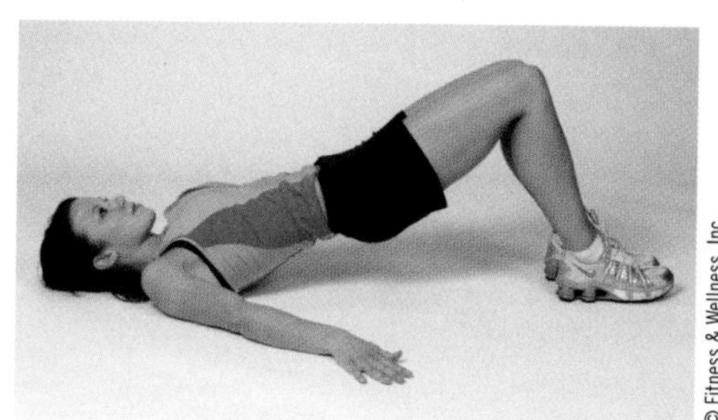

EXERCISE 27 Pelvic Clock

ACTION Lie face up on the floor with the knees bent at about 120°. Fully extend the hips as in the supine bridge (Exercise 26). Now progressively rotate the hips in a clockwise manner (2 o'clock, 4 o'clock, 6 o'clock, 8 o'clock, 10 o'clock, and 12 o'clock), holding each position in an isometric contraction for about 1 second. Repeat the exercise counterclockwise.

AREAS STRENGTHENED Gluteal, abdominal, and hip flexor muscles

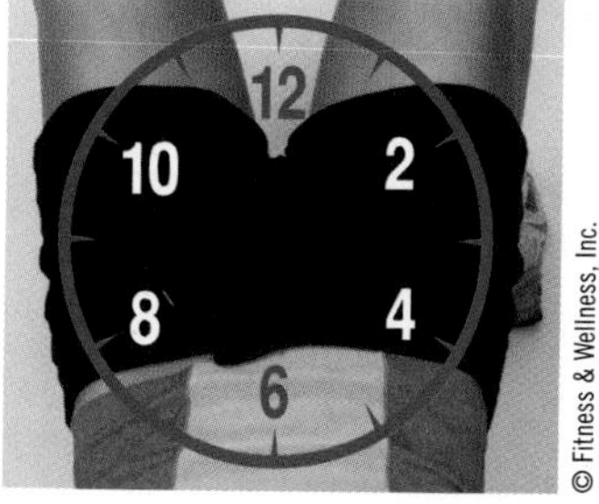

EXERCISE 28 Lateral Bridge

(See Exercise 13 in Chapter 7, page 290)

EXERCISE 29 Prone Bridge

(See Exercise 14 in Chapter 7, page 290)

EXERCISE 30 Leg Press

(See Exercise 16 in Chapter 7, page 291)

EXERCISE 31 **Seated Back**

(See Exercise 20 in Chapter 7, page 293)

EXERCISE 32 **Lat Pull-Down**

(See Exercise 24 in Chapter 7, page 294)

EXERCISE 33 **Back Extension**

(See Exercise 36 in Chapter 7, page 300)

EXERCISE 34 **Lateral Trunk Flex**

(See Exercise 37 in Chapter 7, page 300)

Lab 8A: Muscular Flexibility Assessment

Name ______________________ **Date** ____________ **Grade** ____________

Instructor ______________________ **Course** ____________ **Section** ____________

NECESSARY LAB EQUIPMENT

Acuflex I, Acuflex II, and Acuflex III Flexibility Testers* or homemade flexibility testing equipment as described in Figures 8.1, 8.2, and 8.3.

OBJECTIVE

To assess muscular flexibility and the respective fitness categories.

LAB PREPARATION

The procedures for the flexibility tests* administered in this lab are explained in this chapter (Figures 8.1, 8.2, and 8.3, pages 313–315. It is important that you warm up properly before you perform any of these tests. Do gentle stretching exercises specific to the tests that will be administered. Wear loose exercise clothing for this lab. Be sure to circle either inches or cm, depending on which system you use.

I. Modified Sit-and-Reach Test (page 313)

Trials: 1. __________ inches __________ cm 2. __________ inches __________ cm (circle either inches or cm)

Average score: __________ inches __________ cm Percentile rank: __________ Points: __________

(Table 8.4, page 317)

Fitness category: ______________________

II. Total Body Rotation Test (page 314)

Right Side Left Side (circle one)

Trials: 1. __________ inches __________ cm 2. __________ inches __________ cm (circle either inches or cm)

Average score: __________ inches __________ cm Percentile rank: __________ Points: __________

(Table 8.4, page 317)

Fitness category: ______________________

III. Shoulder Rotation Test (page 315)

Biacromial width: __________ inches __________ cm Rotation score: __________ inches __________ cm

Final score = Rotation score − biacromial width

Final score = __________ − __________ = __________ inches / cm (circle one) Percentile rank: __________

Fitness category: ______________________ Points: __________

(Table 8.4, page 317)

*The Acuflex I, II, and III Flexibility Testers can be obtained from Figure Finder Collection, Novel Products, Inc., P. O. Box 408, Rockton, IL 61072-0408, Phone (800) 323-5143, Fax 815-624-4866.

IV. Overall Flexibility Rating

Test	Points
Modified sit-and-reach:	__________
Total body rotation (right, left — circle one):	__________
Shoulder rotation:	__________
Total Points:	__________

Overall flexibility category (see Table 8.5, page 317): ____________________

V. Flexibility Goals

1. Indicate the flexibility category that you would like to achieve by the end of the term:

   ____

2. Describe your feelings about your current body flexibility and any potential implications that your current flexibility levels may have on your health and wellness. Also, briefly state how you plan to achieve your flexibility objective by the end of the term.

Lab 8B: Posture Evaluation

Name ________________________ Date ____________ Grade ____________

Instructor ________________________ Course ____________ Section ____________

NECESSARY LAB EQUIPMENT

A plumb line, two large mirrors set at about an 85° angle, and a Polaroid camera (the mirrors and the camera are optional—see "Evaluating Body Posture" (pages 313–318).

OBJECTIVE

To determine current body alignment.

LAB PREPARATION

To conduct the posture analysis, men should wear shorts only and women, shorts and a tank top. Shoes should also be removed for this test.

LAB ASSIGNMENT

The class should be divided in groups of four students each. The group should carefully study the posture form given in this lab, then proceed to fill out the form for each member according to the instructions given under "Evaluating Body Posture" (pages 313–318). If no mirrors and camera are available, three members of the group are to rate the fourth person's posture while he/she first stands with the side of the body and then with the back to the plumb line. A final score is obtained by totaling the points given for each body segment and looking up the posture rating according to the total score found in the table provided below.

Results

Total points: ____________

Category: ________________________

Posture Evaluation Standards	
Total Points	Category
≥45	Excellent
40–44	Good
30–39	Average
20–29	Fair
≤19	Poor

Posture Improvement

Indicate how you feel about your posture, identify areas to correct, and specify the steps you can take to make those improvements.

____

____

____

____

____

____

____

____

____

	Good — 5	Fair — 3	Poor — 1	Score
HEAD Left Right	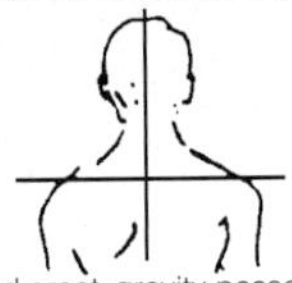 head erect, gravity passes directly through center	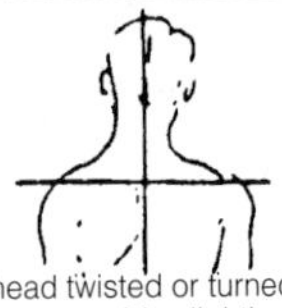 head twisted or turned to one side slightly	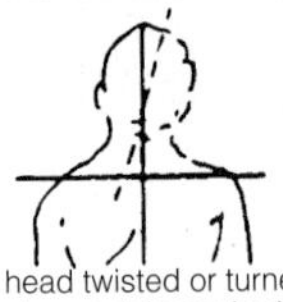 head twisted or turned to one side markedly	
SHOULDERS Left Right	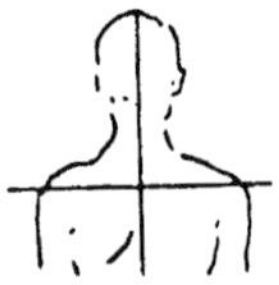 shoulders level horizontally	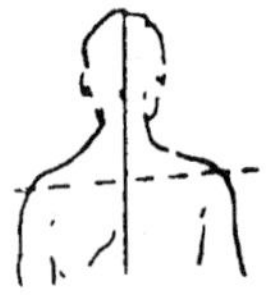 one shoulder slightly higher	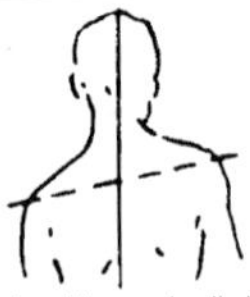 one shoulder markedly higher	
SPINE Left Right	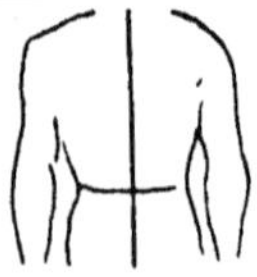 spine straight	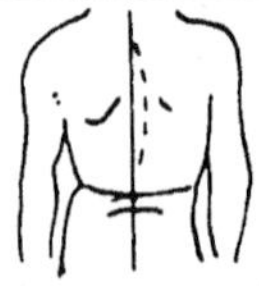 spine slightly curved	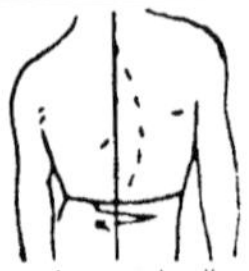 spine markedly curved laterally	
HIPS Left Right	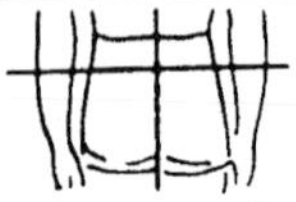 hips level horizontally	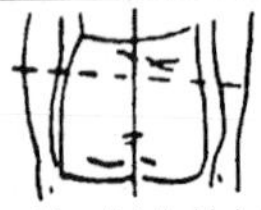 one hip slightly higher	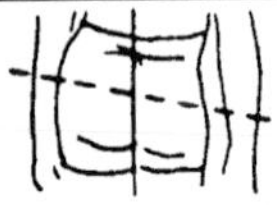 one hip markedly higher	
KNEES and ANKLES	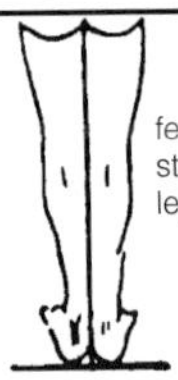 feet pointed straight ahead, legs vertical	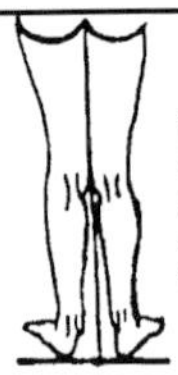 feet pointed out, legs deviating outward at the knee	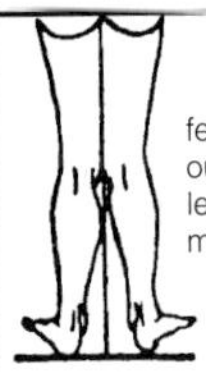 feet pointed out markedly, legs deviate markedly	
NECK and UPPER BACK	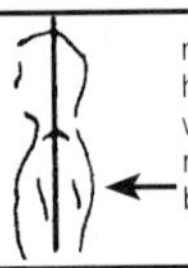 neck erect, head in line with shoulders, rounded upper back	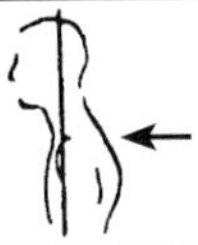 neck slightly forward, chin out, slightly more rounded upper back	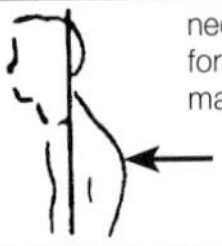 neck markedly forward, chin markedly out, markedly rounded upper back	
TRUNK	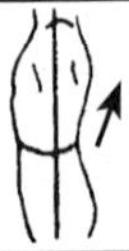 trunk erect	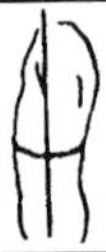 trunk inclined to rear slightly	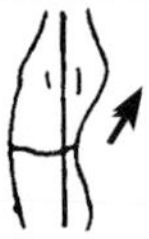 trunk inclined to rear markedly	
ABDOMEN	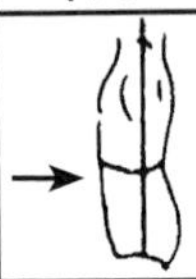 abdomen flat	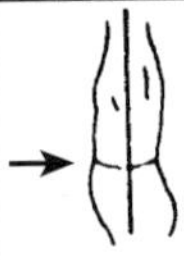 abdomen protruding	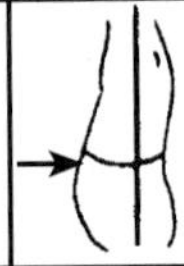 abdomen protruding and sagging	
LOWER BACK	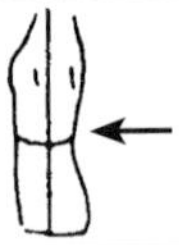 lower back normally curved	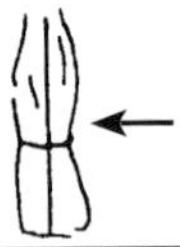 lower back slightly hollow	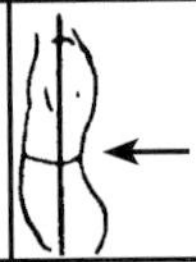 lower back markedly hollow	
LEGS	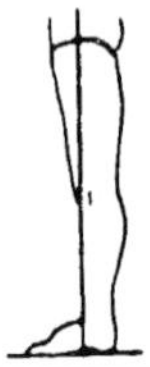 legs straight	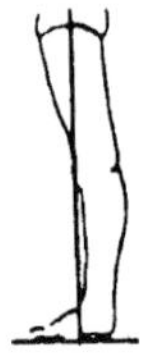 knees slightly hyper-extended	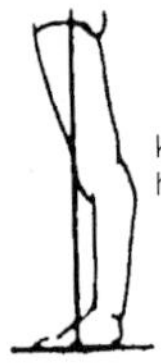 knees markedly hyperextended	
			Total Score	

Adapted from *The New York Physical Fitness Test: A Manual for Teachers of Physical Education*, New York State Education Department (Division of HPER), 1958.

Lab 8C: Flexibility Development and Low Back Conditioning

Name ______________________ Date __________ Grade __________

Instructor ______________________ Course __________ Section __________

NECESSARY LAB EQUIPMENT
Minor implements such as a chair, a table, an elastic band (surgical tubing or a wood or aluminum stick), and a stool or steps.

OBJECTIVE
To develop a flexibility exercise program and a conditioning program for the prevention and rehabilitation of low back pain.

LAB PREPARATION
Wear exercise clothing and prepare to participate in a sample stretching exercise session. All of the flexibility and low back conditioning exercises are illustrated on pages 329–336.

I. Stage of Change for Flexibility Training

Using Figure 2.5 (page 60) and Table 2.3 (page 65), identify your current stage of change for participation in a muscular stretching program:

II. Instruction

Perform all of the recommended flexibility exercises given on pages 329–332. Use a combination of slow-sustained and proprioceptive neuromuscular facilitation stretching techniques. Indicate the technique(s) used for each exercise and, where applicable, the number of repetitions performed and the length of time that the final degree of stretch was held.

Stretching Exercises

Exercise	Stretching Technique	Repetitions	Length of Final Stretch
Lateral head tilt			NA*
Arm circles			NA
Side stretch			
Body rotation			
Chest stretch			
Shoulder hyperextension stretch			
Shoulder rotation stretch			NA
Quad stretch			
Heel cord stretch			
Adductor stretch			
Sitting adductor stretch			
Sit-and-reach stretch			
Triceps stretch			

*Not Applicable

Stretching Schedule (Indicate days, time, and place where you will stretch):

Flexibility-training days: M ☐ T ☐ W ☐ Th ☐ F ☐ Sa ☐ Su ☐ Time of day: ☐ Place: ☐

Low Back Conditioning Program

Perform all of the recommended exercises for the prevention and rehabilitation of low back pain given on pages 332–336. Indicate the number of repetitions performed for each exercise.

Flexibility Exercises	Repetitions
Hip flexor stretch	☐
Single-knee-to-chest stretch	☐
Double-knee-to-chest stretch	☐
Upper- and lower-back stretch	☐
Sit-and-reach stretch	☐
Gluteal stretch	☐
Back extension stretch	☐
Trunk rotation and lower back stretch	☐

Strength/Endurance Exercises	Repetitions	Seconds Held
Pelvic tilt	☐	☐
The cat	☐	☐
Abdominal crunch or abdominal curl-up	☐	
Reverse crunch	☐	
Supine bridge	☐	☐
Pelvic clock	☐	☐
Lateral bridge	☐	☐
Prone bridge	☐	☐
Leg press	☐	
Seated back	☐	
Lat pull-down	☐	
Back extension	☐	☐

Proper Body Mechanics

1. Perform the following tasks using the proper body mechanics given in Figure 8.7 (page 324). Check off each item as you perform the task:

- ☐ Standing position
- ☐ Sitting position
- ☐ Bed posture
- ☐ Resting position for tired and painful back
- ☐ Lifting an object

2. Indicate below actions that you need to work on to improve posture and body mechanics and prevent low back pain.

____

____

____

____

____

____

____

____

____

9

Skill Fitness and Fitness Programming

"If all the benefits of regular physical activity could be packaged in a pill, it would be the most widely prescribed medication in the world today."
—*Anonymous*

OBJECTIVES

- Learn the benefits of good skill-related fitness.
- Identify and define the six components of skill-related fitness.
- Become familiar with performance tests used to assess skill-related fitness.
- Dispel common misconceptions related to physical fitness and wellness.
- Become aware of safety considerations for exercising.
- Learn concepts for preventing and treating injuries.
- Describe the relationship between fitness and aging.
- Be able to write a comprehensive fitness program.

REAL LIFE STORY | Jeremy's Experience

I played varsity basketball in high school. Our conditioning drills seemed really good, and I always became very fit and trim. I stopped playing basketball after high school and started jogging regularly. My first year in college, however, I gained a few pounds. I also ran a few 5K races that year. When training for a race, I would increase my jogging up to 30 miles per week, but my race times weren't really improving. All my training was pretty much done at the same pace. My second year in college, I signed up for the lifetime wellness course. My oxygen uptake placed me in the excellent category, but I was still not doing better in my 5K races. My instructor indicated that I needed to add high-intensity interval training to my running, and she gave me some pointers. I had a good aerobic base because I had been jogging for more than a year, so I started to do speed training (progressing through 100-m, 200-m, 400-m, and mile intervals) twice per week. After just a few weeks, I noticed a substantial improvement in my race pace. I had forgotten that we had done some of that type of training for basketball conditioning. It brought back some good memories. Much to my surprise, by the end of the year I was able to shave more than 2 minutes off my 5K time. A side benefit, I have also lost the extra pounds I gained since I stopped playing varsity basketball. On days when I need a break from running, I now head to the gym and play basketball. I love my exercise program, what I am able to do, and how I feel. It's sort of like reaching the top of the mountain; once you are there, you don't want it any other way.

MyProfile: My Lifetime Fitness Program

Based on your experience with your personal fitness program,

I. What is the most efficient type (mode) of exercise that contributes to good health and contributes to lifetime weight management? ________ Can you explain and justify your answer? ___ Yes ___ No ________________________
____
____

II. Can you name three benefits of cross-training? ___ Yes ___ No ________________________
____
____

III. Have you ever participated in a HIIT program? ___ Yes ___ No If yes, how did you feel at the end of each training session, and what results did you obtain? ___________
____
____

IV. Is it better to (mark one) ___ get fit before playing sports or ___ play sports to get fit? Can you elaborate? ___ Yes ___ No ________________________
____
____
____
____

V. What is your take-home message from Jeremy's experience, and how might it influence your personal fitness program?
____
____
____
____
____
____
____

Skill-related fitness is needed for success in athletics and in lifetime sports and activities, such as basketball, racquetball, golf, hiking, soccer, and water skiing. While most exercise programs are designed to enhance the health-related components of fitness, skill-related sports participation also contributes to health-related fitness, enhances quality of life, and helps people cope more effectively in emergency situations.

Outstanding gymnasts, for example, must achieve good skill-related fitness in all components. A significant amount of agility is necessary to perform a double back somersault with a full twist—a skill during which the athlete must simultaneously rotate around one axis and twist around a different one. Static balance is essential for maintaining a handstand or a scale. Dynamic balance is needed to perform

FAQ

What is the best fitness activity?

No single physical activity, sport, or exercise contributes to the development of overall fitness (see Table 6.10, page 241). Most people who exercise pick and adhere to a single mode, such as walking, swimming, or jogging. Many activities contribute to cardiorespiratory development. The extent of contribution to other fitness components, though, varies among the activities. For total fitness, aerobic activities should be supplemented with strength and flexibility programs. Cross-training—that is, selecting different activities for fitness development and maintenance (jogging, water aerobics, spinning, etc.)—adds enjoyment to the program, decreases the risk of incurring injuries from overuse, and keeps exercise from becoming monotonous.

Is it best not to eat before exercise?

Despite popular belief, research indicates that eating some food, liquid or solid, prior to physical activity provides energy and nutrients that improve endurance and exercise performance. Of course, how long before exercise, how much food, and what type of food you eat depends on the intensity of exercise and your stomach's tolerance to pre-exercise food. The primary fuel for exercise is provided by carbohydrates, which the body converts to glucose and stores as glycogen. Some protein, along with carbohydrates, is recommended (see the next question).

Aim to consume 1 gram of carbohydrate per kilogram of body weight (.5 gram of carbohydrate per pound of body weight) within the hour prior to exercise. For high-intensity aerobic activities, sports drinks consumed 30 to 60 minutes prior to exercise are best, because they are rapidly absorbed by the body. Solid foods (e.g., granola bars, energy bars, bagels, sugar wafers, or crackers) or semiliquid solid foods (e.g., yogurt, gelatin, or pudding) are acceptable for light-intensity aerobic exercise or strength training. Even a snack consumed a few minutes before exercise helps, as long as you exercise longer than 30 minutes. Through trial and error, you will learn which sport snacks best suit your stomach without interfering with exercise performance.

Are there specific nutrient requirements for optimal development and recovery following exercise?

Carbohydrates with some protein appear to be best. A combination of these nutrients is recommended prior to and immediately following high-intensity aerobic or strength-training exercise. A small snack or a protein-containing sports drink 30 to 60 minutes before intense exercise is beneficial. Intense exercise causes microtears in muscle tissue, and the presence of amino acids (the building blocks of proteins) in the blood contributes to the healing process and subsequent development and strengthening of the muscle fibers. Postexercise protein consumption, along with carbohydrates, also accelerates glycogen replenishment in the body after intense or prolonged exercise. Thus, carbohydrates provide energy for exercise and replenishment of glycogen stores after exercise, while protein optimizes muscle repair, growth, glycogen replenishment, and recovery following exercise. Although muscles absorb a greater amount of amino acids up to 48 hours following intense exercise, consumption of the carbohydrate/protein snack immediately following intense exercise, and an hour thereafter, appear to be most beneficial. Aim for a ratio of 4 to 1 grams of carbohydrates to protein. For example, you may consume a snack that contains 40 grams of carbohydrates (160 calories) and 10 grams of protein (40 calories). To optimize development, make sure you consume some protein with snacks or meals for the next 48 hours as well. Examples of good recovery foods include milk and cereal, a tuna fish sandwich, a peanut butter and jelly sandwich, and pasta with turkey meat sauce. Commercial sports drinks and snacks with a four-to-one ratio are now also readily available.

many gymnastics routines (e.g., those on balance beam, parallel bars, and pommel horse).

Coordination is important to successfully integrate multiple skills, each with its own degree of difficulty, into one routine. Power and speed are needed to propel the body into the air, such as when tumbling or vaulting. Quick reaction time is necessary to determine when to end rotation upon a visual clue, such as spotting the floor on a dismount.

The principle of specificity of training applies to skill-related components just as it does to health-related fitness components. The development of agility, balance, coordination, and reaction time is highly task specific. That is, to develop a certain task or skill, the individual must practice that same task many times. There seems to be very little cross-over learning effect.

For instance, properly practicing a handstand (balance) eventually leads to successfully performing the skill, but complete mastery of this skill does not ensure that the person will have immediate success when attempting to perform other static-balance

Skill-related fitness Fitness components important for success in skillful activities and athletic events; encompasses agility, balance, coordination, power, reaction time, and speed.

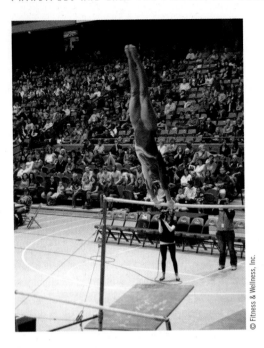
© Fitness & Wellness, Inc.

Successful gymnasts demonstrate high levels of skill fitness.

positions in gymnastics. In contrast, power and speed may improve with a specific strength-training program, frequent repetition of the specific task to be improved, or both.

CRITICAL THINKING

If you are interested in health fitness, should you participate in skill-fitness activities? Explain the pros and cons of participating in skill-fitness activities. Should you participate in skill fitness activities to get fit, or should you get fit to participate in skill-fitness activities?

The rate of learning in skill-related fitness varies from person to person, mainly because these components seem to be determined to a large extent by genetics. Individuals with good skill-related fitness tend to do better and learn faster when performing a wide variety of skills. Nevertheless, few individuals enjoy complete success in all skill-related components. Furthermore, though skill-related fitness can be enhanced with practice, improvements in reaction time and speed are limited and seem to be related to genetic endowment.

Although we do not know how much skill-related fitness is desirable, everyone should attempt to develop and maintain a better-than-average level. As pointed out earlier, this type of fitness is crucial for athletes, and it also enables fitness participants to lead a better and happier life. Improving skill-related fitness not only affords people more enjoyment and success in lifetime sports (e.g., tennis, golf, racquetball, and basketball) but also can help them cope more effectively in emergency situations. Some benefits are as follows:

1. Good reaction time, balance, coordination, agility, or a combination of these can help you avoid a fall or break a fall and thereby minimize injury.
2. The ability to generate maximum force in a short time (power) may be crucial to ameliorate injury or even preserve life if you ever have to lift a heavy object that has fallen on another person or even on yourself.
3. In our society, where the average lifespan continues to expand, maintaining speed can be especially important for elderly people. Many of these individuals—and for that matter, many unfit or overweight young people—no longer have the speed they need to cross an intersection safely before the light changes or run for help if someone else needs assistance.

Regular participation in a health-related fitness program can heighten performance of skill-related components. For example, significantly overweight people do not have good agility or speed. Because participating in aerobic and strength-training programs helps take off body fat, an overweight individual who loses weight through such an exercise program can improve agility and speed. A sound flexibility program decreases resistance to motion about body joints, which may increase agility, balance, and overall coordination. Improvements in strength definitely help develop power. People who have good skill-related fitness usually participate in lifetime sports and games, which in turn help health-related fitness in development, maintenance, or both.

Performance Tests for Skill-Related Fitness

Several performance tests assess the various components of skill-related fitness. Results of the performance tests, expressed in percentile ranks, are given in Table 9.1 (men), on page 350 and Table 9.2 (women) on page 350. Fitness categories for skill fitness components are established according to percentile rankings only. These rankings (see Table 9.3, page 350) fall into categories similar to those given for muscular fitness (strength and endurance) and for flexibility. You can record the results of your skill-related fitness tests in Lab 9A.

Agility

Agility is the ability to quickly and efficiently change body position and direction. Agility is important in sports such as basketball, soccer, and racquetball, in which the participant must change direction rapidly yet maintain proper body control.

Agility Test
SEMO Agility Test[1]

Objective
To measure general body agility

Procedure
The free-throw area of a basketball court or any other smooth area 12 by 19 feet with adequate running space around it can be used for this test. Four plastic cones or similar objects are placed on each corner of the free-throw line, as shown in Figure 9.1.

Start on the outside of the free-throw line at point A, with your back to the free-throw line. When given the "go" command, sidestep from A to B (do not make crossover steps), backpedal from B to D, sprint forward from D to A, again backpedal from A to C, sprint forward from C to B, and sidestep from B to the finish line at A.

During the test, always go outside each corner cone. A stopwatch is started at the "go" command and stopped when you cross the finish line. Take a practice trial, and then use the better of two trials as the final test score. Record the time to the nearest tenth of a second.

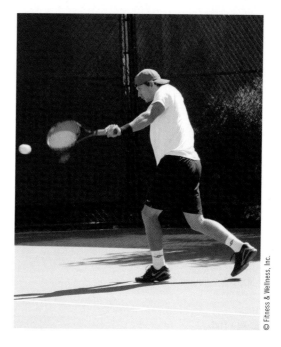

Good tennis players have excellent agility and reaction time.

Balance

The ability to maintain the body in proper equilibrium, or **balance**, is vital in activities such as gymnastics, diving, ice skating, skiing, and even football and wrestling, in which the athlete attempts to upset the opponent's equilibrium.

Balance Test
One-Foot Stand Test

Objective
To measure static balance

Procedure
A flat, smooth floor, not carpeted, is used for this test. Remove your shoes and socks and stand on your preferred foot, placing the other foot on the inside of the supporting knee and the hands on the sides of the hips. When the "go" command is given, raise your heel off the floor and balance yourself as long as possible without moving the ball of the foot from its initial position.

The test is terminated when any of the following occurs:

1. The supporting foot moves (shuffles)
2. The raised heel touches the floor
3. The hands are moved from the hips
4. A minute has elapsed

The test is scored by recording the number of seconds that the testee maintains balance on the selected foot, starting with the "go" command. After a practice trial, use the better of two trials as the final performance score. Record the time to the nearest tenth of a second.

FIGURE 9.1 **SEMO Test for agility.**

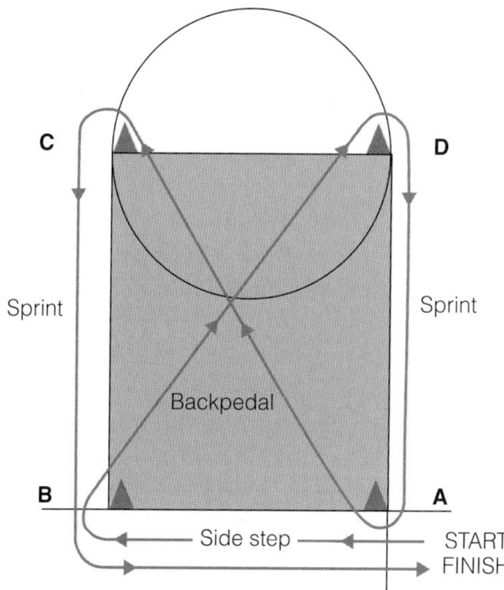

Coordination

Coordination is the integration of the nervous and the muscular systems to produce correct, graceful, and harmonious body movements. This component is important in a wide variety of motor activities, such as golf, baseball, karate, soccer, and racquetball, in which hand–eye movements, foot–eye movements, or both must be integrated.

Coordination Test
Soda Test

Objective
To assess overall motor or muscular control and movement time

Agility The ability to quickly and efficiently change body position and direction.

Balance The ability to maintain the body in proper equilibrium.

Coordination The integration of the nervous and muscular systems to produce correct, graceful, and harmonious body movements.

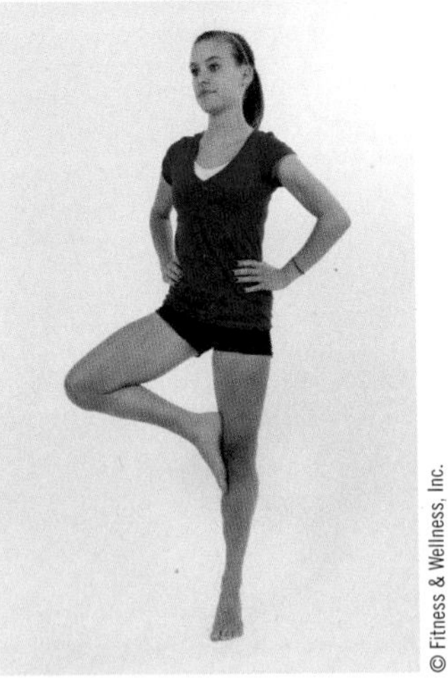

One-Foot Stand Test for balance.

Procedure

Administrator: Homemade equipment is necessary to perform this test. Draw a straight line lengthwise through the center of a piece of cardboard approximately 32 inches long by 5 inches wide. Draw six marks exactly 5 inches away from one another on this line (draw the first mark about $2^1/_2$ inches from the edge of the cardboard). Using a compass, draw six circles, each $3^1/_4$ inches in diameter (a radius of 1 centimeter larger than a can of soda) and centered on the six marks along the line (Figure 9.2).

For the purpose of this test, each circle is assigned a number starting with 1 for the first circle on the right of the test taker and ending with 6 for the last circle on the left.

FIGURE 9.2 Soda Test.

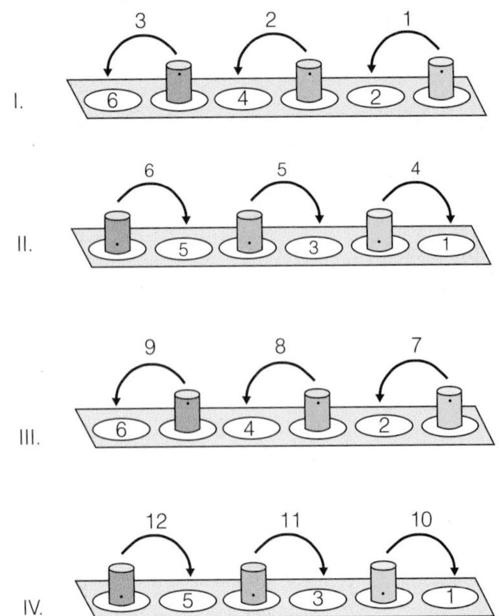

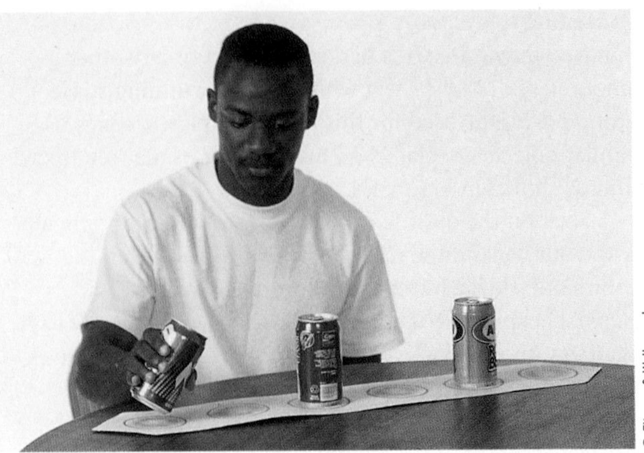

Soda Test for coordination.

The cardboard, three unopened (full) cans of soda, a table, a chair, and a stopwatch are needed to perform the test.

Place the cardboard on a table and have the participant sit in front of it with the center of the cardboard bisecting the body, using the preferred hand for this test. If this is the right hand, place the three cans of soda on the cardboard in the following manner: can one centered in circle 1 (farthest to the right), can two in circle 3, and can three in circle 5.

Participant: To start the test, place the right hand, with the thumb up, on can one with the elbow joint bent about 100 to 120 degrees. When the tester gives the signal and the stopwatch is started, turn the cans of soda upside down, placing can one inside circle 2, followed by can two inside circle 4, and then can three inside circle 6. Immediately return all three cans, starting with can one, then can two, and finally can three, turning them right side up to their original placement. On this "return trip," grasp the cans with the hand in a thumb-down position.

The entire procedure is done twice, without stopping, and is counted as one trial. (Two trips down and up are required to complete one trial.) The watch is stopped when the last can of soda is returned to its original position following the second trip back. The preferred hand (in the example, the right hand) is used throughout the entire task, and the objective of the test is to perform the task as fast as possible, making sure the cans are always placed within each circle.

If you miss a circle at any time during the test (i.e., if a can is placed on a line or outside a circle), the trial must be repeated from the start. A graphic illustration of this test is provided in Figure 9.2.

If using the left hand, follow the same procedure, except the cans are placed starting from the left, with can one in circle 6, can two in circle 4, and can three in circle 2. The procedure is initiated by turning can one upside down onto circle 5, can two onto circle 3, and so on.

Prior to initiating the test, two practice trials are allowed. Two test trials then are administered, and the best time, recorded to the nearest tenth of a second, is used as the test score. If you have a mistrial (misses a circle), the test is repeated until two consecutive successful trials are accomplished.

Power **Power** is defined as the ability to produce maximum force in the shortest time. The two components of power are speed and force (strength). An effective combination of these two components allows a person to produce explosive movements, such as in jumping, putting the shot, and in spiking, throwing, and hitting a ball.

Power is necessary to perform many activities of daily living that require strength and speed, such as climbing stairs, lifting objects, preventing falls, or hurrying to catch a bus. Power is also beneficial in sports such as soccer, tennis, softball, golf, and volleyball.

Power Test
Standing Long Jump Test[2]

Objective
To measure leg power

Procedure
Administrator: Draw a takeoff line on the floor and place a 10-foot-long tape measure perpendicular to this line. Have the participant stand with the feet several inches apart, centered on the tape measure, and the toes just behind the takeoff line (Figure 9.3).

Participant: Prior to the jump, swing your arms backward and bend your knees. Perform the jump by extending your knees and swinging your arms forward at the same time.

The distance is recorded from the takeoff line to the heel or other body part that touches the floor nearest the takeoff line. Three trials are allowed, and the best trial, measured to the nearest inch, becomes the final test score.

Reaction Time **Reaction time** is defined as the time required to initiate a response to a given stimulus. Good reaction time is important for starts in track and swimming, when playing tennis at the net, and in sports such as table tennis, boxing, and karate.

FIGURE 9.3 **Correct placement of the feet for start of the Standing Long Jump Test.**

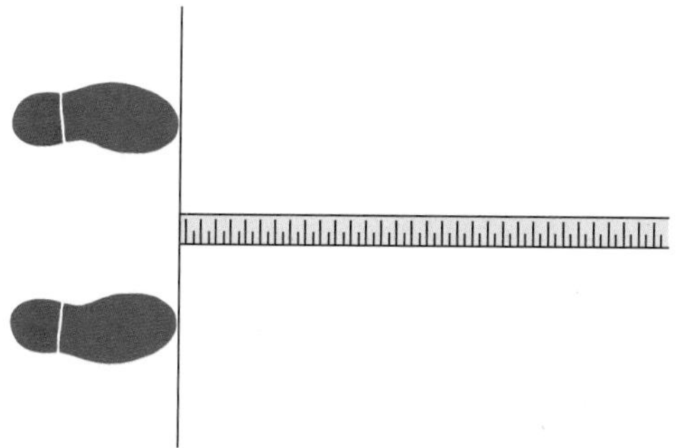

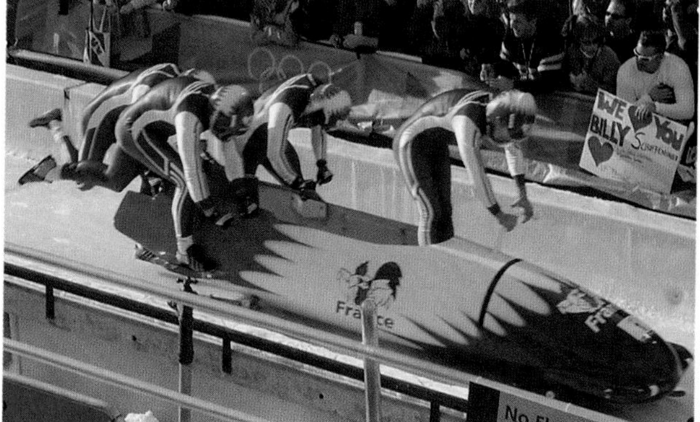

Fast starts in bobsled races require exceptional leg power.

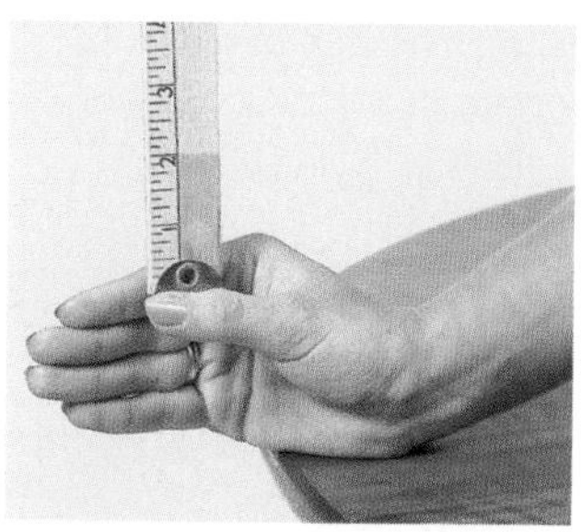

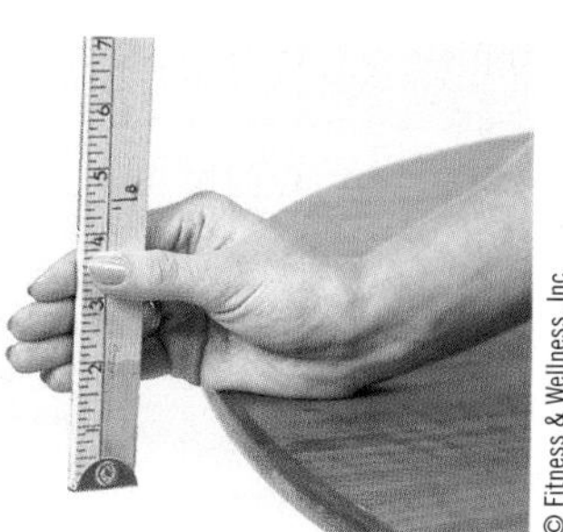

Yardstick Test for reaction time.

Reaction Time Test
Yardstick Test (preferred hand)

Objective
To measure hand reaction time (preferred hand) in response to a visual stimulus

Procedure
Administrator: For this test, you need a regular yardstick with a shaded concentration zone marked on the first 2 inches of the stick (see the photo). Administer the test with the participant sitting in a chair adjacent to a table and the preferred forearm and hand resting on the table.

Participant: Hold the tips of the thumb and fingers in a ready-to-pinch position, about 1 inch apart and 3 inches beyond the edge of the table, with the upper edges of the thumb and index finger parallel to the floor. With the person administering the test holding the yardstick near the upper end and the zero point of the stick even with the upper edge of your thumb and index finger (the administrator may steady the middle of the stick with the other hand), look at the concentration zone and react by catching the stick when it is dropped. Do not look at the administrator's hand

Power The ability to produce maximum force in the shortest time.

Reaction time The time required to initiate a response to a given stimulus.

or move your hand up or down while trying to catch the stick.

Twelve trials make up the test, each preceded by the preparatory command "ready." The administrator makes a random 1- to 3-second count between the "ready" command and each drop of the stick. Each trial is scored to the nearest half inch, read just above the upper edge of the thumb. Three practice trials are given before the actual test to be sure the subject understands the procedure. The three lowest and the three highest scores are discarded, and the average of the middle six is used as the final test score. The testing area should be as free from distractions as possible.

Speed **Speed** is the ability to rapidly propel the body or a part of the body from one point to another. Examples of activities that require good speed for success are soccer, basketball, sprints in track, and stealing a base in baseball. In everyday life, speed can be important in a wide variety of emergency situations.

Speed Test
50-Yard Dash[3]

Objective
To measure speed

Procedure
Two participants take their positions behind the starting line. The starter raises one arm and asks, "Are you ready?" and then gives the "go" command while swinging the raised arm downward as a signal for the timer (or timers) at the finish line to start the stopwatch(es).

The score is the time that elapses between the starting signal and the moment each participant crosses the finish line, recorded to the nearest tenth of a second.

Interpreting Test Results Look up your score for each test in Table 9.1 or 9.2 as relevant, and then use Table 9.3 to see your level of fitness in that particular skill.

Team Sports

Choosing activities that you enjoy will greatly enhance your adherence to exercise. People tend to repeat things they enjoy doing. Enjoyment itself is a reward. In this regard, combining individual activities (e.g., jogging, swimming, and cycling) can deepen commitment to fitness.

People with good skill-related fitness usually participate in lifetime sports and games, which in turn helps develop health-related fitness. Individuals who enjoyed basketball or soccer in their youth tend to stick to those activities later in life. The availability of teams and community leagues may be all that is needed to stop contemplating and start partici-

TABLE 9.1 Percentile Rank and Fitness Category for the Skill-Related Fitness Components: Men

	Agility*	Balance*	Coordination*	Power**	Reaction Time*	Speed**
99	9.5	59.8	5.8	9′10″	3.5	5.4
95	10.3	46.9	7.5	8′5″	4.2	5.9
90	10.6	41.1	7.7	8′2″	4.5	6.0
80	11.1	24.9	8.5	7′10″	4.9	6.3
70	11.5	15.4	8.9	7′7″	5.3	6.4
60	11.7	12.0	9.3	7′5″	5.5	6.5
50	11.9	9.2	9.6	7′2″	5.8	6.6
40	12.1	7.3	9.9	7′0″	6.1	6.8
30	12.4	5.8	10.2	6′8″	6.5	7.0
20	12.9	4.3	10.7	6′4″	6.7	7.1
10	13.7	3.1	11.3	5′10″	7.2	7.5
5	14.0	2.6	11.8	5′3″	7.4	7.9

*Norms developed at Boise State University, Department of Kinesiology.
**From AAHPERD Youth Fitness: Test Manual. 1976.

TABLE 9.2 Percentile Rank and Fitness Category for the Skill-Related Fitness Components: Women

	Agility*	Balance*	Coordination*	Power**	Reaction Time*	Speed**
99	11.1	59.9	7.5	7′6″	3.3	6.4
95	12.0	39.1	8.0	6′9″	4.5	6.8
90	12.2	25.8	8.2	6′6″	4.7	7.0
80	12.5	16.7	8.6	6′2″	5.1	7.3
70	12.9	11.9	9.0	5′11″	5.3	7.5
60	13.2	9.8	9.2	5′9″	5.9	7.6
50	13.4	7.6	9.5	5′5″	6.1	7.9
40	13.9	6.2	9.6	5′3″	6.4	8.0
30	14.2	5.0	9.9	5′0″	6.7	8.2
20	14.8	4.2	10.3	4′9″	7.2	8.5
10	15.5	2.9	10.7	4′4″	7.8	9.0
5	16.2	1.8	11.2	4′1″	8.4	9.5

*Norms developed at Boise State University, Department of Kinesiology.
**From AAHPERD Youth Fitness: Test Manual. 1976.

TABLE 9.3 Skill-Fitness Categories

Percentile Rank	Fitness Category
≥81	Excellent
61–80	Good
41–60	Average
21–40	Fair
≤20	Poor

pating. The social element of team sports provides added incentive to participate. Team sports offer an opportunity to interact with people who share a common interest. Being a member of a team creates responsibility—another incentive to exercise, because you are expected to be there. Furthermore, team sports foster lifetime friendships, strengthening the social and emotional dimensions of wellness.

For those who were not able to participate in youth sports, it's never too late to start (see the discussion of behavior modification and motivation in Chapter 2). Don't be afraid to select a new activity, even if that means learning new skills. The fitness and social rewards will be ample.

Similar to the fitness benefits of the aerobic activities discussed in Chapter 6 (Table 6.10), the contributions of skill-related activities also vary among activities and individuals. The extent to which an activity helps develop each skill-related component varies by the effort the individual makes and, most important, by proper execution (technique) of the skill (correct coaching is highly recommended) and the individual's potential based on genetic endowment. As with aerobic activities, a summary of potential contributions to skill-related fitness for selected activities is provided in Table 9.4.

Table 9.4 Contribution of Selected Activities to Skill-Related Components

Activity	Agility	Balance	Coordination	Power	Reaction Time	Speed
Alpine skiing	4	5	4	2	3	2
Archery	1	2	4	2	3	1
Badminton	4	3	4	2	4	3
Baseball	3	2	4	4	5	4
Basketball	4	3	4	3	4	3
Bowling	2	2	4	1	1	1
Cross-country skiing	3	4	3	2	2	1
Football	4	4	4	4	4	3
Golf	1	2	5	3	1	3
Gymnastics	5	5	5	4	3	3
Ice skating	5	5	5	3	3	3
In-line skating	4	4	4	3	2	4
Judo/karate	5	5	5	4	5	4
Racquetball	5	4	4	4	5	4
Soccer	5	3	5	5	3	4
Table tennis	5	3	5	3	5	3
Tennis	4	3	5	3	5	3
Volleyball	4	3	5	4	5	3
Water skiing	3	4	3	2	2	1
Wrestling	5	5	5	4	5	4

1 = Low, 2 = Fair, 3 = Average, 4 = Good, 5 = Excellent.

CRITICAL THINKING

Sports participation is a good predictor of adherence to exercise later in life. What previous experiences have you had with participation in sports? Were these experiences positive? What effect do they have on your current physical activity patterns?

Specific Exercise Considerations

In addition to the exercise-related issues already discussed in this book, many other concerns require clarification or are somewhat controversial. Let's examine some of these issues.

1. Do People Get a "Physical High" during Aerobic Exercise?

During vigorous exercise, **endorphins** are released from the pituitary gland in the brain. Endorphins can create feelings of euphoria and natural well-being. Higher levels of endorphins often result from aerobic endurance activities and may remain elevated for as long as 30 to 60 minutes after exercise. Many experts believe these higher levels explain the physical high that some people get during and after prolonged exercise.

Endorphin levels also have been shown to increase during pregnancy and childbirth. Endorphins act as painkillers. The higher levels could explain a woman's greater tolerance for the pain and discomfort of natural childbirth and her pleasant feelings shortly after the baby's birth. Several reports have indicated that well-conditioned women have shorter and easier labor. These women may attain higher endorphin levels during delivery, making childbirth less traumatic than it is for untrained women.

2. Can People with Asthma Exercise?

Asthma, a condition that causes difficult breathing, is characterized by coughing, wheezing, and shortness of breath induced by narrowing of the airway passages because of contraction (bronchospasm) of the airway muscles, swelling of the mucous membrane, and excessive secretion of mucus. In a few people, asthma can be triggered by exercise itself, particularly in cool and dry environments. This condition is referred to as exercise-induced asthma (EIA).

People with asthma need to

Speed The ability to rapidly propel the body or a part of the body from one point to another.

Endorphins Morphinelike substances released from the pituitary gland (in the brain) during prolonged aerobic exercise and thought to induce feelings of euphoria and natural well-being.

obtain proper medication from a physician prior to initiating an exercise program. A regular program is best, because random exercise bouts are more likely to trigger asthma attacks. In the initial stages of exercise, an intermittent program (with frequent rest periods during the exercise session) is recommended. Gradual warm-up and cool-down are essential to reduce the risk of an acute attack. Furthermore, exercising in warm and humid conditions (e.g., swimming) is better because it helps moisten the airways and thereby minimizes the asthmatic response. For land-based activities (e.g., walking and aerobics), drinking water before, during, and after exercise helps keep the airways moist, decreasing the risk of an attack. During the winter months, wearing an exercise mask is recommended to increase the warmth and humidity of inhaled air. People with asthma should not exercise alone and should always carry their medication with them during workouts.

3. What Types of Activities Are Recommended for People with Arthritis?

Individuals who have arthritis should participate in a combined stretching, aerobic, and strength-training program. They should do mild stretching prior to aerobic exercise to relax tight muscles. A regular flexibility program following aerobic exercise is encouraged to help maintain good joint mobility. During the aerobic portion of the exercise program, individuals with arthritis should avoid high-impact activities, because these may cause greater trauma to arthritic joints. Low-impact activities such as swimming, water aerobics, and cycling are recommended. A complete strength-training program also is recommended, with special emphasis on exercises that support the affected joint(s). As with any other program, individuals with arthritis should start with light-intensity or resistance exercises and build up gradually to a higher fitness level.

4. What Precautions Should People with Diabetes Take with Respect to Exercise?

As of 2013, there were approximately 26 million people with diabetes in the United States, with more than 1 million new cases being diagnosed each year. Estimates also indicate that 79 million adult Americans (more than one out of every three) have prediabetes. At the current rate, one in three children born in the United States will develop the disease. Type 2 diabetes has been linked to premature mortality and morbidity from cardiovascular disease and to kidney and nerve disease, blindness, and amputation.

There are two types of diabetes: type 1, or insulin-dependent diabetes mellitus (IDDM); and type 2, or non–insulin-dependent diabetes mellitus (NIDDM). In type 1, an autoimmune-related disease found primarily in young people, the pancreas produces little or no insulin. Like everyone else, people with type 1 diabetes benefit from physical activity, but this does not prevent or cure the disease.

Physical activity helps in the prevention and treatment of type 2 diabetes. With type 2, the pancreas may not produce enough insulin or the cells may become insulin resistant, thereby keeping glucose from entering the cell. Type 2 accounts for more than 90 percent of all cases of diabetes, and it occurs mainly in overweight people. (A more thorough discussion of the types of diabetes is given in Chapter 11, pages 441–442.)

If you have diabetes, consult your physician before you start exercising. You may not be able to begin until the diabetes is under control. Never exercise alone, and always wear a bracelet that identifies your condition. If you take insulin, the amount and timing of each dose may have to be regulated with your physician. If you inject insulin, do so over a muscle that won't be exercised, and then wait an hour before exercising.

Both types of diabetes improve with exercise, although the results are more notable in patients with type 2 diabetes. Exercise usually lowers blood sugar and helps the body use food more effectively. The extent to which the blood glucose level can be controlled in overweight people with NIDDM seems to be related directly to how long and how hard they exercise. Normal or near-normal blood glucose levels can be achieved through a proper exercise program.

As with any fitness program, the exercise must be done regularly to be effective against diabetes. The benefits of a single exercise bout on blood glucose are highest between 12 and 24 hours following exercise. These benefits are completely lost within 72 hours after exercise. Thus, regular participation is crucial to derive ongoing benefits. In terms of fitness, all diabetic patients can achieve higher fitness levels, including reductions in weight, blood pressure, and total cholesterol and triglycerides.

The biggest concern for people with diabetes is exercise-induced hypoglycemia during, following, or even a day after the exercise session. Common symptoms of hypoglycemia include weakness, confusion, shakiness, anxiousness, tiredness, hunger, increased perspiration, headaches, and even loss of consciousness. Physical activity increases insulin sensitivity and muscle glucose uptake, thus lowering blood glucose, an effect that may last several hours after exercise. With enhanced insulin sensitivity, a unit of insulin lowers blood glucose to a much greater extent during and following exercise than under nonexercise conditions. Typically, the longer and more intense the exercise bout, the greater the effect on insulin sensitivity.

Both aerobic exercise and strength training are recommended for individuals with type 2 diabetes. According to the American College of Sports Medicine and the American Diabetes Association,[4] patients with type 2 diabetes should adhere to the following guidelines to make their exercise program safe and derive the most benefit:

Aerobic Exercise

- **Intensity.** Exercise should be at a moderate intensity (40 to 60 percent VO_{2max}). Additional benefits, however, are gained through a vigorous-intensity program. The research indicates better blood glucose control by increasing intensity rather than exercise volume. Start your program with 10 to 15 minutes per session, on at least 3 nonconsecutive days, but preferably exercise 5 days per week.

- **Duration.** Aerobic activity duration should be no less than 150 minutes per week or the equivalent of 30 minutes per day at least 5 days per week. As a minimum, each aerobic exercise bout should be at least 10 minutes long and spread throughout the week. Diabetic individuals with a weight problem should build up daily physical activity to 60 minutes per session.
- **Mode.** Any type of aerobic activity, or preferably a combination of aerobic activities that involve large muscle groups and increase oxygen uptake (VO_2), is recommended. Choose activities that you enjoy doing, and stay with them. As you select your activities, be aware of your condition. For example, if you have lost sensation in your feet, swimming or stationary cycling is better than walking or jogging to minimize the risk for injury.
- **Frequency.** Exercise aerobically at least three times per week, and do not allow more than 2 consecutive days between exercise sessions. Five days per week are strongly encouraged.
- **Rate of progression.** A gradual increase in exercise to at least 150 weekly minutes in both intensity and volume (duration and frequency) is strongly encouraged. Progression up to 7 hours per week (420 minutes) has been reported by individuals who have successfully been able to maintain a substantial amount of weight loss.

Muscular Fitness (Strength and Endurance) Training

- **Resistance (intensity).** For optimal insulin action, resistance training should be conducted between 50 and 80 percent of the maximal capacity (1 RM) for each exercise, either on free weights or resistance machines.
- **Sets.** A minimum of one set performed to near fatigue of 5 to 10 exercises involving the body's major muscle groups (upper body, core, and lower body). Initially, each set should consist of 10 to 15 repetitions maximum (RM).
- **Frequency.** Exercise a minimum of twice per week, but preferably three times per week on nonconsecutive days.
- **Rate of progression.** Progression of intensity, sets, and frequency (in that order) are recommended. If you have type 2 diabetes, gradually increase the resistance and aim to work with 8 to 10 RM. Next, sets can progressively be increased up to four sets per exercise. Finally, frequency may be increased from twice weekly to three times per week.

Additional Exercise Guidelines

- Check your blood glucose levels before and after exercise. Do not exercise if your blood glucose is above 300 mg/dL or your fasting blood glucose is above 250 mg/dL and you have ketones in your urine. If your blood glucose is below 100 mg/dL, eat a small carbohydrate snack before exercise.
- If you are on insulin or diabetes medication, monitor your blood glucose regularly and check it at least twice within 30 minutes of starting exercise.
- Schedule your exercise 1 to 3 hours after a meal, and avoid exercise when your insulin is peaking. If you are going to exercise 1 to 2 hours following a meal, you may have to reduce your insulin or blood glucose–reducing medication.
- To prevent hypoglycemia, consume between .15 and .20 gram of carbohydrates per pound of body weight for each hour of moderate-intensity activity. This amount, however, should be adjusted based on your blood glucose monitoring. Up to .25 gram of carbohydrates per pound of body weight may be required for vigorous exercise. Your goal should be to regulate carbohydrate intake and medication dosage so as to maintain blood glucose level between 100 and 200 mg/dL. With physical activity and exercise, you will probably need to reduce your insulin or oral medication, increase carbohydrate consumption, or both.
- Be ready to treat low blood sugar with a fast-acting source of sugar—juice, raisins, or another source recommended by your doctor.
- If you feel that a reaction is about to occur, discontinue exercise immediately. Check your blood glucose level and treat the condition as needed.
- When you exercise outdoors, always do so with someone who knows what to do in a diabetes-related emergency.
- Stay well hydrated. Dehydration can have a negative effect on blood glucose, heart function, and performance. Consume adequate amounts of fluids before and after exercise. Drink about 8 ounces of water before you start each exercise session. If you are going to exercise for longer than an hour, drink 8 ounces (one cup) of a 6 to 8 percent carbohydrate sports drink every 15 to 20 minutes.

People with type 1 diabetes should ingest 15 to 30 grams of carbohydrates during each 30 minutes of intense exercise and follow it with a carbohydrate snack after exercise.

In addition, strength training twice per week using 8 to 10 exercises with a minimum of one set of 10 to 15 repeti-

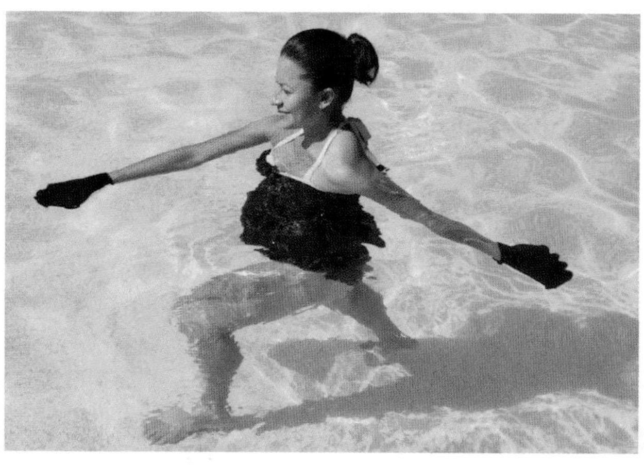

Light- to moderate-intensity exercise is recommended throughout pregnancy.

tions to near fatigue is recommended for individuals with diabetes. A complete description of strength-training programs is provided in Chapter 7.

5. Is Exercise Safe During Pregnancy?

Exercise is beneficial during pregnancy. According to the American College of Obstetricians and Gynecologists (ACOG), in the absence of contraindications, healthy pregnant women are encouraged to participate in regular, moderate-intensity physical activities to continue to derive health benefits during pregnancy.[5] Pregnant women, however, should consult their physicians to ensure that they have no contraindications to exercise during pregnancy.

As a general rule, healthy pregnant women can also accumulate 30 minutes of moderate-intensity physical activity on most, if not all, days of the week. Physical activity strengthens the body and helps prepare for the challenges of labor and childbirth.

The average labor and delivery lasts 10 to 12 hours. In most cases, labor and delivery are highly intense, with repeated muscular contractions interspersed with short rest periods. Proper conditioning better prepares the body for childbirth. Moderate exercise during pregnancy also helps prevent back pain and excessive weight gain, and it speeds recovery following childbirth.

The most common recommendations for exercise during pregnancy for healthy pregnant women with no additional risk factors are as follows:

- Don't start a new or more rigorous exercise program without proper medical clearance.
- Accumulate 30 minutes of moderate-intensity physical activities on most days of the week.
- Instead of using heart rate to monitor intensity, exercise at an intensity level between low and somewhat hard, using the physical activity perceived exertion (H-PAPE) scale in Figure 6.9 (see page 236).
- Gradually switch from weight-bearing and high-impact activities, such as jogging and aerobics, to non–weight-bearing and lower-impact activities, such as walking, stationary cycling, swimming, and water aerobics. The latter activities minimize the risk of injury and may allow exercise to continue throughout pregnancy.
- Avoid exercising at an altitude above 6,000 feet (1,800 meters), as well as scuba diving, because either may compromise the availability of oxygen to the fetus.
- Women who are accustomed to strenuous exercise may continue in the early stages of pregnancy but should gradually decrease the amount, intensity, and exercise mode as pregnancy advances (most healthy pregnant women, however, slow down during the first few weeks of pregnancy until morning sickness and fatigue subside).
- Pay attention to the body's signals of discomfort and distress, and never exercise to exhaustion. When fatigued, slow down or take a day off. Do not stop exercising altogether unless you experience any of the contraindications for exercise listed in the box on the next page.
- To prevent fetal injury, avoid activities that involve potential contact or loss of balance or that cause even mild trauma to the abdomen. Examples of these activities are basketball, soccer, volleyball, cross-country and water skiing, ice skating, road cycling, horseback riding, and motorcycle riding.
- During pregnancy, don't exercise for weight loss purposes.
- Get proper nourishment (pregnancy requires between 150 and 300 extra calories per day), and eat a small snack or drink some juice 20 to 30 minutes prior to exercise.
- Prevent dehydration by drinking a cup of fluids 20 to 30 minutes before exercise, and drink 1 cup of liquid every 15 to 20 minutes during exercise.
- During the first 3 months in particular, don't exercise in the heat. Wear clothing that allows for proper dissipation of heat. A body temperature above 102.6°F (39.2°C) can harm the fetus.
- After the first trimester, avoid exercises that require lying on the back. This position can block blood flow to the uterus and the baby.
- Perform stretching exercises gently, because hormonal changes during pregnancy increase the laxity of muscles and connective tissue. Although these changes facilitate delivery, they also make women more susceptible to injuries during exercise.

6. Does Exercise Help Relieve Dysmenorrhea?

Although exercise has not been shown to either cure or aggravate **dysmenorrhea**, it has been shown to relieve menstrual cramps because it improves circulation to the uterus (see Chapter 3). Less severe menstrual cramps also could be caused by higher levels of endorphins produced during prolonged physical activity, which may counteract pain. Particularly, stretching exercises of the muscles in the pelvic region seem to reduce and prevent painful menstruation that is not the result of disease.[6]

7. Does Participation in Exercise Hinder Menstruation?

In some instances, highly trained athletes develop **amenorrhea** during training and competition. This condition is seen most often in extremely lean women who also engage in sports that require strenuous physical effort over a sustained time. It is by no means irreversible. At present, we do not know whether the condition is caused by physical or emotional stress related to high-intensity training, excessively low body fat, or other factors.

Although women on average, have a lower physical capacity during menstruation, medical surveys at the Olympic Games have shown that women have broken Olympic and world records at all stages of the menstrual cycle. Menstruation should not keep a woman from exercising, and it will not necessarily have a negative effect on performance.

8. Does Exercise Offset the Detrimental Effects of Cigarette Smoking?

Physical exercise often motivates a person to stop smoking, but it does not offset any ill effects of smoking. Smoking

Contraindications to Exercise During Pregnancy

Stop exercise and seek medical advice if you experience any of the following symptoms:

- Unusual pain or discomfort, especially in the chest or abdominal area
- Cramping, primarily in the pelvic or lower back areas
- Muscle weakness, excessive fatigue, or shortness of breath
- Abnormally high heart rate or a pounding (palpitations) heart rate
- Decreased fetal movement
- Insufficient weight gain
- Amniotic fluid leakage
- Nausea, dizziness, or headaches
- Persistent uterine contractions
- Vaginal bleeding or rupture of the membranes
- Swelling of ankles, calves, hands, or face

greatly decreases the ability of the blood to transport oxygen to working muscles.

Oxygen is carried in the circulatory system by hemoglobin, the iron-containing pigment of the red blood cells. Carbon monoxide, a by-product of cigarette smoke, has 210 to 250 times greater affinity for hemoglobin over oxygen. Consequently, carbon monoxide combines much faster with hemoglobin, decreasing the oxygen-carrying capacity of the blood.

Chronic smoking also increases airway resistance, requiring the respiratory muscles to work much harder and consume more oxygen just to ventilate a given amount of air. If a person quits smoking, exercise does help increase the functional capacity of the pulmonary system.

A regular exercise program seems to be a powerful incentive to quit smoking. A random survey of 1,250 runners conducted at the 6.2-mile Peachtree Road Race in Atlanta provided impressive results. The survey indicated that of the men and women who smoked cigarettes when they started running, 81 and 75 percent, respectively, had quit before the date of the race.

9. How Long Should People Wait after a Meal before Exercising Strenuously?

The length of time to wait before exercising after a meal depends on the amount of food eaten. On the average, after a regular meal, people should wait about 2 hours before participating in strenuous physical activity. But a walk or some other light physical activity is fine following a meal. If anything, it helps burn extra calories and may help the body metabolize fats more efficiently.

10. What Type of Clothing Should People Wear When Exercising?

The type of clothing worn during exercise is important. In general, clothing should fit comfortably and allow free movement of the various body parts. Select clothing according to air temperature, humidity, and exercise intensity. Avoid nylon and rubberized materials and tight clothes that interfere with the cooling mechanism of the human body or obstruct normal blood flow. Choose fabrics made of polypropylene, Capilene, Thermax, or any synthetic that draws (wicks) moisture away from the skin, enhancing evaporation and cooling of the body. It's also important to consider exercise intensity, because the harder a person exercises, the more heat the body produces.

When exercising in the heat, avoid the hottest time of the day, between 11:00 a.m. and 5:00 p.m. Surfaces such as asphalt, concrete, and artificial turf absorb heat, which then radiates to the body. Therefore, these surfaces are not recommended. (Also see the discussion about heat and humidity in the section "Why Is Exercising in Hot and Humid Conditions Unsafe?")

Only a minimal amount of clothing is necessary during exercise in the heat, to allow for maximal evaporation. Clothing should be lightweight, light-colored, loose-fitting, airy, and absorbent. Examples of commercially available products that can be used during exercise in the heat are CoolMax and Nike's Dri-FIT. Double-layer acrylic socks are more absorbent than cotton and help prevent blistering and chafing of the feet. A straw-type hat can be worn to protect the eyes and head from the sun. (Clothing for exercise in the cold is discussed in the "What Precautions Must People Take When Exercising in the Cold?" section, page 358.)

For decades, a good pair of shoes has been recommended by most professionals to prevent injuries to lower limbs. Shoes manufactured specifically for the choice of activity have been encouraged. Shoes should have good stability, motion control, and comfortable fit. Purchase shoes in the middle of or later in the day when feet have expanded and might be one half size larger. For increased breathability, shoes with nylon or mesh uppers are recommended. Salespeople at reputable athletic shoe stores can help you select a good shoe that fits your needs.

More recently, a trend has emerged toward barefoot running. For most of human history, people ran either barefoot or with minimal shoes. As in walking, the modern running shoe with its bulky padded heel cushion allows runners to land on the heel and roll forward toward the ball of the foot. The impact-collision force while running is often more than three times the person's body weight. Researchers have observed that joggers and runners who don't wear shoes, or who use minimal footwear, land on the front (ball) or middle of the

Dysmenorrhea Painful menstruation.

Amenorrhea Cessation of regular menstrual flow.

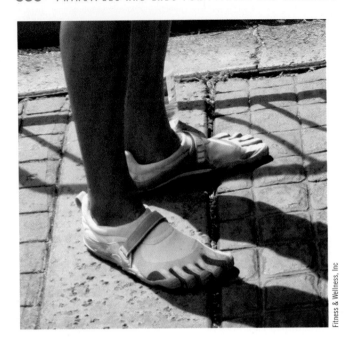
Fitness & Wellness, Inc

Minimalist Running Shoes

foot. This motion induces them to flex the ankle as contact is made with the ground, resulting in smaller impact forces than ankle-strike runners. Such running mechanics are thought to decrease impact-related repetitive stress injuries.

Some experts believe that both the spring in the arch of the foot and the Achilles tendon diminish ground-impact forces. A good illustration is to compare the impact forces generated by landing a jump on the heels versus on the toes.

Shoeless-running proponents believe that wearing cushioned shoes with arch supports alters natural foot-landing actions, weakening muscles and ligaments and rendering feet, ankles, and knees more susceptible to injuries. They recommend wearing a flexible shoe without a heel cushion or arch support. This recommendation has led to the development of barefoot running "shoes." These shoes feature a thin, abrasion-resistant stretch nylon with breathable mesh upper material that wraps around the entire foot to keep rocks and dirt out. At present, the verdict is still out. Data are insufficient to support either recommendation (shoe versus shoeless running). Research is being conducted to determine the best type of footwear to use with repetitive-impact activities. If you decide to give shoeless running a try, be sure to make a gradual transition into the minimal footwear; otherwise, you may end up with a challenging or severe injury (including foot fractures).

11. What Time of the Day Is Best for Exercise?

You can do intense exercise almost any time of the day, with the exception of about 2 hours following a heavy meal or the midday and early afternoon hours on hot, humid days. Moderate exercise seems to be beneficial shortly after a meal, because exercise enhances the **thermogenic response**. A walk shortly after a meal burns more calories than a walk several hours after a meal.

Many people enjoy exercising early in the morning because it gives them a boost to start the day. People who exercise in the morning also seem to stick with it more than others, because the chances of putting off the exercise session for other reasons are minimized. Some prefer the lunch hour for weight-control reasons. By exercising at noon, they do not eat as big a lunch, which helps keep down the daily caloric intake. Highly stressed people seem to like the evening hours because of the relaxing effects of exercise.

12. Why Is Exercising in Hot and Humid Conditions Unsafe?

When a person exercises, only 30 to 40 percent of the energy the body produces is used for mechanical work or movement. The rest of the energy (60 to 70 percent) is converted into heat. If this heat cannot be dissipated properly because the weather is too hot or the relative humidity is too high, body temperature increases; in extreme cases, it can result in death.

The specific heat of body tissue (the heat required to raise the temperature of the body by 1°C) is .38 calorie per pound of body weight (.38 cal/lb). This indicates that if no body heat is dissipated, a 150-pound person has to burn only 57 calories (150 × .38) to increase total body temperature by 1°C. If this person were to conduct an exercise session requiring 300 calories (e.g., running about 3 miles) without any dissipation of heat, the inner body temperature would increase by 5.3°C (300 ÷ 57), which is the equivalent of going from 98.6°F to 108.1°F.

This example illustrates clearly the need for caution when exercising in hot or humid weather. If the relative humidity is too high, body heat cannot be lost through evaporation because the atmosphere is already saturated with water vapor. In one instance, a football casualty occurred when the temperature was only 64°F but the relative humidity was 100 percent. People must be cautious when air temperature is above 90°F and the relative humidity is above 60 percent.

The American College of Sports Medicine recommends avoiding strenuous physical activity when the readings of a wet-bulb globe thermometer exceed 82.4°F. With this type of thermometer, the wet bulb is cooled by evaporation, and on dry days, it shows a lower temperature than the regular (dry) thermometer. On humid days, the cooling effect is less because of less evaporation; hence, the difference between the wet and dry readings is not as great.

Following are descriptions of, and first-aid measures for, the three major signs of heat illness:

- **Heat cramps.** Symptoms include cramps, spasms, and muscle twitching in the legs, arms, and abdomen. To relieve heat cramps, stop exercising, get out of the heat, massage the painful area, stretch slowly, and drink plenty of fluids (water, fruit drinks, or electrolyte beverages).
- **Heat exhaustion.** Symptoms include fainting, dizziness, profuse sweating, cold and clammy skin, weakness, headache, and a rapid, weak pulse. If you incur any of these symptoms, stop and find a cool place to rest. If conscious,

Symptoms of Heat Illness

If any of these symptoms occur, stop physical activity, get out of the sun, and start drinking fluids.

- Decreased perspiration
- Cramping
- Weakness
- Flushed skin
- Throbbing head
- Nausea/vomiting
- Diarrhea
- Numbness in the extremities
- Blurred vision
- Unsteadiness
- Disorientation
- Incoherency

drink cool water. Do not give water to an unconscious person. Loosen or remove clothing and rub your body with a cool, wet towel or apply ice packs. Place yourself in a supine position with the legs elevated 8 to 12 inches. If you are not fully recovered in 30 minutes, seek immediate medical attention.

- **Heat stroke.** Symptoms include serious disorientation; warm, dry skin; no sweating; rapid, full pulse; vomiting; diarrhea; unconsciousness; and high body temperature. As the body temperature climbs, unexplained anxiety sets in. When the body temperature reaches 104°F to 105°F, you may feel a cold sensation in the trunk of the body, goose bumps, nausea, throbbing in the temples, and numbness in the extremities. Most people become incoherent after this stage.

When body temperature reaches 105°F to 107°F, disorientation, loss of fine-motor control, and muscular weakness set in. If the temperature exceeds 106°F, serious neurological injury and death may be imminent.

Heat stroke requires immediate emergency medical attention. Request help and get out of the sun and into a cool, humidity-controlled environment. While you are waiting to be taken to the hospital emergency room, you should be placed in a semiseated position, and your body should be sprayed with cool water and rubbed with cool towels. If possible, cold packs should be placed in areas that receive an abundant blood supply, such as the head, neck, armpits, and groin. Fluids should not be given if you are unconscious; in any case of heat-related illness, if the person refuses water, vomits, or starts to lose consciousness, an ambulance should be summoned immediately. Proper initial treatment of heat stroke is vital.

13. What Should People Do To Replace Fluids Lost during Prolonged Aerobic Exercise?

Starting a workout with the body well-hydrated is important for health and performance prior to prolonged aerobic exercise. Exercise performance is impaired when an individual is dehydrated by as little as 2 percent of body weight. Dehydration at 5 percent of body weight decreases performance by about 30 percent.

Thirst is not an adequate indicator of hydration, as feelings of thirst indicate that dehydration has already begun. In preparation for prolonged exercise, the recommendation is to drink plenty of fluids the day before the activity, 16 to 20 ounces about 4 hours prior to exercise, and another 8 to 12 ounces 15 minutes before the start of the activity.

The main objective of fluid replacement during prolonged aerobic exercise is to maintain the blood volume so that circulation and sweating can continue at normal levels. Adequate water replacement is the most important factor in preventing heat disorders. Drinking about 6 to 8 ounces of cool water every 15 to 20 minutes during exercise is recommended to prevent dehydration. Cold fluids seem to be absorbed more rapidly from the stomach.

Other relevant points are the following:

- Drinking commercially prepared sports drinks is recommended when exercise will be strenuous and carried out for more than an hour. For exercise lasting less than an hour, water is just as effective in replacing lost fluid. The sports drinks you select may be based on your personal preference. Try different drinks at 6 to 8 percent glucose concentration to see which drink you tolerate best and suits your tastes as well.
- Commercial fluid-replacement solutions (e.g., Powerade and Gatorade) contain about 6 to 8 percent glucose, which seems to be optimal for fluid absorption and performance. Sugar does not become available to the muscles until about 30 minutes after consumption of a glucose solution.
- Drinks high in fructose or with a glucose concentration above 8 percent are not recommended, because they slow water absorption during exercise in the heat.
- Most sodas (both cola and noncola) contain between 10 and 12 percent glucose, which is too high for proper rehydration during exercise in the heat.
- Do not overhydrate with just water during a very or ultra–long-distance event, because doing so can

Thermogenic response The amount of energy required to digest food.

Heat cramps Muscle spasms caused by heat-induced changes in electrolyte balance in muscle cells.

Heat exhaustion Heat-related fatigue.

Heat stroke An emergency situation resulting from the body being subjected to high atmospheric temperatures.

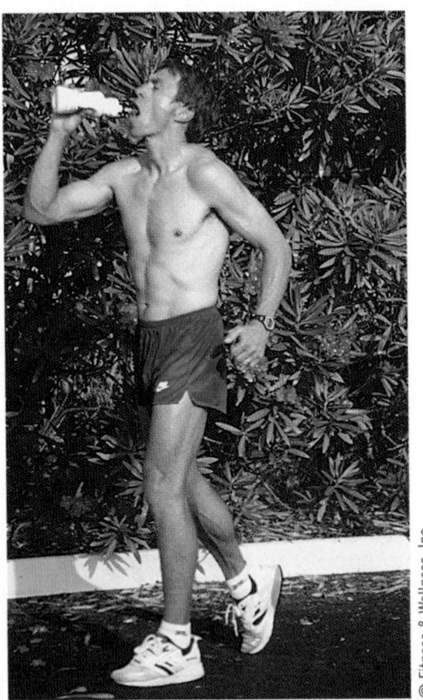

Fluid and carbohydrate replacement are essential when exercising in the heat or for a prolonged period.

lead to hyponatremia (see also "Hyponatremia" in Chapter 3, page 119) or low sodium concentration in the blood. When water loss through sweat during prolonged exercise is replaced by water alone, blood sodium is diluted to the point where it creates serious health problems, including seizures and coma in severe cases.

14. What Precautions Must People Take When Exercising in the Cold?

When exercising in the cold, the two factors to consider are frostbite and **hypothermia**. In contrast to hot and humid conditions, cold weather usually does not threaten health, because clothing can be selected for heat conservation and exercise itself increases the production of body heat.

Most people actually overdress for exercise in the cold. Because exercise increases body temperature, a moderate workout on a cold day makes a person feel that the temperature is 20°F to 30°F warmer than it actually is. Overdressing for exercise can make clothes damp from excessive perspiration. The risk for hypothermia increases when a person is wet or after exercise stops, when the individual is not moving around sufficiently to increase (or maintain) body heat.

Initial warning signs of hypothermia include shivering, losing coordination, and having difficulty speaking. With a continued drop in body temperature, shivering stops, the muscles weaken and stiffen, and the person feels elated or intoxicated and eventually loses consciousness. To prevent hypothermia, use common sense, dress properly, and be aware of environmental conditions.

The popular belief that exercising in cold temperatures (32°F and lower) freezes the lungs is false, because the air is warmed properly in the air passages before it reaches the lungs. Cold is not what poses a threat; wind velocity is what increases the chill factor most.

For example, exercising at a temperature of 25°F with adequate clothing is not too cold to exercise, but if the wind is blowing at 25 miles per hour, the chill factor lowers the actual temperature to 15°F. This effect is even worse if a person is wet and exhausted. When the weather is windy, the individual should exercise (jog or cycle) against the wind on the way out and with the wind upon returning.

Even though the lungs are under no risk when exercising in the cold, the face, head, hands, and feet should be protected because they are subject to frostbite. Watch for signs of frostbite: numbness and discoloration. In cold temperatures, as much as half of the body's heat can be lost through an unprotected head and neck. A wool or synthetic cap, hood, or hat helps hold in body heat. Mittens are better than gloves, because they keep the fingers together so that they lessen the surface area from which the person can lose heat. Inner linings of synthetic material to wick moisture away from the skin are recommended. Avoid cotton next to the skin, because once cotton gets wet, whether from perspiration, rain, or snow, it loses its insulating properties.

Wearing several layers of lightweight clothing is preferable to wearing a single, thick layer, because warm air is trapped between layers of clothes, enabling greater heat conservation. As body temperature increases, the individual can remove layers as necessary.

The first layer of clothes should wick moisture away from the skin. Polypropylene, Capilene, and Thermax are recommended materials. Next, a layer of wool, Dacron, or polyester fleece insulates well even when wet. Lycra tights or sweatpants help protect the legs. The outer layer should be waterproof, wind resistant, and breathable. A synthetic material such as Gore-Tex is best so that moisture can still escape from the body. A ski mask or face mask helps protect the face. In extremely cold conditions, exposed skin, such as the nose, cheeks, and around the eyes, can be insulated with petroleum jelly.

For lengthy or long-distance workouts (cross-country skiing or long runs), exercisers should take a small backpack to carry the removed clothing. Individuals also can carry extra warm and dry clothes in case they stop exercising away from shelter. If people remain outdoors following exercise, added clothing and continuous body movement are essential to maintain body temperature and avoid hypothermia.

15. Can People Exercise When They Have a Cold or the Flu?

The most important considerations are to use common sense and pay attention to symptoms when considering illness and exercise. Usually, people may continue to exercise if symptoms include a runny nose, sneezing, or a scratchy throat. But, if symptoms include fever, muscle ache, vomiting, diarrhea, or a hacking cough, people should avoid exercise. After an illness, it is important to ease back gradually into a program. People should not attempt to return at the same intensity and duration that they were used to prior to the illness.

Exercise-Related Injuries

To enjoy and maintain physical fitness, preventing injury during a conditioning program is essential. Nonetheless, exercise-related injuries are common in individuals who participate in exercise programs. Surveys indicate that more than half of all new participants incur injuries during the first 6 months of the conditioning program.

Most exercise-related injuries, nonetheless, are preventable. The four most common causes of injuries are:

1. High-impact activities
2. Rapid conditioning programs (doing too much too quickly)
3. Improper shoes or training surfaces
4. Anatomical predisposition (i.e., body propensity)

High-impact activities and a significant increase in quantity (duration) of activities are by far the most common causes of injuries. The body requires time to adapt to more intense activities. Most of these injuries can be prevented through a gradual and correct conditioning (low-impact) program. Softer training surfaces, such as artificial turf, grass, or dirt, produce less trauma than wood, asphalt, or concrete.

Because few people have perfect body alignment, injuries associated with overtraining may occur eventually. In case of injury, proper treatment can avert a lengthy recovery process. A summary of common exercise-related injuries and how to manage them follows.

Acute Sports Injuries

The best treatment always has been prevention. If an activity causes unusual discomfort or chronic irritation, you need to treat the cause by decreasing the intensity, switching activities, substituting equipment, or upgrading clothing (e.g., buying proper-fitting shoes).

In cases of acute injury, the standard treatment is rest, ice (cold application), compression (or splinting or both), and elevation of the affected body part. This is commonly referred to as **RICE**.

R = rest

I = ice (cold) application

C = compression

E = elevation

Cold should be applied three to five times a day for 15 minutes at a time during the first 36 to 48 hours by submerging the injured area in cold water, using an ice bag, or applying ice massage to the affected part. An elastic bandage or wrap can be used for compression. Elevating the body part decreases blood flow (and therefore swelling) in that body part.

The purpose of these treatment modalities is to minimize swelling in the area and thus hasten recovery time. After the first 36 to 48 hours, heat can be used if the injury shows no further swelling or inflammation. If you have doubts as to the nature or seriousness of the injury (e.g., suspected fracture), you should seek a medical evaluation.

Obvious deformities (e.g., exhibited by fractures, dislocations, or partial dislocations) call for splinting, cold application with an ice bag, and medical attention. Do not try to reset any of these conditions by yourself, because you could further damage muscles, ligaments, and nerves. Treatment of these injuries should always be left to specialized medical personnel. A quick reference guide for the signs or symptoms and treatment of exercise-related problems is provided in Table 9.5.

Muscle Soreness and Stiffness

Individuals who begin an exercise program or participate after a long layoff from exercise often develop muscle soreness and stiffness. The acute soreness that sets in the first few hours after exercise is thought to be related to general fatigue of the exercised muscles.

Delayed muscle soreness that appears several hours after exercise (usually about 12 hours later) and lasts 2 to 4 days may be related to actual microtears in muscle tissue, muscle spasms that increase fluid retention (stimulating the pain nerve endings), and overstretching or tearing of connective tissue in and around muscles and joints.

Mild stretching before and adequate stretching after exercise help prevent soreness and stiffness. Gradually progressing into an exercise program is also important. A person should not attempt to do too much too quickly. To relieve pain, mild stretching, light-intensity exercise to stimulate blood flow, and a warm bath are recommended.

Exercise Intolerance

When starting an exercise program, you should stay within the safe limits. The best method to determine whether you are exercising too strenuously is to check your heart rate and make sure it does not exceed the limits of your target zone. Exercising above this target zone may not be safe for unconditioned or high-risk individuals. You do not have to exercise beyond your target zone to gain the desired cardiorespiratory benefits.

Several physical signs will tell you when you are exceeding your functional limitations—that is, experiencing **exercise intolerance**. Signs of intolerance include rapid or irregular heart rate, difficult breathing, nausea, vomiting, lightheadedness, headache, dizziness, unusually flushed or pale skin, extreme weakness, lack of energy, shakiness, sore muscles, cramps,

Hypothermia A breakdown in the body's ability to generate heat; a drop in body temperature below 95°F.

RICE An acronym used to describe the standard treatment procedure for acute sports injuries: *r*est, *i*ce (cold application), *c*ompression, and *e*levation.

Exercise intolerance The inability to function during exercise because of excessive fatigue or extreme feelings of discomfort.

and tightness in the chest. Learn to listen to your body. If you notice any of these symptoms, seek medical attention before continuing your exercise program.

Recovery heart rate is another indicator of overexertion. To a certain extent, recovery heart rate is related to fitness level. The higher your cardiorespiratory fitness level, the faster your heart rate decreases following exercise. As a rule, heart rate should be below 120 beats per minute (bpm) 5 minutes into recovery. If your heart rate is above 120 bpm, you most likely have overexerted yourself or could have some other cardiac abnormality. If you lower the intensity of exercise, the duration of exercise, or both and still have a fast heart rate 5 minutes into recovery, consult your physician.

Side Stitch **Side stitch** is a cramplike pain in the rib cage that can develop in the early stages of participation in exercise. It occurs primarily in unconditioned beginners and in trained individuals when they exercise at higher intensities than usual. As their physical condition improves, this condition tends to disappear unless training is intensified.

The exact cause is unknown. Some experts suggest that it could relate to a lack of blood flow to the respiratory muscles during strenuous physical exertion. Some people encounter side stitch during downhill running. If you experience side stitch during exercise, slow down. If it persists, stop altogether. Lying down on your back and gently bringing both knees to the chest and holding that position for 30 to 60 seconds also helps.

Some people get side stitch if they drink juice or eat anything shortly before exercise. Drinking only water 1 to 2 hours prior to exercise sometimes prevents side stitch. Other individuals have problems with commercially available sports drinks during vigorous-intensity exercise. Unless carbohydrate replacement is crucial to complete a long-distance event (more than 60 minutes, such as road cycling, a marathon, or a triathlon), drink cool water for fluid replacement or try a different carbohydrate solution.

Shin Splints **Shin splints**, one of the most common injuries to the lower limbs, usually results from one or more of the following: (1) lack of proper and gradual conditioning, (2) doing physical activities on hard surfaces (wooden floors, hard tracks, cement, or asphalt), (3) fallen foot arches, (4) chronic overuse, (5) muscle fatigue, (6) faulty posture, (7) improper shoes, or (8) participating in weight-bearing activities when excessively overweight.

TABLE 9.5 Reference Guide for Exercise-Related Problems

Injury	Signs/Symptoms	Treatment*
Bruise (contusion)	Pain, swelling, discoloration	Cold application, compression, rest
Dislocations/fracture	Pain, swelling, deformity	Splinting, cold application, seek medical attention
Heat cramp	Cramps, spasms, and muscle twitching in the legs, arms, and abdomen	Stop activity, get out of the heat, stretch, massage the painful area, drink plenty of fluids
Heat exhaustion	Fainting, profuse sweating, cold/clammy skin, weak/rapid pulse, weakness, headache	Stop activity, rest in a cool place, loosen clothing, rub body with cool/wet towel, drink plenty of fluids, stay out of heat for 2–3 days
Heat stroke	Hot/dry skin, no sweating, serious disorientation, rapid/full pulse, vomiting, diarrhea, unconsciousness, high body temperature	**Seek immediate medical attention,** request help and get out of the sun, bathe in cold water/spray with cold water/rub body with cold towels, drink plenty of cold fluids
Joint sprains	Pain, tenderness, swelling, loss of use, discoloration	Cold application, compression, elevation, rest; heat after 36–48 hours (if no further swelling)
Muscle cramps	Pain, spasm	Stretch muscle(s), use mild exercises for involved area
Muscle soreness and stiffness	Tenderness, pain	Mild stretching, low-intensity exercise, warm bath
Muscle strains	Pain, tenderness, swelling, loss of use	Cold application, compression, elevation, rest; heat after 36–48 hours (if no further swelling)
Shin splints	Pain, tenderness	Cold application prior to and following any physical activity, rest; heat (if no activity is carried out)
Side stitch	Pain on the side of the abdomen below the rib cage	Decrease level of physical activity or stop altogether, gradually increase level of fitness
Tendinitis	Pain, tenderness, loss of use	Rest, cold application, heat after 48 hours

*Cold should be applied three to five times a day for 15 minutes. Heat can be applied three times a day for 15–20 minutes.

To manage shin splints, do the following:

1. Remove or reduce the cause (exercise on softer surfaces, wear better shoes or arch supports, or stop exercise until the shin splints heal).
2. Do stretching exercises before and after physical activity.
3. Use ice massage for 10 to 20 minutes before and after exercise.
4. Apply active heat (whirlpool and hot baths) for 15-minute sessions two to three times a day.
5. Use supportive taping during physical activity (a qualified athletic trainer can teach you the proper taping technique).

Muscle Cramps Muscle cramps are caused by the body's depletion of essential electrolytes or a breakdown in the coordination between opposing muscle groups. If you have a muscle cramp, you should first attempt to stretch the muscles involved. In the case of the calf muscle, for example, pull your toes up toward the knees. After stretching the muscle, rub it down gently. Finally, do some mild exercises requiring the use of that muscle.

In pregnant and lactating women, muscle cramps often are related to a lack of calcium. If women get cramps during these times, calcium supplements usually relieve the problem. Tight clothing also can cause cramps by decreasing blood flow to active muscle tissue.

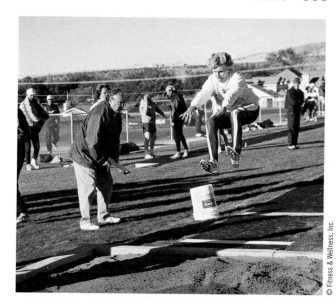

Older adults who exercise enjoy better health, functional capacity, and quality of life and live longer than physically inactive adults.

Exercise and Aging

The elderly constitute the fastest-growing segment of the population. The number of Americans ages 65 and older increased from 3.1 million in 1900 (4.1 percent of the population) to about 40 million (13 percent) in 2010. By 2030, more than 72 million people, or 20 percent of the U.S. population, are expected to be older than 65.

The main objectives of fitness programs for older adults should be to help them improve their functional status and contribute to healthy aging. This implies the ability to maintain independent living status and to avoid disability. Older adults are encouraged to participate in programs that help develop cardiorespiratory endurance, muscular fitness, muscular flexibility, agility, balance, and motor coordination.

Physical Training in the Older Adult

Regular participation in physical activity provides both physical and psychological benefits to older adults. In particular, regular physical activity decreases the risk for cardiovascular disease, stroke, hypertension, type 2 diabetes, osteoporosis, obesity, colon cancer, breast cancer, cognitive impairment, anxiety and depression, and even dementia and Alzheimer's.[7] Physical activity also improves self-confidence and self-esteem. Furthermore, both cardiorespiratory endurance and strength training help increase functional capacity, improve overall health status, improve memory and mental acumen, and increase life expectancy. Strength training also decreases the rate at which strength and muscle mass are lost.

The trainability of older men and women alike and the effectiveness of physical activity in enhancing health have been demonstrated in research. Older adults who increase their physical activity experience significant changes in cardiorespiratory endurance, strength, and flexibility. The extent of the changes depends on their initial fitness level and the types of activities they select for their training (walking, cycling, strength training, etc.).

Improvements in maximal oxygen uptake in older adults are similar to those in younger people, although older people seem to require a longer training period to achieve these changes. Declines in maximal oxygen uptake average about 1 percent per year between ages 25 and 75. A slower rate of decline is seen in people who maintain a lifetime aerobic exercise program.

Results of research on the effects of aging on the cardiorespiratory system of male exercisers versus nonexercisers showed that the maximal oxygen uptake of regular exercisers was almost twice that of the nonexercisers (Table 9.6).[8] The study revealed a decline in maximal oxygen uptake between ages 50 and 68 of only 13 percent in the active group compared with 41 percent in the

Side stitch A sharp pain in the side of the abdomen.

Shin splints Injury to the lower leg characterized by pain and irritation in the shin region of the leg.

inactive group. These changes indicate that about one-third of the loss in maximal oxygen uptake results from aging and that two-thirds of the loss comes from inactivity. Blood pressure, heart rate, and body weight also were remarkably better in the exercising group. Aerobic training seems to decrease high blood pressure in older patients at the same rate as in young hypertensive people.

In terms of aging, muscle strength declines by 10 to 20 percent between ages 20 and 50; between ages 50 and 70, it drops by another 25 to 30 percent. Through strength training, frail adults in their 80s or 90s can double or triple their strength in just a few months. The amount of muscle hypertrophy achieved, however, decreases with age. Strength gains close to 200 percent have been found in previously inactive adults over age 90.[9] In fact, research has shown that regular strength training improves balance, gait, speed, **functional independence**, morale, depression symptoms, and energy intake.[10] Strength-trained older adults are 30 to 50 percent stronger than their sedentary counterparts.

Although muscle flexibility drops by about 5 percent per decade of life, 10 minutes of stretching every other day can prevent most of this loss as people age. Improved flexibility also enhances mobility skills. The latter promotes independence because it helps older adults successfully perform activities of daily living.

In terms of body composition, lean body mass typically declines by 2 to 3 percent per decade starting at age 30. Muscle mass starts to decrease at age 40 and accelerates after age 65, with the legs losing muscle mass at a faster rate. Sedentary adults gain about 20 to 40 pounds of body weight between ages 18 and 55. As a result, body fat continues to increase through adult life, with a greater tendency toward visceral fat accumulation (especially in men) leading to further increase in risk for chronic disease. Regular aerobic activity and strength training have been shown to help older adults properly manage body weight and significantly reduce visceral fat.

TABLE 9.6 Effects of Physical Activity and Inactivity on Older Men

	Exercisers	Nonexercisers
Age (yr)	68.0	69.8
Weight (lb)	160.3	186.3
Resting heart rate (bpm)	55.8	66.0
Maximal heart rate (bpm)	157.0	146.0
Heart rate reserve* (bpm)	101.2	80.0
Blood pressure (mm Hg)	120/78	150/90
Maximal oxygen uptake (mL/kg/min)	38.6	20.3

*Heart rate reserve = maximal heart rate − resting heart rate.
Data from F. W. Kash, J. L. Boyer, S. P. Van Camp, L. S. Verity, and J. P. Wallace, "The Effect of Physical Activity on Aerobic Power in Older Men (A Longitudinal Study)," *The Physician and Sports Medicine* 18, no. 4 (1990): 73–83.

A slight decline in memory is also typically associated with aging. Part of this is due to reduction in the size of the hippocampus, the region of the brain primarily responsible for memory. This region begins to decrease in mass by .5 percent each year, beginning as early as age 40. Recent studies, however, have shown promise in this area that has surpassed the hopes of researchers. Regular physical activity, aerobic exercise, and strength training all have been shown to increase the size of the hippocampus and decrease the rate of brain shrinkage. Maintaining a high level of physical fitness in mid-life can reduce a person's chances of developing Alzheimer's by half and dementia by 60 percent.[11] Even becoming physically active later in life has been shown to produce measurable gains in the weight of the hippocampus following just a few months of training.

Older adults who wish to initiate an exercise program are strongly encouraged to have a complete medical evaluation. Particularly for aging adults, any physical activity program needs to be highly personalized to accommodate health needs and highly varying levels of fitness. An interesting trend among older adults is the growing number of individuals who, once retired, choose to certify as personal trainers to help other older adults develop fitness. Recommended activities for older adults include calisthenics, walking, jogging, swimming, cycling, and water aerobics. Strength training is particularly important for bone health in the absence of weight-bearing aerobic activities.

Older people should avoid isometric and very high-intensity weight-training exercises (see Chapter 7). Activities that require all-out effort or that require participants to hold their breath tend to lessen blood flow to the heart, cause a significant increase in blood pressure, and increase the load placed on the heart. Older adults should participate in activities that require continuous and rhythmic muscular activity (about 40 to 60 percent of heart rate reserve). These activities do not cause large increases in blood pressure or overload the heart.

Mind–body activities such as Tai Chi offer a particular boon in overall mental and physical health. While providing the same cardiorespiratory workout as a moderate-paced walk, Tai Chi also improves posture and strength, promotes healthy breathing habits, trains the body in balance, and can improve sensitivity in the soles of the feet, which helps with balance and increased walking speed.

Preparing for Sports Participation

To enhance your participation in sports, keep in mind that in most cases it is better to get fit before playing sports

Functional independence The ability to carry out activities of daily living without assistance from other individuals.

High Intensity Interval Training (HIIT)

HIIT is a challenging training program that involves high- to very-high-intensity (80 to 90 percent of maximal capacity) intervals, each followed by a low- to moderate-intensity recovery interval. Usually a 1:3 or lower work-to-recovery ratio is used. HIIT provides greater health and fitness benefits than traditional lower-intensity programs. Fitness enthusiasts like HIIT because higher fitness and weight loss goals are reached with this type of training, often with workout sessions of shorter length, as long as caloric intake is carefully monitored and not increased following training. While originally used primarily for cardiorespiratory training, HIIT is increasingly being applied to resistance work, plyometrics, and other types of workouts. One type of HIIT that is growing in popularity is commonly applied to a wide variety of workouts but has exact time prescriptions. It is called the Tabata method. This modality was named after the researcher working with the Japanese speed skating team who tested a variation of workout-to-recovery ratios and honed in on a prescription he found particularly effective: 20 seconds of all-out exertion followed by 10 seconds of rest, repeated in cycles of 4 minutes at a time.[12]

Stability Exercise Balls

Stability exercise balls enhance stability, balance, and muscular fitness. The emphasis is on correct movements and maintenance of proper body alignment while involving the core as much as possible. Additional exercises can be performed to strengthen other body areas. Further information on Stability Exercise Balls and sample exercises are provided in Chapter 7, page 280).

Core Training

The "core" of the body consists of the muscles that stabilize the trunk (spine) and pelvis. Core training emphasizes conditioning of all the muscles around the abdomen, pelvis, lower back, and hips. These muscles enhance body stability, activities of daily living, sport performance, and support the lower back. Core conditioning often incorporates the use of stability balls, foam rollers, and wobble boards, among other pieces of equipment. Further information on Core Strength Training is provided in Chapter 7 (page 279).

Group Personal Training

Personal trainers are increasingly working with small groups of two to three exercisers to continue providing individualized instruction while keeping costs reasonable. The demand for personal trainers will likely be high for years to come as individuals look to personalize workouts and find ways to fit exercise into their schedule. New technology like web-based workout programs and wearable monitors are growing in popularity and are likely to assist personal trainers in their task of supporting customers through a lifestyle change.

Outdoor Training

The lines between indoor and outdoor activities have faded in recent years. While traditional outdoor sports like rock climbing, cycling, and surfing find their indoor fitness audience, many exercisers are taking their workouts outdoors. Spurred especially by the growing popularity of adventure races, people are taking up sports like trail running, cycling, cross country skiing, fast packing, and rowing among others. Triathlons and swimbike races are signing up participants in record numbers. The outdoor setting itself seems to boost mood during exercise, which may explain why even bodyweight training, HIIT, and group sessions with personal trainers are increasingly taking to the open air.

Fitness Boot Camp

A vigorous-intensity outdoor/indoor group exercise program combines traditional calisthenics, running, interval training, bodyweight training (using exercises such as push ups, lunges, pull ups, burpees, squats), plyometrics (see Chapter 7, page 276), and competitive games to develop cardiorespiratory fitness, muscular fitness, muscular flexibility, and lose body fat. This program is based on military-style training and also aims at developing camaraderie and team effort. The program (camp) typically lasts 4 to 8 weeks. Fitness boot camps are challenging, but the group dynamic helps to motivate participants.

Bodyweight Training

Bodyweight training has been around as a strength-training modality for centuries, but fitness enthusiasts are now embracing the concept as they seek to "return to basics." Bodyweight training participants use their own body weight as resistance to develop fitness. Bodyweight exercises are ideal for individuals interested in fitness who do not have access to equipment or facilities. Because body weight provides the only source of resistance, a training session can be conducted anywhere. Exercise examples include pull-ups, push-ups, modified dips, curl-ups, step-ups, prone and lateral bridges, and pelvic tilts. Some of these exercises are provided in the Strength-Training Exercises without Weights (Bodyweight Training) section on pages 286–290. As discussed next under "Circuit Training," bodyweight training can be used to develop both cardiorespiratory endurance and muscular fitness.

Circuit Training

Circuit training has also been around for decades. It was often used to condition elite athletes and military personnel in the

(Continued)

middle of the 20th century. Circuit training involves a combination of 6 to 12 aerobic and bodyweight-training (strength) exercises performed in rapid sequence one after the other, with very limited rest between exercise stations. Each exercise is performed for a given period of time (10 to 30 seconds) or by a specified number of repetitions (10 to 20 repetitions), typically interspaced by short rest periods of 10 to 30 seconds between exercises. Early on, you may use a moderate intensity (less time or repetitions per exercise) and allow longer rest (30 seconds) between exercises. Over the course of several weeks, you can gradually increase the intensity (time and/or repetitions) and decrease the rest interval between exercises. The exercise sequence is set in an order that allows for opposing muscle groups to alternate between exercise stations. For instance, push-ups can be followed by step-ups and abdominal crunches. The circuit training format can make use of strength-training equipment, but it also lends itself well to the body-weight training approach where the person's own body weight provides the resistance rather than using free weights or resistance training machines. Body weight circuit training is an effective and low-cost way to begin and maintain a fitness regimen. For best results, all major muscle groups of the body should be used in each circuit.

Because of the high intensity and limited rest intervals used with this type of training, the exercise modality is often referred to as high-intensity circuit training or HICT. The combination of high-intensity aerobic and bodyweight-strength training, with limited rest between exercises, can elicit similar or greater health and fitness benefits in a much shorter period of time than the traditional 20- to 60-minute sessions. An HICT session involving 12 different exercises can be performed in under 10 minutes per circuit. One to three circuits with 2 to 3 minutes rest between circuits can be performed per training session. When time is of the essence and a traditional training session is not realistic, an HICT session is recommended.

Functional Fitness

Functional fitness involves primarily weight-bearing exercises to develop balance, coordination, good posture, muscular fitness, and muscular flexibility to enhance the person's ability to perform activities of daily living (walking, climbing stairs, lifting, bending) with ease and with minimal risk for injuries. The program's goal is to "train people for real life," rather than a specific fitness component or a given event. Functional fitness training often requires use of fitness equipment such as stability balls, foam blocks, and balancing cushions. Fitness trainers plan classes to target specific everyday activities, even focusing movement around a theme. One class, for example, targeted all the movements used for an evening out to the theater—from side stepping down the aisle to sitting in and rising from the seat to climbing stairs for balcony seating.

Spinning

Spinning is a low-impact aerobic activity performed on specially designed Spinner stationary bicycles in a room or studio with motivational music and under the direction of a certified instructor. Spinning bikes feature racing handlebars, pedals with clips, adjustable seats, and a resistance knob to control workout intensity. Five workout stages, also known as "energy zones" are used to simulate actual cycling training and racing. The workouts are divided into endurance, all-terrain, strength, recovery, and advanced training. New approaches to spinning continue to develop, with cross-discipline classes like spin and swim. New companies are providing online social media support by allowing exercisers to challenge one another to virtual races and to see who is signing up for classes at their gym. Whatever the format, spinning provides a challenging workout for people of all ages and fitness levels.

Yoga

Yoga has proven itself to be more than a trend. Truly it is becoming a permanent institution of fitness. Yoga consists of a system of exercises designed to help align the musculo-skeletal system and develop flexibility, muscular fitness, and balance. Yoga is also used as a relaxation technique for stress management. The exercises involve a combination of postures (known as "asanas") along with diaphragmatic breathing, relaxation, and mediation techniques. Yoga continues to reinvent itself through both new and traditional forms that pop up in studios and gyms across the country. Variations of yoga you may find include anuara, ashtanga, bikram, integral, iyengar, kripalu, kundalini, sivananda, vinyasa, as well as cross-discipline options like yogalates and yogarobics.

Zumba

This dance fitness program was created in Colombia by Alberto "Beto" Perez in the mid-90s. Following great popularity in Colombia, the zumba program was brought to the United States in 1999. The program is now offered globally, and classes are offered at most health fitness clubs in the United States. Zumba combines Latin and international music (cumbia, salsa, merengue, reggaeton, tango, and rock and roll among others) with dance to develop fitness and make exercise fun. The zumba motto has become "Ditch the workout, join the party!" Several types of zumba have been developed, including traditional zumba, zumba gold, zumba toning, aqua zumba, zumbatomic, and zumba marumba.

Bike Commuting

A trend toward bike commuting is beginning to take hold in the United States. Already a transportation staple in Europe and other parts of the world, the bike is becoming the vehicle of choice for a growing number of commuters. Between 2000 and 2012, according to the League of American Bicyclists, the crowd of bike commuters grew by 62 percent, and the trend will only continue to grow in the future. Bike-sharing programs in large cities are helping the trend along and fueling a budding tendency toward building more bike-friendly communities. Arriving at work via bike commute means a start to the workday feeling energetic and positive, as opposed to lethargic and sedentary.

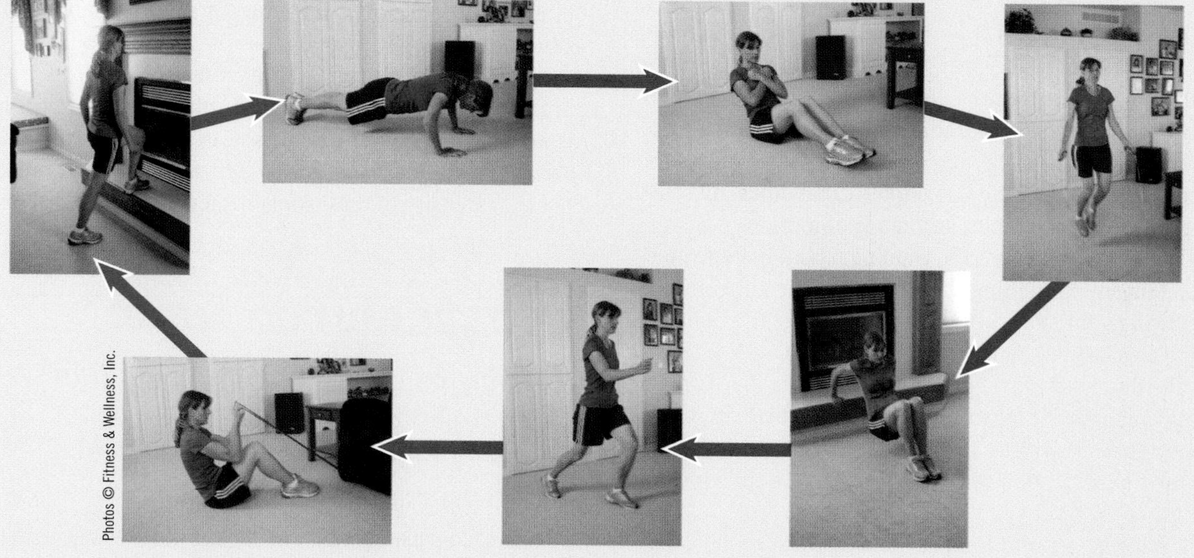

High-Intensity Circuit Training: When properly designed and implemented, a person's own body weight can be used to derive both cardiorespiratory endurance and muscular fitness benefits.

rather than playing sports to get fit.[13] A good preseason training program helps make the season more enjoyable and prevent exercise-related injuries.

Properly conditioned individuals can participate safely in sports and enjoy the activities to their fullest with few or no limitations. Unfortunately, sports injuries are often the result of poor fitness and a lack of sport-specific conditioning. Many injuries occur when fatigue sets in following overexertion by unconditioned individuals.

Base Fitness Conditioning

Preactivity screening that includes a health history (see Lab 1C, "PAR-Q and Health History Questionnaire," page 39), a medical evaluation appropriate to your sport selection, or both is recommended. Once cleared for exercise, start by building a base of general athletic fitness that includes the four health-related fitness components: cardiorespiratory fitness, muscular fitness (strength and endurance), flexibility, and recommended body composition. The base fitness conditioning program should last a minimum of 6 weeks.

As explained in Chapter 6, for cardiorespiratory fitness, select an activity that you enjoy (e.g., walking, jogging, cycling, step aerobics, cross-country skiing, or elliptical training) and train three to five times per week at a minimum of 20 minutes of continuous activity per session. Exercise between 60 and 80 percent intensity for adequate conditioning. You should feel as though you are training somewhat hard to hard at these intensity levels.

Strength (resistance) training helps maintain and increase muscular strength and endurance. Following the guidelines provided in Chapter 7, select 10 to 12 exercises that involve the major muscle groups and train two or three times per week on nonconsecutive days. Select a resistance (weight) that allows you to do 8 to 12 repetitions to near fatigue (8 to 12 RM zone based on your fitness goals—see Chapter 7). That is, the resistance should be heavy enough that when you perform one set of an exercise, you are not able to do more than the predetermined number of repetitions at that weight. Begin your program slowly and perform between one and three sets of each exercise. Recommended exercises include the bench (chest) press, lat pull-down, leg press, leg curl, triceps extension, arm curl, rowing torso, heel raise, abdominal crunch, and back extension.

Flexibility is important in sports participation to enhance the range of motion in the joints. Using the guidelines from Chapter 8, schedule flexibility training 2 or 3 days per week. Perform each stretching exercise four times, and hold each stretch for 10 to 60 seconds. Examples of stretching exercises include the side stretch, body rotation, chest stretch, shoulder hyperextension stretch, sit-and-reach stretch, adductor stretch, quad stretch, heel cord stretch, and single-knee-to-chest stretch.

In terms of body composition, excess body fat hinders sports performance and increases the risk for injuries. Depending on the nature of the activity, fitness goals for body composition range from 12 to 20 percent body fat for men and 17 to 25 percent body fat for most women.

Sport-Specific Conditioning

Once you have achieved the general fitness base, continue with the program but make adjustments to add sport-specific training. This training should match the sport's requirements for aerobic and anaerobic capabilities, muscular strength and/or endurance, and range of motion.

During the sport-specific training, about half of your aerobic/anaerobic training should involve the same muscles used during your sport. Ideally, allocate 4 weeks of sport-specific training before you start participating in the sport. Then continue the sport-specific training on a more limited basis throughout the season. Depending on the nature of the sport (aerobic versus anaerobic), once the season starts, the sports participation can take the place of some or all of your aerobic workouts.

The next step is to look at the demands of the sport. For example, soccer, bicycle racing, cross-country skiing, and snowshoeing are aerobic activities, whereas basketball, racquetball, alpine skiing, snowboarding, and ice hockey are stop-and-go sports that require a combination of aerobic and anaerobic activity. Consequently, aerobic training may be appropriate for cross-country skiing, but it will do little to prepare your muscles for the high-intensity requirements of combined aerobic and anaerobic sports.

High-intensity interval training (HIIT), performed twice per week, is added to the program at this time. HIIT allows you to break your workout into smaller segments so that you can perform a greater training volume at a higher exercise intensity. HIIT has been shown to help improve both aerobic and anaerobic fitness at a faster rate.

Four training variables impact HIIT. The acronym DIRT is frequently used to denote these variables:[14]

D = distance of each speed interval

I = interval or length of recovery between speed intervals

R = repetitions or number of speed intervals to be performed

T = time of each speed interval

Using these four variables, a person can design an unlimited number of HIIT sessions.

The intervals consist of a 1:4 to a 1:1 work-to-recovery ratio. The more intense the speed interval, the longer the required recovery interval. For aerobic intervals (lasting longer than 3 minutes), 1:2, 1:1, or even lower ratios are used. For intense anaerobic speed intervals (30 seconds to 3 minutes), recovery intervals that last two to four times as long as the work period (1:2 to 1:4) are required.

A 1:3 ratio, for example, indicates that you work at a fairly high intensity for, say, 30 seconds and then spend 90 seconds on light- to moderate-intensity recovery. Be sure to keep moving during the recovery phase. Perform four or five intervals at first, and then gradually progress to 10 intervals. As your fitness improves, you can lengthen the high-intensity proportion of the intervals progressively to 60 seconds, decrease the total recovery time, or both.

For aerobic sports, HIIT at least once per week improves performance. Most commonly done at a 1:2 or lower work-to-recovery ratio, you also can do a 5- to 10-minute aerobic work interval followed by 1 to 2 minutes of recovery, but the intensity of these longer intervals should not be as

confidentconsumer

High-intensity interval training (HIIT) programs are becoming very popular, do these programs really help lose weight?

HIIT is a combined aerobic and anaerobic training program that had been used mainly by athletes but is now being embraced by fitness participants seeking better, faster, and more effective development. Following an appropriate warm-up, HIIT includes high- to very high-intensity intervals that are interspersed with a low- to moderate-intensity recovery phase. Typically, a 1:4 or less work-to-recovery ratio is used; the more intense the interval, the longer the recovery period. Research indicates that additional health and fitness benefits are reaped as the intensity of exercise increases. HIIT produces the greatest improvements in aerobic capacity (VO_{2max}) and increases the capability to exercise at a higher percentage of that capacity (anaerobic threshold), thus allowing the participant to burn more calories during the exercise session. The data also show that HIIT increases the capacity for fat oxidation during exercise. Although the fuel used during high-intensity intervals is primarily glucose (carbohydrates), molecular changes occur in the muscle that increase the body's capability for fatty acid oxidation (fat burning). Furthermore, following light- to moderate-intensity aerobic activity, the resting metabolism returns to normal in about 90 minutes. Depending on the volume of training (intensity and number of intervals performed), with HIIT it takes 24 to 72 hours for the body to return to its normal resting metabolic rate. Thus, a greater amount of calories (primarily from fat) are burned up to 3 days following HIIT. Research data indicate that HIIT programs are more effective for weight loss, as long as the individual does not compensate with greater caloric intake following exercise. While the extra calories burned during recovery do make a difference in the long run, keep in mind that the most significant factor is the number of calories actually burned during the HIIT session itself.

BEHAVIOR MODIFICATION PLANNING

Common Signs and Symptoms of Overtraining

- Decreased fitness
- Decreased sports performance
- Increased fatigue
- Loss of concentration
- Staleness and burnout
- Loss of competitive drive
- Increased resting and exercise heart rate
- Decreased appetite
- Loss of body weight
- Altered sleep patterns
- Decreased sex drive
- Generalized body aches and pains
- Increased susceptibility to illness and injury
- Mood disturbances
- Depression

Try It

If following several weeks or months of hard training you experience some of the above symptoms, you need to substantially decrease training volume and intensity for a week or two. This recovery phase will allow the body to recover, strengthen, and prepare for the next training phase. In your Behavior Change Tracker or your Online Journals, modify your training program to allow a light week of training following each 5 to 8 weeks of hard exercise training.

high, and only three to five intervals are recommended. Note that the HIIT workouts are not performed in addition to the regular aerobic workouts; instead, they take the place of one of these workouts.

Consider sport-specific strength requirements as well. Look at the primary muscles used in your sport, and make sure your choice of exercises works those muscles. Try to perform your strength training through a range of motion similar to those used in your sport. Aerobic/anaerobic sports require greater strength; during the season, the recommendation is three sets of 8 to 12 repetitions to near fatigue, two or three times per week. For aerobic endurance sports, the recommendation is a minimum of one set of 8 to 12 repetitions to near fatigue, once or twice per week during the season.

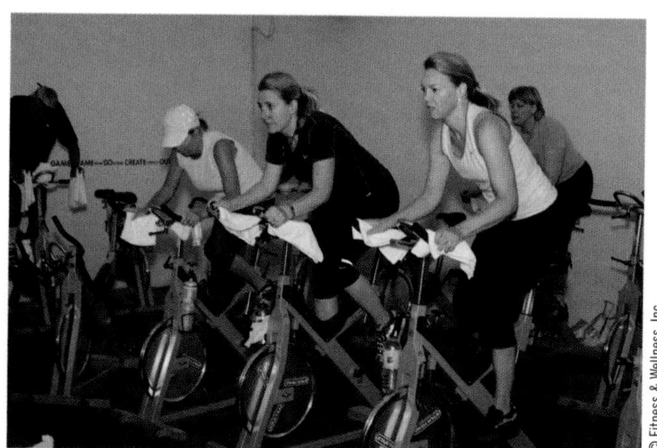

© Fitness & Wellness, Inc.

HIIT promotes fitness, enhances energy expenditure and weight loss, and augments health benefits.

Stop-and-go sports (basketball, racquetball, soccer, etc.) require greater strength than pure endurance sports (triathlon, long-distance running, cross-country skiing, etc.). For example, recreational participants during the sport-specific training phase for stop-and-go sports usually perform three sets of 8 to 12 repetitions to near fatigue, two to three times per week. Competitive athletes and those desiring greater strength gains typically conduct three to five sets of 4 to 12 repetitions to near fatigue three times per week.

For some winter sports, such as alpine skiing and snowboarding, gravity supplies most of the propulsion, and the body acts more as a shock absorber. Muscles in the hips, knees, and trunk are used to control the forces on the body and equipment. Multiple-joint exercises, such as the leg press, squats, and lunges, are suggested for these activities.

Before the season starts, make sure your equipment is in proper working condition. For example, alpine skiers' bindings should be cleaned and adjusted properly so that they release as needed. This is one of the most important things you can do to help prevent knee injuries. A good pair of bindings is cheaper than knee surgery.

The first few times you participate in the sport of your choice, go easy, practice technique, and do not continue once you are fatigued. Gradually increase the length and intensity of your workouts. Consider taking a lesson to have

High-intensity interval training (HIIT) A training program that involves high- to very high-intensity (80 to 90 percent of maximal capacity) intervals, each followed by a low- to moderate-intensity recovery interval. Usually, a 1:3 or lower work-to-recovery ratio is used.

Sample HIIT Programs

The following are sample HIIT programs that you can use. For intensity levels, you should use the H-PAPE scale in Figure 6.9, page 236. Prior to HIIT, be sure to have a sound general aerobic (cardiorespiratory) fitness base—that is, at least 6 weeks of aerobic training, five times per week, for 20 to 60 minutes per session. Once you are ready for HIIT, always have a proper 5- to 10-minute aerobic warm-up prior to the first high-intensity interval. Also, in all cases, follow up the final high-intensity interval with a 5- to 10-minute cooldown phase. You can use the same exercise modality (running, cycling, elliptical training, stair climbing, or swimming) for your entire HIIT, or you can use a combination of these activities with some of the programs listed here, if feasible at your facility. Do not perform back-to-back HIIT on consecutive days. Preferably, depending on the intensity (light, moderate, somewhat hard, vigorous, hard, or very hard) and volume of training, allow 2 to 3 days between HIIT sessions.

Five-Minute Very Hard-Intensity Aerobic Intervals

Exercise at a very hard rate (90 percent of maximal capacity) for 5 minutes, followed by 5 to 10 minutes of recovery at a light to moderate intensity. Start with one interval and work up to three by the third to fifth training session. Initially, use a 1:2 work-to-recovery ratio. Gradually decrease the recovery to a 1:1 ratio or even less.

Stepwise Intensity Interval Training

Using 3- to 5-minute intervals, start at a light-intensity rate of perceived exertion and then progressively step up to the very hard-intensity level. Start with 3-minute intervals; as you become more fit, increase to 5 minutes each. As time allows, and you develop greater fitness, you can add a step-down approach by stepping down to hard, vigorous, somewhat hard, moderate, and finally light.

Fartlek Training

Fartlek training was developed in 1937 by Swedish coach Gösta Holmér. The word *fartlek* means "speed play" in Swedish. It is an unstructured form of interval training, where the intensity (speed) and the distance of each interval are varied as the participant wishes. There is no set structure, and the individual alternates the intensity (from somewhat hard to very hard) and the length of each speed interval with the recovery intervals (light to moderate) and their lengths. Total duration of fartlek training is between 20 and 60 minutes.

Tempo Training

Although no formal intervals are conducted with tempo training, the intensity of training qualifies it as a HIIT program. Following an appropriate warm-up, tempo runs involve continuous training between vigorous (70 percent) and hard (80 percent) for 20 to 60 minutes at a time.

All-Out or Supramaximal Interval Training

All-out interval training involves 10 to 20 supramaximal or "sprint" intervals lasting 30 to 60 seconds each. Depending on the level of conditioning and the length of the speed interval, 2 to 5 minutes of recovery at a light to moderate level are allowed.

Cardio/Resistance Training Program

You may use a combination of aerobic and resistance training for your HIIT. Following a brief aerobic and strength-training warm-up, select about eight resistance training exercises that you can alternate with treadmill running, cycling, elliptical training, or rowing. Perform one set of 8 to 20 RM (based on personal preference) of each exercise followed by 90 seconds of aerobic work after each set. You can pace the aerobic intensity according to the preceding strength-training set. For example, you may choose a light-intensity aerobic interval following a 10 RM for the leg press exercise and a vigorous aerobic interval after a 10 RM arm curl set. Allow no greater recovery time (2 to 5 seconds) between exercise modes than what it takes to walk from the strength-training exercise to the aerobic station (and vice versa).

someone watch your technique and help correct flaws early in the season. Even Olympic athletes have coaches watching them. Proper conditioning allows for a more enjoyable and healthier season.

Overtraining

Rest is important in any fitness conditioning program. Although the term **overtraining** is associated most frequently with athletic performance, it applies just as well to fitness participants. We all know that hard work improves fitness and performance. Hard training without adequate recovery, however, breaks down the body and leads to loss of fitness.

Physiological improvements in fitness and conditioning programs occur during the rest periods following training. As a rule, a hard day of training must be followed by a day of light training. Equally, a few weeks of increased training **volume** are to be followed by a few days of light recovery work. During these recovery periods, body systems strengthen and compensate for the training load, leading to a higher level of fitness. If proper recovery is not built into the training routine, overtraining occurs. Decreased performance, staleness, and injury are frequently seen with overtraining. Thus, to obtain optimal results, training regimens are altered during different phases of the year.

Periodization

Periodization is a training approach that uses a systematic variation in intensity and volume to enhance fitness and performance. This model was designed around the premise that the body becomes stronger as a result of training, but if similar workouts are constantly repeated, the body tires and enters a state of staleness and fatigue.

Periodization is used most frequently for athletic conditioning. Because athletes cannot maintain peak fitness during an entire season, most athletes seeking peak performance use a periodized training approach. Studies have documented that greater improvements in fitness are achieved by using a variety of training loads. Using the same program and attempting to increase volume and intensity over a prolonged time manifest in overtraining.

The periodization training system involves three cycles:

1. Macrocycles
2. Mesocycles
3. Microcycles

These cycles vary in length depending on the requirements of the sport. Typically, the overall training period (season or year) is referred to as a macrocycle. For athletes who need to peak twice a year, such as cross-country and track runners, two macrocycles can be developed within the year.

Macrocycles are divided into smaller weekly or monthly training phases known as mesocycles. A typical season, for example, is divided into the following mesocycles: base fitness conditioning (off-season), preseason or sport-specific conditioning, competition, peak performance, and transition (active recovery from sport-specific training and competition). In turn, mesocycles are divided into smaller weekly or daily microcycles. During microcycles, training follows the general objective of the mesocycle, but the workouts are altered to avoid boredom and fatigue.

The concept behind periodizing can be used in both aerobic and anaerobic sports. In the case of a long-distance runner, for instance, training can start with a general strength conditioning program and cardiorespiratory endurance **cross-training** (jogging, cycling, swimming, etc.) during the off-season. In preseason, the volume of strength training is decreased, and the total weekly running mileage, at moderate intensities, is progressively increased. During the competitive season, the athlete maintains a limited strength-training program but now increases the intensity of the runs while decreasing the total weekly mileage. During the peaking phase, volume (miles) of training is reduced even further, while the intensity is maintained at a high level. At the end of the season, a short transition period of 2 to 4 weeks, involving light- to moderate- intensity activities other than running and lifting weights, is recommended.

Periodization is frequently used for development of muscular strength, progressively cycling through the various components (hypertrophy, strength, and power) of strength training. Research indicates that varying the volume and intensity over time is more effective for long-term progression than either single- or multiple-set programs with no variations. Training volume and intensity are typically increased only for large-muscle or multiple-joint lifts (e.g., bench press, squats, and lat pull-downs). Single-joint lifts (e.g., triceps extension, biceps curls, and hamstring curls) usually remain in the range of three sets of 8 to 12 repetitions.

A sample sequence—one macrocycle—of periodized training is provided in Table 9.7. The program starts with high volume and light intensity. During subsequent mesocycles (divided among the objectives of hypertrophy, strength, and power), the volume is decreased and the intensity (resistance) increases. Following each mesocycle, the recommendation is up to 7 days of very light training. This brief resting period allows the body to fully recuperate, preventing overtraining and risk for injury. Other models of periodization are available, but the example provided is the most commonly used.

For aerobic endurance sports, one to three sets of 8 to 12 repetitions to near fatigue performed once or twice a week are recommended. Although strength training does not enhance maximal oxygen uptake, and strength requirements are not as high with endurance sports, data indicate that strength training helps the individual sustain submaximal exercise for longer periods of time.

In recent years, the practice of altering or cycling workouts has become popular among fitness participants. Research indicates that periodization is not limited to athletes but has been used successfully by fitness enthusiasts who are preparing for special events, such as a 10K run, a triathlon, or a bike race, and by those who are simply aiming for higher fitness. Altering training is also recommended for people who progressed nicely in

Overtraining An emotional, behavioral, and physical condition marked by increased fatigue, decreased performance, persistent muscle soreness, mood disturbances, and feelings of "staleness" or "burnout" as a result of excessive physical training.

Volume (of training) The total amount of training performed in a given work period (day, week, month, or season).

Periodization A training approach that divides the season into three cycles (macrocycles, mesocycles, and microcycles) using systematic variation in intensity and volume of training to enhance fitness and performance

Cross-training A combination of aerobic activities that contribute to overall fitness.

the initial weeks of a fitness program but now feel "stale" and "stagnant." Studies indicate that even among general fitness participants, systematically altering volume and intensity of training is most effective for progress in long-term fitness. Because training phases change continually during a macrocycle, periodization breaks the staleness and the monotony of repeated workouts.

For the nonathlete, a periodization program does not have to account for every detail of the sport. You can periodize workouts by altering mesocycles every 2 to 8 weeks. You can use different exercises, change the number of sets and repetitions, vary the speed of the repetitions, alter recovery time between sets, and even cross-train.

Periodization is not for everyone. People who are starting an exercise program, who enjoy a set routine, or who are satisfied with their fitness routine and fitness level do not need to periodize. For new participants, the goal is to start and adhere to exercise long enough to adopt the exercise behavior.

Personal Fitness Programming: An Example

Now that you understand the principles of fitness assessment and exercise prescription given in Chapters 6 through 8 and this chapter, you can review this program to cross-check and improve the design of your own fitness program. Let's look at an example.

Mary is 20 years old and 5 feet 6 inches tall. She participated in organized sports on and off throughout high school. During the last 2 years, however, she has participated only minimally in physical activity. She was not taught the principles for exercise prescription and has not participated in regular exercise to improve and maintain the various health-related components of fitness.

Mary became interested in fitness and contemplated signing up for a fitness and wellness course. As she was preparing her class schedule for the semester, she noted a Lifetime Fitness and Wellness course. In registering for the course, Mary anticipated some type of structured aerobic exercise. She knew that good fitness was important to health and weight management, but she didn't quite know how to plan and implement a program.

CRITICAL THINKING

In your own experience with personal fitness programs throughout the years, what factors have motivated you and helped you the most to stay with a program? What factors have kept you from being physically active, and what can you do to change these factors?

Once the new course started, she and her classmates received the Stages of Change Questionnaire. Mary learned that she was in the preparation stage for cardiorespiratory endurance, the precontemplation stage for muscular fitness, the maintenance stage for flexibility, and the preparation stage for body composition (see the "Transtheoretical Model" section in Chapter 2, pages 57–61). Various fitness assessments determined that her cardiorespiratory endurance level was fair, her muscular fitness was poor, her flexibility was good, and her percent body fat was 25 (moderate category).

Cardiorespiratory Endurance At the beginning of the semester, the instructor informed the students that the course would require self-monitored participation in activities outside the regularly scheduled class hours. Mary was in the preparation stage for cardiorespiratory endurance. Thus, she knew she would be starting exercise in the next couple of weeks.

While in this preparation stage, Mary chose three processes of change to help her implement her program (see Table 2.1, page 59). She thought she could adopt an aerobic exercise program (the positive outlook process of change) and set a realistic goal to reach the good category for cardiorespiratory endurance by the end of the semester (goal setting). By staying in this course, she committed to go

TABLE 9.7 Periodization Program for Strength

	One Macrocycle			
	Mesocycle 1*	Mesocycle 2*	Mesocycle 3*	Mesocycle 4*
	Hypertrophy	Strength & Hypertrophy	Strength & Power	Peak Performance
Sets per exercise	3–5	3–5	3–5	1–3
Repetitions	8–12	6–9	1–5	1–3
Intensity (resistance)	Low	Moderate	High	Very high
Volume	High	Moderate	Low	Very low
Weeks (microcycles)	6–8	4–6	3–5	1–2

*Each mesocycle is followed by several days of light training.

FIGURE 9.4 Sample starting muscular strength and endurance periodization program.

	Learning Lifting Technique	Muscular Strength	Muscular Endurance	Muscular Strength
Sets per exercise	1–2	2	2	3
Repetitions	10	12	18–20	8–12 (RM)
Intensity (resistance)	Very low	Moderate	Low	High
Volume	Low	Moderate	Moderate	High
Sessions per week	2	2	2	3
Weeks	2	3	2	3

Selected exercises: Bench press, leg press, leg curl, lat pull-down, rowing torso, rotary torso, seated back, and abdominal crunch.

Training days: ☐M ☐T ☐W ☐Th ☐F ☐S ☐S Training time: 3:00 pm

Signature: Mary Johnson Goal: Average Date: 9-10-14

through with exercise (commitment). She prepared a 12-week Personalized Cardiorespiratory Exercise Prescription (see Lab 6D, page 255), wrote down her goal, signed the prescription (now a contract), and shared the program with her instructor and roommates.

As her exercise modalities, Mary selected walking/jogging and aerobics. Initially she walked or jogged twice a week and did aerobics once a week. By the 10th week of the program, she was jogging three times per week and participating in aerobics twice a week. She also selected techniques for monitoring, self-reevaluation, and countering her processes of change (see Table 2.2, page 65). Using the exercise log in Lab 6D (page 255), she monitored her exercise program. At the end of 6 weeks, she scheduled a follow-up cardiorespiratory assessment test (self-reevaluation process of change), and she replaced her evening television hour with aerobic training (countering).

Mary also decided to increase her daily physical activity. She chose to walk 10 minutes to and from school, take the stairs instead of elevators whenever possible, and add 5-minute walks every hour during study time. On Saturdays, she cleaned her apartment and went to a school-sponsored dance at night. On Sundays, she opted to walk to and from church and took a 30-minute leisurely walk after the dinner meal. Mary now was fully in the action stage of change for cardiorespiratory endurance.

Muscular Fitness After Mary started her fitness and wellness course, she wasn't yet convinced that she wanted to strength train. Still, she contemplated strength training because a small part of her grade depended on it. When she read the information on the effect of lean body mass on basal metabolic rate and weight maintenance (consciousness-raising process of change), she thought that perhaps it would be good to add strength training to her program. She also was contemplating the long-term consequences of loss of lean body mass, its effect on her personal appearance, and the potential for decreased independence and quality of life (emotional arousal process of change).

Mary visited her course instructor for additional guidance. Following this meeting, Mary committed herself to strength train. While in the preparation stage, she outlined a 10-week periodized training program (Figure 9.4) and opted to aim for the good strength category by the end of the program.

Because this was the first time Mary had lifted weights, the course instructor introduced her to two other students who were already lifting (helping relationships process of change). She also monitored her program with the form provided in Lab 7B (page 307). Mary promised herself a movie and dinner out if she completed the first 5 weeks of strength training and a new blouse if she made it through 10 weeks (rewards process technique of change).

Muscular Flexibility Good flexibility is not a problem for Mary because she regularly stretched 15 to 30 minutes while watching the evening news on television. She had developed this habit the last 2 years of high school to maintain flexibility as a member of the dance–drill team (environment control—as a team member, she needed good flexibility).

Because Mary had been stretching regularly for more than 3 years, she was in the maintenance stage for flexibility. The flexibility fitness tests revealed that she had good flexibility. These results allowed her to pursue her stretching program, because she thought she would be excellent for this fitness component (self-evaluation process of change).

To gain greater improvements in flexibility, Mary chose slow-sustained stretching and proprioceptive neuromuscular facilitation (PNF). She would need help carrying out the PNF technique. She spoke to one of her lifting classmates; together, they decided to allocate 20 minutes at the end of strength training to stretching (helping relationships process of change), and they chose the sequence of exercises presented in Chapter 8, Lab 8C (consciousness-raising and goal setting).

Body Composition One of the motivational factors to enroll in a fitness course was Mary's desire to learn how to better manage her weight. She had gained a few pounds since entering college. To prevent further weight gain, she thought it was time to learn sound principles for weight management (behavior analysis process of change). She was in the preparation stage of change, because she was planning to start a diet and exercise program but wasn't sure how to get it done. All Mary needed was a little consciousness-raising to get her into the action stage.

With the knowledge she had now gained, Mary planned her program. At 25 percent body fat and 140 pounds, she decided to aim for 23 percent body fat so that she would be in the good category for body composition (goal setting). This meant that she would have to lose about 4 pounds (see Lab 4A, page 159).

Mary's daily estimated energy requirement was about 2,027 calories (see Table 5.3, page 191). Mary also figured out that she was expending an additional 400 calories per day through her newly adopted exercise program and increased level of daily physical activity. Thus, her total daily energy intake would be around 2,427 calories (2,027 + 400).

To lose weight, Mary could decrease her caloric intake by 700 calories per day (body weight × 5; see Lab 5A, page 203), yielding a target daily intake of 1,727 calories. By decreasing the intake by 700 calories daily, Mary should achieve her target weight in about 20 days (4 pounds of fat × 3,500 calories per pound of fat ÷ 700 fewer calories per day = 20 days). Mary picked the 1,800-calorie diet and eliminated one daily serving of grains (80 calories) to avoid exceeding her target 1,727 daily caloric intake.

The processes of change that helped Mary in the action stage for weight management are goal setting, countering (exercising instead of watching television), monitoring, environment control, and rewards. To monitor her daily caloric intake, Mary used the 1,800-calorie diet plan in Lab 5C (page 209). To further exert control over her environment, she gave away all of her junk food. She determined that she would not eat out while on the diet, and she bought only low- to moderate-fat, complex carbohydrate foods during the 3 weeks. As her reward, she achieved her target body weight of 136 pounds.

You Can Get It Done

Once they understand the proper exercise, nutrition, and behavior modification guidelines, people find that implementing a fitness lifestyle program is not as difficult as they thought. With adequate preparation and a personal behavioral analysis, you are now ready to design, implement, evaluate, and adhere to a lifetime fitness program that can enhance your functional capacity and zest for life.

Using the concepts provided thus far in this book and the exercise prescription principles that you have learned, you should now update your personal fitness program in Lab 9B. You also have an opportunity to revise your current stage of change, fitness category for each health-related component of physical fitness, and number of daily steps taken. You have the tools—the rest is up to you!

ASSESS YOUR BEHAVIOR

1. Do you participate in recreational sports as a means to further improve your fitness and add enjoyment to training?
2. Have you been able to meet your cardiorespiratory endurance, muscular fitness, muscular flexibility, and recommended body composition goals?
3. Are you able to incorporate a variety of activities into your fitness program, and do you vary exercise intensity and duration from time to time in your training?

ASSESS YOUR KNOWLEDGE

1. Which of the following is not a skill-related fitness component?
   a. agility
   b. speed
   c. power
   d. strength
   e. balance
2. The ability to quickly and efficiently change body position and direction is known as
   a. agility.
   b. coordination.
   c. speed.
   d. reaction time.
   e. mobility.
3. The two components of power are
   a. strength and endurance.
   b. speed and force.
   c. speed and endurance.
   d. strength and force.
   e. endurance and force.
4. People with diabetes should
   a. not exercise alone.
   b. wear a bracelet that identifies their condition.
   c. exercise at a light- to moderate-intensity level.
   d. check blood glucose levels before and after exercise.
   e. All of the choices are correct.
5. During pregnancy, a woman should
   a. accumulate 30 minutes of moderate-intensity activity on most days of the week.
   b. exercise between low and somewhat hard intensity levels.
   c. avoid exercising at an altitude above 6,000 feet.
   d. All of the choices are correct.
   e. None of the choices are correct.
6. During exercise in the heat, drinking about a cup of cool water every ___ minutes seems to be ideal to prevent dehydration.
   a. 5
   b. 15 to 20
   c. 30
   d. 30 to 45
   e. 60
7. One of the most common causes of activity-related injuries is
   a. high impact.
   b. low level of fitness.
   c. exercising without stretching.
   d. improper warm-up.
   e. All of the choices cause about an equal number of injuries.
8. Improvements in maximal oxygen uptake in older adults (as compared with younger adults) as a result of cardiorespiratory endurance training are
   a. lower.
   b. higher.
   c. difficult to determine.
   d. nonexistent.
   e. similar.
9. To participate in sports, it is recommended that you have
   a. base fitness and sport-specific conditioning.
   b. at least a good rating on skill fitness.
   c. good-to-excellent agility.
   d. basic speed.
   e. All of the choices are correct.
10. Periodization is a training approach that
    a. uses a systematic variation in intensity and volume.
    b. helps enhance fitness and performance.
    c. is commonly used by athletes.
    d. helps prevent staleness and overtraining.
    e. All of the choices are correct.

Correct answers can be found at the back of the book.

NOTES

1. Kirby, R. F. "A Simple Test of Agility," *Coach and Athlete* (June 1971): 30–31.
2. American Alliance for Health, Physical Education, Recreation and Dance. *Youth Fitness: Test Manual.* Reston, VA: AAHPERD, 1976.
3. See note 2.
4. American College of Sports Medicine and American Diabetes Association. "Joint Position Statement: Exercise and Type 2 Diabetes," *Medicine & Science in Sports & Exercise* 42 (2010): 2282–2303.
5. American College of Obstetricians and Gynecologists. "Exercise during Pregnancy and the Postpartum Period," ACOG Committee Opinion No. 267, *International Journal of Gynecology and Obstetrics* 77 (2002): 79–81.
6. University of California at Berkeley. *The Wellness Guide to Lifelong Fitness.* New York, NY: Random House, 1993, p. 198.
7. Chodzko-Zajko,W. J., et al. "Exercise and Physical Activity for Older Adults," *Medicine & Science in Sports & Exercise* 41 (2009): 1510–1530.
8. Kash, F. W., Boyer, J. L., Van Camp, S. P., Verity, L. S., and J. P. Wallace. "The Effect of Physical Activity on Aerobic Power in Older Men (A Longitudinal Study)," *Physician and Sports Medicine* 18, no. 4 (1990): 73–83.
9. Evans, W. S. "Exercise, Nutrition and Aging," *Journal of Nutrition* 122 (1992): 796–801.
10. Walker, J. M., Sue, D., Miles-Elkousy, N., Ford, G., and H. Trevelyan. "Active Mobility of the Extremities in Older Subjects," *Physical Therapy* 64 (1994): 919–923.
11. Elwood, P., et al. "Healthy Lifestyles Reduce the Incidence of Chronic Diseases and Dementia: Evidence from the Caerphilly Cohort Study," *PLoS ONE* 8(12): e81877, (2013).
12. Tabata, I., et al. "Effects of moderate-intensity endurance and high-intensity intermittent training on anaerobic capacity and VO2max," *Medicine and Science in Sports and Exercise* 28, no. 10 (1996):1327–1330.
13. Moore J. M., and W. W. K. Hoeger. "Game On! Preparing Your Clients for Recreational Sports," *ACSM's Health & Fitness Journal* 9, no. 3 (2005): 14–19.
14. Karp, J. R. "Interval Training: The New and Better Way to Train Your Clients?" *IDEA Fitness Journal* 8, no. 2 (2011): 31–34.

SUGGESTED READINGS

American College of Obstetricians and Gynecologists. "Exercise during Pregnancy and the Postpartum Period." ACOG Committee Opinion No. 267. *International Journal of Gynecology and Obstetrics* 77 (2002): 79-81.

Clark, N. *Nancy Clark's Sports Nutrition Guidebook.* Champaign, IL: Human Kinetics, 2008.

Pfeiffer, R. P., and B. C. Mangus. *Concepts of Athletic* Training. Boston: Jones and Bartlett, 2012.

Lab 9A: Assessment of Skill Fitness

Name ______________________ Date ____________ Grade ____________

Instructor ______________________ Course ____________ Section ____________

NECESSARY LAB EQUIPMENT

Agility: Free-throw area of a basketball court (or any smooth area 12 by 19 feet with sufficient running space around it), four plastic cones, and a stopwatch.

Balance: Any flat, smooth floor (not carpeted) and a stopwatch.

Coordination: A 32-inch-long by 5-inch-wide piece of cardboard with six circles drawn on it as explained in Figure 9.2, page 348, three full cans of soda pop (12 oz), and a stopwatch.

Power: A flat, smooth surface, and a 10-foot tape measure (or two standard cloth measuring tapes, each 60 inches long).

Reaction Time: A standard yardstick with a shaded "concentration zone" drawn on the first 2 inches of the stick.

Speed: A school track or premeasured 50-yard straight-away.

OBJECTIVE

To assess the fitness level for each skill-related fitness component.

LAB PREPARATION

Wear exercise clothing, including running shoes. Do not exercise strenuously several hours prior to this lab.

INSTRUCTIONS

Perform all six tests for the fitness-related components as outlined in Chapter 9. Report the results below and answer the questions given at the end of this lab.

Skill-Related Fitness: Test Results

Component				
Agility	Trials:	1. ☐☐.☐	2. ☐☐.☐	
Balance	Trials:	1. ☐☐.☐	2. ☐☐.☐	
Coordination	Trials:	1. ☐☐.☐	2. ☐☐.☐	
Power	Trials:	1. ☐	2. ☐	3. ☐
Reaction Time	Trials:	1. ☐☐.☐	2. ☐☐.☐	3. ☐☐.☐
	4. ☐☐.☐	5. ☐☐.☐	6. ☐☐.☐	7. ☐☐.☐
	8. ☐☐.☐	9. ☐☐.☐	10. ☐☐.☐	11. ☐☐.☐
	12. ☐☐.☐			Average of 6 middle scores = ☐☐.☐
Speed	Trials:	1. ☐☐.☐		

Fitness Component/Test	Percentile Rank*	Category*
Agility: SEMO test		
Balance: One-foot stand		
Coordination: Soda pop test		
Power: Standing long jump		
Reaction Time: Yardstick test		
Speed: 50-yard dash		

*See Tables 9.1, 9.2, and 9.3, page 350, Skill-Related Fitness Categories

Interpretation of Test Results

1. What conclusions can you draw from your test results?

2. Briefly state how you could improve your test results and what activities you could engage in to obtain the desired results.

3. Did you ever participate in organized sports, or have you found success in a particular game or sport? Yes ☐ No ☐

   3a. If your answer is yes, list the sports, games, or events in which you enjoy(ed) success.

   3b. Is there a relationship between your answers to question 3a and your test results in this lab?

Lab 9B: Personal Fitness Plan

Name ______________________ Date ____________ Grade ____________

Instructor ______________________ Course ____________ Section ____________

ASSIGNMENT

This laboratory experience should be carried out as a homework assignment to be completed over the next 7 days.

LAB RESOURCES

Be sure to understand the assessment techniques for the various health-related components of physical fitness; the ACSM exercise prescription guidelines provided in Chapters 6, 7, and 8; the stages of change model and goal setting guidelines explained in Chapter 2; and contributions of different activities to the health-related components of fitness.

OBJECTIVE

To update your personal fitness program according to personal goals, interests, and current exercise prescription guidelines.

I. Exercise Clearance

Is it safe for you to participate in an exercise program? ☐ Yes ☐ No

II. Fitness Evaluation

	Current		Fitness Category Goal		
Component	Test Results	Fitness Category	Training Frequency per Week	Stage of Change	Fitness Goal
Cardiorespiratory endurance					
Muscular fitness (strength and endurance)					
Muscular flexibility					
Body composition			NA		

III. Cardiorespiratory Endurance

Outline your cardiorespiratory endurance program according to ACSM guidelines. Include intensity, frequency, duration, aerobic activities, time of day for training, facility where you will perform the training, and reward for accomplishing your goal.

IV. Muscular Fitness (Strength and Endurance)

Using ACSM guidelines, outline your muscular strength/endurance training program. List the exercises used, sets and repetitions, amount of resistance to be used, frequency per week, training facility, and reward for accomplishing your goal.

V. Muscular Flexibility

Design your flexibility training program to include the selected exercises, technique used, number of repetitions for each exercise, length of final hold, site for training, and reward for accomplishing your goal.

VI. Recreational Activities

List any other sports or recreational activities in which you participate and include how often and how long you participate. Indicate also the primary reason for participation in these activities (physical activity, fitness, competition, skill development, recreation, stress management) and your future goals for these activities.

VII. Daily Physical Activity

Indicate the efforts that you are making to increase daily physical activity, your feelings about your choice of activities, and what future goals you have regarding daily physical activities.

Total number of daily steps:

VIII. Body Composition and Fitness Benefits

List all of the activities in which you participate regularly and rate the respective contribution to body composition and other fitness components. Use the following rating scale: 1 = low, 2 = fair, 3 = average, 4 = good, and 5 = excellent.

Activity	Body Composition	Cardiorespiratory	Musc. Fitness	Musc. Flexibility	Agility	Balance	Coordination	Power	Reaction Time	Speed
Example: Jogging	5	5	2	1	2	2	1	2	1	2

IX. Contract

I hereby commit to carry out the above described fitness plan and complete my goals by ________.

Upon completion of all my fitness goals I will present my results to ________ and will reward myself with ________.

My signature ________ Date ________

Witness signature ________ Date ________

10

Stress Assessment and Management Techniques

"If we all threw our problems in a pile and saw everyone else's, we'd grab ours back."
—*Regina Brett*

OBJECTIVES

- Understand the importance of the mind/body connection in the manifestation of emotions and disease.
- Learn the consequences of sleep deprivation on mental and physical health.
- Define stress, eustress, and distress.
- Explain the role of stress in maintaining health and optimal performance.
- Identify the major sources of stress in your life.
- Define the two major types of behavior patterns.
- Learn to lower your vulnerability to stress.
- Develop time-management skills.
- Define the role of physical exercise in reducing stress.
- Describe and learn to use various stress-management techniques.

CENGAGE brain.com
Visit **www.cengagebrain.com** to access course materials and companion resources for this text, including digital labs, quiz questions designed to check your understanding of the chapter contents, and more! See the preface on page xii for more information.

REAL LIFE STORY | Jose's Experience

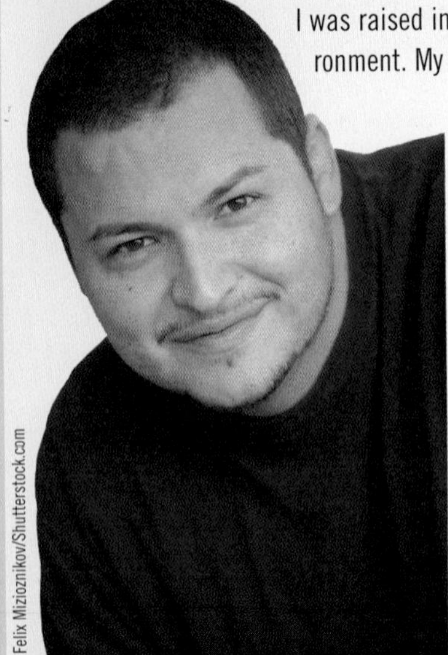
© Felix Mizioznikov/Shutterstock.com

I was raised in a slow pace of life environment. My parents always had time for each other and for us kids. We did a lot of family activities together and we were very involved in sports. Later in high school, my life changed. I became overly competitive as I was trying to excel in both school and sports. I started to skip family outings and time spent together because I was too involved in my own activities. In college, I played intramural sports but also found out that the academic requirements were very demanding. I seemed to have even less time than I had in high school. I always felt pressed for time and would get very upset if anything got in the way or didn't go as I had planned. Getting in the wrong line at fast-food chains and at the supermarket or the wrong traffic lane was extremely upsetting. I became an impatient and aggressive driver. If a friend or even family member called on the phone, I felt quite annoyed and I would try to end the conversation as quickly as possible. I also started to have a difficult time sleeping, I was getting frequent headaches, I was often fatigued, and I noticed that family and friends weren't calling much anymore. I began to feel isolated and couldn't quite figure it all out. I really wasn't happy with myself anymore. My junior year in college I took a *Fitness for Life* class, and the stress chapter really opened my eyes. I never gave stress much consideration, and now the pieces were all coming together. I began to prioritize my activities, did a better job choosing my class schedule, and even set aside daily downtime when I could have time to myself and talk to others. I am still working hard at school, but I have managed to be a little more low key about it all. I try to study, do homework, and exercise with friends as much as possible, and my family feels they have regained their lost son and brother. When I feel that I am getting angry or overstressed, I do deep breathing exercises and tell myself that the only person I stand to hurt by my actions is myself. My change in behavior has helped me be happier and less stressed. I am also sleeping better and no longer suffer recurring headaches.

According to a growing body of evidence, virtually every illness known to modern humanity—from arthritis to migraine headaches, from the common cold to cancer—appears to be influenced for good or bad by our emotions. To a profound extent, emotions affect our susceptibility to and our **immunity** from disease. The way we react to what comes along in life can determine in great measure how we will react to the disease-causing organisms that we face. The feelings we have and the way we express them can either boost our immune system or weaken it.

Emotional health is a key part of total wellness. Most emotionally healthy people take care of themselves physically—they eat well, exercise, and get enough rest. They work to develop supportive personal relationships. In contrast, many people who are emotionally unhealthy are self-destructive. For example, they may abuse alcohol and other drugs or may overwork and lack balance in their lives. Emotional health is so important that it affects what we do, who we meet, who we marry, how we look, how we feel, how the course of our lives unfolds, and even how long we live.

The Mind–Body Connection

Emotions cause physiologic responses that can influence health. Certain parts of the brain are associated with specific emotions and specific hormone patterns. The release of certain hormones is associated with various emotional responses, and those hormones affect health. These responses may contribute to development of disease. Emotions have to be expressed somewhere, somehow. If they are suppressed repeatedly or a person feels conflict about controlling them, they often reveal themselves through physical symptoms. These physiologic responses may weaken the immune system over time.

Immunity The function that guards the body from invaders, both internal and external.

FAQ

Is all stress detrimental to health and performance?

Living in today's world is nearly impossible without encountering stress. The good news is that stress can be self-controlled. Unfortunately, most people have accepted stress as a normal part of daily life, and even though everyone has to face it, few seem to understand it or know how to cope with it effectively. It is difficult to succeed and have fun in life without "runs, hits, and errors." In fact, stress should not be avoided entirely, because a certain amount is necessary for motivation, performance, and optimum health and well-being. When stress levels push people to the limit, however, stress becomes distress and they no longer function effectively.

How can I most effectively deal with distress (negative stress)?

Feelings of stress are the result of the body's instinct to defend itself. If you start to experience mental, social, and physical symptoms such as exhaustion, headaches, sleeplessness, frustration, apathy, loneliness, and changes in appetite, you are most likely under excessive stress and need to take action to overcome the stress-causing event(s). Do not deal with these symptoms through alcohol, drugs, or other compulsive behaviors, which will not get rid of the stressor that is causing the problem. Stress management is best accomplished by maintaining a sense of control when excessive demands are placed on you.

First, recognize when you are feeling stressed. Early warning signs include tension in your shoulders and neck and clenching of your fists or teeth. Now, determine if there is something that you can do to control, change, or remove yourself from the situation. Most importantly, change how you react to stress. Be positive, avoid extreme reactions (anger, hostility, hatred, or depression), try to change the way you see things, work off stress through physical activity, and master one or more stress management techniques to help you in situations in which it is necessary to cope effectively. Finally, take steps to reduce the demands placed on you by prioritizing your activities—"Don't sweat the small stuff." Realize that it is not stress that makes you ill, but the manner in which you react to stress that leads to illness and disease.

MyProfile: Personal Stress Management Survey

Most people fail to recognize the impact stress has on their lives and its effect on health and quality of life.

I. Do you experience mostly eustress or distress in your daily life? Explain. ____________________

____

____

II. Identify a recent life stressor. Can you explain the general adaptation syndrome stage that you are currently experiencing? ___ Yes ___ No ____________________

____

____

III. List significant factors that cause stress in your life, and indicate how you deal with those situations when they arise. ____________________

____

____

IV. Explain personal time management techniques that you use given the many challenges and responsibilities you face in daily life. ____________________

____

____

V. Have you ever used relaxation techniques to effectively manage stress? ___ Yes ___ No If so, explain the experience. ____________________

____

____

The Brain

The brain is the most important part of the nervous system. For the body to survive, the brain must be maintained. All other organs sacrifice to keep the brain alive and functioning when the entire body is under severe stress.

The brain directs nerve impulses that are carried throughout the body. It controls voluntary processes, such as the direction, strength, and coordination of muscle movements; processes involved in smelling, touching, and seeing; and involuntary functions over which you have no conscious control. Among the latter are many automatic, vital functions in the body, such as breathing, heart rate, digestion, control of the bowels and bladder, blood pressure, and release of hormones.

The brain is the cognitive center of the body, the place where ideas are generated, memory is stored, and emotions are experienced. The brain has a powerful influence over the body via the link between the emotions and the immune system. That link is extremely complex.

The emotions that the brain produces are a mixture of feelings and physical responses. Every time the brain manufactures an emotion, physical reactions accompany it. The brain's natural chemicals form literal communication links among the brain, its thought processes, and the cells of the body, including those of the immune system.

Stress and Illness

Chronic distress raises the risk for many health disorders—among them, coronary heart disease (CHD), hypertension, eating disorders, ulcers, diabetes, asthma, depression, migraine headaches, sleep disorders, and chronic fatigue—and may even play a role in the development of certain types of cancers.[1] Recognizing this and overcoming the source of distress quickly and efficiently are crucial in maintaining emotional and physiological stability.

The immune system patrols and guards the body against attackers. This system consists of about a trillion cells called **lymphocytes** (the cells responsible for waging war against disease or infection) and trillions of molecules called **antibodies**. The brain and the immune system are closely linked in a connection that allows the mind to influence both susceptibility and resistance to disease. A number of immune system cells—including those in the thymus gland, spleen, bone marrow, and lymph nodes—are laced with nerve cells.

Cells of the immune system are equipped to respond to chemical signals from the central nervous system. For example, the surface of the lymphocytes contains receptors for a variety of central nervous system chemical messengers, such as catecholamines, prostaglandins, serotonin, endorphins, sex hormones, the thyroid hormone, and the growth hormone. Certain white blood cells possess the ability to receive messages from the brain.

Because of these receptors on the lymphocytes, physical and psychological stress alters the immune system. Stress causes the body to release several powerful neurohormones that bind with the receptors on the lymphocytes and suppress immune function. Stress also causes the nerves to release a molecule known as neuropeptide Y (NPY) that impairs immune-system cells that fight infection. NPY is also believed to cause excessive eating when under stress.

Blood levels of the stress hormone cortisol, inflammatory molecules, and low-density lipoprotein (LDL)-cholesterol all increase during stress episodes. High cortisol levels alone cause inflammation, a condition implicated in many chronic diseases. Inflammatory molecules further promote atherosclerosis and make plaque more likely to rupture, leading to a heart attack or stroke. In a recent review of studies evaluating the effects of tension on heart health, researchers found that chronic stress can increase the risk of CHD by as much as 27 percent. The findings are significant, suggesting that stress can be as threatening as a 50-point increase in LDL cholesterol, or the equivalent of smoking five extra cigarettes per day.[2] Chronic stress is also thought to increase the risk of dementia, in particular Alzheimer's disease. Glucocorticoid hormones released during stressful events are detrimental to neurons and the synapses between them. As age-related mental decline begins, the fewer the number of synapses available, the lower the cognitive reserve, and the greater the risk for Alzheimer's. Furthermore, stress is believed to affect the person's DNA by lowering the cell's ability to divide, leading to premature aging and other age-related diseases.

Sleep and Wellness

Sleep is a natural state of rest that is vital for good health and wellness. It is an anabolic process that allows the body to restore and heal itself. During sleep, we replenish depleted energy levels and allow the brain, muscles, organs, and various body tissues to repair themselves.

Sleep deprivation weakens the immune system, impairs mental function, and has a negative impact on physical, social, academic, and job performance. Lack of sleep also affects stress levels, mood, memory, behavioral patterns, and cognitive performance. Cumulative long-term consequences include an increase in the risk for cardiovascular disease, high blood pressure, obesity, diabetes, and psychological disorders. People who get less sleep have a three-fold increased risk of getting a cold, are more likely to develop CHD earlier in life, have more inflammation in the body, and have higher blood levels of the stress hormone cortisol. What most people notice is a chronic state of fatigue, exhaustion, and confusion.

Stress-wise, getting to bed too late often leads to oversleeping, napping, missing classes, poor grades, and distress. It further increases tension, irritability, intolerance, and confusion, and it may cause depression and life dissatisfaction. Not getting enough sleep can also lead to vehicle accidents with serious or fatal consequences as people fall asleep behind the wheel. More than 40,000 injuries and 1,500 deaths each year are attributed to sleepy drivers (sleepy drivers are just as dangerous as drunk drivers). Irregular sleep patterns, including sleeping in on weekends, also contribute to many of the aforementioned problems.

Although more than 100 sleep disorders have been identified, they can be classified into four major groups:

- Problems with falling and staying asleep
- Difficulties staying awake
- Difficulties adhering to a regular sleep schedule
- Sleep-disruptive behaviors (including sleepwalking and sleep terror disorder)

College students are some of the most sleep-deprived people of all. On average, they sleep about 6 and a half hours per night, and approximately 30 percent report chronic sleep difficulties. Only 8 percent report sleeping 8 or more hours per night. For many students, college is the first time they have complete control of their schedule, including when they go to sleep and how many hours they sleep.

Lack of sleep during school days and pulling all-nighters interferes with the ability to pay attention and to learn, process, and retain new information. You may be able to retain the information in short-term memory, but most likely it will not be there for a cumulative exam or when you need it for adequate job performance. Deep sleep that takes place early in the night and a large portion of the REM (rapid eye movement) dream sleep that occurs near the end of the night have both been linked to learning. The brain has been shown to consolidate new information for long-term memory while you sleep. Convincing sleep-deprived students to get adequate sleep is a real challenge, because they often feel overwhelmed by school, work, and even family responsibilities. Students who go to sleep early and get about 8 hours of sleep per night are more apt to succeed.

Compounding the problem is staying up late Friday and Saturday nights and crashing the next day. Doing so further disrupts the circadian rhythm, the biological clock that controls the daily sleep–wake schedule. Such disruption influences quantity and quality of sleep and keeps people from falling asleep and rising at the necessary times for school, work, or other required activities. In essence, the body wants to sleep and be awake at odd times of the 24-hour cycle.

A term used to describe the cumulative effect of needed sleep that you don't get is sleep debt. Crashing on weekends, although it may help somewhat, does not solve the problem. You need to address the problem behavior by getting sufficient sleep each night so that you can be at your best the next day.

The exact amount of sleep that each person needs varies among individuals. Around 8 hours are required by most people. According to the National Sleep Foundation, currently most people get about 7 hours of sleep per night. Experts believe that the last 2 hours of sleep are the most vital for well-being. Thus, if people need 8 hours of sleep and routinely get 6, they may be forfeiting the most critical sleep hours for health and wellness. Most students do not address sleep disorders until they start to cause mental and physical damage.

While there is no magic formula to determine how much sleep you need, if you don't need an alarm clock to get up every morning, you wake up at about the same time, and you are refreshed and feel alert throughout the day, you most likely have a healthy sleeping habit.

To improve your sleep pattern, you need to exercise discipline and avoid staying up late to watch a movie or leaving your homework or studying for an exam until the last minute. As busy as you are, your health and well-being is your most important asset. You only live once. Keeping your health, and living life to its fullest potential includes a good night's rest. To enhance the quality of your sleep, you should do the following:

- Exercise and be physically active, but avoid vigorous exercise 4 hours prior to bedtime.
- Avoid eating a heavy meal or snacking 2 to 3 hours before going to bed (digestion increases your metabolism).
- Limit the amount of time that you spend (even more so in the evening) surfing and socializing on the Internet, texting, instant messaging (IMing), and watching television.
- Go to bed and rise about the same time each day.
- Keep the bedroom cool, quiet, and dark.
- Develop a bedtime ritual (meditation, prayer, or white noise).
- Use your bed for sleeping only (do not watch television, do homework, or use a laptop in bed).
- Relax and slow down 15 to 30 minutes before bedtime.
- Do not drink coffee or caffeine-containing beverages several hours before going to bed.
- Do not rely on alcohol to fall asleep (alcohol disrupts deep sleep stages).
- Avoid long naps (a 20- to 30-minute "power nap" can be beneficial during an afternoon slump without interfering with night-time sleep).
- Have frank and honest conversations with roommates if they have different sleep schedules.
- Evaluate your mattress every 5 to 7 years for comfort and support; if you wake up with aches and pains or you sleep better when you are away from home, it is most likely time for a new mattress.

Stress

Living in today's world is nearly impossible without encountering **stress**. In an unpredictable world that changes with every new day, most people find

Lymphocytes Immune system cells responsible for waging war against disease or infection.

Antibodies Substances produced by the white blood cells in response to an invading agent.

Stress The mental, emotional, and physiological response of the body to any situation that is new, threatening, frightening, or exciting.

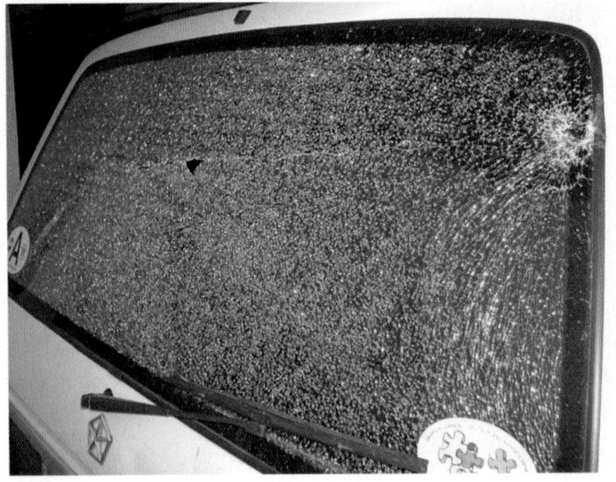

© Fitness & Wellness, Inc.

Vandalism causes distress, or negative stress.

© Fitness & Wellness, Inc.

Marriage is an example of positive stress, also known as eustress.

that working under pressure has become the rule rather than the exception. As a result, stress has become one of the most common problems people face and undermines the ability to stay well. Current estimates indicate that the annual cost of stress and stress-related diseases in the United States exceeds $100 billion, a direct result of health care costs, lost productivity, and absenteeism. Many medical and stress researchers believe that "stress should carry a health warning."

Just what is stress? Dr. Hans Selye, one of the foremost authorities on stress, defined it as "the nonspecific response of the human organism to any demand that is placed upon it."[3] "Nonspecific" indicates that the body reacts in a similar fashion, regardless of the nature of the event that leads to the stress response. In simpler terms, stress is the body's mental, emotional, and physiological response to any situation that is new, threatening, frightening, or exciting.

CRITICAL THINKING

Can you identify sources of eustress and distress in your personal life during this past year? Explain your emotional and physical response to each stressor and how the two differ.

The body's response to stress has been the same since humans were first put on Earth. Stress prepares people to react to the stress-causing event, also called the **stressor**. The problem arises in the way in which people react to stress. Many people thrive under stress; others under similar circumstances are unable to handle it. Their reaction to a stress-causing agent determines whether that stress is positive or negative.

Dr. Selye defined the ways in which we react to stress as either eustress or distress. In both cases, the nonspecific response is almost the same. In the case of **eustress**, health and performance continue to improve even as stress increases. On the other hand, **distress** refers to the unpleasant or harmful stress under which health and performance begin to deteriorate. The relationship between stress and performance is illustrated in Figure 10.1.

Stress is a fact of modern life, and every person needs an optimal level of stress that is most conducive to adequate health and performance. When stress levels reach mental, emotional, and physiological limits, however, stress becomes distress and the person no longer functions effectively.

FIGURE 10.1 Relationship between stress and health and performance.

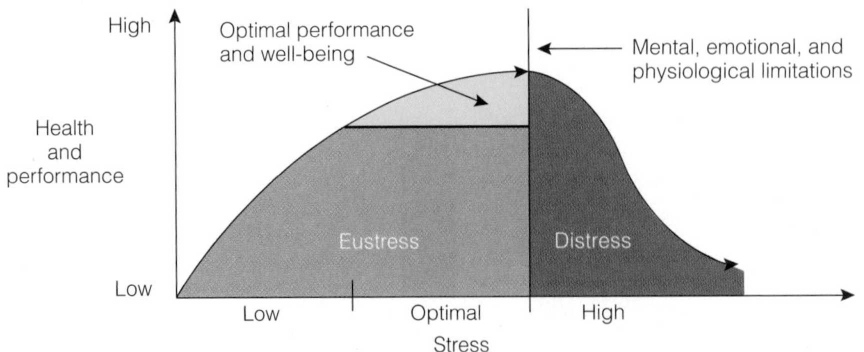

© Cengage Learning

FIGURE 10.2 **GAS, the body's response to stress that can end in exhaustion, illness, or recovery.**

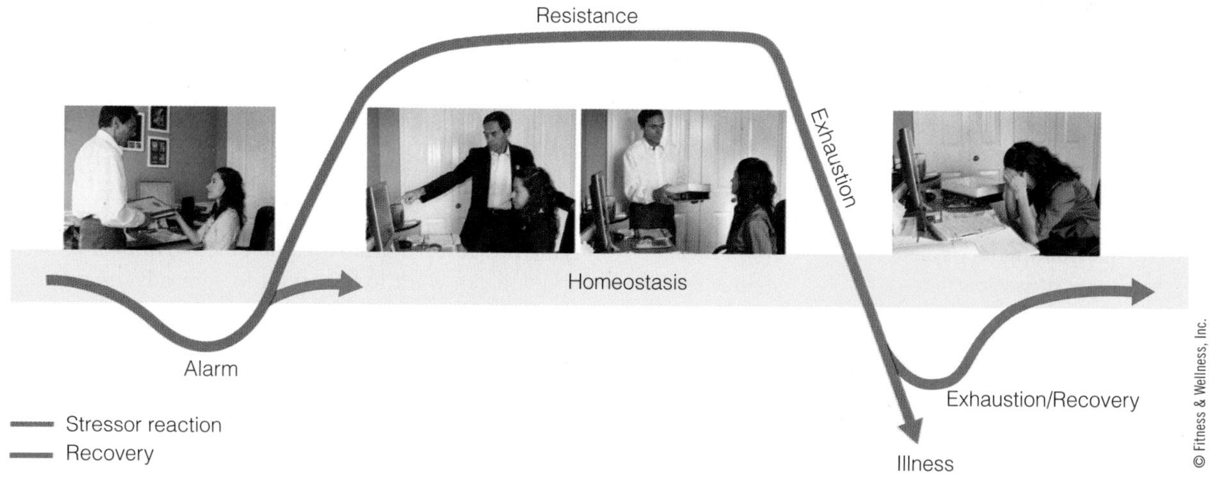

Stress Adaptation

The body continually strives to maintain a constant internal environment. This state of physiological balance, known as **homeostasis**, allows the body to function as effectively as possible. When a stressor triggers a nonspecific response, homeostasis is disrupted. This reaction to stressors, best explained by Dr. Selye through the **general adaptation syndrome (GAS)**, is composed of three stages: alarm reaction, resistance, and exhaustion and recovery.

Alarm Reaction The alarm reaction is the immediate response to a stressor (whether positive or negative). During the alarm reaction, the body evokes an instant physiological reaction that mobilizes internal systems and processes to minimize the threat to homeostasis (see also "Coping with Stress" on pages 394–395). If the stressor subsides, the body recovers and returns to homeostasis.

Resistance If the stressor persists, the body calls upon its limited reserves to build up its resistance as it strives to maintain homeostasis. For a short while, the body copes effectively and meets the challenge of the stressor until it can be overcome (Figure 10.2).

Exhaustion and Recovery If stress becomes chronic and intolerable, the body continues to resist, draining its limited reserves. The body then loses its ability to cope and enters the exhaustion and recovery stage. During this stage, the body functions at a diminished capacity while it recovers from stress. In due time, following an "adequate" recovery period (which varies greatly), the body recuperates and is able to return to homeostasis. If chronic stress persists during the exhaustion stage, however, immune function is compromised, which can damage body systems and lead to disease.

An example of the stress response through the GAS can be illustrated in college test performance. As you prepare to take an exam, you experience an initial alarm reaction. If you understand the material, study for the exam, and do well (eustress), the body recovers and stress is dissipated. If, however, you are not adequately prepared and fail the exam, you trigger the resistance stage. You are now concerned about your grade, and you remain in the resistance stage until the next exam. If you prepare and do well, the body recovers. But, if you fail once again and can no longer bring up

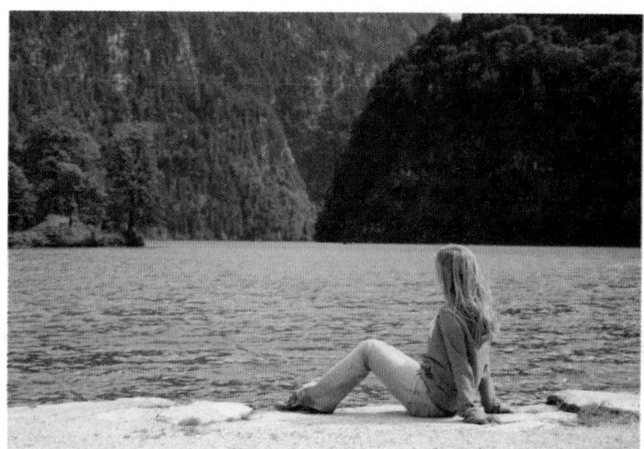

Taking time out during stressful life events is critical for good health and wellness.

Stressor A stress-causing event.

Eustress Positive stress; health and performance continue to improve even as stress increases.

Distress Negative stress; unpleasant or harmful stress under which health and performance begin to deteriorate.

Homeostasis A natural state of equilibrium, which the body attempts to maintain by constantly reacting to external forces that attempt to disrupt this fine balance.

General adaptation syndrome (GAS) A theoretical model that explains the body's adaptation to sustained stress. It includes three stages: alarm reaction, resistance, and exhaustion and recovery.

the grade, exhaustion sets in and physical and emotional breakdowns may occur. Exhaustion may be further aggravated if you are struggling in other courses as well.

The exhaustion stage is often manifested by athletes and the most ardent fitness participants. Staleness is usually a manifestation of overtraining. Peak performance can be sustained for only about 2 to 3 weeks at a time. Any attempts to continue intense training after peaking leads to exhaustion, diminished fitness, and mental and physical problems associated with overtraining (see Chapter 9, page 368). Thus, athletes and some fitness participants also need an active recovery phase following the attainment of peak fitness.

Perceptions and Health

The habitual manner in which people explain the things that happen to them is their **explanatory style**. It is a way of thinking when all other factors are equal and when there are no clear-cut right and wrong answers. The contrasting explanatory styles are pessimism and optimism. People with a pessimistic explanatory style interpret events negatively; people with an optimistic explanatory style interpret events in a positive light—"Every cloud has a silver lining."

A pessimistic explanatory style can delay healing time and worsen the course of illness in several major diseases. For example, it can affect the circulatory system and general outlook for people with CHD. Blood flow actually changes as thoughts, feelings, and attitudes change. People with a pessimistic explanatory style have a higher risk of developing heart disease.

Studies of explanatory style verify that a negative explanatory style also compromises immunity. Blood samples taken from people with a negative explanatory style revealed suppressed immune function, a low ratio of helper-to-suppressor T-cells, and fewer lymphocytes.

In contrast, an optimistic style tends to increase the strength of the immune system. An optimistic explanatory style and the positive attitude it fosters can also enhance the ability to resist infections, allergies, autoimmunities, and even cancer. A change in explanatory style can lead to a remarkable change in the course of disease. An optimistic explanatory style and the positive emotions it embraces—such as love, acceptance, and forgiveness—stimulate the body's healing systems.

Self-Esteem

Self-esteem is a way of viewing and assessing yourself. Positive self-esteem is a sense of feeling good about your capabilities, goals, accomplishments, place in the world, and relationship to others.

People with high self-esteem respect themselves. Self-esteem is a powerful determinant of health behavior and, therefore, of health status. Healthy self-esteem is one of the best things people can develop for overall health, both mental and physical. A good, strong sense of self can boost the immune system, protect against disease, and aid in healing.

Whether people get sick—and how long they stay that way—may depend in part on the strength of their self-esteem. For example, low self-esteem worsens chronic pain. The higher the self-esteem, the more rapid the recovery. If people have strong self-esteem, the outlook is good. If self-esteem is poor, however, their health can decline in direct proportion as their attitude and negative perceptions worsen.

Belief in yourself is one of the most powerful weapons you have to protect your health and live a longer, more satisfying life. It has a dramatic and positive impact on wellness, and you can work to harness it to your advantage.

Fighting Spirit

A **fighting spirit** involves the healthy expression of emotions, whether they are negative or positive. At the other extreme is hopelessness, a surrender to despair. A fighting spirit can play a major role in recovery from disease. People with a fighting spirit accept their disease diagnosis, adopt an optimistic attitude filled with faith, seek information about how to help themselves, and are determined to fight the disease. A fighting spirit makes people take charge.

A fighting spirit may be the underlying factor in what is called **spontaneous remission** from incurable illness. More and more physicians believe that the phenomenon is real and that the patient is the key in spontaneous remission. They believe the patient's attitude, especially the presence of a fighting spirit, is responsible for victory over disease. Fighters are not stronger or more capable than others—they simply do not give up as easily. They enjoy better health and live longer, even when physicians and laboratory tests say they should not. Fighters are intrinsically different from people who give up, and their health status reflects those differences.

Sources of Stress

Several instruments have been developed to assess sources of stress in life. A practical instrument to assess stressors is the **stress events scale**, presented in Lab 10A, which identifies life events within the past 12 months that may have an impact on your physical and psychological well-being.

The stress events scale is divided into two sections. Section 1, to be completed by all respondents, contains a list of potential stress-causing life events with four additional blank spaces for other events experienced but not listed in the survey. Section 2 contains additional statements designed for students only (students should fill out both sections). Common stressors in the lives of college students are depicted in Figure 10.3.

CRITICAL THINKING

Technological advances provide many benefits to our lives. What positive and negative effects do these advances have upon your daily living activities, and what impact are they having on your stress level?

FIGURE 10.3 **Stressors in the lives of college students.**

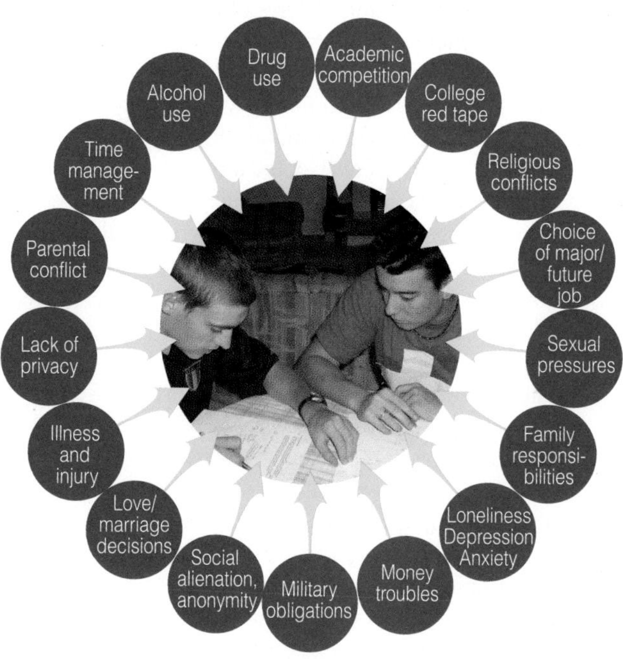

Source: Adapted from W. W. K. Hoeger, L. W. Turner, and B. Q. Hafen. *Wellness Guidelines for a Healthy Lifestyle.* Wadsworth/Thomson Learning, 2007.

The scale requires testees to rate the extent to which life events had a positive or negative impact on their life at the time these events occurred. The ratings are on a 7-point scale. A rating of −3 indicates an extremely undesirable impact (shocked). A zero (0) rating indicates neither a positive nor a negative impact (**neustress**, or indifferent). A rating of +3 indicates an extremely desirable impact (jubilant).

After the person evaluates his or her life events, the negative and the positive points are totaled separately. Both scores are expressed as positive numbers (e.g., positive ratings of 2, 1, 3, and 3 = 9 points of positive score; negative ratings of −3, −2, −2, −1, and −2 = 10 points of negative score). A final "total life change" score can be obtained by adding the positive score and the negative score together as positive numbers (total stress events score = 9 + 10 = 19 points).

Because negative and positive changes alike can produce nonspecific responses, the total life change score is a good indicator of total life stress. Most research in this area, however, suggests that the negative change score is a better predictor of potential physical and psychological illness than the total change score. More research is necessary to establish the role of total change and the role of the ratio of positive to negative stress.

Behavior Patterns

Common life events are not the only source of stress in life. All too often, individuals bring on stress as a result of their behavior patterns. The two main types of behavior patterns, type A and type B, are based on several observable characteristics.

Several attempts have been made to develop an objective scale to identify type A individuals properly, but these questionnaires are not as valid and reliable as researchers would like them to be. Consequently, the main assessment tool to determine behavioral type is still the **structured interview**, during which a person is asked to reply to several questions that describe type A and type B behavior patterns. The interviewer notes not only the responses to the questions but also the individual's mental, emotional, and physical behaviors as he or she replies to each question.

Based on the answers and the associated behaviors, the interviewer rates the person along a continuum, ranging from type A to type B. Along this continuum, behavioral patterns are classified into five categories: A-1, A-2, X (a mix of type A and type B), B-3, and B-4. The type A-1 person exhibits all type A characteristics, and the B-4 person shows a relative absence of type A behaviors. The type A-2 individual does not exhibit a complete type A pattern, and the type B-3 individual exhibits only a few type A characteristics.

Type A behavior characterizes a primarily hard-driving, overambitious, aggressive, and at times hostile and overly competitive person. Type A individuals often set their own goals, are self-motivated, try to accomplish many tasks at the same time, are excessively achievement oriented, and have a high degree of time urgency.

In contrast, **type B** behavior is characteristic of calm, casual, relaxed, and easygoing individuals. Type B people take one thing at a time, do not feel pressured or hurried, and seldom set their own deadlines.

Over the years, experts have indicated that individuals classified as type A are under too much stress and have a significantly higher incidence of CHD. Based on these findings, type A individuals have been counseled to lower their stress level by modifying many of their type A behaviors.

Explanatory style The way people perceive the events in their lives, from an optimistic or a pessimistic perspective.

Self-esteem A sense of positive self-regard and self-respect.

Fighting spirit Determination; the open expression of emotions, whether negative or positive.

Spontaneous remission Inexplicable recovery from incurable disease.

Stress events scale A questionnaire used to assess sources of stress in life.

Neustress Neutral stress; stress that is neither harmful nor helpful.

Structured interview An assessment tool used to determine behavioral patterns that define type A and type B personalities.

Type A The behavior pattern characteristic of a hard-driving, overambitious, aggressive, and at times hostile and overly competitive person.

Type B The behavior pattern characteristic of a calm, casual, relaxed, and easygoing individual.

confidentconsumer

Mastering stress

Managing stress requires self-confidence in the ability to do so and actively working toward this end. Self-confidence is a key attribute of successful people and is critical in almost every aspect of life, yet many people struggle to develop it. As a learned trait, it requires both self-efficacy and self-esteem.

Self-efficacy is people's belief in their own competence and ability to succeed in specific situations. These people see themselves mastering the necessary skills and achieving the goals that matter the most to them. People with a high degree of self-efficacy believe that if they learn and work hard in a particular area, they will be successful despite difficult challenges and setbacks that may lie ahead. The same holds true for stress: Learning what causes stress, decreasing susceptibility to stress, and finding ways to minimize it enhance quality of life.

Self-esteem deals with people's assessment or appraisal of their own worth and how they are viewed by others. It is also related to the sense that they possess high ethical and moral values and that they are able to be successful when they put their minds to it.

Stress management involves changing stressful situations when you can, adjusting your reactions when you can't avoid the stressor, and being on top of your health and overall well-being. To effectively enhance your confidence to manage stress, you need to:

- Decrease stress vulnerability
- Avoid self-defeating thoughts
- Be physically active
- Get adequate rest (sleep) and take time to wind down
- Take control of your health (eat right and avoid drugs, tobacco, and excessive alcohol intake)
- Set and work toward realistic SMART goals (specific, measurable, acceptable, realistic, and time-specific goals)
- Build competence (skills necessary to get the work done)
- Manage time wisely
- Use proper stress management techniques as needed
- Build a strong social network
- Learn to have fun and relax

Many of the type A characteristics are learned behaviors. Consequently, if people can learn to identify the sources of stress and make changes in their behavioral responses, they can move along the continuum and respond more like Type B individuals. The debate, however, has centered on which type A behaviors should be changed, because not all of them are undesirable.

Even though personality questionnaires are not as valid and reliable as the structured interview in identifying type A individuals, Drs. Meyer Friedman and Ray Rosenman, two San Francisco scientists, constructed a type A personality assessment form, adapted from the structured interview method, to give people a general idea of type A behavioral patterns. This assessment form is found in Lab 10B. You can use it to understand your behavioral patterns better. If you obtain a high rating (a low number of points), you are probably type A.

We also know that many individuals perform well under pressure. They typically are classified as type A but do not demonstrate any of the detrimental effects of stress. Drs. Robert and Marilyn Kriegel came up with the term type C to characterize people with these behaviors.[4]

Type C individuals are just as highly stressed as type A people but do not seem to be at higher risk for disease than type B people. The keys to successful type C performance seem to be commitment, confidence, and control. Type C people are highly committed to what they are doing, have a great deal of confidence in their ability to do their work, and are in constant control of their actions. In addition, they enjoy their work and maintain themselves in top physical condition to be able to meet the mental and physical demands of their work.

Type A behavior by itself is no longer viewed as a major risk factor for CHD, but type A individuals who commonly express anger and hostility are at higher risk. Therefore, many behavioral modification counselors now work on changing the latter behaviors to prevent disease. The questionnaire provided in the second part of Lab 10B will help you determine whether you have a hostile personality.

Next time you feel like getting even with someone for what that person may have done to you, you may want to consider that your anger may be more likely to hurt you. Anger increases heart rate and blood pressure and leads to constriction of blood vessels. Over time, these changes can cause damage to the arteries and eventually lead to a heart attack. Studies indicate that hostile people who get angry often, more intensely, and for longer periods of time, have up to a threefold increased risk for CHD and are seven times more likely to suffer a fatal heart attack by age 50.

Many experts also believe that emotional stress is far more likely than physical stress to trigger a heart attack. People who are impatient and readily annoyed when they have to wait for someone or something—an employee, a traffic light, a table in a restaurant—are especially vulnerable.

Type C The behavior pattern of individuals who are just as highly stressed as the type A but do not seem to be at higher risk for disease than the type B individuals.

BEHAVIOR MODIFICATION PLANNING

Changing a Type A Personality

I PLAN TO | I DID IT

- ❑ ❑ Make a contract with yourself to slow down and take it easy. Put it in writing. Post it in a conspicuous spot, then stick to the terms you set up. Be specific. Abstracts ("I'm going to be less uptight") don't work.
- ❑ ❑ Work on only one or two things at a time. Wait until you change one habit before you tackle the next one.
- ❑ ❑ Eat more slowly and eat only when you are relaxed and sitting down.
- ❑ ❑ If you smoke, quit.
- ❑ ❑ Cut down on your caffeine intake, because it increases the tendency to become irritated and agitated.
- ❑ ❑ Take regular breaks throughout the day, even as brief as 5 or 10 minutes, when you totally change what you're doing. Get up, stretch, get a drink of cool water, walk around for a few minutes.
- ❑ ❑ Work on fighting your impatience. If you're standing in line at the grocery store, study the interesting things people have in their carts instead of getting upset.
- ❑ ❑ Work on controlling hostility. Keep a written log. When do you flare up? What causes it? How do you feel at the time? What preceded it? Look for patterns and figure out what sets you off. Then do something about it. Either avoid the situations that cause you hostility or practice reacting to them in different ways.
- ❑ ❑ Plan some activities just for the fun of it. Load a picnic basket in the car and drive to the country with a friend. After a stressful physics class, stop at a theater and see a good comedy.
- ❑ ❑ Choose a role model, someone you know and admire who does not have a Type A personality. Observe the person carefully, then try out some techniques the person demonstrates.
- ❑ ❑ Simplify your life so you can learn to relax a little bit. Figure out which activities or commitments you can eliminate right now, then get rid of them.
- ❑ ❑ If morning is a problem time for you and you get too hurried, set your alarm clock half an hour earlier.
- ❑ ❑ Take time out during even the most hectic day to do something truly relaxing. Because you won't be used to it, you may have to work at it at first. Begin by listing things you'd really enjoy that would calm you. Include some things that take only a few minutes: Watch a sunset, lie out on the lawn at night and look at the stars, call an old friend and catch up on news, take a nap, sauté a pan of mushrooms and savor them slowly.
- ❑ ❑ If you're under a deadline, take short breaks. Stop and talk to someone for 5 minutes, take a short walk, or lie down with a cool cloth over your eyes for 10 minutes.
- ❑ ❑ Pay attention to what your own body clock is saying. You've probably noticed that every 90 minutes or so, you lose the ability to concentrate, get a little sleepy, and have a tendency to daydream. Instead of fighting the urge, put down your work and let your mind wander for a few minutes. Use the time to imagine and let your creativity run free.
- ❑ ❑ Learn to treasure unplanned surprises: a friend dropping by unannounced, a hummingbird outside your window, a child's tightly clutched bouquet of wildflowers.
- ❑ ❑ Savor your relationships. Think about the people in your life. Relax with them and give yourself to them. Give up trying to control others and resist the urge to end relationships that don't always go as you'd like them to.

Try It

If type A describes your personality, pick three of the above strategies and apply them in your life this week. At the end of each day determine how well you have done that day and evaluate how you can improve the next day.

Research is also focusing on individuals who have anxiety, depression, and feelings of helplessness when they encounter setbacks and failures in life. People who lose control of their lives or who give up on their dreams in life, knowing that they could and should be doing better, are probably more likely to have heart attacks than hard-driving people who enjoy their work.

BEHAVIOR MODIFICATION PLANNING

Tips to Manage Anger

I PLAN TO | I DID IT

- ❑ ❑ Commit to change and gain control over the behavior.
- ❑ ❑ Remind yourself that chronic anger leads to illness and disease and may shorten your life.
- ❑ ❑ Recognize when feelings of anger are developing and ask yourself the following questions:
  - Is the matter really that important?
  - Is the anger justified?
  - Can I change the situation without getting angry?
  - Is it worth risking my health over it?
- ❑ ❑ Tell yourself, "Stop, my health is worth it" every time you start to feel anger.
- ❑ ❑ Prepare for a positive response: Ask for an explanation or clarification of the situation, walk away and evaluate the situation, exercise, or use appropriate stress management techniques (breathing, meditation, imagery) before you become angry and hostile.
- ❑ ❑ Manage anger at once; do not let it build up.
- ❑ ❑ Never attack anyone verbally or physically.
- ❑ ❑ Keep a journal and ponder the situations that cause you to be angry.
- ❑ ❑ Seek professional help if you are unable to overcome anger by yourself: You are worth it.

Try It

If you and others feel that anger is disrupting your health and relationships, the above management strategies are critical to help restore a sense of well-being in your life. In your Online Journal or class notebook, list all of the strategies on a separate sheet of paper, study them each morning, and then evaluate yourself every night for the next week. If you gain control over the behavior, continue with the exercise until it becomes a healthy behavior. If you still struggle, professional help is recommended. You are worth it.

Vulnerability to Stress

Researchers have identified a number of factors that can affect the way in which people handle stress. How people deal with these factors can actually increase or decrease vulnerability to stress. The questionnaire provided in Lab 10C lists these factors so that you can determine your vulnerability rating. Many of the items on this questionnaire are related to health, social support, self-worth, and nurturance (sense of being needed). All of these factors are crucial to your physical, social, mental, and emotional well-being and are essential to cope effectively with stressful life events. The more integrated you are in society, the less vulnerable you are to stress and illness.

Positive correlations have been found between social support and health outcomes. People can draw on social support to weather crises. Knowing that someone else cares, that people are there to lean on, and that support is out there is valuable for survival (or growth) in times of need.

The health benefits of physical fitness have already been discussed extensively. The questionnaire in Lab 10C will help you identify specific areas in which you can make improvements to help you cope more efficiently.

As you complete Lab 10C, you will notice that many of the items describe situations and behaviors that are within your control. To make yourself less vulnerable to stress, improve the behaviors that make you more vulnerable to stress. You should start by modifying the behaviors that are easiest to change before undertaking some of the most difficult ones.

Time Management

According to Benjamin Franklin, "Time is the stuff life is made of." The present hurry-up style of American life is not conducive to wellness. The hassles involved in getting through a routine day often lead to stress-related illnesses. People who do not manage their time properly quickly experience chronic stress, fatigue, despair, discouragement, and illness.

Surveys indicate that most Americans think time moves too fast for them, and more than half of those surveyed think they have to get *everything* done. The younger the respondents, the more they struggled with lack of time. Almost half wished they had more time for exercise and recreation, hobbies, and family. Healthy and successful people are good time managers, able to maintain a pace of life within their comfort zone and attribute their success to smart work, not necessarily hard work.

Five Steps to Time Management Trying to achieve one or more goals in a limited time can create a tremendous amount of stress. Many people just don't seem to have enough hours in the day to accomplish their tasks. The

BEHAVIOR MODIFICATION PLANNING

Common Time Killers

I PLAN TO	I DID IT	
❑	❑	Watching television, listening to radio/music
❑	❑	Excessive sleeping
❑	❑	Surfing/socializing on the Internet
❑	❑	Unnecessary texting, IMing, e-mailing
❑	❑	Daydreaming
❑	❑	Shopping
❑	❑	Socializing/parties
❑	❑	Excessive recreation
❑	❑	Talking on the telephone
❑	❑	Worrying
❑	❑	Procrastinating
❑	❑	Drop-in visitors
❑	❑	Confusion (unclear goals)
❑	❑	Indecision (what to do next)
❑	❑	Interruptions
❑	❑	Perfectionism (every detail must be done)

Try It

Using Lab 10D, find the time killers in your life and make the necessary changes as required.

greatest demands on their time, nonetheless, are frequently self-imposed—trying to do too much, too fast, too soon.

Some time killers, such as eating, sleeping, and recreation, are necessary for health and wellness, but in excess, they lead to stress in life. You can follow five basic steps to make better use of your time (also see Lab 10D):

1. Find the time killers. Many people do not know how they spend each part of the day. Keep a 4- to 7-day log and record at half-hour intervals the activities you do. Record the activities as you go through your typical day so that you will remember all of them. At the end of each day, decide when you wasted time. You may be shocked by the amount of time you spent on the phone, on the Internet, sleeping (more than 8 hours per night), or watching television.
2. Set long- and short-range goals. Setting goals requires some in-depth thinking and helps put your life and daily tasks in perspective. What do I want out of life? Where do I want to be 10 years from now? Next year? Next week? Tomorrow? You can use Lab 10D to list these goals.
3. Identify your immediate goals and prioritize them for today and this week (use Lab 10D—make as many copies as necessary). Each day, sit down and determine what you need to accomplish that day and that week. Rank your "today" and "this week" tasks in four categories: (1) top priority, (2) medium priority, (3) low priority, and (4) trash.

   Top-priority tasks are the most important ones. If you were to reap most of your productivity from 30 percent of your activities, which would they be? Medium-priority activities are those that must be done but can wait a day or two. Low-priority activities are those to be done only upon completing all top- and middle-priority activities. Trash activities are not worth your time (e.g., cruising the hallways or channel surfing).
4. Use a daily planner to help you organize and simplify your day. New digital tools have made it easier to have daily tasks and calendared items readily accessible for quick reference from laptops, smart phones, or other mobile devices. In this way, you can access your priority list, appointments, notes, phone numbers, and addresses conveniently from your backpack, pocket, or purse. Many individuals think that planning daily and weekly activities is a waste of time. A few minutes to schedule your time each day, however, may pay off in hours saved.

   As you plan your day, be realistic and find your comfort zone. Determine the best way to organize your day. Which is the most productive time for work, study, and errands? Are you a morning person, or are you getting most of your work done when people are quitting for the day? Pick your best hours for top-priority activities. Be sure to schedule enough time for exercise and relaxation. Recreation is not necessarily wasted time. You need to take care of your physical and emotional well-being to ensure a balanced lifestyle.
5. Conduct nightly audits. Take 10 minutes each night to figure out how well you accomplished your goals that day. Successful time managers evaluate themselves daily. This simple task helps you see the entire picture. Cross off the goals you accomplished, and carry over to the next day those you did not get done. You may realize that some goals can be moved down to low priority or be trashed.

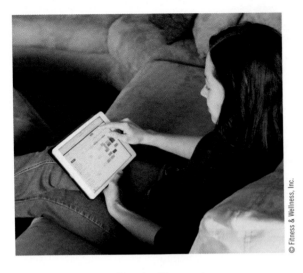
© Fitness & Wellness, Inc.

Planning and prioritizing activities simplifies your days.

Time-Management Skills In addition to the five major steps, the following can help you make better use of your time:

- **Delegate.** If possible, delegate activities that someone else can do for you. Having another person type your paper while you prepare for an exam might be well worth the expense and your time.
- **Say "no."** Learn to say no to activities that keep you from getting your top priorities done. You can do only so much in a single day. Nobody has enough time to do everything he or she would like to get done. Don't overload either. Many people are afraid to say no because they feel guilty if they do. Think ahead, and think of the consequences. Are you doing it to please others? What will it do to your well-being? Can you handle one more task? At some point, you have to balance your activities and look at life and time realistically.
- **Protect against boredom.** Doing nothing can be a source of stress. People need to feel that they are contributing and that they are productive members of society. It is also good for self-esteem and self-worth. Set realistic goals and work toward them each day.
- **Plan ahead for disruptions.** Even a careful plan of action can be disrupted. An unexpected phone call or visitor can change or impede your schedule. Planning your response ahead of time helps you deal with these setbacks.
- **Get it done.** Select only one task at a time, concentrate on it, and see it through. Many people do a little here, do a little there, and then do something else. In the end, nothing gets done. An exception to working on just one task at a time is when you are doing a difficult task. Rather than "killing yourself," interchange with another activity that is not as hard.
- **Eliminate distractions.** If you have trouble adhering to a set plan, remove distractions and trash activities from your eyesight. Television, radio, the Internet, magazines, open doors, or studying in a park might distract you and become time killers.
- **Set aside "overtimes."** Regularly schedule time that you did not think you would need as overtime to complete unfinished projects. Most people underschedule rather than overschedule time. The result is usually late-night burnout. If you schedule overtimes and get your tasks done, enjoy some leisure time, get ahead on another project, or work on other low-priority activities.
- **Plan time for you.** Set aside special time for yourself daily. Life is not meant to be all work. Use your time to walk, read, or listen to your favorite music.
- **Reward yourself.** As with any other healthy behavior, positive change or a job well done deserves a reward. People often overlook the value of rewards, even if they are self-given. Still, they practice behaviors that are rewarded and discontinue those that are not.

One more activity that you should perform weekly is to go through the list of strategies in Lab 10D to determine whether you are becoming a good time manager. Provide a "yes" or "no" answer to each statement. If you are able to answer "yes" to most questions, congratulations: you are becoming a good time manager.

Coping with Stress

The ways in which people perceive and cope with stress seem to be more important in the development of disease than the amount and type of stress. If individuals perceive stress as a definite problem in their lives or if it interferes with their optimal level of health and performance, they can call upon several excellent stress management techniques to help them cope more effectively.

First, of course, the person must recognize the presence of a problem. Many people either do not want to believe that they are under too much stress or they fail to recognize some of the typical symptoms of distress. Noting some of the stress-related symptoms (see the "Common Symptoms of Stress" box) helps a person respond more objectively and initiate an adequate coping response.

When people have stress-related symptoms, they should first try to identify and remove the stressor, or stress-causing agent. This is not as simple as it may seem, because in some situations eliminating the stressor is not possible or people may not know the exact causing agent. If the cause is unknown, keeping a log of the time and days when the symptoms occur, as well as the events preceding and following the onset of symptoms, may be helpful.

For instance, a couple noted that every evening around 6:00 p.m., the wife became nauseated and had abdominal pain. After seeking professional help, both were instructed to keep a log of daily events. It soon became clear that the symptoms did not occur on weekends but always started just before the husband came home from work during the week. Following some personal interviews with the couple,

BEHAVIOR MODIFICATION PLANNING

Common Symptoms of Stress

Check those symptoms you experience regularly.

- ❏ Headaches
- ❏ Muscular aches (mainly in neck, shoulders, and back)
- ❏ Grinding teeth
- ❏ Nervous tic, finger tapping, toe tapping
- ❏ Increased sweating
- ❏ Increase in or loss of appetite
- ❏ Insomnia
- ❏ Nightmares
- ❏ Fatigue
- ❏ Dry mouth
- ❏ Stuttering
- ❏ High blood pressure
- ❏ Tightness or pain in the chest
- ❏ Impotence
- ❏ Hives
- ❏ Dizziness
- ❏ Depression
- ❏ Irritation
- ❏ Anger
- ❏ Hostility
- ❏ Fear, panic, anxiety
- ❏ Stomach pain, flutters
- ❏ Nausea
- ❏ Cold, clammy hands
- ❏ Poor concentration
- ❏ Pacing
- ❏ Restlessness
- ❏ Rapid heart rate
- ❏ Low-grade infection
- ❏ Loss of sex drive
- ❏ Rash or acne

Try It

If you regularly experience some of the above symptoms, use your Online Journal or class notebook to keep a log of when these symptoms occur and under what circumstances. You may find out that a pattern emerges when experiencing distress in life.

it was determined that the wife felt a lack of attention from her husband and responded subconsciously by becoming ill to the point at which she required personal care and affection from her husband. Once the stressor was identified, appropriate behavior changes were initiated to correct the situation.

In many instances, the stressor cannot be removed. Examples of such situations are the death of a close family member, the first year on the job, an intolerable boss, or a change in work responsibility. Nevertheless, stress can be managed through relaxation techniques.

The body responds to stress by activating the **fight-or-flight mechanism**, which prepares a person to take action by stimulating the vital defense systems. This stimulation originates in the hypothalamus and the pituitary gland in the brain. The hypothalamus activates the sympathetic nervous system, and the pituitary activates the release of catecholamines (hormones) from the adrenal glands.

These hormonal changes increase heart rate, blood pressure, blood flow to active muscles and the brain, glucose levels, oxygen consumption, and strength—all necessary for the body to fight or flee. For the body to relax, one of these actions must take place. However, if the person is unable to take action, the muscles tense up and tighten (Figure 10.4). This increased tension and tightening can be dissipated effectively through some coping techniques.

Physical Activity

The benefits of physical activity in reducing the physiological and psychological responses to stress are well established.[5] Exercise is one of the simplest tools to control stress. The value of exercise in reducing stress is related to several factors, the main one being a decrease in muscular tension. For example, a person can be distressed because he or she has had a miserable 8 hours of work with an intolerable boss. To make matters worse, it is late and, on the way home, the car in front is going much slower than the speed limit. The fight-or-flight mechanism—already activated during the stressful day—begins again: catecholamines rise, heart rate and blood pressure shoot up, breathing quickens and deepens, muscles tense, and all systems say "go." However, no

Fight-or-flight mechanism The physiological response of the body to stress that prepares the individual to take action by stimulating the body's vital defense systems.

FIGURE 10.4 Physiological response to stress: fight-or-flight mechanism.

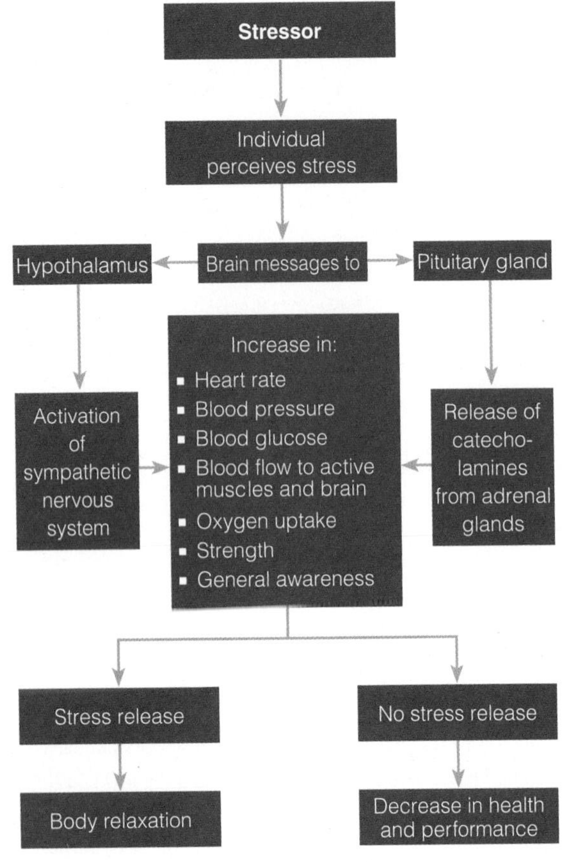

action can be initiated and stress can't be dissipated, because the person cannot just hit the boss or the car in front.

A real remedy would be to take action by "hitting" the swimming pool, the tennis ball, the weight room, or the jogging trail. Engaging in physical activity reduces muscular tension and metabolizes increased catecholamines (which were triggered by the fight-or-flight mechanism and brought about the physiological changes). Furthermore, while the individual is concentrating on the tennis game, there isn't enough time to think about an irrational boss or other undesirable events. Although exercise does not solve problems at work or take care of slow drivers, it certainly helps the person cope with stress and prevents stress from becoming a chronic problem.

Stress management experts often recommend selecting activities like **yoga**, **tai chi**, and Pilates that combine physical activity with additional stress reduction techniques. The latter activities regularly incorporate meditation, breathing, muscle relaxation, or a combination of these techniques—along with physical activity—to help people dissipate stress.

The early evening hours are a popular time to exercise for a lot of highly stressed executives. On the way home from work, they stop at the health club or the fitness center. Exercising at this time helps them to dissipate the stress accumulated during the day. Not only does evening exercise

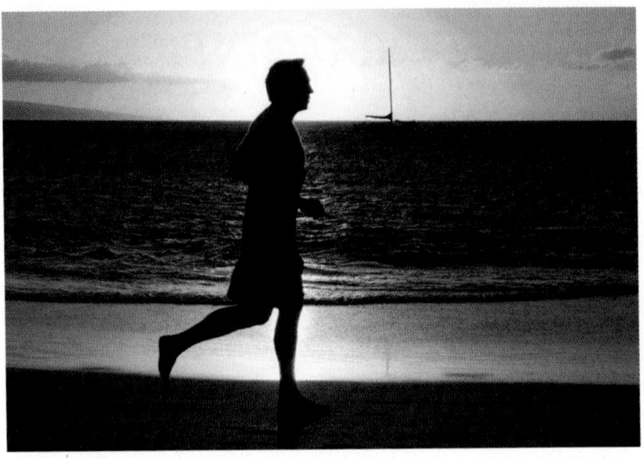

Physical activity is an excellent tool to control stress.

help them get rid of the stress, but it also provides an opportunity to enjoy the evening more. At home, the family appreciates Dad or Mom coming home more relaxed, leaving work problems behind, and being able to dedicate all energy to family activities.

Many people can relate to exercise as a means of managing stress by remembering how good they felt the last time they concluded a strenuous exercise session after a long, difficult day at the office. A fatigued muscle is a relaxed muscle. For this reason, many people have said that the best part of exercise is the shower afterward.

Research also has shown that physical exercise requiring continuous and rhythmic muscular activity, such as aerobic exercise, stimulates alpha-wave activity in the brain. These are the same wave patterns commonly seen during meditation and relaxation.

Further, during vigorous aerobic exercise lasting 30 minutes or longer, morphine-like substances referred to as **endorphins** are thought to be released from the pituitary gland in the brain. These substances not only act as painkillers but also seem to induce the soothing, calming effect often associated with aerobic exercise. Research has also shown that moderate-intensity exercise has an immediate effect on a person's mood and the effects last up to 12 hours following activity. Thus exercise mitigates the daily stress that leads to mood alterations. Exercise is free and easily accessible to everyone. Pick an activity that you enjoy and use it to combat stress, blue moods, anxiety, and depression.

Another way by which exercise helps lower stress is to deliberately divert stress to various body systems. Dr. Selye explains in his book *Stress without Distress* that, when one specific task becomes difficult, a change in activity can be as good or better than rest itself.[6] For example, if a person is having trouble with a task and does not seem to be getting anywhere, jogging or swimming for a while is better than sitting around and getting frustrated. In this way, the mental strain is diverted to the working muscles, and one system helps the other to relax.

Other psychologists indicate that when muscular tension is removed from emotional strain, the emotional strain

BEHAVIOR MODIFICATION PLANNING

Thirty-Second Body Scan

This simple thirty-second exercise helps you scan the body to raise stress awareness.

- ❑ Am I clenching my teeth?
- ❑ Am I furrowing my brow?
- ❑ Are my shoulders tense?
- ❑ Am I breathing rapidly?
- ❑ Am I tapping my fingers?
- ❑ Do I feel knots in my stomach?
- ❑ Are my arms, thighs, or calves tight?
- ❑ Am I nervously bouncing my leg or foot?
- ❑ Am I curling my toes?
- ❑ Do I feel uneasiness anywhere else in my body?

Try It

A body scan can be performed daily or several times a day to help you learn and recognize when you are distressed. People are often unaware of stress signals and activities that are causing excess stress. Increasing awareness allows you to initiate proper actions to more effectively manage stress. An example would be to breathe deeply for 1 to 3 minutes while doing the body scan and repeating positive affirmations (e.g., "I am at peace" or "I am calm and relaxed").

disappears. In many cases, the change of activity suddenly clears the mind and helps put the pieces together.

Researchers have found that physical exercise gives people a psychological boost because exercise does the following:

- Lessens feelings of anxiety, depression, frustration, aggression, anger, and hostility
- Alleviates insomnia
- Provides an opportunity to meet social needs and develop new friendships
- Allows the person to share common interests and problems
- Develops discipline
- Provides the opportunity to do something enjoyable and constructive that leads to better health and total well-being

Beyond the short-term benefits of exercise in lessening stress, a regular aerobic exercise program strengthens the cardiovascular system. Because the cardiovascular system seems to be affected seriously by stress, a stronger system should be able to cope more effectively. For instance, good cardiorespiratory endurance has been shown to lower resting heart rate and blood pressure. Because both heart rate and blood pressure rise in stressful situations, initiating the stress response at a lower baseline counteracts some negative effects of stress. Cardiorespiratory-fit individuals can cope more effectively and are less affected by the stresses of daily living.

Relaxation Techniques

Although benefits are reaped immediately after engaging in any of the several relaxation techniques, several months of regular practice may be necessary for total mastery. The relaxation exercises that follow should not be considered cure-alls. If these exercises do not prove to be effective, more specialized textbooks and professional help are called for. (Some symptoms may not be caused by stress but rather may be related to a medical disorder.)

Biofeedback

Clinical application of **biofeedback** has been used for many years to treat various medical disorders. Besides its successful application in managing stress, it is commonly used to treat medical disorders such as essential hypertension, asthma, heart rhythm and rate disturbances, cardiac neurosis, eczematous dermatitis, fecal incontinence, insomnia, and stuttering. Biofeedback as a treatment modality has been defined as a

Yoga A school of thought in the Hindu religion that seeks to help the individual attain a higher level of spirituality and peace of mind.

Tai chi A self-paced form of exercise often described as "meditation in motion," because it promotes serenity through gentle, balanced, low-impact movements that bring together the mind, body, and emotions.

Endorphins Morphinelike substances released from the pituitary gland in the brain during prolonged aerobic exercise and thought to induce feelings of euphoria and natural well-being.

Biofeedback A stress management technique in which a person learns to influence physiological responses that are not typically under voluntary control or responses that typically are regulated but for which regulation has broken down as a result of injury, trauma, or illness.

technique in which a person learns to influence physiological responses that are not typically under voluntary control or responses that normally are regulated but for which regulation has broken down as a result of injury, trauma, or illness.

In simpler terms, biofeedback is the interaction with the interior self. This interaction enables a person to learn the relationship between the mind and the biological response. The person can "feel" how thought processes influence biological responses (e.g., heart rate, blood pressure, body temperature, and muscle tension) and how biological responses influence thought processes.

As an illustration of this process, consider the association between a strange noise in the middle of a dark, quiet night and the heart rate response. At first, the heart rate shoots up because of the stress the unknown noise induces. The individual may even feel the heart palpitating in the chest and, while still uncertain about the noise, attempt not to panic to prevent an even faster heart rate. Upon realizing that all is well, the person can take control and influence the heart rate to come down. The mind, now calm, is able to exert almost complete control over the biological response.

Complex electronic instruments are required to conduct biofeedback. The process entails a three-stage, closed-loop feedback system:

1. A biological response to a stressor is detected and amplified.
2. The response is processed.
3. Results of the response are fed back to the individual immediately.

The person uses this new input and attempts to change the physiological response voluntarily—this attempt, in turn, is detected, amplified, and processed. The results then are fed back to the person. The process continues with the intent of teaching the person to reliably influence the physiological response for the better (Figure 10.5). The most common methods used to measure physiological responses are monitoring the heart rate, finger temperature, and blood pressure; electromyograms; and electroencephalograms. The goal of biofeedback training is to transfer the experiences learned in the laboratory to everyday living.

FIGURE 10.5 **Biofeedback mechanism.**

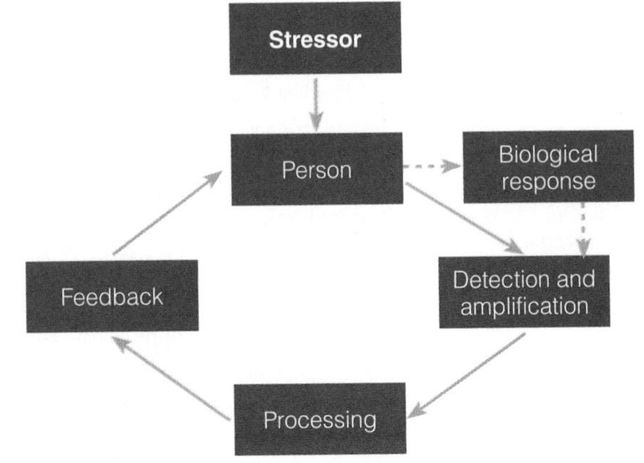

Although biofeedback has significant applications in treating various medical disorders, including stress, it requires adequately trained personnel and, in many cases, costly equipment. Therefore, several alternative methods that yield similar results are frequently substituted for biofeedback. For example, research has shown that exercise and progressive muscle relaxation, used successfully in stress management, seem to be just as effective as biofeedback in treating essential hypertension.

Progressive Muscle Relaxation

Progressive muscle relaxation, developed by Dr. Edmund Jacobsen in the 1930s, enables individuals to relearn the sensation of deep relaxation. The technique involves progressively contracting and relaxing muscle groups throughout the body. Because chronic stress leads to high levels of muscular tension, acute awareness of how progressively tightening and relaxing the muscles feels can release the tension in the muscles and teach the body to relax at will.

Feeling the tension instigated during the exercises also helps the person to be more alert to signs of distress, because this tension is similar to that experienced in stressful situations. In everyday life, these feelings then can cue the person to do relaxation exercises.

Relaxation exercises should be done in a quiet, warm, well-ventilated room. The recommended exercises and the duration of the routine vary from one person to the next. Most important is that the individual pay attention to the sensation he or she feels each time the muscles are tensed and relaxed.

The exercises should encompass all muscle groups of the body. Following is an example of a sequence of progressive muscle relaxation exercises. The instructions for these exercises can be read to the person, memorized, or tape recorded. At least 20 minutes should be set aside to complete the entire sequence. Doing the exercises faster defeats their purpose. Ideally, the sequence should be done twice a day.

The individual performing the exercises stretches out comfortably on the floor, face up, with a pillow under the knees and assumes a passive attitude, allowing the body to relax as much as possible. Each muscle group is to be contracted in sequence, taking care to avoid any strain. Muscles should be tightened to only about 70 percent of the total possible tension to avoid cramping or some type of injury to the muscle.

To produce the relaxation effects, the person must pay attention to the sensation of tensing and relaxing. The person holds each contraction about 5 seconds and then allows the muscles to go totally limp. The person should take enough time to contract and relax each muscle group before going on to the next. An example of a complete progressive muscle relaxation sequence is as follows:

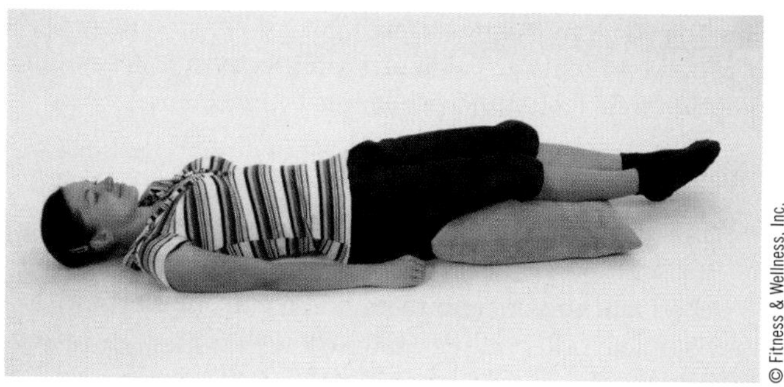

Regularly practicing progressive muscle relaxation helps reduce stress.

1. Point your feet, curling the toes downward. Study the tension in the arches and the top of the feet. Hold, continue to note the tension, and then relax. Repeat once.
2. Flex the feet upward toward the face and note the tension in your feet and calves. Hold and relax. Repeat once.
3. Push your heels down against the floor as if burying them in the sand. Hold and note the tension at the back of the thigh. Relax. Repeat once.
4. Contract the right thigh by straightening the leg, gently raising the leg off the floor. Hold and study the tension. Relax. Repeat with the left leg. Hold and relax. Repeat each leg.
5. Tense the buttocks by raising your hips ever so slightly off the floor. Hold and note the tension. Relax. Repeat once.
6. Contract the abdominal muscles. Hold them tight and note the tension. Relax. Repeat once.
7. Suck in your stomach. Try to make it reach your spine. Flatten your lower back to the floor. Hold and feel the tension in the stomach and lower back. Relax. Repeat once.
8. Take a deep breath, hold it, and then exhale. Repeat. Note your breathing becoming slower and more relaxed.
9. Place your arms at the sides of your body and clench both fists. Hold, study the tension, and relax. Repeat.
10. Flex the elbow by bringing both hands to the shoulders. Hold tight and study the tension in the biceps. Relax. Repeat.
11. Place your arms flat on the floor, palms up, and push the forearms hard against the floor. Note the tension on the triceps. Hold and relax. Repeat.
12. Shrug your shoulders, raising them as high as possible. Hold and note the tension. Relax. Repeat.
13. Gently push your head backward. Note the tension in the back of the neck. Hold and relax. Repeat.
14. Gently bring the head against the chest, push forward, hold, and note the tension in the neck. Relax. Repeat.
15. Press your tongue toward the roof of your mouth. Hold, study the tension, and relax. Repeat.

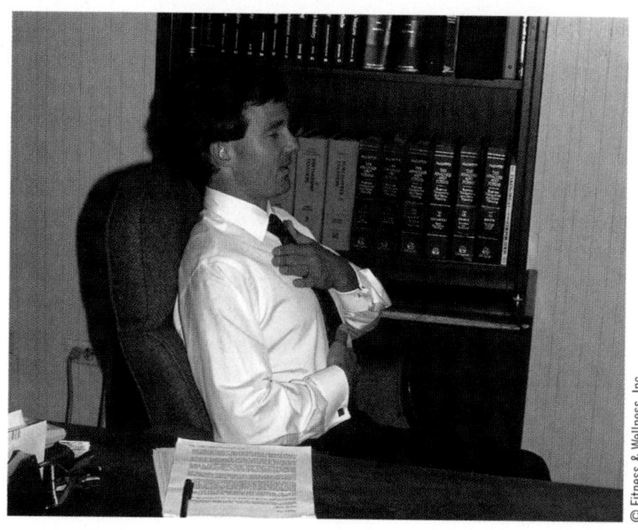

Breathing exercises help dissipate stress.

16. Press your teeth together. Hold, and study the tension. Relax. Repeat.
17. Close your eyes tightly. Hold them closed and note the tension. Relax, leaving your eyes closed. Do this one more time.
18. Wrinkle your forehead and note the tension. Hold and relax. Repeat.

When time is a factor during the daily routine and an individual is not able to go through the entire sequence, he or she may do only the exercises specific to the area that feels most tense. Performing a partial sequence is better than not doing the exercises. Completing the entire sequence, of course, yields the best results.

Breathing Techniques for Relaxation

How often do you pay attention to your breathing? Breathing is among the many physiological functions affected by stress, but even when minimal stress is present, few people maintain a habit of breathing fully and properly. On average, only one-third of an adult's lung capacity is required in normal breathing. Proper breathing is vital to optimal health, as the process of inhaling air feeds life-sustaining oxygen to the lungs and in turn the cardiovascular system feeds it to virtually every part of the body, revitalizing organs, cells, and tissues. A pattern of shallow, quick breathing in reaction to stress restricts the body and brain from receiving the amount of oxygen required for healthy function.

Breathing fully and deeply

Progressive muscle relaxation A stress management technique that involves sequential contraction and relaxation of muscle groups throughout the body.

has been shown to ease anxiety and pain, improve asthma symptoms, burn calories more efficiently, lower blood pressure, strengthen the immune system, and help people with diabetes control blood sugar. Students who practice deep breathing meditation significantly increase academic learning and achievement. One study in particular found that college students who practiced deep-breathing exercises before an exam reported decreased levels of anxiety, nervousness, and loss of concentration.[7] This improvement occurs as deep breathing raises oxygen saturation in cells, increasing energy, cognitive function, and heart-rate variability.

Breathing exercises engage one of your body's most powerful mechanisms for naturally reducing stress. These exercises have been used for centuries in the Orient and India to improve mental, physical, and emotional stamina. In breathing exercises, the person concentrates on "breathing away" the tension and inhaling a large amount of air with each breath. Breathing exercises can be learned in only a few minutes and require considerably less time than the progressive muscle relaxation exercises.

As with any other relaxation technique, these exercises should be done in a quiet, pleasant, well-ventilated room. Any of the three examples of breathing exercises presented here helps relieve tension induced by stress.

1. **Deep breathing.** Lie with your back flat against the floor and place a pillow under your knees. Feet are slightly separated, with toes pointing outward. (The exercise also may be done while sitting in a chair or standing straight.) Place one hand on your abdomen and the other hand on your chest.

   Slowly breathe in and out so that the hand on your abdomen rises when you inhale and falls as you exhale. The hand on the chest should not move much. Repeat the exercise about 10 times. Next, scan your body for tension and compare your present tension with the tension you felt at the beginning of the exercise. Repeat the entire process once or twice.
2. **Sighing.** Using the abdominal breathing technique, breathe in through your nose to a specific count (e.g., 4, 5, or 6). Now exhale through pursed lips to double the intake count (e.g., 8, 10, or 12, respectively). Repeat the exercise 8 to 10 times whenever you feel tense.
3. **Complete natural breathing.** Sit in an upright position or stand straight. Breathing through your nose, gradually fill your lungs from the bottom up. Hold your breath for several seconds. Now exhale slowly by allowing your chest and abdomen to relax, and try to empty your lungs completely. Repeat the exercise 8 to 10 times.

CRITICAL THINKING

List the three most common stressors that you face as a college student. What techniques have you used to manage these situations, and in what way have they helped you cope?

Visual Imagery

Visual or mental **imagery** has been used as a healing technique for centuries in various cultures around the world. In Western medicine, the practice of imagery is relatively new and not widely accepted among health care professionals.

Research is now being done to study the effects of imagery on the treatment of conditions such as cancer, hypertension, asthma, chronic pain, and obesity. Imagery induces a state of relaxation that rids the body of the stress that leads to illness. It improves circulation and increases the delivery of healing antibodies and white blood cells to the site of illness.[8] Imagery also helps a person increase self-confidence, regain control and power over the body, and lessen feelings of hopelessness, fear, and depression.

Visual imagery involves the creation of relaxing visual images and scenes in times of stress to elicit body and mind relaxation. Imagery works by offsetting the stressor with the visualization of relaxing scenes: a sunny beach, a beautiful meadow, a quiet mountaintop, lying in a hammock in a quiet backyard, soaking in a hot tub, or some other peaceful

BEHAVIOR MODIFICATION PLANNING

Five-Minute Destress Technique

The following simple exercise can be used as an effective stress management technique, especially when coming home at the end of the day. Destress by taking five minutes before getting into your evening routine by removing your shoes, lying on the carpet, and placing your feet up on a chair. Use a rolled-up towel at the base of the skull for neck tension or along the middle of the spine for back tension. The lower back should be flat on the floor. Completely relax and practice deep breathing for five minutes.

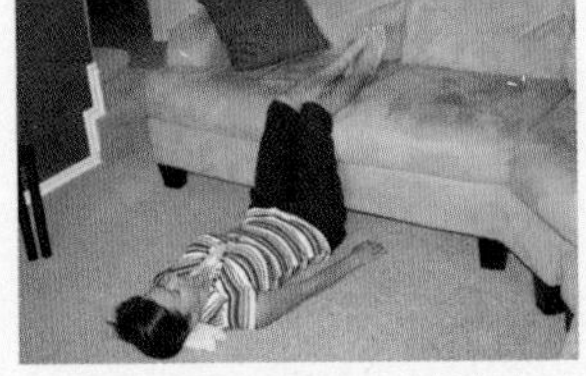

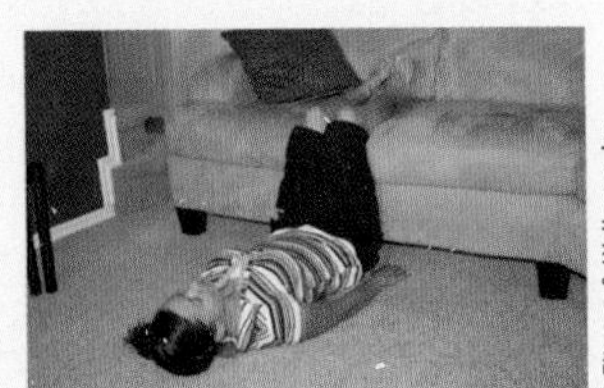

Try It

This simple exercise will help you reduce stress at the end of the day and start your evening right.

BEHAVIOR MODIFICATION PLANNING

Characteristics of Good Stress Managers

Do you have the habits and characteristics of someone who manages stress well?

I PLAN TO	I DID IT	GOOD STRESS MANAGERS...
❑	❑	are physically active, eat a healthy diet, and get adequate rest every day.
❑	❑	believe they have control over events in their life (have an internal locus of control).
❑	❑	understand their own feelings and accept their limitations.
❑	❑	recognize, anticipate, monitor, and regulate stressors within their capabilities.
❑	❑	control emotional and physical responses when distressed.
❑	❑	use appropriate stress management techniques when confronted with stressors.
❑	❑	recognize warning signs and symptoms of excessive stress.
❑	❑	schedule daily time to unwind, relax, and evaluate the day's activities.
❑	❑	control stress when called upon to perform.
❑	❑	enjoy life despite occasional disappointments and frustrations.
❑	❑	look success and failure squarely in the face and keep moving along a predetermined course.
❑	❑	move ahead with optimism and energy and do not spend time and talent worrying about failure.
❑	❑	learn from previous mistakes and use them as building blocks to prevent similar setbacks in the future.
❑	❑	give of themselves freely to others.
❑	❑	have a deep meaning in life.

Try It

Change for many people is threatening, but often required. Pick three of the above strategies and apply them in your life. After several days, determine the usefulness of these strategies to your physical, mental, social, and emotional well-being.

setting. If you are ill, you can also visualize your white blood cells attacking an infection or a tumor. Imagery is also used in conjunction with breathing exercises, meditation, and yoga.

As with other stress management techniques, imagery should be performed in a quiet and comfortable environment. You can either sit or lie down for the exercise. If you lie down, use a soft surface and place a pillow under your knees. Be sure that your clothes are loose and that you are as comfortable as you can be.

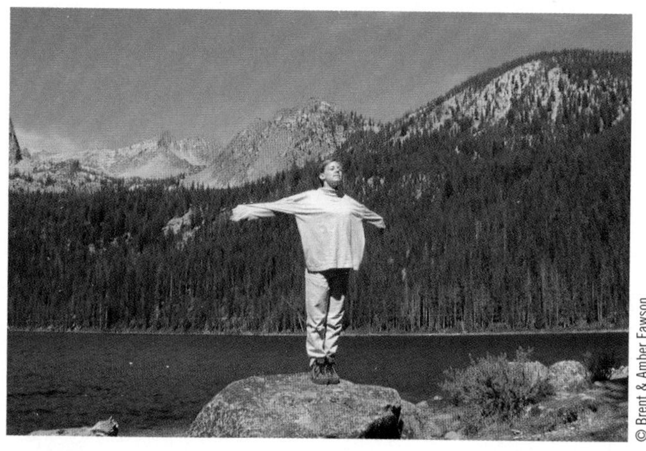

Visual imagery of beautiful and relaxing scenes helps attenuate the stress response.

To start the exercise, close your eyes and take a few breaths using one of the breathing techniques previously described. You then can proceed to visualize one of your favorite scenes in nature. Place yourself into the scene, and visualize yourself moving about and experiencing nature to its fullest. Enjoy the people, the animals, the colors, the sounds, the smells, and even the temperature in your scene. After 10 to 20 minutes of visualization, open your eyes and compare the tension in your body and mind at this point with how you felt prior to the exercise. You can repeat this exercise as often as you deem necessary when you are feeling tension or stress.

You may not always be able to find a quiet and comfortable setting in which to sit or lie down for

Breathing exercises A stress management technique wherein the individual concentrates on "breathing away" the tension and inhaling fresh air to the entire body.

Imagery Mental visualization of relaxing images and scenes to induce body relaxation in times of stress or as an aid in the treatment of certain medical conditions, such as cancer, hypertension, asthma, chronic pain, and obesity.

10 to 20 minutes. If you think imagery works for you, however, you can perform this technique while standing or sitting in an active setting. If you are able, close your eyes, disregard your surroundings for a short moment, and visualize one of your favorite scenes. Once you feel that you have regained some control over the stressor, open your eyes and continue with your assigned tasks.

Autogenic Training

Autogenic training is a form of self-suggestion in which people place themselves in an autohypnotic state by repeating and concentrating on feelings of heaviness and warmth in the extremities. This technique was developed by Johannes Schultz, a German psychiatrist, who noted that hypnotized individuals developed sensations of warmth and heaviness in the limbs and torso. The sensation of warmth is caused by dilation of blood vessels, which increases blood flow to the limbs. Muscular relaxation produces the feeling of heaviness.

In this technique, the person lies down or sits in a comfortable position, eyes closed; concentrates progressively on six fundamental stages; says (or thinks) the following:

1. Heaviness
   My right (left) arm is heavy.
   Both arms are heavy.
   My right (left) leg is heavy.
   Both legs are heavy.
   My arms and legs are heavy.
2. Warmth
   My right (left) arm is warm.
   Both arms are warm.
   My right (left) leg is warm.
   Both legs are warm.
   My arms and legs are warm.
3. Heart
   My heartbeat is calm and regular. (Repeat four or five times.)
4. Respiration
   My body breathes itself. (Repeat four or five times.)
5. Abdomen
   My abdomen is warm. (Repeat four or five times.)
6. Forehead
   My forehead is cool. (Repeat four or five times.)

The autogenic training technique is more difficult to master than any of those mentioned previously. The person should not move too fast through the entire exercise, because this may interfere with learning and relaxation. Each stage must be mastered before proceeding to the next.

Meditation

Meditation helps people draw attention inward and calm the mind. It is a mental exercise that brings about mental, spiritual, and physical benefits, including stress reduction and a feeling of well-being. It encompasses a combination of techniques such as thoughts, breathing, sounds, postures, visualization, and/or movement that help achieve a relaxed state of being. Regular meditation has been shown to decrease blood pressure, stress, anger, anxiety, fear, negative feelings, chronic pain, and increase activity in the brain's left frontal region—an area associated with positive emotions.[9] The objective of meditation is to gain control over one's attention by clearing the mind and blocking out the stressor(s) responsible for the higher tension.

This technique can be learned rather quickly, but first-time users often drop out before reaping benefits because they feel intimidated, confused, bored, or frustrated. In such cases, a group setting is best to get started. Many colleges, community programs, health clubs, and hospitals offer classes.

Initially, the person who is learning to meditate should choose a room that is comfortable, quiet, and free of all disturbances (including telephones). After learning the technique, the person will be able to meditate just about anywhere. A time block of approximately 10 to 15 minutes is adequate to start, but as you become more comfortable with meditation, you can lengthen the time to 30 minutes or longer. To use meditation effectively, meditate daily—just once or twice per week may not provide noticeable benefits.

Meditation "101" Of the several forms of meditation, the following routine is recommended to get started:

1. Sit in a chair in an upright position with the hands resting either in your lap or on the arms of the chair. Close your eyes and focus on your breathing. Allow your body to relax as much as possible. Do not try to consciously relax, because trying means work. Rather, assume a passive attitude and concentrate on your breathing.
2. Allow the body to breathe regularly, at its own rhythm, and repeat in your mind the word "one" every time you inhale, and the word "two" every time you exhale. Paying attention to these two words keeps distressing thoughts from entering your mind.
3. Continue to breathe in this way for about 15 minutes. Because the objective of meditation is to bring about a hypometabolic state leading to body relaxation, do not use an alarm clock to remind you that the 15 minutes have expired. The alarm will only trigger your stress response again, defeating the purpose of the exercise. Opening your eyes once in a while to keep track of the time is fine, but do not rush or anticipate the end of the session. This time has been set aside for meditation, and you need to relax, take your time, and enjoy the exercise.

Mindless Meditation In addition to alleviating stress, mindless meditation is frequently used to help people relieve chronic pain and increase pain tolerance. Chronic pain increases stress hormones that lead a person to think that pain is much worse than it really is. Research indicates that chronic pain sufferers who use this technique not only

Stress-Coping Strategies

- Balance personal, work, and family needs and obligations.
- Have a sense of control and purpose in life.
- Increase self-efficacy.
- Be optimistic.
- Express your emotions.
- Get adequate sleep.
- Eat well-balanced meals.
- Be physically active every day.
- Do not worry about things that you cannot control (the weather, for example).
- Actively strive to resolve conflicts with other people.
- Prepare for stressful events the best possible way (public speaking, job interviews, exams).
- Limit or abstain from alcohol intake.
- Do not use tobacco in any form.
- View change as positive and not as a threat.
- Obtain social support from family members and friends.
- Use stress management programs and counselors available through work and school programs.
- Seek help from church leaders.
- Engage in nonstressful activities (reading, sports, hobbies, and social events).
- Get involved in your community.
- Practice stress management techniques.
- Adopt a healthy lifestyle.

have greater pain tolerance than nonpractitioners, but they also find discomfort is eased by helping the brain stop anticipating the pain. As pain decreases, stress decreases, and the individual is able to sleep better, hurt less, and exercise more, all of which lead to greater comfort and relaxation.

These steps can be followed to use this technique, which is slightly different from the preceding meditation 101:

1. Close your eyes, breathe slowly and naturally, and focus on the feeling of each inhalation and exhalation.
2. Recognize your feelings, thoughts, and body sensations; but do not dwell on them.
3. Continue to focus on your breathing pattern and your feelings for about 15 minutes.
4. Open your eyes and notice your surroundings while maintaining a calm and gentle breathing pattern.
5. You can now proceed to your daily activity schedule with this peaceful, calm, and serene feeling.

Mindfulness Meditation Mindfulness can be defined as awareness of the present moment. In mindfulness meditation, you focus on becoming fully aware and accepting living in the present moment, paying particular attention to your feelings, thoughts, sensations, and emotions without passing judgment or dwelling in the past or projecting yourself into the future. Mindfulness has been successfully used in helping people adhere to medical treatment, improve hypertension and insomnia, more effectively handle pain, and manage anxiety and depression associated with illness.

How these health benefits were attained on a molecular level through mindfulness and relaxation therapy were just discovered in recent years. Researchers have now determined that the relaxation response that counteracts the negative effects of stress can directly affect genes linked to mitochondrial function, energy metabolism, the immune system, and the secretion of insulin.[10] Gene expression is what governs health or illness and is highly susceptible to influences from our environment, diet, and thoughts. Relaxation techniques enhance the expression of those genes, improving the mitochondria and its supporting cell pathways while simultaneously suppressing pathways that channel chronic inflammation, trauma, stress, and cancer. These new findings suggest that in addition to the outward physiological and psychological benefits you enjoy when you practice mindfulness, you can effectively change yourself on the cellular level by means of healthy gene expression. Important during mindfulness meditation is not to worry about things that you have no control over. To live in the present, you must understand that the most significant event that you have control over is *your attitude.* While your confidence may be shaken because of life's challenges and stressors, you can control your attitude. Having a clear understanding that the "storm will pass" and that "there is light at the end of every tunnel," will allow you to navigate through life's stressors and ultimately overcome challenges and enjoy happiness while living in the present.

Let's look at an example. Your roommate agreed to clean up his three-day mess in the kitchen that evening. When you get home from the library that night, the kitchen looks worse and your roommate is sound asleep in the bedroom. You are extremely disappointed and upset. Your thoughts turn to the past and how much worse it may get in the future. The fight-or-flight mechanism kicks in, and you are ready to wake your roommate up and let him have it. Your

Autogenic training A stress management technique using a form of self-suggestion, wherein an individual is able to place himself or herself in an autohypnotic state by repeating and concentrating on feelings of heaviness and warmth in the extremities.

Meditation A stress management technique used to gain control over attention by clearing the mind and blocking out the stressor(s) responsible for the increased tension.

stress level rises with every thought of the past, present, and potential future. If you should act on your impulses, the situation may only get worse, not to mention your relationship with your roommate.

Now put yourself in the same situation, but stay in the present moment. Don't dwell in the past or worry about the future. Instead of allowing greater anger to build up, choose to stay with the uncomfortable feeling of disappointment for a moment. Recognize it, feel it, and acknowledge the disappointment. Maybe your roommate has a valid reason for not getting it done. Perhaps tomorrow you could tell your roommate about your disappointment, but after a night's rest you may choose not to do so. Now turn your attention to another task in the present moment. Eat a healthy meal and savor every bite, listen to your favorite music and enjoy the melody, go for a walk and appreciate the surroundings and beauty of the night, or take a moment to relish your good health. You can now pay attention to your breathing and notice the fresh air and your breathing pattern for a few minutes. Before retiring to bed, conduct your nightly audit and plan the next day's activities. At this point, notice that stress and the fight-or-flight mechanism have dissipated, and the disappointment of the unclean kitchen, over which you had no control, would not have been worth the frustration and anger that you could have experienced. A few years from now, you can have a healthy laugh over the incident.

Yoga

Yoga is an excellent stress-coping technique. It is a school of thought in the Hindu religion that seeks to help the individual attain a higher level of spirituality and peace of mind. Although its philosophical roots can be considered spiritual, yoga is based on principles of self-care.

Practitioners of yoga adhere to a specific code of ethics and a system of mental and physical exercises that promote control of the mind and the body. In Western countries, many people are familiar mainly with the exercise portion of yoga. This system of exercises (postures or asanas) can be used as a relaxation technique for stress management. The exercises include a combination of postures, diaphragmatic breathing, muscle relaxation, and meditation that help buffer the biological effects of stress. Although people are unable to avoid all life stressors, they can definitely change emotional response through performing yoga postures, observing and controlling their breathing pattern, and reflecting on the moment, all of which are actions that help calm the mind and the body.

Western interest in yoga exercises developed gradually over the last century, particularly since the 1970s. The practice of yoga exercises helps align the musculoskeletal system and increases muscular flexibility, muscular strength and endurance, and balance. Research also confirms that yoga can help improve mood and cognition and reduce stress.[11] Yoga exercises help to dispel stress by raising self-esteem, clearing the mind, slowing respiration, promoting neuromuscular relaxation, and increasing body awareness. In addition, the exercises help relieve back pain and control involuntary body functions like heart rate, blood pressure, oxygen consumption, and metabolic rate. Because yoga therapy has shown to be clinically beneficial for rehabilitation after a stroke,[12] yoga is also used in many hospital-based programs for cardiac patients to help manage stress and decrease blood pressure.

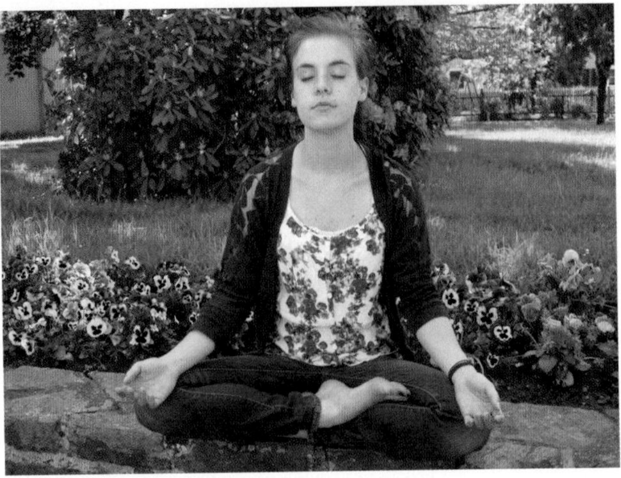

Yoga exercises help induce the relaxation response.

Research on patients with CHD who practiced yoga (among other lifestyle changes) indicates that it slows down or even reverses atherosclerosis. These patients were compared with others who did not use yoga as one of their lifestyle changes.[13] In addition, yoga exercises have been used to help treat chemical dependency, insomnia, and prevent injury.

Of the many styles of yoga, more than 60 are presently taught in the United States. Classes vary according to their emphasis. Some styles of yoga are athletic, while others are passive in nature.

The most popular variety of yoga in the Western world is **hatha yoga**, which incorporates a series of static-stretching postures performed in specific sequences (asanas) that help induce the relaxation response. The postures are held for several seconds while participants concentrate on breathing patterns, meditation, and body awareness.

Today, most yoga classes are variations of hatha yoga, and many typical stretches used in flexibility exercises have been adapted from hatha yoga. Examples include:

1. *Integral yoga* and *viny yoga* that focus on gentle and static stretches
2. *Iyengar yoga*, which promotes muscular strength and endurance
3. *Yogalates*, which incorporates Pilates exercises to increase muscular strength
4. *Power yoga* or *yogarobics*, a high-energy form that links many postures together in a dancelike routine to promote cardiorespiratory fitness

As with flexibility exercises, the stretches in hatha yoga should not be performed to the point of discomfort. Instructors should not push participants beyond their physical limitations. Similar to other stress management techniques, yoga exercises are best performed in a quiet place for 15 to 60 minutes per session. Many yoga participants like to perform the exercises daily.

To appreciate yoga exercises, a person has to experience them. The discussion here serves only as an introduction. Although yoga exercises can be practiced with the instruction of a book or video, most participants take classes. Many of the postures are difficult and complex, and few individuals can master the entire sequence in the first few weeks.

Individuals who are interested in yoga exercises should initially pursue them under qualified instruction. Many universities offer yoga courses, and you can check the phone book or online for a listing of yoga instructors or classes in your area. Yoga courses are offered at many health clubs and recreation centers. Because instructors and yoga styles vary, you may want to sit in on a class before enrolling. The most important thing is to look for an instructor whose views on wellness parallel your own. Instructors are not subject to national certification standards. If you are new to yoga, you are encouraged to compare a couple of instructors before you select a class.

Tai Chi

Tai chi chuan (full name) originated in China centuries ago and is practiced today for defense training and physical and mental health benefits. The martial side, however, is no longer the focus of its practice, so the activity can be performed by young, old, and even very old. In tai chi, the muscles and joints are never extended beyond 70 percent of maximum potential—rather movements are performed with the muscles in a relaxed versus tense state—making it among the safest, low-impact forms of exercise. Surveys show that nearly 3 million people in the United States practice tai chi[14], and many fitness practitioners use it in conjunction with aerobic and strength training.

Tai chi is often described as "meditation in motion," because it is performed with flowing, rhythmic movements that focus heavily on breathing and the slow execution of its movements. The main objective is to promote tranquility and reflection through postures that combine meditation and dance. The postures are performed in sequences known as "sets" that require concentration, coordination, controlled breathing, muscle relaxation, strength, flexibility, gait, and body balance.

Research has attributed many health benefits to tai chi, including diabetes management, arthritis relief, lower blood pressure, faster recovery from heart disease and injury, improved strength and flexibility, better sleep, and improved physical work capacity. Tai chi has gained prevalence with physicians as a supplementary treatment to help prevent or improve medical conditions associated with aging. Among older adults, improved gait and the capability to perform activities of daily living are frequently reported, and some studies have found tai chi to help maintain bone density in elderly women when practiced regularly over time.[15] Tai chi is frequently used for stress management to relieve tension, stress, and anxiety. The mental aspect of having to concentrate on leading the movement and paying attention to detail through the gentle actions dissipates stress. The activity leaves no room to think or worry about other problems, thus calming and relaxing the mind and body.

To master tai chi, you need initial professional guidance. You are encouraged to join the group or class available at many college campuses or community health clubs. The class should emphasize fitness and health benefits rather than combat techniques. Once you have mastered many of the sets available, you can practice the activity on your own.

Which Technique Is Best?

Each person reacts to stress differently. Therefore, the best coping strategy depends mostly on the individual. The technique used does not matter, as long as it works. You may want to experiment with several or all of the techniques presented here to find out which works best for you. A combination of two or more is best for many people.

All of the coping strategies discussed here help to block out stressors and promote mental and physical relaxation by diverting the attention to a different, nonthreatening action. Some of the techniques are easier to learn and may take less time per session. As a part of your class experience, you may participate in a stress management session (see Lab 10E). Regardless of which technique you select, the time spent doing stress management exercises (several times a day, as needed) is well worth the effort when stress becomes a significant problem in life.

Keep in mind that most individuals need to learn to relax and take time for themselves. Stress is not what makes people ill; it's the way they react to the stress-causing agent. Individuals who learn to be diligent and start taking control of themselves find that they can enjoy a better, happier, and healthier life.

Hatha yoga A form of yoga that incorporates specific sequences of static-stretching postures to help induce the relaxation response.

ASSESS YOUR BEHAVIOR

CENGAGE brain .com To access course materials, including companion resources, please visit **www.cengagebrain.com**.

1. Are you able to channel your emotions and feelings to exert a positive effect on your mind, health, and wellness?
2. Do you use time management strategies on a regular basis?
3. Do you use stress management techniques, and do they allow you to be in control over the daily stresses of life?

ASSESS YOUR KNOWLEDGE

1. Positive stress is also referred to as
   a. eustress.
   b. posstress.
   c. functional stress.
   d. distress.
   e. physiostress.
2. Which of the following is *not* a stage of the GAS?
   a. alarm reaction
   b. resistance
   c. compliance
   d. exhaustion and recovery
   e. All are stages of the GAS.
3. The behavior pattern of highly stressed individuals who do not seem to be at higher risk for disease is known as type
   a. A.
   b. B.
   c. C.
   d. E.
   e. X.
4. Effective time managers
   a. delegate.
   b. learn to say "no."
   c. protect from boredom.
   d. set aside overtimes.
   e. All of the choices are correct.
5. Hormonal changes that occur during a stress response
   a. decrease heart rate.
   b. sap the body's strength.
   c. diminish blood flow to the muscles.
   d. induce relaxation.
   e. increase blood pressure.
6. Physical activity decreases stress levels by
   a. deliberately diverting stress to various body systems.
   b. metabolizing excess catecholamines.
   c. diminishing muscular tension.
   d. stimulating alpha-wave activity in the brain.
   e. All of the choices are correct.
7. Biofeedback is
   a. the interaction with the interior self.
   b. the biological response to stress.
   c. the nonspecific response to a stress-causing agent.
   d. used to identify biological factors that cause stress.
   e. most readily achieved while in a state of self-hypnosis.
8. The technique where a person breathes in through the nose to a specific count and then exhales through pursed lips to double the intake count is known as
   a. sighing.
   b. deep breathing.
   c. meditation.
   d. autonomic ventilation.
   e. release management.
9. During autogenic training, a person
   a. contracts each muscle to about 70 percent of capacity.
   b. concentrates on feelings of warmth and heaviness.
   c. visualizes relaxing scenes to induce body relaxation.
   d. learns to reliably influence physiological responses.
   e. notes the positive and negative impacts of frequent stressors on various body systems.
10. Yoga exercises have been successfully used to
    a. stimulate ventilation.
    b. increase metabolism during stress.
    c. slow atherosclerosis.
    d. decrease body awareness.
    e. All of the choices are correct.

Correct answers can be found at the back of the book.

NOTES

1. E. Gullete, et al., "Effects of Mental Stress on Myocardial Ischemia during Daily Life," *Journal of the American Medical Association* 277 (1997): 1521–1525; C. A. Lengacher, et al. "Psychoneuroimmunology and Immune System Link for Stress, Depression, Health Behaviors, and Breast Cancer," *Alternative Health Practitioner* 4 (1998): 95–108.
2. S. Richardson, J. A. Shaffer, L. Falzon, et al., "Meta-Analysis of Perceived Stress and Its Association with Incident Coronary Heart Disease," *The American Journal of Cardiology*, 110, no. 12 (December 2012): 1711–1716.
3. H. Selye, *Stress without Distress* (New York: Signet, 1974).
4. R. J. Kriegel and M. H. Kriegel, *The C Zone: Peak Performance Under Stress* (Garden City, NY: Anchor Press/Doubleday, 1985).
5. See note 2; J. Moses, et al., "The Effects of Exercise Training on Mental Well-Being in the Normal Population: A Controlled Trial," *Journal of Psychosomatic Research* 33 (1989): 47–61; C. Shang, "Emerging Paradigms in Mind–Body Medicine," *Journal of Complementary and Alternative Medicine* 7 (2001): 83–91.
6. See note 1.
7. G. Paul, B. Elam, and S. J. Verhulst, "A Longitudinal Study of Students' Perceptions of Using Deep Breathing Meditation to Reduce Testing Stresses," *Teaching and Learning in Medicine*, 19, no.3 (2007): 287–292.
8. M. Samuels, "Use Your Mind to Heal Your Body," *Bottom Line/Health* 19 (February 2005): 13–14.
9. S. Bodian, "Meditate Your Way to Much Better Health," *Bottom Line/Health* 18 (June 2004): 11–13.
10. M. K. Bhasin, et al., "Relaxation Response Induces Temporal Transcriptome Changes in Energy Metabolism, Insulin Secretion, and Inflammatory Pathways," *PLoS ONE* 8 (May 2013): e62817.
11. A. Lazaridou, P. Philbrook, and A. A. Rzika, "Yoga and Mindfulness as Therapeutic Interventions for Stroke Rehabilitation: A Systematic Review," *Evidence-Based Complementary and Alternative Medicine* (May 2013).
12. See note 10.
13. S. C. Manchanda, et al., "Retardation of Coronary Atherosclerosis with Yoga Lifestyle Intervention," *Journal of the Association of Physicians of India* 48 (2000): 687–694.
14. N. P. Brown, "Easing Ills through Tai Chi," *Harvard Magazine* (January–February 2010).
15. "The Health Benefits of Tai Chi," Harvard *Women's Health Watch* 16, no. 9 (May 2009): 2–4.

SUGGESTED READINGS

Girdano, D. A., D. E. Dusek, and G. S. Everly. *Controlling Stress and Tension*. San Francisco: Benjamin Cummings, 2012.

Greenberg, J. S. *Comprehensive Stress Management*. New York: McGraw-Hill, 2012.

Olpin, M., and M. Hesson. *Stress Management for Life*. Belmont, CA: Wadsworth/Cengage Learning, 2013.

Schwartz, M. S., and F. Andrasik. *Biofeedback: A Practitioner's Guide*. New York: Guilford Press, 2005.

Selye, H. *The Stress of Life*. New York: McGraw-Hill, 1978.

Lab 10A: Stress Events Scale

Name ______________________ Date ____________ Grade ____________

Instructor ______________________ Course ____________ Section ____________

NECESSARY LAB EQUIPMENT
None required.

OBJECTIVE
To determine stressful life events within the past 12 months that may affect your health well-being.

Introduction

The list of stress-causing life events below may have potential adverse effects on your physical and psychological well-being. Check only those events that occurred during the past 12 months and rate the event on a 7-point scale (−3, −2, −1, 0, +1, +2, +3) using the following guidelines:

Negative Effect	Indifferent	Positive Effect
−3 Shocked	0	+3 Jubilant
−2 Dismayed		+2 Delighted
−1 Dissatisfied		+1 Pleased

Section 1: General

	Life Event	Stress Rating
1. Death of a family member	☐	______
2. Death of a close friend or acquaintance	☐	______
3. Substance abuse (addiction to drugs/alcohol)	☐	______
4. Imprisonment	☐	______
5. Law violation (including traffic violations)	☐	______
6. Marriage	☐	______
7. Sexual intimacy	☐	______
8. Pregnancy	☐	______
9. Divorce		
Your own	☐	______
Your parents	☐	______
Other close relative or friend	☐	______

	Life Event	Stress Rating
10. Change/status of		
Self esteem	☐	______
Boyfriend/girlfriend	☐	______
Family relationships	☐	______
Personal health (illness/disease/injury)	☐	______
Family or friend(s) health status	☐	______
Fitness level	☐	______
Sleeping habits	☐	______
Nutrition habits	☐	______
Study habits	☐	______
Friendship(s)	☐	______
Peer acceptance	☐	______
Social activities	☐	______
Recreational activities	☐	______
Mode of transportation	☐	______

Section 1: General (continued)

	Life Event	Stress Rating
11. Ability to laugh and have fun	☐	______
12. Financial status		
Sufficient for needs	☐	______
Increase/decrease in income	☐	______
Mortgage loan	☐	______
Vehicle loan	☐	______
Student loan(s)	☐	______
Other (specify): ______________	☐	______
13. Work responsibilities		
New job	☐	______
Loss of job	☐	______
Change in work responsibilities	☐	______
Change in work hours	☐	______
Relationship with superior(s)	☐	______
Relationship with coworkers	☐	______
14. Time management	☐	______
15. Exceptional personal accomplishment		
Specify: ______________	☐	______
16. Holidays		
Christmas	☐	______
Thanksgiving	☐	______
Other (specify): ______________	☐	______
17. Vacation	☐	______
18. Ability to recoup from trials, tribulations, and challenges	☐	______
19. Spirituality	☐	______
20. Other(s), list: ______________	☐	______
21. ______________	☐	______
22. ______________	☐	______
23. ______________	☐	______

Section 2: Education

	Life Event	Stress Rating
24. Choice of school	☐	______
25. Change in school	☐	______
26. Starting or stopping school	☐	______
27. Loneliness	☐	______
28. Privacy	☐	______
29. Military obligations	☐	______
30. Selecting/changing a major or minor	☐	______
31. School-related activities		
Missed classes	☐	______
Grade(s)	☐	______
Academic probation	☐	______
Course(s)	☐	______
Exam(s)	☐	______
Assignment(s)	☐	______
Academic workload	☐	______
College instructor(s)	☐	______
32. Joining a fraternity/sorority	☐	______
33. Housing		
Satisfied	☐	______
Relationship with roommates	☐	______
Changing roommates	☐	______
Dismissal from dorm or residence	☐	______
Moving	☐	______
34. Graduation	☐	______
35. Career employment	☐	______
36. Other(s), list: ______________	☐	______
37. ______________	☐	______
38. ______________	☐	______

How to Score

Upon completion of the questionnaire, add all the negative and positive scores separately (e.g., positive ratings: 2, 1, 3, and 3 = 9 points positive score; negative ratings: –3, –2, –2, –1, and –2 = 10 points negative score). A final "total stress score" can be obtained by adding the positive score and the negative score together as positive numbers (total stress score: 9 + 10 = 19 points). Stress ratings based on your score are given below. The negative score is the best indicator of stress (distress or negative stress) in your life.

Score Interpretation

Stress Category	Negative Score	Total Score
Poor	≥15	≥30
Fair	9–14	20–29
Average	6–8	15–19
Good	1–5	6–14
Excellent	0	1–5

Stress Events Scale Results

	Points	Stress Category
Negative score:	______	______
Positive score:	______	NA
Total score:	______	______

Lab 10B: Type A Personality and Hostility Assessment

Name ____________ Date ____________ Grade ____________

Instructor ____________ Course ____________ Section ____________

NECESSARY LAB EQUIPMENT
None required.

OBJECTIVE
To determine your Type A personality and hostility ratings.

I. Type A Behavior

Instructions: Please answer "yes" or "no" for each of the items listed below. For questions 7, 15, and 16, give yourself one point for each "yes" answer. For the rest of the questions, give yourself one point for each "no" answer.

Yes	No	
☐	☐	1. Do you feel your job carries heavy responsibility?
☐	☐	2. Would you describe yourself as a hard-driving, ambitious type of person?
☐	☐	3. Do you usually try to get things done as quickly as possible?
☐	☐	4. Would family members and close friends describe you as hard-driving and ambitious?
☐	☐	5. Have people close to you ever asked you to slow down in your work?
☐	☐	6. Do you think you drive harder to accomplish things than most of your associates do?
☐	☐	7. When you play games with people your own age, do you play just for the fun of it?
☐	☐	8. If there's competition in your job, do you enjoy this?
☐	☐	9. When you are driving and there is a car in your lane going much too slowly for you, do you mutter and complain? Would anyone riding with you know you are annoyed?
☐	☐	10. If you make an appointment with someone, are you there on time in almost all cases?
☐	☐	11. If you are kept waiting, do you resent it?
☐	☐	12. If you see someone doing a job rather slowly and you know you could do it faster and better yourself, does it make you restless to watch him or her?
☐	☐	13. Would you be tempted to step in and do it yourself?
☐	☐	14. Do you eat rapidly? Walk rapidly?
☐	☐	15. After you've finished eating, do you like to sit around the table and chat?
☐	☐	16. When you go out to a restaurant and find eight or ten people waiting ahead of you for a table, will you wait?
☐	☐	17. Do you really resent having to wait in line at the bank or post office?
☐	☐	18. Do you always feel anxious to get going and finish whatever you have to do?
☐	☐	19. Do you have the feeling that time is passing too rapidly for you to accomplish all the things you'd like to get done in one day?
☐	☐	20. Do you often feel a sense of time urgency or time pressure?
☐	☐	21. Do you hurry in doing most things?

Form revised from The Structured Interview from the Forum on Type A Behavior, National Heart/Lung/Blood Institute, Ray M. Rosenman, MD, 1981.
This form is reprinted from R. W. Patton, et al., *Implementing Health/Fitness Programs* (Champaign, IL: Human Kinetics Publisher, 1986).

How to Score

Results	Points	
Questions 7, 15, 16:	☐	(1 point for each "yes" answer)
All other questions:	☐	(1 point for each "no" answer)
Total score:	☐	
Your level of Type A:	☐	

Score Interpretation

Rating	Points
High	0–7
Medium	8–13
Low	14–21

II. Hostility Questionnaire

Type A individuals with a hostile personality are at higher risk for disease. This questionnaire can help you identify if you have a hostile personality. Please circle the number of points that best represents your response to each statement.

	Never	Occasionally	Frequently	Always
1. I am impatient.	0	1	2	3
2. I am easily irritated.	0	1	2	3
3. I am argumentative.	0	1	2	3
4. I want to have the final word in every discussion.	0	1	2	3
5. I attack people verbally.	0	1	2	3
6. I am physically aggressive when angry.	0	1	2	3
7. I stop before I act when upset.	3	2	1	0
8. I manage anger at once—I do not let it build up.	3	2	1	0
9. I engage in healthy physical activity when upset or angry.	3	2	1	0
10. I am understanding of unplanned surprises.	3	2	1	0
11. I keep a journal and contemplate what caused me to be angry.	3	2	1	0
12. I give others the benefit of the doubt.	3	2	1	0
13. I am a forgiving person.	3	2	1	0
14. I use positive responses.	3	2	1	0
15. I schedule daily timeouts.	3	2	1	0
16. I sleep 7 to 8 hours per night.	3	2	1	0

Scoring

Any number of points ≥ 1 obtained in items 5, 6, or 7 = ______ = Hostile Personality

Total points for items 1 to 3 and 8 to 16 = ______ A score ≥ 10 points = Hostile Personality

If the scores above indicate that you may have a hostile personality, professional counseling is recommended. The student counseling services at your institution may provide health services to help enhance personal growth, manage stress and hostile behavior, and develop personal effectiveness and resilience. You are strongly encouraged to take steps to control your responses to situations that trigger hostile behavior.

Lab 10C: Stress Vulnerability Questionnaire

Name ______________________ Date ____________ Grade ____________

Instructor ______________________ Course ____________ Section ____________

NECESSARY LAB EQUIPMENT
None required.

OBJECTIVE
To determine your stress vulnerability rating and identify areas where you can reduce your vulnerability to stress.

INSTRUCTIONS
Carefully read each statement and circle the number that best describes your feelings or behavior. Please be completely honest with your answers.

I. Stress Vulnerability Questionnaire

Item	Strongly Agree	Mildly Agree	Mildly Disagree	Strongly Disagree
1. I try to incorporate as much physical activity as possible in my daily schedule.	1	2	3	4
2. I accumulate a minimum of 30 minutes of moderate-intensity physical activity at least five times per week, and I exercise aerobically for 20 minutes or more at least three times per week.	1	2	3	4
3. I regularly sleep 7 to 8 hours per night.	1	2	3	4
4. I take my time eating at least one hot, balanced meal a day.	1	2	3	4
5. I drink fewer than two cups of coffee (or equivalent) per day.	1	2	3	4
6. I am at recommended body weight.	1	2	3	4
7. I enjoy good health.	1	2	3	4
8. I do not use tobacco in any form.	1	2	3	4
9. I limit my alcohol intake to no more than one drink (women) or two (men) per day.	1	2	3	4
10. I do not use hard drugs (chemical dependency).	1	2	3	4
11. There is someone I love, trust, and can rely on for help if I have a problem or need to make an essential decision.	1	2	3	4
12. There is love in my family.	1	2	3	4
13. I routinely give and receive affection.	1	2	3	4
14. I have close personal relationships with other people that provide me with a sense of emotional security.	1	2	3	4
15. There are people close by whom I can turn to for guidance in time of stress.	1	2	3	4
16. I can speak openly about feelings, emotions, and problems with people I trust.	1	2	3	4
17. Other people rely on me for help.	1	2	3	4
18. I am able to keep my feelings of anger and hostility under control.	1	2	3	4
19. I have a network of friends who enjoy the same social activities that I do.	1	2	3	4
20. I take time to do something fun at least once a week.	1	2	3	4
21. My religious beliefs provide guidance and strength in my life.	1	2	3	4
22. I often provide service to others.	1	2	3	4
23. I enjoy my job (or major or school).	1	2	3	4
24. I am a competent worker.	1	2	3	4
25. I get along well with coworkers (or students).	1	2	3	4

Continued

Item	Strongly Agree	Mildly Agree	Mildly Disagree	Strongly Disagree
26. My income is sufficient for my needs.	1	2	3	4
27. I manage time adequately.	1	2	3	4
28. I have learned to say "no" to additional commitments when I already am pressed for time.	1	2	3	4
29. I take daily quiet time for myself.	1	2	3	4
30. I practice stress management as needed.	1	2	3	4

Total Points: ______

Test Interpretation

Rating	Points
Excellent (great stress resistance)	0–30
Good (little vulnerability to stress)	31–40
Average (somewhat vulnerable to stress)	41–50
Fair (vulnerable to stress)	51–60
Poor (very vulnerable to stress)	≥61

This questionnaire helps you identify areas where improvements can be made to help you cope with stress more effectively. As you take this test, you will notice that most of the items describe situations and behaviors that are within your control. To make yourself less vulnerable to stress, improve the behaviors that make you more vulnerable to stress. Start by modifying behaviors that are easiest to change before undertaking the most difficult ones.

II. In the space provided below, list, in order of priority, behaviors that you would like to change to help you decrease your vulnerability to stress. Also, briefly outline how you intend to accomplish these changes.

Lab 10D: Goals and Time Management Skills

Name ______________________ **Date** __________ **Grade** __________

Instructor ______________________ **Course** __________ **Section** __________

NECESSARY LAB EQUIPMENT
None required.

OBJECTIVE
To help you develop time management skills.

INSTRUCTIONS
If you think you don't have enough hours during the day to get everything done, this lab is for you. Be sure to read the Time Management section and fill out all the forms provided with this lab.

I. Long- and Short-Term Goals

In the spaces provided below, list your goals as indicated. You may want to keep this form and review it in years to come.

1. List three goals you wish to accomplish in this life:

____

____

____

2. List three goals you wish to see accomplished 10 years from now:

____

____

____

3. List three goals you wish to accomplish this year:

____

____

____

4. List three goals you wish to accomplish this month:

____

____

____

5. List three goals you wish to accomplish this week:

____

____

____

Signature: ______________________ Date: __________

II. Finding Time Killers

Keep a 4- to 7-day log and record at half-hour intervals the activities you do (make additional copies of this form as needed). Record the activities as you go through your typical day, so you will remember them all. At the end of each day, decide when you wasted time. Using a highlighter, identify the time killers on this form and plan necessary changes for the next day.

Time	Activity
6:00	
6:30	
7:00	
7:30	
8:00	
8:30	
9:00	
9:30	
10:00	
10:30	
11:00	
11:30	
12:00	
12:30	
1:00	
1:30	
2:00	
2:30	
3:00	
3:30	
4:00	
4:30	
5:00	
5:30	
6:00	
6:30	
7:00	
7:30	
8:00	
8:30	
9:00	
9:30	
10:00	
10:30	
11:00	
11:30	
12:00	

III. Daily and Weekly Goals and Priorities

Daily Goals: Take 10 minutes each morning to write down the goals or tasks you wish to accomplish that day. Rank them as top, medium, low, or "trash" priorities. (Make as many copies of this form as needed.) At the end of the day, evaluate how well you accomplished your tasks for the day. Cross off the goals you accomplished and carry over to the next day those you did not get done.

Date: ___/___/___ Day of the Week: ________

Top-Priority Goals

1. ____________
2. ____________
3. ____________
4. ____________

Medium-Priority Goals

1. ____________
2. ____________
3. ____________
4. ____________

Low-Priority Goals

1. ____________
2. ____________
3. ____________
4. ____________

Trash (do only after all other goals have been accomplished)

1. ____________
2. ____________
3. ____________
4. ____________

Weekly Goals: Take a few minutes each Sunday night to write down the goals or tasks you wish to accomplish that week. As with your daily goals, rank them as top, medium, low, or "trash" priorities. (Make as many copies of this form as needed.) At the end of the week, evaluate how well you accomplished your goals. Cross off the goals you accomplished and carry over to the next week those you did not get done.

Week: ___/___/___ to ___/___/___

Top-Priority Goals

1. ____________
2. ____________
3. ____________
4. ____________

Medium-Priority Goals

1. ____________
2. ____________
3. ____________
4. ____________

Low-Priority Goals

1. ____________
2. ____________
3. ____________
4. ____________

Trash (do only after all other goals have been accomplished)

1. ____________
2. ____________
3. ____________
4. ____________

IV. Time Management Evaluation

On a weekly basis, go through the list of strategies below and provide a "yes" or "no" answer to each statement. If you are able to answer "yes" to most questions, congratulations, you are becoming a good time manager.

Strategy Date:															
1. I evaluate my time killers periodically.															
2. I have written down my long-range goals.															
3. I have written down my short-term goals.															
4. I use a daily planner.															
5. I conduct nightly audits.															
6. I conduct weekly audits.															
7. I delegate activities that others can do.															
8. I have learned to say "no" to additional tasks when I'm already in overload.															
9. I plan activities to avoid boredom.															
10. I plan ahead for distractions.															
11. I work on one task at a time until it's done.															
12. I have removed distractions from my work.															
13. I set aside overtimes.															
14. I set aside special time for myself daily.															
15. I reward myself for a job well done.															

Lab 10E: Stress Management

Name ______________________ Date ____________ Grade ____________

Instructor ______________________ Course ____________ Section ____________

NECESSARY LAB EQUIPMENT
None required.

OBJECTIVE
To participate in a stress management session.

I. Stage of Change for Stress Management

Using Figure 2.6 (page 66) and Table 2.3 (page 65), identify your current stage of change for a stress management program:

[ ]

II. Stress Management

Instructions: The class should be divided into groups of about five students per group. Each group should select and go through a minimum of two of the following stress management techniques outlined in Chapter 10:

1. Progressive Muscle Relaxation
2. Breathing Techniques for Relaxation
3. Visual Imagery
4. Autogenic Training
5. Meditation
6. Yoga

A group leader is chosen who will lead the exercise according to the instructions provided for each relaxation technique in Chapter 10. Be sure this experience is conducted in a comfortable room that is as free of noise as possible. If trained personnel or a tape-recording for progressive muscle relaxation exercises is available, the entire class may participate in this experience at once. Institutions that have biofeedback equipment may use it in this laboratory as well.

After completing this lab, answer the four questions given below.

1. Indicate the two relaxation techniques used in your lab:

A. [ ] B. [ ]

2. In your own words, relate your feelings as you were going through exercises A and B above:

Exercise A: ______________________

____

Exercise B: ______________________

____

3. Indicate how you felt mentally, emotionally, and physically after participating in this experience:

____

____

4. Are there situations in your daily life in which you think you would benefit from practicing the selected stress management exercises?

____

____

III. Self-Assessment Stress Evaluation

1. Do you currently perceive stress to be a problem in your life? ☐ Yes ☐ No

2. Do you experience any of the typical stress symptoms listed in the box on page 395? If so, which ones?

3. Indicate any specific events in your life that trigger a stress response.

4. Write specific objectives to either avoid or help you manage the various stress-inducing events listed above, including one or more stress management techniques.

5. Do you have any behavior patterns you would like to modify? List those you would like to change.

6. List specific techniques of change you will use to change undesirable behaviors (see Table 2.2, page 65).

11

Preventing Cardiovascular Disease

"Exercise can be used as a vaccine to prevent disease and a medication to treat disease. If there were a drug with the same benefits as exercise, it would instantly be the standard of care."
—*Robert Sallis*

OBJECTIVES

- Define cardiovascular disease and coronary heart disease.
- Explain the importance of a healthy lifestyle in preventing cardiovascular disease.
- Become familiar with the major risk factors that lead to the development of coronary heart disease, including physical inactivity, an abnormal cholesterol profile, hypertension, elevated homocysteine and C-reactive protein, inflammation, diabetes, and smoking.
- Assess your own risk for developing coronary heart disease.
- Outline a comprehensive program for reducing the risk for coronary heart disease and managing the overall risk for cardiovascular disease.

CENGAGEbrain.com
Visit **www.cengagebrain.com** to access course materials and companion resources for this text, including digital labs, quiz questions designed to check your understanding of the chapter contents, and more! See the preface on page xii for more information.

REAL LIFE STORY | Rita's Experience

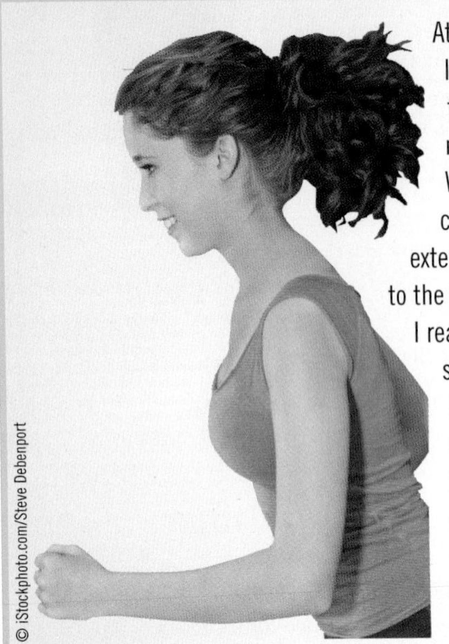
© iStockphoto.com/Steve Debenport

At age 19, cardiovascular disease was the farthest thing from my mind. In my Lifetime Wellness course, we covered the topic quite extensively. When we got to the family history section, I realized that I do have a strong family history. One grandparent on each side of the family died of heart disease. My dad is hypertensive, slightly overweight, and suffered a heart attack in his late 40s. My mother has high cholesterol and is diabetic. No one ever exercised in my family, and I am definitely high strung. After learning about the leading risk factors for heart disease, I decided to have my blood lipids checked at The Wellness Stop on campus. Much to my surprise, my total cholesterol, LDL cholesterol, and triglycerides were borderline high and my HDL cholesterol was low. While at The Wellness Stop, I also checked my blood pressure and found out I was prehypertensive for both systolic and diastolic pressures. Following a frank conversation with my instructor, I decided I needed to start taking better care of my health. I knew I could improve my diet and made significant changes on what I ate. I do a lot of my own cooking now and eat mostly foods that are nutritious and healthy. I have also started to watch salt in my diet. And although I never developed an exercise habit, I thought I'd try aerobics, zumba, and strength training a couple of times per week, plus jogging and elliptical training another two to three times per week. It wasn't easy at first, but I committed to my instructor and knew that my grade depended on my progress. Cross-training also helped, as it is fun to try different activities and meet different people. It took a few months to get into the routine, but it got to the point where I enjoyed the exercise, my increased energy levels, and the "new" person I had become. I have learned to prioritize my schedule and be more patient and tolerable of others. Although I can still do better, I am not as high strung anymore. I plan on still doing better. A healthy lifestyle is part of who I am now. A year later, my blood lipids are in the desirable range and my blood pressure is normal.

MyProfile: My Cardiovascular Disease Risk

For decades, cardiovascular disease has been the leading cause of deaths in the United States. It's primarily a preventable disease, and most of the risk factors are within your control.

I. Do you try daily to incorporate as much physical activity as possible throughout every day of the week and avoid excessive sitting? ___ Yes ___ No Explain how you do so. ____

____

____

II. Do you accumulate a minimum of 30 minutes of moderate-intensity physical activity five times per week or at least 20 minutes of vigorous-intensity exercise three times per week? ___ Yes ___ No

III. Does your diet have ample amounts of grains, fruits, and vegetables, and do you limit the intake of red meats, processed meats, salt, whole-milk products, simple carbohydrates, refined sugars, and processed foods? ___ Yes ___ No

IV. Are you aware of the most significant risk factors that lead to coronary heart disease and the factors that you have control over by the way you choose to live your life? ___ Yes ___ No

V. Have you ever had a blood lipid analysis test done, and what do the results of this test tell you about your current lifestyle, genetics, and potential risk for cardiovascular disease? ______________________________

____

____

VI. Are you familiar with the effects of low-grade inflammation on heart disease and lifestyle factors that increase C-reactive protein levels? ___ Yes ___ No __________

____

____

FAQ

As a young college student, why should I have to worry about heart disease?

Young people should know heart disease can affect them. The process begins early in life, as shown in young American soldiers who have died in wars. Autopsies conducted on soldiers killed at 22 years of age and younger revealed that more than half had early stages of atherosclerosis. Elevated blood cholesterol levels are found in children as young as 10 years old. Overall, risk factor management and positive lifestyle habits are the best ways to prevent disease. The choices you make today will affect your health and well-being in middle age and later.

Trans fat has been debated extensively lately. What foods are most likely to contain trans fat?

With extensive media coverage of their possible harmfulness, the amount of trans fats in foods is decreasing significantly. According to the Centers for Disease Control (CDC), trans fats have decreased by about 60 percent in the last decade, primarily because of its removal from processed foods. Although good news, many foods still contain significant amounts. Trans fats are found primarily in fried foods such as French fries, doughnuts, and apple fritters, but they are also found in baked, packaged, and processed foods, including stick margarine, cookies and pastries, biscuits, crackers, pie crusts, pizza dough, canned frosting, and coffee creamer.

Trans fats increase the risk for heart disease and stroke not only by increasing low-density lipoprotein (LDL, or "bad") cholesterol but also by decreasing cardioprotective high-density lipoprotein (HDL, or "good") cholesterol. To decrease consumption of trans fats, always read the food label for trans fat content and look for "hydrogenated fat/oil" or "partially hydrogenated fat/oil" (i.e., trans fats) on the list of ingredients. The Food and Drug Administration (FDA) does not require food companies to list trans fat content on the label if it is less than .5 gram per serving. The American Heart Association recommends that on average we consume less than 2 grams per day of trans fat. Four servings of a product that contains .49 gram of partially hydrogenated oil, not listed on the food label, provide almost the entire daily allowance of trans fats.

Is resveratrol the "super" nutrient that prevents heart disease?

Resveratrol is a compound found naturally in plant foods, particularly in red and purple grapes (and thus red wine); Japanese knotweed; peanuts; deep blue, red, or purple berries; some juices; and soy. The nutrient is believed to provide many health benefits, including a decreased risk for heart disease. Most of the research, however, has been conducted in animal studies, and there is no definite evidence for health benefits in humans. The media has capitalized on the idea that red wine is good for the heart because of its resveratrol content. There may be other nutrients found in red wine that either alone or in synergy with resveratrol provide benefits. Also, the amount of resveratrol obtained in red wine, juice, or other natural foods is too low in comparison to the therapeutic dose used in the research studies. It is practically impossible, if not foolish, to drink the amount of red wine necessary to approach the therapeutic dose used in the animal studies. More research in humans is clearly needed before definite claims can be made.

Is chocolate heart healthy?

Chocolate is heart healthy because of its content of cocoa antioxidant polyphenol compounds called flavonoids. Chocolate helps lower the risk for heart attacks, strokes, and even type 2 diabetes. Some of the ingredients in chocolate help reduce LDL (bad) cholesterol, increase blood flow to the brain, improve blood sugar absorption and insulin sensitivity, discourage blood clots, and increase nitric oxide levels. Nitric oxide helps relax and dilate arteries and keep them flexible, lowering blood pressure slightly in hypertensive and prehypertensive individuals. Even modest reductions in blood pressure (two to three points on both systolic and diastolic pressure scales) significantly lower coronary artery disease and stroke mortality.

Dark chocolate has a much higher concentration of flavonoids than milk chocolate, while white chocolate has none. Flavonoids enhance activity of special proteins called sterol regulatory element-binding proteins (SREBPs), which are involved in cholesterol metabolism. Activated SREBPs bind to genes on DNA that increase a protein called apolipoprotein A1 in the liver, which is the major protein component of the "good" HDL cholesterol. Flavonoids also decrease liver production of another protein, apolipoprotein B, which is the major protein component of the "bad" LDL cholesterol and increase activity of LDL receptors that induce more cholesterol for removal from the bloodstream. Flavonoids may also fight atherosclerosis (plaque buildup) in the arteries by decreasing the amount of oxidized LDL cholesterol, a major contributor to atherosclerosis.

Dark chocolate with at least 70 percent cocoa content provides the healthiest compounds. The darker the chocolate, the less room for sugar. Milk chocolate contains about twice as much sugar as the darkest chocolate. And although chocolate has saturated fat, it is primarily stearic acid, which has a neutral effect on cholesterol. Unfortunately, the chocolate Americans love most is loaded with sugar, fat, and calories. Do not consume chocolate made with palm, coconut, hydrogenated, or partially hydrogenated oils, and avoid chewy, caramel, marshmallow, or cream-covered chocolates.

High-quality dark chocolate is not a food to be eaten liberally, but it's a health food to be enjoyed in moderation. Keep in mind that chocolate is calorie dense. Eat too much of any type of chocolate, and you will gain weight. Overweightness and obesity are major health problems, with corresponding negative effects on morbidity and mortality. As little as .25 ounce of daily dark chocolate has been shown to provide health benefits. The equivalent of one (26 calories, .6 ounce) to two daily dark-chocolate Hershey's Kisses is all that is needed. Unsweetened cocoa powder with skim or fat-free milk and a touch of sweetener is an even better choice. Chocolate should be viewed as a treat—not a health food. Fruits and vegetables are still better sources of flavonoids.

Prevalence of Cardiovascular Disease

About 30 percent of all deaths in the United States are attributable to **cardiovascular disease (CVD)**, the most prevalent degenerative condition in the United States.[1] More than a third of the adult population has some form of heart and blood vessel disease. According to the Centers for Disease Control and Prevention (CDC), about 60 percent of deaths from heart disease are sudden and unexpected, with no previous symptoms of the disease. Almost half of these deaths occur outside of the hospital, most likely because the individuals failed to recognize early warning symptoms of a heart attack.

Some examples of CVD are coronary heart disease, stroke, **peripheral vascular disease**, congenital heart disease, rheumatic heart disease, atherosclerosis, high blood pressure, and congestive heart failure. According to CDC estimates, if all deaths from major types of CVD were eliminated, life expectancy in the United States would increase by about 7 years.

The American Heart Association (AHA) estimates the cost of heart and blood vessel disease in the United States to be more than $300 billion per year. About 1.5 million people have new or recurrent heart attacks and strokes each year, and more than 40 percent of them die as a result, including some 600,000 deaths from heart disease and 130,000 stroke deaths. More than half of these deaths occur within 1 hour of the onset of symptoms, before the person reaches the hospital.

Stroke

Currently, **stroke** is the fourth-leading cause of death in the United States. About 800,000 new or recurrent strokes are reported each year, and of these, more than a third of these people are left with permanent disabilities. About 20 percent of those who survive require institutional care.

Stroke is the most significant contributor to mental and physical disability in the United States, yet it does not draw the same attention as coronary heart disease, high blood pressure, diabetes, or cancer. Similar to those for coronary heart disease, most risk factors for stroke are preventable. Table 11.1 lists the major risk factors; the first four factors are beyond a person's control, whereas the latter seven are fully manageable.

Signs of Heart Attack and Stroke

Time is extremely critical when suffering a heart attack or stroke. Any or all of the following signs may occur during a heart attack or a stroke. **If you experience any of these and they last longer than a few minutes, call 911 and seek medical attention immediately**. Failure to do so may cause irreparable damage and even result in death.

Warning Signs of a Heart Attack

- Chest pain, discomfort, pressure, or squeezing that lasts for several minutes. These feelings may go away and return later.
- Pain or discomfort in the shoulders, neck, or arms or between the shoulder blades
- Chest discomfort with shortness of breath, lightheadedness, cold sweats, nausea and/or vomiting, a feeling of indigestion, sudden fatigue or weakness, fainting, or sense of impending doom

Warning Signs of Stroke

The acronym **FAST** is commonly used to help recognize and enhance responsiveness for a stroke victim.

- **F**acial dropping. Part of the face is dropping, weak, numb, or hard to move.
- **A**rm weakness. An inability to completely raise one arm.
- **S**peech difficulties. The inability to understand or repeat a simple sentence.
- **T**ime. Time is of the essence when suffering a stroke.
- Other symptoms may include a sudden severe headache, confusion, dizziness, difficulty walking, loss of balance or coordination, or sudden visual difficulty.

Although heart and blood vessel disease is still the number-one health problem in the United States, the incidence declined by almost 46 percent between 1960 and 2010 (Figure 11.1), largely because of health education. People now are aware of the risk factors for CVD and are leading a lifestyle that lowers the risk for these diseases.

Coronary Heart Disease

The heart and the coronary arteries are illustrated in Figure 11.2. The major form of CVD is **coronary heart disease (CHD)**, in which the arteries that supply the heart muscle with oxygen and nutrients are narrowed by fatty deposits, such as cholesterol and triglycerides. Narrowing of the coronary arteries diminishes the blood supply to the heart muscle, which can precipitate a heart attack.

CHD is the single leading cause of death in the United States, accounting for about 20 percent of all deaths and more than half of all deaths from CVD. CHD is also the leading cause of sudden cardiac deaths. More than half of all men and women who die suddenly of CHD have no previous symptoms of the disease. The risk of death is also greater in the least-educated segment of the population. Presently, more than 500,000 coronary bypass operations and more than 1 million coronary **angioplasty** procedures are performed in the United States each year.

TABLE 11.1 Stroke Risk Factors

Unchangeable Factors
Age: Increased risk after age 55
Gender: Higher risk in men
Race: African Americans are at greater risk
Family history
Manageable Factors
Tobacco use: Stop!
Blood pressure: Maintain in normal range
Diet: Decrease fat and sodium consumption and increase potassium, fruit, and vegetable intake
Activity level: Increase frequency and intensity
Weight: Maintain within recommended range
Cholesterol: Aim for normal levels
Diabetes: Prevent or manage condition

FIGURE 11.1 Incidence of cardiovascular disease in the United States for selected years: 1900–2010.

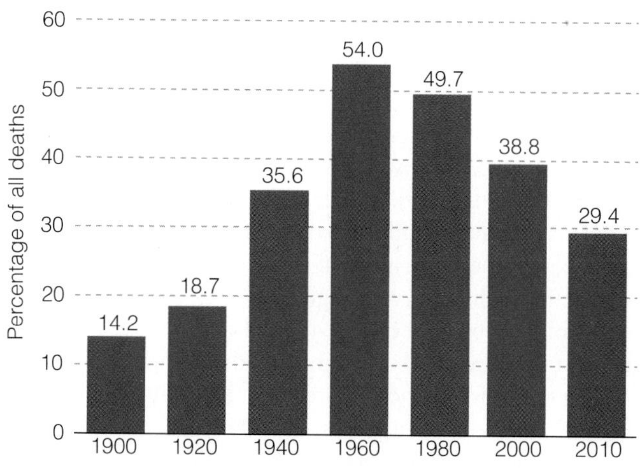

Source: *Centers for Disease Control, Atlanta.*

Coronary Heart Disease Risk Profile

Although genetic inheritance plays a role in CHD, the most important determinant is personal lifestyle. Most of the major **risk factors** for CHD are preventable and reversible. CHD risk factor analyses are administered to evaluate whether a person's lifestyle and genetic endowment are potential contributors to the development of coronary disease. The specific objectives of a CHD risk factor analysis are as follows:

- Screen individuals who may be at high risk for the disease.
- Educate people regarding the leading risk factors for developing CHD.
- Implement programs aimed at reducing the risks.
- Use the analysis as a starting point from which to compare changes induced by the intervention program.

Leading Risk Factors for CHD

The leading risk factors contributing to CHD are listed in Table 11.2. A self-assessment of risk factors for CHD is given in Lab 11A. This analysis can be done even if you have little or no medical information about your cardiovascular health. The guidelines for zero risk are outlined for each fac-

Cardiovascular disease (CVD) The array of conditions that affect the heart and the blood vessels.

Peripheral vascular disease Narrowing of the peripheral blood vessels.

Stroke A condition in which a blood vessel that feeds the brain is clogged, leading to blood flow disruption to the brain.

Coronary heart disease (CHD) A condition in which the arteries that supply the heart muscle with oxygen and nutrients are narrowed by fatty deposits, such as cholesterol and triglycerides.

Angioplasty A procedure in which a balloon-tipped catheter is inserted and then inflated to widen the inner lumen of the artery.

Risk factors Lifestyle and genetic variables that may lead to disease.

FIGURE 11.2 **The heart and its blood vessels.**

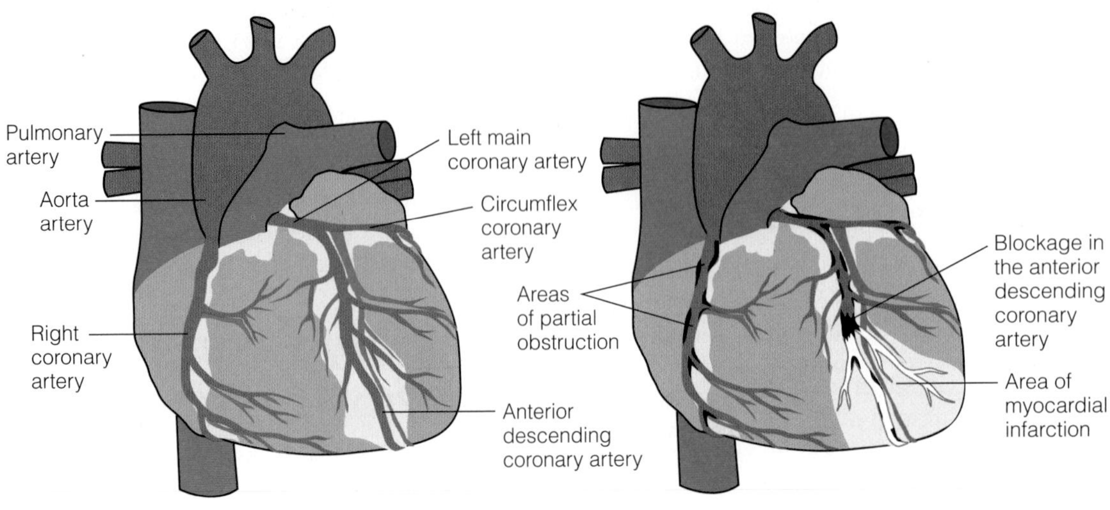

Normal healthy heart

Myocardial infarction (heart attack as a result of acute reduction in blood flow through the anterior descending coronary artery)

TABLE 11.2 **Weighting System for CHD Risk Factors**

Risk Factor	Maximal Risk Points
Unhealthy diet	14
Physical inactivity	8
Smoking	8
Body mass index	8
Hypertension	8
Personal history of heart disease	8
Abnormal heart function	8
Diabetes	6
Family history of heart disease	6
Age	4
Tension and stress	3

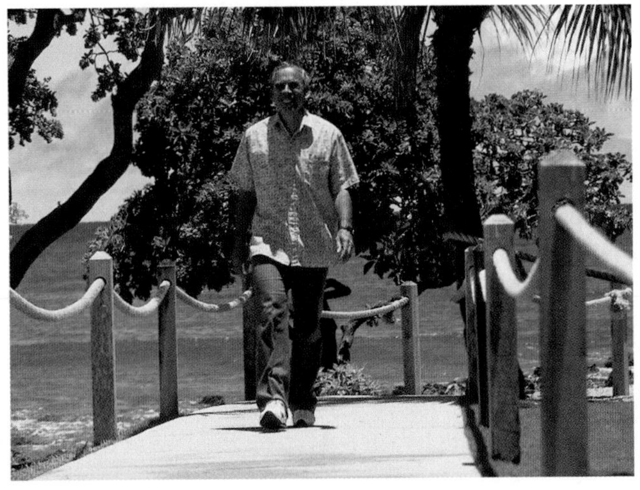

Regular physical activity helps control most major risk factors that lead to heart disease.

tor, making this self-analysis a valuable tool for managing risk factors for CHD.

To provide a meaningful score for CHD risk, a weighting system was developed to show the impact of leading risk factors on developing the disease (Table 11.2 and Lab 11A). The system is based on current research and on the work done at leading preventive medical facilities in the United States. The most significant risk factors are given the heaviest numerical weight.

Based on test results and personal lifestyle, a person receives a score anywhere from zero to the maximum number of points for each factor. When the risk points from all of the risk factors are totaled, the final number is used to place an individual in one of five overall risk categories for potential development of CHD (see Lab 11A).

The very low CHD risk category designates the group at the lowest risk for developing heart disease based on age and gender. The low category suggests that even though these people are taking good care of their cardiovascular health, they can improve it (unless all risk points come from age and family history). Moderate CHD risk means that people can definitely improve their lifestyle to lower the risk for disease; otherwise, medical treatment may be required. A score in the high or very high CHD risk category points to a strong probability of developing heart disease within the next few years and calls for immediate implementation of a personal risk-reduction program, including professional medical, nutritional, and physical activity intervention.

The leading risk factors for CHD are discussed next, along with the general recommendations for risk reduction.

Healthy Lifestyle Cuts Risk of Sudden Cardiac Death

Sudden cardiac death (SCD) is caused by a sudden, unexpected loss of heart function. It is the largest cause of natural death in the United States, responsible for 300,000 to 400,000 adult deaths each year or about half of all heart disease deaths. SCD occurs when the heart's electrical system does not function properly and suddenly becomes very irregular. The heart can beat dangerously fast causing the ventricles to flutter or quiver and blood is not delivered to the body. The greatest concern is the lack of blood flow to the brain during the initial few minutes and the person loses consciousness. Death is almost always imminent unless the person receives immediate emergency treatment. SCD can also take place during an attack itself, as the heart muscle is damaged because it does not receive sufficient oxygen-rich blood.

Research conducted on more than 81,000 women tracked during 26 years showed that adherence to a "low-risk" lifestyle significantly decreases the risk of SCD. The low-risk lifestyle included the following factors:

- Not smoking
- Being physically active for at least 30 minutes a day
- Not being overweight or obese
- Eating a diet rich in fruits, vegetables, whole grains, nuts, beans, and fish; with considerably more monounsaturated than saturated fat, moderate use of alcohol, and low intake of red and processed meats.

The authors concluded that a low-risk lifestyle could prevent as much as 81 percent of the yearly SCDs in the United States.

Source: S. E. Chiuve, (Adherence to a Low-Risk, Healthy Lifestyle and Risk of Sudden Cardiac Death Among Women, Journal of the American Medical Association 306 (2011): 62-69.

Physical Inactivity

Physical inactivity is responsible for low levels of cardiorespiratory endurance (the ability of the heart, lungs, and blood vessels to deliver enough oxygen to the cells to meet the demands of prolonged physical activity). The level of cardiorespiratory endurance (or fitness) is given most commonly by the maximal amount of oxygen (in milliliters) that every kilogram (2.2 pounds) of body weight is able to utilize per minute of physical activity (mL/kg/min). As maximal oxygen uptake (VO_{2max}) increases, so does efficiency of the cardiorespiratory system. Improving cardiorespiratory endurance through aerobic exercise and daily physical activity greatly reduces the overall risk for heart disease.

For habitually sedentary people, sudden heavy-duty physical activity, such as shoveling snow or strenuous yard work, can trigger a cardiovascular event. The research shows that unaccustomed physical exertion increases the risk for a cardiovascular incident 50- to 100-fold.

Although specific recommendations can be followed to improve each risk factor, daily physical activity and a regular aerobic exercise program help to control most of the major risk factors that lead to heart disease. Physical activity and aerobic exercise will:

- Increase cardiorespiratory endurance
- Increase and maintain good heart function, sometimes improving certain electrocardiogram abnormalities
- Improve high-density lipoprotein (HDL) cholesterol
- Lower blood lipids (cholesterol and triglycerides)
- Decrease low-grade (hidden) inflammation in the body
- Prevent and help control diabetes
- Decrease and control blood pressure
- Reduce body fat
- Motivate toward smoking cessation
- Alleviate tension and stress
- Counteract a personal history of heart disease

Data from the research summarized in Figure 1.11 in Chapter 1 clearly show the tie between physical activity and mortality, regardless of age and other risk factors. A higher level of physical fitness benefits even those who exhibit other risk factors, such as high blood pressure and serum cholesterol, cigarette smoking, and a family history of heart disease. In most cases, less fit people in the study without these risk factors had higher death rates than highly fit people with these same risk factors.

The findings show that the higher the level of cardiorespiratory fitness, the longer the life, but the largest drop in premature death is seen between the "unfit" and the "moderately fit" groups. Even small improvements in cardiorespiratory endurance greatly decrease the risk for cardiovascular mortality. Most adults who engage in a moderate exercise program can attain these fitness levels easily. A 2-mile walk in 30 to 40 minutes, 5 to 7 days a week, is adequate to decrease risk.

Subsequent research published in the *New England Journal of Medicine* substantiated the importance of exercise in preventing CHD.[2] The benefits to previously inactive adults of starting a moderate-intensity to vigorous physical activity program were as important as quitting smoking, managing blood pressure, or controlling cholesterol. For relative risk for death from CHD, the increase in physical activity led to the same decrease as giving up cigarette smoking.

The scientific data are quite clear that moderate-intensity physical activity provides substantial benefits in terms of overall cardiovascular risk reduction. The exact amount of aerobic exercise required to decrease the risk for cardiovascular disease is difficult to establish and most likely varies due to genetics, age, gender, body composition, health status, and personal lifestyle, among other factors. What may be sufficient for a low-risk individual may not be enough for someone else with disease risk factors. For example, an apparently healthy individual at recommended body weight may not need more than 30 daily minutes of accumulated moderate-intensity physical activity. Another person with a weight problem and other risk factors such as high blood pressure, cholesterol abnormalities, and borderline high blood sugar may need a much greater amount of activity to counteract these risk factors.

Although research may never indicate the exact amount of aerobic exercise required to lower the risk for cardiovascular disease, pioneer research in this area conducted in the 1980s showed that expending 2,000 calories per week as a result of physical activity yielded the lowest risk for cardiovascular disease among a group of almost 17,000 Harvard University alumni. Expending 2,000 calories per week represents about 300 calories per daily exercise session, or the equivalent of jogging 3 miles in 30 minutes or walking 3 miles in about 45 minutes.

When feasible, scientific studies indicate that vigorous activity is preferable because of greater improvements in aerobic fitness, blood pressure, and glucose control and a larger reduction in CHD risk.[3] Still, do not engage in vigorous exercise without proper clearance and a minimum of 6 weeks of proper conditioning through moderate-intensity activity.

A comprehensive and systematic research review of the effects of physical activity on all-cause mortality was published in 2011. The research included 80 studies that involved more than 1.3 million people. The review concluded that physical activity prolongs life and that premature death risk decreased the most as activity time increased with vigorous exercise.[4] Each weekly hour of light, moderate, or vigorous activity decreased mortality rates by 4, 6, and 9 percent respectively. Furthermore, for every 1,000 weekly calories expanded through exercise, the mortality rate decreased by 11 percent.

In terms of life expectancy, 2012 research involving 654,827 individuals looking at leisure time physical activity of moderate to vigorous intensity and their effects on mortality, the results indicated that higher levels of physical activity are associated with greater gains in life expectancy. People at the highest level of physical activity gained 4.5 years in life expectancy and being active and normal weight (BMI of 18.5 to 24.9) yielded a gain of 7.2 years of life as compared to being inactive and obese.[5]

Also, you should try to minimize total daily sitting time. The data indicate that excessive daily sitting (at a desk, commuting to and from work, eating meals, and watching television) increases the risk for cardiovascular disease, obesity, some chronic disorders, and premature mortality. The risk is increased even if you meet the 30 minutes of moderate-intensity physical activity on most days of the week but still spend a large part of the day sitting. If your job (like most nowadays) requires a large portion of the day to be spent in a sitting position, at least get up and take frequent breaks. Small, creative lifestyle changes make a difference, such as always answering the phone standing; walking to the office next door instead of texting, e-mailing, instant messaging, or using the phone; and using stairs instead of riding elevators and escalators. When watching television, make it a point to get up and walk around during each commercial break. Even better, do dips at the edge of the couch or stand up and sit down 20 times to strengthen your thigh muscles.

While aerobically fit individuals have a lower incidence of cardiovascular disease, regular physical activity and aerobic exercise by themselves do not guarantee a lifetime free of cardiovascular problems. Poor lifestyle habits—such as smoking; eating too many fatty, salty, or sweet foods; being overweight; and having high stress levels—increase cardiovascular risk, and their effects are not eliminated through an active lifestyle.

Overall management of risk factors is the best guideline to lower the risk for CVD. Still, aerobic exercise is one of the most important factors in preventing and reducing cardiovascular problems. Based on the overwhelming amount of scientific data in this area, evidence of the benefits of aerobic exercise in reducing heart disease is far too impressive to be ignored. Low fitness is more dangerous than obesity, smoking, high cholesterol, or diabetes. The basic principles for cardiorespiratory exercise are given in Chapter 6.

As more research studies are conducted, the addition of strength training is increasingly recommended for good heart function. The AHA recommends strength training even for individuals who have had a heart attack or have high blood pressure, as long as they strength train under a physician's advice. Strength training helps control body weight and blood sugar and lowers cholesterol and blood pressure.

Abnormal Electrocardiograms

The **electrocardiogram (ECG or EKG)** is a valuable measure of the heart's function. The ECG provides a record of the electrical impulses that stimulate the heart to contract (Figure 11.3). In reading an ECG, doctors interpret five general areas: heart rate, heart rhythm, axis of the heart, enlargement or hypertrophy of the heart, and myocardial infarction.

During a standard 12-lead ECG, 10 electrodes are placed on the person's chest. From these 10 electrodes, 12 tracings, or "leads," of the electrical impulses as they travel through the heart muscle, or **myocardium**, are studied from 12 different positions. By looking at ECG tracings, medical professionals can identify abnormalities in heart functioning (Figure 11.4). Based on the findings, the ECG may be interpreted as normal, equivocal, or abnormal. An ECG does not always identify problems, so a normal tracing is not an absolute guarantee. Conversely, an abnormal tracing does not necessarily signal a serious condition.

ECGs are taken at rest, during the stress of exercise, and during recovery. A **stress electrocardiogram** is also known as a graded exercise stress test or a maximal exercise tolerance test. Similar to a high-speed test on a car, a stress ECG reveals the tolerance of the heart to increased physical activity. It is a much better test than a resting ECG to discover CHD.

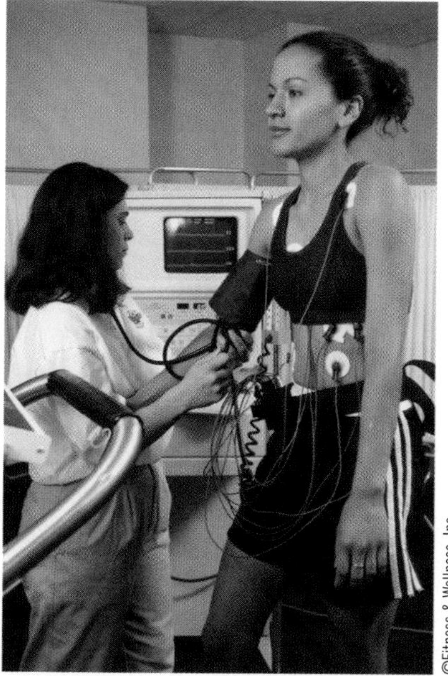

Exercise tolerance test with 12-lead electrocardiograph monitoring (an exercise stress ECG).

FIGURE 11.3 Normal ECG.

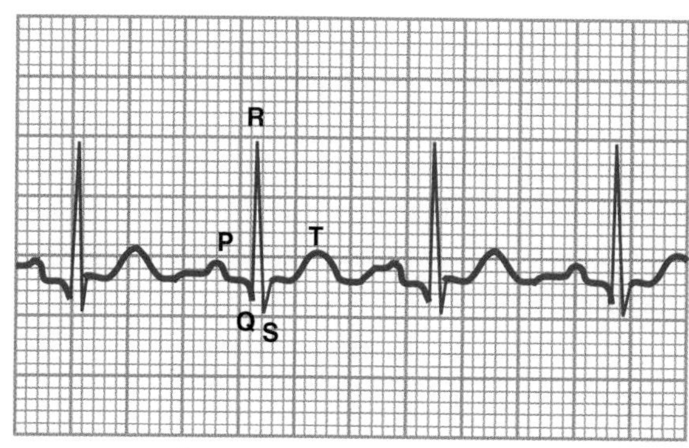

© Cengage Learning

FIGURE 11.4 Abnormal electrocardiogram showing a depressed S-T segment.

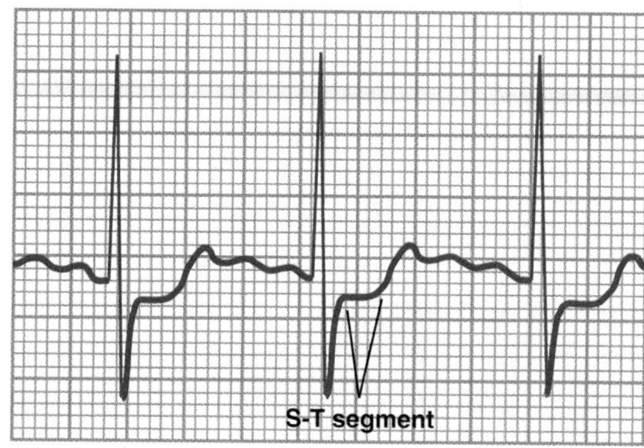

© Cengage Learning

Stress ECGs also are used to assess cardiorespiratory fitness levels, screen individuals for preventive and cardiac rehabilitation programs, detect abnormal blood pressure response during exercise, and establish actual or functional maximal heart rate for exercise prescription. The recovery ECG is another important diagnostic tool to monitor the return of the heart's activity to normal conditions.

Not every adult who wishes to start or continue an exercise program needs a stress ECG. No set of guidelines can cover all cases when a stress electrocardiogram is recommended prior to exercise participation. The test, however, is recommended for individuals who are at high risk or are known to have cardiovascular, pulmonary, renal, or metabolic disease. Moreover, people feeling unusually winded in response to normal exertion, unexplained fatigue, or chest pain, should have the test done.

At times, the stress ECG has been questioned as a reliable predictor of CHD. Nevertheless, it remains the most practical, inexpensive, noninvasive procedure available to diagnose latent (undiagnosed or unknown) CHD. The test is accurate in diagnosing CHD about 65 percent of the time. The sensitivity of the test increases with the severity of the disease, and more accurate results are seen in people who are at high risk for CVD.

Abnormal Cholesterol Profile

Cholesterol receives much attention because of its direct relationship to heart disease. **Blood lipids** (cholesterol and triglycerides) are carried in the bloodstream by protein

Electrocardiogram (ECG or EKG) A recording of the electrical activity of the heart.

Myocardium Heart muscle.

Stress electrocardiogram An exercise test during which the workload is increased gradually until the individual reaches maximal fatigue, with blood pressure and 12-lead electrocardiographic monitoring throughout the test; also known as graded exercise stress test or maximal exercise tolerance test.

Cholesterol A waxy substance, technically a steroid alcohol, found only in animal fats and oil and used in making cell membranes, as a building block for some hormones, in the fatty sheath around nerve fibers, and in other necessary substances.

Blood lipids (fats) Cholesterol and triglycerides.

New Heart Disease and Stroke Prevention Guidelines

In late 2013, the American Heart Association (AHA) and the American College of Cardiology released the much anticipated recommendations for heart disease and stroke prevention. The new guidelines focus on **cholesterol, lifestyle, obesity,** and **risk assessment**.

In terms of **cholesterol**, numeric targets are deemphasized and now focus on treating people who are deemed to be at high risk for cardiovascular disease (CVD), with complete emphasis on statin (drug) therapy. The LDL cholesterol number is no longer the main consideration in treatment. Some experts strongly disagree with these new guidelines. They feel that the recommendations will increase the number of people on statin medications and will not be more effective than the previous target-based guidelines (see Cholesterol Guidelines in Table 11.3, p. 432). The new recommendations specifically target four high-risk groups for whom statin drugs are recommended:

1. People with pre-existing CVD (those who have suffered angina, a heart attack, stroke, a transient ischemic attack or mini stroke, and anyone who has had a cardiovascular procedure such as angioplasty to widen arteries)
2. Type 2 diabetics between 40 and 75 years of age
3. People with very high LDL cholesterol (190 mg/dl or above)
4. People between 40 and 75 without CVD or diabetes who have a 10-year risk of CVD of at least 7.5 percent based on a new *online risk calculator* (see risk assessment in the next column)

Lowering LDL cholesterol, however, is still important. The new guidelines encourage people to consume no more than 5 to 6 percent of total daily calories from saturated fat and less than 1 percent from trans fats.

The **healthy lifestyle** guidelines incorporate adequate physical activity, weight management, and dietary patterns that emphasize vegetables, fruits, whole grains, low-fat dairy products, fish, poultry, and nuts. People should limit red meat, processed foods, saturated and trans fats, sodium, and sugary foods and beverages. Physical activity performed on a regular basis, 40 minutes of exercise 3 to 4 days a week, is also encouraged in the guidelines.

Physicians are encouraged to treat **obesity** as a disease and actively work with obese patients to lose weight. Telling patients that they need to lose weight is not enough. Physicians should prescribe diets that decrease caloric intake by at least 500 calories per day and prescribe a minimum of 2½ hours of physical activity per week. People need to learn to balance caloric intake and physical activity to achieve and maintain a healthy body weight. All Americans should calculate their BMI at least once a year and keep their BMI under 25. Weight loss surgery may be recommended for extremely obese individuals whose health may be at risk.

A newly developed **risk assessment** that calculates the potential 10-year risk for heart attack and stroke is available online at tinyurl.com/cvriskcalculator. The risk calculator helps health care practitioners evaluate people between the ages of 40 and 79. A prediction equation was developed from community-based populations and includes race, gender, age, total cholesterol, HDL cholesterol, blood pressure, blood pressure medication use, diabetes status, and smoking status. People need to aim for normal blood pressure and blood glucose levels and avoid use and exposure to tobacco products. If the 10-year risk is 7.5 or higher, the person is encouraged to take a statin. More than 30 million Americans are believed to exceed this rating, including many who have never had any symptoms of CVD. The 7.5 number does not provide an automatic prescription, but rather is a start to the process, not an end.

According to the AHA, "the goal is not to get more people on statins," but to make sure the drugs are used by the people who can benefit from them. *Some health care experts welcome the new recommendations, while others vigorously oppose them because they deemphasize target numbers for the various cholesterol subcategories.* It remains to be seen how many physicians will adopt the new guidelines, although many doctors will probably use a combination of the two. Regardless of the effectiveness of statins, medications by themselves cannot replace a healthy lifestyle. A multifaceted healthy lifestyle approach has been proven in research studies to be most effective in managing heart disease and stroke risk. Before you consider taking a statin drug, discuss with your physician steps that you can implement to reduce the risk through a healthier lifestyle. If the controversy over the new guidelines and the calculator, however, gets more people in to see their physician, it will be a positive outcome and will have achieved at least some degree of success.

Source: American Heart Association, Understanding the New Prevention Guidelines, http://www.heart.org/HEARTORG/Conditions/Understanding-the-New-Prevention-Guidelines_UCM_458155_Article.jsp. Accessed April 15, 2014.

FIGURE 11.5 The atherosclerotic process.

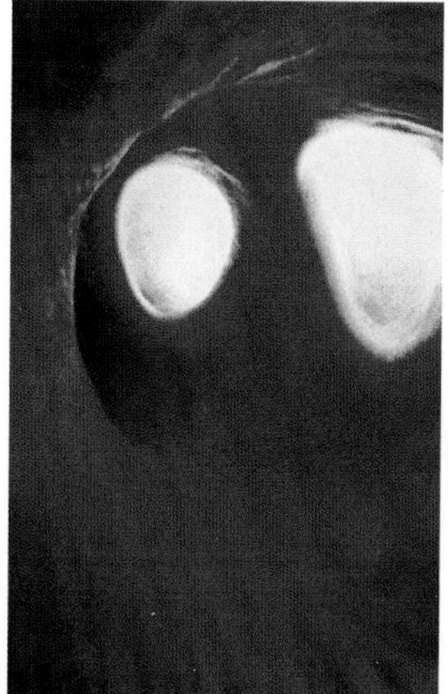
Normal artery

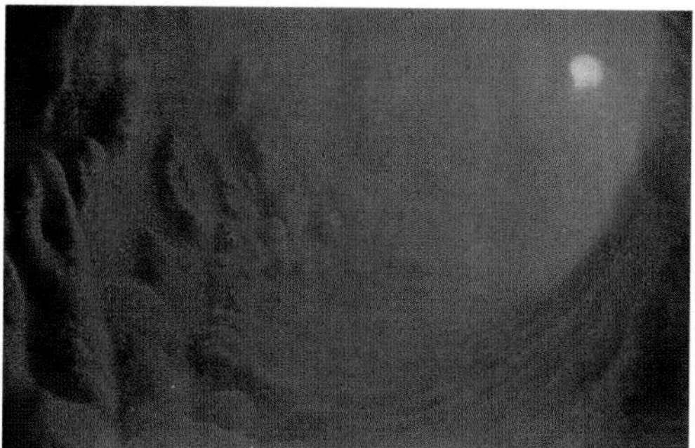
Early stage of atherosclerosis

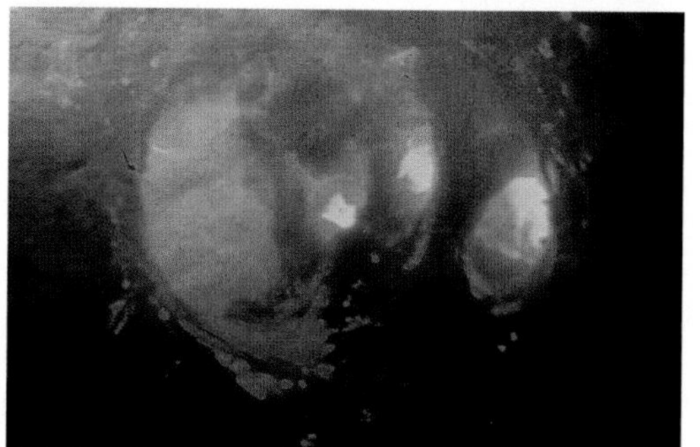
Progression of the atherosclerotic plaque

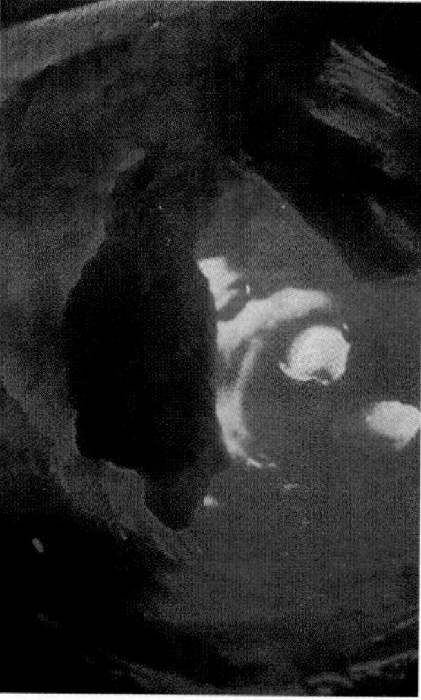
Advanced stage of atherosclerosis

molecules of **high-density lipoproteins (HDLs)**, **low-density lipoproteins (LDLs)**, **very low-density lipoproteins (VLDLs)**, and **chylomicrons**. An increased risk for CHD has been established in individuals with high total cholesterol, high LDL cholesterol, and low HDL cholesterol.

An abnormal cholesterol profile contributes to **atherosclerosis**, the buildup of fatty tissue in the walls of the arteries (Figures 11.5 and 11.6). As the plaque builds up, it blocks the blood vessels that supply the myocardium with oxygen and nutrients (the coronary arteries), and these obstructions can trigger a **myocardial infarction**, or heart attack.

Unfortunately, the heart disguises its problems quite well, and typical symptoms of heart disease, such as **angina pectoris**, do not start until the arteries are about 75 percent blocked. In many cases, the first symptom is sudden death.

The recommendation of the National Cholesterol Education Program (NCEP) is to keep total cholesterol levels below 200 mg/dL. Cholesterol levels between 200 and 239 mg/dL are borderline high, and levels of 240 mg/dL and above indicate high risk for disease (Table 11.3). The risk for heart attack increases 2 percent for every 1 percent increase in total cholesterol.[6] About one-half of U.S. adults have total cholesterol values of 200 mg/dL or higher.

Preventive medicine practitioners often recommend a range between 160 and 180 mg/dL for total cholesterol. Furthermore, in the Framingham Heart Study (a 60-year ongoing project in the community of Framingham, Massachusetts), not a single individual with a total cholesterol level of 150 mg/dL or lower has had a heart attack.

As important as it is, total cholesterol is not the best predictor for cardiovascular risk. Many heart attacks occur in people with only slightly elevated total cholesterol. More significant is the way in which cholesterol is carried in the bloodstream. Cholesterol is transported primarily in the form of LDL and HDL.

LDL ("bad") cholesterol tends to release cholesterol, which then may penetrate the lining of the arteries and speed the process of atherosclerosis. The NCEP guidelines

High-density lipoproteins (HDLs) Cholesterol-transporting molecules in the blood ("good" cholesterol) that help clear cholesterol from the blood.

Low-density lipoproteins (LDLs) Cholesterol-transporting molecules in the blood ("bad" cholesterol) that tend to increase blood cholesterol.

Very low-density lipoproteins (VLDLs) Triglyceride, cholesterol, and phospholipid-transporting molecules in the blood.

Chylomicrons Triglyceride-transporting molecules.

Atherosclerosis Fatty or cholesterol deposits in the walls of the arteries leading to formation of plaque.

Myocardial infarction Heart attack; damage to or death of an area of the heart muscle as a result of an obstructed artery to that area.

Angina pectoris Chest pain associated with CHD.

FIGURE 11.6 Comparison of a normal healthy artery (A) and diseased arteries (B and C).

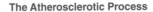

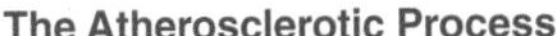

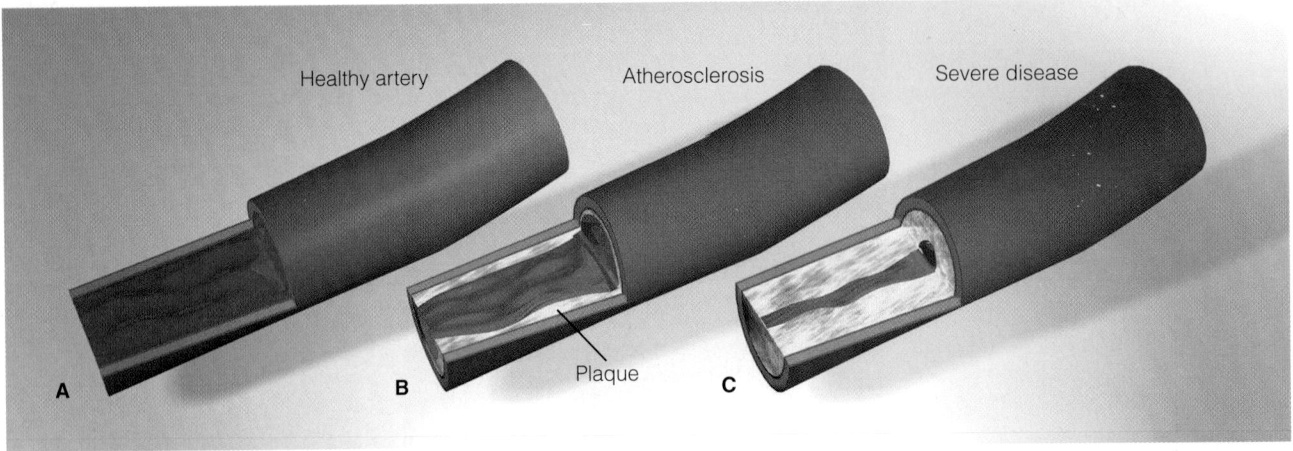

given in Table 11.3 state that an LDL cholesterol value below 100 mg/dL is optimal.

Even when more LDL cholesterol is present than the cells can use, cholesterol seems not to cause a problem until it is oxidized by free radicals (see discussion under "Antioxidants" in Chapter 3, page 110). After cholesterol is oxidized, white blood cells invade the arterial wall, take up the cholesterol, and clog the arteries.

LDL cholesterol particles are of two types: large, or pattern A, and small, or pattern B. Small particles are thought to pass through the inner lining of the coronary arteries more readily, thereby increasing the risk for a heart attack. A predominance of small particles can lead to a sixfold increase in the risk for CHD.

A genetic variation of LDL cholesterol, known as lipoprotein-a or Lp(a), is also noteworthy because a high level of these particles promotes blood clots and earlier development of atherosclerosis. It is thought that certain substances in the arterial wall interact with Lp(a) and lead to premature formation of plaque. About 10 percent of the population has elevated levels of Lp(a). Only medications help decrease Lp(a), and drug options should be discussed with a physician.

Intermediate-density lipoprotein (IDL) is also of concern, because these midsize particles are more likely to cause atherosclerosis than a similar amount of LDL cholesterol. For individuals at risk for heart disease, a comprehensive blood lipid profile that includes total cholesterol, HDL cholesterol, LDL cholesterol, Lp(a), IDL, and size pattern (A and B) is recommended.

In a process known as **reverse cholesterol transport**, HDLs act as "scavengers," removing cholesterol from the body and preventing plaque from forming in the arteries. The strength of HDL is in the protein molecules found in its coating. When HDL comes in contact with cholesterol-filled cells, these protein molecules attach to the cells and take their cholesterol.

The more HDL ("good") cholesterol, the better. HDL cholesterol offers some protection against heart disease. A low level of HDL cholesterol is one of the strongest predictors of CHD at all levels of total cholesterol, including levels below 200 mg/dL. Data suggest that for every 1 mg/dL increase in HDL cholesterol, the risk for CHD drops up to 3 percent in men and 5 percent in women.[7] The recommended HDL cholesterol values to minimize the risk for CHD are at least 40 mg/dL. HDL cholesterol levels above 60 mg/dL help lower the risk for CHD.

Fourteen subgroups of HDL particles have been identified, falling into HDL2 and HDL3 categories. HDL2 are larger particles that carry cholesterol from the arterial wall to the liver for disposal. These particles also have antioxidant and anti-inflammatory effects. In particular, the subgroup HDL2b seems to be most significant because they appear to remove approximately 80 percent of the LDL cholesterol. The HDL3 particles also transport cholesterol out of the arterial wall but may not be as effective as HDL2. HDL3,

TABLE 11.3 Cholesterol Guidelines

	Amount	Rating
Total cholesterol	<200 mg/dL	Desirable
	200–239 mg/dL	Borderline high
	≥240 mg/dL	High risk
LDL cholesterol	<100 mg/dL	Optimal
	100–129 mg/dL	Near or above optimal
	130–159 mg/dL	Borderline high
	160–189 mg/dL	High
	≥190 mg/dL	Very high
HDL cholesterol	<40 mg/dL	Low (high risk)
	≥60 mg/dL	High (low risk)

Source: From the National Cholesterol Education Program.

TABLE 11.4 Cholesterol and Saturated Fat Content of Selected Foods

Food	Serving Size	Cholesterol (mg)	Sat. Fat (g)
Avocado	⅛ med	—	0.5
Bacon	2 slices	30	2.7
Beans, all types	any	—	—
Beef—lean, fat trimmed off	3 oz	75	6.0
Beef heart (cooked)	3 oz	150	1.6
Beef liver (cooked)	3 oz	255	1.3
Butter	1 tsp	12	0.4
Caviar	1 oz	85	—
Cheese			
American	2 oz	54	11.2
Cheddar	2 oz	60	12.0
Cottage, 1% fat	1 cup	10	0.4
Cottage, 4% fat	1 cup	31	6.0
Cream	2 oz	62	6.0
Muenster	2 oz	54	10.8
Parmesan	2 oz	38	9.3
Swiss	2 oz	52	10.0
Chicken, no skin	3 oz	45	0.4
Chicken liver	3 oz	472	1.1
Chicken thigh, wing	3 oz	69	3.3
Egg yolk	1 large	218	1.6
Frankfurter	2	90	11.2
Fruits	any	—	—
Grains, all types	any	—	—
Halibut, flounder	3 oz	43	0.7
Ice cream	½ cup	27	4.4
Lamb	3 oz	60	7.2
Lard	1 tsp	5	1.9
Lobster	3 oz	170	0.5
Margarine, all vegetable	1 tsp	—	0.7
Mayonnaise	1 tbsp	10	2.1
Milk			
Skim	1 cup	5	0.3
Low fat, 2%	1 cup	18	2.9
Whole	1 cup	34	5.1
Nuts	1 oz	—	1.0
Oysters	3 oz	42	—
Salmon	3 oz	30	0.8
Scallops	3 oz	29	—
Sherbet	½ cup	7	1.2
Shrimp	3 oz	128	0.1
Trout	3 oz	45	2.1
Tuna (canned—drained)	3 oz	55	—
Turkey, dark meat	3 oz	60	0.6
Turkey, light meat	3 oz	50	0.4
Vegetables (except avocado)	any	—	—

however, seems to protect against cholesterol oxidation that results in atherosclerosis.

For the most part, HDL cholesterol is determined genetically. Generally, women have higher levels than men. Because the female sex hormone estrogen tends to raise HDL, premenopausal women have a much lower incidence of heart disease. African American children and adult men have higher HDL values than Caucasians. HDL cholesterol also decreases with age.

Increasing HDL cholesterol improves the cholesterol profile and lessens the risk for CHD. Habitual aerobic exercise, a diet high in omega-3 fatty acids, weight loss, no smoking, and modest alcohol intake help raise HDL cholesterol. Drug therapy may also promote higher HDL cholesterol levels. Niacin helps convert HDL3 to HDL2.

Improved HDL cholesterol is clearly related to a regular aerobic exercise program (preferably high intensity, or above 6 metabolic equivalents, for at least 20 minutes three times per week—see Chapter 6). Individual responses to aerobic exercise differ, but generally, the more you exercise, the higher your HDL cholesterol level.

Counteracting Cholesterol The average adult in the United States consumes between 400 and 600 mg of cholesterol daily. The body, however, manufactures more than that. Saturated and trans fats (trans-fatty acids) raise cholesterol levels more than anything else in the diet. These fats produce approximately 1,000 mg of cholesterol per day. Because of individual differences, some people can have a higher-than-normal intake of saturated and trans fats and still maintain normal levels. Others, who have a lower intake, can have abnormally high levels.

Saturated fats are found mostly in meats and dairy products and seldom in foods of plant origin (Table 11.4). Poultry and fish contain less saturated fat than beef does but should be eaten in moderation (about 3 to 6 ounces per day—see Chapter 3). In a 10-year study of more than 500,000 men and women over the age of 50, those who ate the most red meat (an average of 4.5 ounces per day), had a much higher risk of dying from heart disease and cancer.[8] Of the highest red meat eaters, men had a 31 percent higher risk of dying during the study period, whereas women had a 50 percent higher risk of dying from heart disease during this time. Cancer risk was about 20 percent higher among men and women who consumed the most red meat.

Unsaturated fats are mainly of plant origin and cannot be converted to cholesterol. Omega-3-rich fish meals (found in salmon, tuna, and mackerel) also help lower **triglycerides** and increase HDL cholesterol.[9] Because of the cardioprotective benefits of omega-3 fatty

Reverse cholesterol transport A process in which HDL molecules attract cholesterol and carry it to the liver, where it is changed to bile and eventually excreted in the stool.

Triglycerides Fats formed by glycerol and three fatty acids; also called free fatty acids.

acids, the AHA recommends eating oily fish at least twice per week. As illustrated in Figure 11.7, baseline blood levels of omega-3 fatty acids are inversely related to the risk of sudden cardiac death.[10] Individuals in the highest quartile of omega-3 fatty acids (mean = 6.87 percent of total fatty acids) have a 90 percent reduction in sudden cardiac death risk as compared with those in the lowest quartile (mean = 3.58 percent of total fatty acids).

The antioxidant effect of vitamins C and E may provide benefits. Data suggest that a single unstable free radical (an oxygen compound produced during metabolism—see Chapter 3) can damage LDL particles, accelerating the atherosclerotic process. Vitamin C may inactivate free radicals and slow the oxidation of LDL cholesterol. Vitamin E may protect LDL from oxidation, preventing heart disease, but studies suggest that it does not seem to be helpful in reversing damage once it has taken place.

FIGURE 11.7 Relative risk of sudden cardiac death by baseline omega-3 fatty acid (FA) level by quartiles.

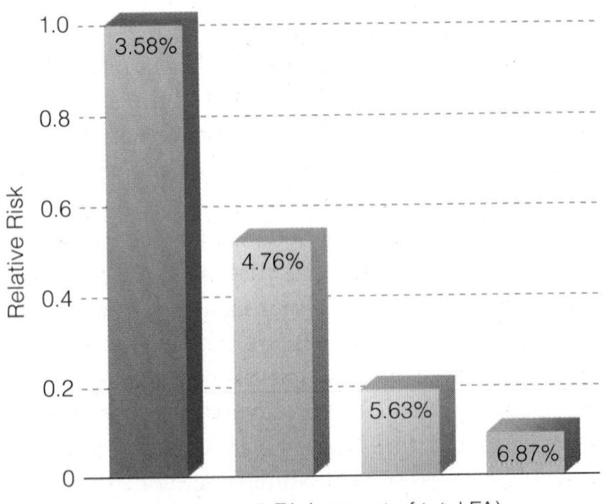

Source: P. Libby, P.M. Ridker, and A. Maseri, "Inflammation and Atherosclerosis," *Circulation* 105 (2002): 1135-1143.

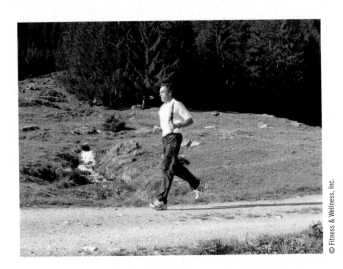

Habitual aerobic exercise helps increase HDL cholesterol ("good" cholesterol).

Trans Fat Foods that contain trans-fatty acids, hydrogenated fat, or partially hydrogenated vegetable oil should be avoided. Studies indicate that these foods elevate LDL cholesterol as much as saturated fats do, but even worse, they lower HDL cholesterol. Trans fat also increases triglycerides, contribute to inflammation, and increase the tendency to form blood clots inside blood vessels. These changes contribute not only to heart disease but also to gallstone formation. Trans fats are found primarily in fried, baked, packaged, and **processed foods**.

Food companies use trans fat because it is inexpensive to produce, is easy to use, lasts a long time, and adds taste and texture to food. Restaurants and fast-food chains have used oils with trans fat because it can be used repeatedly in commercial fryers.

Hydrogen frequently is added to monounsaturated and polyunsaturated fats to increase shelf life and to solidify them so that they are more spreadable. Hydrogenation can change the position of hydrogen atoms along the carbon chain, transforming the fat into a trans-fatty acid. Margarine and spreads, canned frosting, coffee creamer, chips, commercially produced crackers and cookies, and fast foods can contain trans-fatty acids. Small amounts of trans fat are also found naturally in some meats, dairy products, and other animal-based foods.

The AHA has issued dietary guidelines recommending that people limit trans fat intake to less than 1 percent of total daily caloric intake.[11] This amount represents about 1.5 grams of trans fat a day for a 1,500-calorie diet, 2 grams for 2,000 daily calories, and 3 grams for 3,000 daily calories. Because the FDA now requires that all food labels list the trans fat content, people can keep better track of their daily trans fat intake by paying attention to food labels. Additional information on trans fat is found under the "Trans-Fatty Acids" section in Chapter 3 (see page 87).

The FDA allows food manufacturers to label any product that has less than half a gram of trans fat per serving as zero. Be aware that if you eat three or four servings of a particular food near a half a gram of trans fat, you may be getting your maximum daily allowance (1 gram per 1,000 calories of daily caloric intake). Thus, you are encouraged to look at the list of ingredients and search for the words "partially hydrogenated" as an indicator of hidden trans fat.

The labels "partially hydrogenated" and "trans-fatty acids" indicate that the product carries a health risk just as high as or greater than that of saturated fat. Now that trans fats are listed on food labels, companies have reformulated many of their products to reduce or eliminate these fats. Some products once high in trans fats now have none or less than half so they don't have to list them on the label. As a consumer, you are encouraged to check food labels often to obtain current information. Table 11.5 lists the average trans fat content of some foods. These values may vary among brands according to food formulation and ingredients and may change as manufacturers continue to alter food formulations to further decrease or eliminate trans fat content.

TABLE 11.5 **Average Trans Fat Content of Selected Foods***

Food Item	Amount	Grams
Biscuit, breakfast	1	0.5
Bisquick (pancake and baking mix)	1/3 cup mix	1.0
Burrito, steak or ground beef, Taco Bell	1	0.0-1.0
Butter	1 tbsp	0.0–0.3
Country Fried Steak, KFC	1	1.0
Double Quarter Pounder w/cheese, McDonalds	1	2.5
Double Whopper w/cheese, Burger King	1	3.5
Express Taco Salad w/chips	1	1.0
Frosting, canned		0.0–1.5
Margarine, stick	1 tbsp	2.0
Margarine, tub	1 tbsp	0.0–0.5
Milkshakes	1	1.0
Pop Secret Microwave Popcorn	4.5 cups popped	5.0
Tootsie rolls	6 mini	

Note: Trans fat intake should be limited to no more than 1 percent of total daily caloric intake or the equivalent of 1 gram per 1,000 calories of energy intake.
*Trans fat content in food items has been decreasing significantly as food manufacturers have decreased or eliminated the content in their products because of FDA regulations that require trans fats to be listed on food labels. Trans fat content also varies between different brands based on food formulation and ingredients. Check food labels regularly to obtain current information.

Lowering LDL Cholesterol LDL cholesterol levels higher than ideal can be lowered through dietary changes, by losing body fat, by taking medication, and by participating in a regular aerobic exercise program. Research has shown a higher relative risk of mortality in unfit individuals with low cholesterol than fit people with high cholesterol. The lowest mortality rate, of course, is seen in fit people with low total cholesterol levels.

In terms of dietary modifications, a diet lower in saturated fat, trans fats, and cholesterol and high in fiber is recommended. Saturated fat should be replaced with polyunsaturated and monounsaturated fats because the latter tend to decrease LDL cholesterol and increase HDL cholesterol (see the discussion of "Simple Fats" in Chapter 3, pages 86–89). Total saturated fat intake should be less than 5 to 6 percent of the total daily caloric intake, preferably much lower while on a cholesterol-lowering diet. Trans fat intake should be less than 1 percent of daily caloric intake. Exercise is important because dietary manipulation by itself is not as effective in lowering LDL cholesterol as a combination of diet plus aerobic exercise.

Furthermore, "moderate" fat–intake diets (25 to 35 percent of total caloric intake) are better for heart health (as long as most of it is unsaturated fats) than are low-fat diets or highly refined carbohydrate diets. As you increase the intake of unsaturated fats, be sure to substitute these for some other less healthy foods (red meat, sausages, hamburgers, organ meats, butter, margarines, whole-milk products, etc.); otherwise, weight gain will ensue. Excessive carbohydrate intake, especially refined carbohydrates, raises triglycerides, and as triglycerides go up, HDL cholesterol typically decreases. A 12-year follow up study on more than 53,000 men and women indicated that people who cut back on saturated fat but increased intake of whole grains and high-fiber fruits and vegetables were 12 percent less likely to have a heart attack with every 5 percent increase in calories from high-fiber foods. Those who substituted high-glycemic carbohydrates for saturated fat increased heart attack risk by 33 percent for every 5 percent increase in calories from high-glycemic, low-fiber carbohydrates (such as white bread, pasta, potatoes, and sweets).[12] British research published in 2014 points to a decreased risk of dying from CVD by 31 percent by people who consume seven or more servings of fruits and vegetables per day as compared to those who consume less than one (death rates from all causes were down 42 percent and cancer by 25 percent).[13]

Total saturated fat intake should be less than 6 percent of the total daily caloric intake and preferably much lower while on a cholesterol-lowering diet. Trans fat intake should be less than 1 percent of the daily caloric intake. Exercise is important because dietary manipulation by itself is not as effective in lowering LDL cholesterol as a combination of diet plus aerobic exercise.

To lower LDL cholesterol significantly, total daily fiber intake must be in the range of 25 to 38 grams per day (see "Fiber" in Chapter 3), and total fat consumption can be in the range of 25 to 35 percent of total daily caloric intake—as long as most of the fat is unsaturated fat and the average cholesterol consumption is lower than 200 mg. Increasing consumption of cholesterol-lowering foods such as plant sterols (added to some spreads and salad dressings), soy protein, nuts (walnuts, almonds, macadamia nuts, peanuts, pecans, pistachio nuts), vegetables, fruits, whole grains, and foods high in soluble fiber (oats, legumes, and barley), further accelerates the rate of LDL cholesterol reduction. Keep in mind that as you add some of these foods to your diet, you have to take other less healthy foods out.

Among people in the United States, the average fiber intake is less than 15 grams per day. Fiber, in particular the soluble type, has been shown to lower cholesterol. Soluble fiber dissolves in water and forms a gel-like substance that encloses food particles. This property helps bind and excrete fats from the body. Soluble fibers also bind intestinal bile acids that could be recycled into additional cholesterol. Soluble fibers are found primarily in oats, fruits, barley, legumes, and psyllium.

Psyllium, a grain that is added to some multigrain breakfast cereals, also helps lower LDL cholesterol. As little as 3 grams of psyllium daily can lower LDL

Processed foods A food that has been chemically altered from its natural state through additives such as flavors, flavor enhancers, colors, binders, preservatives, stabilizers, emulsifiers, and fillers or has been manufactured through combination or other methods.

cholesterol by 20 percent. Commercially available fiber supplements that contain psyllium (e.g., Metamucil) can be used to increase soluble fiber intake. Three tablespoons daily add about 10 grams of soluble fiber to the diet.

The incidence of heart disease is very low in populations in which daily fiber intake exceeds 30 grams per day. Furthermore, a Harvard University Medical School study of 43,000 middle-aged men who were followed for more than 6 years showed that increasing fiber intake to 30 grams daily resulted in a 41 percent reduction in heart attacks.[14]

When attempting to lower LDL cholesterol, moderate consumption of healthy fats (polyunsaturated and monounsaturated) is encouraged. A drawback of very low-fat diets (less than 25 percent fat) is that they tend to lower HDL cholesterol and increase triglycerides. If HDL cholesterol is already low, polyunsaturated and monounsaturated fats should be added to the diet. Examples of food items that are high in monounsaturated and polyunsaturated fats are nuts and olive, canola, corn, and soybean oils. The table of nutritive values in Appendix A can be used to determine food items that are high in monounsaturated and polyunsaturated fats (see also Figure 3.9, page 101).

The NCEP guidelines for people who are trying to decrease LDL cholesterol allow for a diet with up to 35 percent of calories from fat, including 10 percent from polyunsaturated fats and 20 percent from monounsaturated fats.[15] If you are attempting to lower LDL cholesterol, saturated fats should be kept to an absolute minimum.

Margarines and salad dressings that contain stanol ester, a plant-derived compound that interferes with cholesterol absorption in the intestine, are now also on the market. Make sure, however, that they do not contain significant amounts of saturated fat, trans fat, or partially hydrogenated oils. Over the course of several weeks, daily intake of about 3 grams of margarine or 6 tablespoons of salad dressing containing stanol ester lowers LDL cholesterol by more than 10 percent. Dietary guidelines to lower LDL cholesterol levels are provided in the accompanying box on the next page.

The best prescription for controlling blood lipids is the combination of a healthy diet, a sound aerobic exercise program, and weight control. If this does not work, a physician can recommend appropriate drug therapies based upon a blood test to analyze the various subcategories of lipoproteins.

The NCEP guidelines recommend that people consider drug therapy if, after 6 months on a diet low in cholesterol and trans and saturated fats, cholesterol remains unacceptably high. An unacceptable level is an LDL cholesterol above 190 mg/dL for individuals with fewer than two risk factors and no signs of heart disease. For individuals with more than two risk factors and with a history of heart disease, LDL cholesterol above 160 mg/dL is unacceptable.

Saturated Fat Replacement in the Diet

Although for years we have known that saturated fat raises LDL cholesterol, a review of 21 observational research studies involving almost 350,000 people failed to prove a significant association between saturated fat intake and risk of CHD, stroke, or CVD.[16] Researchers focused on the foods consumed in the American diet that have replaced saturated fat.

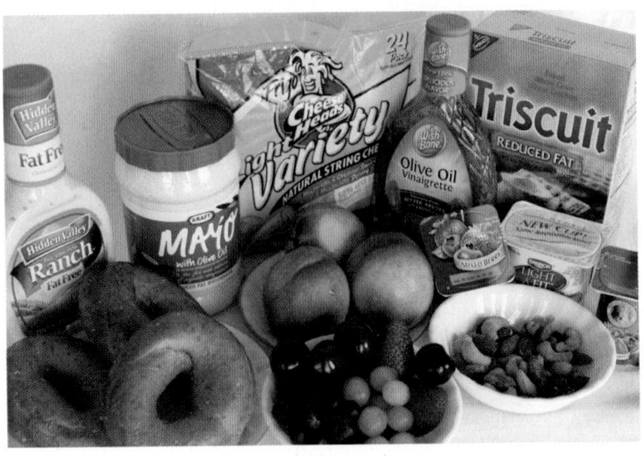

As long as the number of servings and caloric intake are not increased, substituting unsaturated fat, cholesterol-free, and trans fat–free products for calorie-dense high-fat and saturated fat products and simple carbohydrate and refined sugar products in the diet significantly decreases the risk for disease.

Once people learned that saturated fats were unhealthy, instead of consuming more fruits, vegetables, legumes, and grains, many increased consumption of "low-fat" simple carbohydrates and refined sugars (low-fat varieties of breads, rolls, cereals, cookies, ice cream, cakes, and desserts). Although low in fat, simple carbohydrates and refined sugars are high in calories that lead to weight gain. The data show that exchanging refined carbohydrates for saturated fat exacerbates blood lipid problems, including higher LDL cholesterol, a reduction in HDL cholesterol, and higher triglycerides.

The best recommendation is not to limit fat consumption in the diet to the minimum but to maintain a total fat intake of around 25 to 35 percent of total calories, with a primary shift toward polyunsaturated fats.[17] To do so, choose fish, nuts, seeds, and vegetable oils that are liquid at room temperature (with the exception of tropical oils, including coconut, palm, and palm kernel oils).

At present, it is unknown whether the cardioprotective benefits are the result of limiting saturated fat intake or increasing polyunsaturated fat consumption. Another 2010 review found that consumption of polyunsaturated fat in place of saturated fat reduced the incidence of heart attacks and cardiac deaths.[18] Thus, moderate "healthy fat" intake (not low fat)—along with decreased refined carbohydrates and, in most cases, decreased caloric intake—are encouraged. The issue merits further research involving clinical trials (rather than observational studies) before clear answers can be obtained.

BEHAVIOR MODIFICATION PLANNING

Blood Chemistry Test Guidelines

People who have never had a blood chemistry test should do so to establish a baseline for future reference. The blood test should include total cholesterol, LDL cholesterol, HDL cholesterol, triglycerides, and blood glucose.

Following an initial normal baseline test no later than age 20, for a person who adheres to the recommended dietary and exercise guidelines, a blood analysis at least every 5 years prior to age 40 should suffice. Thereafter, a blood lipid test is recommended every year, in conjunction with a regular preventive medicine physical examination.

A single baseline test is not necessarily a valid measure. Cholesterol levels vary from month to month and sometimes even from day to day. If the initial test reveals cholesterol abnormalities, the test should be repeated within a few weeks to confirm the results.

Try It

Blood chemistry tests are available at many wellness centers on college campuses for under $25 for a comprehensive test that includes total cholesterol, LDL cholesterol, HDL cholesterol, triglycerides, and blood glucose levels. Have you had your blood test done, and are you aware of your blood lipid profile?

Dietary Guidelines to Lower LDL Cholesterol

I PLAN TO | I DID IT

❑ ❑ Minimize the use of simple and refined carbohydrates (including sugars) and processed foods.

❑ ❑ Consume between 25 and 38 grams of fiber daily, including a minimum of 10 grams of soluble fiber (good sources are oats, fruits, barley, legumes, and psyllium).

❑ ❑ Increase consumption of vegetables, fruits, whole grains, and beans.

❑ ❑ Do not consume more than 200 mg of dietary cholesterol a day.

❑ ❑ Consume red meats (no more than 3 ounces per serving) fewer than 3 times per week and no organ meats (such as liver and kidneys) and limit (less than 1.5 ounces per serving) processed meats to once per week or none at all.

❑ ❑ Do not consume commercially baked foods.

❑ ❑ Avoid foods that contain trans-fatty acids, hydrogenated fat, or partially hydrogenated vegetable oil.

❑ ❑ Increase intake of omega-3 fatty acids (see Chapter 3) by eating two to three omega-3-rich fish meals per week.

❑ ❑ Consume 25 grams of soy protein a day.

❑ ❑ Drink low-fat milk (1 percent or less fat, preferably) and use low-fat dairy products.

❑ ❑ Do not use coconut oil, palm oil, or cocoa butter.

❑ ❑ Consume nuts (1.5 ounces) on a daily basis (almonds, walnuts, peanuts, hazelnuts, pistachio nuts).

❑ ❑ Limit egg consumption to fewer than three eggs per week (this is for people with high cholesterol only; others may consume eggs in moderation).

❑ ❑ Use margarines and salad dressings that contain stanol ester instead of butter and regular margarine.

❑ ❑ Bake, broil, grill, poach, or steam food instead of frying.

❑ ❑ Refrigerate cooked meat before adding to other dishes. Remove fat hardened in the refrigerator before mixing the meat with other foods.

❑ ❑ Avoid fatty sauces made with butter, cream, or cheese.

❑ ❑ Maintain recommended body weight.

Try It

Dietary guidelines for health and wellness were thoroughly discussed in Chapter 3, "Nutrition for Wellness." How have your dietary habits changed since studying these guidelines, and how well do they support the above recommendations to lower LDL cholesterol?

Elevated Triglycerides

Triglycerides, also known as free fatty acids, make up most of the fat in our diet and most of the fat that circulates in the blood. In combination with cholesterol, triglycerides speed up formation of plaque in the arteries. Triglycerides are carried in the bloodstream primarily by VLDLs and chylomicrons. Triglycerides per se don't end up in the atherosclerotic plaque. Chylomicrons are broken down in the blood into fatty acids and remnant-free, cholesterol-rich particles. Fatty acids are stored in muscle or adipose tissue (fat) and scavenger cells that do contribute to atherosclerosis then take up the remnant particles.

Although they are found in poultry skin, lunch meats, and shellfish, these fatty acids are manufactured mainly in the liver from refined sugars, starches, and alcohol. High intake of alcohol and sugars (honey and fruit juices included) significantly raises triglyceride levels.

To lower triglycerides, avoid pastries, candies, soft drinks, fruit juices, white bread, pasta, and alcohol. In addition, cutting down on overall fat consumption, quitting smoking, reducing weight (if overweight), and doing aerobic exercise are helpful measures. Omega-3 fatty acids also help, but doses higher than those found in fish are required. The AHA recommends two to four grams of fish oil daily under a physician's supervision.

The desirable blood triglyceride level is less than 150 mg/dL (Table 11.6). For people with cardiovascular problems, this level should be below 100 mg/dL. Levels above 1,000 mg/dL pose an immediate risk for potentially fatal sudden inflammation of the pancreas.

LDL Phenotype B Some people consistently have slightly elevated triglyceride levels (above 140 mg/dL) and HDL cholesterol levels below 35 mg/dL. About 80 percent of these people have a genetic condition called LDL phenotype B. Although the blood lipids may not be notably high, these people are at higher risk for atherosclerosis and CHD.

CRITICAL THINKING

Are you aware of your blood lipid profile? If not, what is keeping you from getting a blood chemistry test? What are the benefits of having it done now rather than later in life?

TABLE 11.6 Triglycerides Guidelines

Amount	Rating
<150 mg/dL	Desirable
150–199 mg/dL	Borderline high
200–499 mg/dL	High
≥500 mg/dL	Very high

Source: National Heart, Lung and Blood Institute.

Cholesterol-Lowering Medications Effective medications are available to treat elevated cholesterol and triglycerides. Most notable among them are the statins group (Lipitor, Mevacor, Crestor, Vytorin, Pravachol, Lescol, and Zocor), which can lower cholesterol by up to 60 percent in 2 to 3 months. Statins slow down cholesterol production and increase the liver's ability to remove blood cholesterol. They also decrease triglycerides and produce a small increase in HDL levels. The drug Tricor is commonly used to lower triglycerides.

The new guidelines by the American Heart Association and the American College of Cardiology recommend that people at high risk for CVD disease be treated with statin therapy. Unless at high risk, many experts feel that in general, it is better to lower LDL cholesterol without medication, because drugs often cause undesirable side effects. Many people with heart disease must take cholesterol-lowering medication, but medication is best combined with lifestyle changes to augment the cholesterol-lowering effect. For example, when Zocor was taken alone over 3 months, LDL cholesterol decreased by 30 percent; but when a Mediterranean diet was adopted in combination with Zocor therapy, LDL cholesterol decreased by 41 percent.[19] In 2012 the FDA added safety alerts to the prescribing information of statins. Although rare among the millions of people who take these medications, the adverse effects include memory loss, cognitive impairment like forgetfulness and confusion, higher blood sugar levels that may lead to a diagnosis of diabetes, and muscle pain. Anyone starting treatment with statin drugs should be aware of these side effects.

Other drugs effective in reducing LDL cholesterol are bile acid sequestrans, which bind the cholesterol found in bile acids. Cholesterol subsequently is excreted in the stools. These drugs often are used in combination with statin drugs.

High dosages (1.5 to 3 grams per day) of nicotinic acid or niacin (a B vitamin) also help lower LDL cholesterol, Lp(a), and triglycerides and increase HDL cholesterol (change HDL3 to HDL2). Niacin in combination with some of the aforementioned drugs also exerts positive effects on IDL and pattern size. A fourth group of drugs, known as fibrates, is used primarily to lower triglycerides.

Elevated Homocysteine

Clinical data indicating that many heart attack and stroke victims have normal cholesterol levels have led researchers to look for other risk factors that may contribute to atherosclerosis. Although it is not a blood lipid, one of these factors is a high concentration of the amino acid **homocysteine** in the blood. It is thought to enhance the formation of plaque and the subsequent blockage of arteries.

The body uses homocysteine to help build proteins and carry out cellular metabolism. It is an intermediate amino acid in the interconversion of two other amino acids—methionine and cysteine. This interconversion requires the

B vitamin folate (folic acid) and vitamins B_6 and B_{12}. Typically, homocysteine is metabolized rapidly, so it does not accumulate in the blood or damage the arteries. Still, many people have high blood levels of homocysteine. This might result from either a genetic inability to metabolize homocysteine or a deficiency in the vitamins required for its conversion.

Homocysteine typically is measured in micromoles per liter (μmol/L). Guidelines to interpret homocysteine levels are provided in Table 11.7. A 10-year follow-up study of people with high homocysteine levels showed that those individuals with a level above 14.25 μmol/L had almost twice the risk of stroke compared with individuals whose level was below 9.25 μmol/L.[20] Homocysteine accumulation is theorized to be toxic because it may:

1. Cause damage to the inner lining of the arteries (the initial step in the process of atherosclerosis)
2. Stimulate the proliferation of cells that contribute to plaque formation
3. Encourage clotting, which could completely obstruct an artery and lead to a heart attack or stroke

Keeping homocysteine from accumulating in the blood seems to be as simple as eating the recommended daily servings of vegetables, fruits, grains, and some meat and legumes. Five servings of fruits and vegetables daily can provide sufficient levels of folate and vitamin B_6 to remove and clear homocysteine from the blood. Vitamin B_{12} is found primarily in animal flesh and animal products. Vitamin B_{12} deficiency is rarely a problem, because 1 cup of milk or an egg provides the daily requirement. The body also recycles most of this vitamin; therefore, a deficiency takes years to develop. People who consume five servings of fruits and vegetables daily are unlikely to derive extra benefits from a vitamin-B-complex supplement.

Increasing evidence that folate can prevent heart attacks has led to the recommendation that people consume 400 micrograms (mcg) per day—obtainable from five daily servings of fruits and vegetables. Unfortunately, estimates indicate that more than 80 percent of Americans do not get 400 mcg of folate per day (adequate folate intake also is critical for women of childbearing age to prevent birth defects).

TABLE 11.7 Homocysteine Guidelines

Level	Rating
<9.0 μmol/L	Desirable
9–12 μmol/L	Mild elevation
13–15 μmol/L	Elevated
>15 μmol/L	Extreme elevation

Adapted from K. S. McCully, "What You Must Know Now About Homocysteine," *Bottom Line/Health* 18 (January 2004): 7-9.

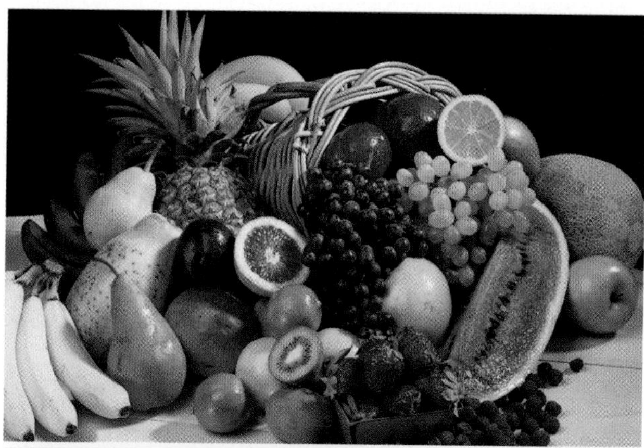

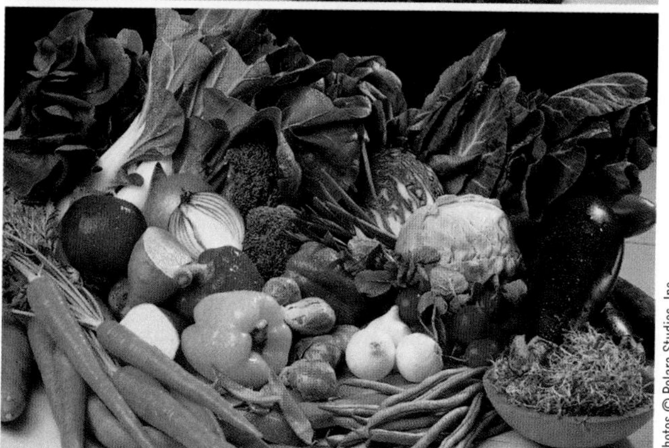

Photos © Polara Studios, Inc.

Ample amounts of fruits and vegetables provide the necessary nutrients to keep homocysteine from causing heart disease or stroke.

Inflammation

In addition to homocysteine, scientists are looking at inflammation as a major risk factor for heart attacks. Low-grade inflammation can occur in a variety of places throughout the body. For years, it has been known that inflammation plays a role in CHD and that inflammation hidden deep in the body is a common trigger of heart attacks, even when cholesterol levels are normal or low and arterial plaque is minimal.

To evaluate ongoing inflammation in the body, physicians have turned to **C-reactive protein (CRP)**, a protein produced in the liver whose levels in the blood increase with injury or irritation (inflammation) anywhere in the body. Physical inactivity, smoking, excessive body weight, a diet high in saturated fat, chronic stress, periodontal disease, and infections can all cause inflammation.

Individuals with elevated CRP are more prone to cardiovascular events, even in the absence of elevated LDL cholesterol. The evidence shows that CRP blood levels elevate years before a first

Homocysteine An amino acid that, when allowed to accumulate in the blood, may lead to plaque formation and blockage of arteries.

C-reactive protein (CRP) A protein whose blood levels increase with inflammation, at times hidden deep in the body; elevation of this protein is an indicator of potential cardiovascular events.

heart attack or stroke and that individuals with elevated CRP have twice the risk of a heart attack. The risk of a heart attack is even higher in people with both elevated CRP and cholesterol, resulting in an almost ninefold increase in risk (see Figure 11.8).

Because high CRP levels might be a better predictor of future heart attacks than high cholesterol alone, a test known as high-sensitivity CRP (hs-CRP), which measures inflammation in the blood vessels, has been approved by the FDA. The term "high sensitivity" was derived from the test's capability to detect small amounts of CRP in the blood.

Results of the hs-CRP test provide a good measure of the probability of plaque rupturing within the arterial wall. The two main types of plaque are soft and hard. Soft plaque is the most likely to rupture. Ruptured plaque releases clots into the bloodstream that can lead to a heart attack or a stroke. Other evidence has linked high CRP levels to high blood pressure and colon cancer.

Excessive intake of alcohol and high protein diets also increases CRP. Evidence further indicates that high-fat fast food increases CRP levels for several hours following the meal. And cooking meat and poultry at high temperatures creates damaged proteins called advanced glycosylation end products, which trigger inflammation. Several studies have also indicated that high intake of omega-6 fatty acids may cause inflammation (also see Chapter 3, page 88). The current American diet is too high in omega-6 foods, and obesity increases inflammation. With weight loss, CRP levels decrease proportional to the amount of fat lost.

An hs-CRP test is relatively inexpensive, and it is highly recommended for individuals at risk for heart attack. A level above 2 mg/L appears to be a better predictor of a heart attack than an LDL cholesterol level above 130 mg/dL. General guidelines for hs-CRP levels are given in Table 11.8.

A weakness of the hs-CRP test is that it does not detect differences between acute and chronic inflammation, and results may not be stable from day to day. An acute inflammation, for example, could be the result of a pulled muscle or a passing cold. It is chronic inflammation that increases heart disease risk. Thus, a new test that specifically detects chronic inflammation, lipoprotein phospholipase A2 (PAL2), may soon replace the hs-CRP test.

CRP levels decrease with statin drugs, which also lower cholesterol and reduce inflammation. A study on 17,802 apparently healthy men and women with LDL cholesterol below 130 mg/dL but CRP levels above 2.0 mg/L showed that a daily dose of the statin drug Crestor reduced LDL cholesterol by 50 percent, CRP by 37 percent, and the risk of heart attack, stroke, and death by 54, 48, and 47 percent, respectively.[21] The results were so impressive that researchers stopped the trial halfway through the study.

Exercise, weight loss, proper nutrition, and quitting smoking are helpful in reducing hs-CRP. Omega-3 fatty acids inhibit proteins that cause inflammation. Aspirin therapy also helps by controlling inflammation.

FIGURE 11.8 Relationships among CRP, cholesterol, and risk of CVD.

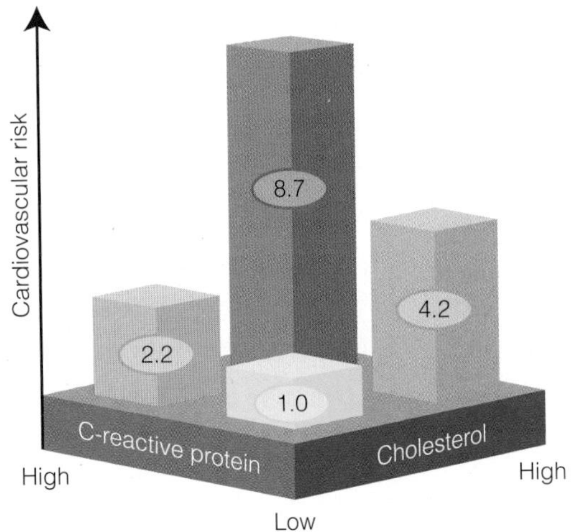

Source: Adapted from P. Libby, P. M. Ridker, and A. Maseri, "Inflammation and Atherosclerosis," *Circulation* 105 (2002): 1135-1143.

TABLE 11.8 Hs-CRP Guidelines

Amount	Rating
<1 mg/L	Low risk
1–3 mg/L	Average risk
>3 mg/L	High risk

Source: T.A. Pearson et al., "Markers of Inflammation and Cardiovascular Disease," *Circulation* 107 (2003): 499-511.

Diabetes

Diabetes mellitus is a condition in which blood glucose is unable to enter the cells because the pancreas totally stops producing **insulin**, or it does not produce enough to meet the body's needs, or the cells develop **insulin resistance**. The role of insulin is to "unlock" the cells and escort glucose into the cell.

Currently, diabetes affects more than 27 million people in the United States; 7 million are undiagnosed, and another 80 million people are prediabetic. Between 1980 and 2003, the prevalence of diabetes more than doubled. By 2020, diabetes and prediabetes are projected to account for 10 percent of total health care spending, with an estimated yearly cost of $500 billion. At the present rate of escalation, the CDC predicts that by 2050 one of every three Americans will have diabetes.

The incidence of CVD and death in the diabetic population is quite high. Two of three people with diabetes will die from CVD. People with chronically elevated blood glucose levels may have problems metabolizing fats, which can make them more susceptible to atherosclerosis, CHD, heart attacks, high blood pressure, and stroke. People with diabetes also have lower HDL cholesterol and higher triglyceride levels.

Furthermore, chronic high blood sugar can lead to stroke, nerve damage, vision loss, kidney damage, sexual dysfunction, and decreased immune function (making people more susceptible to infections). Compared with those who do not have diabetes, diabetic patients are four times more likely to become blind and 20 times more likely to develop kidney failure. Nerve damage in the lower extremities decreases awareness of injury and infection, and a small, untreated sore can result in severe infection and gangrene, which can even lead to an amputation.

An 8-hour fasting blood glucose level above 125 mg/dL on two separate tests confirms a diagnosis of diabetes (Table 11.9). A level of 126 mg/dL or higher should be brought to the attention of a physician.

Types of Diabetes Diabetes is one of two types: **type 1 diabetes**, or insulin-dependent diabetes mellitus, and **type 2 diabetes**, or non-insulin-dependent diabetes mellitus. Type 1 also has been called "juvenile diabetes," because it is found mainly in young people. With type 1 diabetes, the pancreas produces little or no insulin. With type 2 diabetes, either the pancreas does not produce sufficient insulin or it produces adequate amounts but the cells become insulin resistant, thereby keeping glucose from entering the cell. Type 2 diabetes accounts for 90 to 95 percent of all cases of diabetes.

Presently, more than 1 in 10 American adults have diabetes. Although diabetes has a genetic predisposition, 60 to 80 percent of type 2 diabetes is related closely to overeating, obesity, and lack of physical activity. Type 2 diabetes, once limited primarily to overweight adults, now accounts for almost half of the new cases diagnosed in children. According to the CDC, 1 in 3 children born in the United States today will develop diabetes.

More than 80 percent of all people with type 2 diabetes are overweight or have a history of excessive weight. In most cases, this condition can be corrected through regular exercise, a special diet, and weight loss.

Aerobic exercise helps prevent type 2 diabetes. The protective effect is even greater in those with risk factors such as obesity, high blood pressure, and family propensity. The preventive effect is attributed to less body fat and to better sugar and fat metabolism resulting from the regular exercise program. At 3,500 calories of energy expenditure per week through exercise, the risk is cut in half versus that of a sedentary lifestyle.

Both moderate- and vigorous-intensity physical activity are associated with increased insulin sensitivity and decreased risk for diabetes. The key to increase and maintain

TABLE 11.9 Blood Glucose Guidelines

Amount	Rating
≤100 mg/dL	Normal
101–125 mg/dL	Prediabetes
≥126 mg/dL	Diabetes*

*Confirmed by two tests on different days.

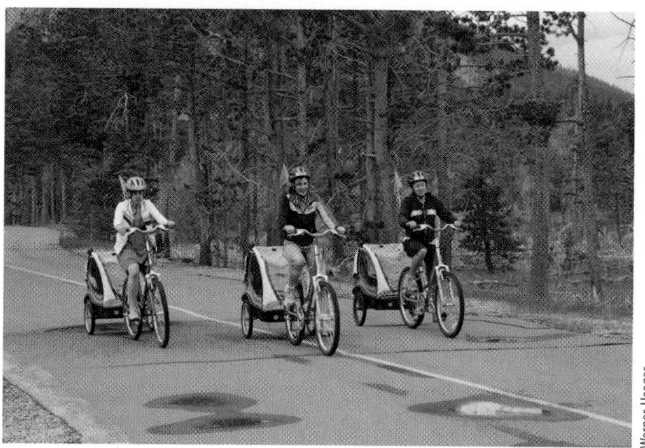

Regular physical activity increases insulin sensitivity and decreases the risk for diabetes.

proper insulin sensitivity is regularity of the exercise program. Failing to maintain habitual physical activity voids these benefits. Thus, a simple aerobic exercise program (walking, cycling, or swimming four or five times per week) often is prescribed because it increases the body's sensitivity to insulin. Exercise guidelines for diabetic patients are discussed in detail in Chapter 9.

In fact, accumulating evidence indicates that increasing physical activity, losing excess weight, and improving nutrition is more effective to control diabetes and lower CVD risk than relying on drugs to manage the disease.[22] Furthermore, research suggests that diabetic patients are worse off when medications are used to decrease blood sugar levels and blood pressure to *normal or below normal* levels. Accordingly, diabetic patients are strongly encouraged to adopt healthy lifestyle factors even if glucose levels are controlled with medication.

A diet high in complex carbohydrates (unrefined whole grains and whole foods) and water-soluble fibers (found in fruits, vegetables, oats, beans, and psyllium), low in saturated fat, low in sugar, and including a small amount of lean protein with meals is helpful in treating diabetes. Weight loss, even if only a 5 to 10 percent reduction in weight, can make a notable

Diabetes mellitus A disease in which the body doesn't produce or utilize insulin properly.

Insulin A hormone secreted by the pancreas; essential for proper metabolism of blood glucose (sugar) and maintenance of blood glucose level.

Insulin resistance The inability of the cells to respond appropriately to insulin.

Type 1 diabetes Insulin-dependent diabetes mellitus, a condition in which the pancreas produces little or no insulin; also known as juvenile diabetes.

Type 2 diabetes Non-insulin-dependent diabetes mellitus, a condition in which insulin is not processed properly; also known as adult-onset diabetes.

BEHAVIOR MODIFICATION PLANNING

Guidelines to Prevent and Manage Type 2 Diabetes

Experts agree that the following healthy lifestyle strategies are effective in type 2 diabetes management:

I PLAN TO | I DID IT

❏ ❏ Follow an overall healthful dietary pattern that includes

- A minimum of five daily servings of fruits and vegetables; even better, at least seven daily servings for greater protection
- At least three daily servings of whole grains
- Consumption of at least two 3-oz servings of fatty fish per week
- A few small portions of nuts each week
- Skim milk and low-fat dairy products in your daily diet

❏ ❏ Maintain recommended body weight

❏ ❏ Increase daily physical activity to at least 30 minutes of daily moderate-intensity activity and strength training two to three times per week.

Try It

Review your Behavior Change Plan and your Online Journal or class notebook. Are you following these guidelines? Are there changes you need to make to your Behavior Change Plan to bring yourself into closer compliance?

difference in controlling blood sugar. These lifestyle changes (proper nutrition, physical activity, and weight loss) often allow diabetic patients to normalize their blood sugar level without the use of medication.

Finally, evidence also suggests that consumption of low-fat dairy products lowers the risk for type 2 diabetes. Research on more than 41,000 men showed that those who consumed the most dairy products had a 23 percent lower incidence of the disease. Furthermore, each additional daily serving of dairy products was associated with a 9 percent decrease in type 2 diabetes risk.[23]

Glycemic Index Although complex carbohydrates are recommended in the diet, people with diabetes need to pay careful attention to the glycemic index (explained in Chapter 5 and detailed in Table 5.1, page 172). Refined and starchy foods (small-particle carbohydrates, which are quickly digested) rank high on the glycemic index, whereas grains, fruits, and vegetables are low-glycemic foods.

Foods high on the glycemic index cause a rapid increase in blood sugar. A diet that includes many high-glycemic foods increases the risk for CVD in people with high insulin resistance and **glucose intolerance**. Combining a moderate amount of high-glycemic foods with low-glycemic foods or with some fat and protein, however, can bring down the average index.

Hemoglobin A1$_c$ Test Individuals who have high blood glucose levels should consult a physician to decide on the best treatment. They also might obtain information about the hemoglobin A1$_c$ (HbA1$_c$) test, which measures the amount of glucose that has been in a person's blood over the last 3 months. Blood glucose can become attached to hemoglobin in the red blood cells. Once attached, it remains there for the life of the red blood cell, which is about 3 months. The higher the blood glucose, the higher the concentration of glucose in the red blood cells. Results of this test are given in percentages.

The HbA1$_c$ goal for diabetic patients is to keep it under 7 percent. At this level and below, diabetic patients have a lower risk of developing diabetes-related problems of the eyes, kidneys, and nerves. Because the test tells a person how well blood glucose has been controlled over the last 3 months, a change in treatment is almost always recommended if the HbA1$_c$ results are above 8 percent. All people with type 2 diabetes should have an HbA1$_c$ test twice per year.

Diagnosis of Metabolic Syndrome

	Men	Women
Waist circumference	>40 in	>35 in
Blood pressure	>130/85 mm Hg	>130/85 mm Hg
Fasting blood glucose	>100 mg/dL	>100 mg/dL
Fasting HDL cholesterol	<40 mg/dL	<50 mg/dL
Fasting triglycerides	>150 mg/dL	>150 mg/dL

Metabolic Syndrome

As the cells resist the actions of insulin, the pancreas releases even more insulin in an attempt to keep blood glucose from rising. A chronic rise in insulin seems to trigger a series of abnormalities referred to as the **metabolic syndrome**. These abnormal conditions include abdominal obesity (see Figure 4.9, page 151), elevated blood pressure, high blood glucose, low HDL cholesterol, high triglycerides, and an increased blood-clotting mechanism. All of these conditions increase the risk for CHD and other diabetes-related conditions (blindness, infection, nerve damage, kidney failure, etc.). Currently, more than 30 percent of Americans 20 years of age and older (about 50 million Americans) have metabolic syndrome. And according to World Health Organization estimates, one-fifth of the world adult population is afflicted by this condition.

People with metabolic syndrome have an abnormal insulin response to carbohydrates, in particular high-glycemic foods. Research on metabolic syndrome indicates that a low-fat, high-carbohydrate diet may not be the best for preventing CHD and actually could increase the risk for the disease in individuals with high insulin resistance and glucose intolerance. It might be best for these people to distribute daily caloric intake so that 45 percent of the calories are derived from carbohydrates (primarily low-glycemic carbohydrates), 40 percent from fat, and 15 percent from protein.[24] Of the 40 percent fat calories, most of the fat should come from mono- and poly-unsaturated fats and less than 7 percent from saturated fat.

Individuals with metabolic syndrome also benefit from weight loss (if overweight), exercise, and smoking cessation. Insulin resistance drops by about 40 percent in overweight people who lose 20 pounds. A total of 45 minutes of daily aerobic exercise enhances insulin efficiency by 25 percent. Quitting smoking also decreases insulin resistance.

Hypertension

Some 60,000 miles of blood vessels run through the human body. As the heart forces the blood through these vessels, the fluid is under pressure. **Blood pressure** is measured in milliliters of mercury (mm Hg), usually expressed in two numbers—**systolic blood pressure** is the higher number, and **diastolic blood pressure** is the lower number. Ideal blood pressure is 120/80 or lower.

Standards Statistical evidence indicates that damage to the arteries starts at blood pressures above 120/80. The risk for CVD doubles with each increment of 20/10, starting with a blood pressure of 115/75.[25] All blood pressures of at least 140/90 are considered to be **hypertension** (Table 11.10) Blood pressures ranging from 120/80 to 139/89 are referred to as prehypertension.

Based on estimates, approximately 1 in every 3 adults is hypertensive. The incidence is higher among African Americans—in fact, it is among the highest in the world. Approximately 30 percent and 20 percent of all deaths in African American men and women, respectively, may be caused by high blood pressure.

TABLE 11.10 Blood Pressure Guidelines (in mm Hg)

Rating	Systolic	Diastolic
Normal	<120	<80
Prehypertension	121–139	81–89
Stage 1 hypertension	140–159	90–99
Stage 2 hypertension	≥160	≥100

Source: *National High Blood Pressure Education Program.*

Although the threshold for hypertension has been set at 140/90, many experts believe that the lower the blood pressure, the better. Even if the pressure is around 90/50, as long as that person does not have any symptoms of **hypotension**, he or she need not be concerned. Typical symptoms of hypotension are dizziness, lightheadedness, and fainting.

Blood pressure also may fluctuate during a regular day. Many factors affect blood pressure, and one single reading may not be a true indicator of the real pressure. For example, physical activity and stress increase blood pressure, and rest and relaxation decrease blood pressure. Consequently, several measurements should be taken before diagnosing high pressure.

Incidence and Pathology

Based on estimates by the AHA, about 78 million Americans are hypertensive and more than 60,000 Americans die each year as a direct result of high blood pressure. Hypertension, however, is a contributing factor to many other ailments, and it has been linked to as

Glucose intolerance A condition characterized by slightly elevated blood glucose levels.

Metabolic syndrome An array of metabolic abnormalities that contribute to the development of atherosclerosis triggered by insulin resistance. These conditions include low HDL cholesterol, high triglycerides, high blood pressure, and an increased blood-clotting mechanism.

Blood pressure A measure of the force exerted against the walls of the vessels by the blood flowing through them.

Systolic blood pressure Pressure exerted by the blood against walls of arteries during forceful contraction (systole) of the heart; the higher of the two numbers in blood pressure readings.

Diastolic blood pressure Pressure exerted by the blood against walls of arteries during relaxation phase (diastole) of the heart; the lower of the two numbers in blood pressure readings.

Hypertension Chronically elevated blood pressure.

Hypotension Low blood pressure.

many as 350,000 annual deaths from all causes. The dramatic increase in hypertension seems to be linked to the growing obesity epidemic and the aging of the U.S. population. Unless appropriate, healthy lifestyle strategies are implemented, people who do not have high blood pressure at age 55 have a 90 percent chance of developing it at some point in their lives.

Hypertension has been referred to as "the silent killer." It does not hurt, it does not make you feel sick, and unless you check it, years may go by before you even realize you have a problem. High blood pressure is a risk factor for CHD, congestive heart failure, stroke, kidney failure, and osteoporosis.

All inner walls of arteries are lined by a layer of smooth endothelial cells. Blood lipids cannot penetrate the healthy lining and start to build up on the walls unless the cells are damaged. High blood pressure is thought to be a leading contributor to destruction of this lining. As blood pressure rises, so does the risk for atherosclerosis. The higher the pressure, the greater the damage to the arterial wall, making the vessels susceptible to fat deposits, especially if serum cholesterol is also high. Blockage of the coronary vessels decreases blood supply to the heart muscle and can lead to heart attacks. When brain arteries are involved, a stroke may follow.

A clear example of the connection between high blood pressure and atherosclerosis can be seen by comparing blood vessels in the human body. Even when atherosclerosis is present throughout major arteries, fatty plaques rarely are seen in the pulmonary artery, which goes from the right part of the heart to the lungs. The pressure in this artery normally is below 40 mm Hg, and at such a low pressure, significant deposits do not occur. This is one of the reasons that people with low blood pressure have a lower incidence of CVD.

Constantly elevated blood pressure also causes the heart to work much harder. At first the heart does well, but in time this continual strain produces an enlarged heart, followed by congestive heart failure. Furthermore, high blood pressure damages blood vessels to the kidneys and eyes, which can result in kidney failure and loss of vision.

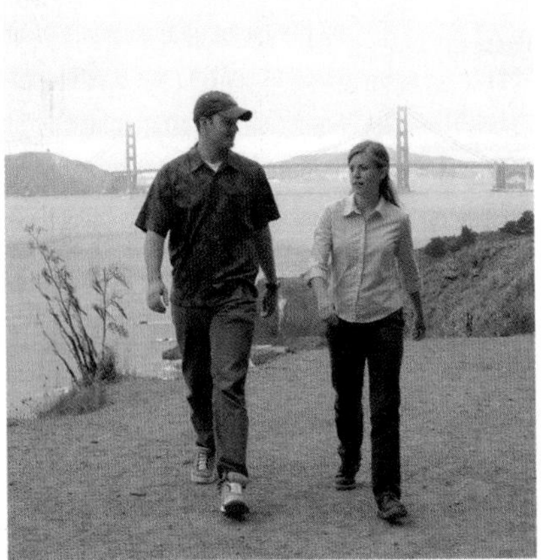

Lifetime physical activity helps maintain healthy blood pressure.

Treatment Of all cases of hypertension, 90 percent have no definite cause. Called "essential hypertension," this type of hypertension is treatable. Aerobic exercise, weight reduction, a diet low in salt and fat and high in potassium and calcium, lower alcohol and caffeine intake, smoking cessation, stress management, and antihypertensive medication all have been used effectively to treat essential hypertension.

The remaining 10 percent of hypertensive cases are caused by pathological conditions, such as narrowing of the kidney arteries, glomerulonephritis (a kidney disease), tumors of the adrenal glands, and narrowing of the aortic artery. With this type of hypertension, the pathological cause has to be treated before the blood pressure problem can be corrected.

CRITICAL THINKING

Do you know what your most recent blood pressure reading was, and did you know at the time what the numbers meant? How would you react if your doctor were to instruct you to take blood pressure medication?

Antihypertensive medicines often are the first choice of treatment for these cases, but they produce many side effects. These include lethargy, sleepiness, sexual difficulties, higher blood cholesterol and glucose levels, lower potassium levels, and elevated uric acid levels. A physician may end up treating these side effects as much as the hypertension. Because of the many side effects, about half of the patients stop taking the medication within the first year of treatment.

Another factor contributing to elevated blood pressure is too much sodium in the diet (salt, or sodium chloride, contains approximately 40 percent sodium). With a high sodium intake, the body retains more water, which increases the blood volume and, in turn, drives up the pressure. High intake of potassium seems to regulate water retention and lower the pressure slightly. According to the Institute of Medicine of the National Academy of Sciences, people need to consume at least 4,700 mg of potassium per day. Most Americans get only half that amount. Foods high in potassium include vegetables (especially leafy green ones), citrus fruit, dairy products, fish, beans, and nuts.

Although sodium is essential for normal body functions, the body can function with as little as 200 mg, or a tenth of a teaspoon, daily. Even under strenuous conditions in jobs and sports that incite heavy perspiration, the amount of sodium required is seldom more than 3,000 mg per day. Yet, sodium intake in the typical U.S. diet is about 4,000 mg per day.[26] The upper limit of sodium intake has been set at 2,300 mg per day, and *Dietary Guidelines for Americans 2010* recommends a daily sodium intake of less than 2,300 mg. Adults over age 51, African Americans, and all individuals with high blood pressure, diabetes, and chronic kidney disease are encouraged to keep daily intake below 1,500 mg. Among Americans, about 95 percent of men and 75 percent of women exceed these guidelines.

Salt-sensitive people, even in the absence of high blood pressure, are encouraged to decrease sodium intake because they have death rates similar to those of people with hypertension. The AHA has issued guidelines calling for everyone to reduce daily sodium intake to less than 1,500 mg. Estimates indicate that if Americans were to follow these guidelines, heart attacks and strokes would decrease by 155,000 cases each year.

Two other studies corroborate previous concerns. First, a review of 13 sodium consumption-related studies shows that decreasing sodium intake by about 2,000 mg per day is associated with a 23 and 17 percent reduction in the risk of stroke and CVD, respectively.[27] A second large study projected that reducing sodium intake by 1,200 mg per day would prevent as many as 92,000 deaths a year in the United States.[28] To either prevent or postpone the onset of hypertension and to help some hypertensive people control their blood pressure, consumption of even less sodium than previously recommended is encouraged.[29] Lower sodium intake may also reduce the risk of left ventricular hypertrophy, congestive heart failure, gastric cancer, end-stage kidney disease, osteoporosis, and bloating. Research data support the notion that daily sodium intake should be reduced as much as possible.

Where does all the sodium come from? Part of the answer is given in Table 11.11 (the list does not include salt added at the table). Most of the sodium that people consume comes from packaged and prepared foods, over whose ingredients the consumer has no control.

When treating high blood pressure (unless it is extremely high), before recommending medication, many sports medicine physicians suggest a combination of aerobic exercise, weight loss, and less sodium in the diet. In most instances, this treatment brings blood pressure under control. Prepackaged, canned, and frozen foods are often loaded with added salt. Among the worst offenders are soups, spaghetti sauces, lunch meats, pickled foods, soy sauce, salad dressings, cheeses, and crackers.

As a consumer, you need to always read food labels and pick only those items that are low in sodium content. When eating out, request that your dish be prepared with less salt. Some restaurant dishes contain up to 6,000 mg of sodium per serving. You will do best by downsizing your portion (taking the rest home), sharing the dish with someone else, or trying to find the lower-sodium dishes. You can also retrain your taste buds to enjoy food with less salt.

The relative risk for mortality based on blood pressure and fitness levels is similar to that of physical fitness and cholesterol. In men and women alike, the relative risk for early mortality is lower in fit people with high systolic blood pressure (140 mm Hg or higher) than in unfit people with a healthy systolic blood pressure (120 mm Hg or lower).

The link between hypertension and obesity seems to be quite strong. Blood volume increases with excess body fat, and each additional pound of fat requires an estimated extra mile of blood vessels to feed this tissue. Furthermore, blood capillaries are constricted by the adipose tissues because

TABLE 11.11 Sodium and Potassium Levels of Selected Foods

Food	Serving Size	Sodium (mg)	Potassium (mg)
Apple	1 med	1	182
Asparagus	1 cup	2	330
Avocado	½	4	680
Banana	1 med	1	440
Beans			
Kidney (canned)	½ cup	436	330
Lima (cooked)	½ cup	2	478
Pinto (cooked)	½ cup	2	398
Refried (canned)	½ cup	377	336
Bologna	3 oz	1,107	133
Bouillon cube	1	960	4
Cantaloupe	¼	17	341
Carrot (raw)	1	34	225
Cheese			
American	2 oz	614	93
Cheddar	2 oz	342	56
Muenster	2 oz	356	77
Parmesan	2 oz	1,056	53
Chicken, light meat	6 oz	108	700
Frankfurter	1	627	136
Haddock	6 oz	300	594
Ham (honey/smoked)	2 oz	495	91
Hamburger, reg	1	500	321
Marinara pasta sauce	½ cup	527	406
Milk, skim	1 cup	126	406
Nuts			
Brazil	1 nut	1	120
Walnuts	½ cup	1	327
Orange	1 med	1	263
Peach	1 med	2	308
Pickle, dill	2 oz	550	26
Pizza, cheese—14″ diam.	⅛	456	85
Potato	1 med	6	763
Salami	3 oz	1,047	170
Salmon (baked)	4 oz	75	424
Salmon (canned)	6 oz	198	756
Salt	1 tsp	2,132	0
Soups			
Chicken Noodle	1 cup	979	55
Cream of Mushroom	1 cup	955	98
Vegetable Beef	1 cup	1,046	162
Soy sauce	1 tsp	1,123	22
Spaghetti, tomato sauce and cheese	6 oz	648	276
Spinach (cooked, fresh)	1 cup	126	838
Strawberries	1 cup	1	244
Tomato (raw)	1 med	3	444
Tomato juice	1 cup	680	430
Tuna (drained)	3 oz	38	255
Whopper with cheese	1	1,432	534

Source: *National High Blood Pressure Education Program.*

these vessels run through them. As a result, the heart muscle must work harder to pump the blood through a longer, constricted network of blood vessels.

Regular physical activity plays a large role in managing blood pressure. On average, fit individuals have lower blood pressure than unfit people. Aerobic exercise of moderate intensity supplemented by strength training is recommended for individuals with high blood pressure.[30]

Comprehensive reviews of the effects of aerobic exercise on blood pressure have found that, in general, people can expect exercise-induced reductions of approximately 4 to 5 mm Hg in resting systolic blood pressure and 3 to 4 mm Hg in resting diastolic blood pressure.[31] Although these reductions do not seem large, a decrease of about 5 mm Hg in resting diastolic blood pressure has been associated with a 40 percent decrease in the risk for stroke and a 15 percent reduction in the risk for CHD.[32] Even in the absence of any decrease in resting blood pressure, hypertensive individuals who exercise have a lower risk for all-cause mortality compared with hypertensive or sedentary individuals. Research data also show that exercise, not weight loss, is the major contributor to the lower blood pressure of exercisers. If they discontinue aerobic exercise, they do not maintain these changes.

Another extensive review of research studies on the effects of at least 4 weeks of strength training on resting blood pressure yielded similar results.[33] Both systolic and diastolic blood pressures decreased by an average of 3 mm Hg. Participants in these studies, however, were primarily individuals with normal blood pressure. Of greater significance, the results showed that strength training did not cause an increase in resting blood pressure. More research remains to be done on hypertensive subjects.

The effects of long-term participation in exercise are apparently much more remarkable. An 18-year follow-up study on exercising and nonexercising subjects showed much lower blood pressures in the active group.[34] The exercise group had an average resting blood pressure of 120/78 compared with 150/90 for the nonexercise group (Table 11.12).

Aerobic exercise programs for hypertensive patients should be of moderate intensity. Training at 40 to 60 percent intensity seems to have the same effect in lowering blood pressure as training at 70 percent intensity. High-intensity training (above 70 percent) in hypertensive patients may not lower the blood pressure as much as moderate-intensity exercise. Even so, people may be better off being highly fit and having high blood pressure than being unfit and having low blood pressure. The death rates for unfit individuals with low systolic blood pressure are much higher than those for highly fit people with high systolic blood pressure. Strength training for hypertensive individuals calls for a minimum of one set of 10 to 15 repetitions that elicit a "somewhat hard"

BEHAVIOR MODIFICATION PLANNING

Guidelines to Stop Hypertension

I PLAN TO | I DID IT

❑ ❑ Participate in a moderate-intensity aerobic exercise program (50% intensity) for 30 to 45 minutes 5 to 7 times per week.

❑ ❑ Participate in a moderate-resistance strength-training program (use 12 to 15 repetitions to near-fatigue on each set) 2 times per week (seek your physician's approval and advice for this program).

❑ ❑ Lose weight if you are above recommended body weight.

❑ ❑ Limit sodium intake to less than 1,500 mg/day.

❑ ❑ Do not smoke cigarettes or use tobacco in any other form.

❑ ❑ Practice stress management.

❑ ❑ Do not consume more than two alcoholic beverages a day if you are a man or one if you are a woman.

❑ ❑ Consume more potassium-rich foods.

❑ ❑ Follow the Dietary Approach to Stop Hypertension (DASH) diet:

Food Group	Servings
Whole grains	7–8 per day
Fruits and vegetables	8–10 per day
Low-fat or fat-free dairy foods	2–13 per day
Meat, poultry, or fish	2 or less per day
Beans, peas, nuts, or seeds	4–15 *per week*
Fats and oils	2–3 servings per day
Snacks and sweets	4–5 *per week*

Try It

In your Online Journal or class notebook, make a comparison of the goals of the DASH diet and Dietary Guidelines for Americans. How do they differ?

TABLE 11.12 Effects of Long-Term (14–18 years) Aerobic Exercise on Resting Blood Pressure

	Initial	Final
Exercise Group		
Age (yr)	44.6	68.0
Blood Pressure (mm Hg)	120/79	120/78
Nonexercise Group		
Age (yr)	51.6	69.7
Blood Pressure (mm Hg)	135/85	150/90

Note: The aerobic exercise program consisted of an average of four training sessions per week, each 66 minutes long, with about 76 percent of heart rate reserve.
Based on data from F. W. Kash, J. L. Boyer, S. P. Van Camp, L. S. Verity, and J. P. Wallace, "The Effect of Physical Activity on Aerobic Power in Older Men (A Longitudinal Study)," *The Physician and Sports Medicine* 18, no. 4 (1990): 73-83.

perceived exertion rating, using 8 to 10 multijoint exercises two or three times per week.

Most important is a preventive approach. Keeping blood pressure under control is easier than trying to bring it down once it is high. Regardless of your blood pressure history, high or low, you should have it checked routinely. To keep your blood pressure as low as possible, exercise regularly, lose excess weight, eat less sodium-containing foods, do not smoke, practice stress management, do not consume more than two alcoholic beverages a day if you are a man or one if you are a woman, and consume more potassium-rich foods, such as potatoes, bananas, orange juice, cantaloupe, tomatoes, and beans (see the box "Guidelines to Stop Hypertension"). An alcoholic drink is defined as 5 ounces of wine, 12 ounces of beer, or 1.5 ounces of 80-proof liquor. The Dietary Approaches to Stop Hypertension (DASH)—which emphasizes fruits, vegetables, grains, and dairy products—lowers systolic blood pressure by 11 points and diastolic pressure by 5.5 points.[35]

Those who are taking medication for hypertension should not stop without the approval of the prescribing physician. If it is not treated properly, high blood pressure can kill. By combining medication with the other treatments, people might eventually reduce or eliminate the need for drug therapy.

Excessive Body Fat

Excessive body fat is an independent risk factor for CHD, but disease risk may actually be augmented by other risk factors that usually accompany excessive body fat. Risk factors such as high blood lipids, hypertension, and diabetes typically are seen in conjunction with obesity. All of these risk factors usually improve with increased physical activity.

Attaining recommended body composition helps improve several CHD risk factors and helps people reach a better state of health and wellness. While data indicate that a 10 percent weight loss results in significant improvements in CHD risk factors, some studies have shown reduction in chronic disease risk factors with only a 2 to 3 percent weight loss.[36]

DIVERSITY CONSIDERATIONS: CARDIOVASCULAR DISEASE AND ETHNICITY

Cardiovascular diseases are the leading cause of death in the United States. Disparities, however, exist based on racial or ethnic background and gender. Risk factor awareness is lower among African American and Hispanic women than among white women. This discrepancy has not changed over the last few years. Data also indicate that the prevalence of having two or more risk factors is highest among African Americans and among American Indian and Alaska Natives and lowest among Asians. The prevalence of obesity is highest among Mexican American males and African American women. Hypertension is highest among African Americans, while blood cholesterol levels are highest among white and Mexican American men and white women. Cardiovascular mortality rates at all ages are highest in African Americans.

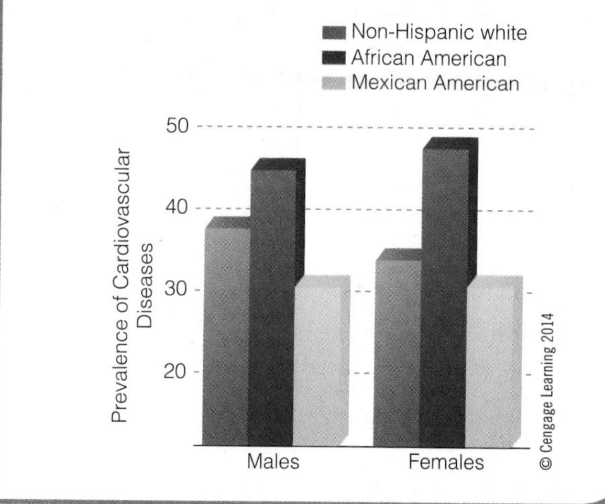

For years, we have known that where people store fat affects risk for disease. People who store body fat in the abdominal area as opposed to in the hips and thighs are at higher risk for disease. Furthermore, when abdominal fat is stored primarily around internal organs (visceral fat—also see Figure 4.9, page 151), disease risk is greater than when abdominal fat is stored subcutaneously or retroperitoneally.

The best approach to prevent increases in visceral fat is through regular exercise. Data on men and women who were followed for 6 months showed no visceral fat gains in groups that either walked (178 minutes per week) or jogged (120 minutes per week) an average of 12 miles per week.[37] A sedentary group in this same study actually gained 8.6 percent visceral fat during the six months, while a 20-mile-per-week jogging group (173 min/week) lost 7 percent visceral fat. Thus, it appears that 30 minutes of vigorous exercise six times per week is best to properly manage visceral fat. Of significant concern, just six months of inactivity further increased visceral fat and the concomitant increase in disease risk.

TABLE 11.13 Relationship Among Body Weight, Physical Activity, and Heart Failure Risk

Body Weight and Activity Status	Percent Risk Increase*
Lean** and inactive	19%
Overweight and active	49%
Overweight and inactive	78%
Obese and active	168%
Obese and inactive	293%

*As compared with lean and active men.
**Lean = BMI ≤25, Overweight = BMI >25 and <30, Obese = BMI ≥30.
Source: S. Kenchaiah et al., "Body Mass Index and Vigorous Physical Activity and the Risk of Heart Failure Among Men," *Circulation* 119 (2009): 44-52.

Data on 21,094 men followed for more than 20 years indicated that an elevated body mass index (BMI) of greater than 25 was associated with an increased risk of heart failure.[38] Furthermore, the data showed that as BMI increased in both active and inactive men, so did the risk for heart failure. The increased risk for heart failure improved proportionally with increased BMI or decreased physical activity (Table 11.13).

If you have a weight problem and want to get down to recommended weight, you must do the following:

1. Increase daily physical activity up to 90 minutes a day, including aerobic and strength-training programs
2. Follow a diet lower in fat, refined sugars, and processed foods and high in complex carbohydrates and fiber
3. Reduce total caloric intake moderately while getting the necessary nutrients to sustain normal body functions.

A comprehensive weight reduction and weight control program is discussed in detail in Chapter 5.

Cigarette Smoking

More than 57 million adults and 3.5 million adolescents in the United States smoke cigarettes. Smoking is the single largest preventable cause of illness and premature death in the United States. It has been linked to CVD, cancer, bronchitis, emphysema, and peptic ulcers. In relation to coronary disease, smoking speeds the process of atherosclerosis and carries a threefold increase in the risk of sudden death after a myocardial infarction.

According to estimates, about 20 percent of all deaths from CVD are attributable to smoking. Smoking prompts the release of nicotine and another 1,200 toxic compounds into the bloodstream. Similar to hypertension, many of these substances are destructive to the inner membrane that protects the walls of the arteries. Once the lining is damaged, cholesterol and triglycerides can be deposited readily in the arterial wall. As the plaque builds up, it obstructs blood flow through the arteries.

Furthermore, smoking encourages the formation of blood clots, which can completely block an artery already narrowed by atherosclerosis. In addition, carbon monoxide, a by-product of cigarette smoke, decreases the blood's oxygen-carrying capacity. A combination of obstructed arteries, less oxygen, and nicotine in the heart muscle heightens the risk for a serious heart problem.

Smoking also increases heart rate, raises blood pressure, and irritates the heart, which can trigger fatal cardiac **arrhythmias**. Another harmful effect is a decrease in HDL cholesterol, the "good" type that helps control blood lipids. Smoking actually presents a much greater risk of death from heart disease than from lung disease.

Pipe and cigar smoking and tobacco chewing also increase the risk for heart disease. Even if the tobacco user inhales no smoke, he or she absorbs toxic substances through the membranes of the mouth, and these end up in the bloodstream. Individuals who use tobacco in any of these three forms also have a much greater risk for cancer of the oral cavity.

The risks for both CVD and cancer start to decrease the moment a person quits smoking. One year after quitting, the risk for CHD decreases by half, and within 15 years, the relative risk of dying from CVD and cancer approaches that of a lifetime nonsmoker. A more thorough discussion of the harmful effects of cigarette smoking, the benefits of quitting, and a complete program for quitting are detailed in Chapter 13.

Tension and Stress

Tension and stress have become part of contemporary life. Everyone has to deal daily with goals, deadlines, responsibilities, and pressures. Almost everything in life (whether positive or negative) can be a source of stress. What creates the health hazard is not the stressor itself but, rather, the individual's response to it.

The human body responds to stress by producing more **catecholamines**, which prepare the body for quick physical action—often called fight or flight. These hormones increase heart rate, blood pressure, and blood glucose levels, enabling the person to take action. If the person actually fights or

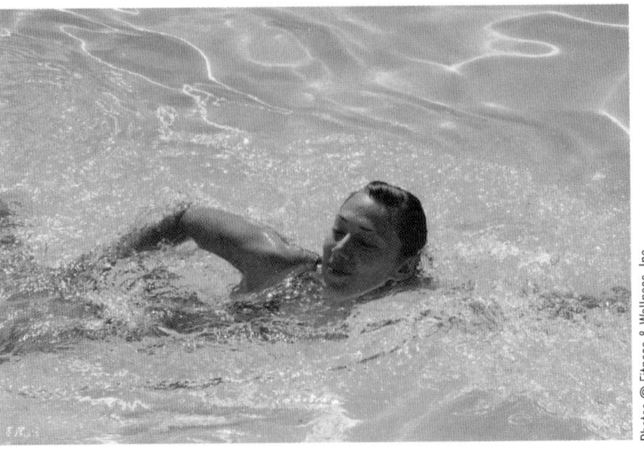

Physical activity is one of the best ways to relieve stress.

flees, the higher levels of catecholamines are metabolized and the body can return to a normal state. If, however, a person is under constant stress and unable to take action (as in the death of a close relative or friend, loss of a job, trouble at work, or financial insecurity), the catecholamines remain elevated in the bloodstream.

People who are not able to relax place a constant low-level strain on the cardiovascular system that could manifest as heart disease. Higher levels of the hormones epinephrine and cortisol in highly stressed people may raise blood pressure and cholesterol by 20 to 50 percent.[39] In addition, when people are in a stressful situation, the coronary arteries that feed the heart muscle constrict, reducing the oxygen supply to the heart. If the blood vessels are largely blocked by atherosclerosis, arrhythmias or even a heart attack may follow. The research indicates that people who feel too much stress too often significantly increase their risk for a deadly heart attack.

A little known fact is that the risk of sudden cardiac death is twice as high on Mondays, most likely because of the stress of having to go back to work after the weekend. Heart attacks are also more common in the morning because cortisol levels and stress hormones are highest, on average, at that time of the day.

Anger and hostility also contribute to heart disease by increasing heart rate, blood pressure, blood glucose, cholesterol, and interleukin-6 (a marker for arterial inflammation). Angina risk increases following an outburst of anger and doubles the risk for a heart attack in the first 2 hours thereafter.[40] Depression and isolation have also been linked to higher death rates from heart disease.

Weight gain is often the end result of excessive stress. That is because most people tend to eat more when distressed and the choice is typically "comfort foods" that are calorie dense and promote weight gain with the subsequent increased risk for cardiovascular disease.

Individuals who are under a lot of stress and do not cope well with stress need to take measures to counteract the effects of stress in their lives. One way is to identify the sources of stress and learn how to cope with them. People need to take control of themselves, examine and act upon the things that are most important in their lives, and ignore less meaningful details.

Physical activity is one of the best ways to relieve stress. When a person takes part in physical activity, the body metabolizes excess catecholamines and is able to return to a normal state. Exercise also steps up muscular activity, which contributes to muscular relaxation after completing the physical activity.

Many executives in large cities are choosing the evening hours for their physical activity programs, stopping after work at the health or fitness club. In doing this, they are able to "burn up" the excess tension accumulated during the day and enjoy the evening hours. This has proved to be one of the best stress management techniques. More information on stress management techniques is presented in Chapter 10.

Personal and Family History

Individuals who have had cardiovascular problems are at higher risk than those who have never had a problem. People with this history should control other risk factors as much as they can. Many of the risk factors are reversible, so this greatly decreases the risk for future problems. The more time that passes after the occurrence of the cardiovascular problem, the lower the risk for recurrence.

A genetic predisposition to heart disease has been demonstrated clearly. All other factors being equal, a person with blood relatives who now have or did have premature heart disease runs a greater risk than someone with no such history. Premature CHD is defined as a heart attack before age 55 in a close male relative or before age 65 in a close female relative. The younger the age at which the relative incurred the cardiovascular incident, the greater the risk for the disease.

In some cases, there is no way of knowing whether the heart problem resulted from a person's genetic predisposition or simply poor lifestyle habits. A person may have been physically inactive, been overweight, smoked, and had bad dietary habits—all of which contributed to a heart attack. Regardless, blood relatives fall in the "family history" category. Because we have no reliable way to differentiate all the factors contributing to CVD, a person with a family history should watch all other factors closely and maintain the lowest risk level possible. In addition, the person should have a blood chemistry analysis annually to make sure the body is handling blood lipids properly.

Age

Age is a risk factor because of the higher incidence of heart disease as people get older. This tendency may be induced partly by other factors stemming from changes in lifestyle as we get older—less physical activity, poorer nutrition, obesity, and so on. Young people should not think they are exempt from heart disease, though. The process begins early in life. Autopsies conducted on American soldiers killed at age 22 and younger revealed that approximately 70 percent had early stages of atherosclerosis. Other studies found elevated blood cholesterol levels in children as young as 10 years old.

Although the aging process cannot be stopped, it certainly can be slowed. Physiological age versus chronological age is important in preventing disease. Some individuals in their 60s and older have the body of a 30-year-old. And 30-year-olds often are in such poor condition and health that they almost seem to have the body of a 60-year-old. The best ways to slow the natural aging process are to engage in risk factor management and positive lifestyle habits.

Arrhythmias Irregular heart rhythms.

Catecholamines Fight-or-flight hormones, including epinephrine and norepinephrine.

Other Risk Factors for Coronary Heart Disease

Additional evidence points to a few other factors that may be linked to coronary heart disease. One of these factors is gum disease. The oral bacteria that build up with dental plaque can enter the bloodstream and contribute to inflammation, formation of blood vessel plaque, and blood clotting and thus increase the risk for heart attack. Data on women who have periodontal disease indicate that these women also have higher blood levels of CRP and lower HDL cholesterol. Daily flossing, using an electric toothbrush, scraping the tongue, and irrigating the gums with water are all preventive measures that help protect from gum disease.

Another factor that has been linked to CVD is loud snoring. People who snore heavily may suffer from sleep apnea, a sleep disorder in which the throat closes for a brief moment, causing breathing to stop. Individuals who snore heavily may triple their risk of a heart attack and quadruple their risk of a stroke.

Sudden emotional-related increases in heart rate often also trigger heart problems.[41] For example, the risk of a heart attack is highest on the day and the first few weeks after receiving unexpected bad news. Sports fans who get overly excited about their team can experience a twofold or higher increase in heart rate. A person with a resting heart rate of 80 to 90 bpm can easily reach near or maximal heart rate in these situations. Heart attacks occur in these cases because the unconditioned heart is unable to sustain the sudden/drastic increase in heart rate.

An extramarital affair can also contribute to a cardiac event. Data indicates that 80 percent of post-sex heart attack deaths occur in people following sex in a hotel room with someone other than their spouse. Researchers believe that such encounters lead to higher levels of arousal, resulting in a sudden and sustained heart rate that an unconditioned heart is unable to tolerate.

Low birth weight, considered to be less than 5.5 pounds, also has been linked to heart disease, hypertension, and diabetes. Individuals with low birth weight should bring this information to the attention of their personal physician and regularly monitor the risk factors for CHD.

Aspirin therapy is recommended to prevent heart disease. For individuals at moderate risk or higher, an aspirin dosage of about 81 mg per day (the equivalent of a baby aspirin) can prevent or dissolve clots that cause heart attack or stroke. With such daily use, the incidence of nonfatal heart attack decreases by about a third.

Cardiovascular Risk Reduction

Most of the risk factors are reversible and preventable. Having a family history of heart disease and some of the other risk factors because of neglect in lifestyle does not mean you are doomed. A healthier lifestyle—free of cardiovascular problems—is something over which you have extensive control. Be persistent! Willpower and commitment are required to develop patterns that eventually turn into healthy habits and contribute to your total well-being and longevity.

ASSESS YOUR BEHAVIOR

1. Do you make a conscious effort to increase daily physical activity, and are you able to accumulate at least 30 minutes of moderate-intensity activity a minimum of 5 days per week?
2. Is your diet fundamentally low in saturated fat, trans fat, refined carbohydrates, and processed foods, and do you meet the daily suggested amounts of fruits, vegetables, and fiber, and do you use primarily unsaturated fats?
3. Have you recently had your blood pressure measured and established your blood lipid profile? Do you know what the results mean, and are you aware of strategies to manage them effectively?

ASSESS YOUR KNOWLEDGE

1. CHD
   a. is the single leading cause of death in the United States.
   b. is the leading cause of sudden cardiac deaths.
   c. is a condition in which the arteries that supply the heart muscle with oxygen and nutrients are narrowed by fatty deposits.
   d. accounts for approximately 16 percent of all deaths in the United States.
   e. All of the choices are correct.
2. The incidence of cardiovascular disease during the past 50 years in the United States has
   a. increased.
   b. decreased.
   c. remained constant.
   d. increased in some years and decreased in others.
   e. fluctuated according to medical technology.

3. Regular aerobic activity helps
  a. lower LDL cholesterol.
  b. lower HDL cholesterol.
  c. increase triglycerides.
  d. decrease insulin sensitivity.
  e. All of the choices are correct.

4. The risk of heart disease increases with
  a. high LDL cholesterol.
  b. low HDL cholesterol.
  c. high concentration of homocysteine.
  d. high levels of hs-CRP.
  e. All of the choices are correct.

5. An optimal level of LDL cholesterol is
  a. between 200 and 239 mg/dL.
  b. about 200 mg/dL.
  c. between 150 and 200 mg/dL.
  d. between 100 and 150 mg/dL.
  e. below 100 mg/dL.

6. As a part of a CHD prevention program, saturated fat intake should be kept below
  a. 35 percent.
  b. 30 percent.
  c. 22 percent.
  d. 15 percent.
  e. 6 percent.

7. Statin drugs
  a. increase the liver's ability to remove blood cholesterol.
  b. decrease LDL cholesterol.
  c. slow cholesterol production.
  d. help reduce inflammation.
  e. All of the choices are correct.

8. Type 2 diabetes is closely related to
  a. overeating.
  b. obesity.
  c. lack of physical activity.
  d. insulin resistance.
  e. All of the choices are correct.

9. Metabolic syndrome is related to
  a. low HDL cholesterol.
  b. high triglycerides.
  c. an increased blood-clotting mechanism.
  d. an abnormal insulin response to carbohydrates.
  e. All of the choices are correct.

10. Comprehensive reviews on the effects of aerobic exercise on blood pressure found that, in general, an individual can expect exercise-induced reductions of approximately
  a. 3 to 5 mm Hg.
  b. 5 to 10 mm Hg.
  c. 10 to 15 mm Hg.
  d. more than 15 mm Hg.
  e. There is no significant change in blood pressure with exercise.

Correct answers can be found at the back of the book.

NOTES

1. U.S. Department of Health and Human Services, Centers for Disease Control and Prevention, National Center for Health Statistics, *National Vital Statistics Reports, Deaths: Preliminary Data for 2011, 61*, no. 6 (October 10, 2012).
2. R. S. Paffenbarger, Jr., R. T. Hyde, A. L. Wing, I. Lee, D. L. Jung, and J. B. Kampert, "The Association of Changes in Physical-Activity Level and Other Lifestyle Characteristics with Mortality Among Men," *New England Journal of Medicine* 328 (1993): 538–545.
3. D. P. Swain and B. A. Franklin, "Comparative Cardioprotective Benefits of Vigorous vs. Moderate Intensity Aerobic Exercise," *American Journal of Cardiology* 97, no. 1 (2006): 141–147.
4. G. Samitz, M. Egger, and M. Zwahlen, "Domains of Physical Activity and All-Cause Mortality: Systematic Review and Dose-Response Meta-Analysis of Cohort Studies," *International Journal of Epidemiology* 40 (2011):1382–1400.
5. S. C. Moore, et al., "Leisure Time Physical Activity of Moderate to Vigorous Intensity and Mortality: A Large pooled Cohort Analysis," *PLOS Medicine* 9, no. 11 (2012): e1335. doi:10.1371/journal.pmed.001001335.
6. "Lipid Research Clinics Program: The Lipid Research Clinic Coronary Primary Prevention Trial Results," *Journal of the American Medical Association* 251 (1984): 351–364.
7. "HDL on the Rise," *HealthNews* (September 10, 1999).
8. R. Singa, et al., "Meat Intake and Mortality: A Prospective Study of Over Half a Million People," *Archives of Internal Medicine* 169 (2009): 562–571
9. A. E. Buyken, et al., "Modifications in Dietary Fat Are Associated with Changes in Serum Lipids of Older Adults Independently of Lipid Medication," *Journal of Nutrition* 140 (2010): 88–94.
10. C. M. Albert, et al., "Blood Levels of Long-Chain n-3 Fatty Acids and the Risk of Sudden Death," *New England Journal of Medicine* 346 (2002): 1113–1118.
11. A. H. Lichtenstein, et al., "Diet and Lifestyle Recommendations Revision 2006: A Scientific Statement from the American Heart Association Nutrition Committee," *Circulation* 114 (2006): 82–96.
12. M. U. Jacobsen, et al., "Intake of Carbohydrates Compared with Intake of Saturated Fatty Acids and Risk of Myocardial Infarction: Importance of the Glycemic Index." *American Journal of Clinical Nutrition* 91 (2010): 1764–1768.
13. O. Oyebode, et al., "Fruit and Vegetable Consumption and All-cause Cancer and CVD Mortality: Analysis for Health Survey for English data," *Journal of Epidemiology and Community Health,* Published Online First: 31 March 2014 doi:10.1136/jech-2013-203500.
14. E. B. Rimm, A. Ascherio, E. Giovannucci, D. Spiegelman, M. J. Stampfer, and W. C. Willett, "Vegetable, Fruit, and Cereal Fiber Intake and Risk of Coronary Heart Disease Among Men," *Journal of the American Medical Association* 275 (1996): 447–451.
15. National Cholesterol Education Program Expert Panel, "Summary of the Third Report of the National Cholesterol Education Program (NCEP) Expert Panel on Detection, Evaluation, and Treatment of High Blood Choles-

terol in Adults (Adult Treatment Panel III)," *Journal of the American Medical Association* 285 (2001): 2486–2497.

16. P. W. Siri-Tarino, Q. Sun, F. B. Hu, and R. M. Krauss, "Meta-Analysis of Prospective Cohort Studies Evaluating the Association of Saturated Fat with Cardiovascular Disease," *American Journal of Clinical Nutrition* 91 (2010): 535–546.
17. P. W. Siri-Tarino, Q. Sun, F. B. Hu, and R. M. Krauss, "Saturated Fat, Carbohydrate, and Cardiovascular Disease," *The American Journal of Clinical Nutrition* 91 (2010): 502–509.
18. D. Mozaffarian, R. Micha, and S. Wallace, "Effects on Coronary Heart Disease of Increasing Polyunsaturated Fat in Place of Saturated Fat: A Systematic Review of Meta-Analysis of Randomized Controlled Trials," *PLoS Medicine* 7 (2010): 7:e1000252.
19. A. Jula, et al., "Effects of Diet and Simvastatin on Serum Lipids, Insulin, and Antioxidants in Hypercholesterolemic Men," *Journal of the American Medical Association* 287 (2002): 598–605.
20. "The Homocysteine-CVD Connection," *HealthNews* (October 25, 1999).
21. P. M. Ridger, et al., "Rosuvastatin to Prevent Vascular Events in Men and Women with Elevated C-Reactive Protein," *New England Journal of Medicine* 359 (2008): 2195–2207.
22. D. M. Nathan, "Navigating the Choices for Diabetes Prevention," *New England Journal of Medicine* 362 (2010): 1533–1535; The Accord Study Group, "Effects of Combination Lipid Therapy in Type 2 Diabetes Mellitus," *New England Journal of Medicine* 362 (2010): 1563–1574; The Accord Study Group, "Effects of Intensive Blood Pressure Control in Type 2 Diabetes Mellitus," *New England Journal of Medicine* 362 (2010): 1575–1585.
23. H. K. Choi, et al., "Dairy Consumption and Risk of Type 2 Diabetes Mellitus in Men," *Archives of Internal Medicine* 165 (2005): 997–1003.
24. G. M. Reaven, T. K. Strom, and B. Fox, *Syndrome X: Overcoming the Silent Killer That Can Give You a Heart Attack* (Englewood Cliffs, NJ: Simon & Schuster, 2000).
25. A. V. Chobanian, et al., "The Seventh Report of the Joint National Committee on Prevention, Detection, Evaluation, and Treatment of High Blood Pressure," *Journal of the American Medical Association* 289 (2003): 2560–2571.
26. "Shake the Salt Habit to Reduce Your Risk of Stroke and Heart Disease," *Health & Nutrition Letter* (March 2010).
27. P. Strazzullo, L. D'Elia, N-B Kandala, and F. P. Cappuccio, "Salt Intake, Stroke, and Cardiovascular Disease: Meta-Analysis of Prospective Studies," *British Medical Journal* 339 (2009): b4567.
28. K. Bibbins-Domingo, et al., "Projected Effect of Dietary Salt Reductions on Future Cardiovascular Disease," *New England Journal of Medicine* 362 (2010): 590–599.
29. "Salt Takes a Licking," *University of California at Berkeley Wellness Letter* (April 2010).
30. L. S. Pescatello, et al., "Exercise and Hypertension Position Stand," *Medicine and Science in Sports and Exercise* 36 (2004): 533–553.
31. G. Kelley, "Dynamic Resistance Exercise and Resting Blood Pressure in Adults: A Meta-analysis," *Journal of Applied Physiology* 82 (1997): 1559–1565; G. A. Kelley and Z. Tran, "Aerobic Exercise and Normotensive Adults: A Meta-Analysis," *Medicine and Science in Sports and Exercise* 27 (1995): 1371–1377; G. Kelley and P. McClellan, "Antihypertensive Effects of Aerobic Exercise: A Brief Meta-Analytic Review of Randomized Controlled Trials," *American Journal of Hypertension* 7 (1994): 115–119.
32. R. Collins, et al., "Blood Pressure, Stroke, and Coronary Heart Disease; Part 2, Short-term Reductions in Blood Pressure: Overview of Randomized Drug Trials in Their Epidemiological Context," *Lancet* 335 (1990): 827–838.
33. G. A. Kelley and K. S. Kelley, "Progressive Resistance Exercise and Resting Blood Pressure: A Meta-Analysis of Randomized Controlled Trials," *Hypertension* 35 (2000): 838–843.
34. F. W. Kash, J. L. Boyer, S. P. Van Camp, L. S. Verity, and J. P. Wallace, "The Effect of Physical Activity on Aerobic Power in Older Men (A Longitudinal Study)," *Physician and Sports Medicine* 18, no. 4 (1990): 73–83.
35. S. G. Sheps, "High Blood Pressure Can Often Be Controlled Without Medication," *Bottom Line/Health* (November 1999).
36. J. E. Donnelly, et al., "Appropriate Physical Activity Intervention Strategies for Weight Loss and Prevention of Weight Regain for Adults," *Medicine and Science in Sports and Exercise* 41 (2009): 459–471.
37. C. A. Slentz, et al., "Inactivity, Exercise, and Visceral Fat. STRRIDE: A Randomized, Controlled Study of Exercise Intensity and Amount," *Journal of Applied Physiology* 99 (2005): 1613–1618.
38. S. Kenchaiah, et al., "Body Mass Index and Vigorous Physical Activity and the Risk of Heart Failure among Men," *Circulation* 119 (2009): 44–52.
39. M. Guarneri, "What Most People Don't Know about Heart Disease," *Bottom Line/Health* 21 (July 2007): 11–12.
40. B. A. Franklin, "Sex Can Cause a Heart Attack," *Bottom Line/Health* 27 (March 2013): 1–3.
41. See note 39.

SUGGESTED READINGS

American Heart Association. *Heart Disease and Stroke Statistics.* Dallas, TX: AHA, 2014 Update.

American Heart Association, "Understanding the New Prevention Guidelines," http://www.heart.org/HEARTORG/Conditions/Understanding-the-New-Prevention-Guidelines_UCM_458155_Article.jsp. Accessed April 15, 2014.

National Cholesterol Education Program Expert Panel. "Summary of the Third Report of the National Cholesterol Education Program (NCEP) Expert Panel on Detection, Evaluation, and Treatment of High Blood Cholesterol in Adults (Adult Treatment Panel III)," *Journal of the American Medical Association* 285 (2001): 2486–2497.

Lab 11A: Self-Assessment Coronary Heart Disease Risk Factor Analysis

Name ______________________ Date __________ Grade __________

Instructor ______________________ Course __________ Section __________

NECESSARY LAB EQUIPMENT
Basic lab equipment to repeat the body composition and blood pressure tests.

OBJECTIVE
To assess your current risk for coronary heart disease (CHD) and develop a behavior modification program.

I. Instructions

The disease process for cardiovascular disease starts early in life, primarily as a result of poor lifestyle habits. Studies have shown beginning stages of atherosclerosis and elevated blood lipids in children as young as 10 years old. Consequently, the purpose of this activity is to establish a baseline CHD risk profile and to point out the "zero-risk" level for each coronary risk factor.

		Score
1. Physical Activity	Do you get 30 or more minutes of daily moderate-intensity physical activity: Fewer than 3 times per week........8 Between 3 and 4 times per week........3 5 or more times per week........0	
2. Abnormal Heart Function	Do you ever feel your heart beat irregularly, skipping beats, fluttering, or palpitating........2–8	
3. Diet (use the highest score if all apply)	Does your regular diet include: 1 or more daily servings of red meat; 7 or more eggs/week; daily butter, cheese, whole milk, refined carbohydrates, alcohol, processed foods; and frequent grilling or cooking meat and poultry at high temperatures........10–14 3 to 6 servings of red meat/week; 1% or 2% milk; some cheese, refined carbohydrates, processed foods, and alcohol; some whole grains, fruits, vegetables, and cold-water fish........4–10 Red meat fewer than two times/week; skim milk and skim milk products; limited refined carbohydrates, processed foods, and alcohol; ample daily amounts of whole-grain products, fruits, and vegetables; cold-water fish at least 2 times/week........0–3	
4. Diabetes	Are you pre-diabetic........3 Are you diabetic........6	

Factor			Score
5. Blood Pressure Add scores for both readings (e.g., 144/88 score = 4)	**Systolic** <120 .... (0) 121–139 .... (1) 140–159 .... (3) ≥160 .... (4)	**Diastolic** <80 .... (0) 0 81–89 .... (1) 1–2 90–99 .... (3) 3–6 ≥100 .... (4) 4–8	
6. Body Mass Index (BMI)	≤25.0 .... 0 25.0–29.99 2	30.0–39.99 .... 4 ≥40.0 8	
7. Smoking	Lifetime non-smoker .... 0 Ex-smoker more than 1 year .... 0 Ex-smoker less than 1 year .... 1 Non-smoker, but live or work in smoking environment .... 2 Pipe or cigar smoker, or chew tobacco 3	Smoke 1–9 cigarettes/day .... 3 Smoke 10–19 cigarettes/day .... 4 Smoke 20–29 cigarettes/day .... 5 Smoke 30–39 cigarettes/day .... 6 Smoke 40 or more cigarettes/day 8	
8. Tension and Stress Are you:	Sometimes tense .... 1 Often tense 2	Always tense 3	
9. Personal History	Have you ever had a heart attack, stroke, coronary disease, or any known heart problem: During the last year .... 8 1–2 years ago 5	2–5 years ago .... 3 More than 5 years ago 2	
10. Family History	Have any of your blood relatives (parents, uncles, brothers, sisters, grandparents) suffered from cardiovascular disease: One or more before age 51 .... 6 One or more between 51 and 60 4	One or more after age 60 .... 2 None had cardiovascular disease 0	
11. Age	29 or younger .... 0 30–39 .... 1 40–49 2	50–59 .... 3 ≥60 4	

Total Risk Score:

How to Score

Risk Category	Total Risk Score
Very Low	5 or fewer points
Low	Between 6 and 15 points
Moderate	Between 16 and 25 points
High	Between 26 and 35 points
Very High	36 or more points

II. Stage of Change for Cardiovascular Disease Prevention

Using Figure 2.6 (page 66) and Table 2.3 (page 65), identify your current stage of change for participation in a cardiovascular disease risk-reduction program:

III. In a few sentences, using a separate sheet of paper, discuss your family and personal risk for cardiovascular disease. Also, discuss lifestyle changes that you have already implemented in this course, as well as additional changes that you can make to decrease your own risk for cardiovascular disease.

IV. Physical Activity Rating

Number of daily steps at the beginning of the term: ______ Current number of daily steps: ______

Current physical activity rating (use Table 1.2, page 12): ______

12

Cancer Prevention

"Our science looks at a substance-by-substance exposure and doesn't take into account the multitude of exposures we experience in daily life. If we did, it might change our risk paradigm. The potential risks associated with extremely low-level exposure may be underestimated or missed entirely."
—*Heather Logan*

OBJECTIVES

- Define cancer and understand how it starts and spreads.
- Cite guidelines for preventing cancer.
- Delineate the major risk factors that lead to specific types of cancer.
- Assess the risk for developing certain types of cancer.
- Learn everyday lifestyle strategies that you can use immediately to decrease overall cancer risk.

CENGAGE**brain**.com
Visit **www.cengagebrain.com** to access course materials and companion resources for this text, including digital labs, quiz questions designed to check your understanding of the chapter contents, and more! See the preface on page xii for more information.

REAL LIFE STORY | Yolanda's Experience

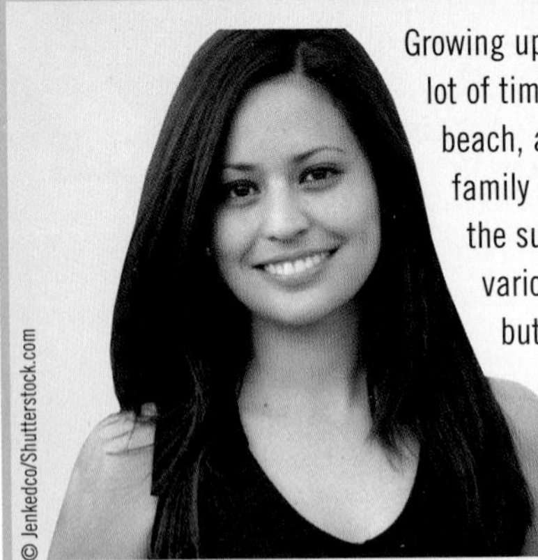
© Jenkedco/Shutterstock.com

Growing up in the 90s, we spent a lot of time outdoors and at the beach, and at times our entire family spent too much time in the sun. On and off we had various degrees of sunburn, but we didn't think much of it. I remember one particular time when my mother was so badly sunburned that she couldn't move very effectively for several days. The past few years she has had several precancerous skin growths removed from her skin. I didn't worry much about them, as I felt that physicians would just take care of it. Then in my Health and Wellness class, we got into the cancer-prevention unit. We learned about skin cancer and the effects of excessive unprotected sun exposure on our health. I also saw a poster by the American Cancer Society that said "Fry Now, Pay Later." It really hit home. My mother is in her 40s now, and on top of her precancerous lesions, her skin is pretty wrinkled and leathery. The skin has aged beyond her years. I am happy that she's taking care of her health now, but she wishes she knew better then. I know I have had my share of excessive sun exposure in my youth. I will do better in the future, and I trust that I can avoid what has happened to her. The extra suntan is not worth it to me, and I plan to practice safe sun-exposure recommendations from here on out. As I learned, the suntan fades at the end of the summer but the skin damage does not.

MyProfile: Personal Cancer-Prevention Program

To the best of your ability, answer the following questions. If you do not know the answer(s), this chapter will guide you through them.

I. Do you have a family history of cancer? ___ Yes ___ No If yes, are you taking any preventive measures to decrease your personal risk for cancer? ___ Yes ___ No

II. What role do nutrition, physical activity, and exercise play in your personal cancer-prevention program? __________

III. Explain lifestyle factors that you are aware of that increase cancer risk and factors that decrease such risk. __________

IV. Are you aware of environmental contaminants that may cause cancer? ___ Yes ___ No Can you list some of them? ___ Yes ___ No __________

V. Are tanning and personal appearance worth the potential risk of developing skin cancer? ___ Yes ___ No Explain your thoughts on the topic. __________

VI. Are you familiar with cancer-prevention self-exams and warning signals to look for in a cancer-prevention program? ___ Yes ___ No

Under normal conditions, the 100 trillion cells in the human body reproduce themselves in an orderly way. Cell growth (cell reproduction) takes place to repair and replace old, worn-out tissue. Cell growth is controlled by **deoxyribonucleic acid (DNA)** and **ribonucleic acid (RNA)**, found in the nucleus of each cell. When nuclei lose their ability to regulate and control cell growth, cell division is disrupted and mutant cells can develop (Figure 12.1). Some of these cells might grow uncontrollably and abnormally, forming a mass of tissue called a tumor, which can be either **benign** or **malignant**. Benign tumors do not invade other tissues. Although they can interfere with normal bodily functions, they rarely cause death. A malignant tumor is a **cancer**. Cancer is not a single disease, but rather a category of diseases that share similar traits including gene mutation and uncontrolled cell growth. More than 100 types of cancer can develop in any tissue or organ of the human body.

The process of cancer actually begins with an alteration in DNA. An individual starts life with every cell in the body having identical DNA. Within that DNA are three key genes that are involved in cancer development if they become defective: proto-oncogenes, tumor suppressor genes, and DNA repair genes. Proto-onconogenes control the type of cell being created from the DNA instructions (kidney cell, skin cell, etc.) and the frequency of cell division. In cell division, these genes act like the gas pedal does in a car, spurring the process on. Tumor suppressor genes slow cell growth during specified points of the cell lifecycle and therefore act like the

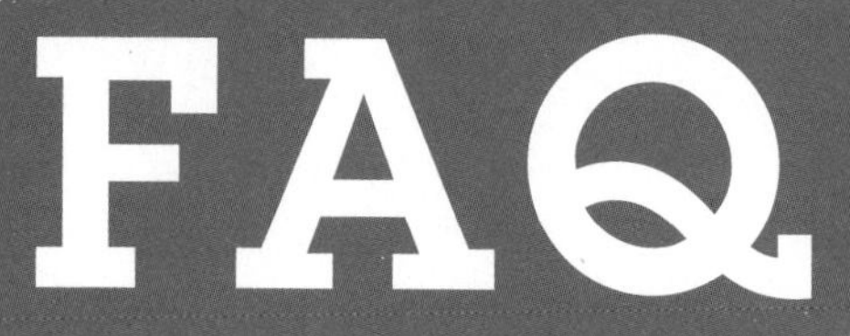

Can a healthy diet reduce cancer risk?

Much research is currently under way to examine the effects of foods in preventing and fighting off cancer. There is strong scientific evidence that a healthy diet and maintenance of recommended body weight reduce cancer risk. The current state of knowledge, however, cannot indicate that a certain dietary pattern will absolutely reduce your cancer risk. Years of research will be required to unravel most of this knowledge. Moreover, because we have so many environmental factors at play in our lives every day, science may never be able to provide conclusive evidence that a certain diet will prevent cancer in most cases.

An emerging field of study called epigenetics is revolutionizing the way we understand our genetic inheritance of cancer risks and other genetic predispositions. Researchers have discovered that the choices we make in our everyday lives can turn certain genes on or off, thereby delaying or hastening the onset of disease. Many of the foods that are currently recommended in a cancer-prevention diet are similar to those encouraged to decrease disease risk and enhance health and overall well-being. If you are truly adhering to healthy dietary guidelines (see the Behavior Modification Planning box on page 463), you are most likely eating the right foods to decrease your cancer risk.

Does regular physical activity affect cancer risk?

Regular physical activity has been shown to decrease the risk for developing certain types of cancer, in particular cancers of the colon, breast, endometrium, lungs, and prostate gland. Research shows that as little as 15 minutes of exercise three times per week decreases breast cancer risk by up to 40 percent in people of all races and ethnicities. Other research suggests that strength training at least twice per week cuts the risk of dying from cancer in men up to 40 percent. Physical activity also prevents type 2 diabetes and obesity. The latter have been linked to colon, pancreatic, gallbladder, ovarian, endometrium, thyroid, cervical, kidney, esophagus, breast and possibly other types of cancers. The American Cancer Society recommends aiming for at least 30 minutes of moderate-intensity to vigorous physical activity five or more days per week, although 60 to 90 minutes of intentional activity are preferable. For most nontobacco users, a healthy dietary pattern and regular physical activity are the two most significant lifestyle behaviors that reduce cancer risk.

Does aspirin therapy protect against cancer?

A 2011 study published in the journal *The Lancet* indicated that a regular daily dose of aspirin may decrease cancer risk up to 58 percent in some cases (esophageal cancer) and reduced total cancer deaths by 34 percent after 5 years. Even 15 years later, death rates were still lower by 20 percent among aspirin users, with the biggest drop in cancer deaths seen in esophageal, colorectal, lung, and prostate cancers. Low-dose therapy (75 to 81 mg) was as effective as a larger dose. It is believed that aspirin inhibits the effects of enzymes (COX-2) that promote potential cancer-causing cell damage. Aspirin also decreases low-grade inflammation, thought to play a role in cancer development and growth. Aspirin therapy, however, is not recommended for healthy people because of the small risk of gastrointestinal (GI) bleeding and ulcers. About 50,000 yearly deaths in the United States are attributed to GI bleeding, caused partially by aspirin and other nonsteroidal anti-inflammatory drug (NSAID) use. Aspirin-therapy damage to the GI tract may not cause any noticeable symptoms, and a fecal occult blood test may be necessary to detect possible bleeding. Hemorrhagic strokes have also been linked to low-dose aspirin therapy. If you are at high risk for cancer (and cardiovascular disease), you are encouraged to talk to your doctor before starting aspirin therapy. If you take aspirin, do so with warm water, which helps dissolve the tablet faster, making it less likely to cause serious bleeding.

brake pedal in a car. DNA repair genes fix any mistakes that occur during cell division using enzymes they code for this purpose. In a healthy cell, these genes all work together to repair and replace cells. Defects in these genes—caused by external factors such as radiation, chemicals, and viruses, as well as internal factors such as immune conditions, hormones, and genetic mutations—ultimately allow the cell to grow into a tumor. Proto-oncogenes mutate to become **oncogenes** and act like a gas pedal that is stuck down, speeding cell growth. Mutated **tumor suppressor genes** act like brakes that have gone out, allowing uncontrolled growth. Most tumors have errant copies of more than one of these genes. Mutations in other types of genes can also aid in the

Deoxyribonucleic acid (DNA) The genetic substance of which genes are made; the molecule that contains a cell's genetic code.

Ribonucleic acid (RNA) The genetic material that guides the formation of cell proteins.

Benign Noncancerous.

Malignant Cancerous.

Cancer A group of diseases characterized by uncontrolled growth and spread of abnormal cells.

Oncogenes Genes that initiate cell division.

Tumor suppressor genes Genes thatt deactivate the process of cell division.

FIGURE 12.1 **Normal vs cancerous cell division.**

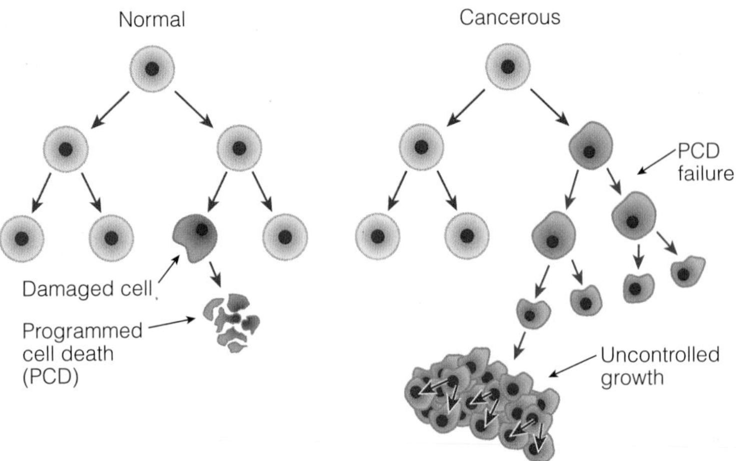

onset of cancer—for example, mutations in cells that recruit a new blood supply to the tumor or target new sites in the body for spreading cancer.

A healthy cell will duplicate, on average, 52 times in its lifetime. Normally, the DNA molecule is duplicated perfectly during cell division. When the DNA molecule is not replicated exactly, specialized enzymes make repairs quickly. Occasionally, however, a cell will divide without being repaired. The two new cells will both carry the resulting defect. Usually damaged cells are sensed and are instructed to carry out programmed cell death (PCD). But when conditions allow abnormal cells to survive, they will continue to divide and pass on the defect. Precancerous cells tend to have mutations that let them proliferate faster than healthy cells (think of the broken brake pedal or gas pedal stuck down). Thus, it becomes more likely that future cell divisions will result in an additional mutation and pass along both mutations. It is not known how many mutations are necessary, but eventually, after several generations of cells have passed on a collection of accumulated mutations, a cancerous cell will develop. That one cell will proliferate and ultimately form a small tumor. Cancer is a slow developing disease. A decade or more might pass between the initial mutations (as a result of carcinogenic exposure or genetics) and the time that cancer is diagnosed.

The process of abnormal cell division is related indirectly to chromosome segments called **telomeres** (Figure 12.2). Chromosomes are the threadlike package of DNA in the nucleolus of each cell. Telomeres are protective end caps on chromosomes, similar to the plastic tips on shoelaces. Each time a cell divides, telomeres shorten. After many cell divisions, the telomeres become critically short and the cell either stops functioning properly or dies.

Recent research has found that each person is born with varying lengths of telomeres, but only the critically short telomeres are a point of concern. Short telomeres are associated with a variety of diseases and mortality risks. Telomeres shorten naturally as a part of aging. Telomere shortening is accelerated, however, by negative lifestyle factors including acute stress, obesity, toxins such as those that result from smoking, and inflammation, among others. Telomeres are preserved and possibly lengthened by positive lifestyle factors, including stress management, exercise, and good nutrition.

An enzyme known as **telomerase** can restore telomeres after each cell division, so telomeres don't shorten. Most cells in the human body do not have enough telomerase to maintain telomere length. Only a select few cells, such as cells associated with our immune system, have enough telomerase to allow the division process to continue. Cancer cells are another exception; they maintain their telomeres indefinitely (Figure 12.3). Almost all cancer cells rely on telomerase for this preservation. As a result, cells continue to reproduce, creating a malignant tumor. Telomeres and telomerase are a relatively recent discovery. While researchers can use telomere length as an indicator of a person's "real age" and disease risk, scientists are just beginning to understand the complex role telomeres have in the growth of cancerous tumors and their role in the aging process.

FIGURE 12.2 **Erosion of chromosome telomeres in normal cells.**

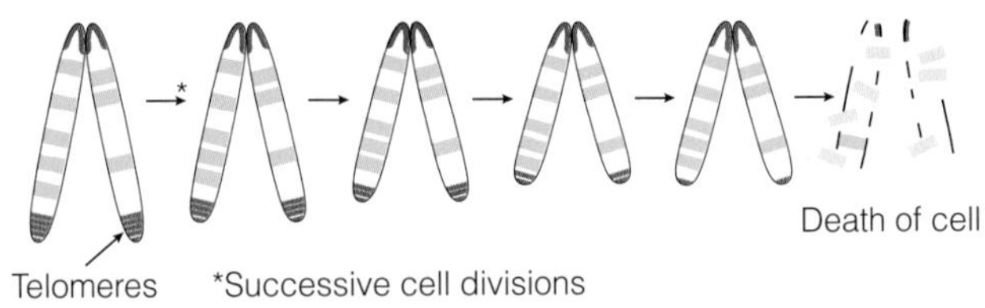

FIGURE 12.3 **Action of the enzyme telomerase.**

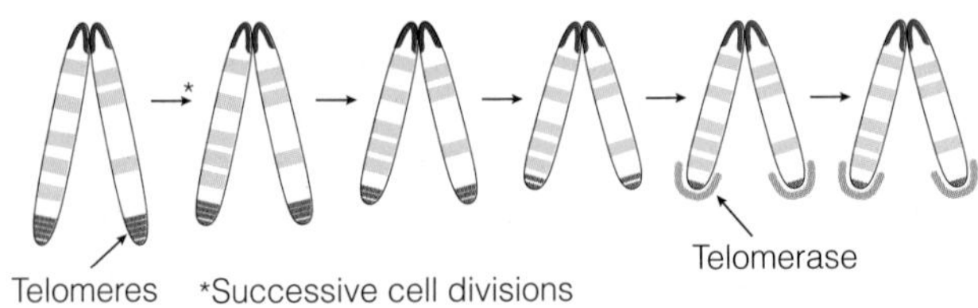

FIGURE 12.4 **How cancer starts and spreads.**

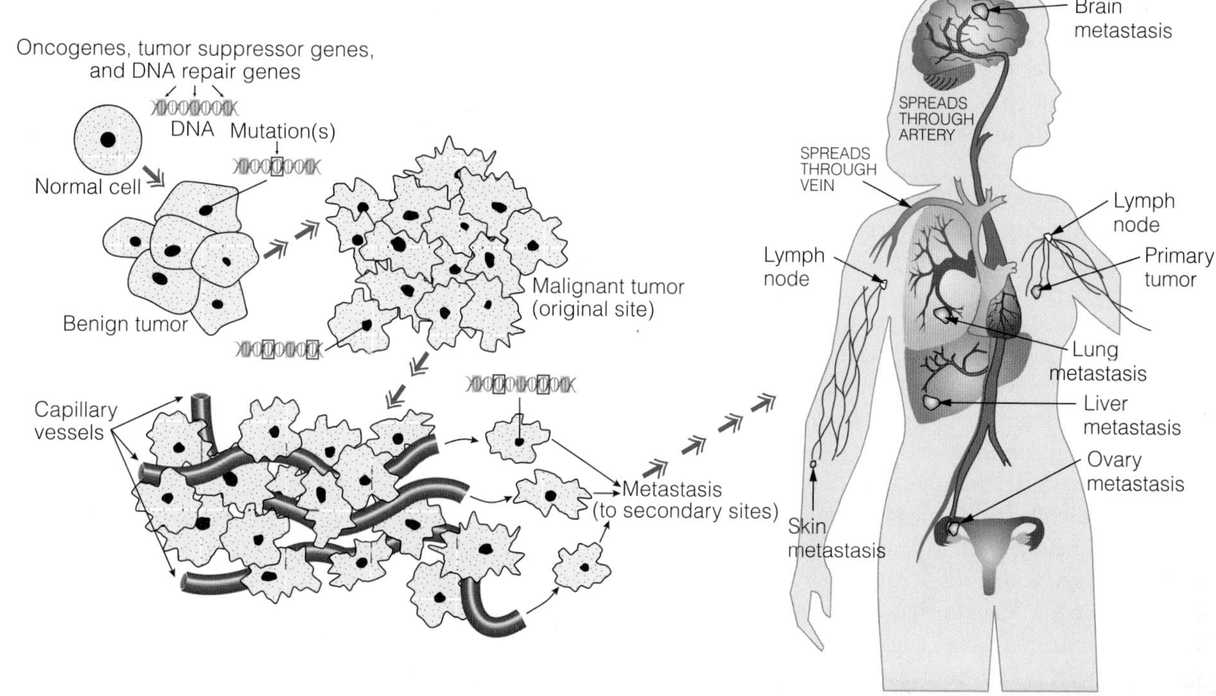

Cancer starts with the abnormal growth of one cell, which can then multiply into billions of cancerous cells. A critical turning point in the development of cancer is when a tumor reaches about a million cells. At this stage, it is referred to as **carcinoma in situ**. The undetected tumor may go for months or years without significant growth. While it remains encapsulated, it does not pose a serious threat to human health. To grow, however, the tumor requires more oxygen and nutrients.

In time, a few of the cancer cells start producing chemicals that signal the body to start **angiogenesis**, or the growth of a new network of capillaries (blood vessels) that penetrate the tumor and help it grow by delivering oxygen and nutrients and carrying away waste products. During normal healthy processes, angiogenesis is limited to a few infrequent functions such as healing wounds or development during pregnancy. During cancer, angiogenesis is the precursor of **metastasis**. Through the new blood vessels formed by angiogenesis, cancerous cells now can break away from a malignant tumor and migrate to other parts of the body, where they can cause new cancer (Figure 12.4).

Most adults have precancerous or cancerous cells in their bodies. By middle age, the human body contains millions of precancerous cells. Adults have had more time to be exposed to carcinogens or the occasional accidental mutations during some of the billions of cell divisions that take place over a person's lifetime. The immune system and blood turbulence destroy most cancer cells, but only one abnormal cell lodging elsewhere is enough to start a new cancer. These cells grow and multiply uncontrollably, invading and destroying normal tissue. The rate at which cancer cells grow varies from one type to another. Some types grow quickly, and others take years.

Once cancer cells metastasize, treatment becomes more difficult. Although therapy can kill most cancer cells, a few cells might become resistant to treatment. These cells then can grow into a new tumor that will not respond to the same treatment.

Genetic vs Environmental Risk

The complex ways that our inherited traits and our external environment interplay may never fully be understood. In recent years, researchers have made great strides in understanding how our genes and environment interact to prevent or trigger cancer.

Genetics play the primary role in susceptibility in about 5 to 10 percent of all cancers. In the majority of cancer cases,

Telomeres A strand of molecules at both ends of a chromosome.

Telomerase An enzyme that allows cells to reproduce indefinitely.

Carcinoma in situ An encapsulated malignant tumor that has not spread.

Angiogenesis The formation of blood vessels (capillaries).

Metastasis The movement of cells from one part of the body to another.

cancerous mutations are sporadic and acquired during a person's lifespan.

Effects of genetically caused cancer can be seen in the early childhood years or may result in multiple, independent cancers in different sites during a person's lifetime. Some cancers are a combination of genetic and environmental liability. Genetics may add to the environmental risk for certain types of cancers.

Even without environmental effects, genetic risk factors are a complex web of interplaying forces. Two people who have the same type of cancer could have developed it through different forms of mutations and changes. In many cases, when a family is found to have above average rates of a certain type of cancer, no genetic alteration can be found. Scientists are then left to speculate if the cancer is a result of combined genetic risk factors or environmental exposures the family has had in common.

One person may start accumulating random precancerous gene changes, while family members and neighbors in the same environment do not. When both the affected individual and someone lacking those changes are exposed to a cancer-causing agent in the same environment, the individual who has accumulated these changes will be the only one to develop disease. It is known that the environment works with genetics to trigger precancerous cells. Research is now opening doors in this field of study.

For most of the 20th century, a person's genetic traits were thought to be unalterable. Once a person inherited risk of disease, it was believed that there was little that could be done to change that risk. The field of **epigenetics** has drastically disrupted our understanding of genetics and has shown that environmental choices change the way our genes work and that certain genes can be turned off and on by lifestyle choices. This happens on the molecular level through one of two processes.

Chemical tags called methyl groups can be added directly to DNA to switch genes off. Meanwhile other chemical tags can be added to the proteins (called histones) around which DNA wraps itself, like spool on a thread. These tags then turn genes off by coiling the bundle of protein and DNA tightly away so they cannot be reached for transcription, or turn genes on by unfurling DNA for open transcription. These tags are added or removed depending on lifestyle choices. Whether the gene is available to be expressed depends on these tags sitting on top of the gene. The word epigenetics means "on top of" genetics. A person's genome has been compared to computer hardware, while the epigenome has been compared to computer software, telling the genome how to work.

Epigentic processes can encourage tumor-friendly changes that do not involve amutation, or they can help deter tumor development. Epigenetics is already used in some cancer treatments that silence certain genes and reactivate others.

Perhaps even more ground-breaking, researchers have discovered that epigentic changes acquired by the environment can be passed down from parent to offspring. While these changes are reversible, they can be detected in offspring two or three generations later. For example, traumatic experiences in one generation may produce fearful associations in offspring. Food choices, in particular, affect our epigenetic code. You may be answering for food choices your grandparents made. Equally, your grandchildren may someday answer for the food choices you make.

Incidence of Cancer

According to the most recent mortality statistics from the National Center for Health Statistics, cancer causes about 23 percent of all deaths in the United States. It is the second-leading cause of death in the country and is expected to be the leading cause by 2030. It is currently the leading cause of death in children between ages 1 and 14. The major contributor to the increase in incidence of cancer during the past five decades is lung cancer. Tobacco use alone is responsible for 30 percent of all deaths from cancer. Another third of all deaths from cancer are related to unhealthy nutrition, physical inactivity, and excessive body weight (fat).

For the first time, in 2014, cancer was announced as the number-one worldwide cause of death. The global rise in cancer deaths is due primarily to the large increase in tobacco use in developing countries, particularly in India and China, home to 40 percent of the world's smokers. Developing countries face additional affronts as they have higher rates of cancers caused by infections, while still facing growing rates of obesity as they adopt a more sedentary western lifestyle.

CRITICAL THINKING

Have you ever had, or do you now have, family members with cancer? Can you identify lifestyle or environmental factors as possible contributors to the disease? If not, are you concerned about your genetic predisposition, and, if so, are you making lifestyle changes to decrease your risk?

Cancer is predicted to develop in approximately 1 of every 2 men and 1 of 3 women in the United States, affecting approximately 3 of every 4 families. The incidence is also higher in African Americans than in any other racial or ethnic group. About 585,720 Americans died from cancer in 2014, and more than1.6 million new cases were diagnosed that same year.[1] The U.S. death rates for the major cancer sites are given in Figure 12.5.

Like coronary heart disease, cancer is largely preventable. As much as 90 percent of all human cancer is related to lifestyle or environmental factors. The American Cancer Society released updated guidelines on nutrition and physical activity for cancer prevention.[2] These guidelines recommend that people:

1. Maintain healthy body weight throughout life
2. Adopt a physically active lifestyle, which should include exercise and limited time spent doing sedentary activities

FIGURE 12.5 **U.S. death rates for major cancer sites, 2011.**

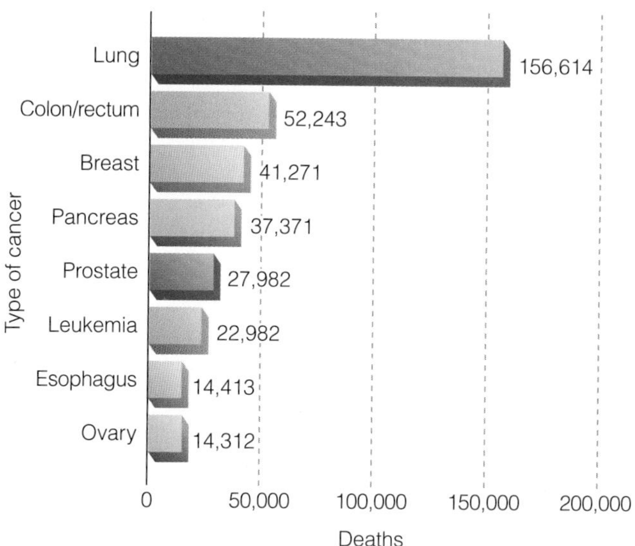

Source: U.S.Department of Health and Human services, Centers for Disease Control and Prevention, National Center for Health statistics, National Vital Statistics Reports, Deaths: preliminary data for 2011 61, no. 6 (October 10, 2012)

3. Adopt a healthy diet with emphasis on plant foods
4. Limit alcohol consumption if they drink alcoholic beverages

Additional general guidelines for cancer prevention that have existed for several decades now indicate that people should not use tobacco in any form and avoid exposure to secondhand smoke and occupational hazards (Figure 12.6). Most cancers could be prevented by following the previously listed positive lifestyle habits and reducing environmental contaminants that may cause cancer (see box on the next page).

Research sponsored by the American Cancer Society and the National Cancer Institute showed that individuals who have a healthy lifestyle have some of the lowest cancer mortality rates ever reported in scientific studies. In a landmark study, a group of about 10,000 members of the Church of Jesus Christ of Latter-Day Saints (commonly referred to as the Mormon church) in California was reported to have only about one-third (men) to one-half (women) the rate of cancer mortality of the general white population[3] (Figure 12.7). In this study, investigators looked at three general health habits in the participants: lifetime abstinence from smoking, regular physical activity, and sufficient sleep. Healthy lifestyle guidelines (encouraged by the church since 1833) include abstaining from all forms of tobacco, alcohol, and drugs and adhering to a well-balanced diet based on grains, fruits, and vegetables, and moderate amounts of poultry and red meat.

FIGURE 12.6 **Estimates of the relative role of the major cancer-causing factors.**

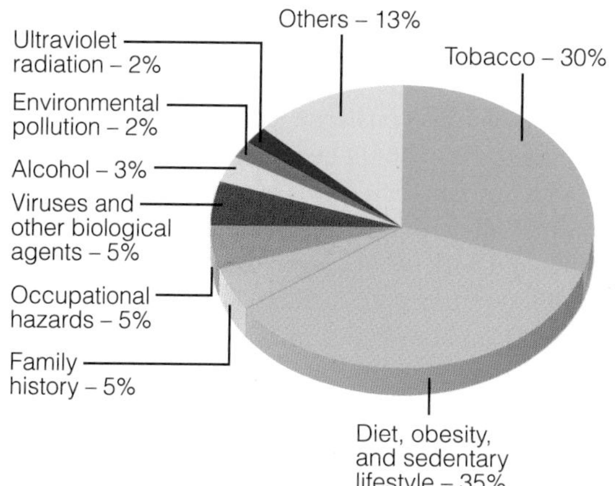

Source: Adapted from data from the 10 Commandments of Cancer Prevention, *Harvard's Men's Health Watch*, April 2009.

FIGURE 12.7 **Effects of a healthy lifestyle on cancer mortality rate.**

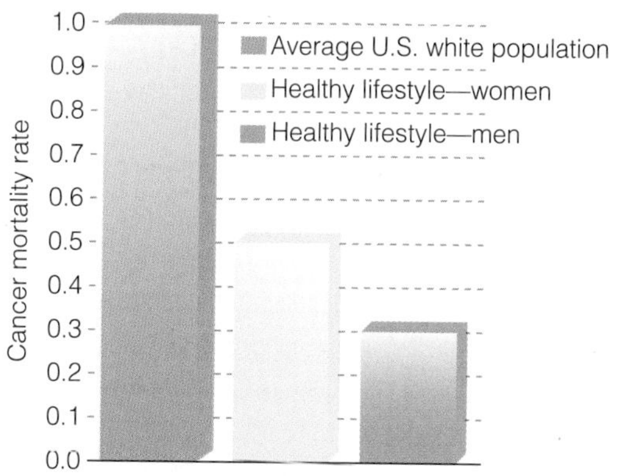

Source: "Health Practices and Cancer Mortality Among Active California Mormons," *Journal of the National Cancer Institute* 81 (1989): 1807-1814.

Additional 2009 data from more than 23,000 German participants indicated that people who never smoked, had a body mass index (BMI) lower than 30, exercised at least 3.5 hours per week, and consumed a diet rich in fruits and vegetables and low in meat had a 36 percent lower risk for cancer. The conclusion of the latter two studies is that lifestyle is definitely an important factor in the risk for cancer.[4]

Equally important is that approximately 13.7 million Americans with a history of cancer were alive in 2012. Currently, almost 7 in 10 people diagnosed with cancer are expected to be alive 5 years after their initial diagnosis.[5]

Guidelines for Preventing Cancer

The biggest factor in fighting cancer today is health education. A survey conducted by the American Institute for Cancer Research (AICR) published in 2014 revealed alarming results about our understanding of the link between lifestyle and cancer

Epigenetics The study of differences in an organism caused by changes in gene expression rather than changes in the genome itself.

Reducing Environmental Contaminants That May Cause Cancer

Since its creation in 1971, the U.S. President's Cancer Panel has monitored exposure by the public to potential environmental cancer risks in daily life. The public remains by and large unaware of most of these widespread and underestimated risks, factors that are critical in any cancer prevention efforts. Exposure to environmental contaminants poses a threat to health because they may alter or interfere with a variety of biologic processes. Among the recommendations released in 2010 by the presidential panel are:

1. Filter tap water or well water and whenever possible use filtered water instead of commercially bottled water.
2. Properly dispose of pharmaceuticals, household chemicals, paints, and other products to minimize drinking water and soil contamination.
3. Eliminate exposure to secondhand smoke and tobacco use in general.
4. Use stainless steel, glass, or BPA-free plastic water bottles.
5. Microwave in ceramic or glass instead of plastic containers.
6. Remove shoes before entering a home to avoid bringing in toxic chemicals, including pesticides.
7. Limit the consumption of food that is grown with pesticides and meats from animals raised with antibiotics and growth hormones.
8. Limit the consumption of processed, charred, or well-done meats, which are high in heterocyclic amines and polyaromatic hydrocarbons.
9. Practice safe-sun exposure and avoid over exposure to ultraviolet light when the sunlight is most intense.
10. Reduce radiation exposure (x-rays) from medical sources.
11. Avoid exposure to three highly carcinogenic chemicals: formaldehyde, benzene, and radon.*
12. Use headsets and text, instead of talking on cell phones, and keep cell phone calls brief to reduce exposure to electromagnetic energy. Although not scientifically proven, there is concern that frequent exposure to electromagnetic energy from cell phone use increases cancer risk.
13. Contaminant exposure in children is of significant concern because per pound of body weight they take in more food, water, air, and other substances than adults do. Toxic chemicals remain active longer in their developing brain and organs, placing them at far greater risk through chemical exposure.

*Formaldehyde is used in particle board, plywood, carpet, draperies, foam insulation, furniture, toiletries, and permanent press fabrics. Exposure is highest when newly installed. Benzene exposure is widespread and found primarily in vehicle exhaust. Radon exposure, which forms naturally and collects in homes, should be checked on a regular basis.

risk. Fewer than half of the respondents were aware that body weight is linked to cancer risk or of the link between processed meat consumption and cancer development. Worse, only one in five respondents agreed that genetics is not the main cause of developing cancer.

Cancer prevention education is an urgent concern because of the real control people have over their own cancer risk. A recent study by the AICR assessed lifestyle choices of 58,000 people and determined how many of the AICR's recommendations for reducing cancer each individual was successfully living. With each recommendation adopted by the individual, cancer risk decreased. The AICR found that people who followed a minimum of five recommendations halved their risk of dying from cancer as compared to people who followed none.[6]

People need to be informed about the risk factors for cancer and the guidelines for early detection. The most effective way to protect against cancer is to change negative lifestyle habits and behaviors. Following are some guidelines for preventing cancer. For most Americans who do not use tobacco, increased physical activity and dietary choices are the most important modifiable risk factors.

Dietary Changes

The American Cancer Society estimates that one-third of all cancer incidents in the United States could be related to nutrition and lack of physical activity. A healthy diet, therefore, is crucial to decrease the risk for cancer. The diet should be predominately vegetarian. Dietary fiber, nutrients, and phytonutrients appear to work in synergy during metabolic processes to prevent and slow cancer development at various stages. **Cruciferous vegetables**, tea, vitamin D, soy products, calcium, and omega-3 fats are encouraged. If alcohol and sugar are used, they should be used in moderation. Also important to a nutrient-rich diet is avoiding obesity. Excess weight, especially around the waist, increases cancer risk.

Green and dark yellow vegetables, cruciferous vegetables (cauliflower, broccoli, cabbage, kale, Brussels sprouts, and kohlrabi), and beans (legumes) seem to protect against cancer. Folate—found naturally in dark green leafy vegetables, dried beans, and orange juice—may reduce the risk for colon and cervical cancers. Brightly colored fruits and vegetables also contain **carotenoids** and vitamin C. Lycopene, one of the many carotenoids (a phytonutrient—see the following discussion), has been linked to lower risk for cancers

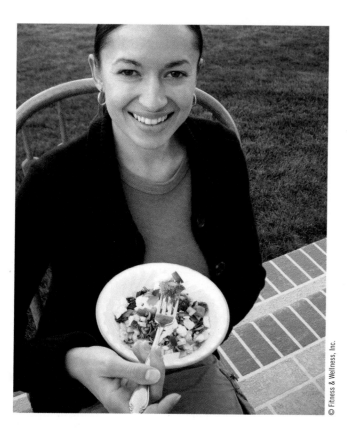

© Fitness & Wellness, Inc.

Cruciferous vegetables are recommended in a cancer-prevention diet.

of the prostate, colon, and cervix. Lycopene is especially abundant in cooked tomato products.

The evidence for vitamin D in protecting against cancer continues to be the focus of research. Vitamin D appears to be the most powerful regulator of cell growth and seems to keep cells from becoming malignant. Researchers are still working to understand the cause and effect relationship between health and vitamin D levels, but the protective effect of vitamin D appears to be strongest against breast, colon, and prostate cancers and possibly lung and digestive cancers. People should strive for "safe sun" exposure, that is, 10 to 20 minutes of unprotected sun exposure, on most days of the week between 10:00 a.m. and 4:00 p.m. For people living in the northern United States and Canada with limited sun exposure during the winter months, a vitamin D_3 supplement of up to 2,000 IUs per day is strongly recommended.

Cruciferous vegetables Plants that produce cross-shaped leaves (cauliflower, broccoli, cabbage, Brussels sprouts, and kohlrabi), which seem to have a protective effect against cancer.

Carotenoids Pigment substances in plants that are often precursors to vitamin A. More than 600 carotenoids are found in nature, about 50 of which are precursors to vitamin A, the most potent one being beta-carotene.

BEHAVIOR MODIFICATION PLANNING

Tips for a Healthy Cancer-Fighting Diet

I PLAN TO | I DID IT

I. Increase intake of phytonutrients, fiber, cruciferous vegetables, and more antioxidants by

❑ ❑ Eating a predominantly vegetarian diet

❑ ❑ Eating more fruits and vegetables every day (six to eight servings per day maximize anticancer benefits)

❑ ❑ Increasing the consumption of broccoli, cauliflower, kale, turnips, cabbage, kohlrabi, Brussels sprouts, hot chili peppers, red and green peppers, carrots, sweet potatoes, winter squash, spinach, garlic, onions, dried beans, strawberries, apples, grapes, tomatoes, pineapple, and citrus fruits in the regular diet

❑ ❑ Eating vegetables raw or quickly cooked by steaming or stir-frying

❑ ❑ Substituting tea and fruit and vegetable juices for coffee and soda

❑ ❑ Eating whole-grain breads

❑ ❑ Including calcium in the diet (or from a supplement)

❑ ❑ Including soy products in the diet

❑ ❑ Using whole-wheat flour instead of refined white flour in baking

❑ ❑ Using brown (unpolished) rice instead of white (polished) rice

II. Limit saturated and trans fats by

❑ ❑ Using primarily unsaturated fats (olive oil, canola oil, nuts, seeds, avocado, fish, flaxseeds, and flaxseed oil)

III. Balancing caloric input

❑ ❑ Balancing caloric input with caloric output to maintain recommended body weight

Try It

Make a copy of these cancer-fighting diet tips and each week incorporate into your lifestyle two additional dietary behaviors from the above list.

The cancer-protective benefits of this vitamin have already been discussed in detail in Chapter 3 (see "Vitamin D," page 112).

Some researchers believe that the antioxidant effect of vitamins help protect the body. Proteins that require the mineral selenium also appear to have a protective effect. During normal metabolism, most oxygen in the human body is converted into stable forms of carbon dioxide and water. A small amount, however, ends up in an unstable form known as oxygen free radicals, which are thought to attack and damage the cell membrane and DNA, leading to the formation of cancers. Antioxidants are thought to absorb free radicals before they can cause damage and to interrupt the sequence of reactions once damage has begun. Research is still required in this area, because a clear link has not been established.

Phytonutrients **Phytonutrients** are compounds found in abundance in fruits, vegetables, beans, nuts, and seeds. These nutrients may prevent cancer by blocking the formation of cancerous tumors and perhaps even disrupting the process once it has started. Each plant contains hundreds of phytonutrients. New phytonutrients are continually being discovered and our understanding of the way combinations of phytonutrients work in synergy with each other and with dietary fiber and nutrients is continually growing. Examples of these nutrients and their effects are found in Table 12.1. To obtain the best possible protection, a minimum of five servings of a variety of fruits and vegetables should be consumed each day. Fruits and vegetables should be consumed several times a day (instead of in one meal) to maintain phytonutrients at effective levels throughout the day. Phytonutrient blood levels drop within 3 hours of consuming foods containing these nutrients.

TABLE 12.1 **Selected Phytonutrients: Their Effects and Sources**

Phytonutrient	Effect	Good Sources
Sulforaphane	Removes carcinogens from cells	Broccoli
PEITC	Keeps carcinogens from binding to DNA	Broccoli
Genistein	Prevents small tumors from accessing capillaries to get oxygen and nutrients	Soybeans
Flavonoids	Helps keep cancer-causing hormones from locking onto cells	Most fruits and vegetables
p-Coumaric and chlorogenic acids	Disrupts the chemical combination of cell molecules that can produce carcinogens	Strawberries, green peppers, tomatoes, pineapple
Capsaicin	Keeps carcinogens from binding to DNA	Hot chili peppers

Fiber Initial studies linked low intake of fiber to increased risk for colorectal cancer. Other data, however, have been inconclusive.[7] While high fiber intake may not decrease the risk for colorectal cancer, a high fiber diet is still encouraged because it decreases the risk for other chronic conditions, such as cardiovascular disease and diabetes. Daily consumption of 25 grams (women) to 38 grams (men) of fiber is recommended. Whole grains are high in fiber and contain vitamins and minerals (folate, selenium, and calcium). Calcium may protect against colon cancer by preventing the rapid growth of cells in the colon, especially in people with colon polyps.

Tea Polyphenols (a group of phytonutrients) are potent cancer-fighting antioxidants found in fresh fruits and vegetables and many grains. A prime source is tea. White, green, and black tea are all created from the same plant and all seem to provide protection. Teas derived from other plants, such as red tea, appear to have benefits as well. Evidence also points to certain components in tea that can inhibit cancer at various stages. Polyphenols are known to block the formation of **nitrosamines** and quell the activation of **carcinogens**. Polyphenols also are thought to fight cancer by shutting off the formation of cancer cells, turning up the body's natural detoxification defenses, and thereby suppressing progression of the disease. Tea polyphenols specifically have been shown to cause some types of cancer cells to die much like normal cells do, preventing tumor formation, reducing cancer cell proliferation, and possibly suppressing angiogenesis. Different types of tea contain different mixtures of polyphenols depending on the specific variety of the plant, the growing location, and the way the tea is processed. White tea, which is harvested in the spring and uses young leaves and white buds, appears to have the highest amount. Green tea, which is minimally processed by steaming and drying, is next. And black tea, which is withered and fermented, comes in third. Herbal teas do not provide the same benefits as regular tea.

Observational data on tea-drinking habits in China showed that people who regularly drank green tea had about half the risk for chronic gastritis and stomach cancer, and the risk decreased further as the number of years of drinking green tea increased.[8] In Japan, where people drink green tea regularly but smoke twice as much as people in the United States, the incidence of lung cancer is half that of the United States.

The antioxidant effect of one of the polyphenols in green tea, epigallocatechin gallate (EGCG), is at least 25 times more effective than vitamin E and 100 times more effective than vitamin C at protecting cells and DNA from damage believed to cause cancer, heart disease, and other diseases associated with free radicals.[9] EGCG also is twice as strong as the red wine antioxidant resveratrol in helping prevent heart disease. Because it is easily extractable, EGCG is the subject of continued studies, with hopes that it could be added to milk or functional foods for wider reaching cancer protection.

Many benefits of regular tea consumption warrant further investigation. Optimistic results in animal studies are still unclear in humans. Drinking two or more cups of tea daily, preferably white or green, in place of popular high-sugar, nutrient-deficient sodas is encouraged.

Spices Although still in the early stages, research is uncovering cancer-fighting phytonutrients in many traditional spices. These phytonutrients may alter damaging carcinogenic pathways, provide antioxidant effects, promote cancer-fighting enzymes, decrease inflammation, stimulate the immune system, and suppress the development of tumors.[10] Ginger, garlic, oregano, curry, pepper, cloves, fennel, rosemary, turmeric, and black pepper are all encouraged for use in cooking and at the table.

Sugar Although the scientific evidence linking cancer to high sugar intake is not yet conclusive, evidence indicates that frequent consumption of sugar and high-sugar foods may be associated with an increased risk and faster progression of some types of cancer. Sugar is rapidly absorbed into the blood, quickly raising blood glucose and insulin levels. Not only does high blood glucose lead to diabetes, but it also suppresses immune function and becomes a readily available energy substrate for cancer cells to grow.

At this point, the data point to a link between high glucose levels and an increased risk of developing pancreatic, liver, gallbladder, colon, and respiratory tract cancers and dying of pancreatic, stomach, uterus, and cervix cancers. Decreasing sugar consumption also appears to enhance the outcome of cancer treatment in patients with the disease.

The evidence is strongest for the development of pancreatic cancer, one of the most deadly forms of cancer.[11] Researchers theorize that excessive glucose poisons and kills pancreatic cells, increasing cancer risk. Excessive insulin results in insulin-like growth factor, believed to increase cell proliferation and cancer. The data showed that people who consumed the most sugar, including creamed fruit, syrup-based drinks, soft drinks, and foods such as coffee, tea, and cereal to which sugar is added, had almost a 70 percent higher risk of developing pancreatic cancer compared to those with the lowest sugar consumption. Individuals who drank more than two soft drinks a day almost doubled the risk for pancreatic cancer.

Dietary Fat Although previously viewed as a risk factor, minimal evidence exists that total fat intake affects cancer risk. There is far greater evidence that being overweight or obese increases cancer risk. Excessive caloric intake leads to weight gain, and high-fat foods are typically calorie dense. Thus, indirectly, a high-fat diet can increase cancer risk through excessive body weight.

In any healthy diet, fat intake should be primarily monounsaturated and omega-3 polyunsaturated fats (found in flaxseed and several types of cold-water fish). These types of fat seem to offer protection against colorectal, pancreatic, breast, oral, esophageal, and stomach cancers. Omega-3 fats also block the synthesis of prostaglandins, bodily compounds that promote growth of tumors.

Processed Meat and Protein Salt-cured, smoked, and nitrite-cured foods have been associated with cancers of the esophagus, stomach, colon, and rectum. Processed meats (hot dogs, ham, bacon, sausage, and lunch meats) should be consumed sparingly and always with vitamin C-rich foods, such as orange juice, because vitamin C seems to discourage the formation of nitrosamines. These potentially cancer-causing compounds are formed when nitrites and nitrates, which are used to prevent the growth of harmful bacteria in processed meats, combine with other chemicals in the stomach. According to the American Cancer Society, a daily intake of 1 ounce per day of processed meat 5 to 6 times per week for men and 2 to 3 times for women increases colorectal cancer risk by 50 percent.

The combination of the heme protein with iron, both found abundantly in red meat (but not poultry and fish), also contributes to the formation of nitrosamines in the large intestine, increasing the risk for colorectal cancer.

Furthermore, nutritional guidelines discourage the excessive intake of protein. Too much animal protein appears to decrease blood enzymes that prevent precancerous cells from developing into tumors. According to the National Cancer Institute, eating substantial amounts of red meat may increase the risk for colorectal, pancreatic, breast, prostate, and renal cancer.

Cooking protein at high temperatures should be avoided or done only occasionally. The data suggest that grilling, broiling, or frying meat, poultry, or fish at high temperatures to medium well or well done leads to the formation of carcinogenic substances known as heterocyclic amines (HCAs) and polycyclic aromatic hydrocarbons (PAHs). Individuals who prefer their meat medium well or well done have a much higher risk for colorectal, stomach, breast, and prostate cancers. Cancer risk seems to correlate to the amount of well-done meat an individual consumes, but even small amounts each day add up.

When proteins are cooked at high temperatures, amino acids are changed into HCAs that collect on the surface of meats. Charring meat increases their formation to

Phytonutrients Compounds found in fruits and vegetables that block formation of cancerous tumors and disrupt the progress of cancer.

Nitrosamines Potentially cancer-causing compounds formed when nitrites and nitrates, which prevent the growth of harmful bacteria in processed meats, combine with other chemicals in the stomach.

Carcinogens Substances that contribute to the formation of cancers.

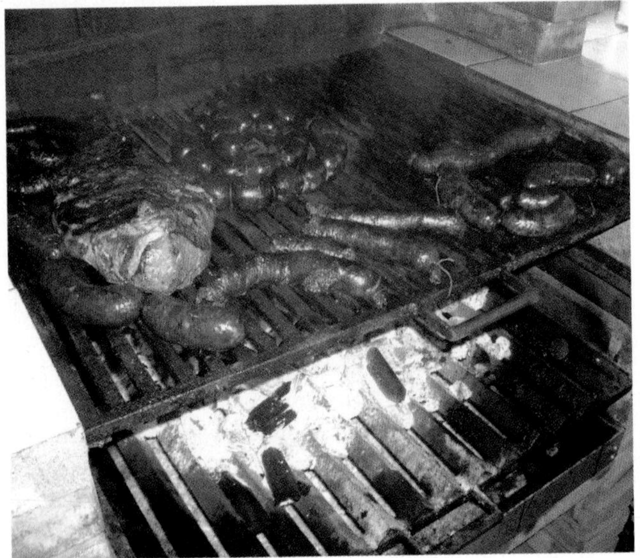

Cooking protein at high temperatures to medium well or well done should be done only occasionally, because it leads to the formation of carcinogenic substances on the surface of meats.

an even greater extent. PAHs are formed when fat drips onto the rocks or coals of the grill. The subsequent fire flare-up releases smoke that coats the food with PAHs.

An electric contact grill such as a George Foreman grill is preferable when cooking meats, because cooking temperatures are easily controlled. When cooking on an outdoor grill, line the grill with foil to minimize flare-up damage. Microwaving meat for a couple of minutes before barbecuing also decreases the risk, as long as the fluid released by the meat is discarded. Most potential carcinogens collect in this solution. Precooking in the microwave also decreases grilling time.

For an occasional outdoor barbecue, what you grill and how you grill are the most important factors. Animal products (both red and white meat) are the culprits, whereas grilling fruits and vegetables does not produce HCAs or PAHs. When grilling meats, the following approach can decrease HCAs and PAHs up to 90 percent.

- Cook meats with natural antioxidants as such decrease or eliminate HCAs and PAHs. Always marinate meat for at least 4 hours using some combination of vinegar, lemon juice, oil (preferably olive oil), and herbs and condiments including rosemary, red and black pepper, paprika, allspice, garlic, mustard, turmeric, thyme, chives, oregano, basil, sage, or parsley, among others. The marinade is believed to act as a barrier against the heat.
- Keep the meat moist and trim off all excess fat to avoid flare-ups.
- Microwave meat, poultry, and fish for 90 seconds to 2 minutes prior to grilling as such eliminates most of the HCAs.
- Cook at lower heat, under 350°F, to "medium" rather than "well" or "well done."
- Cook over aluminum foil with small holes cut in the foil so that drippings can pass through.
- Opt for kabobs or smaller cuts of meat that need less time on the grill.
- Turn the meat over frequently, every three to four minutes.
- Remove all skin before serving.
- Consider grilling on a water-soaked cedar plank or in an aluminum foil packet.
- Add broccoli to your meal. Broccoli has been shown to break down HCAs.
- Eat less meat as such increases your risk for cancer.

Soy Soy protein seems to decrease the formation of carcinogens during cooking of meats. Soy foods may help because soy contains chemicals that prevent cancer. Although further research is merited, isoflavones (phytonutrients) found in soy are structurally similar to estrogen and may prevent breast, prostate, lung, and colon cancers. Isoflavones, frequently referred to as phytoestrogens or plant estrogens, also block angiogenesis. Presently, it is not known whether the health benefits of soy are derived from isoflavones by themselves or in combination with other nutrients found in soy.

One drawback of soy was found in studies in which animals with tumors were given large amounts of soy. The estrogen-like activity of soy isoflavones actually led to the growth of estrogen-dependent tumors. Experts, therefore, caution women with breast cancer or a history of this disease to limit their soy intake, because it could stimulate cancer cells by closely imitating the actions of estrogen.

No specific recommendations are available as to the recommended amount of daily soy protein intake to prevent cancer. Based on the traditional diets of people (including children) in China and Japan who consume soy foods regularly, there doesn't seem to be an unsafe natural level of consumption. Soy protein powder supplementation, however, may elevate intake of soy protein to an unnatural (and perhaps unsafe) level.

Alcohol Consumption The general recommendation has been that people should consume alcohol in moderation, because too much alcohol raises the risk for developing certain cancers, especially when it is combined with tobacco smoking or smokeless tobacco. In combination, these substances significantly increase the risk for cancers of the mouth, larynx, throat, esophagus, and liver. The combined action of heavy alcohol and tobacco use can increase the odds of developing cancer of the oral cavity 15-fold.

A 2009 study of almost 1.3 million women between the ages of 45 and 75, however, indicated that as little as one drink of alcohol per day increases a women's risk for cancer by 13 percent, including cancers of the breast, esophagus, larynx, rectum, and liver.[12] The researchers concluded that even low-to-moderate alcohol consumption increases cancer risk in women, and the risks outweigh any potential cardioprotective benefits. Based on these data, it is estimated that about 30,000 yearly female cancers in the United States are due to these low levels of alcohol consumption. For women with a family history of breast cancer, the estimated risks are even higher. Thus, experts recommend that such women are better off abstaining from alcohol intake.

Nutrient Supplements An expert panel of the World Cancer Research Fund and the American Institute of Cancer Research stated that unless recommended by your doctor, you should not use supplements to protect against cancer. There is strong evidence that high-dose supplements of certain nutrients increase the risk for certain cancers. The best source of nutrients is a healthy diet.

Excessive Body Weight

Following tobacco abstention, the next most important action you can take for cancer prevention is to maintain recommended body weight. Based on estimates, the lethal combination of excess weight, physical inactivity, and poor nutrition account for one-third of deaths from cancer.[13] Furthermore, obese men and women have a more than 50 percent increased risk for dying from any form of cancer.[14] Adult weight gain increases the risk for many cancers, including those of the breast, colon and rectum, endometrium, esophageal, pancreas, and kidney. Obesity may also increase the risk for gallbladder, liver, prostate, ovarian, thyroid, and cervical cancers. For each of these types of cancer, the American Institute for Cancer Research has released the number of cases that could be prevented by diet, physical activity, and weight management. For example, 89,311 cases of breast cancer, 68,415 cases of colorectal cancer, and 25,630 cases of prostate cancer in the United States would have never occurred.[15] The AICR emphasizes that these numbers are legitimate and reachable goals for preventing cancer through better food choices and weight management. Investigators theorize that fat tissue produces excess hormone levels, causes chronic inflammation, effects tumor growth regulators, and increases blood levels of insulin and insulin-like growth factor-1 in the body that stimulate tumor growth.

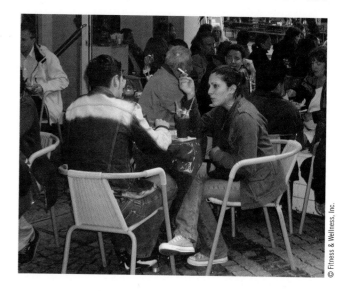

© Fitness & Wellness, Inc.

Heavy drinking, smoking, and tobacco use in general greatly increase the risk of oral cancer.

TABLE 12.2 Estimated Cancer Cases Preventable by Diet, Activity, and Weight Management in the United States per Year

Number of Cases Prevented	
Breast, female	89,311
Lung	80,716
Colorectal	68,415
Endometrial	31,052
Prostate	25,630
Mouth, Pharyngeal & Laryngeal	24,545
Kidney	15,341
Esophageal	12,537
Stomach	10,443
Pancreatic	8,820
Liver	4,979
Gallbladder	2,237
Total Cases Prevented	

Adapted from http://www.aicr.org/research/research_science_policy_report.html, downloaded April 30, 2014; AICR/WRCF, *Policy and Action for Cancer Prevention* 2009; Continuous Update Project reports; Rebecca Siegel et al. "Cancer statistics, 2014." *CA: A Cancer Journal for Clinicians Volume 64*, January/February 2014.

Abstaining from Tobacco

Cigarette smoking by itself is a major health hazard. The biggest carcinogenic exposure in the environment without question is tobacco use and exposure to secondhand smoke. If we include all related deaths, smoking is responsible for more than 443,000 unnecessary deaths and 159,000 lung cancer deaths in the United States each year. Smoking causes 6 million deaths worldwide annually, and that figure is expected to reach 8 million by 2030. The average life expectancy for a chronic smoker is about 13 to 14 years shorter than for a nonsmoker.[16]

Of all cancers, at least 30 percent are tied to smoking, and 87 percent of lung cancers are linked to smoking. Cigarette smoking contributes to at least 15 additional types of cancer, including oral, lip, nasal, pharyngeal, laryngeal, esophageal, uterine, stomach, and pancreatic. Use of smokeless tobacco can also lead to nicotine addiction and dependence, as well as increased risk for cancers of the mouth, larynx, throat, and esophagus. If you smoke or use any other tobacco products, *stop now!* If you do not smoke, don't ever start. If you are ever around people who are smoking, claim your right to clean air, or distance yourself from them as much as you possibly can.

The death of Hall of Fame baseball player Tony Gwynn from oral cancer at the age of 54 in 2014 has many users rethinking the use of chewing tobacco as a safer mode of tobacco use. Oral cancers are usually not discovered until they have spread to another part of the body. About 40,000 people are diagnosed yearly with oral cancer in the United States and almost half of these patients will die within the first five years of the diagnosis. Those who survive end up totally disfigured. While cigarette smoking rate has decreased, chewing tobacco rate has actually increased. Smokeless tobacco should be regulated just as aggressively as cigarette use, with strong warning labels and a ban on all flavored forms.

Avoiding Excessive Exposure to Sun

Near-daily safe-sun exposure, that is, 10 to 20 minutes of unprotected exposure during peak hours of the day, is beneficial to health. However, too much exposure to ultraviolet (UV) radiation is a major contributor to skin cancer. The most common sites of skin cancer are the areas exposed to the sun most often (face, neck, and back of the hands). UV rays are strongest when the sun is high in the sky. Therefore, you should avoid prolonged sun exposure between 10:00 a.m. and 4:00 p.m. Take the shadow test: If your shadow is shorter than you, the UV rays are at their strongest.

The three types of skin cancer are

1. Basal cell carcinoma
2. Squamous cell carcinoma
3. Malignant melanoma

Nearly 90 percent of the almost 1 million cases of basal cell or squamous cell skin cancers reported yearly in the United States could have been prevented by protecting the skin from excessive sun exposure. **Melanoma**, the most deadly type, caused approximately 9,710 deaths in 2014. About 20 percent of Americans will develop skin cancer in their lifetime. Treatment for non-melanoma skin cancer increased by more than 75 percent between 1992 and 2006. Melanoma increased 800 and 400 percent in young women and young men respectively between 1970 and 2009.

One to two blistering sunburns can double the lifetime risk for melanoma, even more so if the sunburn takes place prior to age 18, when cells divide at a faster rate than later in life. Furthermore, nothing is healthy about a "healthy tan." Tanning of the skin is the body's natural reaction to permanent and irreversible damage from too much exposure to the sun. Even small doses of sunlight add up to a greater risk for skin cancer and premature aging. The tan fades at the end of the summer season, but the underlying skin damage does not disappear.

The stinging sunburn comes from **ultraviolet B (UVB) rays**, which are also thought to be the main cause of premature wrinkling and skin aging; roughened, leathery, and sagging skin; and skin cancer. Unfortunately, the damage may not become evident until up to 20 years later. By comparison, skin that has not been overexposed to the sun remains smooth and unblemished and, over time, shows less evidence of aging.

Sunlamps and tanning parlors provide mainly **ultraviolet A (UVA) rays**. Once thought to be safe, they too are now known to be damaging and have been linked to melanoma. As little as 15 to 30 minutes of exposure to UVA rays can be as dangerous as a day spent in the sun. Similar to regular exposure to sun, short-term exposure to recreational tanning at a salon causes DNA alterations that can lead to skin cancer.[17]

Sunscreen lotion should be applied about 30 minutes before lengthy exposure to the sun, because the skin takes that long to absorb the protective ingredients. Select sunscreens labeled "broad spectrum," because these products block both UVA and UVB rays. A **sun protection factor (SPF)** of at least 15 is recommended. SPF 15 means that the skin takes 15 times longer to burn than it would with no lotion. If you ordinarily get a mild sunburn after 20 minutes of noonday sun, an SPF 15 allows you to remain in the sun about 300 minutes before burning. Sunscreens with stronger SPF factors are not necessarily better. They should be applied just as often, and they block only an additional 3 to 4 percent of UV rays. SPF 15 is adequate for most people.

Medical experts are also concerned about hormone-mimicking active ingredients in some sunscreens that are absorbed into the skin and possibly the bloodstream. Under particular scrutiny are the ingredients oxybenzone and retinyl palmitate. Although the jury is still out on any potential harmful health effects of these ingredients, preferably choose a sunscreen that contains zinc oxide, titanium dioxide, or both. These are finely crushed minerals in sunscreens that shield the skin from the sun's ultraviolet rays.

When swimming or sweating, you should reapply sunscreens more often, because all sunscreens lose strength when they are diluted. Look for "water resistant" or "very water resistant" sunscreens, which adhere to the skin for

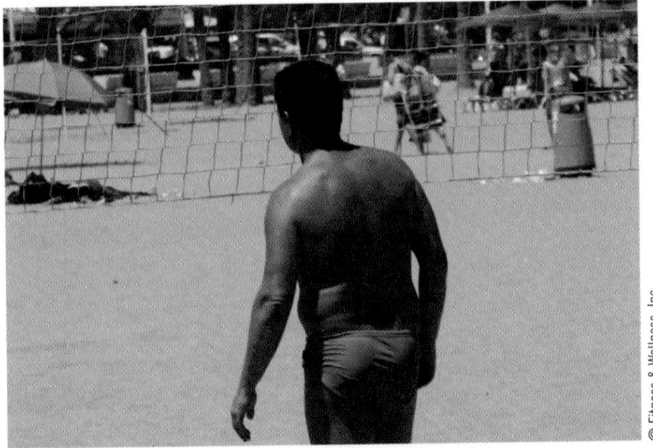

Tanned skin is the body's natural reaction to permanent and irreversible damage—a precursor to skin cancer.

40 to 80 minutes, respectively, even if the sunscreen promises "continuous protection."

If you plan on being out in the sun for a lengthy period, even better than sunscreen is wearing protective clothing, including long-sleeved shirts, long pants, and a hat with a two- to three-inch brim all the way around. This sun-protection strategy is even more critical for fair-skinned individuals who burn readily or turn red after only a few minutes of unprotected sun exposure, have a large number of moles, or have a personal or family history of skin cancer risk. Sun-protective fabrics, such as those manufactured by Coolibar or Sun Precautions, offer additional protection. You can also use RIT Sun Guard, a laundry additive that when used in washing penetrates the fibers and subsequently absorbs UV rays during sun exposure. The additive blocks up to 96 percent of UVA and UVB rays.

Monitoring Estrogen, Radiation Exposure, and Potential Occupational Hazards

Estrogen use has been linked to endometrial and breast cancer in some studies. Estrogen produced by excess fat in women after menopause is of particular concern. Exposure to radiation, although it increases the risk for cancer through x-rays, may have benefits that outweigh the risk involved, and most medical facilities use the lowest dose possible to keep the risk to a minimum. Occupational hazards—such as exposure to asbestos fibers, nickel and uranium dusts, chromium compounds, vinyl chloride, and bischlormethyl ether—increase the risk for cancer. The Federal Government updates a list of environmental exposures every two years. The current list includes over 220 substances, and while each carcinogen should be considered individually, keep in mind that each person will have an individualized reaction to the combined exposures of their genetic expression and their lifetime environment. Cigarette smoking magnifies the risk from occupational hazards.

Physical Activity

An active lifestyle has been shown to have a protective effect against cancer. Although the mechanism is not clear, physical fitness and cancer mortality in men and women may have a graded and consistent inverse relationship (Figure 12.8). Regular physical activity is known to reduce chronic low-grade inflammation that can cause DNA damage and promotes unhealthy cell growth that may cause cancer. It also decreases hormone levels of estrogen and insulin that at unhealthy levels encourage cancer development.

We now know that a daily 30-minute, moderate-intensity exercise program lowers the risk for colon, breast, and uterine cancers between 20 and 50 percent. Vigorous

FIGURE 12.8 Association between physical fitness and cancer mortality.

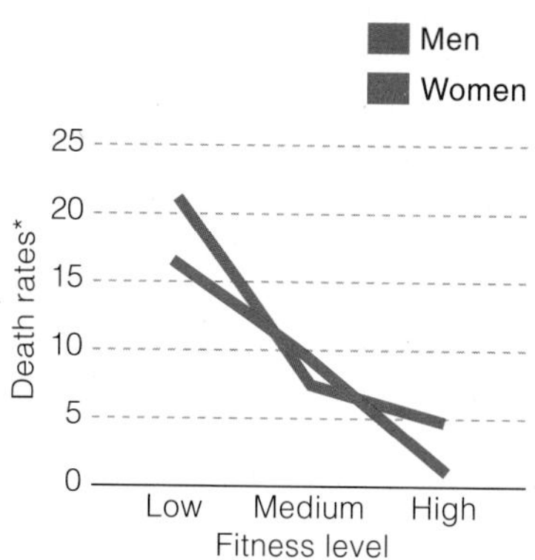

*Age-adjusted per 10,000 person-year at follow-up

Adapted from S.N. Blair, H.W. Kohl, III, R.S. Paffenbarger, Jr., D.B. Clark, D.H. Cooper, and L.W. Gibbons, "Physical Fitness and All-Cause Mortality: A Prospective Study of Healthy Men and Women," *Journal of the American Medical Association* 262 (1989): 2395-2401.

physical activity may lower the risk for more aggressive and fatal types of prostate cancer.[18]

Research among 38,410 men followed for an average period of 17.2 years indicated a strong inverse relationship between cardiorespiratory fitness and cancer mortality; that is, the less fit men had greater cancer deaths rates than the more fit men.[19] A 2009 study on more than 2,200 men 49 years of age and older that were followed for more than 35 years found that at least 30 minutes a day of moderate- to high-intensity physical activity is inversely associated with the risk of premature death from cancer in men.[20] The researchers concluded that the activity needed to be at least moderate intensity to achieve the benefit of reducing overall cancer mortality. After 10 years, men who switched from low- or medium- to high-intensity physical activity (greater than 5.2 metabolic equivalent task levels) were found to have half the risk of dying from cancer. There were no changes in mortality rate when switching from low- to medium-level physical activity. Other data suggest that in men 65 or older, exercising vigorously at least three times per week decreases the risk for advanced or fatal prostate cancer by 70 percent.[21]

In one study, data on more than 6,300 women indicated that regular exercise lowers the risk for breast cancer by up to 40 percent, regardless of race or ethnicity.[22] Other studies have

Melanoma The most virulent, rapidly spreading form of skin cancer.

Ultraviolet B (UVB) rays Ultraviolet rays that cause sunburn and lead to skin cancers.

Ultraviolet A (UVA) rays Ultraviolet rays that pass deeper into the skin and are believed to cause skin damage and skin cancers.

Sun protection factor (SPF) The degree of protection offered by ingredients in sunscreen lotion; at least SPF 15 is recommended.

found similar results. Women who are active throughout life also cut their risk for endometrial cancer by about 40 percent. Those who started exercise in adulthood cut their risk by about 25 percent.[23] Among women diagnosed with breast cancer, those who walk 2 to 3 miles per hour one to three times per week are 20 percent less likely to die of the disease. Those who walk three to five times per week cut their risk in half.[24] Researchers believe that the decreased levels of circulating ovarian hormones through physical activity decrease breast cancer risk. Physical activity also decreases inflammation and body fat, both risk factors for cancer.

Regular strength training also contributes to lower cancer mortality. A total of 8,677 men between the ages of 20 and 82 were tracked for more than two decades. The data indicated that men who regularly worked out with weights and had the highest muscle strength were up to 40 percent less likely to die from cancer, even among men with a higher waist circumference and BMI.[25]

The risk for other forms of cancer may also decrease, but additional research is necessary before definite statements can be made. Growing evidence suggests that the body's autoimmune system may play a role in preventing cancer and that moderate-intensity exercise improves the autoimmune system.

Early Detection

Fortunately, many cancers can be controlled or cured through early detection. The real problem comes when cancerous cells spread, because they become more difficult to destroy. Therefore, effective prevention, or at least early detection, is crucial. Herein lies the importance of periodic screening. Once a month, women should practice breast self-examination (BSE) and men should undertake testicular self-examination (TSE). Men should pick a regular day each month (e.g., the first day of each month) to practice TSE, and women should perform BSE two or three days after the menstrual period is over.

Other Factors

The contributions of many other much-publicized factors are not as significant as those just pointed out. Intentional food additives, saccharin, processing agents, pesticides, and packaging materials currently used in the United States and other developed countries seem to have minimal consequences.

High levels of tension and stress and poor coping may affect the autoimmune system negatively and render the body less effective in dealing with the various cancers. Chronic stress increases cortisol and inflammatory chemicals that sustain cancer growth.[26]

Warning Signals of Cancer

Everyone should become familiar with the following warning signals for cancer and bring those present to a physician's attention:

1. Change in bowel or bladder habits
2. Sore that does not heal
3. Unusual bleeding or discharge
4. Thickening or lump in the breast or elsewhere
5. Indigestion or difficulty in swallowing

BEHAVIOR MODIFICATION PLANNING

Do you currently avoid the following cancer promoters?

I PLAN TO	I DID IT	
❑	❑	Physical inactivity
❑	❑	Being more than 10 pounds overweight
❑	❑	Frequent consumption of red meat
❑	❑	Any form of tobacco use
❑	❑	Charred/burned foods
❑	❑	Frequent consumption of nitrate-/nitrite-cured, salt-cured, or smoked foods
❑	❑	Alcohol consumption
❑	❑	Excessive sun exposure
❑	❑	Estrogens
❑	❑	Methyleugenol (flavoring agent in packaged foods)
❑	❑	Radon, formaldehyde, and benzene
❑	❑	Wood dust (high levels)

Try It

In your Online Journal or class notebook, make a list of cancer promoters around you and note whether you take necessary actions to avoid them. If you do not, note what it would take for you to do so.

6. Obvious change in wart or mole
7. Nagging cough or hoarseness
8. Unexplained weight loss
9. Ongoing pain or fatigue

In Lab 12A, you can determine how well you are doing in terms of a cancer-prevention program. Lab 12B provides a questionnaire to alert you to symptoms that may indicate a health problem. Although in most cases nothing serious will be found, any symptoms calls for a physician's attention as soon as possible. Scientific evidence and testing procedures for the prevention and early detection of cancer do change. Studies continue to provide new information. The intent of cancer-prevention programs is to educate and guide people toward a lifestyle that helps prevent cancer and enables early detection of malignancy.

Treatment of cancer should always be left to specialized physicians and cancer clinics. Current treatment modalities include surgery, radiation, radioactive substances, chemotherapy, hormones, and immunotherapy.

Cancer: Assessing Your Risks

Figure 12.9 provides a self-testing questionnaire to help you assess your cancer risk. The factors listed in the questionnaire are the major risk factors for specific cancer sites and by no means represent the only ones that might be involved. Check your status against the factors contained in this questionnaire. Based on the number of risk factors that apply to you, rate yourself on a scale from 1 to 3 (1 for low risk, 2 for moderate risk, and 3 for high risk) for each cancer site. Explanations of the risk factors for each type of cancer follow. If you are at higher risk, you are advised to discuss the results with your physician. Record your risk level totals for each cancer site in Lab 12C.

Common Sites of Cancer

Lung Cancer

Risk Factors

1. Smoking status. Tobacco smoke causes nearly 9 out of 10 cases of lung cancer (includes cigarette, cigar, and pipe smoking). Smoking low tar or "light" cigarettes increases lung cancer risk as much as regular cigarettes. The rates for ex-smokers who have not smoked for 10 years is half that of nonsmokers.
2. Amount and length of time smoked. The risk increases with the number of cigarettes smoked per day and years the individual has smoked.
3. Secondhand smoke. Exposure to secondhand smoke increases lung cancer risk. For example, nonsmoking spouses who live with a smoker have a 20 percent greater risk of developing lung cancer than do spouses of nonsmokers. Some individuals have a greater susceptibility to lung cancer as a result of secondhand smoke exposure.
4. Radon gas exposure. Radon, a radioactive gas that tends to build up indoors, is a potential cancer risk. The risk is also much greater for smokers. Homes and buildings should be tested periodically for radon content. State and local U.S. Environmental Protection Agency offices provide information on radon testing.
5. Type of industrial work. Exposure to certain mining materials, uranium and radioactive products, or asbestos has been demonstrated to be associated with lung cancer. Exposure to materials in other industries also carries a higher risk. Smokers who work in these industries have greatly increased risks. Exposure to arsenic; radiation from occupational, medical, or environmental sources; and air pollution increase the risk for lung cancer.

Colon and Rectum Cancer

Risk Factors

1. Age. Colon cancer occurs more frequently after 50 years of age.
2. Family predisposition. Colon cancer is more common in families that have a previous history of this disease. Also, families who are predisposed to carry hereditary nonpolyposis colon cancer (HNPCC, or Lynch syndrome) are at a higher risk of developing colon cancer. HNPCC also increases the risk for several other cancers, and individuals who are susceptible should talk to their doctor about regular screenings.
3. Personal history. Polyps and bowel diseases are associated with colon cancer.
4. Physical inactivity. Strong scientific evidence points to a higher risk for colorectal cancer in physically inactive individuals.
5. Race or ethnicity. African Americans and Jews of Eastern European descent have some of the highest colorectal cancer rates in the world.

In addition to the previously mentioned risk factors, smoking; alcohol consumption; a diet high in saturated fat, red meat, or both; a diet low in fiber; inadequate consumption of fruits and vegetables; type 2 diabetes; and inflammatory bowel disease increase the risk for colon or rectal cancer. Regular screening is an important measure in catching and removing polyps before they can turn into tumors and is recommended beginning at age 50.

Skin Cancer

Risk Factors

1. UV light exposure. Excessive UV light is a culprit in skin cancer. Always practice safe sun exposure, that is, only 10 to 20 minutes of daily unprotected sun exposure. For longer exposure, protect yourself with a sunscreen medication.

FIGURE 12.9 **Cancer questionnaire: assessing your risks.**

Name:____________________ Date:______________

Course:__________ Section:__________ Gender:__________ Age:__________

Assessing Your Risks for Cancer

Read each question concerning each site and its specific risk factors. Be honest in your responses. Your risk increases as you move beyond item 1 for each factor. For example, the risk for lung cancer increases progressively as the number of cigarettes smoked per day increases. If none of the answers apply, skip to the next question. Based on the number of risk factors that apply to you, rate yourself on a scale from 1 to 3 (1 for low risk, 2 for moderate risk, and 3 for high risk) for each cancer site. Record your results in Lab 12B.

Lung Cancer

■ Smoking status
1. Nonsmoker
2. Smoker

■ Amount of cigarettes smoked per day
1. NA
2. Less than 1 pack
3. 1–2 packs
4. 2+ packs

■ Years smoked
1. None
2. 1–15
3. 15–25
4. >25

■ Radon gas exposure
1. No
2. Yes
3. Yes and smoker

■ Type of industrial work
1. Mining
2. Uranium and radioactive products
3. Asbestos

Colon/Rectum Cancer

■ Age
1. ≤40
2. 41–60
3. >60

■ Family predisposition
1. No
2. Yes

■ Personal history
1. No
2. Polyps
3. Bowel diseases

■ Are you physically active?
1. Yes
2. No

■ Are you African American or a Jew of Eastern European descent?
1. No
2. Yes

■ Family history of HNPCC (or Lynch Syndrome)?
1. No
2. Yes

Skin Cancer

■ Do you practice safe sun exposure?
1. Yes
2. No

■ Complexion—fair and/or light skin
1. No
2. Yes

■ Personal or family history
1. No
2. Yes

■ Work in mines, around coal tar, radioactive materials, or arsenic?
1. No
2. Yes

■ Radiation treatment
1. No
2. Yes

Breast Cancer

■ Age
1. ≤35
2. 36–50
3. ≥51

■ Are you Caucasian?
1. No
2. Yes

■ Family history
1. No
2. One family member
3. Two or more family members

■ Personal history of breast or ovarian cancer
1. No
2. Yes

■ Maternity
1. First pregnancy before age 30
2. First child after age 30
3. No children

■ Hormone replacement therapy
1. No
2. Short-term use
3. Long-term use

■ Are you physically active?
1. Yes
2. No

■ Alcohol
1. No alcohol
2. <1 drink per day
3. 1 drink per day
4. >1 drink per day

■ Are you significantly overweight?
1. No
2. Yes and premenopausal
3. Yes and postmenopausal

Cervical Cancer

■ Human papilloma virus (HPV) infection
1. Never been infected
2. Previously or currently infected

■ Smoking status
1. Nonsmoker
2. Ex-smoker
3. Current smoker

■ HIV and chlamydia infections
1. Neither one
2. HIV
3. Chlamydia
4. Both

■ Fruits and vegetables
1. ≥5 servings per day
2. 3-4 servings per day
3. 1–2 servings per day
4. <1 serving per day

■ Are you overweight?
1. No
2. Yes

■ Are you using birth control pills?
1. No
2. Yes

■ Pregnancy
1. Two or fewer
2. Prior to age 17
3. Multiple pregnancies

■ Family history
1. No
2. Yes

Endometrial Cancer

■ Estrogen therapy
1. No
2. Yes

■ Age
1. ≤40
2. 41–49
3. ≥50

■ Are you Caucasian?
1. No
2. Yes

■ Pregnancy
1. Yes
2. No

■ Body weight
1. At recommended weight
2. Overweight
3. Obese

■ Diabetes
1. No
2. Yes

■ Total years of menstrual cycles
1. "Normal"
2. Greater than "normal" (early start and/or late cessation)

■ Are you hypertensive?
1. No
2. Yes

■ Are you physically active?
1. Yes
2. No

■ Family predisposition
1. No
2. Yes

Prostate Cancer

■ Age
1. ≤64
2. ≥65

■ Family history
1. No
2. Yes

■ Are you African American?
1. No
2. Yes

■ Diet
1. Low in saturated fat
2. High in saturated fat

■ Are you physically active?
1. Yes
2. No

Testicular Cancer

■ Did you have an undescended testicle?
1. No
2. Yes

■ Did you have abnormal testicular development?
1. No
2. Yes

■ Do you have a family history of testicular cancer?
1. No
2. Yes

■ Are you Caucasian?
1. No
2. Yes

Pancreatic Cancer

■ Age
1. ≤55
2. ≥56

(continued)

FIGURE 12.9 Cancer questionnaire: assessing your risks. (Continued)

- Tobacco use
  1. No
  2. Yes
- Sugar intake
  1. Low
  2. Moderate
  3. Excessive
- Are you obese?
  1. No
  2. Yes
- Do you now have or have you had chronic pancreatitis, cirrhosis, or diabetes?
  1. No
  2. Yes
- Are you physically active?
  1. Yes
  2. No
- Are you African American?
  1. No
  2. Yes
- Family history
  1. No
  2. Yes
- Family history of HNPCC (or Lynch Syndrome)?
  1. No
  2. Yes

Kidney and Bladder Cancer

- Smoking history
  1. Nonsmoker
  2. Ex-smoker
  3. Cigarette smoker
- Were you diagnosed with congenital (inborn) abnormalities of the kidneys or bladder?
  1. No
  2. Yes
- Have you been exposed to aniline dyes, naphthalenes, or benzidines?
  1. No
  2. Yes
- Do you have a history of schistosomiasis (a parasitic bladder infection)?
  1. No
  2. Yes
- Do you suffer from frequent urinary tract infections?
  1. No
  2. Yes
- Family predisposition
  1. No
  2. Yes
- Are you overweight?
  1. No
  2. Yes
- High blood pressure
  1. No
  2. Yes

Oral Cancer

- Tobacco use
  1. Nonuser
  2. Ex-user
  3. Pipe, cigar, or smokeless tobacco
  4. Cigarettes
- Alcohol use
  1. Do not drink alcohol
  2. Less than 1 drink per day (women) or 2 drinks per day (men)
  3. More than 1 drink per day (women) or 2 drinks per day (men)
- Do you practice safe sun exposure?
  1. Yes
  2. No

Esophageal and Stomach Cancer

- How many servings of fruits and vegetables do you consume daily?
  1. >8
  2. 5–8
  3. 3–5
  4. <3
- How often do you consume salt-cured, smoked, or nitrate-cured foods?
  1. Rarely
  2. Less than once per week
  3. 1–3 times per week
  4. >3 times per week
- Have you been told that you have an imbalance in stomach acid?
  1. No
  2. Yes
- Do you have a history of pernicious anemia?
  1. No
  2. Yes
- Have you been diagnosed with chronic gastritis or gastric polyps?
  1. No
  2. Yes
- Family history of esophageal or stomach cancer?
  1. No
  2. Yes
- Are you overweight?
  1. No
  2. Yes
- Do you use alcohol or tobacco in any form?
  1. No
  2. Yes

Ovarian Cancer

- Age
  1. <50
  2. 51–60
  3. 61–70
  4. >70
- Do you have a personal history of ovarian problems?
  1. No
  2. Yes
- Have you had estrogen postmenopausal hormone therapy?
  1. No
  2. Yes
- Do you have an extensive history of menstrual irregularities?
  1. No
  2. Yes
- Family history
  1. None
  2. Colon/Rectum cancer
  3. Endometriosis
  4. Breast cancer
  5. Ovarian cancer
- Do you have a personal history of breast cancer?
  1. No
  2. Yes
- Have you had a child?
  1. Yes
  2. No
- Body weight
  1. Normal
  2. 10–50 pounds overweight
  3. >50 pounds overweight
- Do you have a family history of nonpolyposis colon cancer?
  1. No
  2. Yes
- Family history of HNPCC (or Lynch Syndrome)?
  1. No
  2. Yes

Thyroid Cancer

- Age
  1. <35
  2. 35–55
  3. 56–70
  4. >70
- Sex
  1. Male
  2. Female
- Did you receive radiation therapy to the head and neck region in childhood or adolescence?
  1. No
  2. Yes
- Do you have a family history of thyroid cancer?
  1. No
  2. Yes

Liver Cancer

- Do you have a family history of cirrhosis of the liver?
  1. No
  2. Yes
- Do you have a personal history of hepatitis B or hepatitis C virus?
  1. No
  2. Yes
- Have you been exposed to vinyl chloride (industrial gas used in plastics manufacturing)?
  1. No
  2. Yes
- Have you been exposed to aflatoxin (natural food contaminant)?
  1. No
  2. Yes
- Alcohol
  1. None
  2. ≤2 drinks per day
  3. ≥3 drinks per day
- Are you Asian American or Pacific Islander?
  1. No
  2. Yes

Leukemia

- Family history
  1. No
  2. Yes
- Do you suffer from Down syndrome or other genetic abnormalities?
  1. No
  2. Yes
- Have you had excessive exposure to ionizing radiation?
  1. No
  2. Yes
- Are you exposed to environmental chemicals?
  1. No
  2. Yes

Lymphomas

- Are you physically active?
  1. Yes
  2. No
- Do you have a family history of lymphomas?
  1. No
  2. Yes
- Are you exposed to
  1. Herbicides
  2. Organic solvents
- Have you had an organ transplant?
  1. No
  2. Yes
- Have you been diagnosed with any of the following?
  1. Epstein-Barr virus
  2. HIV
  3. Human T-cell leukemia/lymphoma virus-I (HTLV-1) virus

2. Complexion. Risk factors vary for different types of skin. Individuals with light complexions, people with natural blond or red hair, and those who burn easily are at greater risk.
3. Personal and family history of melanoma and moles. Of particular note are large or unusual moles or a large number of moles.
4. Work environment. Work in mines and around coal tar, radioactive materials, or arsenic (used in some insecticides) can cause cancer of the skin.
5. Radiation. Individuals who have undergone radiation treatment run a much higher risk for skin cancer in the treated area.

Risks for skin cancer are difficult to state. For instance, a person with a dark complexion can work longer in the sun and be less likely to develop cancer than a light-skinned person. Furthermore, a person wearing a long sleeved shirt and a wide-brimmed hat who spends hours working in the sun has less risk than a person wearing a swimsuit who sunbathes for only a short time. The risk increases greatly with age, and family history also plays a role.

If any of the previous risk factors apply to you, you need to protect your skin from the sun or any other toxic material. Changes in moles, warts, or skin sores are important and should be evaluated by your doctor (Figure 12.10).

FIGURE 12.10 Warning signs of melanoma: ABCDE rule for moles.

A. *Asymmetry:* One half of a mole or lesion doesn't look like the other half.

B. *Border:* A mole has an irregular, scalloped, or not clearly defined border.

C. *Color:* The color varies or is not uniform from one area of a mole or lesion to another, whether the color is tan, brown, black, white, red, or blue.

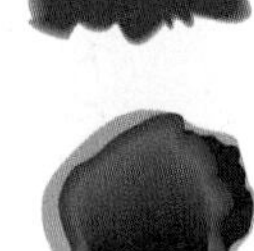

D. *Diameter:* The lesion is larger than 6 millimeters (1⁄4 inch) or larger than a pencil eraser.

E. *Elevation:* Does it raise off the skin?

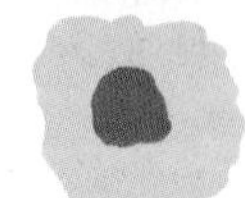

Source: Adapted from FDA Consumer, May 1991. From Family Practice Recertification 14, no. 3 (March 1992).

Skin Self-Exam

One of the easiest and quickest self-exams is a brief survey to detect possible skin cancers (see Figure 12.11). A simple skin self-exam can reduce deaths from melanoma by as

FIGURE 12.11 Skin self-examination

The American Cancer Society recommends you stand in front of a mirror and

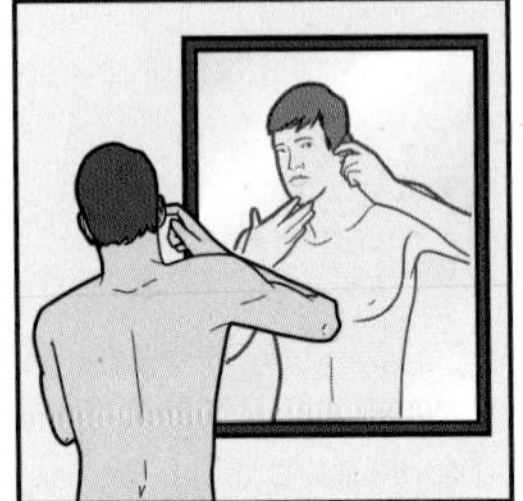

Examine your face (especially the nose, mouth, and lips), front and back of the ears, neck, chest, abdomen, and upper back. Women should also lift their breasts to examine the skin underneath.

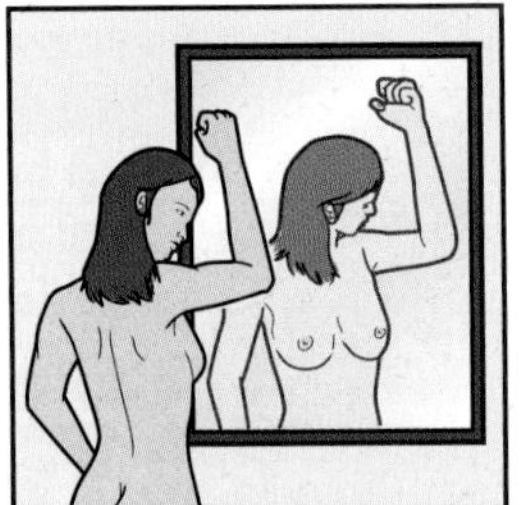

Check both sides of your arms, underarms, both sides of the hands, between the fingers, and under the fingernails.

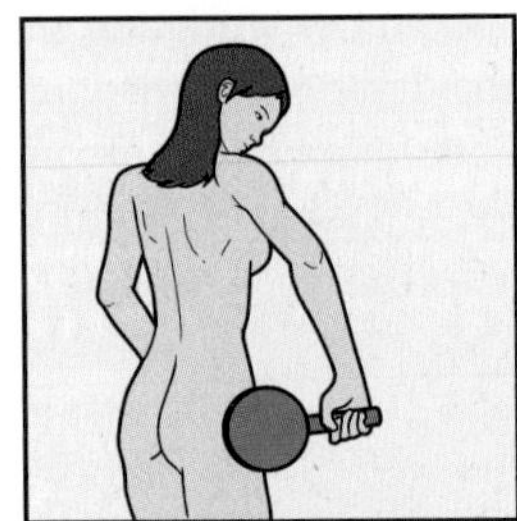

With the aid of a handheld mirror, scan your lower back, buttocks, and genital area.

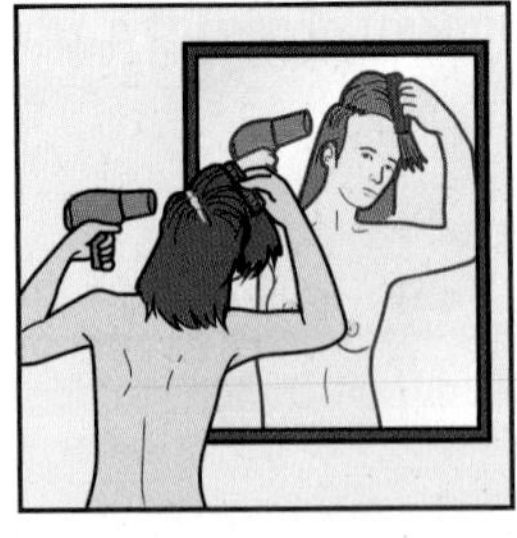

Using a comb, a hair blow dryer, and if possible, the assistance of a friend or family member, thoroughly examine the entire scalp.

Sit down on a chair or bench and

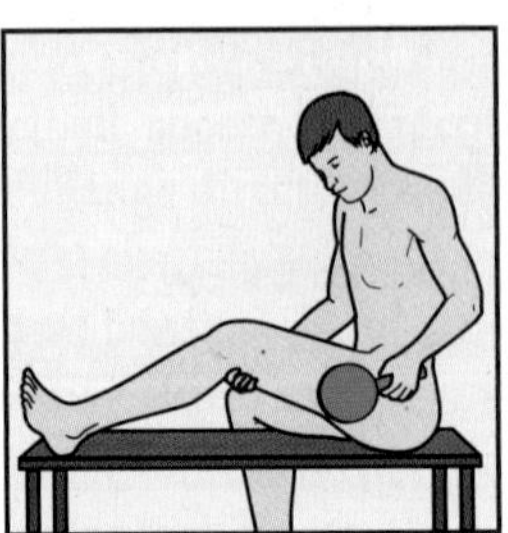

Inspect the front of your thighs, lower legs, the top and soles of your feet, between the toes, and under the toenails. Using a handheld mirror, inspect the back of your thighs and the lower legs.

much as 63 percent, saving as many as 4,500 lives in the United States each year:

- Make a drawing of yourself. Include a full frontal view, a full back view, and close-up views of your head (both sides), the soles of your feet, the tops of your feet, and the backs of your hands.

CRITICAL THINKING

What significance does a "healthy tan" have in your social life? Are you a "sun worshiper," or are you concerned about skin damage, premature aging, and potential skin cancer in your future?

- After you get out of the bath or shower, examine yourself closely in a full-length mirror. On your sketch, note any moles, warts, or other skin marks you find anywhere on your body. Pay particular attention to areas that are exposed to the sun constantly, such as your face, the tops of your ears, and your hands.
- Briefly describe each mark on your sketch—its size, color, texture, and so on.
- Repeat the exam about once a month. Watch for changes in the size, texture, or color of moles, warts, or other skin marks. If you notice any difference, contact your physician. You also should contact a doctor if you have a sore that does not heal.

Breast Cancer

Risk Factors

1. Age. The risk for breast cancer increases significantly after 50 years of age.
2. Race. Breast cancer occurs slightly more frequently in white women than African American women. The latter, however, are more likely to die from the disease.

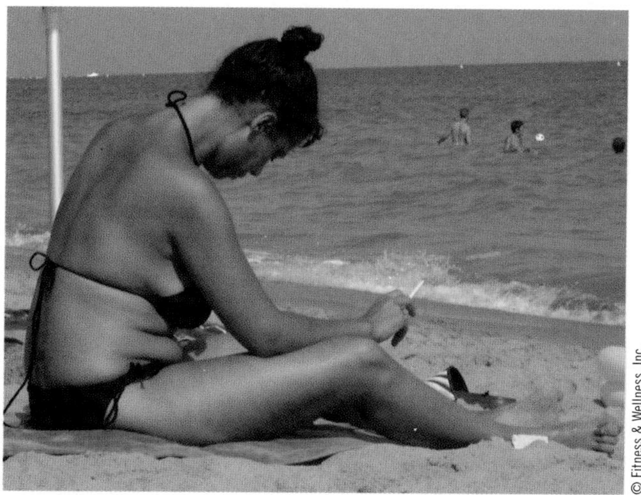

Cigarette smoking and excessive body weight and sun exposure are major risk factors for cancer.

3. Family history. The risk for breast cancer is higher in women with a family history of breast and ovarian cancers. The risk is even higher if more than one family member has developed these cancers, and is further enhanced by the closeness of the relationship (e.g., a mother or sister with breast cancer indicates a higher risk than a cousin with breast cancer).
4. Genes. Inherited mutations in genes (breast cancer gene 1 or BRCA1 and breast cancer gene 2 or BRCA2) are found in families with high rates of breast cancer. Women who carry this genetic mutation have as much as an 80 percent greater chance of developing breast cancer and 50 percent higher chance of ovarian cancer. Prophylactic removal of the breasts and/or ovaries significantly decreases the risk of breast cancer. Not all women who opt to have the surgery necessarily indicates that they would develop breast cancer. As an extremely emotional and personal decision, women who are contemplating preventive surgery should seek professional counseling prior to undertaking this option.
5. Personal history. A previous history of breast or ovarian cancer indicates a higher risk.
6. Maternity. The risk is higher in women who have never had children and in women who bear children after 30 years of age. Women are encouraged to breastfeed their babies at least six months, which also reduces the risk for breast cancer.
7. Physical inactivity. Physically inactive women are at higher risk. Regular aerobic exercise has consistently been associated with a lower risk of breast cancer. Some research even indicates that the risk of dying from breast cancer decreases by more than 40 percent in women with high aerobic fitness as compared to less fit women. Vigorous aerobic activity at least three times per week seems most effective. Adding strength training twice a week is also helpful.
8. Hormone replacement therapy (HRT). Long-term use of a combination of progesterone and estrogen increases the risk. The risk seems to apply to current and recent users.
9. Alcohol. Even one alcoholic drink per day slightly enhances breast cancer risk in women. Two or more drinks per day clearly enhance the risk.
10. Obesity. Adipose tissue increases estrogen levels. Higher estrogen levels, particularly following menopause, increase the risk.

About 5 to 10 percent of breast cancers may be related to gene mutations, the most common are BRCA1 and BRCA2. These are tumor suppressor genes located on chromosomes 17 and 13. Researchers believe that the majority of breast cancer cases that run in families are a result of environmental influences combined with more common gene mutations that result in only a slight increase in breast cancer risk.

Women with low to moderate risk should practice monthly BSE (Figure 12.12) and have their breasts examined by a doctor as a part of a cancer-related checkup.

Periodic mammograms should be included as recommended. Women at high risk should practice monthly BSE and have their breasts examined regularly by a doctor. See your doctor for the recommended examinations (including mammograms and physical exam of breasts).

Clinical breast exams by a physician are recommended every 3 years for women between ages 20 and 40 and every year for women over age 40. The American Cancer Society also recommends an annual **mammogram** for women over age 40. The 2009 guidelines by the U.S. Preventive Service Task Force, although heatedly debated by many health care practitioners, recommended that women get a mammogram every 2 years starting at age 50. According to Otis Brawley, chief medical officer of the American Cancer Society, "This is one screening test I recommend unequivocally, and would recommend to any woman 40 and over." Frequency of mammograms is currently an area of debate among health care practitioners, and personal risk factors should be considered to determine when to start and how often they should be done.

Other possible risk factors for breast cancer that are not listed in the questionnaire are high breast tissue density (a mammographic measure of the amount of glandular breast tissue relative to fatty breast tissue), a long menstrual history (onset of menstruation prior to age 13 and ending later in life), postmenopausal hormone therapy, recent use of oral contraceptives or postmenopausal estrogens, high saturated fat intake, atypical hyperplasia or carcinoma in situ, high refined carbohydrate intake, chronic cystic disease, and ionizing radiation. To decrease the risk, increase fiber, folic acid, monounsaturated fat, and vegetable consumption and increase daily physical activity.

FIGURE 12.12 Breast self-examination.

Looking

Stand in front of a mirror with your upper body unclothed. Look for changes in the shape and size of the breast, and for dimpling of the skin or "pulling in" of the nipples. Any changes in the breast may be made more noticeable by a change in position of the body or arms. Also look for changes in shape from one breast to the other.

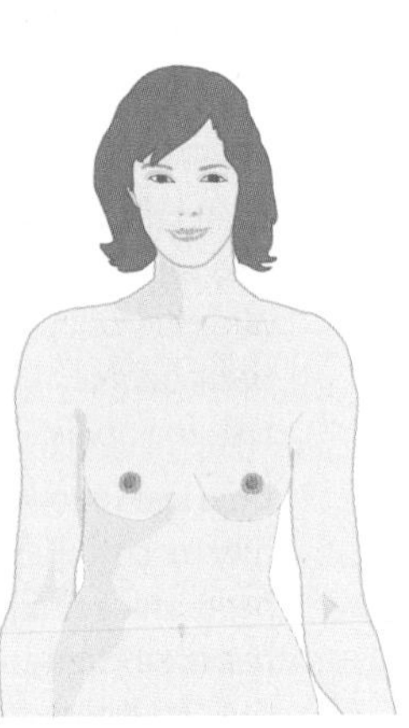

1. Stand with your arms down.

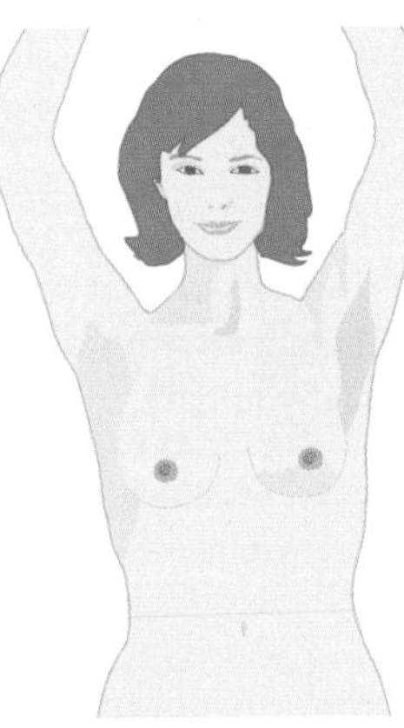

2. Raise your arms overhead.

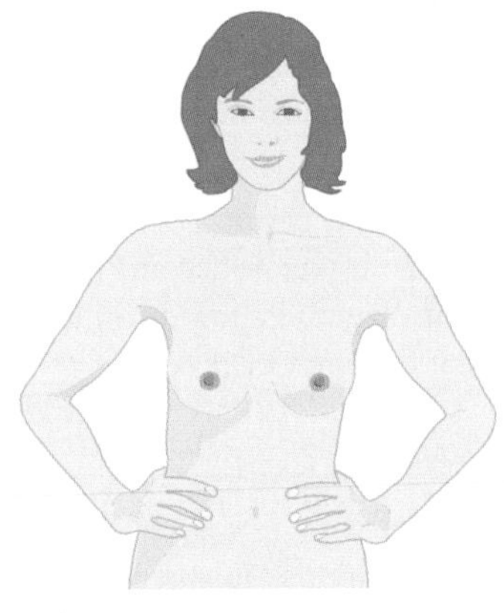

3. Place your hands on your hips and tighten your chest and arm muscles by pressing firmly.

Feeling

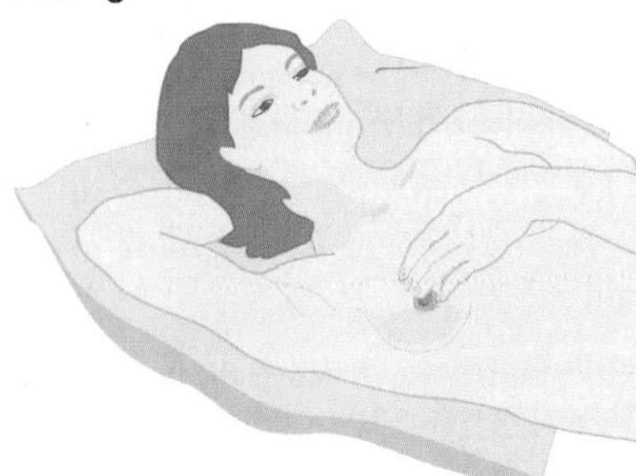

1. Lie flat on your back. Place a pillow or towel under one shoulder, and raise that arm over your head. With the opposite hand, you'll feel with the pads, not the fingertips, of the three middle fingers, for lumps or any change in the texture of the breast or skin.

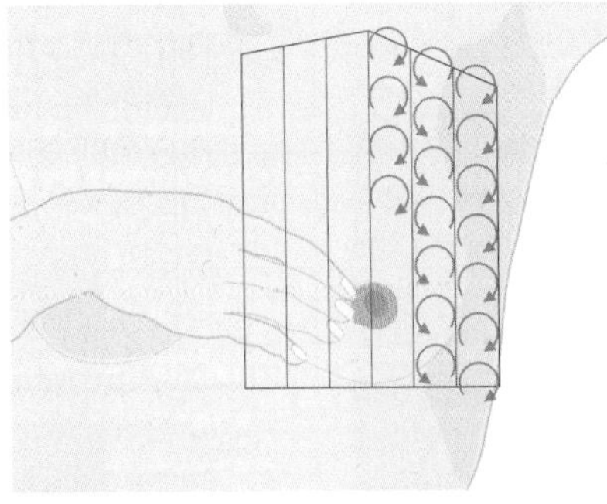

2. The area you'll examine is from your collarbone to your bra line and from your breastbone to the center of your armpit. Imagine the area divided into vertical strips. Using small circular motions (the size of a dime), move your fingers up and down the strips. Apply light, medium, and deep pressure to examine each spot. Repeat this same process for your other breast.

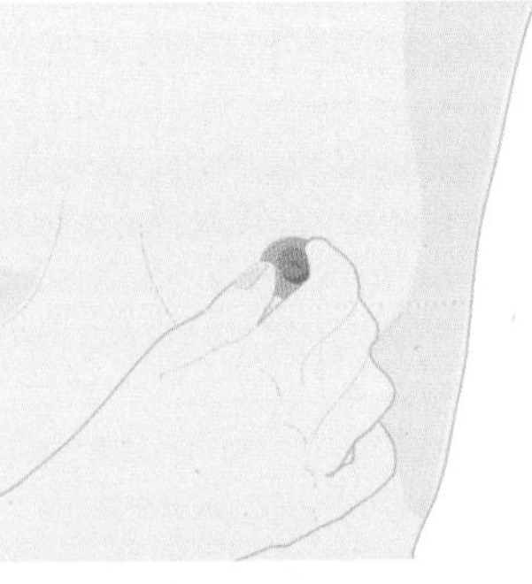

3. Gently squeeze the nipple of each breast between your thumb and index finger. Any discharge, clear or bloody, should be reported to your doctor immediately.

Source: From Hales, (with Profile Plus 2005, Health, Fitness and Wellness Explorer, and InfoTrac), 11e © 2005 Cengage Learning.

Men should not feel immune to breast cancer. Although not common in men, each year approximately 2,000 men in the United States are diagnosed with breast cancer and 400 die from it.

Cervical Cancer (Women)

Risk Factors

1. Human papilloma virus (HPV). The most significant risk factor for cervical cancer is infection with HPV, a group of more than 100 related viruses, some of which can cause cervical cancer. The virus is frequently transmitted through vaginal, anal, or oral sex; or simply by skin-to-skin contact with a body area infected with HPV. Most infected women do not develop cervical cancer, but other factors (described next) must be present for the cancer to develop.
2. Smoking. The risk doubles in women who smoke. Tobacco byproducts are found in cervical mucus of women who smoke.
3. Infections. Both human immunodeficiency virus (HIV) and chlamydia (bacterial infection—see Chapter 14) infections increase the risk for cervical cancer.
4. Diet. Low consumption of fruits and vegetables has been linked to higher cervical cancer risk.
5. Overweight. Women who are overweight are at higher risk.
6. Birth control pills. Long-term use of birth control pills increases the risk. The risk decreases once their use is stopped.
7. Pregnancies. Multiple pregnancies (three or more) increase the risk. Pregnancy prior to age 17 also increases the risk.
8. Family history. Cervical cancer may run in families, because women in families that have had this cancer are less able to fight off HPV.

Early detection through a Pap test during a pelvic exam should be performed annually in women who are or have been sexually active or who have reached the age of 18. Following three normal tests during three consecutive years, the Pap test may be done less frequently, at the discretion of the physician.

Endometrial Cancer (Women)

Risk Factors

1. Estrogen use. Cancer of the endometrium is associated with high cumulative exposure to estrogen. Obesity, a long menstral history, and hormone replacement therapy all increase estrogen exposure. You should consult your physician before starting or stopping any estrogen therapy.
2. Age. Endometrial cancer is seen in older age groups.
3. Race. White women have a higher occurrence but African American women have a higher incidence of death.
4. Family History. While the genetic source has not yet been identified, there are families with an increased risk for endometrial cancer. Other women who carry the genetic abnormalities for HNPCC (or Lynch syndrome) have a 40 to 60 percent risk of developing endometrial cancer.
5. Pregnancy. The fewer children the woman has delivered, the greater the risk for endometrial cancer.
6. Excessive weight. Women who are significantly overweight or obese are at greater risk.
7. Diabetes. Cancer of the endometrium is associated with diabetes.
8. Total number of menstrual cycles (periods). The greater the number of lifetime menstrual cycles (periods), the greater the risk.
9. Hypertension. Cancer of the endometrium is associated with high blood pressure.
10. Physical inactivity. The risk for endometrial cancer is higher among physically inactive women.

Prostate Cancer (Men) The prostate gland is actually a cluster of smaller glands that encircle the top section of the urethra (urinary channel) at the point where it leaves the bladder. Although the function of the prostate is not entirely clear, the muscles of these small glands help squeeze prostatic secretions into the urethra.

Risk Factors

1. Age. The highest incidence of prostate cancer is found in men over age 65 (more than 60 percent of cases).
2. Family history.
3. Race. African American men have the highest rate in the world.
4. Diet. A diet high in red meat or high-fat dairy products may increase the risk.
5. Physical inactivity. The risk may be greater in physically inactive men.

Prostate cancer is difficult to detect and control because the causes are not known. Death rates can be lowered through early detection and awareness of the warning signals. Detection is done by a digital rectal exam of the gland and a prostate-specific antigen (PSA) blood test once a year after the age of 50. Possible warning signals include difficulties in urination (especially at night), painful urination, blood in the urine, and constant pain in the lower back or hip area.

Factors that may decrease the risk include increasing the consumption of tomato-rich foods and fatty fish in the diet two or three times per week, avoiding a high-fat (especially animal fat) diet, increasing daily consumption of produce and grains, and maintaining

Mammogram Low-dose x-rays of the breasts used as a screening technique for the early detection of breast tumors.

recommended vitamin D intake (obtained through supplements, multivitamins, and fortified milk and manufactured by the body when exposed to sunlight). Vigorous exercise such as jogging or swimming has been shown to lower risk of advanced prostate cancer by as much as 70 percent in older men, and even brisk walking has been shown to halt the cancer's progression.

Testicular Cancer (Men) Testicular cancer accounts for only 1 percent of all male cancers, but it is the most common type of cancer seen in men between ages 15 and 34. The incidence is higher in Caucasians than in African Americans. If diagnosed early, this type of cancer is highly curable.

Risk Factors

1. Undescended testicle.
2. Abnormal testicle development.
3. Family history of testicular cancer.
4. Race. White American men have the highest rate (five times greater than African American and three times greater than Asian American and Native American men).

The incidence of testicular cancer is quite high in males born with an undescended testicle. Therefore, this condition should be corrected before puberty. The risk, however, remains high and individuals who had this condition should be vigilant.

Some warning signals associated with testicular cancer are a small lump on the testicle, slight enlargement (usually painless) and change in consistency of the testis, sudden buildup of blood or fluid in the scrotum, pain in the groin and lower abdomen or discomfort accompanied by a sensation of dragging and heaviness, breast enlargement or tenderness, and enlarged lymph glands.

Early diagnosis of testicular cancer is essential, because this type of cancer spreads rapidly to other parts of the body. Because in most cases no early symptoms or pain is associated with testicular cancer, most people do not see a physician for months after discovering a lump or a slightly enlarged testis. Unfortunately, this delay allows almost 90 percent of testicular cancer to metastasize (spread) before a diagnosis is made. TSE once a month following a warm bath or shower (when the scrotal skin is relaxed) is recommended. Guidelines for performing a TSE are given in Figure 12.13.

FIGURE 12.13 **Testicular self-examination.**

How to Examine the Testicles

You can increase your chances of early detection of testicular cancer by regularly performing a testicular self-examination (TSE). The following procedure is recommended:

- Perform the self-exam once a month. Select an easy day to remember such as the first day or first Sunday of the month.
- Learn how your testicle feels normally so that it will be easier to identify changes. A normal testicle should feel oval, smooth, and uniformly firm, like a hard-boiled egg.
- Perform TSE following a warm shower or bath, when the scrotum is relaxed.
- Gently roll each testicle between your thumb and the first three fingers until you have felt the entire surface. Pay particular attention to any lumps, change in size or texture, pain, or a dragging or heavy sensation since your last self-exam. Do not confuse the epididymis at the rear of the testicle for an abnormality.
- Bring any changes to the attention of your physician. A change does not necessarily indicate a malignancy, but only a physician is able to determine that.

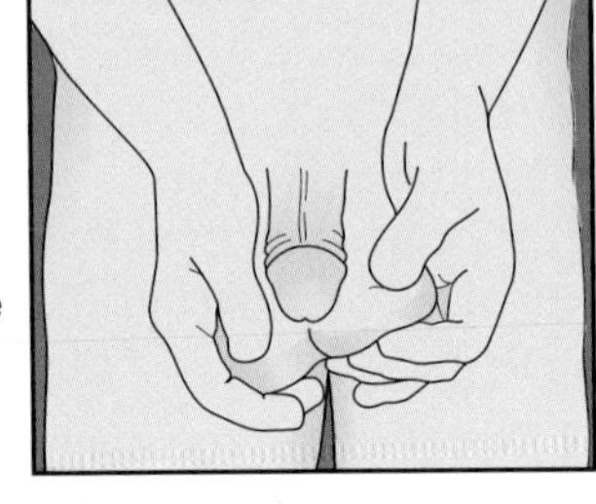

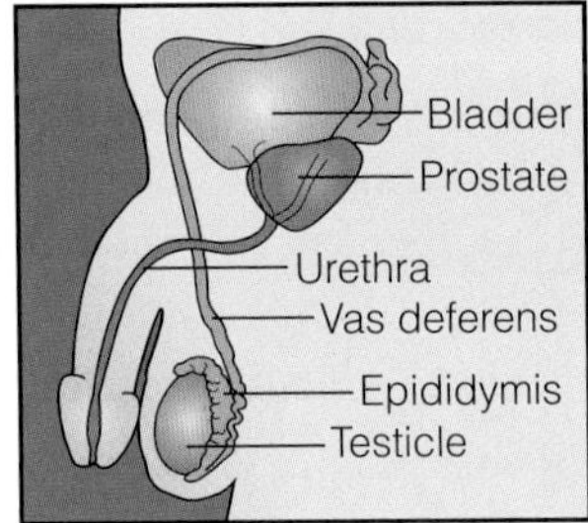

Pancreatic Cancer The pancreas is a thin gland that lies behind the stomach. This gland releases insulin and pancreatic juice. Insulin regulates blood sugar, and pancreatic juice contains enzymes that aid in digesting food.

Possible Risk Factors

1. The risk increases with age. Almost 90 percent of cases are seen in people older than 55.
2. BRCA2 mutations.
3. A family history of other cancers and syndromes, including melanoma and HNPCC or Lynch syndrome that share genes that could also cause pancreatic cancer.
4. Cigarette smoking, cigar smoking, and smokeless tobacco use significantly increase the risk.
5. Excessive sugar intake, which may increase the risk of developing pancreatic cancer by 70 percent.
6. Obesity.
7. Physical inactivity.
8. Chronic pancreatitis.
9. Cirrhosis.
10. Diabetes.
11. Family history.
12. African American race.

Detection of pancreatic cancer is difficult because (1) no symptoms are apparent in the early stages and (2) advanced disease symptoms are similar to those of other diseases. Only a biopsy can provide a definite diagnosis, but because pancreatic cancer is primarily a "silent" disease, the need for a biopsy is apparent only when the disease is already in an advanced stage.

Warning signals that may be related to pancreatic cancer include pain in the abdomen or lower back; jaundice; loss of weight and appetite; nausea; weakness, weariness, and loss of energy; agitated depression; dizziness; chills; muscle spasms; double vision; and coma.

Kidney and Bladder Cancer The kidneys are the organs that filter the urine, and the bladder stores and empties the urine. Most cases of these two types of cancer are caused by environmental factors. Bladder cancer occurs most frequently between the ages of 50 and 70. Of all bladder cancers, 80 percent are seen in men, and the incidence among Caucasian males is twice that among African American males.

Possible Risk Factors

1. Heavy cigarette smoking is responsible for almost half of all deaths from bladder cancer in men and one-third of deaths from bladder cancer in women.
2. Congenital abnormalities of either organ, detectable by a physician.
3. Exposure to certain chemical compounds, such as aniline dyes, naphthalenes, or benzidines, cadmium, some herbicides, and asbestos.
4. History of schistosomiasis, a parasitic bladder infection.
5. Frequent urinary-tract infections, particularly after age 50.
6. High blood pressure.
7. Family history.
8. Obesity.
9. The rate is higher in men.

Avoiding cigarette smoking and occupational exposure to cancer-causing chemicals is important to decrease the risk. Bloody urine, especially in repeated occurrences, is always a warning sign and requires immediate evaluation. Bladder cancer is diagnosed through urine analysis and examination of the bladder with a cystoscope (a small tube that is inserted into the tract through the urethra).

Oral Cancer

Oral cancer affects the mouth, lips, tongue, salivary glands, pharynx, larynx, and floor of the mouth. Most of these cancers seem to be related to cigarette smoking, tobacco use in general, and excessive consumption of alcohol.

Risk Factors

1. Heavy use of tobacco (cigarette, cigar, pipe, or smokeless).
2. Excessive alcohol consumption.
3. Excessive exposure to sunlight.

Regular examinations and good dental hygiene help prevention and early detection of oral cancer. Warning signals include a sore that doesn't heal or a white patch in the mouth, a lump in the mouth, problems with chewing and swallowing, loose teeth, or a constant feeling of having "something" in the throat. A person with any of these conditions should be evaluated by a physician or a dentist. A tissue biopsy normally is conducted to diagnose the presence of cancer.

Esophageal and Stomach Cancer The incidence of gastric cancer in the United States has dropped significantly the past few decades. Cancer experts attribute this drastic decrease to changes in dietary habits and refrigeration. This type of cancer is more common in men, and the incidence is higher in African American males than in Caucasian males.

Risk Factors

1. A diet low in fresh fruits and vegetables.
2. High consumption of salt-cured, smoked, and nitrate-cured foods.
3. Imbalance in stomach acid, heartburn, or gastroesophageal reflex disease.
4. History of pernicious anemia.
5. Chronic gastritis or gastric polyps.
6. Bacterial infection of *Helicobacter pylori* (*H. pylori*), which is also a cause of stomach ulcers.
7. Excessive body weight.
8. Tobacco and alcohol use.
9. Family history of these types of cancer.

Prevention is accomplished primarily by increasing dietary intake of complex carbohydrates and fiber and decreasing the intake of salt-cured, smoked, and nitrate-cured foods. In addition, regular guaiac testing for occult blood (hemoccult test) is recommended. Warning signals for this type of cancer include indigestion for 2 weeks or longer, blood in the stools, vomiting, and rapid weight loss.

Ovarian Cancer (Women) The ovaries are part of the female reproductive system that produces and releases the egg and the hormone estrogen. Ovarian cancer develops more frequently after menopause.

Risk Factors

1. Higher risk with age.
2. History of ovarian problems.
3. Inherited BRCA1 or BRCA2 mutations.
4. Estrogen postmenopausal hormone therapy.
5. Extensive history of menstrual irregularities.
6. Family history of ovarian or breast cancer as well as of cancers of the colon, rectum, or endometriosis.
7. Personal history of breast cancer.
8. Nulliparity (no pregnancies).
9. Excessive body weight.
10. HNPCC or Lynch syndrome

In most cases, ovarian cancer has no signs or symptoms. Therefore, regular pelvic examinations to detect signs of enlargement or other abnormalities are highly recommended.

Some warning signals may be bloating, an enlarged abdomen, lower abdominal or pelvic pressure or pain, abnormal vaginal bleeding, unexplained digestive disturbances, trouble eating or feeling full quickly, "normal"-size (premenopause-size) ovaries after menopause, and frequent or urgent urination without infection. The previous symptoms may happen sporadically, but if they are a change from "normal," occur more often, or worsen, consult your doctor. Mutations to the BRCA1 and BRCA2 genes are also a significant risk factor.

Thyroid Cancer The thyroid gland, located in the lower portion of the front of the neck, helps regulate growth and metabolism. Thyroid cancer occurs almost three times as often in women as in men. The incidence also is higher in Caucasians than African Americans.

Risk Factors

1. Age.
2. Radiation therapy of the head and neck region received in childhood or adolescence or exposure to high levels of radiation.
3. Family history of thyroid cancer.
4. Being female increases your risk.

Regular inspection for thyroid tumors is done by palpating the gland and surrounding areas during a physical examination. Thyroid cancer grows slowly; therefore, it is highly treatable. Nevertheless, any unusual lumps in front of the neck should be reported promptly to a physician. Although thyroid cancer does not have many warning signals (besides a lump), difficulty swallowing, choking, labored breathing, and persistent hoarseness are some potential signs.

Liver Cancer The incidence of liver cancer in the United States is low. Men are more prone than women to this cancer, and the disease is more common after age 60.

Risk Factors

1. History of cirrhosis of the liver.
2. History of hepatitis B or hepatitis C virus.
3. Exposure to vinyl chloride (industrial gas used in plastics manufacturing) and aflatoxin (a natural food contaminant).
4. Excessive alcohol consumption.
5. Race/ethnicity. Asian Americans and Pacific Islanders have the highest rate.

Prevention consists primarily of avoiding the risk factors and being aware of warning signals. Possible signs and symptoms are a lump or pain in the upper right abdomen (which may radiate into the back and shoulder), fever, nausea, rapidly deteriorating health, jaundice, and tenderness of the liver.

Leukemia Leukemia is a type of cancer that interferes with blood-forming tissues (bone marrow, lymph nodes, and spleen) by producing too many immature white blood cells. People who have leukemia cannot fight infection very well. The causes of leukemia are mostly unknown, although suspected risk factors have been identified.

Possible Risk Factors

1. Inherited susceptibility, but not transmitted directly from parent to child.
2. Greater incidence in individuals with Down syndrome (mongolism) and a few other genetic abnormalities.
3. Excessive exposure to ionizing radiation.
4. Environmental exposure to chemicals such as benzene, found in gasoline and cigarette smoke.

Detection is not easy because early symptoms can be associated with other serious ailments. When leukemia is suspected, the diagnosis is made through blood tests and a bone marrow biopsy.

Early warning signals include fatigue, pallor, weight loss, easy bruising, nosebleeds, loss of appetite, repeated infections, hemorrhages, night sweats, bone and joint pain, and fever. At a more advanced stage, fatigue increases, hemorrhages become more severe, pain and high fever continue, the gums swell, and various skin disorders occur.

Lymphoma Lymphomas are cancers of the lymphatic system. The lymphatic system consists of lymph nodes found throughout the body and a network of vessels that link these nodes. The lymphatic system participates in the body's immune reaction to foreign cells, substances, and infectious agents.

Possible Risk Factors

As with leukemia, the causes of lymphomas are unknown. Age is a strong risk factor. Because of the weakened immune system, the majority of cases are seen in people over 60. Individuals who have received organ transplants are at higher risk. Some researchers suspect that a form of herpesvirus (called Epstein-Barr virus) is active in the initial stages of lymphosarcomas. Risk for non-Hodgkin's lymphoma is higher in people who carry HIV and human T-cell leukemia/lymphoma virus I (HTLV-I). A family history increases the risk as well.

> **CRITICAL THINKING**
>
> You have learned about many of the risk factors for major cancer sites. How will this information affect your health choices in the future? Will it be valuable to you, or will you quickly forget all you have learned and remain in a contemplation stage of change at the end of this course?

Other researchers suggest that certain external factors may alter the immune system, making it more susceptible to the development and multiplication of cancer cells. Exposure to radiation, herbicides, organic solvents, and other chemicals may also increase risk, as may poor diet and insufficient physical inactivity.

BEHAVIOR MODIFICATION PLANNING

Lifestyle Factors That Decrease Cancer Risk

Do you have these healthy lifestyle factors working in your favor?

I PLAN TO	I DID IT	Factor	Function
❑	❑	Physical activity	Controls body weight, may influence hormone levels, strengthens the immune system.
❑	❑	Fiber	Contains anti-cancer substances, increases stool movement, blunts insulin secretion.
❑	❑	Fruits and vegetables	Contain phytonutrients and vitamins that thwart cancer.
❑	❑	Recommended weight	Helps control hormones that promote cancer.
❑	❑	Healthy grilling	Prevents formation of heterocyclic amines (HCAs) and polycyclic aromatic hydrocarbons (PAHs), both carcinogenic substances.
❑	❑	Tea	Contains polyphenols that neutralize free radicals, including epigallocatechin gallate (EGCG), which protects cells and the DNA from damage believed to cause cancer.
❑	❑	Spices	Provide phytonutrients and strengthen the immune system.
❑	❑	Vitamin D	Disrupts abnormal cell growth.
❑	❑	Monounsaturated fat	May contribute to cancer cell destruction.

Try It

In your Online Journal or class notebook, note ways you can incorporate all of these factors into your everyday lifestyle.

Prevention of lymphoma is limited because little is known about its causes. Enlargement of a lymph node or a cluster of lymph nodes is the first sign of lymphoma. Other signs and symptoms are an enlarged spleen or liver, weakness, fever, back or abdominal pain, nausea or vomiting, unexplained weight loss, unexplained itching and sweating, and fever at night that lasts a long time.

What Can You Do?

If you are at high risk for any form of cancer, you are advised to discuss this with your physician. "An ounce of prevention is worth a pound of cure." Although cardiovascular disease is the number-one killer in the United States, cancer is the number-one fear. Of all cancers, 60 to 80 percent are preventable, and about 50 percent are curable. Most cancers are lifestyle related, so being aware of the risk factors and following basic recommendations for preventing cancer will greatly decrease your risk for developing it.

ASSESS YOUR BEHAVIOR

CENGAGE brain.com To access course materials, including companion resources, please visit **www.cengagebrain.com**.

1. Are you physically active on most days of the week?
2. Does your diet include ample amounts of colorful fruits and vegetables and of fiber, and is it low in red and processed meats?
3. Are you aware of your family history of cancer?
4. Do you practice monthly breast self-examination (women) or testicular self-examination (men)?
5. Do you respect the sun's rays? Do you use sunscreen lotion or wear protective clothing when you are in the sun for extended periods of time? Do you perform regular skin self-examinations?
6. Do you avoid all forms of tobacco and exposure to secondhand smoke?
7. Are you familiar with the seven warning signals of cancer?

ASSESS YOUR KNOWLEDGE

1. Cancer can be defined as
   a. a process whereby some cells invade and destroy the immune system.
   b. uncontrolled growth and spread of abnormal cells.
   c. the spread of benign tumors throughout the body.
   d. interference of normal body functions through blood flow disruption caused by angiogenesis.
   e. All of the choices are correct.
2. Cancer treatment becomes more difficult when
   a. cancer cells metastasize.
   b. angiogenesis is disrupted.
   c. a tumor is encapsulated.
   d. cells are deficient in telomerase.
   e. cell division has stopped.
3. The leading cause of deaths from cancer in women is
   a. lung cancer.
   b. breast cancer.
   c. ovarian cancer.
   d. skin cancer.
   e. endometrial cancer.
4. Cancer
   a. is primarily a preventable disease.
   b. is often related to tobacco use.
   c. has been linked to dietary habits.
   d. has risk that increases with obesity.
   e. All of the choices are correct.
5. About 60 percent of cancers are related to
   a. genetics.
   b. environmental pollutants.
   c. viruses and other biological agents.
   d. UV radiation.
   e. diet, obesity, and tobacco use.
6. A cancer-prevention diet should include
   a. ample amounts of fruits and vegetables.
   b. cruciferous vegetables.
   c. phytonutrients.
   d. soy products.
   e. All of the choices are correct.
7. The biggest carcinogenic exposure in the workplace is to
   a. asbestos fibers.
   b. cigarette smoke.
   c. biological agents.
   d. nitrosamines.
   e. pesticides.
8. Which of the following is not a warning signal for cancer?
   a. Change in bowel or bladder habits
   b. Nagging cough or hoarseness
   c. A sore that does not heal
   d. Indigestion or difficulty in swallowing
   e. All of the choices are warning signals for cancer.
9. The risk for breast cancer is higher in
   a. women under age 50.
   b. women with more than one family member with a history of breast cancer.
   c. minority groups than in white women.
   d. women who had children prior to age 30.
   e. All of the choices are correct.
10. The risk for prostate cancer can be decreased by
   a. being physically active.
   b. adding fatty fish to the diet.
   c. avoiding a high-fat diet.
   d. increasing daily consumption of produce and grains.
   e. All of the choices are correct.

Correct answers can be found at the back of the book.

NOTES

1. American Cancer Society, *2014 Cancer Facts and Figures* (New York: ACS, 2014).
2. L. H. Kushi et al., "American Cancer Society Guidelines on Nutrition and Physical Activity for Cancer Prevention," *CA: A Cancer Journal for Clinicians* 62, no. 5 (2012): 30–67.
3. J. E. Enstrom, "Health Practices and Cancer Mortality among Active California Mormons," *Journal of the National Cancer Institute* 81 (1989): 1807–1814.
4. A. S. Ford et al., "Healthy Living is the Best Revenge: Findings from the European Prospective Investigation into Cancer and Nutrition—Potsdam Study," *Archives of Internal Medicine* 169 (2009): 1355–1362.
5. See note 1.
6. American Institute for Cancer Reasearch, "Halving Cancer Deaths with AICR Recommendations for Prevention," *Cancer Research Update,* March 5, 2014.
7. Y. Park et al., "Dietary Fiber Intake and Risk of Colorectal Cancer," *Journal of the American Medical Association* 294 (2005): 2849–2857.
8. V. W. Setiawan et al., "Protective Effect of Green Tea on the Risks of Chronic Gastritis and Stomach Cancer," *International Journal of Cancer* 92 (2001): 600–604.
9. L. Mitscher and V. Dolby, *The Green Tea Book—China's Fountain of Youth* (New York: Avery Press, 1997).
10. "Curbing Cancer's Reach: Little Things That Might Make a Big Difference," *Environmental Nutrition* 29, no. 6 (2006): 1, 6; American Institute for Cancer Reasearch, "The Spices of Cancer Prevention," *Cancer Research Update,* August 21, 2013.
11. S. C. Larsson, L. Bergkvist, and A. Wolk, "Consumption of Sugar-Sweetened Foods and the Risk of Pancreatic Cancer in a Prospective Study," *American Journal of Clinical Nutrition* 84 (2006): 1171–1176.
12. N. E. Allen et al., "Moderate Alcohol Intake and Cancer Incidence in Women," *Journal of the National Cancer Institute* 101 (2009): 296–305.
13. See note 1.

14. E. E. Calle, C. Rodriguez, K. Walker-Thurmond, and M. J. Thun, "Overweight, Obesity, and Mortality from Cancer in a Prospectively Studied Cohort of U.S. Adults," *New England Journal of Medicine* 348 (2003): 1625–1638.

15. American Institute for Cancer Reasearch, "As Cancer Increases, New Estimates on Preventability," *Cancer Research Update,* February 5, 2014.

16. See note 1.

17. S. E. Whitmore, W. L. Morison, C. S. Potten, and C. Chadwick, "Tanning Salon Exposure and Molecular Alterations," *Journal of the American Academy of Dermatology* 44 (2001): 775–780.

18. C. A. Thomson and P. A. Thomson, "Healthy Lifestyle and Cancer Prevention," *ACSM's Health & Fitness Journal* 12, no. 3 (2008): 18–26.

19. S. W. Farrell et al., "Cardiorespiratory Fitness, Different Measures of Adiposity, and Cancer Mortality in Men," *Obesity* 15 (2007): 3140–3149.

20. L. Byberg et al., "Total Mortality After Changes in Leisure Time Physical Activity in 50 Year Old Men: 35 Year Follow-up of Population Based Cohort," *British Medical Journal* (2009): 338, doi 10.1136.

21. E. L. Giovannucci, "A Prospective Study of Physical Activity and Incident and Fatal Prostate Cancer," *Archives of Internal Medicine* 165 (2005): 1005–1010.

22. L. Ratnasinghe et al., *Exercise and Breast Cancer Risk: A Multinational Study* (Beltsville, MD: Genomic Nanosystems, BioServe Biotechnologies, 2009).

23. C. W. Matthews et al., "Physical Activity and Risk of Endometrial Cancer: A Report from the Shanghai Endometrial Cancer Study," *Cancer Epidemiology Biomarkers & Prevention* 14 (2005): 779–785.

24. M. D. Holmes et al., "Physical Activity and Survival after Breast Cancer Diagnosis," *Journal of the American Medical Association* 293 (2005): 2479–2486.

25. J. R. Ruiz, "Muscular Strength and Adiposity as Predictors of Adulthood Cancer Mortality in Men," *Cancer Epidemiology, Biomarkers & Prevention* 18 (2009): 1468–1476.

26. D. Servan-Schreiber, "The Anticancer Life Plan," *Bottom Line Health* 23, no. 5 (May 2009).

SUGGESTED READINGS

American Cancer Society. *2012 Cancer Facts and Figures.* New York: ACS, 2012.

"Dietary Do's and Don'ts from the Latest Research on Cancer Prevention." *Tufts University Health & Nutrition Letter* 27, no. 5 (July 2009).

"Eating to Beat Cancer." Special Supplement to the *Tufts University Health & Nutrition Letter* 25, no. 3 (May 2007).

U.S. Department of Health and Human Services, National Institutes of Health, National Cancer Institute. *Reducing Environmental Cancer Risk: What We Can Do Now.* Washington, DC: President's Cancer Panel, April 2010.

World Cancer Research Fund and American Institute for Cancer Research. *Food, Nutrition, Physical Activity and the Prevention of Cancer: A Global Perspective.* Washington, DC: WCRF/AICR, 2007.

Lab 12A: Cancer Prevention Guidelines

Name ______________________ Date __________ Grade __________

Instructor ______________________ Course __________ Section __________

NECESSARY LAB EQUIPMENT
None required.

OBJECTIVE
To encourage healthy lifestyle practices that will help decrease the risk for cancer.

I. Cancer Prevention: Are You Taking Control?

Today, scientists think most cancers may be related to lifestyle and environment—what you eat and drink, whether you smoke, and where you work and play. The good news, then, is that you can help reduce your own cancer risk by taking control of things in your daily life.

12 Steps to a Healthier Life and Reduced Cancer Risk	Yes	No
1. **Are you eating more cabbage-family vegetables?** They include broccoli, cauliflower, Brussels sprouts, all cabbages, and kale.	☐	☐
2. **Does your diet include high-fiber foods?** Fiber is found in whole grains, fruits, and vegetables including peaches, strawberries, potatoes, spinach, tomatoes, wheat and bran cereals, rice, popcorn, and whole-wheat bread.	☐	☐
3. **Do you choose foods with vitamin A?** Fresh foods with beta-carotene, including carrots, peaches, apricots, squash, and broccoli, are the best source—not vitamin pills.	☐	☐
4. **Is vitamin C included in your diet?** You'll find it naturally in lots of fresh fruits and vegetables, including grapefruit, cantaloupe, oranges, strawberries, red and green peppers, broccoli, and tomatoes.	☐	☐
5. **Are you physically active for at least 30 minutes every day and do you avoid excessive sitting on most days of the week?** Total number of daily steps: ☐ Total minutes of daily physical activity: ☐	☐	☐
6. **Do you maintain healthy weight (a BMI between 18.5 and 25)?**	☐	☐
7. **Do you limit salt-cured, smoked, nitrite-cured foods?** Choose bacon, ham, hot dogs, or salt-cured fish only occasionally if you like them a lot.	☐	☐
8. **If you smoke, have you tried quitting?**	☐	☐
9. **If you drink alcohol at all, is your intake moderate (no more than two drinks per day for men and one per day for women)?**	☐	☐
10. **Do you get almost daily "safe sun" exposure, and yet respect the sun's rays?** "Safe sun" exposure means 10 to 20 minutes of unprotected sun exposure (without sunscreen) to the face, arms, and hands during peak daylight hours on most days of the week. If not, do you take a daily vitamin D_3 supplement?	☐	☐
Do you protect yourself with sunscreen (at least SPF 15) and wear long sleeves and a hat, especially during midday hours (10 a.m. to 4 p.m.) if you are going to be exposed to the sun for a prolonged period?	☐	☐
11. **Do you have a family history of any type of cancer? If so, have you brought this to the attention of your personal physician?**	☐	☐
12. **Are you familiar with the seven warning signals for cancer?**	☐	☐

If you answered "yes" to most of these questions, **congratulations.** You are taking control of simple lifestyle factors that will help you feel better and reduce your risk for cancer.

Source: Adapted from the American Cancer Society, Texas Division.

Lab 12B: Early Signs of Illness

Name ______________________ Date ____________ Grade ____________

Instructor ______________________ Course ____________ Section ____________

NECESSARY LAB EQUIPMENT
None required.

OBJECTIVE
To encourage early recognition of symptoms to improve the chances for cure or control

Major illnesses often begin with minor symptoms that if recognized early, allow you to control or cure the condition. In many cases, nothing is seriously wrong. Should you experience any of the following symptoms, however, you are strongly encouraged to bring them to the attention of your physician as soon as possible. In the following statements, please check only the conditions that apply.

- ☐ 1. Persistent unusual fatigue.
- ☐ 2. Sudden change in sleeping habits or feeling sleepy most of the day.
- ☐ 3. Sudden unexplained weight gain or loss (about 6 to 10 lb. in 10 weeks).
- ☐ 4. Pain or discomfort anywhere in the body that is not easily explained.
- ☐ 5. Severe headaches with no apparent reason.
- ☐ 6. A sore anywhere in the body that does not heal within a month.
- ☐ 7. Changes in moles, warts, or a skin blemish that begin to bleed, itch, or change in color, shape, or size.
- ☐ 8. Difficulty in swallowing, sudden vomiting occurrences, vomiting blood, or blood in coughed-up phlegm.
- ☐ 9. Shortness of breath or pain in the chest that may radiate to the jaw, shoulders, arms, or between the shoulder blades.
- ☐ 10. Fainting spells without reason.
- ☐ 11. Blurred vision or changes in vision such as seeing haloes.
- ☐ 12. Hoarseness or loss of voice without apparent reason that lasts several days.
- ☐ 13. A nagging cough that is getting worse.
- ☐ 14. Excessive thirst.
- ☐ 15. Swelling in the limbs/ankles or abdomen.
- ☐ 16. Persistent indigestion or abdominal pain.
- ☐ 17. A significant change in bowel habits, interchanging attacks of diarrhea and constipation.
- ☐ 18. Bowel movements that look unusually dark or rectal bleeding.
- ☐ 19. In men, discomfort/difficulty urinating, cloudy or reddish-looking urine, or discharge from the tip of the penis.
- ☐ 20. In women, vaginal bleeding or spotting between regular menstrual periods or following menopause.
- ☐ 21. In women, a lump or unusual thickening in a breast, changes in the shape or size of the breast, dimpling of the skin, "depression" of the nipples, any alteration in the breast noticeable by a change in position of the body, or any clear or bloody discharge after gently squeezing each nipple between your thumb and index finger .
- ☐ 22. Excessive sweating.

Source: Fitness & Wellness, Inc.

Lab 12C: Cancer Risk Profile

Name ______________________ Date ____________ Grade ____________

Instructor ______________________ Course ____________ Section ____________

NECESSARY LAB EQUIPMENT
None required.

OBJECTIVE
To determine your risk for selected cancer sites.

I. Cancer Risk Profile

Instructions—Read the section "Cancer: Assessing Your Risks" (beginning on page 471) and complete the Cancer Questionnaire: Assessing Your Risks in Figure 12.9 (pages 472–73). Rate yourself on a scale from 1 to 3 (1 = low risk, 2 = moderate risk, 3 = high risk) according to the risk factors provided for each site and write the scores and risk categories in the blanks provided below.

Cancer Site	Total Points		Risk Category
	Men	Women	
Lung	☐	☐	☐
Colon-Rectum	☐	☐	☐
Skin	☐	☐	☐
Breast		☐	☐
Cervical		☐	☐
Endometrial		☐	☐
Prostate	☐		
Testicular	☐		
Pancreatic	☐	☐	☐
Kidney and Bladder	☐	☐	☐
Oral	☐	☐	☐
Esophageal and Stomach	☐	☐	☐
Ovarian		☐	
Thyroid	☐	☐	☐
Liver	☐	☐	☐
Leukemia	☐	☐	☐
Lymphomas	☐	☐	☐

II. Stage of Change for Cancer Prevention

Using Figure 2.6 (page 66) and Table 2.3 (page 65), identify your current stage of change for participation in a cancer-prevention program:

III. Personal Interpretation

In the space provided below, discuss your results for the various cancer sites. State your feelings about cancer and comment on any experiences that you may have had with cancer patients.

IV. Cancer Prevention

Discuss lifestyle habits that you should eliminate and habits that you need to adopt to reduce your own risk of cancer. Also indicate how you can best implement and adhere to these changes.

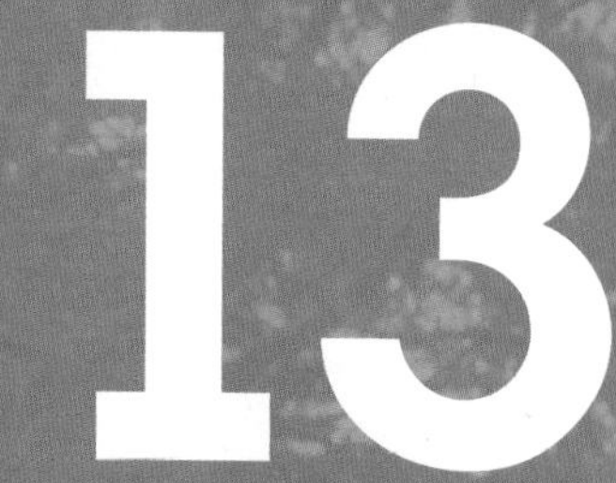

Addictive Behavior

Addictive behaviors are lifetime nightmares that focus on immediate self-gratification without thought or concern for one's well-being or that of others. Ultimately, it takes away the control the person has over life itself.

OBJECTIVES

- Address the detrimental effects of addictive substances, including psychotherapeutics, inhalants, marijuana, cocaine, methamphetamine, MDMA (Ecstasy), heroin, new psychoactive substances (NPS), and alcohol.
- List the detrimental health effects of tobacco use.
- Recognize cigarette smoking as the largest preventable cause of premature illness and death in the United States.
- Enumerate the reasons people smoke.
- Explain the benefits and the significance of a smoking-cessation program.
- Learn how to implement a smoking-cessation program to help yourself (if you smoke) or someone else go through the quitting process.

CENGAGE brain.com

Visit **www.cengagebrain.com** to access course materials and companion resources for this text, including digital labs, quiz questions designed to check your understanding of the chapter contents, and more! See the preface on page xii for more information.

REAL LIFE STORY | Jose's Experience

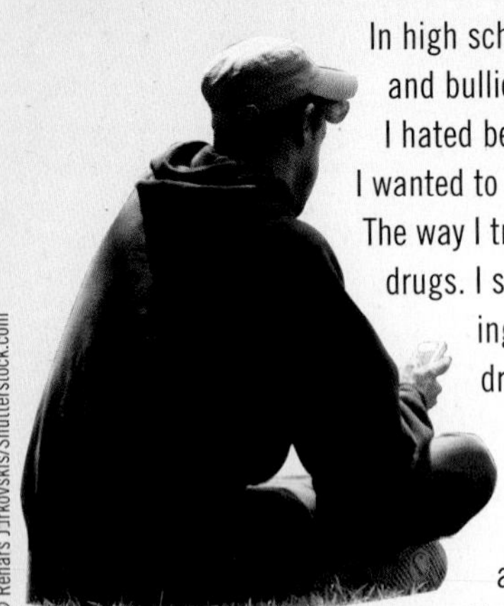
© Renars Jurkovskis/Shutterstock.com

In high school I used to get teased and bullied a lot. It was so bad that I hated being the person I was, and I wanted to become somebody else. The way I tried to do that was through drugs. I started out drinking and doing marijuana. When I was drunk or high, I felt calm, confident, and popular. My self-doubts and self-hatred would go away for a while. The problem was, the bad feelings always came back. Eventually, some friends offered me meth, so I tried it. For me, the effects of meth were very intense. When I was using it, I felt like the king of the world. As soon as it wore off, I felt so horrible; I would do pretty much anything just to feel better again. That began a period of a couple years where meth crowded out everything else in my life. I stopped caring about school and about any goals I had for the future. I didn't care if I disappointed my parents or my friends. I didn't even care anymore about my younger brother, and he has always been my best friend and one of the people I love most in the world. Meth just completely took over my life. I dropped out of school and left home for several months. I camped out with several other addicts where we set up our own meth lab. We lived in really filthy conditions. Eventually I got disgusted with the way I was living, and I became terrified by the fact that I needed bigger and bigger doses of meth for a high that lasted only a fraction of the amount of time it used to. No matter how much I used, I was miserable much more often than I felt good. I finally moved back home and reached out for help to overcome my addiction. At first, I attended 12-step meetings almost constantly, and I finally managed to get clean. Now, the fact that I was able to go back and get my high school diploma, and now am in college, is a miracle to me. I have a second chance to make something of my life. That chance could easily have been lost forever due to drugs.

Substance abuse remains one of the most serious health problems afflicting society. Chemical dependency is extremely destructive, having ruined and ended millions of lives. When addictive behaviors are an issue, education is vital—more, perhaps, than with any other unhealthy behavior. Education concerning addiction may assist in the search for answers, treatment, and a more productive and better life. The information in this chapter will help you make informed decisions. The time to make healthy choices is *now*.

Addiction

When most people think of **addiction**, they probably think of dark and dirty alleys, an addict shooting drugs into a vein, or a wino passed out next to a garbage can after having spent an evening drinking alcohol. Psychotherapists have described addiction as a problem of imbalance or unease within the body and mind.

Almost anything can be addicting. Of the many types of addiction, some addictive behaviors are more detrimental than others. The most serious form is chemical dependency on drugs such as tobacco, alcohol, cocaine, methamphetamine, MDMA (Ecstasy), heroin, marijuana, or prescription drugs. Less serious are addictions to work, coffee, shopping, and even exercise.

People who are addicted to food eat to release stress or boredom, or to reward themselves for every small personal achievement. Many people are addicted to television and the Internet. Others become so addicted to their jobs that all they think about is work. It may start out as enjoyable, but when it totally consumes a person's life, work can become an unhealthy behavior. If you find that you are readily irritated, moody, grouchy, constantly tired, not as alert as you used to be, or making more mistakes than usual, you may be becoming a workaholic and need to slow down or take time off work.

Even though exercise has enhanced the health and quality of life of millions of people, a relatively small number become obsessed with exercise, which has the potential for overuse and addiction. Compulsive exercisers feel guilty and uncomfortable when they miss a day's workout. Often, they continue to exercise even when they have injuries and sicknesses that require proper rest for adequate recovery. People who exceed the recommended guidelines to develop and maintain fitness (see Chapters 6–9) are exercising for reasons other than health—including addictive behavior.

Addiction to caffeine can have undesirable side effects. Caffeine is the most widely consumed psychoactive drug, and according to the FDA, 80 percent of adults in the United States consume caffeine daily. In some individuals, caffeine doses in excess of 200 to 500 milligrams (mg) can produce an abnormally rapid heart rate, abnormal heart rhythms, higher blood pressure, and increased secretion of gastric acids, leading to stomach problems and possible birth defects in offspring. Too much caffeine can cause jitteriness and insomnia, and induce symptoms of anxiety, depression, nervousness, and dizziness.

The caffeine content of drinks

Addiction Compulsive and uncontrollable behavior(s) or use of substance(s).

MyProfile: Addictive Behavior Survey

To the best of your ability, answer the following questions. If you do not know the answer(s), this chapter will guide you through them.

I. Have you ever suffered from addiction to any legal or illicit drug? ___ Yes ___ No What helped you overcome the addictive behavior? If you have not yet overcome it, are you ready to do so? ___ Yes ___ No Do you know where to turn for assistance? ___ Yes ___ No ____________________

____

____

II. Do you regularly—weekly or nearly weekly—exceed the recommended one to two alcoholic beverages per day? ___ Yes ___ No Do you understand potential health, personal, and family implications associated with alcohol abuse? ___ Yes ___ No

III. Have you decided to forgo instant gratification and peer pressure by saying "no" to substance abuse (legal or illicit) that may or will harm your health and long-term life satisfaction? ___ Yes ___ No What led to this decision, and how long ago did you make this choice? ____________________

____

____

____

IV. What are your feelings about tobacco use in general and exposure to secondhand smoke in particular? ____________

____

____

____

V. If you smoked cigarettes, have you quit? ___ Yes ___ No If you never smoked, have you helped someone else successfully kick the habit? ___ Yes ___ No If you answered "yes" to either, what approach did you use? Why were you successful in accomplishing this goal?____________

____

____

____

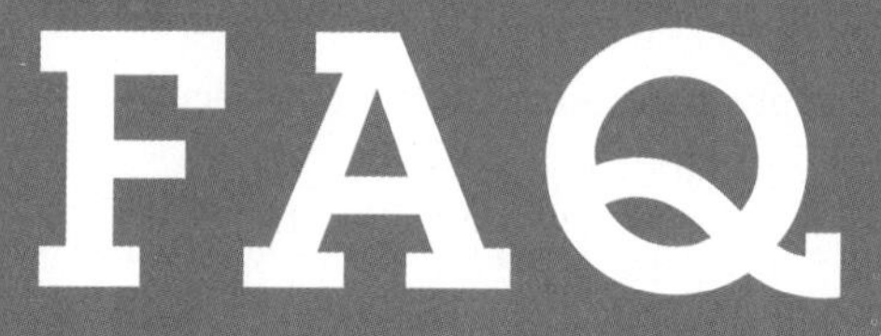

What is drug addiction, and how quickly can someone become addicted to drugs?

Drug addiction (addictive behavior, substance abuse, or chemical dependency) is a complex brain disease that over time can alter brain structure and function, and is characterized by compulsive and uncontrollable drug cravings even at the peril of serious negative consequences. How quickly addictive behavior develops cannot be predicted. There are vast individual differences among people in sensitivity to different drugs.

Psychological and physiological factors, as well as the type of drug used, influence a person's response to the drug and subsequent addiction to it. Whereas one individual may use a certain drug several times without harmful effects, someone else may seriously overdose the first time the same drug is used. All drugs have potentially damaging effects, and some have life-threatening consequences. One moment of weakness, or caving in to peer pressure, can easily result in a lifetime nightmare, not just for users but for everyone around them as well.

How can I tell if someone is addicted to drugs?

People with addictive behavior compulsively seek and use drugs despite potential serious repercussions, such as physical and family problems, loss of a job, or problems with the law. Some individuals realize that they need to cut down on their drinking or drug use, or they are told to do so by others. At times, they crave alcohol or drugs when they first get up in the morning and they feel bad or guilty about their addictive behavior. If you see any of these signs in someone you know, that person most likely has an addiction.

How is drug addiction treated?

In the early stages of substance abuse, most people believe that they can stop using the drug(s) on their own. Most of these attempts, however, fail to achieve long-term abstinence. Long-term drug use results in altered brain functions that linger long after the person stops using drugs. Effective treatment of drug addiction is rarely accomplished without professional help. Treatment modalities are behavioral-based therapies, oftentimes combined with medication to help the body detoxify and effectively manage symptoms of withdrawal. Responses to these therapies vary among individuals, and several courses of rehab may be necessary to overcome the problem. For some individuals, it becomes a lifetime battle, and relapses are possible even after prolonged periods of abstinence.

varies according to the product. In 8 ounces of coffee, for example, the content varies from 93 mg in instant coffee to as high as 133 mg in brewed coffee. Soft drinks, mainly colas, range in caffeine content from about 58 to 90 mg per 20-ounce bottle. The Food and Drug Administration (FDA) states that 400 mg of caffeine per day—the amount in about 4 to 5 cups of coffee—is safe as a stimulant for most healthy adults.

For energy drinks, the FDA requires caffeine to be listed on the label, but it does not mandate that the amount of caffeine be specified. Top-selling energy drinks on the market, such as Red Bull, Full Throttle, Monster, NOS, Amp, and Rockstar, have a caffeine content in the range of 71 to 224 mg per serving (about 8 ounces). Be aware that the larger 16-ounce cans contain two servings and twice the amount of caffeine. Popular 2 to 2.5-ounce five-hour energy shots range from 78 to 242 mg per serving,[1] which, on the high end, is about the amount of caffeine in two cups of coffee.

Emergency room (ER) visits involving energy drink consumption doubled between 2007 to 2011, and the trend continues to escalate. In 2011, there were some 20,000 energy drink–related ER visits, a 36 percent increase over 2010. More than half of these ER visits (58 percent) were directly attributed to energy drink consumption only. Reported symptoms in the ER include lightheadedness, headaches, dizziness, and heart palpitations.

Teens who consume energy drinks—about one-third of adolescents in the United States—report higher rates of drug, alcohol, and cigarette use.[2] Among college students, research indicates that consumption of energy drinks is linked to precarious behaviors such as illicit drug use, violence, smoking, prescription drug use, and sexual risk taking. Mixing energy drinks with alcohol is also a concerning college trend. A common misconception among young people is that energy drinks allow them to consume more alcohol because the energy drinks keep them awake longer. High consumption of caffeine can conceal the sedative effects of intoxication, making people who mix energy drinks with alcohol more likely to drive while drunk. Some erroneously believe that caffeine can help counteract the effects of drinking, making it safe to drive. Data also indicate that men are more likely to mix energy drinks with alcohol and illicit drugs, whereas women mix alcohol with pharmaceuticals.

Caffeine is now advertised as an energy booster and is added to a variety of other food items such as energy bars, candy, gum, waffles, syrup, and even oatmeal. This trend is quite alarming to the FDA. Individuals who are caffeine sensitive should read all food labels for potential caffeine in those items.

Although previous examples may be the first addictions you think of, they are by no means the only forms. Other addictions can be to gambling, pornography, sex, people, places, and more.

According to the 2012 National Survey on Drug Use and Health (NSDUH) by the U.S. Department of Health and Human Services, more than 23.9 million Americans use illicit drugs, including marijuana, prescription-type psychotherapeutics used non-medically, cocaine, hallucinogens, inhalants, and heroin[3] (Figure 13.1). North America has the world's largest illicit drug market, and for most drugs, has use rates much higher than the global average. The U.S. Office of National Drug Control Policy reports that each year, Americans spend nearly $100 billion on illegal drugs, with an additional cost to taxpayers of $193 billion in lost productivity, health care, criminal justice, and drug enforcement costs.[4]

Risk Factors for Addiction

Although addictive behaviors cover a wide spectrum, they have factors in common that predispose people to addiction. Among these factors are the following[5]:

- The behavior is reinforced.
- The addiction is an attempt to meet basic human needs, such as physical needs, the need to feel safe, the need to belong, the need to feel important, or the need to reach one's potential.
- The addiction seems to relieve stress temporarily.
- The addiction results from peer pressure.
- The addiction can be present within the person's value system (for example, a person whose values wouldn't let him or her shoot heroin may be able to rationalize compulsive eating or obsessive playing of computer games).
- A serious physical illness is present, and the addiction may provide escape from pain or fear of disfigurement.
- The addict feels pressured to perform or succeed.
- The addict has self-hate.
- A genetic link is present. Heredity might dictate susceptibility to some addictions.
- Society allows addiction. Advertising even encourages it (you can sleep better with a pill, snacking helps you enjoy life more fully, parties and sports are more fun with alcohol, shop 'til you drop, and so on).

FIGURE 13.1 Illicit drug use among Americans age 12 and older, 2012.

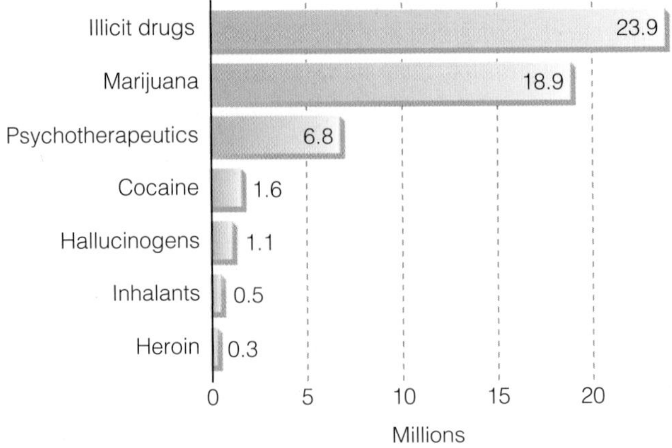

Source: http://www.samhsa.gov/data/NSDUH/2012SummNatFindDetTables/NationalFindings/NSDUHresults2012.htm#fig2.1, downloaded April 1, 2014.

The same general traits and behaviors are involved in all kinds of addictions, whether they involve food, sex, gambling, shopping, or drugs.

Most people with addictions deny their problem. Even when the addiction is clear to people around them, addicts continue to deny that they are addicted. Instead, they tend to get angry when someone tries to talk about the behavior and are likely to make excuses for their actions. Many addicts blame others for their problem. In some cases, addicts admit their problem but fail to take any steps to change.

Recognizing that all forms of addiction are unhealthy, this chapter focuses on some of today's most self-destructive addictive substances: psychotherapeutics, inhalants, marijuana, cocaine, methamphetamine, MDMA (Ecstasy), heroin, new psychoactive substances (NPS), alcohol, and tobacco. About half a million Americans die each year from tobacco, alcohol, and illegal drug use.

Drugs and Dependence

A drug is any substance that alters the user's ability to function. Drugs encompass over-the-counter drugs, prescription medications, and illegal substances. Many drugs lead to physical and psychological dependence.

Any drug can be misused and abused. "Drug misuse" implies the intentional and inappropriate use of over-the-counter or prescribed medications.[6] Examples include taking more medication than prescribed, mixing drugs, not following prescription instructions, or discontinuing a drug prior to a physician's approval. "Drug abuse" is the intentional and inappropriate use of a drug, resulting in physical, emotional, financial, intellectual, social, spiritual, or occupational consequences of the abuse.[7] Many substances, if used in the wrong manner, can be abused.

When drugs are used regularly, they integrate into the body's chemistry, increasing the user's tolerance to the drug and forcing the user to increase the dosage constantly to obtain similar results. Drug abuse leads to serious health problems, and more than half of all adolescent suicides are drug related. Often, drug abuse opens the gate to other illegal activities. According to the National Center on Addiction and Substance Abuse, the majority of convicted criminals—about 85 percent of federal and state inmates—have abused drugs.

According to the U.S. Department of Education, today's drugs are stronger and more addictive, and they pose a greater risk than ever before. Alcohol, tobacco, and illegal drug use lead to many negative health-related consequences—including cancers, cardiovascular diseases, stroke, bacterial endocarditis, fatal and nonfatal overdose, hepatitis, human immunodeficiency virus (HIV) infection and acquired immune deficiency syndrome (AIDS), and other sexually transmitted infections. Substance abuse is also linked to increased risk of intentional and unintentional injuries, complications in pregnancy and delivery, and psychiatric disturbances, ranging from acute panic attacks to chronic mood disturbances. Furthermore, illegal drug use is associated with negative effects on employment, school achievement, socioeconomic status, and family stability; if only because illegal drug use, once detected, can lead to school suspension or expulsion and to arrest, conviction, and incarceration for drug-related crimes.[8]

If you are uncertain about addictive behavior(s) in your life, the Addictive Behavior Questionnaire in Lab 13A can help you identify a potential problem. Some of the most commonly abused drugs in our society are discussed next.

DIVERSITY CONSIDERATIONS

Evidence exists of disparities in illegal drug use among different racial and ethnic-minority groups. Caucasians have the highest rate of alcohol and smokeless tobacco use. Hispanics are more likely to abuse alcohol and engage in binge drinking. African Americans are more likely than Caucasians or Hispanics to use cocaine and heroin. It is difficult to assess all of the complex and sometimes reciprocal linkages between the illegal drug use and the many negative health and social experiences, but there is little doubt that illegal drug use contributes to an increased probability of arrest, conviction, and incarceration for members of racial and ethnic-minority populations in the United States and to associated health and social disparities. As such, illegal drug use is linked either directly or indirectly to these disparities.

Source: U.S. Department of Health and Human Services, (Bethesda, MD: DHHS, National Institutes of Health, National Institute on Drug Abuse, Division of Epidemiology, Services & Prevention Research, 2003).

Nonmedical Use of Prescription Drugs

Fifty-four million Americans aged 12 or older have reported nonmedical use of psychotherapeutic drugs at some point in their lifetime. Psychotherapeutic drugs include any prescription pain reliever, tranquilizer, stimulant, or sedative (but not over-the-counter drugs). In 2012, more than 16 million Americans abused prescription drugs, with thousands dying from a drug overdose. Currently, drug poisoning is the second leading cause of unintentional injury deaths in the United States, killing more Americans than car accidents in over half of the nation. America's drug problem has been expanding to not only include illicit drug use, but also abuse of prescription drugs. As a result, the CDC has classified prescription drug abuse in the United States as an epidemic. Nearly 16,500 yearly deaths are attributed to overdose of prescription pain relievers, more than overdoses of cocaine and heroin combined. The most commonly abused prescription medications are:

- Opioids, commonly prescribed to treat pain. These include codeine, morphine, oxycodone (OxyContin), and hydrocodone (Vicodin).

- Central nervous system depressants, used to treat anxiety and sleep disorders. Examples include Mebaral, Nembutal, Valium, Xanax, Ambien, and Lunesta.
- Stimulants, prescribed to treat the sleep disorder narcolepsy, attention-deficit hyperactivity disorder (ADHD), and obesity. Examples include Dexedrine, Adderall, Ritalin, and Concerta.

Most individuals, in particular young people, obtain these drugs with or without consent from friends and family members. A major concern is that many abusers believe these substances are safer than illicit drugs because they are prescribed by a healthcare professional and dispensed by a pharmacist and cause no serious or life-threatening consequences. The risks associated with psychotherapy drug misuse or abuse vary depending on the drug. Some of the risks include respiratory depression or cessation, decreased or irregular heart rate, high body temperature, seizures, and cardiovascular failure. Abuse of prescription drugs, or using them in a manner other than exactly as prescribed, can lead to addictive behavior.

Inhalant Abuse

Inhalant abuse involves common household products—including whipped cream canisters, cooking sprays, deodorant and hair sprays, glues, nail polish remover, spray paints, gasoline, and lighter and cleaning fluids—whose vapors or aerosol gases are inhaled to get high. Also referred to as "huffing" or "sniffing glue," these drugs are taken by volatilization and not following burning and heating, as is the case with tobacco, marijuana, or crack cocaine.

Based on estimates, about 23 million Americans have used inhalants at least once in their lifetime. Approximately 2.6 percent of youth ages 12 to 17 currently abuse inhalants.[9] Even occasional or a single instance of inhalant abuse can be extremely dangerous. The effects include alcohol-like intoxication, euphoria, hallucinations, drowsiness, disinhibition, lightheadedness, headaches, dizziness, slurred speech, agitation, loss of sensation, belligerence, depressed reflexes, impaired judgment, and unconsciousness. As with other drug abuse, users can be injured by the harmful effects of the vapors and detrimental intoxication behavior. More serious consequences include suffocation due to lack of oxygen supply, pneumonia, vomit aspiration, organ damage (including the brain, liver, and kidneys), abnormal heart rhythms, and sudden cardiac death. Inhalants are especially risky because they can be deadly at any time, even the very first time they are used. Inhalant abuse leads to a strong need to continue their use, and individuals abusing inhalants are more likely to initiate other drug use and have a higher lifetime prevalence of substance abuse.

Marijuana

Marijuana (pot, grass, or weed as it is commonly called) is the most widely used illegal drug in the United States. Estimates by the Office of National Drug Control Policy indicate that 42 percent of Americans have smoked marijuana. Most users smoke loose marijuana that has been rolled into a joint or packed into a pipe. A few users bake it into foods such as brownies or use it to brew a tea. Marijuana cigarettes are often laced with other drugs, such as crack cocaine.

In small doses, marijuana has a sedative effect. Larger doses produce physical and psychological changes. Studies in the 1960s indicated that the potential effects of marijuana were exaggerated and that the drug was relatively harmless. The drug as it is used today, however, is much stronger than when the initial studies were conducted.

The main and most active psychoactive constituent in marijuana is delta-9-tetrahydrocannabinol (THC), a naturally occurring compound in the *Cannabis sativa* plant from which marijuana is derived. In the 1960s, THC content in marijuana ranged from 0.02 to 2 percent. Users called the latter "real good grass." Today's THC content averages 11 percent, although it has been reported as high as 27 percent. The average potency has tripled over the past three decades.

THC reaches the brain within a few seconds after marijuana smoke is inhaled, and the psychic and physical changes reach their peak in about 2 or 3 minutes. THC then is metabolized in the liver to waste metabolites, but 30 percent of it remains in the body a week after the marijuana was smoked. THC is not completely eliminated until 30 days or more after an initial dose of the drug. The drug always remains in the system of regular users.

Some short-term effects of marijuana are **tachycardia**, dryness of the mouth, reddened eyes, stronger appetite, decrease in coordination and tracking (the eyes' ability to follow a moving stimulus), difficulty in concentration, intermittent confusion, impairment of short-term memory and continuity of speech, interference with the physical and mental learning process during periods of intoxication, and increased risk for heart attack for a full day after smoking the drug. Another common effect is the **amotivational syndrome**. This syndrome persists after periods of intoxication but usually disappears a few weeks after the individual stops using the drug.

Long-term harmful effects include atrophy of the brain (leading to irreversible brain damage), less resistance to infectious diseases, chronic bronchitis, lung cancer (marijuana smoke may contain as much as 50 to 70 percent more cancer-producing hydrocarbons than cigarette smoke), and possible sterility and impotence.

CRITICAL THINKING

The legalization of marijuana is being heatedly debated across the United States. Do you think this decision should rest with the government, medical personnel, or the individuals themselves?

One of the most common myths about marijuana use is that it is not addictive. Marijuana use in the United States has increased over the past few years, and recent

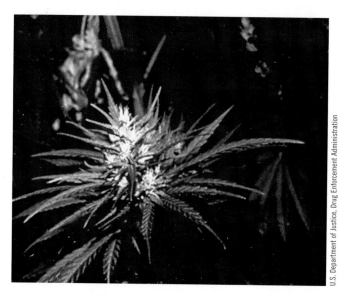
U.S. Department of Justice, Drug Enforcement Administration

The flowering top of *Cannabis sativa.*

surveys report that more than 60 percent of high school seniors don't believe the use of natural marijuana is harmful.[10] Scientific evidence shows that regular users of marijuana do develop physical and psychological dependence. As with cigarette smokers, when regular users go without the drug, they crave the substance, go through mood changes, are irritable and nervous, and develop an obsession to get more. Over half of illicit drug users begin experimenting with marijuana.

Lobbyists continue to work to convince the federal government to legalize marijuana. Though the sale and possession of marijuana continues to be illegal under federal law, the government has allowed states to amend possession offences and decriminalize or legalize marijuana under individual state laws. As of January 2014, marijuana has been legalized in 20 states—for medical use in 18 states and for both medical and recreational use in Colorado and Washington.

The use of marijuana for medical purposes appears to be beneficial in selected conditions such as neuralgia, convulsive disorders, emaciation, and post-traumatic stress disorder (PTSD). A substantial amount of research is necessary, however, before we can fully understand its medicinal use.

Cocaine

Similar to marijuana, **cocaine** was thought for many years to be relatively harmless. This misconception came to an abrupt halt when two well-known athletes in their 20s—Len Bias (basketball) and Don Rogers (football)—died suddenly following cocaine overdoses. Over the years, cocaine has been given several different names, including, among others, coke, C, snow, blow, nose candy, toot, flake, Peruvian lady, white dragon, and happy dust. This drug can be sniffed or snorted, smoked, or injected.

When cocaine is snorted, it is absorbed quickly through the mucous membranes of the nose into the bloodstream. The drug is usually arranged in fine powder lines 1 to 2 inches long. Each line stimulates the autonomic nervous system for about 30 minutes. When cocaine is injected intravenously, larger amounts of cocaine can enter the body in a shorter time. The popularity of cocaine is based on the almost universal guarantee that users find themselves in an immediate state of euphoria and well-being. The addiction begins with a desire to get high, often at social gatherings and usually with the assurance that "occasional use is harmless." Many of these first-time users will become addicted, and for most it is the beginning of a lifetime nightmare.

Animal research with cocaine has shown that all laboratory animals can become compulsive cocaine users. Animals work more persistently at pressing a bar for cocaine than bars for other drugs, including opiates. In one instance, an addicted monkey pressed the bar almost 13,000 times until it finally got a dose of cocaine. People respond in a similar way. Cocaine addicts prefer drug usage to any other activity and use the drug until the supply or the user is exhausted.

Cocaine users also exhibit unusual behaviors compared with their previous conduct, even to the point at which a user has been known to sell a child to obtain more cocaine. It is an expensive drug—$1,000 to $2,600 per ounce for powdered cocaine. Educated people are not immune to cocaine addiction. Cocaine use is common in upper middle class communities and professions—daily habits can cost addicts hundreds to thousands of dollars, with binges in the $20,000 to $50,000 range. Cocaine addiction can lead to loss of a job and career, loss of family, bankruptcy, and death. Though intervention in the chain of supply of cocaine by law enforcement has helped considerably decrease cocaine use in the past decade, the United States remains the world's largest cocaine market.

Crack cocaine is a smokable form of cocaine that is processed with baking soda or ammonia to make it into a more concentrated and solid "rock" form. The name comes from the cracking sound it makes when heated and smoked. Crack cocaine is many times more potent than powdered or injected cocaine and is highly addictive. Two-thirds of users in the United States who are addicted to cocaine use crack. Because it is so potent, crack doses are smaller and, therefore, less expensive ($8 to $40 each), although users still spend hundreds of

Marijuana A psychoactive drug prepared from a mixture of crushed leaves, flowers, small branches, stems, and seeds from the hemp plant *Cannabis sativa;* also called pot, grass, or weed.

Tachycardia Faster-than-normal heart rate.

Amotivational syndrome A condition characterized by loss of motivation, dullness, apathy, and no interest in the future.

Cocaine 2-beta-carbomethoxy-3-betabenozoxytropane, the primary psychoactive ingredient derived from coca plant leaves.

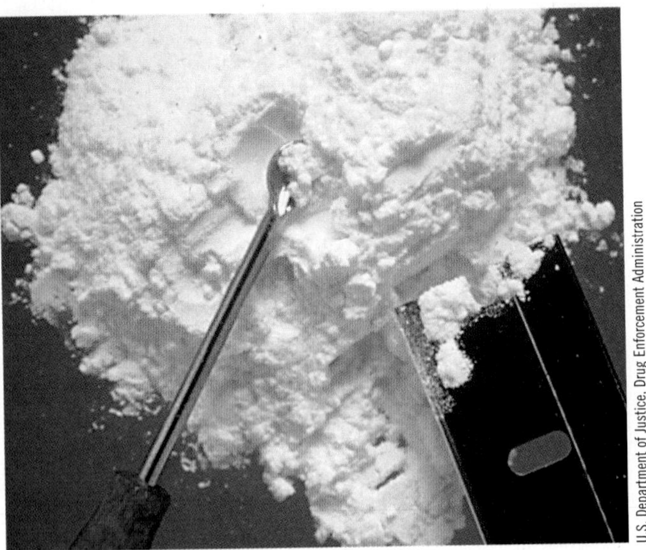

U.S. Department of Justice, Drug Enforcement Administration

Powdered cocaine.

dollars a day to support their addiction. The crack high lasts about 12 minutes, which is shorter than the high from snorted or injected cocaine. Choosing to use cocaine in this form heightens the risk for emphysema and heart attack.

Cocaine seems to alleviate fatigue and raise energy levels, as well as lessen the need for food and sleep. Following the high comes a "crash," a state of physiological and psychological depression, often leaving the user with the desire to get more. This can produce a constant craving for the drug. Similar to alcoholics, cocaine users recover only by abstaining completely from the drug. A single backslide can result in renewed addiction.

Light to moderate cocaine use is typically associated with feelings of pleasure and well-being. Sustained cocaine snorting can lead to a constant runny nose, nasal congestion and inflammation, and perforation of the nasal septum. Long-term consequences of cocaine use include loss of appetite, digestive disorders, weight loss, malnutrition, insomnia, confusion, anxiety, and cocaine psychosis, characterized by paranoia and hallucinations. In one type of hallucination, referred to as formication, or "coke bugs," the chronic user perceives imaginary insects or snakes crawling on or underneath the skin.

High doses of cocaine can cause nervousness, dizziness, blurred vision, vomiting, tremors, seizures, strokes, angina, cardiac arrhythmias, and high blood pressure. As with smoking marijuana, there is an increased risk for heart attack following cocaine use. The user's risk may be 24 times higher than normal for up to three hours following cocaine use. Almost one-third of cocaine users who incurred a heart attack had no symptoms of heart disease prior to taking cocaine. In addition, users are at risk for hepatitis, HIV, and other infectious diseases because of the risky behaviors they engage in to obtain the drug.

Large overdoses of cocaine can precipitate sudden death from respiratory paralysis, cardiac arrhythmias, and severe convulsions. If individuals lack an enzyme used in metabolizing cocaine, as few as two to three lines of cocaine may be fatal.

Chronic users who constantly crave the drug often turn to crime, including murder, to sustain their habit. Some users view suicide as the only solution to this sad syndrome.

Methamphetamine

Methamphetamine, or meth, is a more potent form of amphetamine. **Amphetamines** in general are part of a large group of synthetic agents used to stimulate the central nervous system. A powerfully addictive drug, methamphetamine falls under the same category of psychostimulant drugs as amphetamines and cocaine. It is also known as a "club drug," a group of illegal substances used at dance clubs, rock concerts, and raves (all-night dance parties). Other club drugs include MDMA, LSD, GHB, Rohypnol, and ketamine.

Methamphetamine typically is a white, odorless, and bitter-tasting powder that dissolves readily in water or alcohol. The drug is a potent central nervous system stimulant that produces a general feeling of well-being, decreases appetite, increases motor activity, and decreases fatigue and the need for sleep.

Unlike most other drugs, methamphetamine reaches rural and urban populations alike. Young people especially prefer methamphetamine because of its low cost and long-lasting effects—up to 12 hours following use.

In the past, methamphetamine was easily manufactured in clandestine meth "labs" using over-the-counter pseudoephedrine, typically found in cold medications. Because of the ease of accessibility to methamphetamine ingredients, in March 2006 the federal Combat Methamphetamine Epidemic Act of 2005 was signed into law. This law requires retailers to keep cold medications behind the counter, and consumers are limited as to the amount they can purchase.

Despite legislative efforts, reports of methamphetamine labs within the United States remain high as faster ways to produce the drug in smaller batches allow for increased proliferation. Mexico is the primary foreign source of methamphetamine for the United States. Production in Canada, however, has increased significantly, primarily by Canadian-based Asian drug trafficking organizations. These organizations run large-capacity superlabs.

Methamphetamine labs are set up almost anywhere, including garages, basements, or hotel rooms. The abundance of potential meth lab sites makes it difficult for drug enforcement agencies to locate many of these facilities. The risk of injury in a meth lab, however, is high, because potentially explosive environmental contaminants are discarded during production of the drug.

Methamphetamine can be snorted, swallowed, smoked, or injected. It is commonly referred to as speed or crystal when snorted or taken orally, ice or glass when smoked, and crank when injected. Depending on how it is taken, methamphetamine affects the body differently. Smoked or in-

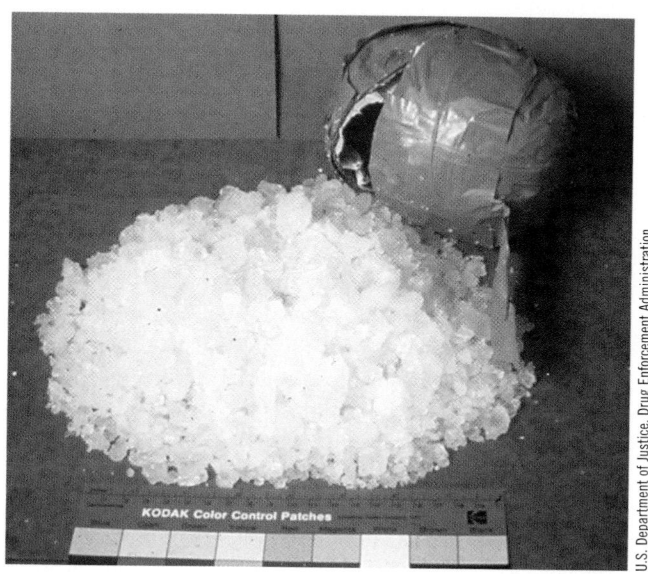

U.S. Department of Justice, Drug Enforcement Administration

"Ice," so named for its appearance, is a smokable form of methamphetamine.

jected methamphetamine provides an immediate intense, pleasurable rush that lasts only a few minutes. Nonetheless, negative effects can continue for several hours. When the drug is snorted or taken orally, the user does not experience a rush but develops a feeling of euphoria that lasts up to 16 hours.

Users of methamphetamine experience increases in body temperature, blood pressure, heart rate, and breathing rate; a decrease in appetite; hyperactivity; tremors; and violent behavior. High doses produce irritability, paranoia, irreversible damage to blood vessels in the brain (causing strokes), and risk for sudden death from hypothermia and convulsions if not treated at once.

Chronic abusers experience insomnia, confusion, hallucinations, inflammation of the heart lining, schizophrenia-like mental disorder, and brain cell damage similar to that caused by a stroke. Physical changes to the brain may last months or perhaps become permanent. Over time, methamphetamine use may reduce brain levels of **dopamine**, which can lead to symptoms similar to those of Parkinson's disease. In addition, users frequently are involved in violent crime, homicide, and suicide. Using methamphetamine during pregnancy may cause prenatal complications, premature delivery, and abnormal physical and emotional development of the child.

Similar to other stimulants, methamphetamine is often used in a binge cycle. Addiction takes hold quickly because the person develops tolerance to methamphetamine within minutes of using it. The high disappears long before blood levels of the drug drop significantly. The user then attempts to maintain the pleasurable feelings by taking in more of the drug, and a binge cycle ensues.

The binge cycle, which can last for a couple of weeks, consists of several stages. The initial rush lasts 5 to 30 minutes. During this stage, heart rate, blood pressure, and metabolism increase and the user receives a great sense of pleasure. The high follows, lasting up to 16 hours. During this stage, users become arrogant and more argumentative. The binge stage sets in next and lasts between 2 and 14 days. Addicts continue to use the drug in an attempt to maintain the high as long as possible.

When addicts no longer can achieve a satisfying high, they enter the tweaking stage, the most dangerous stage in the cycle. At this point, users may have gone without food for several days and without sleep anywhere from 3 to 15 days. They become paranoid, irritable, and violent. Tweakers crave more of the drug, but no amount of amphetamines restores the pleasurable, euphoric feelings they achieved during the high. Thus, the addicts become increasingly frustrated, unpredictable, and dangerous to those around them (including police officers and medical personnel) and to themselves. Once they finally crash, they are no longer dangerous. The users now become lethargic and sleep for 1 to 3 days.

Following the crash, addicts fall into a 1-to 3-month period of withdrawal. During this stage, they can be paranoid, aggressive, fatigued, depressed, suicidal, and filled with an intense craving for another high. Reuse of the drug relieves these feelings. Therefore, the incidence of relapse in users who seek treatment is high.

MDMA (Ecstasy)

MDMA, also known as Ecstasy, became popular among teenagers and young adults in the United States in the mid-1980s, when it evolved into the most common club drug. Although its use already constituted a serious drug problem in Europe, MDMA was not illegal in the United States until 1985. Prior to 1985, few Americans abused this drug. In the 1970s, some therapists used MDMA as a tool to help patients open up and feel at ease. MDMA is named for its chemical structure: 3,4-methylenedioxymethamphetamine. Street names for the drug are X-TC, E, Adam, and love drug.

MDMA use, once popular primarily among Hispanic Americans and Caucasians, has spread to a range of demographic subgroups. Typically, dealers push the drug as a way to increase energy, pleasure, and self-confidence. MDMA is now available in numerous settings, including high schools, private homes, malls, and other popular gathering places for teenagers and young adults.

In recent years, MDMA use has increased

Methamphetamine A potent form of amphetamine; also called meth.

Amphetamines A class of powerful central nervous system stimulants.

Dopamine A neurotransmitter that affects emotional, mental, and motor functions.

MDMA 3,4-methylenedioxymethamphetamine, a synthetic hallucinogen drug with a chemical structure that closely resembles MDA and methamphetamine; also known as Ecstasy.

dramatically in a powder or capsule form known as Molly, marketed as a pure crystalline MDMA that is purportedly safer and purer than Ecstacy, which is routinely mixed with other drugs and contaminates. Molly has been glamorized in current music and pop culture, making it a popular drug with teens and college students at raves, dance clubs, and music festivals. Its claim to be a "pure" or "organic" MDMA has bolstered the drug into reaching a broader demographic of users—the U.S. Drug Enforcement Administration (DEA) has reported that Molly's newest users are middle-aged professionals. Law enforcement officials warn users to beware of claims that Molly offered to them is pure MDMA. Molly most often contains a toxic mixture of other drugs and lab-created chemicals that users ingest unknowingly when they take the drug. The DEA has found that only a small percentage of Molly seized in recent years actually contained any MDMA.

The trafficking of MDMA is increasing at an alarming rate, and multiple agencies have reported large seizures of the drug. In 2012 the United States Customs and Border Protection reported 2,670 confiscations of MDMA, up from 186 in 2008. Most of the supply comes from Canada. All Canadian labs combined are believed to produce more than 2 million tablets per week.

Although MDMA usually is swallowed in the form of one or two pills in doses of up to 120 mg per pill, it can also be smoked, snorted, or occasionally, injected. Because the drug often is prepared with other substances, users have no way of knowing the exact potency of the drug or additional substances found in each pill. Furthermore, many users combine MDMA with alcohol, marijuana, or other drugs, which makes it even more dangerous.

MDMA shares characteristics with stimulants and hallucinogens. Its chemical structure closely parallels the hallucinogen **methylenedioxyamphetamine (MDA)** and methamphetamine, both man-made stimulants that damage the brain. The addictive properties of MDMA and stimulation of hyperactivity have been compared to stimulants such as amphetamines and cocaine. The chemical structure of MDMA and its appeal, however, are similar to hallucinogens, but with milder psychedelic effects.

Among young people, MDMA has a reputation for being fun and harmless as long as it is used sensibly. But it is not a harmless drug. Research is uncovering many negative side effects. The pleasurable effects peak about an hour after a pill is swallowed and last for 2 to 6 hours. Users claim to feel enlightened and introspective, accepting of themselves and trustful of others. Because they tend to act and feel closer to, or more intimate with, the people around them, some believe this drug to be an aphrodisiac, even though MDMA actually hampers sexual ability. MDMA also acts as a stimulant by increasing brain activity and making users feel more energetic.

Like most addictive drugs, the effects of MDMA are said to diminish with each use. MDMA users may experience rapid eye movement, faintness, blurred vision, chills, sweating, nausea, muscle tension, and teeth grinding. Users often bring infant pacifiers to raves to combat the latter side effect. Individuals with heart, liver, or kidney disease or high blood pressure are especially at risk, because MDMA increases blood pressure, heart rate, and body temperature. Thus, its use may lead to seizures, kidney failure, a heart attack, or a stroke. The hot, crowded atmosphere at raves and dance clubs also heightens the risk to the user. Deaths are more likely when water is unavailable, because the crowded atmosphere, combined with the stimulant effects of MDMA, causes dehydration (bottled water is often sold at inflated prices at raves). Other evidence suggests that a pregnant woman using MDMA may find long-term learning and memory difficulties in her child.

The damaging effects of the drug can be long lasting and are possible after only a few uses. Long-term side effects, lasting for weeks after use, include confusion, depression, sleep disorders, anxiety, aggression, paranoia, and impulsive behavior. Questions still remain about other potential long-term effects. Verbal and visual memory may be significantly impaired for years after prolonged use. Researchers are focusing on these lasting side effects, which may be the result of depleted serotonin, a neurotransmitter that is released with each dose of MDMA. The short-term effect of serotonin release is increased brain activity. Serotonin helps regulate sleep cycles, pain, emotion, and appetite. Because MDMA may damage the neurons that release serotonin, long-term effects could be dangerous.

Advocates of MDMA are attempting to get approval to study medical uses of the drug. For example, MDMA could relieve suffering in terminally ill cancer patients. It also could help people in therapy for marital problems by encouraging introspection and conversation. Because MDMA is heralded as an instant antidepressant, it may help people who are in mourning. Opponents, meanwhile, question the value of MDMA as an effective treatment modality, because its effects diminish with continued use.

Heroin

Heroin use has increased in recent years. Although the most common users are those in suburban, middle-class neighborhoods and lower-income populations, its use is starting to appear in more affluent communities as well. Common nicknames for heroin include diesel, dope, dynamite, white death, nasty boy, china white, H. Harry, gumball, junk, brown sugar, smack, tootsie roll, and chasing the dragon.

In 2005, a heroin-based recreational drug referred to as cheese became popular among middle and high school students, and has since attracted a wider base of older users. Cheese is a combination of heroin with crushed tablets of over-the-counter medications that contain acetaminophen and the antihistamine diphenhydramine. Law enforcement has dubbed the drug "starter" or "gateway" heroin.

Most recently, Mexican drug dealers have found a way to produce a purer (and therefore more potent) form of heroin known as Mexican tar heroin or black tar. Named after its black, gooey consistency, this ultrapotent form of heroin (reported as high as 60 to 80 percent potency) is known to kill unsuspecting users before they even have a chance to remove the syringe or are done snorting the substance. The potency and cheap price of the drug has broadened its appeal, resulting in an increase in both use and reports of overdose among a wide range of users.

Heroin is classified as a narcotic drug. It is synthesized from morphine, a natural substance found in the seedpod of several types of poppy plants. In its purest form, heroin is a white powder, but on the streets it is typically available in yellow or brown powders. The latter colors are attained when pure heroin is combined with other drugs or substances, such as sugar, cornstarch, chalk, brick dust, or laundry soap. Heroin also is sold in a hardened or solid form (black tar), which usually is dissolved with other liquids for use in injectable form. Many users combine heroin with cocaine, a risky process commonly called speedballing.

Today's heroin is more pure, powerful, and affordable than ever before. Highly dangerous, heroin is a significant health threat to users in that they have no way of determining the strength of the drug purchased on the street, which places them at a constant risk for overdose and death.

Heroin can be injected intravenously or intramuscularly, sniffed or snorted, or smoked. Although injection has been the predominant method of heroin use, users are turning from intravenous injections because of the risk for HIV infection. The availability of relatively low-priced, high-purity heroin further contributes to the number of people who smoke or snort the drug. Some users have the misconception that heroin is less addictive when it is snorted or smoked. Whether injected, snorted, or smoked, heroin is an extremely addictive drug, and both physical and psychological dependence develop rapidly. Drug tolerance sets in quickly, and each time the drug is used, a higher dose is required to produce the same effects. Use of heroin induces a state of euphoria that comes within seconds of intravenous injection or within 5 to 15 minutes with other methods of administration. Because the drug is a sedative, during the initial rush people have a sense of relaxation and do not feel any pain. In users who inhale the drug, however, the rush may be accompanied by nausea, vomiting, intense itching, and at times severe asthma attacks. As the rush wears off, users experience drowsiness, confusion, slowed cardiac function, and decreased breathing rate.

A heroin overdose can cause convulsions, coma, and death. During an overdose, heart rate, breathing, blood pressure, and body temperature drop dramatically. These physiological responses can induce vomiting and tight muscles and cause breathing to stop. Death is often the result of lack of oxygen or choking to death on vomit.

About 4 to 5 hours after taking the drug, withdrawal sets in. Heroin withdrawal is painful and usually lasts up to 2 weeks—but could go on for several months. Symptoms of short-term use include red or raw nostrils, bone and muscle pains, muscle spasms and cramps, sweating, hot and cold flashes, runny nose and eyes, drowsiness, sluggishness, slurred speech, loss of appetite, nausea, diarrhea, restlessness, and violent yawning. Heroin use can also kill a developing fetus or cause a spontaneous abortion.

Symptoms of long-term use of heroin include hallucinations, nightmares, constipation, sexual difficulties, impaired vision, reduced fertility, boils, collapsed veins, and a significantly elevated risk for lung, liver, and cardiovascular diseases, including bacterial infections in blood vessels and heart valves. The additives used in street heroin can clog vital blood vessels, because these additives do not dissolve in the body, leading to infections and death of cells in vital organs. Sudden infant death syndrome (SIDS) also is seen more frequently in children born to heroin-addicted mothers.

Heroin addiction is treated with behavioral therapies and pharmaceutical agents. Medication suppresses withdrawal symptoms, which makes it easier for patients to stop using heroin. The combination of these two treatment modalities helps people learn to lead a more stable, productive, and drug-free lifestyle.

New Psychoactive Substances (NPS)

The 2013 World Drug Report, compiled by the United Nations Office on Drugs and Crime, has warned of the rapid emergence of **new psychoactive substances (NPS)**, a term coined by the Commission on Narcotic Drugs in March 2012 to refer to unregulated substances of abuse whose effects are made to mimic that of controlled drugs.[11] The term "new" does not necessarily mean that the substance itself is new, but rather that the misuse of the substance or mixture of substances is newly introduced to a specific market. The largest numbers of NPS worldwide were identified in the United States, with a total of 158 NPS identified in 2012 alone, double the amount of the European Union. NPS is also more than twice as widespread in American youth than in those of Europe. Among students, NPS use is more common than all other drugs except marijuana. Though the highest concentration of NPS is in Europe and North America, most NPS originate in regions with advanced chemical and pharmaceutical industries, particularly Asia.

The trend of increased creativity in the preparation of synthetic substances or spinoffs of known substances is fueled by widespread access to drug formulas via the Internet and by the urgency of dealers to escape legislation that is constantly adapting in an effort to control known

Methylenedioxyamphetamine (MDA) A hallucinogenic drug that is structurally similar to amphetamines.

Heroin A potent drug that is a derivative of opium.

New psychoactive substances (NPS) Unregulated substances of abuse whose effects are made to mimic that of controlled drugs.

drugs. The United States Congress signed into law the Synthetic Drug Abuse Prevention Act (SDAPA) in July 2012, which identified 26 substances as Schedule I controlled substances, establishing drug codes for enforcement. Despite legislative efforts, however, small alterations in formulas by drug designers consistently outpace efforts to control or ban NPS.

Until they are placed under regulatory control, these substances are often marketed as legal alternatives to controlled drugs, said to be "legal highs" or "herbal highs," to emphasize a seemingly safe and natural origin. Substances are also masked under the name of ordinary household products to imply that they are both harmless and legal, such as bath salts, plant food, herbal incense, potpourri, or jewelry cleaner.

NPS are commonly referred to by both the general population and national associations as "synthetic drugs" or "designer drugs." Because of the vast quantity of NPS that can each contain a mixture of many substances, it's difficult to determine or speculate the long-term health implications of NPS use. NPS include a broad range of synthetic and plant-based psychoactive substances, including synthetic cannabinoids (synthetic marijuana, Spice), synthetic cathinones (mephedrone sold as bath salts, plant food, or meow meow), piperazines ("ecstacy substitutes"), phenethylamines (4-MMA, methyl-MA), ketamine (Special K, vitamin K, jet), and other plant-derived substances such as kratom, khat, and *Salvia divinorum*. The most prevalent forms of NPS in the United States are synthetic cannabinoids.

Synthetic Cannabinoids (Fake Pot or Spice) Synthetic cannabinoids are currently the most widely used NPS in the United States and worldwide.[12] More commonly known as "fake pot," synthetic cannabinoids are man-made chemicals that have compounds similar to the chemical THC found in the natural *Cannabis sativa* plant used for marijuana, though synthetic versions are generally more potent. Users claim that the substances provide a marijuana-like high and are popular among teenagers and young adults. The 2013 Monitoring the Future survey of youth drug-use trends found that 7.9 percent of high school seniors used synthetic cannabinoids in the past year, placing it as the second most common illicit drug used by seniors after marijuana.[13]

Synthetic cannabinoids are often sprayed onto a mixture of herbs and are sold as Spice, K2, Moon Rocks, Skunk, Kind, Genie, Summit, potpourri, herbal incense, Yucatan Gold, Purple Passion, Train Wreck, or Ultra (among other names). According to the federal Drug Enforcement Agency (DEA), the adverse effects of synthetic cannabinoids are far more dangerous than the side effects of marijuana, including seizures, high blood pressure, anxiety attacks, hallucinations, nausea, loss of consciousness, and chemical dependency. Some samples tested have been shown to be 100 times more potent than marijuana.

Between 2010 and 2011, the number of calls that poison control centers received for "synthetic marijuana" rose from 2,900 to 7,000.[14] However, this trend was curbed in 2012 by 25 percent, primarily due to timely legislative efforts to control compounds used to manufacture the drugs. Using its emergency scheduling authority—which grants the temporary control of emerging substances that pose a potential health risk—the DEA made the possession and sale of five types of synthetic cannabinoids no longer legal in 2011, retaining all but one of the five under control as designated Schedule I substances under the July 2012 Synthetic Drug Abuse Prevention Act. Subsequent laws expanded the list to include three more types of synthetic cannabinoids in 2013, and four more were temporarily scheduled as of January 2014. Though usage rates of synthetic cannabinoids among young people remain high, these legislative efforts have helped decrease the sale and use of these substances in recent years.

Alcohol

Drinking **alcohol** has been a socially acceptable behavior for centuries. Alcohol is an accepted accompaniment at parties, ceremonies, dinners, sport contests, the establishment of kingdoms or governments, and the signing of treaties between nations. Alcohol also has been used for medical reasons as a mild sedative or as a painkiller for surgery.

For a short period of 14 years, from 1920 to 1933, by constitutional amendment, the sale and use of alcohol were declared illegal in the United States. This amendment was repealed because drinkers and nondrinkers alike questioned the right of government to pass judgment on individual moral standards. In addition, organized crime activities to smuggle and sell alcohol illegally expanded enormously during this period.

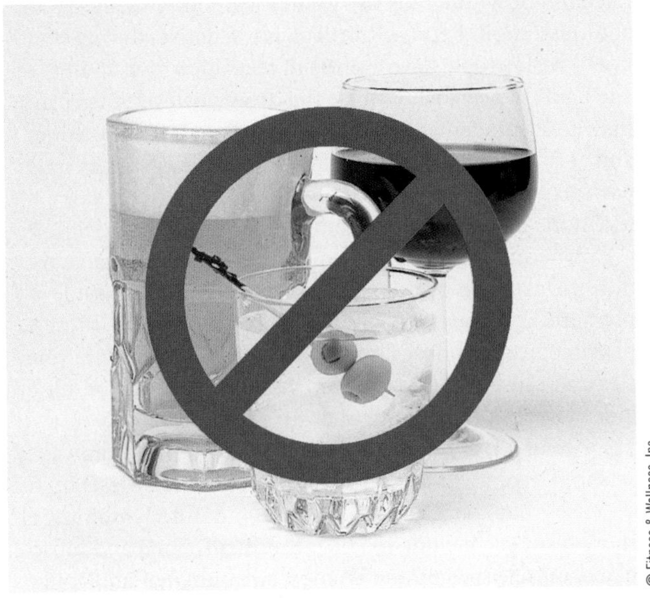

The sale of alcohol was illegal in the United States between 1920 and 1933.

Alcohol is the most abused substance in the United States and the cause of one of the most significant health-related drug problems in the country today. According to *Dietary Guidelines for Americans 2010,* 79,000 yearly deaths in the United States are due to excessive drinking.

Based on the 2012 NSDUH, more than 135 million people 12 years and older (52.1 percent) used alcohol within a month of the survey and 59.6 million (23 percent) participated in binge drinking at least once in the 30 days prior to the survey. About 17 million people (6.5 percent) were heavy drinkers, and 1 in 9 people drove under the influence of alcohol at least once in the 12 months prior to the interview. The highest prevalence is among 21-to 25-year-olds, with 70 percent of this age group using alcohol within a month of the survey.

Alcohol drinkers are also more likely to misuse other drugs. More than half of lifetime drinkers have used one or more illicit drugs at some time in their lives, compared with less than 10 percent of lifetime nondrinkers.

Although modest health benefits are derived from moderate alcohol consumption, the media have extensively exaggerated these benefits. The press likes to discuss this topic because it seems to be "a vice that's good for you." Research supports the assertion that consuming no more than two alcoholic beverages a day for men and one for women provides modest benefits in decreasing the risk for cardiovascular disease.

The benefits of modest alcohol use can be equated to those obtained through a small daily dose of aspirin (about 81 mg per day, or the equivalent of a baby aspirin) or eating a few nuts each day. Aspirin or a few nuts do not lead to impaired judgment or actions that you may later regret or have to live with for the rest of your life.

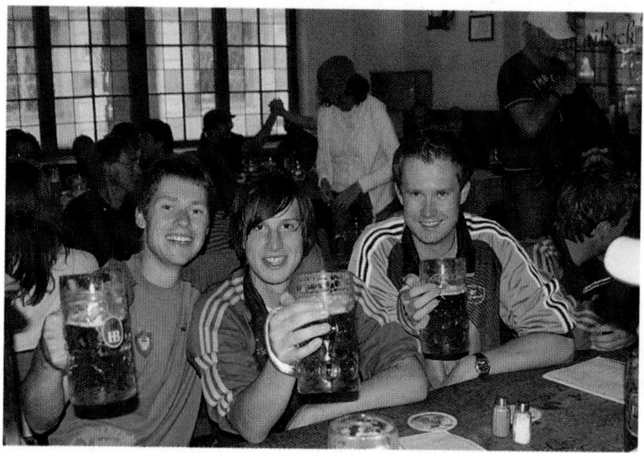

Approximately 14 million Americans will develop a drinking problem during their lifetime.

Consequences of Drinking Alcohol Alcohol is not for everyone. **Alcoholism** seems to have both a genetic and an environmental component. The reasons some people can drink for years without becoming addicted, whereas others follow the downward spiral of alcoholism, are not understood. The addiction to alcohol develops slowly. Most people think they are in control of their drinking habits and do not realize they have a problem until they become alcoholics, when they find themselves physically and emotionally dependent on the drug. This addiction is characterized by excessive use of, and constant preoccupation with, drinking. Alcohol abuse, in turn, leads to mental, emotional, physical, and social problems.

The effects of alcohol intake include impaired peripheral vision, decreased visual and hearing acuity, slower reaction time, reduced concentration and motor performance (including increased swaying), and impaired judgment of distance and speed of moving objects. Furthermore, alcohol alleviates fear, increases risk taking, stimulates urination, and induces sleep. A single large dose of alcohol also may decrease sexual function. Two of the most serious consequences of alcohol abuse are increased risks of accidents and violent behavior. Excessive drinking has been linked to more than half of all deaths from car accidents. The risk for rape, domestic violence, child abuse, suicide, and murder also increases with alcohol abuse.

One of the most unpleasant, dangerous, and life-threatening effects of drinking is the **synergistic action** of alcohol when combined with other drugs, particularly central nervous system depressants. Each person reacts to a combination of alcohol and other drugs in a different way. The effects range from loss of consciousness to death.

Long-term effects of alcohol abuse are serious and often life threatening (Figure 13.2). Some of these detrimental effects are lower resistance to disease; **cirrhosis** of the liver; higher risk for breast, oral, esophageal, larynx, stomach, colon, and liver

What Constitutes a Standard Drink

In the United States, a drink is considered 14 grams of pure alcohol (ethanol), or the equivalent of

- 5 ounces of wine
- 12 ounces of beer
- 1.5 ounces of 80-proof liquor

Alcohol Ethyl alcohol, a depressant drug that affects the brain, slows central nervous system activity, and has strong addictive properties.

Alcoholism A disease in which an individual loses control over drinking alcoholic beverages.

Synergistic action The effect of mixing two or more drugs, which can be much greater than the sum of two or more drugs acting by themselves.

Cirrhosis A disease characterized by scarring of the liver.

cancer; **cardiomyopathy**; irregular heartbeat; elevated blood pressure; greater risk for stroke; osteoporosis; inflammation of the esophagus, stomach, small intestine, and pancreas; stomach ulcers; sexual impotence; birth defects; malnutrition; brain cell damage leading to loss of memory; depression; psychosis; and hallucinations.

Social Consequences of Alcohol Abuse

Alcohol abuse further leads to social problems that include loss of friends and jobs, separation of family members, child abuse, domestic violence, divorce, and problems with the law. Heavy drinking also contributes to decreased performance at work and school, because drinkers are more likely to arrive late, make more mistakes, leave assignments incomplete, encounter problems with fellow workers or students, get lower grades and job evaluations, and flunk out of school or lose jobs. Alcohol abuse also worsens financial concerns, because drinkers have less money for needed items such as food and clothing, fail to pay bills, and may have additional medical expenses, insurance premiums, and fines.

Alcohol on Campus Alcohol is the number-one drug problem among college students. According to national surveys, about 60 percent of full-time college students report using alcohol within the past month, and 40 percent have engaged in binge drinking (consumed five or more drinks in a row). Alcohol is a factor in about 25 percent of all college dropouts, and of the more than 18 million college students in the United States, between 2 and 3 percent eventually will die from alcohol-related causes.

The statistics are sobering. For college students between the ages of 18 and 24,[15]

- 1,825 die from alcohol-related unintentional injuries
- Almost 700,000 are assaulted by another student who has been drinking
- 599,000 are unintentionally injured under the influence of alcohol
- More than 150,000 develop alcohol-related health problems
- About 97,000 are victims of alcohol-related sexual assault or date rape
- 400,000 have unprotected sex
- More than 100,000 were too intoxicated to know whether they'd consented to having sex
- Almost 3.4 million drive under the influence of alcohol

In terms of academic work, a national survey involving about 94,000 college students from 197 colleges and universities conducted over three years showed that grade point average (GPA) was related to average number of drinks per week (Figure 13.3).[16] Students with a D-or F-level GPA reported a weekly consumption of almost 10 drinks. Students with A-level GPAs consumed about 4 drinks per week.

The National Institute on Alcohol Abuse and Alcoholism states that about one-quarter of college students report having academic problems due to alcohol abuse, including missing classes, falling behind, and receiving lower grades on exams and papers. Students tend to be most susceptible to drinking during the first six weeks of their freshman year when they encounter new social and academic pressures. In fact, college students enrolled full time have higher rates of alcohol use, binge and heavy drinking, and driving under the influence than their peers ages 18 to 22 that are part

FIGURE 13.2 **Long-term risks associated with alcohol abuse.**

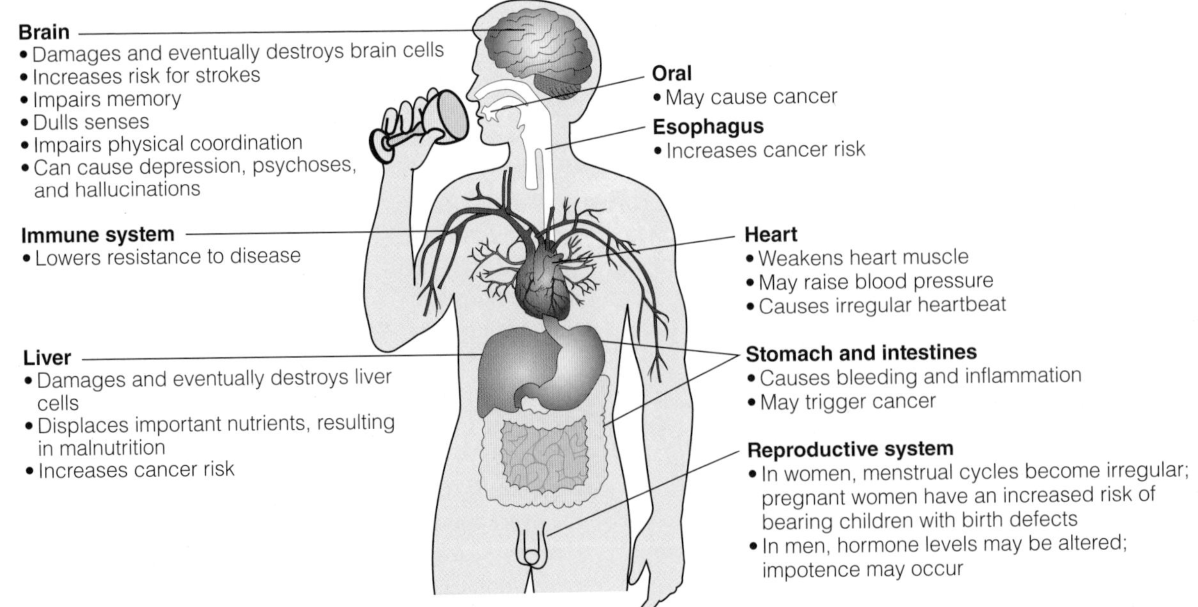
Brain
• Damages and eventually destroys brain cells
• Increases risk for strokes
• Impairs memory
• Dulls senses
• Impairs physical coordination
• Can cause depression, psychoses, and hallucinations
Immune system
• Lowers resistance to disease
Liver
• Damages and eventually destroys liver cells
• Displaces important nutrients, resulting in malnutrition
• Increases cancer risk
Oral
• May cause cancer
Esophagus
• Increases cancer risk
Heart
• Weakens heart muscle
• May raise blood pressure
• Causes irregular heartbeat
Stomach and intestines
• Causes bleeding and inflammation
• May trigger cancer
Reproductive system
• In women, menstrual cycles become irregular; pregnant women have an increased risk of bearing children with birth defects
• In men, hormone levels may be altered; impotence may occur

BEHAVIOR MODIFICATION PLANNING

When Your Date Drinks.

- **Don't** make excuses for his/her behavior, no matter how embarrassing.
- **Don't** allow embarrassment to put you in a situation with which you are uncomfortable.
- **Do** be sure that body language and tone of voice match verbal messages you send.
- **Do** leave as quickly as you can, without your date. **Don't** stop to argue. Intoxicated people can't listen to reason.
- **Do** call a cab, a friend, or your parents. **Don't** ride home with your date.

For women:

- **Do** make your position clear. "No!" is much more effective than "Please stop!" or "Don't!"
- **Do** make it clear that you will call the police if rape is attempted.

Try It

In your Online Journal or class notebook, write down strategies you can incorporate today to ensure your health and wellness.

time students or who don't attend college. College students who develop habits of heavy and binge drinking in their first year put their health and academic potential at risk during their college years and into early adulthood.

Another major concern is that more than half of college students participate in games that involve heavy drinking (consuming five or more drinks in one sitting). Often, students take part because of peer pressure and fear of rejection. Data show that one night of binge drinking results in an extra intake of around 2,000 calories from alcoholic beverages alone, plus another 800 calories from food and munchies consumed during the drinking episode. Some students even binge drink three days in a row on weekends.

Excessive drinking can also precipitate unplanned and unprotected sex (risking HIV infection), date rape, and alcohol poisoning. When some young people turn 21, they "celebrate" by having 21 drinks. Unaware of the risks of excessive alcohol intake in a relatively short period, drinking friends then try to let them "sleep it off," only to find that they never wake up but rather suffer death from alcohol poisoning. Each year, thousands of college students are taken to the emergency room for alcohol poisoning, which can result in permanent brain damage or death. Signs of alcohol poisoning include inability to wake or rouse a person, vomiting, slow or irregular breathing, low body temperature or hypothermia, bluish or pale skin, or mental confusion. Of the more than 18 million college students in the United States, between 2 and 3 percent eventually will die from alcohol-related causes.

FIGURE 13.3 Average number of drinks by college students per week by GPA.

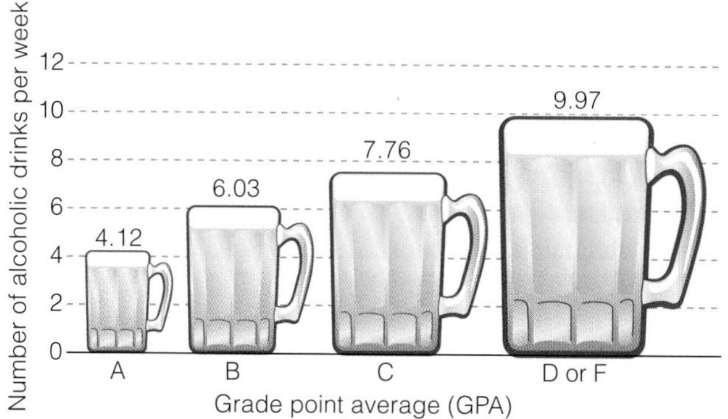

Source: C.A. Presley, J.S. Leichliter, and P. W. Meilman, Alcohol and Drugs on American College Campuses: Findings from 1995, 1996, and 1997 (A Report to College Presidents) (Carbondale, IL: Southern Illinois University, 1999).

How to Cut Down on Drinking

To find out whether drinking is a problem in your life, refer to the questionnaire in Lab 13A, developed by the American Medical Association. A "yes" answer to any of these questions can be regarded as a warning sign to potential future problems. If you have answered three or more of them with a "yes," your drinking habits can be harmful to your well-being and may indicate that you are alcohol dependent or an alcoholic. An evaluation by a health care professional is highly recommended.

If a person is determined to control the problem, it is not that difficult. The first and most important step is to want to cut down. If you want to do this but cannot seem to do so, you need to accept the probability that alcohol is becoming a serious problem for you, and you should seek guidance from your physician or from an organization such as Alcoholics Anonymous. The next few suggestions also may help you cut down your alcohol intake:

- **Set reasonable limits for yourself.** Decide not to exceed a certain number of drinks on a given occasion, and stick to your decision. No more than two beers or two cocktails a day is a reason-

Cardiomyopathy A disease affecting the heart muscle.

able limit. If you set a target such as this and consistently do not exceed it, you have proven to yourself that you can control your drinking.

- **Learn to say "no."** Many people have "just one more" drink because others in the group are doing this or because someone puts pressure on them, not because they want a drink. When you reach the sensible limit you have set for yourself, politely but firmly refuse to exceed it. If you are being the generous host, pour yourself a glass of water or juice "on the rocks." Nobody will notice the difference.
- **Drink slowly.** Don't gulp a drink. Choose your drinks for their flavor, not their "kick," and savor the taste of each sip.
- **Dilute your drinks.** If you prefer cocktails to beer, try tall drinks: Instead of downing gin or whiskey straight or nearly so, drink it diluted with a mixer such as tonic water or soda water in a tall glass. That way, you can enjoy both the flavor and the act of drinking but take longer to finish each drink. Also, you can make your two-drink limit last all evening or switch to the mixer by itself.
- **Do not drink on your own.** Confine your drinking to social gatherings. You may have a hard time resisting the urge to pour yourself a relaxing drink at the end of a hard day, but many formerly heavy drinkers have found that a soft drink satisfies the need as well as alcohol did. What may help you really unwind, even with no drink, is a comfortable chair, loosened clothing, and perhaps soothing music, a television program, a good book to read, or even some low-to moderate-intensity physical activity.
- **Try a smartphone app to help control your drinking.** More and more smartphone applications are being developed that offer great tools to help you monitor and control drinking habits. Some features include tracking tools to help calculate blood alcohol levels as you drink, the ability to set up messaging from your personal support team to check your progress, profiles from a network of peers also trying to cut down to provide motivation, and links to helpful resources about addiction and recovery. One recent study found that recovery patients who used a smartphone app after treatment for alcohol abuse were 12 percent more likely to abstain from alcohol and also have fewer relapses.[17]

Treatment of Addictions

Recovery from any addiction is more likely to be successful with professional guidance and support. The first step is to recognize the reality of the problem. The Addictive Behavior Questionnaire in Lab 13A will help you recognize possible addictive behavior in yourself (or someone you know). If the answers to five or more of these questions is positive, you may have a problem, in which case you should contact a physician, your institution's counseling center, or the local mental health clinic for a referral.

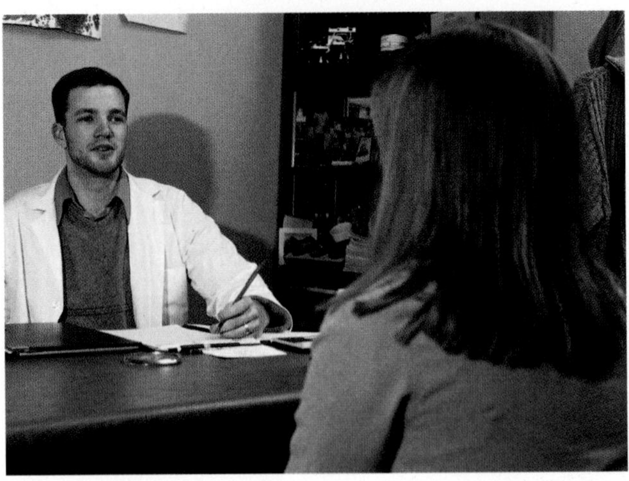

The sooner treatment for addiction is started, and the longer the user stays in treatment, the better the chances for recovery and a more productive life.

You also may contact the Substance Abuse and Mental Health Services Administration at 1-800-662-HELP (1-800-662-4357) for referral to 24-hour substance abuse treatment centers in your local area. All information discussed during a phone call to this center is kept strictly confidential. Information is also available on the Internet at www.samhsa.gov. The national center provides printed information on drug abuse and addictive behavior.

About 4 million Americans received treatment for illicit drug or alcohol abuse in 2012. An additional 20 million people in the United States were estimated to need treatment for illicit drug or alcohol abuse but did not receive such treatment at any specialty facility.[18]

Among intervention and treatment programs for addiction are psychotherapy, medical care, and behavior modification. If addiction is a problem in your life, you need to act upon it without delay. Addicts do not have to resign themselves to a lifetime of addiction. The sooner you start, and the longer you stay in treatment, the better your chances of recovering and leading a healthier and more productive life.

Tobacco Use

People throughout the world have used tobacco for hundreds of years. Before the 18th century, they smoked tobacco primarily in the form of pipes or cigars. Cigarette smoking per se did not become popular until the mid-1800s, and its use started to increase dramatically in the 20th century.

An estimated 69 million Americans aged 12 and older use tobacco products, including 57.5 million cigarette smokers, 13 million cigar smokers, 9 million using smokeless tobacco, and 2.5 million pipe smokers.[19] As depicted in Figure 13.4, tobacco use in general declines with education.

When tobacco leaves are burned, hot air and gases containing **tar** (chemical compounds) and **nicotine** are released in the smoke. More than 7,000 chemicals, hundreds of them

FIGURE 13.4 **Tobacco use among adults age 18 or older, 2012.**

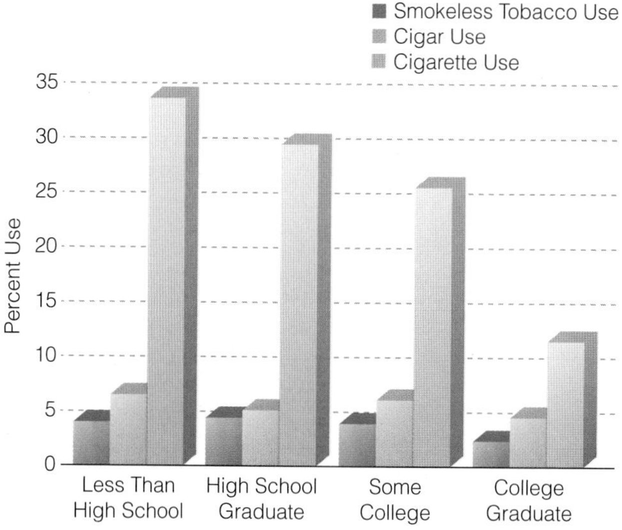

Source: http://www.samhsa.gov/data/NSDUH/2012SummNatFindDetTables/NationalFindings/NSDUHresults2012.htm#fig2.1, downloaded April 1, 2014.

toxic, have been found in tobacco smoke. About 70 are proven carcinogens. The harmful effects of cigarette smoking and tobacco use in general were not exactly known until the early 1960s, when research began to show a link between tobacco use and disease.

In 1964, the U.S. Surgeon General issued the first major report presenting scientific evidence that cigarettes were a major health hazard in American society. More than 40 percent of the U.S. adult population smoked cigarettes at the time. Since the report in 1964, more than 15 million premature deaths in the United States alone are attributed to smoking.

In 2012, 22 percent of Americans 12 years and older smoked cigarettes. Young people who smoke are also more likely to abuse other illicit drugs. Smokers between the ages of 12 and 17 are nine times more likely to use drugs than nonsmokers in this same age group.

Morbidity and Mortality Tobacco use in all its forms is considered a significant threat to life. Up to half of tobacco users will die from its use. World Health Organization estimates indicate that 10 percent of the 7 billion people presently living will die as a result of smoking-related illnesses, which kill more than 6 million people each year. At the present rate of escalation, this figure is expected to climb to 8 million deaths annually by 2030. A total of 100 million tobacco-related deaths occurred in the 20th century, and based on estimates, there will be 1 billion deaths in the 21st century.

CRITICAL THINKING

Do you think the government should outlaw the use of tobacco in all forms? Or does the individual have the right to engage in self-destructive behavior?

To gain some perspective on the seriousness of the tobacco problem, CDC statistics indicate that drug overdoses and drug-related murders kill more than 40,000 people per year in the United States. By comparison, tobacco, a legal drug, kills about 12 times as many people as all illegal drugs combined.

Cigarette smoking is the largest preventable cause of illness and premature death in the United States. Death rates from heart disease, cancer, stroke, aortic aneurysm, chronic bronchitis, emphysema, and peptic ulcers all increase with cigarette smoking.

In pregnant women, cigarette smoking has been linked to retarded fetal growth, higher risk for spontaneous abortion (miscarriage), and prenatal death. Smoking is also the most prevalent cause of injury and death from fire. The average life expectancy for chronic smokers is 10 years shorter than that for nonsmokers, and the death rates among chronic smokers during their most productive years of life, between ages 25 and 65, is twice the national average. If we consider all related deaths, smoking is responsible for more than 480,000 U.S. deaths each year—enough deaths to wipe out the entire population of Miami in a single year. For every tobacco-related death, there are 30 others, or 16 million people in the United States, who suffer from at least one serious illness associated with cigarette smoking. More deaths are caused each year by tobacco use than by all deaths from HIV, illegal drug use, motor vehicle injuries, alcohol use, suicides, and murders combined.

Based on a report by U.S. government physicians, each cigarette shortens life by 7 to 11 minutes. This figure represents 5.5 million years of potential life that Americans lose to smoking each year.

Effects on Cardiovascular System Each year approximately 180,000 heart disease deaths are attributed to cigarette smoking. The CDC states that smoking increases the risk of coronary heart disease two- to four-fold. The mortality rate following heart attacks is higher for smokers because their attacks usually are more severe and their risk for deadly arrhythmias is much greater.

Cigarette smoking affects the cardiovascular system by increasing heart rate, blood pressure, and susceptibility to atherosclerosis, blood clots, coronary artery spasm, cardiac arrhythmia, and arteriosclerotic peripheral vascular disease. Evidence also indicates that smoking decreases high-density lipoprotein (HDL) cholesterol, the "good" cholesterol that lowers the risk for heart disease. Smoking further increases the amount of fatty acids, glucose, and various hormones in the blood. The carbon monoxide in smoke hinders the capacity of the blood to carry oxygen to body tissues. Both carbon monoxide and nicotine can damage the inner walls of the arter-

Tar A chemical compound that forms during the burning of tobacco leaves.

Nicotine An addictive compound found in tobacco leaves.

ies and thereby encourage the buildup of fat on them. Smoking also causes increased adhesiveness and clustering of platelets in the blood, decreases platelet survival and clotting time, and increases blood thickness. Any of these effects can precipitate a heart attack.

Smoking and Cancer The American Cancer Society reports that 87 percent of lung cancer is attributable to smoking. Lung cancer is the leading cancer killer, accounting for approximately 160,000 deaths in the United States in 2012, or about 30 percent of all deaths from cancer.[20] Cigarette smoking also leads to chronic lower respiratory disease, the third-leading cause of death in the United States (see also Chapter 1). Figure 13.5 illustrates normal and diseased **alveoli**.

The most common carcinogenic exposure in the workplace is cigarette smoke. Both fatal and nonfatal cardiac events are increased greatly in people who are exposed to passive smoke. About 42,000 additional deaths result each year in the United States from secondhand smoke (also known as environmental tobacco smoke, or ETS), which includes death from cardiovascular diseases, lung cancer, and SIDS.[21] Furthermore, almost 22 million children between the ages of 3 and 11 are exposed to secondhand smoke, and approximately 30 percent of the indoor workforce is not protected by smoke-free workplace policies. According to the U.S. Surgeon General, the evidence clearly shows that there is no risk-free level of exposure to ETS, prompting Dr. Richard Carmona, U.S. Surgeon General from 2002–2006, to state: "Based on the science, I wouldn't allow anyone in my family to stand in a room with someone smoking."[22]

FIGURE 13.5 **Normal and diseased alveoli in lungs.**

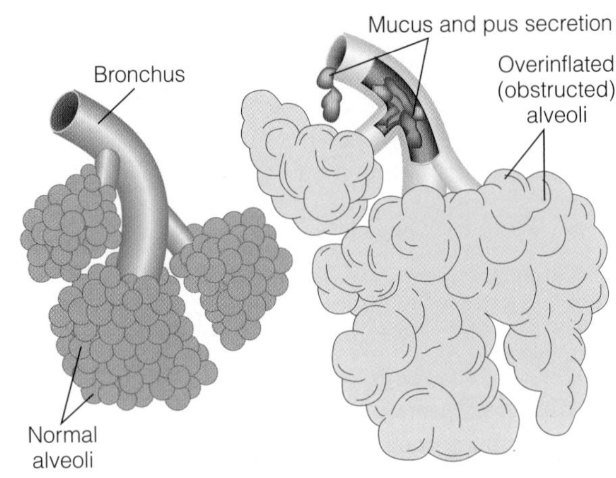

Two large-scale reviews of research studies on American, Canadian, and European communities that have passed laws to curb secondhand smoke by banning it in public places, including bars and restaurants, have shown an average drop of 17 percent in heart attacks in the first year compared to levels in communities without such a ban. There is a further 26 percent decline in heart attacks for at least three years each year thereafter. Within 20 minutes of secondhand smoke inhalation, chemical changes can be detected in the body's blood clotting mechanism, increasing the risk for heart attack or stroke. Research also indicates that lifetime exposure to secondhand smoke (which in adults is defined as 20 years or more for home exposure or 10 years or more

FIGURE 13.6 **The health effects of smoking.**

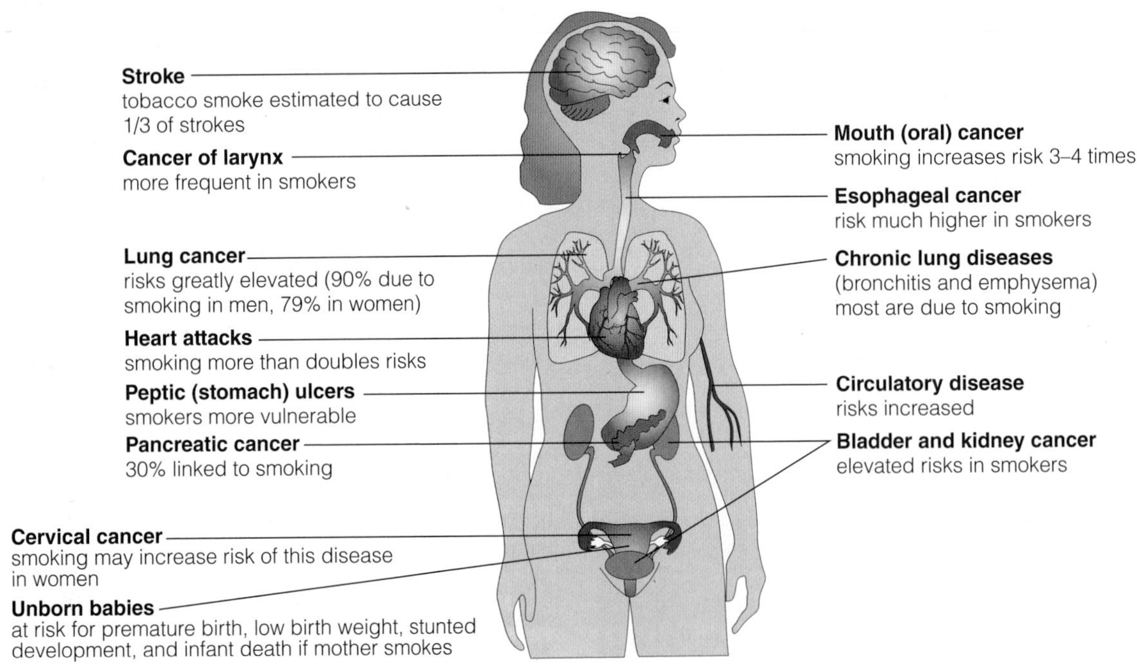

of work exposure) increases the risk of stillbirth, miscarriage, or tubal ectopic pregnancy in women regardless of whether they ever smoked personally. Nonsmokers exposed to secondhand smoke at home or at the office have up to a 30 percent greater risk of suffering a heart attack. Furthermore, exposure to thirdhand smoke—tobacco smoke contamination that saturates carpets, wallpaper, paint, fabrics, and furniture upholstery—also increases the risk of cancer and is particularly damaging for infants and young children that have the most contact with floors, surfaces, furniture, toys, and other objects in the home.

CRITICAL THINKING

You are in a designated nonsmoking area and the person next to you lights up a cigarette. What can you say to this person to protect your right to clean air?

Although the five-year survival rate for all cancers in the United States, Canada, and Europe is now at 68 percent (up from 49 percent in 1977), the five-year survival rate for lung cancer is about 17 percent. In addition to lung cancer, cigarette smoking increases the risk for oral cavity, lip, nasopharynx, nasal cavity and paranasal sinus, pharynx, larynx, esophagus, stomach, colorectum, pancreas, uterine cervix, ovary, kidney, bladder, liver, and acute myeloid leukemia cancers (also see Figure 13.6).

Other Forms of Tobacco Many tobacco users are aware of the health consequences of cigarette smoking but may fail to realize the risks of pipe smoking, cigar smoking, and tobacco chewing. As a group, pipe and cigar smokers have lower risks for heart disease and lung cancer than cigarette smokers. Nevertheless, blood nicotine levels in pipe and cigar smokers have been shown to approach those of cigarette smokers, because nicotine is still absorbed through the membranes of the mouth. Therefore, these tobacco users still have a higher risk for heart disease than nonsmokers do.

Cigarette smokers who substitute pipe or cigar smoking for cigarettes usually continue to inhale the smoke, which results in more nicotine and tar being brought into their lungs than they inhale through cigarette smoke. Consequently, the risk for disease is even higher if pipe or cigar smoke is inhaled. The risk and mortality rates for lip, mouth, and larynx cancer for pipe smoking, cigar smoking, and tobacco chewing are higher than those for cigarette smoking.

Smokeless Tobacco

Smokeless tobacco has been promoted in the past as a safe alternative to cigarette smoking. However, the Advisory Committee to the U.S. Surgeon General has stated that smokeless tobacco represents a significant health risk and is just as addictive as cigarette smoking.

Over 9 million Americans use smokeless tobacco. The greatest concern is the increase in use of smokeless tobacco among young people. Surveys indicate that about 15 percent of high school males use smokeless tobacco. The average starting age for smokeless tobacco use is 10 years old.

Adverse Effects of Secondhand Smoke

- A 30 percent increase in coronary heart disease risk (some adverse effects begin within minutes to hours of exposure).
- Increases blood clotting, enhancing the risk of heart attacks and strokes.
- Lowers HDL (good) cholesterol.
- Increases oxidation of LDL cholesterol, enhancing atherosclerosis.
- Increases oxygen-free radicals.
- Decreases levels of antioxidants.
- Increases chronic inflammation.
- Increases insulin resistance, leading to higher blood sugar levels and risk for diabetes.
- Increases lung and overall cancer risk.
- Increases risk for pulmonary diseases.
- Increases risk for adverse effects during pregnancy.
- Increases sudden infant death syndrome (SIDS) risk.

Using smokeless tobacco can lead to gingivitis and periodontitis. It carries a fourfold increase in oral cancer and in some cases even premature death. People who chew or dip also have a higher rate of cavities, sore gums, bad breath, and stained teeth. Their senses of smell and taste diminish; consequently, they tend to add more sugar and salt to food. These practices alone increase the risk for being overweight and having high blood pressure. Nicotine addiction and its related health risks also hold true for smokeless tobacco users. Nicotine blood levels approach those of cigarette smokers, increasing the risk for diseases of the cardiovascular system. Furthermore, research has revealed changes in heart rate and blood pressure similar to those of cigarette smokers.

Using tobacco in any form can be addictive and poses a serious threat to health and well-being. Eliminating its use is the most important lifestyle change a tobacco user can make to improve health, quality of life, and longevity.

Health Care Costs of Tobacco Use Heavy smokers use the health care system, especially hospitals, twice as much as nonsmokers do. The American Cancer Society reports that for every time smokers

Alveoli Air sacs in the lungs where gas exchange (oxygen and carbon dioxide) takes place.

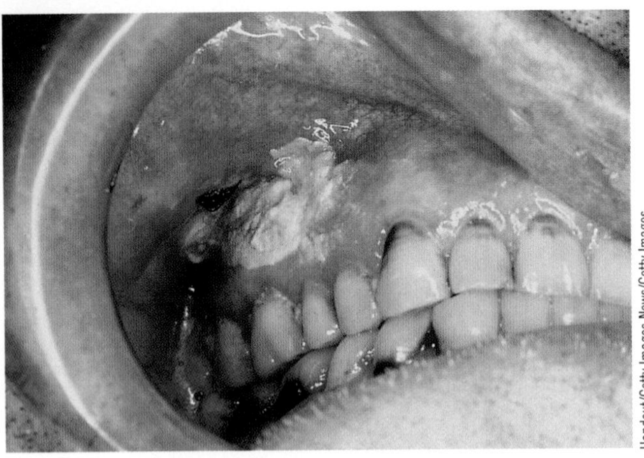

Handout/Getty Images News/Getty Images

Smokeless tobacco can lead to gum and teeth damage, as well as oral cancer (pictured).

purchase a pack of cigarettes in the United States at an average price of $6.36, they create $35 of future health-related costs for themselves. The yearly cost to a given company has been estimated to be up to $6,000 per smoking employee. This cost includes employee health care, absenteeism, additional health insurance, morbidity or disability and early mortality, on-the-job time lost, property damage or maintenance and depreciation, worker compensation, and the impact of secondhand smoke.

If every U.S. smoker were to give up cigarettes, in 1 year alone sick time would drop by approximately 90 million days, heart conditions would decrease by 280,000, chronic bronchitis and emphysema would number 1 million fewer cases, and total death rates from cardiovascular disease, cancer, and peptic ulcers would fall off drastically.

Every day, more than 1,300 Americans die from smoking-related illnesses. That is the equivalent of three fully loaded jumbo jets crashing every day with no survivors. Imagine what the coverage and concern would be if 480,000 people each year were to die in the United States alone because of airplane accidents. People would not even consider flying anymore. Most people would think of it as a form of suicide.

Smoking kills more Americans in a single year than died in battle during World War II and the Vietnam War combined. Think of the public outrage if 480,000 Americans were to die annually in a meaningless war. What if a single nonprescription drug were to cause more than 160,000 deaths from cancer and 180,000 deaths from heart disease? The U.S. public would not tolerate these situations. We would mount an intense fight to prevent the deaths.

Yet, aren't people committing slow suicide by smoking cigarettes? Isn't tobacco a nonprescription drug available to almost anyone who wishes to smoke, killing some 480,000 Americans each year? If cigarettes were invented today, the tobacco industry would be put on trial for mass murder.

Trends The fight against all forms of tobacco use is stronger than ever. This was not always the case. It has been difficult to fight an industry that wields such enormous financial and political influence as does the tobacco industry in the United States. Tobacco is one of the top 10 cash crops in the United States. The tobacco industry has influenced elections cleverly by emphasizing the individual's right to smoke, avoiding that so many people die because of it.

Philip Morris International, a.k.a Altria, one of the largest tobacco-producing companies in the world, receives nearly 90 percent of its revenues from the sale of cigarettes. Philip Morris has donated millions of dollars to prominent organizations, which no longer question the detrimental effects of tobacco use. Among the organizations that have received donations from Philip Morris are the United Way, YMCA, Salvation Army, Pediatric AIDS Foundation, Red Cross, Cystic Fibrosis Foundation, March of Dimes, Easter Seals, Muscular Dystrophy Association, Multiple Sclerosis Society, Hemophilia Foundation, United Cerebral Palsy, American Civil Liberties Union, American Bar Association, Task Force for Battered Women, Boy Scouts, Boys and Girls Club, and Big Brothers Big Sisters. We call drug runners unprincipled scum, yet we welcome Philip Morris with glee and call it civic pride.[23]

Tobacco was socially accepted for many years. Cigarette smoking, however, is no longer acceptable in most social circles. Smoking is prohibited in most public places as a result of nonsmokers and ex-smokers alike fighting for their rights to clean air and health.

Many smokers are unaware of, or simply do not care to realize, how much cigarette smoke bothers nonsmokers. Smokers sometimes think that blowing the smoke off to the side is enough to get it out of the way. It is not enough. Smokers do not comprehend this until they quit and later find themselves in that situation. Suddenly they realize why cigarette smoke is so unpleasant and undesirable to most people.

The FDA Drug Abuse Advisory Committee has taken a strong stance against the use of all forms of tobacco products. Although the AHA commends the work initiated by the FDA, the AHA has further stated that the FDA and the federal government have an obligation to take regulatory action against the national problem of nicotine addiction and abuse of cigarettes and tobacco products in general. The U.S. Surgeon General's office has stated that health education, combined with social, economic, and regulatory approaches, is imperative to offset the tobacco industry's marketing and promotion and to promote nonsmoking environments.

Why People Smoke

People typically begin to smoke without realizing its detrimental effects on their health and life in general. Although people start to smoke for many reasons, the three fundamental instigators are peer pressure, desire to appear "grown up," and rebellion against authority. Smoking only three packs of cigarettes can lead to physiological addiction, turning smoking into a nasty habit that has become the most widespread example of drug dependency in the United States.

Smoking Addiction and Dependency

The drug nicotine has strong addictive properties. Within seconds of inhalation, nicotine affects the central nervous system and can act simultaneously as a tranquilizer and a stimulant. The stimulating effect produces strong physiological and psychological dependency. The physical addiction to nicotine is six to eight times more powerful than the addiction to alcohol and most likely greater than that of some hard drugs currently used.

Psychological dependency develops over a longer time. People smoke to aid relaxation, and they gain a certain amount of pleasure from the ritual of smoking. Smokers automatically associate many activities of daily life with cigarettes—coffee drinking, alcohol drinking, being part of a social gathering, relaxing after a meal, talking on the telephone, driving, reading, and watching television. In many cases, the social rituals of smoking are the most difficult to eliminate. The dependency is so strong that years after people have stopped smoking, they may still crave cigarettes when they engage in certain social activities.

Most of the remaining information in this chapter is written directly to smokers. Nonsmokers, however, will gain a better understanding of smokers by reading it. The following material also provides valuable information to help others implement a smoking-cessation program.

Why Do You Smoke? Test

Most people smoke for a variety of reasons. To find out why people smoke, the National Clearinghouse for Smoking and Health developed the simple Why Do You Smoke? Test. This test, contained in Lab 13B, lists some statements by smokers describing what they get out of smoking cigarettes. Smokers are asked to indicate how often they have the feelings described in each statement when they are smoking.

The scores obtained on this test assess smokers for each of six factors that describe individuals' feelings when they smoke. The first three highlight the positive feelings that people derive from smoking. The fourth factor relates to reducing tension and relaxing. The fifth reveals the extent of dependence on cigarettes. The sixth factor differentiates habit smoking and purely automatic smoking. Each of the remaining factors fits one of the six reasons for smoking discussed next. A score of 11 or above on any factor indicates that smoking is an important source of satisfaction for you. The higher you score (15 is the highest), the more important a given factor is in your smoking, and the more useful a discussion of that factor can be in your attempt to quit.

If you do not score high on any of the six factors, chances are that you do not smoke much or have not been smoking for long. If so, giving up smoking, and staying off, should be fairly easy.

1. **Stimulation.** If you score high or fairly high on the stimulation factor, you are among those smokers stimulated by the cigarette. You think it helps wake you up, organize your energies, and keep you going. If you try to give up smoking, you may want a safe substitute—a brisk walk or moderate exercise, for example—whenever you feel the urge to smoke.
2. **Handling.** Handling things can be satisfying, but you can keep your hands busy in many ways without lighting up or playing with a cigarette. Why not toy with a pen or pencil? Try doodling. Play with a coin, a piece of jewelry, or some other harmless object.
3. **Pleasure/Relaxation.** Finding out whether you use the cigarette to feel good—you get real, honest pleasure from smoking—or to keep from feeling bad (factor 4) is not always easy. About two-thirds of smokers score high or fairly high on accentuation of pleasure, and about half of those also score as high or higher on reduction of negative feelings. Those who get real pleasure from smoking often find that honest consideration of the harmful effects of their habit is enough to help them quit. They substitute social and physical activities and find that they do not seriously miss cigarettes.
4. **Crutch: Tension Reduction**. Many smokers use cigarettes as a crutch during moments of stress or discomfort. Ironically, the heavy smoker—the person who tries to handle severe personal problems by smoking many times a day—is apt to discover that cigarettes do not help deal with problems effectively. This kind of smoker may stop smoking readily when everything is going well but may be tempted to start again in a time of crisis. Again, physical exertion or social activity may be a useful substitute for cigarettes, especially in times of tension.
5. **Craving: Psychological Addiction.** Quitting smoking is difficult for people who score high on this factor. The craving for a cigarette begins to build the moment the previous cigarette is put out, so tapering off is not likely to work. Such smokers must go **cold turkey**. If you are dependent on cigarettes, you might try smoking more than usual for a day or two to spoil your taste for cigarettes and then isolating yourself from cigarettes until the craving is gone.
6. **Habit.** If you are smoking from habit, you no longer get much satisfaction from cigarettes. You light them frequently without even realizing you are doing it. You may have an easy time quitting and staying off if you can break the habitual patterns you have built up. Cutting down gradually may be effective if you change the way you smoke cigarettes and the conditions under which you smoke them. The key to success is to become aware of each cigarette you smoke. You can do this by asking yourself, "Do I really want this cigarette?" You might be surprised at how many you do not want.

Cold turkey Eliminating a negative behavior all at once.

Smoking Cessation

If you are contemplating a smoking-cessation program or are preparing to stop cigarette smoking, you need to know that quitting smoking is not easy. Annually, only about 20 percent of smokers who try to quit the first time succeed. The addictive properties of nicotine and smoke make quitting difficult.

The American Psychiatric Association and the National Institute on Drug Abuse have indicated that nicotine is perhaps the most addictive drug known to humans. The U.S. Surgeon General has concluded that [24]

- Cigarettes and other forms of tobacco are addicting.
- Nicotine is the drug responsible for the addictive behavior.
- Pharmacological and behavioral traits that determine addiction to tobacco are similar to those that determine addiction to drugs such as heroin and cocaine.

Smokers develop a tolerance to nicotine and tobacco smoke. They become dependent on both and get physical and psychological withdrawal symptoms when they stop smoking. Even though giving up smoking can be extremely difficult, it is by no means impossible, as attested by the many people who have quit. During the past four decades, cigarette smoking in the United States had declined gradually among smokers of all ages.

Surveys have shown that approximately 70 percent of all smokers would like to quit. In 1964 (when the U.S. Surgeon General first reported the link between smoking and increased risk for disease and mortality), 40 percent of the adult population—53 percent of men and 32 percent of women—smoked. In 2012, only 26.7 percent of adult men and 21.1 percent of adult women smoked. Almost 50 million Americans have given up cigarettes.

Furthermore, more than 91 percent of successful ex-smokers have been able to do it on their own, either by quitting cold turkey or by using self-help kits available from organizations such as the American Cancer Society, the AHA, and the American Lung Association. Smokers' information and treatment centers can be readily found online.

Do You Want to Quit? Test

The most important factor in quitting cigarette smoking is the person's sincere desire to do so. Although a few smokers can simply quit, this usually is not the case. Those who can quit easily are primarily light or casual smokers. They realize that the pleasure of an occasional cigarette is not worth the added risk for disease and premature death. For heavy smokers, quitting most likely will be a difficult battle. Even though many do not succeed the first time around, the odds of quitting are better for those who repeatedly try to stop.

If you are a smoker and want to find your readiness to quit, the Do You Want to Quit? Test, developed by the National Clearinghouse for Smoking and Health contained in Lab 13B, will measure your attitude toward the four primary reasons you want to quit smoking. The results indicate whether you are ready to start the program. On this test, the higher you score in any category, say, the Health category, the more important that reason is to you. A score of 9 or above in one of these categories indicates that this is one of the most important reasons you may want to quit.

1. **Health.** Knowing the harmful consequences of cigarettes, many people have stopped smoking and many others are considering doing so. If your score on the Health factor is 9 or above, the health hazards of smoking may be enough to make you want to quit now. If your score on this factor is low (6 or below), consider the hazards of smoking. You may be lacking important information or may even have incorrect information. If so, health considerations are not playing the role they should in your decision to keep smoking or to quit.
2. **Example.** Some people stop smoking because they want to set a good example for others. Parents quit to make it easier for their children to resist starting to smoke. Doctors quit so that they can be role models for their patients. Teachers quit to discourage their students from smoking. Sports stars want to set an example for their young fans. Husbands quit to influence their wives to quit, and vice versa. Examples have a significant influence on behavior. Surveys show that almost twice as many high school students smoke if both parents are smokers compared with those whose parents are nonsmokers or former smokers. If your score is low (6 or lower), you might not be interested in giving up smoking to set an example for others. Perhaps you do not realize how important your example could be.
3. **Aesthetics.** People who score high (9 or above) in this category recognize and are disturbed by some of the unpleasant aspects of smoking. The smell of stale smoke on your clothing, bad breath, and stains on your fingers and teeth might be reason enough to consider quitting.
4. **Mastery.** If you score 9 or above on this factor, you are bothered by knowing that you cannot control your desire to smoke. You are not your own master. Awareness of this challenge to your self-control may make you want to quit.

Breaking the Habit

The following seven-step plan has been developed as a guide to help you quit smoking. You should complete the total program in 4 weeks or less. Steps 1 through 4 combined should take no longer than 2 weeks. A maximum of 2 additional weeks is allowed for the rest of the program.

Step 1 Decide positively that you want to quit. Avoid negative thoughts of how difficult this can be. Think positive. You can do it.

Now prepare a list of the reasons you smoke and the reasons you want to quit (see Lab 13B). Make several copies

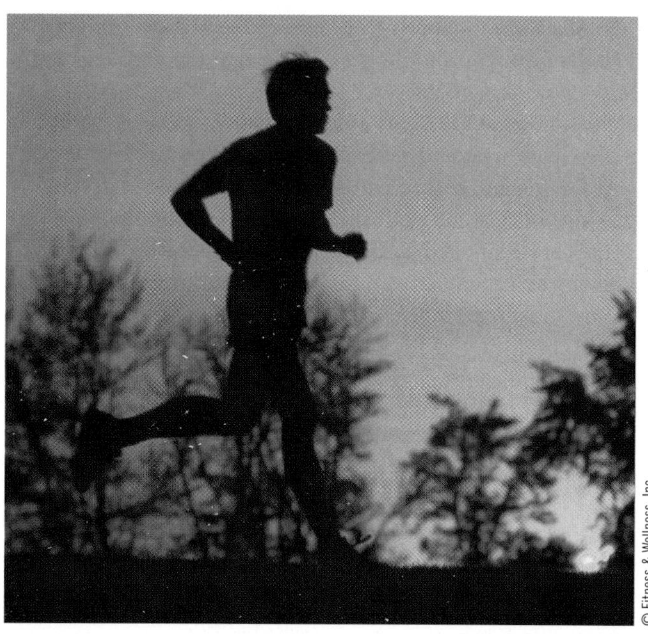

Starting an exercise program prior to giving up cigarettes encourages cessation and helps with weight control during the process.

of the list, and keep them in places where you commonly smoke. Frequently review the reasons for quitting, because this will motivate and prepare you psychologically to quit.

When the reasons for quitting outweigh the reasons for smoking, you will have an easier time quitting. Read as much information as possible on the detrimental effects of tobacco and the benefits of quitting.

Step 2

Initiate a personal diet and exercise program. About one-third of the people who quit smoking gain weight. This could be caused by one or a combination of the following reasons:

1. Food becomes a substitute for cigarettes.
2. Appetite increases.
3. Basal metabolism may slow.

If you start an exercise and weight-control program prior to quitting smoking, weight gain should not be a problem. If anything, exercise and lower body weight create more awareness of healthy living and strengthen the motivation for giving up cigarettes.

Even if you gain some weight, the harmful effects of cigarette smoking are much more detrimental to human health than a few extra pounds of body weight. Experts have indicated that as far as the extra load on the heart is concerned, giving up one pack of cigarettes a day is the equivalent of losing between 50 and 75 pounds of excess body fat.

Step 3 Decide on the approach you will use to stop smoking. You may quit cold turkey or gradually cut down the number of cigarettes you smoke daily. Base your decision on your scores obtained on the Why Do You Smoke? Test. If you score 11 points or higher in either the Crutch: Tension Reduction or the Craving: Psychological Addiction category, your best chance for success is quitting cold turkey. If your highest scores occur in any of the other four categories, you may choose either approach.

People still argue about which approach is more effective. Quitting cold turkey may cause fewer withdrawal symptoms than tapering off gradually. When you are cutting down slowly, the fewer cigarettes you smoke, the more important each one becomes. Therefore, you have a greater chance for relapse and returning to the original number of cigarettes you smoked. But when the cutting-down approach is accompanied by a definite target date for quitting, the technique has been shown to be quite effective. Smokers who taper off without a target date for quitting are the most likely to relapse.

Step 4 Keep a daily log of your smoking habit for a few days. This will help you understand the situations in which you smoke. To assist this process, make copies of Lab 13B or develop your own form. Keep this form with you, and every time you smoke, record the required information. Keep track of the number of cigarettes you smoke, times of day you smoke them, events associated with smoking, amount of each cigarette smoked, and a rating of how badly you needed that cigarette. Rate each cigarette from 1 to 3:

1. = desperately needed
2. = moderately needed
3. = no real need

This daily log will assist you in three ways:

1. You will get to know your habit.
2. It will help you eliminate cigarettes you do not crave.
3. It will help you find positive substitutes for situations that trigger your desire to smoke.

Step 5 Set the target date for quitting. If you are going to taper off gradually, read the instructions in the "Cutting Down Gradually" section (see page 514) before you proceed to step 6. When you set the target date, choose a special date to add extra incentive. An upcoming birthday, anniversary, vacation, graduation, family reunion—all are examples of good dates to free yourself from smoking. Dates when you are going to be away from events and environments that trigger your desire to smoke may be especially helpful. Once you have set the date, do not change it. Do not let anyone or anything interfere with this date.

Let your friends and relatives know of your intentions and ask for their support. Consider asking someone else to quit with you. That way, you can support each other in your efforts to stop. Avoid anyone who will not support you in your effort to quit. When you are attempting to quit, other people can be a prime obstacle. Many smokers are intolerable when they first stop smoking, so some friends and relatives prefer that they continue to smoke.

Step 6 Stock up on low-calorie foods—carrots, broccoli, cauliflower, celery, popcorn (butter and salt free), fruits, sunflower seeds (in the shell), sugarless gum, and so on—and drink plenty of water. Keep the food handy on the day you stop and the first few days following cessation. Substitute this food for a cigarette when you want one.

Step 7 On your quit day and the first few days thereafter, do not keep cigarettes handy. Stay away from friends and events that trigger your desire to smoke, and drink a lot of water and fruit juices. To replace the old behavior with new behavior, replace smoking time with new, positive substitutes that make smoking difficult or impossible.

When you want a cigarette, take a few deep breaths and then occupy yourself by doing any of a number of things, such as talking to someone else, washing your hands, brushing your teeth, eating a healthy snack, chewing on a straw, doing dishes, playing sports, going for a walk or a bike ride, or going swimming. Engage in activities that require the use of your hands. Try gardening, sewing, writing letters, drawing, doing household chores, or washing the car. Visit nonsmoking places such as libraries, museums, stores, and theaters. Plan an outing or a trip away from home. Any of these activities can keep your mind off cigarettes. Record your choice of activity or substitute under the Remarks/Substitutes column in Lab 13B.

Quitting Cold Turkey Many people have found that quitting all at once is the easiest way to stop smoking. Most smokers have tried this approach at least once. Even though it might not work the first time, they don't allow themselves to get discouraged, and they eventually succeed. Many times, after several attempts, all of a sudden they are able to overcome smoking without too much difficulty.

On average, as few as three smokeless days are sufficient to break the physiological addiction to nicotine. The psychological addiction may linger for years but will get weaker as time goes by.

Cutting Down Gradually Tapering off cigarettes can be done in several ways:

1. Eliminate cigarettes you do not strongly crave (those ranked 3 and 2 on your daily log).
2. Switch to a brand lower in nicotine, tar, or both every few days.
3. Smoke less of each cigarette.
4. Smoke fewer cigarettes each day.

Most people prefer a combination of these four suggestions.

Before you start cutting down, set a target date for quitting. Once the date is set, don't change it. The total time until your quit date should be no longer than 2 weeks. Reduce the total number of cigarettes you smoke each day by 10 to 25 percent. As you smoke less, be careful not to take more puffs or inhale more deeply as you smoke, because this offsets the principle of cutting down.

As an aid in tapering off, make several copies of Lab 13B. By now, you should have completed the first daily log of your smoking habit—see step 4 under "Breaking the Habit" on page 513. Start a new daily log, and every night review your data and set goals for the following day.

Decide and record which cigarettes will be easiest to give up, what brand you will smoke, the total number of cigarettes to be smoked, and how much of each you will smoke. Log any comments or situations you want to avoid, as well as any substitutes you could use to help you in the program. For example, if you always smoke while drinking coffee, substitute juice for coffee. If you smoke while driving, arrange for a ride or take a bus to work. If you smoke with a certain friend at lunch, avoid having lunch with that friend for a week or so. Continue using this log until you have stopped smoking completely.

Nicotine-Substitution Products

Nicotine-substitution drug products such as nicotine transdermal patches and nicotine gum were developed to help people kick the tobacco habit. These products are thought to be most effective when used in a physician-supervised cessation program. As with tapering off, these products gradually decrease the amount of nicotine used until their users no longer crave the drug.

Nicotine patches supply a steady dose of nicotine through the skin. According to a nicotine-replacement patch website, the program consists of a 10-week plan with three levels of nicotine patches. The person is asked to stop smoking before beginning the program; otherwise, the individual ends up with a very high blood nicotine level. A 21-mg patch is used during the first 6 weeks of the program, followed by a 14-mg patch for 2 weeks, and a final 7-mg patch for the last 2 weeks. The intent is to simulate a gradual weaning from the nicotine with fewer side effects. The instructions are specific, and the individual must carefully follow the instructions for the program to be effective. The site is clear that the program only works if the person is committed to quit the habit, because the patch does not override the mind.

At present, evidence shows that patches are not more effective for quitting smoking than doing so without patches. However, one study showed that patches are more effective when used in conjunction with exercise.[25] About 8 out of 10 smokers who exercised along with the use of nicotine-replacement therapy successfully quit smoking.

Nicotine-replacement patches are available in various dosages, delivering anywhere from about 5 to 21 mg of nicotine in a 24-hour period. The retail cost for a 10-week program ranges from $100 to $200, significantly cheaper than smoking a pack a day for 10 weeks. Public safety concerns regarding the use of nicotine patches, including indications, precautions, warnings, contraindications, potential abuse, and marketing and labeling issues are monitored and regulated by the FDA. People contemplating their use should pay careful attention to contraindications and potential side effects. Pregnant and lactating women and people with heart disease or high blood pressure or who have had a recent heart attack should check with their physician prior to using nicotine-substitution products. Skin redness, swelling, or rashes are sometimes associated with the use of nicotine patches. Other undesirable side effects are listed on the label and should be monitored closely.

Electronic Cigarettes Electronic cigarettes, more commonly known as e-cigarettes, personal vaporizers, or simply VP, were introduced to the U.S. market in 2007 as alternative devices to simulate the act of tobacco smoking. The electronic inhaler heats up a liquid nicotine solution into an aerosol mist that smokers inhale. Although e-cigarettes don't produce secondhand smoke, they do produce secondhand vapor. Because the vapor can contain many of the same toxic chemicals found in cigarette smoke, there is a growing national trend to regulate the devices. E-cigarettes have been banned on aircrafts and in many cities and restaurants where traditional smoking is not allowed. Health risks are unknown at this time because limited research is available on these products. Although e-cigarettes are marketed as safer alternatives because they have far fewer of the toxic chemical compounds found in cigarette smoke, the FDA warns of potential addiction and abuse of these products. The amount of nicotine an e-cigarette delivers depends on the strength of the liquid nicotine cartridge a smoker installs, which can contain nicotine comparable to light or ultra light cigarettes, or as much nicotine as regular cigarettes or more. Some cartridges also contain liquid without nicotine to help users continue to experience the sensation of smoking without the detrimental effects.

Though distributors are not allowed to market e-cigarettes as aids to smoking cessation, e-cigarettes are commonly being used as an alternative to nicotine patches. The CDC reports that one-fifth of traditional-cigarette adult smokers had tried e-cigarettes. The real concern is that if smokers use both traditional and e-cigarettes, rather than using e-cigarettes to quit cigarettes completely, the health consequences could be exponentially greater. Authorities also fear candy-flavored e-cigarettes may cause young people to use the devices as a "gateway" to conventional cigarettes. Federal surveys show that 1 in 10 high school students tried e-cigarettes in 2012, double the rate of use in 2011. Though teen cigarette use has declined in recent years, the numbers are unfortunately offset in part by the growing use of alternative tobacco products, including e-cigarettes, cigars, dissolvable tobacco, snus, and hookahs.

CRITICAL THINKING

If you ever smoked or now smoke cigarettes, discuss your perceptions of how others accepted your behavior. If you smoked and have quit, how did you accomplish the task, and has it changed the way others view you? If you never smoked, how do you perceive smokers?

Life after Cigarettes

When you first quit smoking, you can expect a series of withdrawal symptoms for a few days; among them are lower heart rate and blood pressure, headaches, gastrointestinal discomfort, mood changes, irritability, aggressiveness, and difficulty sleeping.

The physiological addiction to nicotine is broken only 3 days following your last cigarette. Thereafter, you should not crave cigarettes as much. For the habitual smoker, the psychological dependency could be the most difficult to break. The first few days probably will not be as difficult as the first few months. Any of the activities of daily life that you have associated with smoking—either stress or relaxation, joy or unhappiness—may trigger a relapse even months, or at times years, after quitting.

Ex-smokers should realize that even though some harm may have been done already, it is never too late to quit. The greatest early benefit is a lower risk for sudden death. Furthermore, the risk for illness starts to decrease the moment you stop smoking. You will have fewer sore throats and sores in the mouth, less hoarseness, no more cigarette cough, and lower risk for peptic ulcers.

Circulation to the hands and feet will improve, as will gastrointestinal and kidney and bladder functions. Everything will taste and smell better. You will have more energy, and you will gain a sense of freedom, pride, and well-being. You no longer will have to worry whether you have enough cigarettes to last through a day, a party, a meeting, a weekend, or a trip.

BEHAVIOR MODIFICATION PLANNING

Tips to Help Stop Smoking

Check the suggestions that may work for you and incorporate them into your own retraining program.

I PLAN TO | I DID IT

Preparing to Quit

- ❑ ❑ Create a personal list of reasons to quit. Keep the list handy, review it frequently, and add to it as needed.
- ❑ ❑ Know what to expect. Information is available from government sources, health organizations, doctors, hospitals, or on the web. Talk with people who have quit or contact a local group or a hotline.
- ❑ ❑ Review any past attempts to quit. Determine what worked and what didn't work for you.
- ❑ ❑ Get a physical examination and discuss your desire to quit smoking with your doctor. Ask whether medication may help you quit.
- ❑ ❑ Create a stop-smoking plan customized to your personality, preferences, and schedule. If you are tapering off, set intermediate goals. Make sure to plan for times of intense desire for a cigarette. Be prepared and determine what you can use as a substitute for that cigarette. Is there anyone you can call for assistance or to help you distract your mind? Do not forget to include rewards for your success. Sign a contract and ask a friend to sign it as a witness.
- ❑ ❑ Determine your quit day. Choose a special day, such as a birthday, an anniversary, or a holiday. Select a day on which you will not feel a strong temptation to smoke—for instance, a stressful work day. Once you pick a date, do not alter this date.
- ❑ ❑ Enlist the support of friends, loved ones, team members, coworkers—as many people as you can. Ask others not to smoke around you or leave cigarettes in view. If you can, find someone else who wants to quit with you.
- ❑ ❑ Inquire about counseling. Individual, group, and telephone counseling can improve your chances of success.
- ❑ ❑ Consider starting a weight loss and exercise program before you quit. Such positive action will increase your confidence in your ability to quit and can keep you from gaining weight when you stop smoking.
- ❑ ❑ Stage a farewell activity to cigarettes and smoking; perhaps by overindulging so that the idea of smoking is no longer appealing or with a ceremony to destroy all cigarettes, lighters, and ashtrays.
- ❑ ❑ Change your environment. Clean your room or house, clothes, and car to remove the scent of tobacco smoke. Rearrange the furniture, paint the walls a different color, open windows to freshen the air, and buy plants or flowers.
- ❑ ❑ Plan changes in your routine. Reschedule regular activities, use different routes to get to places you normally go, go to bed earlier and get up earlier, and avoid being rushed.
- ❑ ❑ Start a new hobby or other activity, for example, dancing, making videos, painting, acting, or learning to cook ethnic foods—something enjoyable that you've wanted to do for a long time.
- ❑ ❑ Stock up on healthy, low-calorie snacks.

While Tapering Off

- ❑ ❑ Make cigarettes as hard to get as possible. Leave them with someone else, lock them up, wrap them up like gifts with lots of tape or ribbon.
- ❑ ❑ Don't store cigarettes—wait until one pack is finished before buying another.
- ❑ ❑ Never carry matches or a lighter.
- ❑ ❑ Each time you want to smoke, write down what you are doing and feeling and how important the cigarette is to you—before you light up.
- ❑ ❑ Smoke only in uninteresting or uncomfortable places.
- ❑ ❑ Put off the first cigarette of the day for as long as possible.
- ❑ ❑ Smoke just half a cigarette.

After Quitting

- ❑ ❑ To help prevent relapse, rather than saying "I quit smoking," say "I don't want to smoke."
- ❑ ❑ Get plenty of sleep.
- ❑ ❑ Eat regular, healthy, appetizing meals; pay attention to the flavors and textures of the foods.
- ❑ ❑ Be mindful of negative thoughts and replace them with positive actions—from "I can't stand this" to "What else can I do right now to keep my mind off cigarettes?" for example.

BEHAVIOR MODIFICATION PLANNING

- ❑ ❑ Spend time in places where smoking is not allowed—libraries, museums, churches, malls, and movie theaters.
- ❑ ❑ Tune in to the sights and scents around you.
- ❑ ❑ Drink plenty of water and other low-calorie drinks (but avoid caffeine).
- ❑ ❑ Deal with one minute, one hour, and one day at a time.
- ❑ ❑ Plan something that will bring you pleasure every day.
- ❑ ❑ Be aware of life stressors and plan a variety of ways to relax without cigarettes.
- ❑ ❑ Avoid situations in which you used to smoke, including being with people who smoke.
- ❑ ❑ Be wary of alcohol: Drinking lowers your chances of success.
- ❑ ❑ Use your lungs more by increasing daily physical activity and sports participation. Try to notice how clean the air feels flowing in and out of your lungs.
- ❑ ❑ Celebrate and reward yourself for each success.
- ❑ ❑ Visit your dentist and have your teeth cleaned and whitened.
- ❑ ❑ Calculate how much money you are saving and use this money to reward yourself or someone else with a small luxury.
- ❑ ❑ Consult your doctor if you are concerned about your physical or emotional feelings.
- ❑ ❑ If you gain weight, don't attempt to lose the weight until after you get over the craving for cigarettes.

Instead of Smoking a Cigarette

- ❑ ❑ Take several deep breaths, focusing on your breathing and the fresh air that you are inhaling.
- ❑ ❑ Tell yourself to wait three minutes; redirect your thoughts by visualizing a serene landscape or planning a dream vacation or weekend away from home.
- ❑ ❑ Go for a walk. If you have a dog, take the dog for a walk.
- ❑ ❑ Chew gum or suck on hard, sugarless candy—always carry some with you.
- ❑ ❑ Talk to someone you can easily reach for support.
- ❑ ❑ Munch on carrots, celery sticks, or other healthy snacks.
- ❑ ❑ Use your hands: Wash dishes, sweep the floor, brush your teeth, write in a journal, sketch a cartoon, or play a musical instrument.
- ❑ ❑ Go swimming or take a shower.

If You Relapse

- ❑ ❑ Don't be discouraged—most people try several times before they are finally able to kick the habit.
- ❑ ❑ Instead of berating yourself, remember your successes and recommit to quitting.
- ❑ ❑ Re-evaluate your smoking-cessation plan and modify it as necessary.
- ❑ ❑ Remember that relapse doesn't mean failure. Failure comes to those who give up. Instead, learn from your mistake and reach once more for your goal.

Try It

Nicotine is believed to be the most addictive drug we know. Smokers who are trying to kick the habit need behavioral change strategies to enhance their rate of success. From the above strategies, prepare a list of those that may work for you. Conduct nightly audits on how well you have done that day. Every third day, review all of the above strategies and make changes to your list as necessary.

When you first quit and you think how tough it is and how miserable you feel because you cannot have a cigarette, try the opposite: Think of the benefits and how great it is not to smoke. The ex-smoker's risk for heart disease approaches that of a lifetime nonsmoker 10 years following cessation and for cancer, 15 years after quitting.

If you have been successful and stopped smoking, a lot of events can still trigger your urge to smoke. When confronted with these events, some people rationalize and think, "One cigarette won't hurt. I've been off for months (years in some cases)" or "I can handle it. I'll smoke just today." It won't work. Before you know it, you will be back to the regular nasty habit. Be prepared to take action in those situations by finding substitutes, such as those provided in the "Tips to Help Stop Smoking" box that begins on page 516.

Start thinking of yourself as a nonsmoker—no "butts" about it. Remind yourself how difficult it has been and how long it has taken you to get to this point. If you have come this far, you certainly can resist brief moments of temptation. It will get easier rather than harder as time goes on.

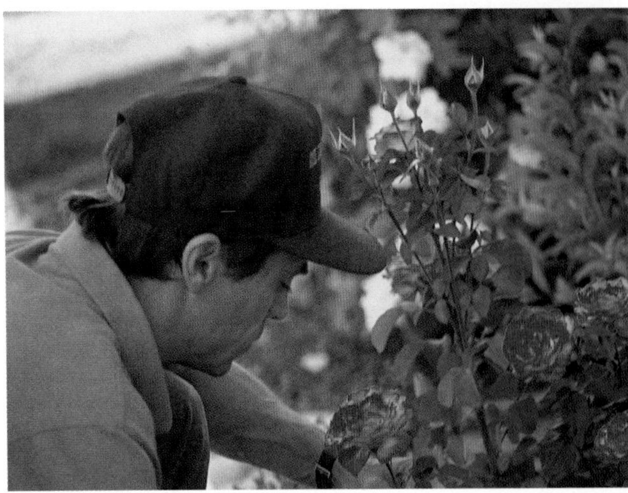

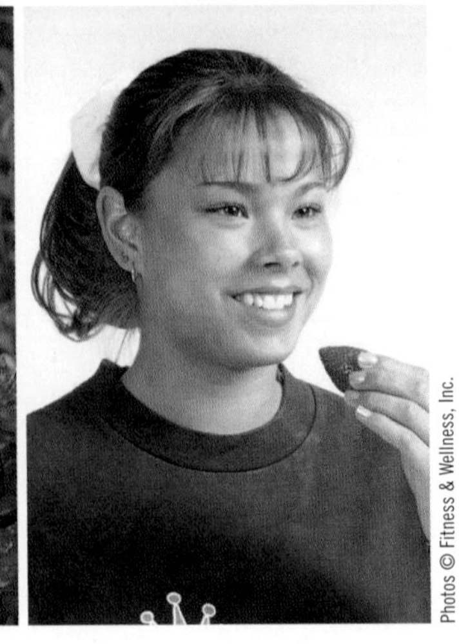

Photos © Fitness & Wellness, Inc.

The simple pleasures of life, such as taste and smell, improve with smoking cessation.

ASSESS YOUR BEHAVIOR

CENGAGE brain .com To access course materials, including companion resources, please visit **www.cengagebrain.com**.

1. Is your life free of addictive behavior? If not, will you commit right now to seek professional help at your institution's counseling center? Addictive behavior destroys health and lives—don't let it waste yours.
2. Are you prepared to walk away, even at the peril of losing close friendships and relationships, if you are put in a situation in which you are pressured to drink, smoke, or engage in any other form of drug (legal or illegal) abuse?

ASSESS YOUR KNOWLEDGE

1. The following substance is not an object of chemical dependency:
   a. Ecstasy
   b. alcohol
   c. cocaine
   d. heroin
   e. All choices are objects of chemical dependency.
2. The most widely used illegal drug in the United States is
   a. marijuana.
   b. alcohol.
   c. cocaine.
   d. heroin.
   e. Ecstasy.
3. Cocaine use
   a. causes lung cancer.
   b. leads to atrophy of the brain.
   c. can lead to sudden death.
   d. causes amotivational syndrome.
   e. All of the choices are correct.
4. Methamphetamine
   a. is less potent than amphetamine.
   b. increases fatigue.
   c. helps a person relax.
   d. is a central nervous system stimulant.
   e. increases the need for sleep.
5. Ecstasy
   a. is popular among middle-aged people.
   b. is a relatively harmless drug.
   c. is used primarily by African American males.
   d. increases heart rate and blood pressure.
   e. All of the choices are correct.
6. Treatment of chemical dependency is
   a. accomplished primarily by the individual alone.
   b. most successful when there is peer pressure to stop.
   c. best achieved with the help of family members.
   d. seldom accomplished without professional guidance.
   e. usually done with the help of friends.

7. Cigarette smoking is responsible for about ___ deaths in the United States each year.
   a. 12,000
   b. 87,000
   c. 255,000
   d. 480,000
   e. 850,000

8. Cigarette smoking increases death rates from
   a. heart disease.
   b. cancer.
   c. stroke.
   d. aortic aneurysm.
   e. All of the choices are correct.

9. The percentage of lung cancer attributed to cigarette smoking is
   a. 25 percent.
   b. 43 percent.
   c. 58 percent.
   d. 64 percent.
   e. 87 percent.

10. Smoking cessation results in
   a. a decrease in sore throats.
   b. improved gastrointestinal function.
   c. a decrease in risk for sudden death.
   d. better tasting of foods.
   e. All of the choices are correct.

Correct answers can be found at the back of the book.

NOTES

1. *Consumer Reports,* December 2012, "The buzz on energy drink caffeine," http://*www.consumerreports.org/cro/magazine/2012/12/the-buzz-on-energy-drink-caffeine/index.htm*; downloaded March 30, 2014.
2. Y. M. Terry-McElrath, P. M. O'Malley, L. D. Johnston, "Energy Drinks, Soft Drinks, and Substance Use Among United States Secondary School Students," *Journal of Addiction Medicine* 8, no.1 (2014): 6.
3. U.S. Department of Health and Human Services, Office of Applied Studies, *Results from the 2012 National Survey on Drug Use and Health: National Findings*, http://nsduhweb.rti.org, downloaded April 1, 2014.
4. U.S. Office of National Drug Control Policy, *What America's Users Spend on Illegal Drugs: 2000–2010,* (February 2014), http://www.whitehouse.gov/ondcp/research-and-data/estimation-drug-expenditures-consumption-supply, downloaded April 1, 2014.
5. W. W. K. Hoeger, L. W. Turner, and B. Q. Hafen, *Wellness: Guidelines for a Healthy Lifestyle* (Belmont, CA: Wadsworth/Thomson Learning, 2007).
6. R. Goldberg, *Drugs Across the Spectrum* (Belmont, CA: Wadsworth/Cengage Learning, 2014).
7. See note 6.
8. U.S. Department of Health and Human Services, *Drug Use Among Racial/Ethnic Minorities* (Bethesda, MD: DHHS, National Institutes of Health, National Institute on Drug Abuse, Division of Epidemiology, Services & Prevention Research, 2003).
9. Substance Abuse and Mental Health Services Administration, Center for Behavioral Health Statistics and Quality. (March 18, 2014). *The NSDUH Report: Recent Declines in Adolescent Inhalant Use.* Rockville, MD.
10. L. D. Johnston, P.M. O'Malley, J.G. Bachman, & J.E. Schulenberg, *Monitoring the Future National Results on Drug Use: 1975-2013 Overview, Key Findings on Adolescent Drug Use.* Ann Arbor: Institute for Social Research, The University of Michigan.
11. United Nations Office on Drugs and Crime (UNODC), *World Drug Report 2013,* http://www.unodc.org/wdr/, downloaded April 1, 2014.
12. See note 11.
13. See note 10.
14. See note 11.
15. "A Snapshot of Annual High-Risk College Drinking Consequences," http://www.collegedrinkingprevention.gov/statssummaries/snapshot.aspx, downloaded April 1, 2014.
16. C. A. Presley, J. S. Leichliter, and P. W. Meilman, *Alcohol and Drugs on American College Campuses: Findings from 1995, 1996, and 1997* (A Report to College Presidents) (Carbondale, IL: Southern Illinois University, 1999).
17. D.H. Gustafson et al., "A Smartphone Application to Support Recovery From Alcoholism: A Randomized Clinical Trial," *JAMA Psychiatry* (March 2014): doi:10.1001/jamapsychiatry.2013.4642.
18. See note 3.
19. See note 3.
20. American Cancer Society, 2014 Cancer Facts and Figures (New York: ACS, 2014).
21. U.S. Department of Health and Human Services. *The Health Consequences of Smoking—50 Years of Progress: A Report of the Surgeon General.* Atlanta: U.S. Department of Health and Human Services, Centers for Disease Control and Prevention, National Center for Chronic Disease Prevention and Health Promotion, Office on Smoking and Health, 2014.
22. U.S. Public Health Service, *The Health Consequences of Involuntary Exposure to Tobacco Smoke: A Report of the Surgeon General—Executive Summary* (Rockville, MD: U.S. Department of Health and Human Services, 2006).
23. American Cancer Society, *World Smoking & Health* (Atlanta, GA: ACS, 1993).
24. See note 21.
25. R. H. Zwick et al., "Exercise in Addition to Nicotine Replacement Therapy Improves Success Rates in Smoking Cessation," *Chest* 130, no. 4 (2006): 145S.

SUGGESTED READINGS

American Cancer Society. *2014 Cancer Facts and Figures.* New York: ACS, 2014.

Doweiko, H. E. *Concepts of Chemical Dependency.* Belmont, CA: Wadsworth/Cengage, 2015.

Goldberg, R. *Drugs across the Spectrum.* Belmont, CA: Wadsworth/Cengage, 2014.

U.S. Department of Health and Human Services. The Health Consequences of Smoking—50 Years of Progress: A Report of the Surgeon General. Atlanta: U.S. Department of Health and Human Services, Centers for Disease Control and Prevention, National Center for Chronic Disease Prevention and Health Promotion, Office on Smoking and Health, 2014.

U.S. Public Health Service. *The Health Consequences of Involuntary Exposure to Tobacco Smoke: A Report of the Surgeon General—Executive Summary.* Rockville, MD: DHHS, 2006.

Lab 13A: Addictive Behavior Questionnaires

Name ____________________ Date __________ Grade __________

Instructor ____________________ Course __________ Section __________

NECESSARY LAB EQUIPMENT
None required.

OBJECTIVE
To determine possible addictive behavior.

INSTRUCTION
The following questionnaires are for your own personal information. Answer all questions on a separate sheet of paper and keep that sheet for yourself. Turn in only this page to your instructor as proof that you have read and completed the questionnaire. If you wish to do so, you may personally discuss the results of these questionnaires with your course instructor.

I. Stage of Change for Addictive Behavior

If chemical dependency is a problem in your life, use Figure 2.6 (page 66) and Table 2.3 (page 65) to identify your current stage of change for participation in a treatment program for addictive behavior.

II. Recognizing Addictive Behavior

The following questionnaire has been designed to identify possible addictive behavior (chemical dependency). This test is not designed to determine if you have an addictive disease, but rather to help recognize potential addictive behavior in yourself or the people around you. The term "drug" may imply illicit substances or drugs (such as marijuana, cocaine, heroin, Ecstasy, or methamphetamine), misuse of prescription drugs (painkillers, sleeping pills), or alcohol abuse.

1. Are you a compulsive person?
2. Are you a person of excesses?
3. Do you depend heavily on others or are you completely independent of others?
4. Do you spend a lot of time thinking about a drug(s)?
5. Do you use drugs other than for medical reasons?
6. Do you misuse prescription drugs?
7. Are you unable to stop using drugs or limit their use to required situations only?
8. Can you get through a week without misusing drugs?
9. Do friends or relatives sense or mention that you have a drug problem?
10. Has drug misuse ever created a problem between you and friends or relatives?
11. Have family members or friends ever sought help for problems associated with your misuse of drugs?
12. Have you ever sought help for drug misuse?
13. Do you deny or lie about the misuse of drugs?
14. Do you tend to associate with people who exhibit the same behaviors or take the same drugs you do?
15. Do you get angry at people who try to keep you from getting the drugs you desire?
16. Do you have a difficult time stopping the use of a drug when you start misusing it?
17. Do you experience withdrawal symptoms if you do not take the drugs you wish to have?
18. Has the misuse of drugs affected the way you function in life (school, work, recreation)?
19. Have you put yourself or others at risk by your actions while misusing drugs?
20. Have you unsuccessfully tried to cut back or stop the misuse of drugs?

Interpretation

If you answered "yes" to five or more of these questions, you may have an addictive behavior and should seek further evaluation by a physician, your institution's counseling center, or contact a local mental health clinic for a referral. You may also contact the National Center for Substance Abuse Treatment at 1-800-662-4357 for 24-hour substance abuse treatment centers in your area. Depending on the question (for example, 7, 8, 12, 15, 16, 17, 18, 20), note that even fewer than five "yes" answers may already be indicative of chemical dependency.

III. Alcohol Abuse

Use a separate sheet of paper to answer the following questions. This questionnaire can help you determine if your drinking (alcohol) patterns are a problem for you. If you do not consume alcohol, skip this questionnaire, as drinking does not interfere with your health and well-being.

	Yes	No
1. Do you consume more than one (women) or two (men) drinks per day?	☐	☐
2. Does drinking interfere with your short- or long-term goals?	☐	☐
3. Does drinking interfere with your school or work productivity?	☐	☐
4. Have you missed school or work because of drinking?	☐	☐
5. Do you skip workouts because of drinking?	☐	☐
6. Do you drink to increase self-confidence?	☐	☐
7. Do you drink to feel more at ease with others?	☐	☐
8. Do you drink to be socially accepted by others?	☐	☐
9. Are you annoyed by other people's comments about your drinking habits?	☐	☐
10. Are you untruthful about the number of drinks you have had when questioned by others?	☐	☐
11. To drink, do you associate with people who are not a good influence on you or that you normally don't relate to?	☐	☐
12. Do you drink alone?	☐	☐
13. At social gatherings, do you actively look for a refill before being offered one?	☐	☐
14. Do you frequently serve yourself a more generous drink than the "going" amount for others?	☐	☐
15. Do you drink to relieve stress, forget worries, or life's problems?	☐	☐
16. Has drinking affected your reputation?	☐	☐
17. Have you missed appointments due to drinking?	☐	☐
18. Do you participate in binge drinking episodes?	☐	☐
19. Do you have difficulty remembering what you have done because of drinking?	☐	☐
20. Does drinking affect your family life or relationship with roommates?	☐	☐
21. Are you ever abusive to others when drinking?	☐	☐
22. Have you experienced financial difficulties as a result of drinking?	☐	☐
23. Do you feel physically deprived if you cannot drink daily?	☐	☐
24. Do you need a drink early in the day to get going?	☐	☐
25. Do you need a drink at certain times of the day?	☐	☐
26. Has drinking disrupted your sleeping pattern?	☐	☐
27. Do you ever feel that you need to cut down on drinking?	☐	☐
28. Do you ever feel bad or guilty about your drinking pattern?	☐	☐
29. Have you been treated by a physician or health professional for drinking?	☐	☐
30. Have you ever been treated in a hospital or other institution for drinking?	☐	☐

A "yes" answer to any of these questions can be regarded as a warning sign to potential future problems. If you have answered three or more of them with a "yes," your drinking habit can be harmful to your well-being and may indicate that you are alcohol dependent or an alcoholic. An evaluation by a healthcare professional is highly recommended.

IV. Changing Addictive Behavior

Using a separate sheet of paper, specifically indicate the steps that you are going to take to correct addictive behavior(s) and identify people or organizations that you will contact to help you get started.

Lab 13B: Smoking Cessation Questionnaires

Name ______________________ Date ____________ Grade ____________

Instructor ______________________ Course ____________ Section ____________

NECESSARY LAB EQUIPMENT
None required.

OBJECTIVE
To develop a smoking cessation program either for yourself or for friends and relatives.

I. Introduction

The forms provided in this lab have been designed to help smokers identify reasons why they smoke and their readiness to initiate a smoking cessation program. These forms should be filled out prior to initiating a smoking cessation program. Interpretation of the results is given in this chapter ("Why Do You Smoke?" Test, page 511). The daily cigarette smoking log, Part V of this lab, has been developed to help smokers get to know their habit, cut down on cigarettes not really needed, and find positive substitutes when confronted with situations that trigger their desire to smoke.

II. "Why Do You Smoke?" Test

	Always	Fre-quently	Occa-sionally	Seldom	Never
A. I smoke cigarettes to keep myself from slowing down.	5	4	3	2	1
B. Handling a cigarette is part of the enjoyment of smoking it.	5	4	3	2	1
C. Smoking cigarettes is pleasant and relaxing.	5	4	3	2	1
D. I light up a cigarette when I feel angry about something.	5	4	3	2	1
E. When I have run out of cigarettes, I find it almost unbearable until I can get them.	5	4	3	2	1
F. I smoke cigarettes automatically without even being aware of it.	5	4	3	2	1
G. I smoke cigarettes for stimulation, to perk myself up.	5	4	3	2	1
H. Part of the enjoyment of smoking a cigarette comes from the steps I take to light up.	5	4	3	2	1
I. I find cigarettes pleasurable.	5	4	3	2	1
J. When I feel uncomfortable or upset about something, I light up a cigarette.	5	4	3	2	1
K. I am very much aware of the fact when I am not smoking a cigarette.	5	4	3	2	1
L. I light up a cigarette without realizing I still have one burning in the ashtray.	5	4	3	2	1
M. I smoke cigarettes to give me a "lift."	5	4	3	2	1
N. When I smoke a cigarette, part of the enjoyment is watching the smoke as I exhale it.	5	4	3	2	1
O. I want a cigarette most when I am comfortable and relaxed.	5	4	3	2	1
P. When I feel "blue" or want to take my mind off cares and worries, I smoke cigarettes.	5	4	3	2	1
Q. I get a real gnawing hunger for a cigarette when I haven't smoked for a while.	5	4	3	2	1
R. I've found a cigarette in my mouth and didn't remember putting it there.	5	4	3	2	1

How to Score: (See page 511 to interpret your test results.)
Enter the numbers you have circled on the test questions in the spaces provided below, putting the number you have circled to question A on line A, to question B on line B, and so on. Add the three scores on each line to get a total for each factor. For example, the sum of your scores over lines A, G, and M gives you your score on "Stimulation"; lines B, H, and N give the score on "Handling." Scores can vary from 3 to 15. Any score 11 and above is high; any score 7 and below is low.

A	____	+ G	____	+ M	____	= ____	Stimulation
B	____	+ H	____	+ N	____	= ____	Handling
C	____	+ I	____	+ O	____	= ____	Pleasure/Relaxation
D	____	+ J	____	+ P	____	= ____	Crutch: Tension Reduction
E	____	+ K	____	+ Q	____	= ____	Craving: Psychological Addiction
F	____	+ L	____	+ R	____	= ____	Habit

From *A Self-Test for Smokers,* U.S. Department of Health and Human Services, 1983.

III. "Do You Want to Quit?" Test

	Strongly Agree	Mildly Agree	Mildly Disagree	Strongly Disagree
A. Cigarette smoking might give me a serious illness.	4	3	2	1
B. My cigarette smoking sets a bad example for others.	4	3	2	1
C. I find cigarette smoking to be a messy kind of habit.	4	3	2	1
D. Controlling my cigarette smoking is a challenge to me.	4	3	2	1
E. Smoking causes shortness of breath.	4	3	2	1
F. If I quit smoking cigarettes, it might influence others to stop.	4	3	2	1
G. Cigarettes cause damage to clothing and other personal property.	4	3	2	1
H. Quitting smoking would show that I have willpower.	4	3	2	1
I. My cigarette smoking will have a harmful effect on my health.	4	3	2	1
J. My cigarette smoking influences others close to me to take up or continue smoking.	4	3	2	1
K. If I quit smoking, my sense of taste or smell will improve.	4	3	2	1
L. I do not like the idea of feeling dependent on smoking.	4	3	2	1

How to Score: (See page 512, "Do You Want to Quit?" Test, to interpret your results.)

Write the number you have circled after each statement on the test in the corresponding space to the right. Add the scores on each line to get your totals. For example, the sum of your scores A, E, and I gives you your score for the Health factor. Scores can vary from 3 to 12. Any score of 9 or over is high; any score 6 or under is low.

A ______ + E ______ + I ______ = ______ Health
B ______ + F ______ + J ______ = ______ Example
C ______ + G ______ + K ______ = ______ Aesthetics
D ______ + H ______ + L ______ = ______ Mastery

From *A Self-Test for Smokers,* U.S. Department of Health and Human Services, 1983.

IV. Reasons to Smoke, Reasons to Quit

Reasons to Smoke Cigarettes

1. ______
2. ______
3. ______
4. ______
5. ______

Reasons to Quit Cigarette Smoking

1. ______
2. ______
3. ______
4. ______
5. ______

V. Daily Cigarette Smoking Log

Today's Date: ____________ Quit Date: ____________ Decision Date: ____________

Cigarettes to be smoked today: ____________ Brand: ____________

No.	Time	Activity	Rating[a]	Amount Smoked[b]	Remarks/Substitutes
1.					
2.					
3.					
4.					
5.					
6.					
7.					
8.					
9.					
10.					
11.					
12.					
13.					
14.					
15.					
16.					
17.					
18.					
19.					
20.					

[a]Rating: 1 = desperately needed, 2 = moderately needed, 3 = no real need
[b]Amount Smoked: entire cigarette, two-thirds, half, etc.

Additional comments, list of friends and/or activities to avoid.

____

____

____

____

____

____

VI. Conclusion

In a few sentences, indicate your feelings about cigarette smoking and what you have learned from the previous questionnaires.

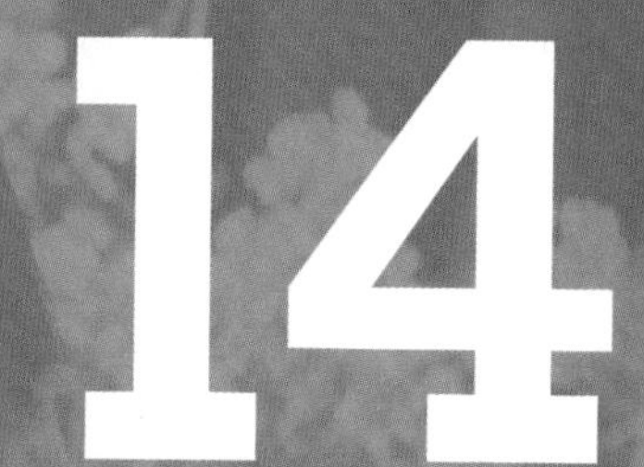

Preventing Sexually Transmitted Infections

Anyone who has unprotected sexual contact can acquire a sexually transmitted infection (STI). More than half of all Americans will be infected during their lifetime. Infections are most common among teens and young adults, with about half of all infections occurring in people younger than 25. One in four college students has had or has an STI. Multiple sex partners and unsafe sexual practices greatly increase the risk of acquiring an STI.

OBJECTIVES

- Name and describe the most common sexually transmitted infections (STIs).
- Outline the health consequences of STIs.
- Define the difference between human immunodeficiency virus (HIV) and acquired immune deficiency syndrome (AIDS).
- Explain the seriousness of the AIDS epidemic in the United States and worldwide.
- Describe ways to prevent acquiring STIs.

CENGAGEbrain.com

Visit **www.cengagebrain.com** to access course materials and companion resources for this text, including digital labs, quiz questions designed to check your understanding of the chapter contents, and more! See the preface on page xii for more information.

REAL LIFE STORY | Darlene's Experience

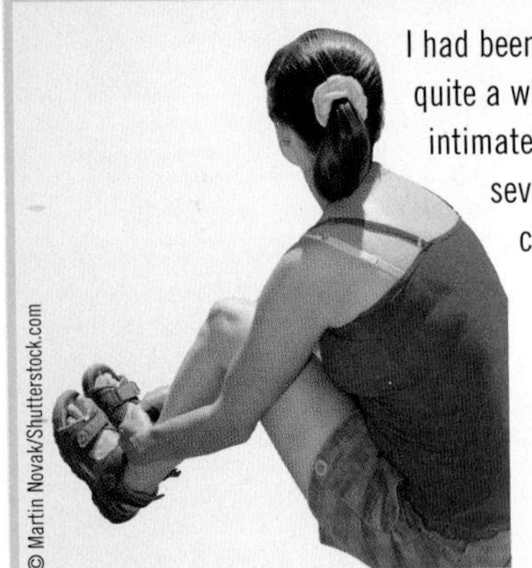

© Martin Novak/Shutterstock.com

I had been dating my boyfriend for quite a while and we had been in an intimate sexual relationship for several months. One day he came down with a cold sore (herpes simplex virus type 1, or HSV-1), and I didn't think much of it. Not knowing any potential ramifications, we slept together a couple of times during his outbreak. I was shocked when a few days later I came down with a case of genital herpes. I have now learned that one out of every six adults is infected with genital herpes. From my physician, I learned that a "simple" cold sore can cause genital herpes, and vice versa. Simply touching the cold sore and then the genital area can lead to this infection. I now have a lifetime chronic disease, as herpes is presently incurable and I have to live with recurrent herpes outbreaks. The sad thing is that I had no understanding of the risk I was taking. Had I known better, of course I would have made a different choice.

Based on estimates by the World Health Organization, more than 1 million people worldwide are infected daily with **sexually transmitted infections (STIs)**. STIs have also reached epidemic proportions in the United States. According to the American Social Health Association, more than half of all Americans will acquire at least one STI in their lifetime. Each year, about 20 million people in the United States are newly infected with STIs, costing Americans almost $16 billion in direct health care expenses. Half of all new STI infections affect young people between the ages of 15 and 24.[1] Young people are most at risk because they are more likely to have multiple sex partners. According to estimates, one in four college students has had or has an STI. To avoid embarrassment, stigma, or concerns about confidentiality, young people are reluctant to discuss their risky sexual behavior with a physician. Though the private nature of STIs make people less willing to talk about them openly, early education about STI prevention and honest communication between sexual partners is crucial for both individual health and the health of the nation.

The CDC reports that there are over 110 million STIs among men and women in the United States. The infection rate is about the same among young men and young women, but the health consequences of untreated STIs is

FIGURE 14.1 **Young people ages 15–24 represent 50% of all new STIs.**

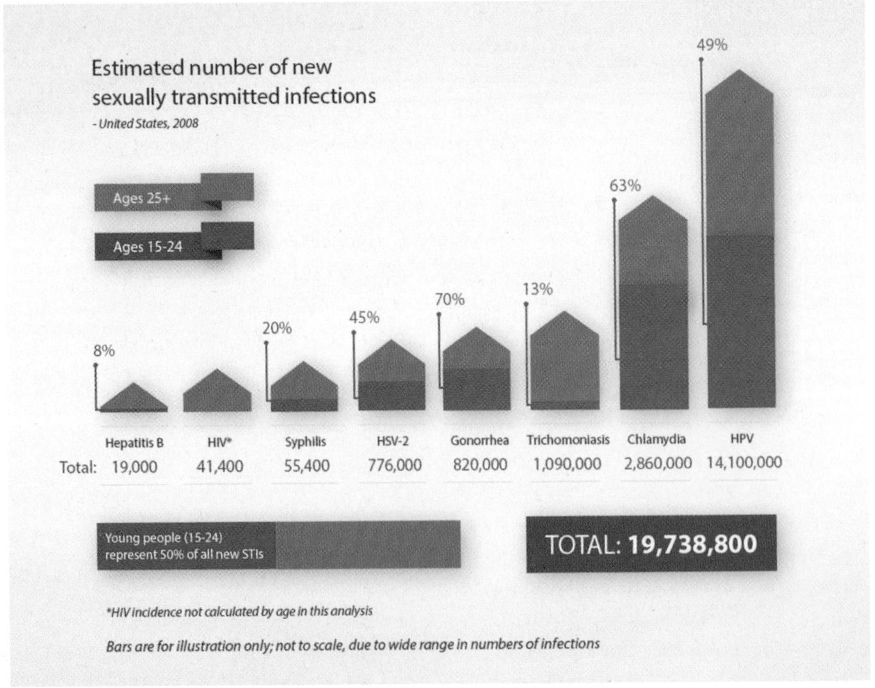

Source: http://www.cdc.gov/std/stats/sti-estimates-fact-sheet-feb-2013.pdf Downloaded April 15, 2014.

more serious for women, including infertility. About 24,000 women in the United States become infertile each year because of an STI they may not have even known they had. Because the majority of STIs exist without obvious symptoms, a person can have an STI that goes unnoticed for years. Most STIs do not cause significant harm, but if not diagnosed or treated early, some STIs can lead to serious health problems, including cervical cancer, pelvic inflammatory disease, ectopic pregnancy, and an increased risk of HIV. As early detection is critical, the CDC has released general screening recommendations for all sexually active people.

Center for Disease Control and Prevention's (CDC) STI Screening Recommendations Because STIs are preventable, significant reductions in new infections are not only possible, they are urgently needed. Prevention can minimize the negative, long-term consequences of STIs and also reduce health care costs. The high incidence and overall prevalence of STIs in the general population suggests that many Americans are at substantial risk of exposure to STIs, underscoring the need for STI prevention.

Abstaining from sex, reducing the number of sexual partners, and consistently and correctly using condoms are all effective STI prevention strategies. Safe, effective vaccines are also available to prevent hepatitis B virus (HBV) and some types of HPV that cause disease and cancer. And for all individuals who are sexually active—particularly young people—STI screening and prompt treatment (if infected) are critical to protect a person's health and prevent transmission to others. If you are sexually active, the CDC encourages you to talk to your health care provider about STI testing and which tests may be right for you. The following are the CDC guidelines:

- All adults and adolescents should be tested at least once for HIV.
- Annual chlamydia screening for all sexually active women age 25 and younger, as well as older women with risk factors such as new or multiple sex partners.
- Yearly gonorrhea screening for at-risk sexually active women (e.g., those with new or multiple sex partners, and women who live in communities with a high burden of disease).
- Syphilis, HIV, chlamydia, and hepatitis B screening for all pregnant women, and gonorrhea screening for at-risk pregnant women at the first prenatal visit, to protect the health of mothers and their infants.
- Trichomoniasis screening should be conducted at least annually for all HIV-infected women.
- Screening at least once a year for syphilis, chlamydia, gonorrhea, and HIV for all sexually active gay men, bisexual men, and other men who have sex with men (MSM). MSM who have multiple or anonymous partners should be screened more frequently for STIs (e.g., at 3 to 6 month intervals). In addition, MSM who have sex in conjunction with illicit drug use (particularly methamphetamine use) or whose sex partners participate in these activities should be screened more frequently.

Types and Causes of STIs

Of the more than 30 known pathogens that are transmitted through sexual contact, 8 are responsible for most STIs. Four of those eight infections are caused by bacteria and other parasitical organisms and can be readily treated and cured if diagnosed early, including: chlamydia, gonorrhea, syphilis, and trichomoniasis. Bacterial infections are often cured with antibiotics. The other four infections are caused by viruses and currently have no cure, including human papillomavirus (HPV)/genital warts, genital herpes, hepatitis, and human immunodeficiency virus (HIV). These viral infections are often referred to as the four "H"s. Hepatitis B is the only STI that can be prevented if a person is vaccinated before being exposed to the virus, though for HIV, some evidence has shown that early antiretroviral drug therapy may help reduce the chance of infection even after exposure (see HIV treatment). Symptoms from all viral STIs can also be alleviated with corresponding forms of treatment.

Currently, the United States has the highest rate of sexually transmitted infections of any country in the industrialized world. Following are brief descriptions of the leading STIs, their symptoms, and their treatments (if any).

Chlamydia

Chlamydia is a bacterial infection that spreads during vaginal, anal, or oral sex or from the vagina to a newborn baby during childbirth. Chlamydia can seriously damage the reproductive system. This infection is considered a major factor in male and female infertility. Because symptoms are usually mild or absent, 3 out of 4 people with the infection don't know they're ill until the infection has become quite serious. Infertility often occurs "silently," because the individual is unaware of the infection until it is too late to prevent the irreversible damage.

Chlamydia is the most commonly reported STI. In any given year, there may be as many as 2.8 million cases of chlamydia in the United States. Almost 55 percent of these cases are reported in women between the ages of 15 and 24. Only about 1.4 million cases are reported each year because most people are not aware of their infection.[2] Testing is frequently skipped because

Sexually transmitted infections (STIs) Communicable diseases spread through sexual contact.

Chlamydia An STI, caused by a bacterial infection, that can significantly damage the reproductive system.

patients are mistreated for symptoms that mimic other STIs. The CDC recommends that sexually active women age 25 or younger be tested every year for chlamydia and that all women who are pregnant be tested at their first prenatal visit. Those treated for chlamydia should be tested again after 3 months, even if their sex partner was also treated, as it is common to be reinfected with chlamydia.

Symptoms of serious infection include abdominal pain, fever, nausea, vaginal bleeding, and arthritis. Although chlamydia can be treated successfully with oral antibiotics, its damage to the reproductive system is irreversible.

MyProfile: STIs Survey

To the best of your ability, answer the following questions. If you do not know the answer(s), this chapter will guide you through them.

I. Are you aware that there are more than 30 STIs and that some are incurable? ___ Yes ___ No

II. Do you understand that more than 50 percent of all Americans will acquire at least one STI in their lifetime and that almost half of them are seen in people between the ages of 15 and 24? ___ Yes ___ No

III. Can you explain the difference between HIV infection and AIDS? ___ Yes ___ No ______________________________
____
____

IV. Do you understand the concept of "safe sex" and guidelines to follow to prevent STIs? ___ Yes ___ No

V. If you choose not to have sex, have you thought out an appropriate response in the event that you are asked or are pressured to have sex? ___ Yes ___ No

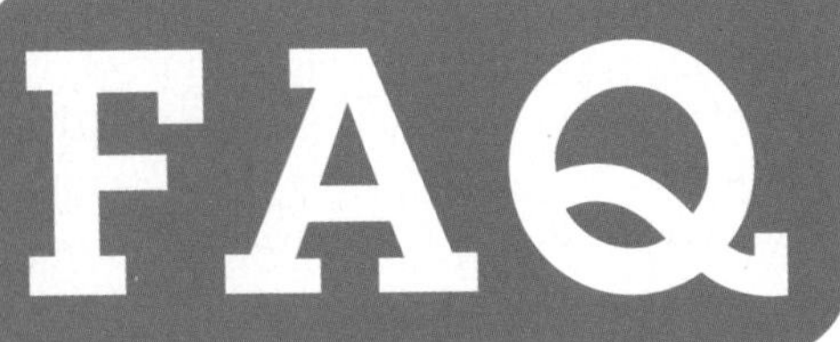

What is the difference between a sexually transmitted infection (STI) and a sexually transmitted disease (STD)?

Health experts are beginning to replace the acronym STD with STI. The concept of disease implies a clear medical condition that manifests itself through signs or symptoms that define a specific disease. In terms of STIs, once infected, a person may or may not develop signs or symptoms indicative of disease. The unfortunate reality is that in the early stages of infection, many individuals with STIs exhibit no signs or symptoms or ones that are so mild that they are often ignored.

What is "safe" sex?

Safe sex means taking precautions during sexual intercourse or other form of sexual contact, designed to prevent the exchange of blood, semen, vaginal fluids, or breast milk that can keep you or your partner from getting an STI. These infections include chlamydia, gonorrhea, pelvic inflammatory disease, syphilis, trichomoniasis, human papillomavirus (HPV)/genital warts, genital herpes, hepatitis, and human immunodeficiency virus (HIV). When unsure about your partner, use a lubricated latex condom from start to finish for each sexual act. If you think your partner should use a condom but refuses to do so, say "no" to sex with that person. While a condom definitely reduces the risk for infection, you need to realize that even with condom use you may acquire an STI. Condoms may not totally cover surrounding infected areas, and sometimes they rupture.

How does HIV damage the immune system?

Upon HIV infection, the virus attacks and starts killing CD4 cells in the immune system. CD4 cells are a special type of white blood cell that fights off infections (viral, fungal, and parasitic). Initially, the body can make more CD4 cells to replace the cells damaged by HIV. Eventually, however, the body is unable to replace all damaged cells. As the number of CD4 cells decreases, the immune system weakens and the person is more susceptible to sickness, illness, and infections, including the development of acquired immune deficiency syndrome (AIDS).

Am I at risk for contracting HIV in a medical or dental office?

HIV transmission in a health care setting is extremely rare. The implementation of strict infection control procedures protects both the patient and the health care provider. Only one such case, of a Florida dentist in 1990, has been reported by the Centers for Disease Control and Prevention of patients having been infected. Data on more than 22,000 patients treated by 63 HIV-infected health care providers reveal no cases of transmission from provider to patient in a health care setting.

Gonorrhea

One of the oldest STIs, **gonorrhea** is caused by a bacterial infection. Gonorrhea is transmitted through contact with the vagina, penis, anus, or mouth of an infected person. Mothers can also pass the infection to their babies during childbirth. According to the CDC, approximately 820,000 individuals get new gonorrheal infections each year in the United States, less than half of the cases are reported, and about 570,000 are in the 15 to 24 age group.[3] Typical symptoms in men include a pus-like secretion from the penis and painful urination. Infected women may have discharge and painful urination as well. Up to 80 percent of infected women, however, don't experience any symptoms until the infection has become fairly serious. At this stage, women develop fever, severe abdominal pain, and pelvic inflammatory disease (discussed next).

If untreated, gonorrhea can produce widespread bacterial infection, infertility, heart damage, and arthritis in men and women, as well as blindness in children born to infected women. At present, gonorrhea is treated with penicillin and other antibiotics, but these will not repair any damage already done. There are signs from the CDC surveillance systems, however, that this disease may become resistant to the only available treatment option because drug-resistant strains are increasing and successful treatment is becoming more difficult.

Pelvic Inflammatory Disease

Estimates indicate that each year in the United States more than 1 million women experience an acute episode of a condition known by the umbrella term **pelvic inflammatory disease (PID)**.[4] PID is not an STI but, rather, refers to complications resulting from STIs, especially chlamydia and gonorrhea. PID often develops when the STI spreads to the fallopian tubes, uterus, and ovaries. Sexually active women are at higher risk for developing PID—especially those younger than age 25—because the cervix is not yet fully matured, increasing the risk for STIs that lead to PID. The more sex partners a woman has, the greater the risk for PID.

Complications associated with PID typically include scarring and obstruction of the fallopian tubes (which may lead to infertility), ectopic pregnancies, and chronic pelvic pain. If a woman with PID becomes pregnant, she could have an ectopic (tubal) pregnancy, which destroys the embryo and can kill the woman. Yearly, more than 100,000 women in the United States become infertile as a result of PID.

Typical symptoms of PID are fever, nausea, vomiting, chills, spotting between menstrual periods, heavy bleeding during periods, and pain in the lower abdomen during sexual intercourse, between menstrual periods, or during urination. Many times, however, women do not know they have PID, because these symptoms are not always present.

PID is treated with antibiotics, bed rest, and sexual abstinence. Furthermore, surgery may be required to remove infected or scarred tissue or to repair or remove the fallopian tubes or uterus.

Syphilis

Another common type of STI, also caused by bacterial infection, is **syphilis**. It is referred to as "the great imitator," because signs and symptoms are often indistinguishable from other diseases.

Once on the verge of elimination, syphilis began reappearing as a public health threat in 2001. More than 55,000 new cases are reported each year.[5] The incidence is highest in men between 20 and 29 years of age. A troubling statistic released in 2012 is that 75 percent of primary and secondary stage syphilis (see following discussion) cases occurred among men who have sex with men.

Syphilis is transmitted through direct contact with a syphilis sore during vaginal, anal, or oral sex. In the primary stage, between 10 and 90 days following infection (average of 21 days), a painless sore appears where the bacteria entered the body (sometimes multiple sores appear). A sore also can appear on the lips or in the mouth and can infect another person through kissing. This sore disappears on its own in 3 to 6 weeks. If untreated, the infection progresses to the secondary stage.

During the secondary stage, as the initial sore is healing or several weeks thereafter, skin rashes and mucous membrane lesions appear. A rough, reddish-brown rash can be seen on the palms of the hands and the bottoms of the feet, although types of rashes can appear on other parts of the body. Additional sores may also appear within 6 months of the initial outbreak. Signs and symptoms of the secondary stage disappear with or without treatment. Untreated, the infection progresses into the latent stage.

A latent stage, during which the victim is not contagious, may last up to 30 years, lulling victims into thinking they are healed. During the last stage of the infection, some people develop paralysis, crippling, gradual blindness, heart disease, brain and organ damage, or dementia; others die as a direct result of the infection. Syphilis can also spread from an infected mother to her unborn baby in pregnancy and cause serious health issues in a developing fetus, including premature birth and stillbirth.

Syphilis is diagnosed by microscopic examination of material from a sore or through a simple blood test. One of the oldest known STIs, syphilis once killed its victims, but now penicillin and other antibiotics are used to treat it. A single injection of penicillin cures individuals who have been infected for less than a year. Additional treatments are necessary for people infected longer than a year. Antibiotics are also available for individuals aller-

Gonorrhea An STI caused by a bacterial infection.

Pelvic inflammatory disease (PID) An overall designation referring to the effects of other STIs, primarily chlamydia and gonorrhea.

Syphilis An STI caused by a bacterial infection.

gic to penicillin. People infected with syphilis must abstain from sexual activity until all syphilis sores have disappeared. Sexual partners must be informed of potential infection so that they can seek treatment if necessary.

Trichomoniasis

Although not as well known as other STIs, **trichomoniasis** or "trich" is a very common STI caused by infection with a protozoan parasite called *Trichomonas vaginalis.* Although symptoms of the disease vary, most women and men who have the parasite cannot tell they are infected. It is considered the most common curable STI. About 3.7 million people in the United States are infected, about 70 percent do not have any signs or symptoms of infection, and the incidence is more common in women than men. Presently it is unknown why some people with the infection get symptoms while others don't. Most likely it is related to the person's age and overall health. Asymptomatic infected individuals can still pass the infection on to others.

Men with trichomoniasis can experience itching or irritation inside the penis, a burning sensation after urination or ejaculation, or discharge from the penis. Women may also feel itching or burning, redness or soreness of the genitals, uncomfortable urination, or an unusual discharge that can be clear, white, yellowish, or greenish. Having trichomoniasis can make sex quite uncomfortable. Without treatment, the infection can last for months or even years.

Trichomoniasis increases the risk of getting or spreading other STIs. For example, trichomoniasis can cause genital inflammation that makes it easier to become HIV-infected or to pass the virus on to others.

Trichomoniasis can be cured with a single dose of prescription antibiotics, either metronidazole or tinidazole. Pregnant women can also be treated with these medications. Drinking alcohol within 24 hours of taking the medication can lead to uncomfortable side effects.

People who have been treated for trichomoniasis can get reinfected. About 20 percent of people get infected again within 3 months of antibiotic treatment. To avoid reinfection, be sure that all sex partners get treated as well, and do not engage in sexual activity until all of your symptoms have disappeared (about a week). See your physician if the symptoms return.

Human Papillomavirus and Genital Warts

Human papillomavirus (HPV) is the most common sexually transmitted infection. There are more than 100 strains of HPV, and about 40 are sexually transmitted. "Low-risk" strains are wart-causing, whereas "high-risk" are cancer causing. Some strains of HPV infect the genital area, including the skin of the penis, the vulva, anus, lining of the vagina, cervix, and rectum, but they can also infect the mouth and throat as well. Others are known as "high risk" types and can lead to cancers of the cervix, vulva, vagina, anus, or penis.

Most HPVs have no signs or symptoms, and the body's immune system clears them up within two years of infection without any form of treatment, while some forms persist. Presently, experts do not know why that is the case. When the body's immune system can't clear up a high-risk HPV infection, over time it turns normal cells into abnormal cells and subsequently cancer. Thirteen HPV types can cause cancer of the cervix; one of these types can cause cancers of the vulva, vagina, penis, anus, and certain head and neck cancers (specifically, the oropharynx, which includes the back of the throat, base of the tongue, and tonsils). HPV is responsible for nearly all cases of cervical cancer, 90 percent of anal, 60 to 70 percent of oropharyngeal, and more than 50 percent of vaginal, vulvar, and penile cancers.

Approximately 14 million new cases of HPV are reported each year and at least 79 million Americans are currently infected.[6] Most sexually active people acquire HPV infection during their lifetime. At least 80 percent of women will acquire HPV infection by age 50. Most women are diagnosed with HPV through an abnormal Pap test. Infection is spread through genital or oral contact. Because most people have no signs or symptoms, they are unaware of the infection and can transmit the virus to a sex partner.

One of the potential health problems of HPV is **genital warts**, which show up between weeks or months after exposure. These warts may be flat or raised and usually are found on the penis or around the vulva and the vagina. They also can appear in the mouth, throat, rectum, on the cervix, or

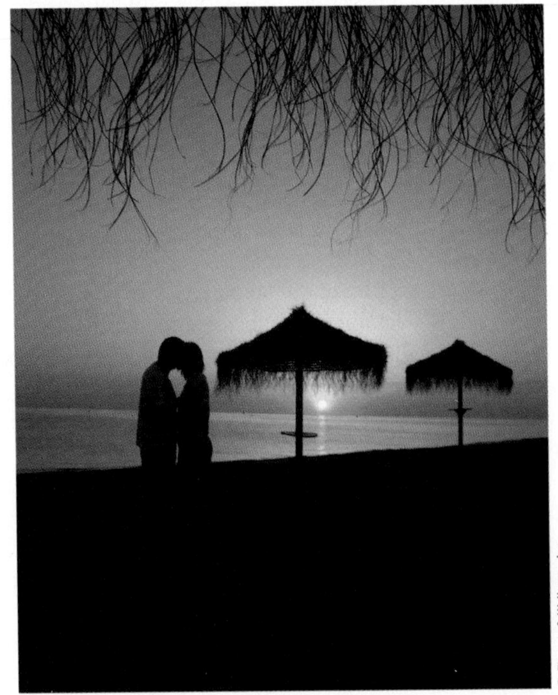

More than 25 infections are spread through sexual contact. About 1 in 4 adults in the United States has an STI.

around the anus. Based on data from the CDC, as many as 360,000 new cases of genital warts are diagnosed yearly in the United States. In some cities, nearly half of all sexually active teenagers have genital warts.

Health problems associated with genital warts include increased risk for cancers of the cervix, vulva, vagina, anus, penis, and enlargement and spread of the warts, leading to obstruction of the urethra, vagina, and anus. Because babies born to infected mothers commonly develop warts over their bodies, cesarean section is recommended for childbirth.

Treatment requires completely removing all warts. This can be done by freezing them with liquid nitrogen, dissolving them with chemicals, or removing them through electrosurgery or laser surgery. Infected patients may have to be treated more than once, because genital warts can recur.

Prevention of HPV infection is best accomplished through a mutually monogamous sexual relationship with an uninfected partner. It is difficult to know, however, if a person who has been sexually active in the past is currently infected.

Two HPV vaccines, Gardasil and Cervarix, are available to prevent cervical cancer and other diseases caused by HPV. Both vaccines protect against HPV types 16 and 18, which cause most cervical cancers. Additionally, Gardasil protects against HPV types 6 and 11 and most genital warts. To derive the benefits provided, a three-dose series of HPV vaccination is routinely recommended for 11- and 12-year-old girls and boys and is highly recommended for all girls and women between the ages of 13 and 26 if they did not receive all doses when they were younger. Gardasil has also been approved for males between 9 and 26. To get the full benefits of the vaccine, people should get vaccinated before they become sexually active. The vaccines are most effective in women who have not been infected with any of the HPV types covered. Few women, however, are infected with all HPV types, thus vaccination still offers protection against those viruses that have not been acquired. The vaccine has not been widely tested in people older than 26. Licensing for this group may become available if the vaccine proves to be safe and effective for the older age group as well.

The HPV vaccines have surpassed all expectations in terms of disease prevention and is considered an "anti-cancer vaccine." Since the introduction of the vaccines in 2006, vaccine-type HPV prevalence decreased 56 percent among female teenagers 14 to 19 years of age. According to CDC Director Tom Frieden, "This report shows that HPV vaccine works well, and the report should be a wake-up call to our nation to protect the next generation by increasing HPV vaccination rates. Unfortunately only one-third of girls aged 13 to 17 have been fully vaccinated with HPV vaccine. Countries such as Rwanda have vaccinated more than 80 percent of their teen girls. Our low vaccination rates represent 50,000 preventable tragedies—50,000 girls alive today will develop cervical cancer over their lifetime that would have been prevented if we reach 80 percent vaccination rates. For every year we delay in doing so, another 4,400 girls will develop cervical cancer in their lifetimes."[7]

Genital Herpes

One of the most common STIs, **genital herpes** is caused by the herpes simplex virus (HSV). There are several types of HSV that produce different ailments, including genital herpes, oral herpes, shingles, and chicken pox. The two most common forms of HSV are types 1 and 2. In type 1—the HSV most often known to cause oral herpes—cold sores or fever blisters appear on the lips and mouth. HSV-2 is better known as the virus that causes genital herpes.

The fundamental difference between the two main types of HSV lies in their preferred "site of residence." The HSV-1 virus typically establishes latency in a collection of nerve cells near the ear known as trigeminal ganglion. HSV-2 usually establishes latency at the base of the spine in the sacral ganglion. The virus can remain dormant for a long time, but repeated outbreaks are common. The number of outbreaks tends to decrease over the years. Excessive fatigue, stress, cold, wind, wetness, heat, sun, sweating, rubbing, chafing, and friction, as well as lack of sleep, illness, restrictive clothing, and diet can precipitate new outbreaks. Some foods such as popcorn, coffee, peanuts, chocolate, and alcohol may trigger outbreaks.

Unknown to most people, HSV-1 also causes genital herpes, and an increasing number of genital herpes caused by HSV-1 has been found worldwide. Approximately 100 million Americans older than the age of 12 are infected with HSV-1. Most of these individuals acquired the virus as children. By age 50, more than 80 percent of the population has been exposed to HSV-1. Another 40 million are infected with HSV-2. One out of six people 14 to 49 years old are infected with the type 2 virus.[8] One in five women, one in nine men, and one in five adolescents are currently infected with genital herpes (HSV-2).

HSV is a highly contagious virus. Victims are most contagious during an outbreak, but the virus can also spread through virus-containing secretions. A few days following infection, a tingling sensation and lesions appear on the infected areas, most notably the mouth, genitals, and rectum, but can also surface on other parts of the body. Lesions can be somewhat painful.

Individuals infected with oral HSV-1 may shed the virus about 5 percent of the time, when they have no other symptoms of infection or visible lesions. In persons with asymptomatic HSV-2 infections, infected individuals can shed the virus up to 10 percent of days when they show no symptoms. At

Trichomoniasis An STI caused by a parasitical infection.

Human papillomavirus (HPV) A group of viruses that can cause STIs.

Genital warts An STI caused by a viral infection.

Genital herpes An STI caused by a viral infection of HSV-1 or HSV-2. The virus can attack different areas of the body but typically causes blisters on the genitals.

present, HSV-2 transmission most often occurs from an infected person who does not have a visible sore and may not even be aware of such an infection.

In conjunction with the lesions, victims usually have mild fever, swollen glands, and headaches. The symptoms disappear within a few weeks, causing some people to believe they are cured. Presently, though, herpes is incurable, and its victims remain infected for life.

Society has typically labeled HSV-1 infection (cold sores) an "acceptable" viral infection, whereas infection with HSV-2 is viewed as a "bad" infection. The social stigma and emotional perspective of genital herpes make it difficult to objectively compare it with an oral infection, labeled as "just a cold sore" and acceptable to most people. HSV types 1 and 2, nonetheless, both cause oral and genital herpes. People who have an outbreak of oral herpes should not touch their own or someone else's genitals after touching the oral cold sores. Doing so can lead to a herpes infection of the genitals (genital HSV-1 infection). Oral sex can also result in transmission of HSV from the lips to the genitals. Thirty percent of *all new cases* of genital herpes result from HSV-1 infection. A 2011 study involving college students showed that HSV-1 accounts for 78 percent of female and 85 percent of male genital herpes infections.[9]

CRITICAL THINKING

A "cold sore" or "fever blister" caused by an HSV-1 infection is highly contagious and can lead to the development of genital herpes either by direct contact through oral sex or if the person with the outbreak touches the sore and then their own or their partner's genitals. What can you do to protect yourself, loved ones, and others from a wider spread of the virus?

This startling finding is because of changing beliefs in what constitutes "safe" sex. The primary mode of HSV-1 transmission is by direct contact. College students assume that oral sex is safer and thus have vaginal intercourse and oral sex at about the same rate; giving HSV-1 a greater opportunity to spread.

The opposite is true as well: Oral sex with a genital HSV-2-infected person can cause oral HSV-2 infection (although there seems to be some degree of immunity against oral HSV-2 in people already infected with oral HSV-1). People with oral or genital sores should take care not to touch these sores. Following hand contact with cold or herpes sores, individuals should carefully wash themselves with soap. Avoid touching the eyes as such can cause vision damage as well.

During an outbreak, genital lesions may appear in areas that can be covered by a latex condom, but they can also appear in areas that cannot be covered. Use of a latex condom may protect against genital herpes only when the infected area is completely covered. Condoms, however, may not cover all infected areas. Thus genital herpes infections still occur. Individuals with HSV infection should abstain from sexual activity when lesions or other herpes symptoms are present. Sex partners of infected individuals should always be informed that they may become infected even if no lesions or symptoms are present. The best preventive approach is a mutually monogamous sexual relationship with an uninfected partner. Blood tests are available to determine HSV infection.

Hepatitis

Hepatitis is a general term that means inflammation of the liver but also refers to a group of viruses (A, B, C, D, and E) that cause liver inflammation through infection. Viral hepatitis is the leading cause of liver cancer and the need for liver transplants. About 4.4 million Americans live with chronic hepatitis and don't know they are infected.

Hepatitis viruses spread through physical contact with the blood or bodily fluid of an infected person. Of the five viruses, B and C are the two most frequently transmitted through sexual activity, with Hepatitis B being the most prevalent. Most people don't think of hepatitis as an STI; however, it is estimated that as much as 30 percent of infections result from sexual transmission.

Hepatitis B (HBV) is a very common infection, affecting 350 million people worldwide. In the United States, an estimated 43,000 new cases are reported each year, with most infections occurring between 20 and 39 years.[10] Hepatitis B is transmitted when blood, semen, or other bodily fluid enters the body through kissing and vaginal, anal, or oral sex. HBV can also be passed from an infected mother to her baby during pregnancy or through blood contact via intravenous drug use, body piercings, and tattoos.

Hepatitis viruses travel through infected tissue into the blood and then to the liver, where it causes inflammation and cell damage. Hepatitis B can cause both acute and chronic liver inflammation. Only 50 percent of newly acquired infections produce symptoms, which include yellow coloration of the skin or eyes (jaundice), fever, abdominal pain, loss of appetite, tiredness, and nausea. The initial (acute) phase of infection lasts only a few weeks and then clears for the majority of people. Those who recover from the initial infection develop immunity to HBV, protecting them from future infection. Only a small number of people who do not recover from the infection develop chronic inflammation that can lead to disease and cancer in the liver. Infection from HBV can be diagnosed by laboratory tests detecting the virus or antibodies against the virus in the blood.

Hepatitis B is the only viral STI that can be successfully prevented through vaccination. Since 1990, implementation of routine vaccination at birth has resulted in a drastic 82 percent decline in rates of acute Hepatitis B, especially among children. The vaccine is administered in a three-dose series of injections to the muscle tissue of the shoulder over a period of months. It is recommended that all babies be vaccinated at birth, as well as at risk groups, including sexually active men and women, illicit drug users, health-care workers, adoptees from countries were hepatitis B is common, international travelers, and welfare volunteers.

DIVERSITY CONSIDERATIONS: STIs among Minority Groups

Many social and economic factors that place African Americans and Latinos at risk for other diseases also fuel the spread of STIs in these communities. For example, people who don't have the means to see a doctor may not get an STI test or treatment until it's too late—and poverty, high school drop-out, and unemployment rates are considerably higher among African Americans and Latinos. Other factors, such as greater STI prevalence in communities of racial and ethnic minorities, can increase individuals' risk of infection, even with similar levels of risk behavior. Distrust of the medical system may also cause some African Americans to access health services less, and language barriers may affect quality of and access to care for some Latinos. These factors provide an important reminder that while people have a personal responsibility to protect their own health, it is also critical to address the root causes of these disparities.

Source: Centers for Disease Control and Prevention, "2012 Sexually Transmitted Diseases Surveillance," http://www.cdc.gov/std/stats12/minorities.htm, downloaded April 15, 2014.

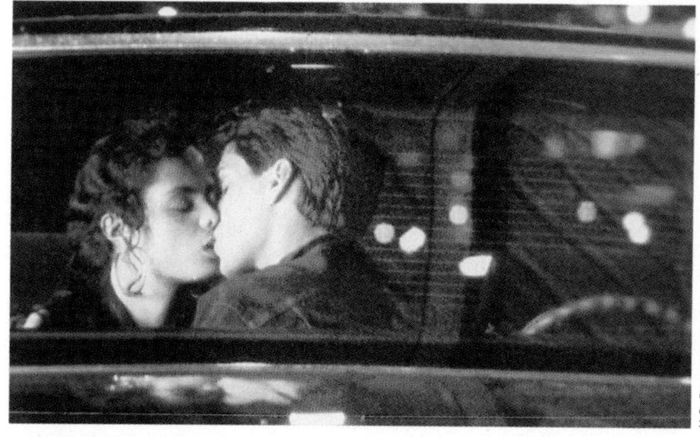

U.S. Department of Health & Human Services

Drug and alcohol use can make people more willing to have unplanned and unprotected sex, thereby risking HIV infection.

CRITICAL THINKING

Many individuals who have STIs withhold this information from potential sexual partners. Do you think it should be considered a criminal action if an individual knowingly transmits an STI to someone else?

HIV and AIDS

Of all STIs, **human immunodeficiency virus (HIV)** infection is the most frightening because in most cases it is fatal and it has no known cure. **AIDS**—which stands for **acquired immune deficiency syndrome**—is the end stage of infection by HIV. In Lab 14A, you have the opportunity to evaluate your basic understanding of HIV and AIDS.

HIV is a chronic infectious disease that is passed from one person to another through blood-to-blood and sexual contact. The virus spreads most commonly among individuals who engage in risky behavior, such as having unprotected sex or sharing hypodermic needles. When a person becomes infected with HIV, the virus multiplies, then attacks and destroys white blood cells. These cells are part of the immune system, and their function is to fight off infections and diseases in the body.

As the number of white blood cells that are killed increases, the body's immune system gradually breaks down or may be destroyed. Without an immune system, a person becomes susceptible to various **opportunistic infections** and to cancers.

The only means to determine whether someone has HIV is through an HIV antibody test. Being HIV-positive does not mean that the person has AIDS. HIV is a progressive infection. At first, people who become infected with HIV might not know they are infected. An incubation period of weeks, months, or years may pass during which no symptoms appear. The virus may live in the body 10 years or longer before disease symptoms emerge. HIV infection can produce neurological abnormalities, leading to depression, memory loss, slower mental and physical response time, and sluggishness in limb movements that may progress to a severe disorder known as HIV dementia.

When the infection progresses to a point at which certain diseases develop, the person is said to have AIDS. HIV itself doesn't kill. Nor do people die from AIDS. "AIDS" is the term designating the final stage of HIV infection, and death is the result of a weakened immune system that is unable to fight off these opportunistic infections.

Earliest symptoms of AIDS include unexplained weight loss, constant fatigue, mild fever, swollen lymph glands, diarrhea, and sore throat. Advanced symptoms include loss of appetite, skin diseases, night sweats, and deterioration of mucous membranes.

Most of the illnesses that AIDS patients

Hepatitis B (HBV) An STI caused by a viral infection that affects the liver.

Human immunodeficiency virus (HIV) A virus that leads to AIDS.

Acquired immune deficiency syndrome (AIDS) Any of a number of diseases that arise when the body's immune system is compromised by HIV; the final stage of HIV infection.

Opportunistic infections Infections that arise in the absence of a healthy immune system, which would fight them off in healthy people.

develop are harmless and rare in the general population but are fatal to AIDS victims. Two of the fatal conditions in AIDS patients, for example, are Pneumocystis jiroveci pneumonia (a parasitic infection of the lungs) and Kaposi's sarcoma (a type of skin cancer). HIV also attacks the nervous system, causing damage to the brain and spinal cord. An unsettling finding is that brain damage is seen even in patients who are on drug therapy. The brain appears to provide a haven for HIV where drugs cannot follow, leading to a selective destruction pattern of brain regions that control motor, language, and sensory functions. This finding may explain why individuals often display slower reflexes and disruption of balance and gait in the early stages of AIDS. Patients also frequently exhibit mild vocabulary loss, judgment problems, and difficulty planning.

On becoming infected, the immune system forms antibodies that bind to the virus. Most infected individuals will show these antibodies within 3 months of infection, the average being 25 days. In rare cases, they are not detectable until after 6 months or longer.

If HIV infection is suspected, seek medical attention *immediately*. Some evidence indicates that an immediate course of antiretroviral drugs reduces the chances that a person will be infected. This is referred to as post-exposure prophylaxis (PEP), frequently used to prevent transmission in health care workers injured by needle sticks. Less information is available about the effectiveness of PEP for people exposed to HIV through sexual activity or drug-use injections, but it also appears to be effective. If you think you were exposed, discuss the possibility with an HIV specialist (local AIDS organizations provide the most recent information) as soon as possible. Sexual assault victims should consider the potential effects and benefits of PEP.

Following the initial consultation with a medical specialist, the individual may still need to wait 3 months to be tested. If the test is negative and the person still suspects infection, the test should be repeated 3 months later. During this time, and from then on, individuals should refrain from further endangering themselves and others through risky behaviors. Some people are tested to reassure themselves that their behaviors are acceptable. Even if the test turns up negative for HIV, this does not represent a "license" to continue risky behaviors.

No one has to become infected with HIV. At present, once infected, with the exception of a handful of rare cases, a person cannot become uninfected. There is no second chance. Everyone must protect himself or herself against this chronic infection. If people do not—and are so ignorant as to believe it cannot happen to them—they are putting themselves and their partners at risk.

New therapies are preventing AIDS from developing in a growing number of HIV-infected individuals. Professionals, however, disagree as to how many HIV carriers actually will develop AIDS. Even if individuals have not developed AIDS, they can pass on the virus to others, who then could easily develop AIDS.

Transmission of HIV

HIV is transmitted by the exchange of cellular body fluids, including blood and other body fluids containing blood, semen, vaginal secretions, and maternal milk.

The most recent data available on HIV infection diagnoses among adults and adolescents in the United States by race/ethnicity are given in Figure 14.2. The percentage of adults and adolescents currently living with a diagnosis of HIV infection, by gender and transmission category, as of the end of 2010, are provided in Figure 14.3. Further, approximately 50,000 new infections are presently being reported each year. Of all new infections, about 63 percent are reported in men who had sex with men, 25 percent in men and women through heterosexual sex, 8 percent by injection drug use, 3 percent in male-to-male sexual contact and injection drug use combined, and less than 1 percent in other unidentified categories. Currently about 47 percent of the new infections occur in African Americans, followed by Caucasians (28 percent), Hispanics (21 percent), Asians (2 percent), and multiple races (2 percent). American Indians/Alaska Natives and Native Hawaiians/Pacific Islanders each account for 1 percent or less of diagnosis.

Today, the risk of being infected with HIV from a blood transfusion is slight. Prior to 1985, several cases of HIV infection came from blood transfusions because the blood had been donated by HIV-infected individuals. Now, all individuals who donate blood are first tested for HIV. To be absolutely safe, people who are planning to have surgery might consider storing their own blood in advance, so safe blood will be available if a transfusion becomes necessary.

FIGURE 14.2 Adult and adolescent diagnoses of HIV infection, by race or ethnicity, 2008–2011—United States and 6 U.S.-dependent areas.

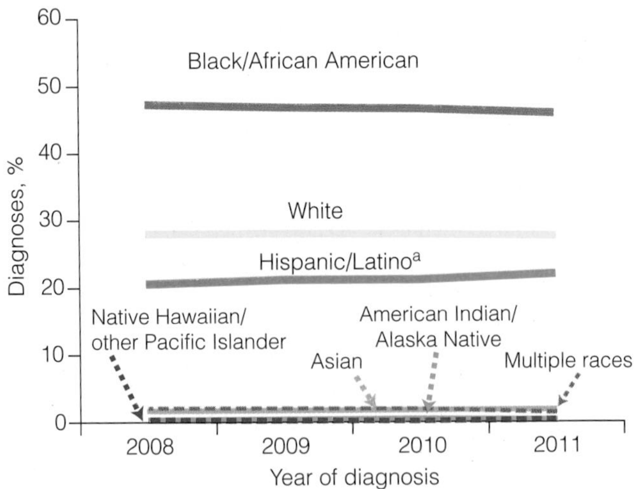

Note: Data include persons with a diagnosis of HIV infection regardless of stage of disease at diagnosis. All displayed data have been statistically adjusted to account for reporting delays, but not for incomplete reporting.

[a]Hispanics/Latinos can be of any race.

Source: http://www.cdc.gov/hiv/pdf/statistics_surveillance_raceEthnicity.pdf, downloaded April 15, 2014.

FIGURE 14.3 Adults and adolescents living with a diagnosis of HIV infection, by gender and transmission category, 2010—United States and 6 U.S.-dependent areas.

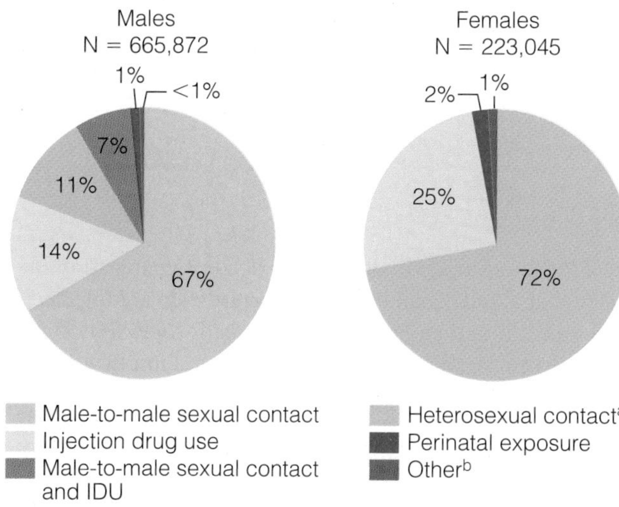

Note: Data include persons with a diagnosis of HIV infection regardless of stage of disease at diagnosis. All displayed data have been statistically adjusted to account for reporting delays and missing transmission category, but not for incomplete reporting.
[a]Heterosexual contact with a person known to have, or to be at high risk for, HIV infection.
[b]Includes hemophilia, blood transfusion, and risk factor not reported or not identified.

Source: http://www.cdc.gov/std/stats/sti-estimates-fact-sheet-feb-2013.pdf Downloaded April 15, 2014.

A myth regarding HIV is that it can be transmitted by donating blood. People cannot get HIV from giving blood. Health professionals use a brand-new needle every time they withdraw blood from a person. They use these needles only once and destroy them immediately after each person has donated blood.

People do not get HIV because of who they are but, rather, because of what they do. HIV and AIDS can threaten anyone, anywhere: men, women, children, teenagers, young people, older adults, Caucasians, African Americans, Hispanic Americans, Asian Americans, Native Americans, Africans, Europeans, homosexuals, heterosexuals, bisexuals, drug users. Nobody is immune to HIV. HIV can be transmitted between males, between females, from male to female, or from female to male. Although HIV and AIDS are preventable, nearly all of the people who get HIV do so because they engage in risky behaviors.

Risky Behaviors

You cannot tell whether people are infected with HIV or have AIDS by simply looking at them or taking their word. Not you, not a nurse, not even a doctor can tell without an HIV antibody test. Therefore, every time you engage in risky behavior, you run the risk of contracting HIV. There are two basic risky behaviors:

1. Having unprotected vaginal, anal, or oral sex with an HIV-infected person. Unprotected sex means having sex without using a condom properly. A person should select only latex (rubber or prophylactic) condoms that state "disease prevention" on the package. Although you might have unprotected sex with an infected person and not get the virus, you can get it by having unprotected sex only once with an infected individual.

   Rubbing during sexual intercourse often damages mucous membranes and causes unseen bleeding (even in the mouth). During vaginal, anal, or oral sexual contact, infected blood, semen, or vaginal fluids can penetrate the mucous membranes that line the vagina, the penis, the rectum, the mouth, or the throat. From the membrane, HIV then travels into the previously uninfected person's blood.

   Health experts believe that unprotected anal sex is the riskiest type of sex. Even though bleeding is not visible in most cases, anal sex almost always causes tiny tears and bleeding in the rectum. This happens because the rectum does not stretch easily, the mucous membrane is quite thin, and small blood vessels lie directly beneath the membrane. Condoms also are more likely to break during anal intercourse, because more friction is produced in a smaller cavity. All of these factors greatly enhance the risk of transmitting HIV.

   Although latex condoms, if used correctly, provide for "safer" sex, they are not foolproof. Abstaining from sex is the only 100 percent assurance that you are protecting yourself from HIV infection and other STIs.

2. Sharing hypodermic needles or other drug paraphernalia with someone who is infected. Following an injection, a small amount of blood remains in the needle and sometimes in the syringe. If the person who used the syringe is infected with HIV and you use that same syringe to shoot up, regardless of the drug used (legal or illegal), that small amount of blood is sufficient to spread the virus. All used syringes should be destroyed and disposed of immediately.

   In addition, you must be cautious when getting acupuncture, getting a tattoo, or having the ears or other

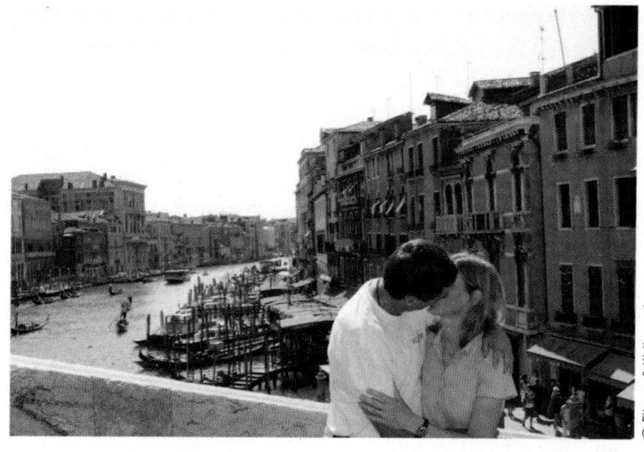

A monogamous sexual relationship almost completely removes people from risking HIV infection and the danger of developing other STIs.

body parts pierced. If the needle was used previously on an HIV-infected person and was not disinfected properly, you risk getting HIV.

Otherwise-prudent people often act irrationally and engage in risky behaviors when they are under the influence of drugs. Getting high can make you willing to have sex when you didn't plan to—thereby running the risk of contracting HIV.

Small concentrations of the virus have been found in saliva and teardrops. In principle, if two people have open cuts on the lips or in the mouth or gums, HIV could be transmitted through open-mouth kissing. Prolonged open-mouth kissing can damage the mouth or lips and allow HIV to be transmitted from an infected person to a partner through cuts or sores in the mouth. These cases, however, are rare.

Myths about HIV Transmission

HIV cannot be transmitted through perspiration. Sporting activities with no physical contact pose no risk to uninfected individuals unless they both have open wounds through which blood from an infected person can come in direct contact with the open wound of the uninfected person. The skin is an excellent line of defense against HIV. Blood from an infected person cannot penetrate the skin except through an opening in the skin. As an extra precaution, a person should use vinyl or latex gloves when performing work that requires direct contact with someone else's blood or open wound.

HIV is not transmitted through casual contact. HIV cannot be caught by spending time with, shaking hands with, or hugging an infected person; from a toilet seat, dishes, or silverware used by an HIV patient; or by sharing a drink, food, a towel, or clothes with a person who has HIV.

Some people fear getting HIV from health care professionals. The chances of getting infected during physical or medical procedures are practically nil. Health care workers take extra care to protect themselves and their patients from HIV.

Another myth regarding HIV transmission is that you can get it from insects or animals. The H in HIV stands for "human." You cannot catch HIV from insects or animals. Animals do not contract HIV.

Trends in HIV Infection and AIDS

As of 2012, estimates by the World Health Organization indicate that about 35 million people worldwide are infected with HIV. More than 36 million have died from AIDS since the epidemic began in 1981. Close to 2.3 million new worldwide infections were reported in 2012. And women and children are becoming increasingly affected, with 17.7 million women and 3.3 million children now living with HIV.[11]

About 1.1 million people in the United States are infected with HIV, and almost 16 percent are unaware of the infection. One in every four newly reported cases are in youth ages 13 to 24, and because most don't know they are infected, they are not receiving treatment and have a high risk of passing the virus to others unknowingly. African Americans, Latinos, and gay and bisexual men of all races remain the most disproportionately affected by HIV. Although men who have sex with men (MSM) represent only 4 percent of American males, this group accounts for 78 percent of new HIV infections among males as well as 63 percent of new infections overall.

Through the end of 2010, an estimated 636,000 people diagnosed with AIDS have died from diseases caused by HIV. Though annual AIDS diagnoses and deaths within the United States and dependent areas have subsided since their peak in the early 90s (Figure 14.4), the number of people living with AIDS in the United States continues to increase

FIGURE 14.4 AIDS diagnoses, deaths, and persons living with AIDS, 1985–2009—United States and 6 U.S.-dependent areas.

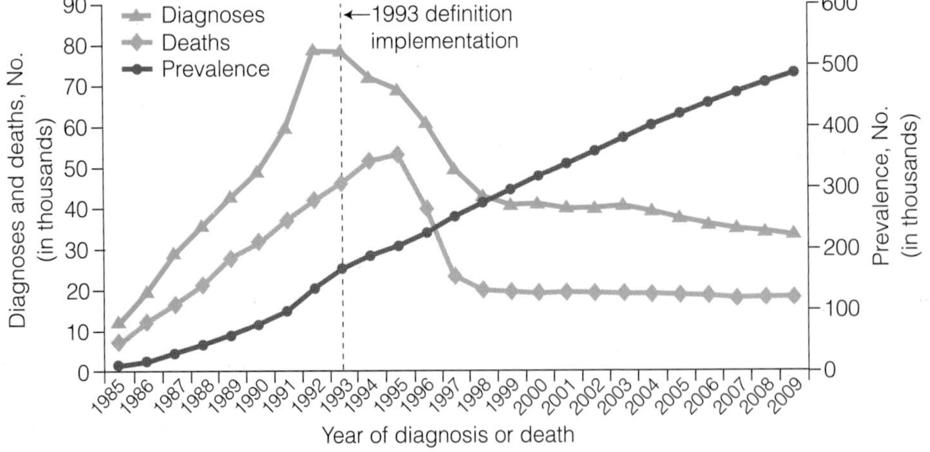

Note: All displayed data have been statistically adjusted to account for reporting delays, but not for incomplete reporting. Death may be due to any cause.

Source: http://www.cdc.gov/std/stats/sti-estimates-fact-sheet-feb-2013.pdf Downloaded April 15, 2014.

over time, escalating the need for better treatment methods and assistance for those that are victimized by the disease.

As with any other serious illness, HIV-infected people and AIDS patients deserve respect, understanding, and support. Rejection and discrimination are traits that come from immaturity, hate, and ignorance. Education, knowledge, and responsible behaviors are the best ways to minimize fear and discrimination.

HIV Testing

A person can be tested for HIV in several ways. You may look up your local Public Health Department or AIDS Information Service (or related names) on the Internet or visit the student health clinic at your local educational institution. Testing results are kept confidential.

Many states also conduct anonymous testing. Your name is never recorded. You can call several toll-free hotlines or access the CDC website (www.cdc.gov/hiv) for more information on anonymous testing, treatment programs, support services, and information about HIV, AIDS, and STIs in general. All information discussed during a phone call to these hotlines is kept confidential. The numbers to call are:

- National AIDS Hotline: 1-800-CDC-INFO (1-800-232-4636) in English and Spanish
- National AIDS Hotline for the hearing impaired (TTY): 1-888-232-6348
- STI Hotline: 1-800-227-8922

Information on local testing facilities is also available online at www.hivtest.org.

The CDC recommends HIV testing for all patients in health care settings ages 13 to 64, including pregnant women during the routine panel of prenatal screening tests. The recommendations further include annual screening for people at high risk for infection. Consent for HIV testing is now included in the general consent form for medical care. Patients, however, can decline testing if they choose to do so.

HIV Treatment

Even though several drugs are being tested to treat and slow the infection process, AIDS still has no known cure. To date, one leukemia patient, "the Berlin patient," is known to have been cured of HIV infection after undergoing a bone marrow transplant from a donor who had a rare genetic mutation that makes a person resistant to HIV infection. Other patients using a similar treatment, however, have not been as fortunate. At least 40 approaches to an AIDS vaccine are being explored. The best advice at this point is to take a preventive approach.

Antiretroviral drugs are available that delay the progress of HIV infection and even keep many people from developing AIDS. Antiretroviral drugs have turned HIV infection from an almost imminent predecessor of death to a lifelong chronic disease. Thanks to advances in the development of these drugs, many HIV-infected people can now look forward to decades of life. HIV-infected individuals, however, must take the drugs every day for the rest of their life. In most cases, failure to do so results in the virus coming back with full strength. The drugs don't eradicate HIV but rather suppress the virus and make it almost undetectable in the blood. The world, unfortunately, does not have the resources to make the drugs available to most HIV-infected people for decades to come.

About 30 drugs are available that suppress HIV. The drugs are usually used in combinations, commonly referred to as highly active antiretroviral therapy or "AIDS cocktails." Because the virus mutates rapidly and because some individuals don't tolerate some of the drugs, physicians often switch drug combinations to keep HIV under control.

A study sponsored by the National Institutes of Health that was set to conclude in 2015 was stalled in early in May 2011when a data review by a federal monitoring agency called for immediate release of its findings because of its significance in the prevention of HIV transmission. The study found that early treatment with antiretroviral drugs, at the time of HIV diagnosis, greatly decreased the risk of transmitting the virus to an uninfected partner. The research was conducted on 1,763 couples in nine countries throughout the world. Only one of the partners in each couple was infected with HIV. The results showed a 96 percent reduction in HIV infection risk only among patients who received the early drug treatment. (All couples in the study were urged to use condoms, which are still critical for protection.) Early treatment is thus critical to decrease transmission risk. HIV-infected individuals, nonetheless, cannot make the assumption that they will not pass on the virus simply because they are on antiretroviral medication.

The value of early treatment has been further substantiated with two recent cases of newborn babies whose infections were effectively suppressed for several years by early and aggressive drug therapy that began just hours after birth. The stunning success of the two cases has fueled international measures to reconsider general treatment methods for infected newborns. A federally funded clinical trial began in 2014 to test the viability of early treatment on a larger scale, with as many as 60 HIV-infected babies put on an antiretroviral drug regimen within 48 hours after birth. Up until now, aggressive drug treatment in babies has been avoided due to potential toxicity; however, the results of the upcoming trial could alter the way HIV-infected newborns are treated by health care professionals. Other reports have also shown success in long-term suppression of the virus to extremely low levels in some adults who were treated immediately after diagnoses, giving researchers hope that a "functional cure" for HIV may be possible in the future.

For the majority of cases, however, antiretroviral drugs do not cure HIV infection or AIDS. They suppress the virus (decrease the viral load), even to undetectable levels, but they do not eliminate the virus. The sooner the treatment is initiated, the better the prognosis for a longer life.

For HIV-infected individuals, viral load tests are available to detect the amount of virus present in the blood. These tests measure HIV ribonucleic acid, the part of HIV that knows how to make more of the virus. Following drug therapy, an undetectable viral load does not mean the person is cured. It means that the amount of HIV in the blood is so low that it cannot be detected. Because there is no known cure, the person is still infected with HIV and can infect others. Although undetectable in the blood, the virus is still present in other body tissues and in the lymph system.

Development of a vaccine to prevent HIV infection or AIDS seems highly unlikely in the near future. People should not expect a medical breakthrough, although researchers are cautiously optimistic about finding a cure. Treatment modalities, however, continue to improve and allow HIV-infected individuals and AIDS patients to live longer and more productive lives.

Several AIDS clinical trials are available in the United States. These projects are cosponsored by the CDC, the FDA, the National Institute of Allergy and Infectious Diseases, the National Library of Medicine, and the National Institutes of Health. The purpose of AIDS clinical trials is to evaluate experimental drugs and various therapies for people at all stages of HIV infection. Interested individuals can call 1-800-TRIALS-A (1-800-874-2572). As with all HIV testing, calls are confidential. Eligibility to participate in an AIDS clinical trial varies, and all applicants are evaluated individually. By calling the telephone number, an interested person receives information on the purpose and location of the trials (studies) that are open, eligibility requirements and exclusion criteria, and names and telephone numbers of people to contact.

Preventing STIs

The good news is that you can do things to prevent the spread of STIs and take precautions to keep yourself from becoming a victim. The CDC recommends sexual abstinence in dating followed by a long-term mutually monogamous relationship with an uninfected partner as the most reliable way to avoid STI infection.[12]

Wise Dating

With the advent of the Internet, it has become common to search for sex partners online. Surveys have shown that people who seek sex partners over the Internet are at greater risk of contracting an STI. These people also are more likely to have characteristics that increase their chances of transmitting STIs.

Dating and getting to know other people are normal aspects of life. Dating, however, does not mean the same thing as having sex. Sexual intercourse as a part of dating can be risky, and one of the risks is infection. You can't tell whether someone you are dating or would like to date has been exposed to HIV or other STIs. Avoiding sexual activity in dating keeps you virtually risk free from STI infection.

Monogamous Sexual Relationship The facts are in: The best long-term prevention technique is a mutually **monogamous** sexual relationship. Mutual monogamy means both you and your partner agree to only have sex with each other. Committing to this one behavior removes you almost completely from any risk for developing an STI in your lifetime.

Unfortunately, in today's society, trust is elusive. You may be led to believe you are in a safe, monogamous rela-

BEHAVIOR MODIFICATION PLANNING

Protecting Yourself and Others from STIs

Are you sexually active? If you are not, read the following items to better educate yourself regarding intimacy. If you are sexually active, continue through all the questions below.

- ❑ Do you plan ahead before you get into a sexual situation?
- ❑ Do you know whether your partner now has or has ever had an STI? Are you comfortable asking your partner this question?
- ❑ Are you in a mutually monogamous sexual relationship, and do you know that your partner does not have an STI?
- ❑ Do you have multiple sexual partners? If so, do you *always* practice safe sex?
- ❑ Do you avoid alcohol and drugs in situations where you may end up having planned or unplanned sex?
- ❑ Do you abstain from sexual activity if you know or suspect that you have an STI? Do you seek medical care and advice as to when you can safely resume sexual activity?

Try It

Taking chances during sexual contact is not worth the risk of an STI. Sex lasts a few minutes; the STI can last a lifetime, with potentially fatal consequences. Think ahead, know the facts, and don't place yourself in a situation where you may no longer be able to or have the desire to say no. Keep in mind that more than half of all Americans will acquire at least one STI in their lifetime. A few minutes of sexual pleasure can easily have consequences that you may regret for the rest of your life.

tionship when your partner actually (1) may cheat on you and get infected, (2) has a one-night stand with someone who is infected, (3) got infected several years ago before the current relationship and still doesn't know about the infection, (4) may choose not to tell you about the infection, or (5) shoots up drugs and becomes infected. In any of these cases, an STI, including HIV, can be passed on to you.

Because your future and your life are at stake, and because you may never know if your partner is infected, you should give serious and careful consideration to postponing sex until you believe you have found an uninfected person with whom you can have a lifetime monogamous relationship. In doing so, you do not have to live with the fear of catching HIV or other STIs or deal with an unplanned pregnancy.

Many people postpone sexual activity until they are married. This is the best guarantee against HIV. Young people should understand that married life provides plenty of time for fulfilling and rewarding sex.

If you choose to delay sex, don't let peers pressure you into changing your mind. Some people would have you believe that you aren't a "real" man or woman if you don't have sex. Manhood and womanhood are proven not during sexual intercourse but, instead, through mature, responsible, and healthy choices.

Other people may lead you to believe that love doesn't exist without sex. Sex in the early stages of a relationship is not the product of love. It is simply the fulfillment of a physical, and often selfish, drive. A loving relationship develops over a long time with mutual respect for each other.

Having sexual encounters with multiple partners may be considered commonplace by peers or even encouraged to gain popularity. The reality is that nearly 50 percent of young women and over 40 percent of young men ages 15 to 19 years old have not had any sexual partners, with about 20 percent reporting only one sexual partner between the ages of 20 to 24.[13]

Teenagers are especially susceptible to peer pressure leading to premature sexual intercourse. The result? More than 750,000 teen girls in the United States get pregnant each year, which means three in ten girls will get pregnant at least once before age 20. Presently, the U.S. teen pregnancy, teen birth, and abortion rates are among the highest of all industrialized nations. Too many young people wish they had postponed sex and silently admire those who do. Sex lasts only a few minutes. The consequences of irresponsible sex may last a lifetime. And in some cases, they are fatal!

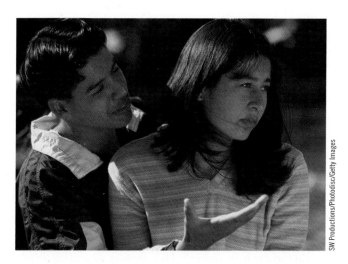

SW Productions/Photodisc/Getty Images

If someone does not respect your choice to wait, he or she does not deserve your friendship—or anything else.

Sexual promiscuity never leads to a trusting, loving, and lasting relationship. Mature people respect others' choices. If someone doesn't respect your choice to wait, he or she certainly doesn't deserve your friendship—or anything else.

There is no greater sex than that between two loving and responsible individuals who mutually trust, admire, and love each other. Contrary to many beliefs, these relationships are possible. They are built upon unselfish attitudes and behaviors.

As you look around, you will find that many people hold these values. Seek them out, and build your friendships and future around people who respect you for who you are and what you believe. You don't have to compromise your choices or values. In the end, you will reap the greater rewards of a lasting relationship free of HIV and other STIs.

Also, be prepared so that you know your course of action before you get into an intimate situation. Look for common interests, and work together toward them. Express your feelings openly: "I'm not ready for sex; I just want to have fun, and kissing is fine with me." If your friend doesn't accept your answer and isn't willing to stop the advances, be prepared with a strong response. Statements like, "Please stop" or "Don't!" are mostly ineffective. Use a firm statement such as, "No, I'm not willing to have sex" or "I've already thought about this and I'm not going to have sex." If this still doesn't work, inform them that their forceful behavior is considered rape and say, "This is rape, and I'm going to call the police."

CRITICAL THINKING

Discuss how the information presented in this chapter has affected your feelings and perceptions about sex. What impact will this information have on your wellness lifestyle?

Reducing the Risk for STIs and HIV Infection

Based upon recommendations from health experts, observing the following precautions can reduce your risk for STIs, including HIV infection and, subsequently, AIDS:

1. Postpone sex until you and your uninfected partner are prepared to enter into a lifetime monogamous relationship.
2. Unless you are in a monogamous relationship and you know your

Monogamous A sexual relationship in which two people have sexual relations only with each other.

partner isn't infected (which you may never know for sure), practice safer sex every time you have sex and don't have sexual contact with anyone who doesn't practice safe sex. This means you should use a latex condom from start to finish for each sexual act. If your partner refuses to use a condom, say "no" to sex with that person.

3. Use "barrier" methods of contraception to help prevent the infection from spreading. Condoms, diaphragms, and spermicidal suppositories, foams, and jellies can all deter the spread of certain STIs. Spermicidal agents may act as a disinfectant as well. Young people are especially susceptible. Traditionally, teenagers have not used birth-control methods and therefore remain at high risk for STIs and unwanted pregnancies. At this time, take a few minutes and list at least three ways you might bring up the subject of condoms with your partner. Also, think of ways you might convince a person to use a condom. If your partner refuses to use a condom, your answer should be quite simple: "No condom, no sex."
4. Know your partner and limit your sexual relationships. The days are gone when sex was thought to be safe with anonymous encounters at a bathhouse or a singles bar. Having only one partner lowers your chances of becoming infected. Although you can still become infected by having unprotected sex with one person only, the more partners you have, the greater your chances for infection.
5. Don't have sex with prostitutes.
6. Determine the conditions under which you will allow sex. Ask yourself: "Am I willing to have sex with this person?" If you decide to have sex, practice safer sex. There is no reason to accept anything else. You will feel better about yourself.
7. Plan before you get into a sexual situation. Discuss STIs with the person you are contemplating having sex with before you do so. Even though talking about STIs might be awkward, the short-lived embarrassment of addressing intimate questions can keep you from contracting or spreading infection. If you don't know the person well enough to address this issue or you are uncertain about the answers, don't have sex with this individual.
8. Negotiate safer sex. Focus on the problem, not the person. Describe your feelings about the problem, using "I" or "we" instead of "you." For example, you might say, "I'm feeling awkward and uncomfortable. The only way I can feel comfortable is by using a condom." You also can offer options and provide alternative solutions. You might indicate to your partner, "We can work this out together. Let's go for a drive and get a condom. We'll feel better about what we're doing."
9. If you are sexually promiscuous, have periodic physical checkups. You can easily get exposed to an STI from a person who does not have any symptoms and who is unaware of the infection. Sexually promiscuous men and women between ages 15 and 35 are a particularly high-risk group for developing STIs.
10. Avoid sexual contact with anyone who has had sex with one or more individuals at risk for getting HIV, even if they are now practicing safer sex.
11. If you do have sex with someone who might be infected with HIV or whose history is unknown to you, avoid exchanging body fluids.
12. Don't share toothbrushes, razors, or other implements that could become contaminated with blood with anyone who is, or who might be, infected with HIV.
13. If you suspect that your partner is infected with an STI, ask. He or she may not be aware of the infection, so look for signs, such as sores, redness, inflammation, a rash, growths, warts, or a discharge. If you are unsure, abstain.
14. If you know you have an infection, be responsible enough to abstain from sexual activity. Go to a physician or a clinic for treatment, and ask your doctor when you can safely resume sexual activity. Abstain until it is safe. Just as you want to be protected in a sexual relationship, you should want to protect your partner. If you are diagnosed with an STI and you believe you know the person who gave it to you, think of ways you might bring up the subject of STIs with this person. You need to take responsibility and discuss this matter with your partner. As a result of your conversation, medical treatment can be initiated and other people can be protected from infection.
15. Wear loose-fitting clothes made from natural fibers. Tight-fitting clothing made from synthetic fibers (especially underwear and nylon pantyhose) can create conditions that encourage the growth of bacteria and can actually aggravate STIs.
16. Consider abstaining from sexual relations if you have any kind of an illness or disease, even a common cold. Any kind of illness makes you more susceptible to other illnesses, and lower immunity can make you more vulnerable to STIs. The same holds true for times when you are under extreme stress, fatigued, or overworked. Drugs and alcohol also can lower your resistance to infection.
17. Thoroughly wash immediately after sexual activity. Although washing with hot, soapy water does not guarantee safety against STIs, it can prevent you from spreading certain germs on your fingers and might wash away bacteria and viruses that have not entered the body yet.
18. Be cautious regarding procedures (e.g., acupuncture, tattooing, and ear piercing) in which needles or other nonsterile instruments may be used repeatedly to pierce the skin or mucous membranes. These procedures are safe if proper sterilization methods are followed or disposable needles are used. Before undergoing the procedure, ask what precautions are being taken.
19. If you plan to undergo artificial insemination, insist that frozen sperm be obtained from a laboratory that tests all donors for infection with HIV. Donors should be tested twice before the lab accepts the sperm—once at the time of donation and again a few months later.

20. If you know you will be having surgery soon, and if you are able, consider donating blood for your own use. This eliminates the already-small risk of contracting HIV through a blood transfusion. It also eliminates the more substantial risk for contracting other blood-borne diseases, such as hepatitis, from a transfusion.

Avoiding risky behaviors that destroy quality of life and life itself is crucial to a healthy lifestyle. Learning the facts and acting upon your personal values so that you can make responsible choices can protect you and those around you from painful, embarrassing, startling, unexpected, or fatal conditions.

ASSESS YOUR BEHAVIOR

CENGAGE brain.com To access course materials, including companion resources, please visit **www.cengagebrain.com**.

1. Do you believe that a mutually monogamous sexual relationship is the best way to prevent STIs? If not, do you always take precautions to practice safer sex?
2. If you are not prepared to have a sexual relationship, are you prepared to say so? Have you prepared exactly what to say if you are asked to have sex?
3. Have you carefully considered the consequences of engaging in a sexual relationship, including the risk for STIs, HIV infection, your partner being untruthful about his or her sexual history and STIs, and the potential of an unplanned pregnancy?
4. Are you capable of discussing your and your partner [illegible] ual history prior to engaging in a sexual relationship th[illegible] ld bring about detrimental consequences for the rest o[illegible] r life?
5. If you have an STI or a history of STIs, are you suff[illegible] ly responsible to have an open and honest discussion w[illegible] potential partner about the risk for infection and conse[illegible] es thereof?

ASSESS YOUR KNOWLEDGE

1. What percentage of Americans will develop at least one STI in their lifetime?
   a. 30 to 40 percent
   b. 20 to 30 percent
   c. More than 50 percent
   d. 15 to 20 percent
   e. 40 to 50 percent
2. Which of the following STIs is not caused by a bacterial infection?
   a. Chlamydia
   b. Genital warts
   c. Syphilis
   d. Gonorrhea
   e. All of the choices are caused by bacterial infections.
3. Chlamydia
   a. can cause damage to the reproductive system that cannot be reversed by treatment, even if successful.
   b. can cause infertility.
   c. may occur without symptoms.
   d. may cause arthritis.
   e. All of the choices are correct.
4. Gonorrhea can cause
   a. widespread bacterial infection.
   b. infertility.
   c. heart damage.
   d. arthritis.
   e. All of the choices are correct.
5. Treatment of genital warts is done by
   a. dissolving the warts with chemicals.
   b. electrosurgery.
   c. freezing the warts with liquid nitrog[illegible]
   d. All of the choices are correct.
   e. None of the choices are correct.
6. Herpes
   a. is incurable.
   b. causes sores that are treate[illegible] ectrosurgery.
   c. requires antibiotics for su[illegible] l treatment and cure.
   d. is caused by a bacterial i[illegible] tion.
   e. is not a serious STI, bec[illegible] e the person becomes uninfected once the sores heal.
7. Cold sores or fever blisters
   a. can cause genital herpes.
   b. are not highly contagious.
   c. are treatable if caused by bacterial infection.
   d. All of the choices are correct.
   e. None of the choices are correct.
8. The only way to determine whether someone is infected with HIV is through
   a. an AIDS outbreak.
   b. a physical exam by a physician.
   c. a bacterial culture test.
   d. an HIV antibody test.
   e. All of the choices are correct.

9. HIV
   a. attacks and destroys white blood cells.
   b. readily multiplies in the human body.
   c. breaks down the immune system.
   d. increases the likelihood of developing opportunistic infections and cancers.
   e. All of the choices are correct.

10. The best way to protect yourself against STIs is
   a. through the use of condoms for all sexual acts.
   b. by knowing about the people who have previously had sex with your partner.
   c. through a mutually monogamous sexual relationship.
   d. by having sex only with an individual who has no symptoms of STIs.
   e. All of the choices provide equal protection against STIs.

Correct answers can be found at the back of the book.

NOTES

1. Centers for Disease Control and Prevention, "Incidence, Prevalence, and Cost of Sexually Transmitted Infections in the United States," available at http://www.cdc.gov/std/stats/.htm (downloaded April 15, 2014).
2. Centers for Disease Control and Prevention, "Sexually Transmitted Diseases," available at http://www.cdc.gov/STD/(downloaded April 15, 2014).
3. See note 2.
4. See note 2.
5. See note 2.
6. See note 2.
7. Centers for Disease Control and Prevention, "Press Release: New Study shows HPV vaccine helping lower HPV infection rates in teen girls," available at http://www.cdc.gov/media/releases/2013/p0619-hpv-vaccinations.html (downloaded April 15, 2014).
8. See note 2.
9. R. Horowitz, et al., "Herpes Simplex Virus Infection in a University Health Population: Clinical Manifestations, Epidemiology, and Implications. *The Journal of American College Health,* 59, no. 2 (2011): 69–74.
10. See note 2.
11. World Health Organization, "Global Epidemiology," http://www.who.int/hiv/data/en/ (downloaded April 15, 2014).
12. See note 2.
13. A. Chandra, et al., Sexual Behavior, Sexual Attraction, and Sexual Identity in the United States: Data from the 2006–2008 National Survey of Family Growth. *National Health Statistics Reports*; no 36. Hyattsville, MD: National Center for Health Statistics, March 2011.

SUGGESTED READINGS

Blona, R., and J. Levitan. *Healthy Sexuality.* Belmont, CA: Wadsworth/Thomson Learning, 2006.

Centers for Disease Control and Prevention. "Sexually Transmitted Diseases Treatment Guidelines 2010," *Morbidity and Mortality Weekly Report, Recommendations and Reports* 59, no. RR-12 (December 17, 2010): 1–110.

Hoeger, W. W. K., L. W. Turner, and B. Q. Hafen. *Wellness: Guidelines for a Healthy Lifestyle.* Belmont, CA: Wadsworth/Thomson Learning, 2007.

Lab 14A: Self-Quiz on HIV and AIDS

Name ______________________ Date ____________ Grade ____________

Instructor ______________________ Course ____________ Section ____________

NECESSARY LAB EQUIPMENT
None required.

OBJECTIVE
To evaluate basic understanding of HIV and AIDS.

INSTRUCTION
Please answer all of the following questions.

Indicate whether the following statements are true or false, then turn the page to see how well you understand HIV and AIDS.

	True	False
1. AIDS—acquired immunodeficiency syndrome—is the end stage of infection caused by the human immunodeficiency virus, HIV.	☐	☐
2. HIV is a chronic infectious disease that spreads among individuals who choose to engage in risky behavior such as unprotected sex or the sharing of hypodermic needles.	☐	☐
3. AIDS is curable.	☐	☐
4. Abstaining from sex is the only 100 percent sure way to protect yourself from HIV infection.	☐	☐
5. A person infected with HIV can look and feel healthy.	☐	☐
6. Condoms are 100 percent effective in protecting you against HIV infection.	☐	☐
7. Using drugs and alcohol makes a person less likely to use a condom and use it correctly.	☐	☐
8. If you're sexually active, latex condoms provide the best protection against HIV infection.	☐	☐
9. Using drugs and alcohol can make you more likely to have unplanned and unprotected sex.	☐	☐
10. A pregnant woman who has HIV can transmit the virus to her baby during childbirth.	☐	☐
11. You can become HIV-infected by donating blood.	☐	☐
12. HIV can be transmitted by spending time with or through casual contact (shaking hands, hugging) with an infected person.	☐	☐
13. The only means to determine whether someone has HIV is through an HIV antibody test.	☐	☐
14. HIV can completely destroy the immune system.	☐	☐
15. The HIV virus may live in the body 10 years or longer before AIDS symptoms develop.	☐	☐
16. People infected with HIV have AIDS.	☐	☐
17. HIV infection is preventable.	☐	☐
18. Early treatment can reduce the symptoms of HIV-infected people.	☐	☐
19. Drugs are now available that can lengthen the life of an HIV-infected person.	☐	☐
20. Antiretroviral drugs delay the progress of HIV infection and can keep many people from developing AIDS.	☐	☐

(continued)

Selected items on this questionnaire are adapted from *Test Your Survival Smarts: Self-Quiz on Drugs and AIDS,* National Institute on Drug Abuse, U. S. Department of Health & Human Services.

Answers:

1. True. AIDS is the term used to define the manifestation of opportunistic diseases and cancers that occur as a result of HIV infection (also referred to as "HIV disease").
2. True. People do not get HIV because of who they are, but because of what they do. Almost all of the people who get HIV do so because they choose to engage in risky behaviors.
3. False. There is no cure for AIDS, although some medications are now available that delay the progress of HIV and keep some people from developing AIDS.
4. True. Abstinence will protect you from HIV infection. But you may still get the disease by sharing hypodermic needles.
5. True. The symptoms of HIV are often not noticeable until several years after a person has been infected. That's why—no matter who your partner is—it is important to always protect yourself against HIV and the risk of developing AIDS, either by abstaining from sex or by *always* practicing safe sex.
6. False. Only abstaining from sex gives you 100 percent protection, but condoms, if used correctly, are effective in protecting against HIV infection.
7. True. Teens who are drunk or high are less likely to use condoms because, under the influence, they forget or believe that nothing "bad" can happen.
8. True. Proper use is necessary to minimize the risk of infection, but condoms are not 100 percent foolproof as sometimes they do break.
9. True. Otherwise-prudent people often act irrationally and engage in risky behaviors when they are under the influence of drugs and alcohol.
10. True. HIV transmission can occur between a pregnant woman and her baby during childbirth. A baby can also be infected through breast-feeding, although this occurs less frequently.
11. False. A myth regarding HIV is that it can be transmitted by donating blood. People cannot get HIV from giving blood. A brand-new needle is used by health professionals every time they draw blood. These needles are used only once and are destroyed and thrown away immediately after each individual has donated blood.
12. False. HIV is transmitted by the exchange of cellular body fluids, including blood and other body fluids containing blood, semen, vaginal secretions, and maternal milk. These fluids are most often exchanged during sexual intercourse, by using hypodermic needles previously used by infected individuals, or by contact with open wounds, cuts, or sores.
13. True. Not you, not a nurse, not even a doctor, can tell without an HIV antibody test. Upon HIV infection, the immune system's line of defense against the virus is the formation of antibodies that bind to the virus. On the average it takes 3 months for the body to manufacture enough antibodies to show positive in an HIV antibody test. Sometimes it takes 6 months or longer.
14. True. The virus multiplies, then attacks and destroys white blood cells. These cells are part of the immune system, and their function is to fight off infections and diseases in the body. As the number of white blood cells killed increases, the body's immune system gradually breaks down or may be completely destroyed.
15. True. Ten years or longer may go by before the person develops AIDS.
16. False. Being HIV-positive does not necessarily mean that the person has AIDS. It may be 10 years or longer following infection before the individual develops the symptoms that fit the case definition of AIDS. From that point on, the person may live another 2 to 3 years. In essence, from the point of infection, the individual may endure a chronic disease for about 12 or more years.
17. True. The best prevention technique is abstaining from sex until the time comes for a mutually monogamous sexual relationship (two people having a sexual relationship only with each other). That one behavior will almost completely remove you from any risk of HIV infection or developing any other sexually transmitted infection.
18. True. The sooner treatment is initiated, the better the prognosis is for a longer life.
19. True. Available antiretroviral drugs can delay the progress of infection.
20. True. Antiretroviral drugs allow HIV-infected individuals to live healthier and longer lives and even keep some people from developing AIDS. However, these drugs do not cure HIV infection or AIDS.

15

Lifetime Fitness and Wellness

The human body is extremely resilient during young age—not so during middle and older age. Thus, lifestyle choices you make today will affect your health, well-being, and quality of life tomorrow.

OBJECTIVES

- Understand the effects of a healthy lifestyle on longevity.
- Learn to differentiate between physiological and chronological age.
- Estimate your life expectancy and determine your real physiological age.
- Learn about complementary and alternative medicine practices.
- Learn guidelines for preventing consumer fraud.
- Understand factors to consider when selecting a health or fitness club.
- Know how to select appropriate exercise equipment.
- Review health and fitness accomplishments and chart a wellness program for the future.

REAL LIFE STORY | James' Experience

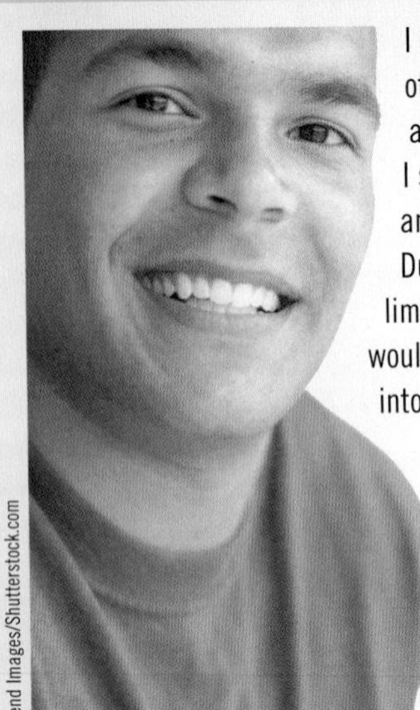
Blend Images/Shutterstock.com

I participated in sports on and off during my youth. I didn't really love competitive sports, but I sure enjoyed all the attention and recognition we received. During the summers, other than limited yard work my parents would ask me to do, I would turn into a couch potato. I spent my days playing video games and watching TV with friends and surfing the net. Come fall, I always had to work hard to get back in shape for sports, often having to diet to get the summer weight off. To this date, I still hate to go hungry. My sophomore year in college I took the required Lifetime Fitness & Wellness course. We learned sound exercise, nutrition, weight management, and healthy lifestyle guidelines. We also walked, jogged, swam, cycled, and lifted weights, and a few times we did interval training. I don't think I was ever as fit through sports as I was at the end of that course. I even learned to use moderation in all things. I no longer overeat or overindulge, not even during the Thanksgiving and Christmas seasons. It is much easier to stay at the recommended weight than trying to lose weight following summers of being a couch potato. I learned to think in terms of long-term gratification rather than instant gratification. I feel so much better about myself now: the way I look, the energy I have, and my newfound increased functional capacity. I love my life now, and I know I can maintain this feeling by adhering to a lifetime fitness and wellness program.

FAQ

How does regular physical activity affect chronological versus physiological age?

Chronological age is your actual age—that is, how old you are. Physiological age is used in reference to your functional capacity to perform physical work at any stage of your life. Data on individuals who have taken part in systematic physical activity throughout life indicate that these people maintain a higher level of functional capacity and do not experience the declines typical in later years. From a functional point of view, typical sedentary people in the United States are about 25 years older than their chronological age indicates. Thus, an active 60-year-old person can have a physical capacity similar to that of an inactive 35-year-old person. Similarly, a sedentary 20-year-old college student most likely has the physical capacity of a 45-year-old active individual.

What are the differences among conventional medicine, complementary and alternative medicine (CAM), and integrative medicine?

Conventional medicine implies the practice of traditional medicine by medical doctors, osteopaths, and allied health professionals, such as registered nurses, physical therapists, and psychologists. CAM comprises a group of diverse medical and health care systems, practices, and products that are not presently considered part of conventional medicine. The safety and effectiveness of many of these practices have not been rigorously tested through well-designed scientific studies. Integrative medicine is a growing trend among health care providers that uses a combination of conventional medicine and CAM treatments for which there is some scientific evidence of safety and effectiveness.

What is the greatest benefit of a lifetime wellness lifestyle?

There are many benefits derived from an active wellness lifestyle, including greater functional capacity, good health, less sickness, lower health care expenses and time under medical supervision, and a longer and more productive life. Without question, these benefits altogether translate into one great benefit: an optimum quality of life. That is, the combined benefit is the freedom to live life to its fullest without functional and health limitations. Most people go through life merely wishing that they could live without such limitations. But the power is within each of us to do so. And it is accomplished only by taking action today and living a wellness way of life for the rest of our lives.

MyProfile: Lifetime Fitness and Wellness

To the best of your ability, answer the following questions. If you do not know the answer(s), this final chapter will guide you through them.

I. Have you considered how long you would like to live and what type of health and well-being you desire to enjoy throughout life? ___ Yes ___ No Explain lifestyle habits you have implemented that contribute to this end. ______

II. Do you understand the difference between chronological and physiological age? ___ Yes ___ No What is your current physiological age? ___ years List changes that you can still work on to add years to your life and life to your years. ______

III. Have you ever sought complementary or alternative medical treatment? ___ Yes ___ No If you have done so and feel comfortable talking about it, what was it for and what results did you obtain? ______

IV. Have you ever been the victim of quackery and fraud? ___ Yes ___ No If so, how were you entrapped? Can you discuss precautions that a person can take to prevent such occurrences? ______

V. Have you planned and written out short-term and long-range SMART goals to attain now that you are about to finish this course? ___ Yes ___ No What arrangements have you made to maintain your exercise program and healthy lifestyle habits? What can you do to stay up-to-date on fitness and wellness concepts and future developments in the field? Elaborate on your answer. ______

Better health, higher quality of life, and longevity are the three most important benefits derived from a lifetime fitness and wellness program. You have learned that physical fitness in itself does not always lower the risk for chronic diseases and ensure better health. Thus, implementation of healthy behaviors is the only way to attain your highest potential for well-being. The real challenge comes now that you are about to finish this course: maintaining your lifetime commitment to fitness and wellness. Adhering to a program in a structured setting is a lot easier, but from now on, you will be on your own.

In this chapter, you have an opportunity to evaluate how well you are adhering to health-promoting behaviors and how these behaviors affect your **physiological age** and length of life. You will also learn how to chart a personal wellness program for the future.

Research data indicate that healthy (and unhealthy) lifestyle actions you take today have an impact on health and quality of life in middle and advanced age. Whereas most young people don't seem to worry much about health and longevity, you may want to take a closer look at the quality of life of your parents or other middle-aged and older friends and relatives that you know. Though you may have a difficult time envisioning yourself at that age, their health status and **functional capacity** may help you determine how you would like to live when you reach your fourth, fifth, and subsequent decades of life.

Although previous research has documented declines in physiological function and motor capacity as a result of aging, no hard evidence at present proves that large declines in physical work capacity are related primarily to aging alone.

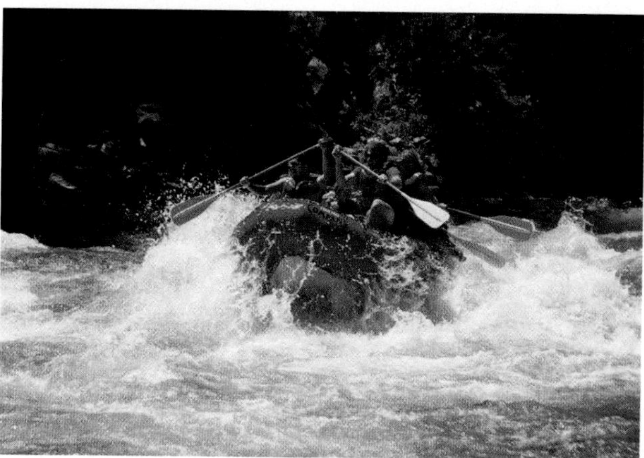

Good physical fitness provides freedom to enjoy many of life's recreational and leisure activities without limitations.

Lack of physical activity—a common phenomenon in today's society as people age—is accompanied by decreases in physical work capacity that are greater by far than the effects of aging.

Physiological age The biological and functional capacity of the body as it should be in relation to the person's maximal potential at any given age in the lifespan.

Functional capacity The ability to perform ordinary and unusual demands of daily living without limitations and excessive fatigue or injury.

FIGURE 15.1 Relationships among physical work capacity, aging, and lifestyle habits.

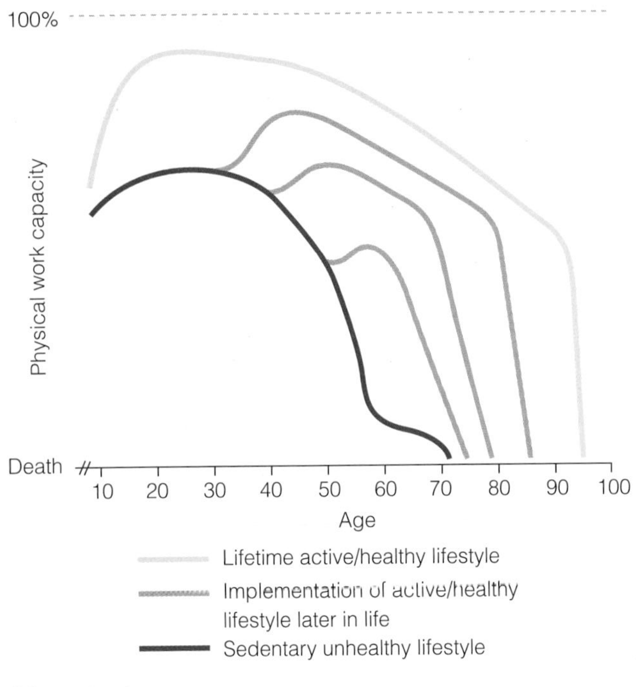

Unhealthy behaviors precipitate premature aging. For sedentary people, any type of physical activity is seriously impaired by age 40 and productive life ends before age 60. Most of these people hope to live to be age 65 or 70 and often must cope with serious physical ailments. These people "stop living at age 60 but are buried at age 70" (see the theoretical model in Figure 15.1).

Scientists believe that a healthy lifestyle allows people to live a vibrant life—a physically, intellectually, emotionally, socially active, and functionally independent existence—to age 95. Such are the rewards of a wellness way of life. When death comes to active people, it usually is rather quick and not as a result of prolonged illness. In Figure 15.1, note the low, longer slope of the "sedentary/unhealthy lifestyle" before death.

Life Expectancy and Physiological Age

Aging is a natural process, but some people seem to age better than others. Most likely, you know someone who looks younger than his or her **chronological age** indicates, and vice versa—that is, someone who appears older than his or her chronological age indicates. For example, you may have an instructor who you would have guessed was about 40 but in reality is 52 years old. On the other hand, you may have a relative who looks 60 but is actually 50 years old. Why the differences?

During the aging process, natural biological changes occur within the body. Although no single measurement can predict how long you will live, the rate at which aging changes take place depends on a combination of genetic and lifestyle factors. Your lifestyle habits determine to a great extent how your genes affect your aging process. Hundreds of research studies point to critical lifestyle behaviors that determine your statistical chances of dying at a younger age or living a longer life. Research also shows that lifestyle behaviors have a far greater impact on health and longevity than genes alone.

> **CRITICAL THINKING**
>
> Have you examined the quality of life that older people around you have, and have you considered what life will be like for you at that age?

Throughout this book, you have studied many of these factors. The question that you now need to ask yourself is, are your lifestyle habits accelerating or decelerating the rate at which your body is aging? To help you determine how long and how well you may live the rest of your life, the **life expectancy** and physiological age prediction questionnaire provided in Lab 15A can help answer this question. By looking at 48 critical genetic and lifestyle factors, you will be able to estimate your life expectancy and your real physiological age. Of greater importance, most of these factors are under your control, and you can do something to make them work for you instead of against you.

As you fill out the questionnaire, you must be honest with yourself. Your life expectancy and physiological age prediction are based on your present lifestyle habits, should you continue those habits for life. Using the questionnaire, you will review factors you can modify or implement in daily living that may add years and health to your life. The questionnaire is not a precise scientific instrument but rather an estimated life expectancy analysis according to the impact of lifestyle factors on health and longevity. Also, the questionnaire is not intended as a substitute for advice and tests conducted by medical and health care practitioners.

Conventional Western Medicine

Conventional Western medicine, also known as allopathic medicine, has seen major advances in care and treatment modalities during the past few decades. Conventional medicine is based on scientifically proven methods, wherein medical treatments are tested through rigorous scientific trials. In addition to a **primary care physician** (medical doctor), people seek advice from other practitioners of conventional medicine, including **osteopaths**, **dentists**, **oral surgeons**, **orthodontists**, **ophthalmologists**, **optometrists**, **physician assistants**, and **nurses**.

Finding a physician

Invariably there are times when you will need medical attention. Finding the right physician can be a challenging task because there are few resources available to do so. Preventive health care professionals caution that you should shop for a doctor the same way you do research to shop for other items and get the best quality care for your investment. Having a primary care physician is important to establish a relationship with your doctor while you are in good health and subsequently get the best possible care you deserve when truly needed. Attempting to get an appointment on short notice is often difficult for new patients, and the choices can be limited.

Most people select a physician by a referral from family and friends, but your search requires more than that. You ought to be comfortable with your doctor, and a few questions and skepticism on your part may help. If you trust your doctor, you can be completely open about your health care concerns. If a follow-up consultation is needed, your physician can help direct you to the appropriate specialist to coordinate your care.

First determine your medical needs, and then start your search by taking a look at the list of doctors in your health care plan and cross-checking the list with the top doctors in the area where you live. Location and hospital affiliations are important to consider as well. Having to travel a long distance discourages patients from seeking medical care when recommended or needed. Next, inquire about education, qualifications, skills, residency, and experience so that they meet your expectations. Additionally, because your association with your physician may become a lifetime relationship, you want to make sure that your personalities agree.

Other considerations include gender and age. Many women prefer female physicians for certain conditions, whereas men are more open to either gender. Older physicians are typically more experienced, while younger ones may be more in tune with recent advances and new medical procedures and technologies. You need to decide for yourself about your comfort zone and potential treatment options for your condition.

Finally, performing an Internet search provides valuable information about the physician's practice, friendliness, and availability to patients. Some sites provide information regarding board certification and possible disciplinary actions. Once you have narrowed your search, an introductory phone conversation is fully within your right. Most physicians are open to such a conversation. A physician's choice not to do so gives you information about the doctor's personality, time constraints, or openness with patients.

Searching for a Hospital Another point to consider is the choice of hospital if a medical procedure is needed. An alarming statistic in the United States is that almost 100,000 hospital patients die each year from medical errors.[1] This figure represents more than double the number of people killed in automobile accidents each year. The data shows that about 5 percent of all hospital patients develop an infection while hospitalized. Selecting the appropriate facility is just as important as finding a good physician. Research has shown that patients get better medical care in some hospitals, experience fewer medical complications, and receive better attention for their needs. To decide on a hospital, follow these simple steps:

1. Does the hospital routinely handle your medical procedure? Check the hospital's record of treating patients with your condition in a safe and effective way. As with the physician of your choice, the more experienced the staff is with your procedure, the better the outcome for you.
2. Is the hospital accredited by The Joint Commission? The Joint Commission is an independent foundation that administers accreditation programs for hospitals and other health care organizations.
3. Does your doctor have privileges at the hospital (is he permitted to admit patients)?
4. Is the hospital covered by your health care plan?
5. What is the hospital readmission or bounce back rate? The bounce back rate is a medical term used to look at how many patients require rehospitalization within 30 days of the procedure. The higher the rate, the higher the risk for post-medical care complications. At present, one in five admissions results in readmission within 30 days. You can

Chronological age Calendar age.

Life expectancy How many years a person is expected to live.

Conventional Western medicine A traditional medical practice based on methods that are tested through rigorous scientific trials; also called allopathic medicine.

Primary care physician A medical practitioner who provides routine treatment of ailments; typically, the patient's first contact for health care.

Osteopath A medical practitioner with specialized training in musculoskeletal problems who uses diagnostic and therapeutic methods of conventional medicine, in addition to manipulative measures.

Dentists Practitioners who specialize in diseases of the teeth, gums, and oral cavity.

Oral surgeons Dentists who specialize in surgical procedures of the oral–facial complex.

Orthodontists Dentists who specialize in the correction and prevention of tooth irregularities.

Ophthalmologists Medical specialists concerned with diseases of the eye and prescription of corrective lenses.

Optometrists Health care practitioners who specialize in the prescription and adaptation of lenses.

Physician assistants Health care practitioners trained to treat most standard cases of care.

Nurses Health care practitioners who assist in the diagnosis and treatment of health problems and provide many services to patients in a variety of settings.

find out about the hospital bounce back rating at www.HospitalCompare.HHS.gov.

6. How well does the hospital check and improve its own safety record? Hospitals with effective staff communication, good team work, and regular patient care discussions have lower rates of infection than hospitals with a poor culture of safety. Although such data isn't readily available to the consumer, you can ask the hospital staff if they would trust their health care to their place of employment. Don't just accept a "yes" response, but evaluate the behavior, character, and choice of words in their response.
7. Have you discussed with former patients, family members, and friends their experience at the hospital? They can provide information on the treatment, response, friendliness, care, and helpfulness of the personnel, as well as privacy, comfort, and condition of the hospital.
8. Do you have a choice of procedures? If you do, always select a minimally invasive procedure. Discuss with your doctor all available options. If needed, opt for a second opinion. About one-third of second opinions differ from the initial diagnosis. Minimally invasive procedures have a lower risk of infection and involve shorter hospital stays and less pain.
9. What is the surgeon's experience? Death rates for any given surgical procedure are greatly reduced by the surgeon's experience with the procedure. Therein lies the importance of selecting a physician with ample experience in treating your condition.
10. Is the facility a teaching hospital with medical interns and residents? If so, inquire as to who will provide and oversee your care. If possible, avoid teaching hospitals during the month of July, when new interns and residents arrive and your medical care may not be as safe and efficient as the rest of the year.
11. Is the hospital a for-profit or not-for-profit hospital? For-profit hospitals may discharge you early or skip out on proper treatment because you are either uninsured or your health care plan only allows a certain amount of time in the hospital. If such is an issue, some consumer groups feel that you should think twice before going to a for-profit hospital.
12. Have you obtained a copy of your medical records? Request a copy of the physician's notes taken during your visit or procedure. Reviewing the notes can help clarify a diagnosis and the prescribed follow-up treatment. It will also allow you to correct any errors in information you provided your doctor. Under federal law, you have the right to obtain your records.

Complementary and Alternative Medicine

Notwithstanding modern technological and scientific advancements, many medical treatments either do not improve the patient's condition or cause other ailments. Only about 20 percent of conventional treatments have proved to be clinically effective in scientific trials.[2] Thus, approximately 38 percent of adults (Figure 15.2) and 12 percent of children in the United States are turning to **complementary and alternative medicine**, or **CAM** (also called "unconventional," "nonallopathic," or "integrative" medicine) in search of answers to their health problems.[3] Unconventional medicine is referred to as complementary or alternative because patients use it to either augment their regular medical care or to replace conventional practices, respectively.

The reasons for seeking complementary and alternative treatments are diverse. Among the reasons commonly given by patients who seek unconventional treatments are lack of progress in curing illnesses and disease, frustration and dissatisfaction with physicians, lack of personal attention, testimonials about the effectiveness of alternative treatments, and rising health care costs. People who use CAM tend to be more educated and believe that body, mind, and spirit all contribute to good health.

The National Center for Complementary and Alternative Medicine (NCCAM) was established under the National Institutes of Health (NIH) to examine methods of healing previously unexplored by science. CAM includes treatments and health care practices not widely taught in medical schools, not generally used in hospitals, and not usually reimbursed by medical insurance companies. Many physicians now endorse complementary and alternative treatments, and an ever-increasing number of medical schools are offering courses in this area.

The NCCAM classifies CAM therapies into three categories:[4]

- **Natural products.** This includes the use of a variety of herbal medicines (also known as botanicals), vitamins, and minerals. Many are sold over-the-counter as dietary supplements. (Some uses of dietary supplements—for

FIGURE 15.2 Complementary and alternative medicine use in the United States, by age, 2007.

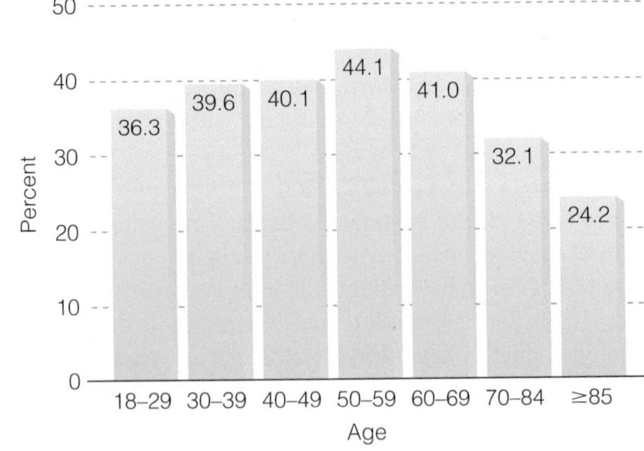

Source: P. M. Barnes, B. Bloom, and R. Nahin, CDC National Health Statistics Report #12. Complementary and Alternative Medicine Use Among Adults and Children: United States, 2007. December 2008.

example, taking a multivitamin to meet minimum daily nutritional requirements or taking calcium to promote bone health—are not considered CAM.) CAM natural products include probiotics—live microorganisms (usually bacteria) that are similar to microorganisms normally found in the human digestive tract.

Interest in and use of CAM natural products have grown considerably in recent decades. Approximately 17.7 percent of American adults use a nonvitamin or nonmineral natural product. The most commonly used product was fish oil or omega-3, reported by 37.4 percent of all adults who said they use natural products.

- **Mind–body medicine.** This practice focuses on the interactions among the brain, mind, body, and behavior, with the intent to use the mind to affect physical functioning and promote health. Many CAM practices embody this concept in different ways. The most common are meditation, yoga, and acupuncture. Other examples of mind–body practices include deep-breathing exercises, guided imagery, progressive muscle relaxation, qigong, and tai chi.

  Several mind–body approaches ranked among the top 10 CAM practices reported by adults. Data indicate that 12.7 percent of adults use deep-breathing exercises, 9.4 percent practice meditation, and 6.1 percent practice yoga. Progressive relaxation and guided imagery are also among the top 10 CAM therapies for adults.

- **Manipulative and body-based practices.** This practice focuses primarily on the structures and systems of the body, including the bones and joints, soft tissues, and circulatory and lymphatic systems. Among the therapies within this category are spinal manipulation and massage therapy.

  Spinal manipulation is performed by chiropractors and by other health care professionals, such as physical therapists, osteopaths, and some conventional medical doctors. Practitioners use their hands or a device to apply a controlled force to a joint of the spine, moving it beyond its passive range of motion. The amount of force applied depends on the form of manipulation used. Spinal manipulation is among the treatment options used by people with low back pain—a common condition that can be difficult to treat. Massage therapy encompasses many techniques. In general, therapists manipulate the muscles and other soft tissues of the body. People use massage for a variety of health-related purposes, including to relieve pain, rehabilitate sports injuries, reduce stress, increase relaxation, address anxiety and depression, and aid general well-being. About 8.6 percent of adults use chiropractic or osteopathic manipulation and 8.3 percent of adults use massage therapy.

Alternative medical practices have not gone through the same standard scrutiny as conventional medicine. Nonallopathic treatments are often based on theories that have not been scientifically proven. This does not imply that unconventional medicine practices do not help people. Many people have found relief from ailments or been cured through unconventional treatments. In time, however, these theories will need to be investigated using scientific trials similar to those common in conventional medicine.

CAM includes a range of healing philosophies, approaches, and therapies. The practices most often associated with nonallopathic medicine are **acupuncture**, **chiropractics**, **herbal medicine**, **homeopathy**, **naturopathic medicine**, **ayurveda**, **magnetic therapy**, and **massage therapy**. Each of these practices offers a different approach to treatments based on its beliefs about the body, some of which are hundreds or thousands of years old.

Many practitioners of these treatments believe that their modality aids the body as it performs its natural healing process. Because of their approach, alternative treatments usually take longer than conventional allopathic medical care. Nonallopathic treatments are usually less harsh on the patient, and practitioners tend to avoid surgery and extensive use of medications.

Unconventional therapies are frequently viewed as holistic, implying that the practitioner looks at all dimensions of wellness when evaluating a person's condition. Practitioners often persuade patients to adopt healthier lifestyle habits that not only help improve current conditions but also prevent other ailments. CAM also allows patients to better

Complementary and alternative medicine (CAM) A group of diverse medical and health care systems, practices, and products that are not presently considered part of conventional medicine; also called unconventional, nonallopathic, or integrative medicine.

Acupuncture A Chinese medical system that requires body piercing with fine needles during therapy to relieve pain and treat ailments and diseases.

Chiropractics A health care system that proposes many diseases and ailments are related to misalignments of the vertebrae and emphasizes manipulation of the spinal column.

Herbal medicine An unconventional system that uses herbs to treat ailments and disease.

Homeopathy A system of treatment based on the use of minute quantities of remedies that in large amounts produce effects similar to the disease being treated.

Naturopathic medicine An unconventional system of medicine that relies exclusively on natural remedies to treat disease and ailments.

Ayurveda A Hindu system of medicine based on herbs, diet, massage, meditation, and yoga to help the body boost its natural healing process.

Magnetic therapy Unconventional treatment that relies on magnetic energy to promote healing.

Massage therapy The rubbing or kneading of body parts to treat ailments.

understand treatments, and patients are often allowed to administer self-treatment.

Costs for CAM practices are typically lower than conventional medicine costs. With the exception of acupuncture and chiropractic care, most nonallopathic treatments are not covered by health insurance. Typically, patients pay directly for these services. Estimates indicate that almost $34 billion is spent out-of-pocket a year on complementary and alternative medical treatments.[5] These costs account for about 11.2 percent of total out-of-pocket health care expenses in the United States. If you are considering alternative medical therapies, consult with your health care insurance provider to determine which therapies are reimbursable.

CAM does have shortcomings, including the following:

1. Many practitioners do not have the years of education given to conventional medical personnel and often know less about physiological responses that occur in the body.
2. Some practices are devoid of science; hence, the practitioner can rarely explain the specific physiological benefits of the treatment used. Much of the knowledge is based on experiences with previous patients.
3. The practice of CAM is not regulated like that of conventional medicine. The training and certification of practitioners, malpractice liability, and evaluation of tests and methods used in treatments are not routinely standardized. Many states, however, license practitioners in the areas of chiropractic services, acupuncture, naturopathy, homeopathy, herbal therapy, and massage therapy. Other therapies are usually unmonitored.
4. Unconventional medicine lacks regulation of natural and herbal products. The word "natural" does not imply that the product is safe. Many products, including some herbs, can be toxic in large doses.
5. About one-third of all adults in the United States combine multivitamins, antacids, and other herbal and dietary supplements with their prescriptions.[6] Combinations such as these can yield undesirable side effects. Therefore, individuals should always let their health care practitioners know which medications and alternative (including vitamin and mineral) supplements are being taken in combination.

Herbal medicine has been around for centuries. Through trial and error, by design, or by accident, people have found that certain plant substances have medicinal properties. Today, products that are safer and more effective and have fewer negative side effects have replaced many of these plant products. Although science has found the mechanisms whereby some herbs work, much research remains to be done.

Many herbs or herbal remedies are not safe for human use and continue to meet resistance from the scientific community. One of the main concerns is that active ingredients in drug therapy must be administered in accurate dosages. With herbal medicine, the potency cannot always be adequately controlled.

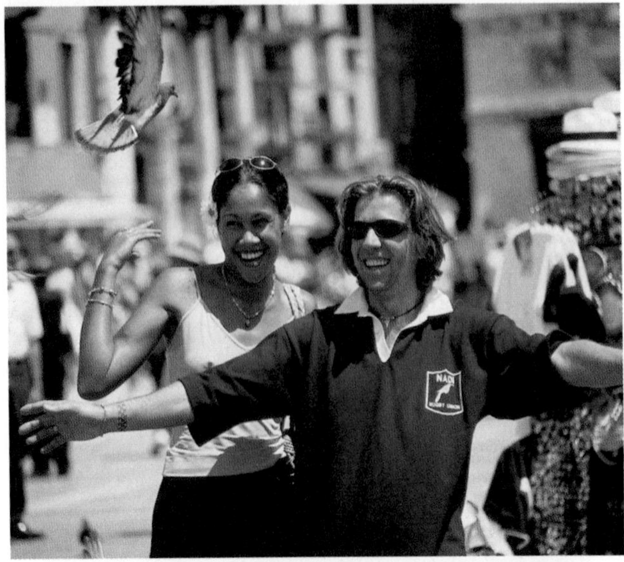

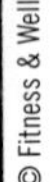

© Fitness & Wellness, Inc.

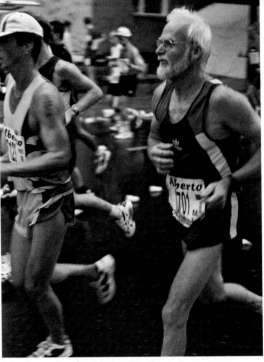

© Fitness & Wellness, Inc.

A healthy lifestyle enhances functional capability, quality of life, and longevity.

Also, some herbs produce undesirable side effects. For example, ephedra (ma huang), a popular weight loss and energy supplement, can cause high blood pressure, rapid heart rate, tremor, seizures, headaches, insomnia, stroke, and even death. About 1,400 reports of adverse effects linked to

DIVERSITY CONSIDERATIONS: CAM USE BY GENDER, RACE, AND ETHNICITY

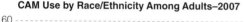

People of all backgrounds use CAM. In general, CAM utilization among adults is greater among women, those with higher levels of education, and people with higher incomes. The figure below shows overall CAM use by race or ethnicity. Lack of insurance coverage and access to conventional medical care and physicians also play significant roles in the use of CAM among racial and ethnic groups. CAM is often used for chronic pain control, but unlike the general trend in CAM use by race or ethnicity, data show no difference among the various groups in CAM use when seeking relief for chronic pain.

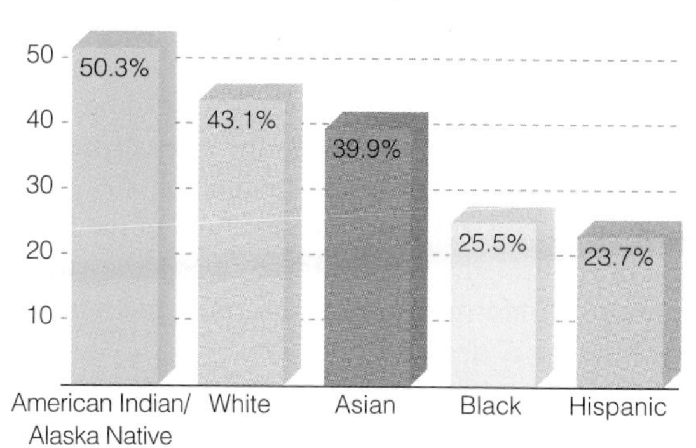

Source: P. M. Barnes, B. Bloom, and R. Nahin, CDC National Health Statistics Report #12. Complementary and Alternative Medicine Use Among Adults and Children: United States, 2007. December 2008.

herbal products containing ephedra, including 81 ephedra-related deaths, prompted its removal from the marketplace. Saint-John's-wort, commonly taken as an antidepressant, can produce serious interactions with drugs used to treat heart disease. Ginkgo biloba impairs blood clotting; thus, it can cause bleeding in people already on regular blood-thinning medication or aspirin therapy. Other herbs, like yohimbe, kava, chaparral, comfrey, and jin bu huan, have been linked to adverse events.

Conventional health care providers are becoming more willing to refer patients to someone who is familiar with alternative treatments, but you need to be an informed consumer. Ask your primary care physician to obtain valid information regarding the safety and effectiveness of a particular treatment.

Nonetheless, the medical community at times resists and rejects unconventional therapies. If your physician is unable or unwilling to provide you with valid information about a treatment, medical, college, or public libraries and popular bookstores are good places to search for this information. You need to educate yourself about the advantages and disadvantages of alternative treatments, risks, side effects, expected results, and length of therapy.

Information on a range of medical conditions or specific diseases can also be obtained by calling the NIH at 1-301-496-4000. Ask the operator to direct you to the appropriate NIH office. The NCCAM office also provides a website (http://www.nccam.nih.gov) with access to federal databases hosting hundreds of thousands of bibliographic records of research published on CAM during the past four decades.

When you select a primary care physician or a nonallopathic practitioner, consult local and state medical boards, other health regulatory boards and agencies, and consumer affairs departments for information about a given practitioner's education, accreditation, and license and about complaints that may have been filed against this health care provider. Many unconventional medical fields also have a national organization that provides guidelines for practitioners and health consumers. These organizations can guide you to the appropriate regulatory agencies within your state where you can obtain information regarding a specific practitioner.

You may also talk to individuals who have undergone similar therapies and learn about the competence of the practitioner in question. Keep in mind, however, that patient testimonials do not adequately assess the safety and effectiveness of alternative treatments. Whenever possible, search for results of controlled scientific trials of the therapy in question and use this information in your decision process.

When undergoing any type of treatment or therapy, always disclose this information with all of your health care providers, whether conventional or unconventional. Adequate health care management requires that health care providers be informed of all concurrent therapies, so that they have a complete picture of the treatment plan. Lack of knowledge by one health care provider regarding treatments by another provider can interfere with the healing process or even worsen a given condition.

Millions of Americans have benefited from CAM practices. You may also benefit from such services, but you need to make careful and educated decisions about the available options. By finding well-trained (and preferably licensed) practitioners, you increase your chances for recovery from ailments and disease.

Integrative Medicine

Integrative medicine involves a combination of the practices and methods of conventional Western medicine and of CAM. Physicians and other health care professionals may use an integrative approach to help patients

Integrative medicine The combination of the practices and methods of alternative medicine with conventional Western medicine.

manage symptoms or improve the effectiveness of a conventional treatment. For example, many cancer treatment centers have instituted integrative programs that offer acupuncture, massage, meditation, and other forms of counseling or therapies to ease pain and side effects from conventional treatments like chemotherapy.

Integrative medicine is a preventative and proactive approach to health and wellness that encompasses all aspects of the individual's lifestyle, taking into account the whole person, not just the disease or illness. It is based on a partnership between the patient and the doctor, where the ultimate goal is to treat the body, mind, and spirit. It can further involve principles of preventive medicine and therapies not accepted as typical medical practice, including prayer, meditation, social support, and recreation.

Many patients are turning to integrative medicine because of dissatisfaction with their health care providers, reporting scheduling frustrations, unclear communication, lack of involvement in treatment decisions, or limited time with physicians to adequately discuss health concerns. As a result, integrative medicine has become a growing trend among physicians and health care systems within the United States, with integrative medicine departments being instituted at several universities, hospitals, and various treatment centers. The concept is not without its critics, as the practice is driven by market forces that tout benefits that may or may not be backed by reliable scientific data, making it hard for patients to make informed decisions about using integrative care options.

Quackery and Fraud

The growth of the fitness and wellness industry during the past few decades has spurred the promotion of fraudulent products that deceive consumers into miraculous, quick, and easy ways to achieve total well-being. **Quackery and fraud** have been defined as the conscious promotion of unproven claims for profit.

Today's market is saturated with "special" foods, diets, supplements, pills, cures, equipment, books, and videos that promise quick, dramatic results. Advertisements for these products often are based on testimonials, unproven claims, secret research, half-truths, and quick-fix statements that the uneducated consumer wants to hear. In the meantime, the organization or enterprise making the claims stands to reap a large profit from consumers' willingness to pay for astonishing and spectacular solutions to problems related to their unhealthy lifestyles.

Television, magazine, online, and newspaper advertisements are not necessarily reliable. For instance, one piece of equipment sold through television and newspaper advertisements promised to "bust the gut" through five minutes of daily exercise that appeared to target the abdominal muscle group. This piece of equipment consisted of a metal spring attached to the feet on one end and held in the hands on the other end. According to handling and shipping distributors, the equipment was "selling like hotcakes," and companies could barely keep up with consumer demands.

Three problems became apparent to the educated consumer: First, there is no such thing as spot reducing; therefore, the claims could not be true. Second, five minutes of daily exercise burn hardly any calories and therefore have no effect on weight loss. Third, the intended abdominal (gut) muscles were not really involved during the exercise. The exercise engaged mostly the gluteal and lower back muscles. This piece of equipment could then be found at garage sales for about a tenth of its original cost.

Although people in the United States tend to be firm believers in the benefits of physical activity and positive lifestyle habits as a means to promote better health, most do not reap these benefits because they simply do not know how to put into practice a sound fitness and wellness program that gives them the results they want. Unfortunately, many uneducated wellness consumers are targets of deception by organizations making fraudulent claims for their products.

Deception is not limited to advertisements. Deceit is all around us: in newspaper and magazine articles, the Internet, trade books, radio, and television shows. To make a profit, popular magazines occasionally exaggerate health claims or leave out pertinent information to avoid offending advertisers. Some publishers print books on diets or self-treatment approaches that have no scientific foundation. Consumers should even be cautious about news reports of the latest medical breakthroughs. Reporters have been known to overlook important information or give certain findings greater credence than they deserve.

Precautions must also be taken when seeking health advice on the Internet. The Internet is full of both credible and dubious information. The following tips can help as you conduct a search on the Internet:

- Look for government, university, non-profit, or well-known medical school websites. Sites ending in ".gov" are produced and maintained by federal agencies and typically publish information based on the most reliable and up-to-date research. University and non-profit websites typically end in ".edu" or ".org" respectively. Be aware, however, that sites containing these endings in their web addresses may not always be reputable, as scammers often set up deceptive sites with addresses that look credible to target consumers.
- Look for credentials of the person or organization sponsoring the site.
- Check when the site was last updated. Credible sites are updated often.
- Check the appearance of the information on the site. It should be presented in a professional manner. If every sentence ends with an exclamation point, you have a good cause for suspicion.
- Exercise caution if the site's sponsor is trying to sell a product. If so, be leery of opinions posted on the site. They could be biased, given that the company's main objective is to sell a product. Credible companies trying to sell a product on the Internet usually reference their

BEHAVIOR MODIFICATION PLANNING

Healthy Lifestyle Guidelines

I PLAN TO | I DID IT

- ❑ ❑ Accumulate a minimum of 30 minutes of moderate-intensity physical activity at least five days per week.
- ❑ ❑ Exercise aerobically in the proper cardiorespiratory training zone at least three times per week for a minimum of 20 minutes.
- ❑ ❑ Accumulate at least 10,000 steps on a daily basis.
- ❑ ❑ Strength train at least once per week (preferably twice per week) using a minimum of eight exercises that involve all major muscle groups of the body.
- ❑ ❑ Perform flexibility exercises that involve all major joints of the body at least two to three times per week.
- ❑ ❑ Avoid excessive sitting throughout the day: Take intermittent 10-minute breaks for every hour that you are sitting (at the computer, studying, playing table games, or watching television).
- ❑ ❑ Eat a healthy diet that is rich in whole-wheat grains, fruits, and vegetables; includes cold water fish two to three times per week; and is low in saturated and trans fats.
- ❑ ❑ Eat a healthy breakfast every day.
- ❑ ❑ Do not use tobacco in any form, avoid secondhand smoke, and avoid all other forms of substance abuse.
- ❑ ❑ Maintain healthy body weight (achieve a range between the high-physical fitness and health-fitness standards for percent body fat).
- ❑ ❑ Get 7 to 8 hours of sleep per night.
- ❑ ❑ Practice safe sex every time you have sex and don't have sexual contact with anyone who doesn't practice safe sex.
- ❑ ❑ Get 10 to 20 minutes of safe sun exposure on most days of the week.
- ❑ ❑ Manage stress effectively.
- ❑ ❑ Limit daily alcohol intake to two or less drinks per day if you are a man or one drink or less per day if you are a woman (or do not consume any alcohol at all).
- ❑ ❑ Have at least one close friend or relative in whom you can confide and to whom you can express your feelings openly.
- ❑ ❑ Be aware of your surroundings and take personal safety measures at all times.
- ❑ ❑ Seek continued learning on a regular basis.
- ❑ ❑ Subscribe to a reputable health/fitness/nutrition newsletter to stay up-to-date on healthy lifestyle guidelines.
- ❑ ❑ Seek proper medical evaluations as necessary.

Try It

Now that you are about to complete this course, evaluate how many of the healthy lifestyle guidelines have become part of your personal wellness program. Prepare a list of those that you still need to work on and use Lab 15C to write SMART goals and specific objectives that will help you achieve the desired behaviors. Remember that each one of the guidelines will lead to a longer, healthier, and happier life.

sources of health information and provide additional links that support their product.

- Compare a site's content to other credible sources. The content should be similar to that of other reputable sites or publications.
- Note the address and contact information for the company. A reliable company lists more than a post office box, an 800 number, and the company's e-mail address. When only the latter information is provided, consumers may never be able to locate the company for questions, concerns, or refunds.
- Be on the alert for companies that claim to be innovators while criticizing competitors or the government for being close minded or trying to keep them from doing business.
- Watch for advertisers that use valid medical terminology in an irrelevant context or use vague pseudomedical jargon to sell their product.

Not all people who promote fraudulent products, however, know they are doing so. Some may be convinced that the product is effective. If you have questions or concerns about a health product, you can search the Federal Trade Commission's website at www.consumer.ftc.gov under the topic "Health & Fitness" to get credible information on the latest market claims concerning healthy living, treatment and cures, weight loss,

Quackery and fraud The conscious promotion of unproven claims for profit.

and fitness. As the nation's consumer protection agency, you can also file a complaint with the FTC about scams and/or dubious health claims at www.ftc.gov/complaint or call 1-877-382-4357.

Other consumer protection organizations also offer to follow up on complaints about quackery and fraud. The existence of these organizations, however, should not give the consumer a false sense of security. The overwhelming number of complaints made each year makes it impossible for these organizations to follow up on each case individually. The U.S. Food and Drug Administration's (FDA's) Center for Drug Evaluation Research, for example, has developed a priority system to determine which health fraud product it should regulate first. Products are rated on how great a risk they pose to the consumer. With this in mind, you can use the following list of organizations to make an educated decision before you spend your money. You can also report consumer fraud to these organizations:

- Food and Drug Administration. The FDA regulates safety and labeling of health products and cosmetics. You can search for the office closest to you in the federal government listings (blue pages) of the phone book or on the Internet at www.fda.gov.
- Better Business Bureau (BBB). The BBB can tell you whether other customers have lodged complaints about a product, a company, or a salesperson. You can find a listing for the local office in the business section of the phone book, or you can check the organization's website at www.bbb.com.
- Consumer Product Safety Commission. This independent federal regulatory agency targets products that threaten the safety of American families. Unsafe products can be researched and reported on their website at www.cpsc.gov.
- Your state Attorney General. Attorney Generals govern state consumer protection divisions to enforce local laws and investigate claims that protect consumers and businesses from deceptive acts and practices. Find a list of state Attorney Generals at www.naag.org.
- Your local Consumer Protection Office. Find your local consumer protection office to report frauds and scams or get help with a consumer complaint at www.consumeraction.gov.

Another way to get informed before you make your purchase is to seek the advice of a reputable professional. Ask someone who understands the product but does not stand to profit from the transaction. As examples, a physical educator or an exercise physiologist can advise you regarding exercise equipment; a registered dietitian can provide information on nutrition and weight control programs; a physician can offer advice on nutrition supplements. Also, be alert to those who bill themselves as "experts." Look for qualifications, degrees, professional experience, certifications, and reputation.

Keep in mind that if it sounds too good to be true, it probably is. Fraudulent promotions often rely on testimonials or scare tactics and promise that their products will cure a long list of unrelated ailments; they use words like "quick fix," "time-tested," "newfound," "miraculous," "special," "secret," "all natural," "mail-order only," and "money-back guarantee." Deceptive companies move often so that customers have no way of contacting the company to ask for reimbursement.

When claims are made, ask where the claims are published. Refereed, or peer-reviewed, scientific journals are the most reliable sources of information. When a researcher submits information for publication in a refereed journal, at least two qualified and reputable professionals in the field conduct blind reviews of the manuscript. A blind review means the author does not know who will review the manuscript and the reviewers do not know who submitted the manuscript. Acceptance for publication is based on this input and relevant changes.

Reliable Health Websites

- American Cancer Society www.cancer.org
- American College of Sports Medicine www.acsm.org
- American Heart Association www.heart.org
- Centers for Disease Control and Prevention www.cdc.gov
- Clinical Trials Listing Service www.centerwatch.com
- Food and Drug Administration www.fda.gov
- Healthfinder—Your Guide to Reliable Health Information www.healthfinder.gov
- Medical Matrix (requires subscription) www.medmatrix.org
- MedlinePlus—Trusted Health Information for You www.medlineplus.gov
- National Cancer Institute www.cancer.gov
- National Center for Complementary and Alternative Medicine www.nccam.nih.gov
- National Institutes of Health www.nih.gov
- National Library of Medicine www.nlm.nih.gov
- National Women's Health Information Center www.womenshealth.gov
- WebMD www.webmd.com
- World Health Organization www.who.int/en/

Looking at Your Fitness Future

Once you've decided to pursue a lifetime wellness program, you face several more decisions about exactly how to accomplish it. Following are a few issues you are likely to encounter.

Health and Fitness Club Memberships

You may want to consider joining a health or fitness facility. Or, if you have mastered the contents of this book and your choice of fitness activity is one you can pursue on your own (walking, jogging, cycling, etc.), you may not need to join a health club. Barring injuries, you may continue your exercise program outside the walls of a health club for the rest of your life. You also can conduct strength-training and stretching programs in your home (see Chapters 7 and 8). Nonetheless, exercising in a health or fitness center provides not only social support but also professional guidance and multiple exercise choices, all three of which are strong motivators for exercise maintenance and adherence.

To stay up-to-date on fitness and wellness developments, you should buy a reputable and updated fitness and wellness book every four to five years. You may subscribe to a credible health, fitness, nutrition, or wellness newsletter to stay current. You can also surf the web, but be sure that the sites you are searching are run by credible and reliable organizations.

If you are contemplating membership in a fitness facility, do all of the following:

- Make sure that the facility complies with the standards established by the American College of Sports Medicine (ACSM) for health and fitness facilities. These standards are given in Figure 15.3.
- Examine all exercise options in your community: health clubs and spas, YMCAs, gyms, colleges, schools, community centers, senior centers, and the like.
- Check to see whether the facility's atmosphere is pleasant and nonthreatening to you. Will you feel comfortable with the instructors and other people who go there? Is it clean and well kept? If the answers are no, this may not be the right place for you.

FIGURE 15.3 ACSM standards for health and fitness facilities.

1. A facility must have an appropriate emergency plan.
2. A facility must offer each adult member a preactivity screening that is relevant to the activities that will be performed by the member.
3. Each person who has supervisory responsibility must be professionally competent.
4. A facility must post appropriate signs in those areas of a facility that present potential increased risk.
5. A facility that offers services or programs to the youth must provide appropriate supervision.
6. A facility must conform to all relevant laws, regulations, and published standards.

Adapted from ACSM's Health/Fitness Facility Standards and Guidelines (Champaign, IL: Human Kinetics, 2012).

- Analyze costs across facilities, equipment, and programs. Take a look at your personal budget. Will you really use the facility? Will you exercise there regularly? Many people obtain memberships and permit dues to be withdrawn automatically from a credit card or local bank account, yet seldom attend the fitness center.
- Find out what types of spaces and features are available: walking and running track; basketball, tennis, or racquetball courts; aerobic exercise room; strength-training room; pool, locker rooms; saunas; hot tubs; handicapped access; and so on.
- Check the aerobic, strength-training, and stretching equipment available. Does the facility have treadmills, bicycle ergometers, elliptical trainers, a swimming pool, free weights, and strength-training machines? Make sure that the features and equipment meet your activity interests.
- Consider the location. Is the facility close, or do you have to travel several miles to get there? Distance often discourages participation.
- Check on times the facility is accessible. Is it open during your preferred exercise time (e.g., early morning or late evening)?
- Work out at the facility several times before becoming a member. Does it have ample space amid all the equipment and people in the facility? Are people standing in line to use equipment, or is it readily available during your exercise time?
- Evaluate the facility for cleanliness and hygiene. Is the equipment and facility regularly cleaned and disinfected? Sweat and body fluids are great environments for bacterial growth. The facility should also provide hand sanitizers, paper towels, facial tissue, and clean towels for members.
- Inquire about the instructors' knowledge and qualifications. Do the fitness instructors have college degrees or professional training certifications from organizations such as the ACSM, the American Council on Exercise (ACE), the National Strength and Conditioning Association (NSCA), or the National Academy of Sports Medicine (NASM)? These organizations have rigorous standards to ensure professional preparation and quality of instruction.
- Consider the approach to fitness (including all health-related components of fitness). Is it well rounded? Do the instructors spend time with members, or do members have to seek them out constantly for help and instruction?
- Ask about supplementary services. Does the facility provide or contract out for regular health and fitness assessments (cardiovascular endurance, body composition, blood pressure, blood chemistry analysis, etc.)? Are wellness seminars (e.g., nutrition, weight control, and stress management) offered? Do these have hidden costs?

Reliable Sources of Health, Fitness, Nutrition, and Wellness Information

Newsletter	Approx. Yearly Issues	Annual Cost
Consumer Reports on Health www.ConsumerReports.org/health 800-234-2188	12	$24
Environmental Nutrition www.environmentalnutrition.com 800-829-5384	12	$20
Tufts University Health & Nutrition Letter www.tuftshealthletter.com 800-274-7581	12	$24
University of California Berkeley Wellness Letter www.berkeleywellness.com 386-447-6328	12	$24

Personal Trainers

The current way of life has opened an entire job market for personal trainers, who are presently in high demand by health and fitness participants. A **personal trainer** is a health or fitness professional who evaluates, motivates, educates, and trains clients to help them meet individualized healthy lifestyle goals. Rates typically range between $20 and $50 an hour, or more for trainers that are highly specialized or in high demand. Some trainers offer reduced rates for extended packages or prepaid sessions. For most people, using the expertise of a personal trainer is an investment in fitness, health, and quality of life.

Exercise sessions are usually conducted at a health or fitness facility or at the client's home. Experience and the ability to design safe and effective programs based on the client's current fitness level, health status, and fitness goals are important. Personal trainers also recognize their limitations and refer clients to other health care professionals as necessary.

Popular reality shows featuring trainers using "tough love" and "no pain-no gain" approaches to exercise for weight loss have led to an increase in high-intensity programs such as CrossFit, boot camp, Insanity, and others. Though this type of training has its benefits, be aware that extreme, military-type conditioning programs can result in injury or adverse health problems for those unconditioned for high-intensity training. The ACSM recommends that personal trainers have prospective clients undergo pre-exercise screening to identify any cardiac or injury risk factors before enrolling in a new exercise program. When choosing a potential trainer that may use a challenging approach, be sure to discuss any health restrictions with your trainer to ensure you receive instruction that is both safe and well-tailored to your personal fitness level.

Currently, anyone who prescribes exercise can make the claim to be a personal trainer without proof of education, experience, or certification. Although good trainers need to strive to maximize their health and fitness, a good physique and previous athletic experience do not certify a person as a personal trainer.

Because of the high demand for personal trainers, more than 200 organizations now certify fitness specialists. This has led to great confusion by clients on how to evaluate the credentials of personal trainers. Certification and a certificate are different. Certification implies that the individual has met educational and professional standards of performance and competence. A certificate typically is awarded to an individual who attended a conference or workshop but is not required to meet any professional standards.

Presently, no licensing body is in place to oversee personal trainers, making the process of becoming a personal trainer relatively easy. Some states have proposed bills that would require potential trainers to apply for a state-issued license before offering services to the public, though no legislation has yet been signed into law. At a minimum, personal trainers should have an undergraduate degree and certification from a reputable organization such as the ACSM, ACE, NSCA, or NASM. Undergraduate (and graduate) degrees should be conferred in a fitness-related area such as exercise science, exercise physiology, kinesiology, sports medicine, or physical education. When looking for a personal trainer, always inquire about the trainer's education and certification credentials.

Before selecting a trainer, you must establish your program goals. Following are sample questions to ask yourself and consider when interviewing potential trainers prior to selecting one:

- Can the potential personal trainer provide you with a resume?
- What type of professional education and certification does the potential trainer possess?
- How long has the person been a personal trainer, and are references available upon request?
- Are you looking for a male or female trainer?
- What are the fees? Are multiple sessions cheaper than a single session? Can individuals be trained in groups? Are there cancellation fees if you are not able to attend a given session?
- How long will you need the services of the personal trainer: one session, multiple sessions, periodically, or indefinitely?
- What goals do you intend to achieve with the guidance of the personal trainer: weight loss, cardiorespiratory fitness,

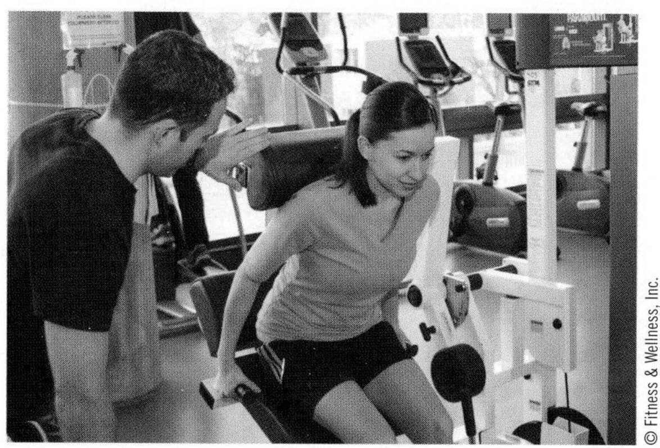

A personal trainer provides valuable guidance and helps motivate individuals to achieve fitness goals.

strength fitness, flexibility fitness, improved health, sport fitness conditioning, or a combination of these?

- What type of personality are you looking for in the trainer—a motivator, a hard-challenging trainer, a gentle trainer, or professional counsel only?

When seeking fitness advice from a health or fitness trainer online, here's a final word of caution: Be aware that certain services cannot be provided over the Internet. An Internet trainer is not able to directly administer fitness tests, motivate, observe exercise limitations, or respond effectively in an emergency situation (spotting or administering first aid or cardiopulmonary resuscitation [CPR]) and thus is not able to design the safest and most effective exercise program for you.

Purchasing Exercise Equipment

A final consideration is that of purchasing your own exercise equipment. The first question you need to ask yourself is, do I really need this piece of equipment? Most people buy on impulse because of television advertisements or because a salesperson has convinced them it is a great piece of equipment that will do wonders for their health and fitness. Ignore claims that an exercise device or machine can provide "easy" or "no sweat" results in a few minutes only. Keep in mind that the benefits of exercise are obtained only if you do exercise. With some creativity, you can implement an excellent and comprehensive exercise program with little, if any, equipment (see Chapters 6–9).

Many people buy expensive equipment only to find they do not enjoy that mode of activity. They do not remain regular users. Stationary bicycles (lower body only) and rowing ergometers were among the most popular pieces of equipment a few years ago. Most of them now are seldom used and have become "fitness furniture" somewhere in the garage or basement. Furthermore, be skeptical of testimonials and before-and-after pictures from "satisfied" customers. These results may not be typical, and it doesn't mean that you will like the equipment.

Exercise equipment has its value for people who prefer to exercise indoors, especially during winter months. It supports some people's motivation and adherence to exercise. The convenience of having equipment at home also allows for flexible scheduling. You can exercise before or after work or while you watch your favorite television show.

If you are going to purchase equipment, the best recommendation is to try it out several times before buying it. Ask yourself several questions: Did I enjoy the workout? Is the unit comfortable? Am I too short, tall, or heavy for it? Is it stable, sturdy, and strong? Do I have to assemble the machine? If so, how difficult is it to put together? How durable is it? Ask for references—people or clubs that have used the equipment extensively. Are they satisfied? Have they enjoyed using the equipment? Talk with professionals at colleges, sports medicine clinics, or health clubs.

Another consideration is to look at used units for signs of wear and tear. Quality is important. Cheaper brands may not be durable, so your investment would be wasted.

Finally, watch out for expensive gadgets. Monitors that provide exercise heart rate, work output, caloric expenditure, speed, grade, and distance may help motivate you, but they are expensive, need repairs, and do not enhance the actual fitness benefits of the workout. Look at maintenance costs and check for service personnel in your community.

CRITICAL THINKING

Do you admire some people around you whom you would like to emulate in their wellness lifestyle? What behaviors do these people exhibit that would help you adopt a healthier lifestyle? What keeps you from emulating these behaviors, and how can you overcome these barriers?

Self-Evaluation and Behavioral Goals for the Future

The main objective of this book is to provide the information and experiences necessary to implement your personal fitness and wellness program. If you have implemented the programs in this book, including exercise, you should be convinced that a wellness lifestyle is the only way to attain a higher quality of life.

Most people who engage in a personal fitness and wellness program experience this new quality of life after only a few weeks of

Personal trainer A health or fitness professional who evaluates, motivates, educates, and trains clients to help them meet individualized, healthy, lifestyle goals.

training and practicing healthy lifestyle patterns. In some instances, however—especially for individuals who have led a poor lifestyle for a long time—a few months may be required to establish positive habits and feelings of well-being. In the end, though, everyone who applies the principles of fitness and wellness reaps the desired benefits.

Prior to the completion of this course, you need to identify community resources available to you that will support your path to lifetime fitness and wellness. Lab 15B provides a road map to initiate your search for this support. You will find the process beneficial, one that will help you maintain your new wellness way of life.

Self-Evaluation Throughout this course, you have had an opportunity to assess various fitness and wellness components and write goals to improve your quality of life. You now should take the time to evaluate how well you have achieved your goals. Ideally, if time allows and facilities and technicians are available, reassess the health-related components of physical fitness. If you are unable to reassess these components, determine subjectively how well you accomplished your goals. You will find a self-evaluation form in part I of Lab 15C.

Behavioral Goals for the Future If you have not yet achieved all of your goals during this course, or if you need to reach beyond your current achievements, a final assignment should be conducted to help you chart the future. To complete this assignment, fill out the wellness compass shown in part II of Lab 15C. This compass displays various wellness components, each illustrating a scale from 5 to 1. A 5 indicates a low or poor rating; a 1 indicates an excellent or wellness rating for that component. Using the wellness compass, rate yourself for each component according to the following instructions:

1. Color in red a number from 5 to 1 to indicate where you stood on each component at the beginning of the semester. For example, if at the start of this course you rated poor in cardiorespiratory endurance, color the number 5 in red for that component.
2. Color in blue a second number from 5 to 1 to indicate where you stand on each component at the present time. If your level of cardiorespiratory endurance improved to average by the end of the semester, color the number 3 in blue for that component. If you were not able to work on a given component, simply color in blue on top of the previous red.
3. Select one or two components you intend to work on in the next two months. Developing new behavioral patterns takes time, and trying to work on too many components at once most likely will lower your chances for success. Start with components in which you think you have a high chance for success.

   Next, color in yellow the intended goal (number) to accomplish by the end of the two months. If your goal is to achieve a good level of cardiorespiratory endurance, color the number 2 in yellow for that component. When you achieve this level, you may later color the number 1 for that component, also in yellow, to indicate your next goal.

After you have completed the previous exercise, write goals and objectives for the one or two components you intend to work on during the next two months (use the form in part III of Lab 15C). As you write and work on these goals, review the SMART goals section in Chapter 2, pages 64–65.

One final assignment that you should complete is to summarize your feelings about your past and present lifestyle, what you have learned in this course, and the changes that you were able to successfully implement. Use part IV of Lab 15C for this evaluation, and keep this summary where you can review it in months and years to come.

The Fitness and Wellness Experience and a Challenge for the Future

Patty Neavill is a typical example of someone who often tried to change her life but was unable to do so because she did not know how to implement a sound exercise and weight control program. At age 24 and at 240 pounds, she was discouraged with her weight, level of fitness, self-image, and quality of life in general. She had struggled with her weight most of her life. Like thousands of other people, she had made many unsuccessful attempts to lose weight.

Patty put her fears aside and decided to enroll in a fitness course. As part of the course requirement, a battery of fitness tests was administered at the beginning of the semester. Patty's cardiovascular endurance and muscular (strength) fitness ratings were poor, her flexibility classification was average, and her percent body fat was 41 percent.

Following the initial fitness assessment, Patty met with her course instructor, who prescribed an exercise and nutrition program like the one in this book. Patty fully committed to carry out the prescription. She walked or jogged five times a week. She enrolled in a weight-training course that met twice a week. Her daily caloric intake was set in the range of 1,500 to 1,700 calories.

Determined to increase her level of activity further, Patty signed up for recreational volleyball and basketball courses. Besides being fun, these classes provided four additional hours of activity per week.

She took care to meet the minimum required servings from the basic food groups each day, which contributed about 1,200 calories to her diet. The remainder of the calories came primarily from complex carbohydrates.

At the end of the 16-week semester, Patty's cardiovascular endurance, muscular fitness, and flexibility ratings had all improved to the good category, she had lost 50 pounds, and her percent body fat had decreased to 22.5 percent.

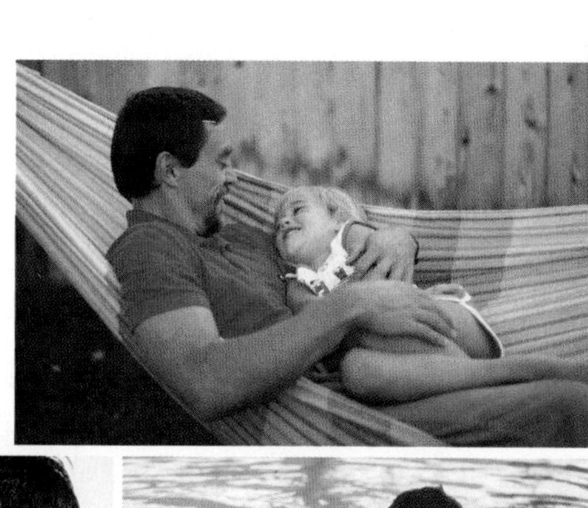
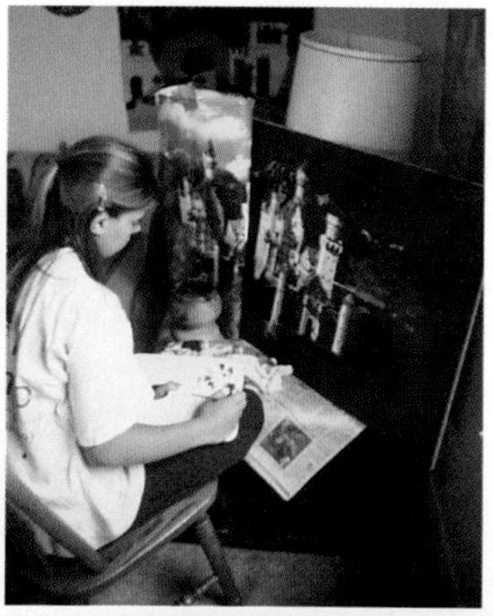
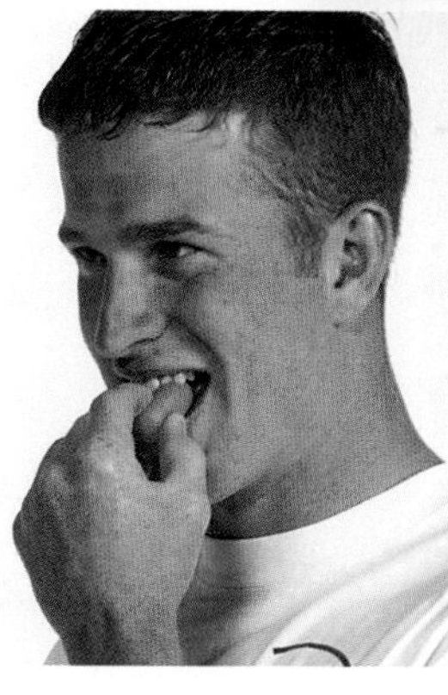
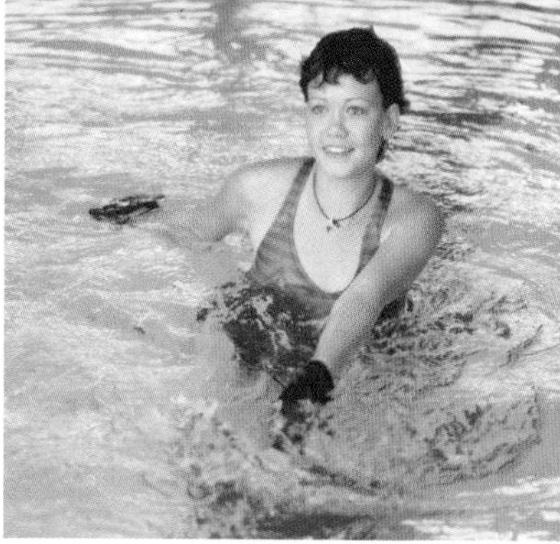
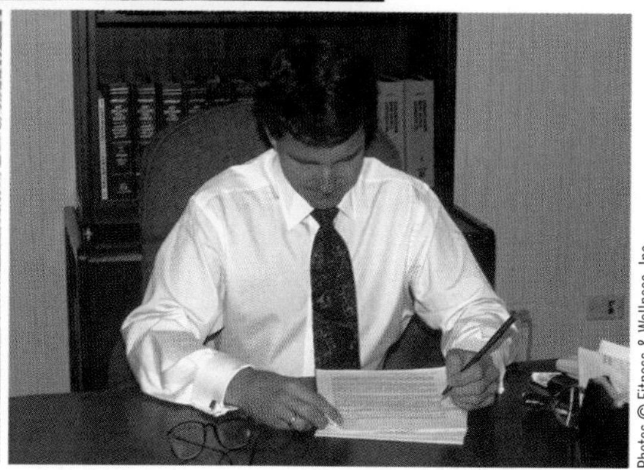

Fitness and healthy lifestyle habits lead to improved health, quality of life, and wellness.

Patty was tall. At 190 pounds, most people would have thought she was too heavy. Her percent body fat, however, was lower than the average for college female physical education major students (about 23 percent body fat).

A thank-you note from Patty to the course instructor at the end of the semester read:

> *Thank you for making me a new person. I truly appreciate the time you spent with me. Without your kindness and motivation, I would have never made it. It is great to be fit and trim. I've never had this feeling before, and I wish everyone could feel like this once in their life.*
> *Thank you,*
> *Your trim Patty!*

Patty had never been taught the principles governing a sound weight loss program. She not only needed this knowledge but, like most Americans who never have experienced the process of becoming physically fit, also needed to be in a structured exercise setting to truly feel the joy of fitness.

Even more significant was that Patty maintained her aerobic and strength-training programs. A year after ending her calorie-restricted diet, her weight increased by 10 pounds, but her body fat decreased from 22.5 to 21.2 percent. As you may recall from Chapter 5, this weight increase is related mostly to changes in lean tissue, that is lost during the weight-reduction phase.

In spite of only a slight drop in weight during the second year following the calorie-restricted diet, a two-year follow-up revealed a further decrease in body fat, to 19.5 percent. Patty understood the new quality of life reaped through a sound fitness program, and at the same time, she finally learned how to apply the principles that regulate weight maintenance.

If you have read and successfully completed all of the assignments set out in this book, including a regular exercise program, you should be convinced of the value of exercise and healthy lifestyle habits in achieving a new quality of life.

Perhaps this new quality of life was explained best by the late Dr. George Sheehan, when he wrote[7]:

> *For every runner who tours the world running marathons, there are thousands who run to hear the leaves and listen to the rain, and look to the day when it is all suddenly as easy as a bird in flight. For them, sport is not a test but a therapy, not a trial but a reward, not a question but an answer.*

The real challenge comes now: a lifetime commitment to fitness and wellness. To make the commitment easier, enjoy yourself and have fun along the way. If you implement your program based on your interests and what you enjoy doing most, then adhering to your new lifestyle will not be difficult.

Your activities over the past few weeks or months may have helped you develop "positive addictions" that will carry on throughout life. If you truly experience the feelings Dr. Sheehan expressed, there will be no looking back. If you don't get there, you won't know what it's like. Fitness and wellness is a process, and you need to put forth a constant and deliberate effort to achieve and maintain a higher quality of life. Improving the quality of your life, and most likely your longevity, is in your hands. Only you can take control of your lifestyle and thereby reap the benefits of wellness.

ASSESS YOUR BEHAVIOR

1. Has your level of physical activity increased compared with the beginning of the term?
2. Do you participate in a regular exercise program that includes cardiorespiratory endurance, muscular fitness, and muscular flexibility training?
3. Is your diet healthier now compared with a few weeks ago?
4. Are you able to take pride in the lifestyle changes that you have implemented over the past several weeks? Have you rewarded yourself for your accomplishments?

ASSESS YOUR KNOWLEDGE

1. From a functional point of view, typical sedentary people in the United States are about ___ years older than their chronological age indicates.
   a. 2
   b. 8
   c. 15
   d. 20
   e. 25
2. Which one of the following factors has the greatest impact on health and longevity?
   a. genetics
   b. the environment
   c. lifestyle behaviors
   d. chronic diseases
   e. gender
3. Your real physiological age is determined by
   a. your birthdate.
   b. lifestyle habits.
   c. amount of physical activity.
   d. your family's health history.
   e. your ability to obtain proper medical care.
4. CAM is
   a. also known as allopathic medicine.
   b. referred to as "Western" medicine.
   c. based on scientifically proven methods.
   d. a method of unconventional medicine.
   e. All of the choices are correct.
5. CAM health care practices and treatments are
   a. not widely taught in medical schools.
   b. endorsed by many physicians.
   c. not generally used in hospitals.
   d. not usually reimbursed by medical insurance companies.
   e. All of the choices are correct.
6. In CAM,
   a. practitioners believe that their treatment modality aids the body as it performs its natural healing process.
   b. treatments are usually shorter than with typical medical practices.
   c. practitioners rely extensively on the use of medications.
   d. patients are often discouraged from administering self-treatment.
   e. All of the choices are correct.
7. When the word "natural" is used with a product,
   a. it implies that the product is safe.
   b. it cannot be toxic, even when taken in large doses.
   c. it cannot yield undesirable side effects when combined with prescription drugs.
   d. there will be no negative side effects with its use.
   e. None of the choices are correct.
8. To protect yourself from consumer fraud when buying a new product,
   a. get as much information as you can from the salesperson.
   b. obtain details about the product from another salesperson.
   c. ask someone who understands the product but does not stand to profit from the transaction.
   d. obtain all research information from the manufacturer.
   e. All of the choices are correct.
9. Which of the following should you consider when looking to join a health or fitness center?
   a. location
   b. instructor's certifications
   c. type and amount of equipment available
   d. verification that the facility complies with ACSM standards
   e. All of the choices are correct.

10. When you purchase exercise equipment, the most important factor is
   a. to try it out several times before buying it.
   b. a recommendation from an exercise specialist.
   c. cost effectiveness.
   d. that it provides accurate exercise information.
   e. to find out how others like this piece of equipment.

Correct answers can be found at the back of the book.

NOTES

1. M. Makary, "Surprising Dangers in the Hospital," *Bottom Line Health* 27, no. 2 (2013): 5–6
2. R. J. Donatelle, *Access to Health* (San Francisco: Benjamin Cummings, 2008).
3. National Institutes of Health, National Center for Complementary and Alternative Medicine, *2007 Statistics on CAM Use in the United States*, available at http://nccam.nih.gov/news/camstats/2007/camsurvey_fs1.htm (downloaded May 7, 2014).
4. National Center for Complementary and Alternative Medicine, National Institutes of Health, *CAM Basics: What Is Complementary and Alternative Medicine?*, available at http://nccam.nih.gov/sites/nccam.nih.gov/files/D347_05-25-2012.pdf (downloaded May 7, 2014).
5. National Institutes of Health, National Center for Complementary and Alternative Medicine, *Statistics on CAM Costs*, available at http://nccam.nih.gov/news/camstats/costs (downloaded May 7, 2014).
6. E. K. Farina et al., "Concomitant Dietary Supplement and Prescription Medication Use Is Prevalent among US Adults with Doctor-Informed Medical Conditions," *Journal of the Academy of Nutrition and Dietetics*, no. 7 (April 2014).
7. *Dynamics of Fitness: The Body in Action*, Film (Pleasantville, NY: Human Relations Media, 1980).

SUGGESTED READINGS

American College of Sports Medicine. *ACSM's Health/Fitness Facility Standards and Guidelines*. Champaign, IL: Human Kinetics, 2012.

American College of Sports Medicine. *ACSM's Resources for Guidelines for Exercise Testing and Prescription*. Philadelphia: Wolters Kluwer/Lippincott Williams & Wilkins, 2014.

American College of Sports Medicine. *ACSM's Resources for the Personal Trainer*. Philadelphia: Lippincott Williams & Wilkins, 2014.

Roizen, M. F. *Real Age: Are You as Young as You Can Be?* New York: Cliff Street Books, 1999.

Lab 15A: Life Expectancy and Physiological Age Prediction Questionnaire

Name ______________________ **Date** ____________ **Grade** ____________

Instructor ______________________ **Course** ____________ **Section** ____________

NECESSARY LAB EQUIPMENT

None required.

OBJECTIVE

To estimate the total number of years that you will live and your real physiologic age based on your present lifestyle habits.

INSTRUCTIONS

Circle the points to the correct answer to each question. At the end of each page, obtain a net score for that page. Be completely honest with yourself. Your age prediction is based on your lifestyle habits, should you continue those habits for life. Using this questionnaire, you will learn about factors that you can modify or implement that can add years and health to your life. The scoring system is provided at the end of the questionnaire. Please note that the questionnaire is not a precise scientific instrument, but rather an estimated life expectancy analysis according to the impact of lifestyle factors on health and longevity. This questionnaire is not intended to substitute for advice and tests conducted by medical and healthcare practitioners.

Questionnaire

1. What is your current health status?
   - A. Excellent +2
   - B. Good +1
   - C. Average 0
   - D. Fair −1
   - E. Poor −2
   - F. Bad −3

2. How many days per week do you accumulate 30 minutes of moderate-intensity physical activity (at least 40 percent of heart rate reserve–see Chapter 6)?
   - A. More than 7 times per week +3
   - B. 3 to 5 +1
   - C. 1 or 2 0
   - D. Less than once per week −3

3. How often do you participate in a vigorous-intensity cardio-respiratory exercise (more than 60 percent of heart rate reserve) for at least 20 minutes?
   - A. 3 or more times per week +2
   - B. 2 times per week +1
   - C. Once per week −1
   - D. Less than once per week −2

4. How often do you perform strength-training exercises per week (a minimum of 8 exercises using 8 to 12 repetitions to near-fatigue on each exercise)?
   - A. 1–2 times +2
   - B. Less than once or less than 8 exercises with 8 to 12 reps per session 0
   - C. Do not strength train −1

5. How many times per week do you perform flexibility exercises (at least 15 minutes per stretching session)?
   - A. 3 or more +1
   - B. 1 to 3 times +.5
   - C. 1 time 0
   - D. Do not perform flexibility exercises −.5

6. How many servings of fruits and vegetables do you eat on a daily basis?
   - A. 9 or more +3
   - B. 6 to 8 +2
   - C. 5 +1
   - D. 3 or 4 0
   - E. 2 or less −2

7. How many grams of fiber do you consume on an average day?
   - A. 25 or more +1
   - B. Between 13 and 24 0
   - C. 10 to 12 or don't know −1
   - D. Less than 10 −2

8. As a percentage of total calories, what is your average fat intake daily?
   - A. 30% or less (mostly unsaturated) +1
   - B. 30% to 35% (mostly unsaturated) 0
   - C. More than 35% −2

9. As a percentage of total calories, what is your average saturated fat intake daily?
   - A. 5% or less +1
   - B. More than 5% but less than 7% 0
   - C. Don't know −1
   - D. More than 7% −2

10. How many servings of red meat (3 to 6 ounces) do you consume weekly?
    - A. 1 or none +1
    - B. 2 or 3 0
    - C. 4 to 7 −2
    - D. More than 7 −3

Page score: ______

11. How many servings of omega-3-rich fish (3 to 6 ounces) do you consume weekly?
   A. 2 or more +2
   B. 1 0
   C. None −1

12. As a percentage of total calories, what is your average daily trans fatty acid intake?
   A. No trans fat intake +1
   B. Less than 1% 0
   C. 1% to 2% −1
   D. More than 2% −2

13. How many alcoholic drinks (a 12-ounce bottle of beer, a 4-ounce glass of wine, or a 1.5-ounce shot of 80-proof liquor) do you consume per day?
   A. Men 2 or less, women 1 or none +1
   B. None 0
   C. Men 3–4, women 2–4 −1
   D. 5 or more −3

14. How many milligrams of vitamin C do you get from food daily?
   A. Between 250 and 500 +1
   B. More than 90 but less than 250 +.5
   C. Less than 90 −1

15. How many micrograms of selenium do you get daily (preferably from food)?
   A. Between 100 and 200 +1
   B. Between 50 and 99 +.5
   C. Less than 50 −1

16. How many milligrams of calcium and how many international units of vitamin D do you get from food and supplements on an average day?
   A. Calcium = 1,200, vitamin D = 1,000 or more +1
   B. Calcium = 1,200, vitamin D = less than 1,000 +.5
   C. Calcium = 800 to 1,200, vitamin D = less than 1,000 0
   D. Calcium = less than 800, vitamin D = less than 1,000 −1

17. How many times per week do you eat breakfast?
   A. 7 +1
   B. 5 or 6 +.5
   C. 3 or 4 0
   D. Less than 3 −.5

18. How many cigarettes do you smoke each day?
   A. Never smoked cigarettes or more than 15 years since giving up cigarettes +2
   B. None for 5 to 14 years +1
   C. None for 1 to 4 years 0
   D. None for 0 to 1 year −1
   E. Smoker, less than 1 pack per day −3
   F. Smoker, 1 pack per day −5
   G. Smoker, up to 2 packs per day −7
   H. Smoker, more than 2 packs per day −10

19. Do you use tobacco products other than cigarettes?
   A. Never have 0
   B. Less than once per week −1
   C. Once per week −2
   D. 2 to 6 times per week −3
   E. More than 6 times per week −5

20. How often are you exposed to secondhand smoke or other environmental pollutants?
   A. Less than 1 hour per month 0
   B. Between 1 and 5 hours per month −1
   C. Between 5 and 29 hours per month −2
   D. Daily −3

21. Do you use addictive drugs, other than tobacco or alcohol?
   A. None 0
   B. 1 −3
   C. 2 or more −5

22. What is the age of your parents (or how long did they live)?
   A. Both older than 76 +3
   B. Only one older than 76 +1
   C. Both are still alive and younger than 76 0
   D. Only one younger than 76 −1
   E. Neither one lived past 76 −3

23. What is your body composition classification (see Table 4.11 on page 156)?
   A. Excellent +2
   B. Good +1
   C. Average 0
   D. Overweight −1
   E. Obese −2

24. What is your blood pressure?
   A. 120/80 or less (both numbers) +2
   B. 120–140 or 80–90 (either number) −1
   C. Greater than 140/90 (either number) −3

25. What is your HDL cholesterol?
   A. Men greater than 45, women greater than 55 +2
   B. Men 35 to 44, women 45 to 54 0
   C. Don't know −1
   D. Men less than 35, women less than 45 −2

26. What is your LDL cholesterol?
   A. Less than 100 +2
   B. 100 to 130 0
   C. 130 to 159 −1
   D. 160 or higher +2
   E. Don't know −2

27. Do you floss and brush your teeth regularly?
   A. Every day +.5
   B. 3 to 6 days per week 0
   C. Less than 3 days per week −.5

28. Are you a diabetic?
   A. No 0
   B. Yes, well-controlled −1
   C. Yes, poorly or not controlled −3

Page score: ______

29. How often do you get 10 to 20 minutes of unprotected ("safe") sun exposure between 10:00 a.m. and 4:00 p.m.?
    A. Almost daily +3
    B. 4 to 5 times per week +1
    C. 3 times per week 0
    D. 1 to 2 times per week −1
    E. Less than once per week −3

30. How often do you tan?
    A. Not at all +1
    B. Less than 3 times per year −1
    C. More than 3 times per year −2

31. How often do you wear a seat belt?
    A. All the time +1
    B. Most of the time −.5
    C. Less than half the time −1

32. How fast do you drive?
    A. Always at or less than the speed limit 0
    B. Up to 5 mph above the speed limit −.5
    C. Between 5 and 10 mph above the speed limit −1
    D. More than 10 mph above the speed limit −2

33. Do you drink and drive?
    A. Never 0
    B. Yes (even if only once) −5

34. Do you suffer from addictive behavior (misuse or abuse of alcohol, prescription and/or hard drugs)?
    A. No 0
    B. Yes −10

35. In terms of your sexual activity:
    A. I am not sexually active or I am in a monogamous sexual relationship +1
    B. I have more than one sexual partner but I always practice safe sex −1
    C. I have multiple sexual partners and I do not practice safe sex techniques −3

36. What is your marital status?
    A. Happily married +1
    B. Single and happy 0
    C. Single and unhappy −.5
    D. Divorced −1
    E. Widowed with a belief in life hereafter −1
    F. Widowed −2
    G. Married and unhappy −2

37. On the average, how many hours of sleep do you get each night?
    A. 8 +2
    B. 7 to 8 0
    C. 6 to 7 −1
    D. Less than 6 −2

38. Your stress rating according to the Stress Events Scale (see Lab 10A, page 409) is:
    A. Excellent +1
    B. Good 0
    C. Average −.5
    D. Fair −1
    E. Poor −2

39. Your Type A behavior rating is:
    A. Low 0
    B. Medium −1
    C. High −2

40. When under stress (distress), how often do you practice stress management techniques?
    A. Always +1
    B. Most of the time +.5
    C. Not applicable (don't suffer from stress) 0
    D. Sometimes −1
    E. Never −2

41. Do you suffer from depression?
    A. Not at all 0
    B. Mild depression −1
    C. Severe depression −2

42. How often do you associate with people who have a positive attitude about life?
    A. Always +.5
    B. Most of the time 0
    C. About half of the time −.5
    D. Less than half the time −1

43. Do you have close family or personal relationships whom you can trust and rely on for help in times of need?
    A. Yes +1
    B. No −1

44. Do you feel loved and can you routinely give affection and love?
    A. Yes +1
    B. No −1

45. Do you have a good sense of humor?
    A. Yes +1
    B. No −1

46. How satisfied are you with your schoolwork?
    A. Satisfied +.5
    B. It's okay 0
    C. Not satisfied −.5

47. How do you rate your present job satisfaction?
    A. Love it +1
    B. Like it 0
    C. It's okay −.5
    D. Don't like it −1
    E. Hate it −2
    F. Not applicable 0

48. How do you rate yourself spiritually?
    A. Very spiritual +1
    B. Spiritual 0
    C. Somewhat spiritual −.5
    D. Not spiritual at all −1

Page score: ______

Net score for all questions: ______

Source: *Life Expectancy and Physiological Age Prediction Questionnaire.* (Fitness & Wellness, Inc., Boise, Idaho, 2010).

How to Score

To estimate the total number of years that you will live, (a) determine a net score by totaling the results from all 46 questions, (b) obtain an age change score by multiplying the net score by the age correction factor given next, and (c) add or subtract this number from your base life expectancy age (76 for men and 81 for women–the current life expectancies in the United States). For example, if you are a 20-year-old male and the net score from the answers to all questions was –16, your estimated life expectancy would be 71.2 years (age change score = –16 × .3 = – 4.8, life expectancy = 76 – 4.8 = 71.2).

You also can determine your real physiological age by subtracting a positive age-change score or adding a negative age-change score to your current chronological (calendar) age. For instance, in the previous example, the real physiological age would be 24.8 years (20 + 4.8). If the age change score had been +4.8, the real physiological age would have been 15.2 years (20 – 4.8). Thus, a healthy lifestyle will always make your physiological age younger than your chronological age. Your real physiological age will have much greater significance in middle and older age, when real-age reductions of 10 to 25 years occur in people who lead unhealthy lifestyles. Thus a 50-year-old person could easily have a real physiological age of 30.

Age Correction Factor (ACF)*

Age	ACF
≤30	.3
31–40	.4
41–50	.5
51–60	.6
61–70	.6
71–80	.5
81–90	.4
≥9	.3

*Adapted from M. F. Roizen, *RealAge* (New York: Cliff Street Books, 1999).

Age Change Score (ACS) = ______ (net score) × ______ (ACF) = ______

Life Expectancy

Men = 76 ± ______ (ACS) = ______ years

Women = 81 ± ______ (ACS) = ______ years

Real Physiological Age**

Men = ______ (your age) ± ______ (ACS) = ______ years

Women = ______ (your age) ± ______ (ACS) = ______ years

**Subtract a positive ACS from, or add a negative ACS to, your current age.

Behavior Modification

State your feelings about the experience of taking this questionnaire, analyze your results, and list lifestyle factors that you can work on that will positively affect your health and longevity.

Lab 15B: Fitness and Wellness Community Resources

Name ______________________ **Date** ____________ **Grade** ____________

Instructor ______________________ **Course** ____________ **Section** ____________

NECESSARY LAB EQUIPMENT
None required.

OBJECTIVE
To identify community resources available for you to continue your path toward lifetime fitness and wellness.

INSTRUCTION
Using a community directory, identify a minimum of three fitness, recreational, or wellness facilities that will allow you to maintain and further develop your personal fitness and wellness program. Initially, contact all three facilities by phone to obtain the pertinent information (see Item I). On completion of this task, make an appointment to personally visit at least one of the facilities during a time when you would work out, and evaluate the equipment, equipment availability, personnel, and programs that would be available to you. Keep in mind that one of the options available to you may be your own campus health/fitness/recreation center. College alumni, for a fee, often have the option to continue to use such a facility.

I. Initial Contact

	Facility I	Facility II	Facility III
Facility Name:	________	________	________
Address:	________	________	________
Distance from home:	________	________	________
Mode of transportation to the facility:	________	________	________
Travel time to the facility:	________	________	________
Monthly fee:	________	________	________
Hours of operation:	________	________	________
Cardio equipment:	________	________	________
	________	________	________
	________	________	________
Strength training:	________	________	________
	________	________	________
	________	________	________
Flexibility equipment:	________	________	________
	________	________	________
	________	________	________
Personal trainers, availability and costs:	________	________	________
Personal trainers' certifications:	________	________	________
Fitness tests, availability and costs:	________	________	________
Exercise classes:	________	________	________
	________	________	________
	________	________	________
Other services (nutrition,	________	________	________
stress management, smoking	________	________	________
cessation, cardiac profiles, etc.):	________	________	________
Free trial of facility available?	________	________	________

II. Facility Visit and Evaluation

1. Provide an overall impression of the facility:

____

____

2. Was the staff knowledgeable, accessible, and friendly?

____

____

3. Were you able to work out at the facility? ___ Yes ___ No
   If so, was the equipment available and suitable to your preferences?

____

____

   Did you feel comfortable with other individuals using the facility (please indicate why or why not)?

____

____

4. Provide an overall evaluation of the locker facilities and other amenities available to you.

____

____

5. Overall letter grade for the facility: A B C D E F

III. Ongoing Educational Program

1. Are there any other community resources available to you that would benefit your personal health, fitness, and wellness lifestyle program? Please list:

____

____

2. Contact at least one reliable health, fitness, nutrition, or wellness newsletter that you may subscribe to (see page 560) for a free copy and list the newsletter in the space provided. Also indicate if there are any other fitness/wellness materials that have provided valuable information to you.

____

____

3. List at least three reliable and helpful websites that you accessed this term and indicate why these sites were useful to you.

____

____

____

Lab 15C: Self-Evaluation and Future Behavioral Goals

Name ______ Date ______ Grade ______

Instructor ______ Course ______ Section ______

NECESSARY LAB EQUIPMENT

None required unless fitness tests are repeated.

OBJECTIVE

To conduct a self-evaluation of the goals achieved in this course and to write behavioral goals for the future.

INSTRUCTION

Review the section on SMART Goals in Chapter 2 (pages 64–65) prior to completing this lab. If time allows and technicians are available, repeat the assessments for the health-related components of fitness.

I. Fitness Evaluation

Conduct a self-evaluation of the fitness goals you accomplished in this course. Fill in the required information on the health-related fitness components below. If you were unable to repeat your fitness assessments, subjectively determine how well you reached your goals.

1. Did you accomplish your goal for:

Cardiorespiratory Endurance (see Lab 6A) ☐ Yes ☐ No

Pre-assessment VO_{2max}: ☐ mL/kg/min Fitness Category: ☐

Post-assessment VO_{2max}: ☐ mL/kg/min Fitness Category: ☐

Body Composition (see Labs 4A and 4B) ☐ Yes ☐ No

Pre-assessment Percent Body Fat: ☐ Body Composition Category: ☐

Post-assessment Percent Body Fat: ☐ Body Composition Category: ☐

Muscular Fitness (strength and endurance—see Lab 7A) ☐ Yes ☐ No

Pre-assessment Percentile Total Points: ☐ Fitness Category: ☐

Post-assessment Percentile Total Points: ☐ Fitness Category: ☐

Muscular Flexibility (see Lab 8A) ☐ Yes ☐ No

Pre-assessment Percentile Total Points: ☐ Fitness Category: ☐

Post-assessment Percentile Total Points: ☐ Fitness Category: ☐

Current Number of Daily Steps: ☐

Activity category (see Table 1.2, page 12): ☐

II. Wellness Evaluation

Using the Wellness Compass, rate yourself for each component and plan goals for the future according to the following instructions:

1. Color in red a number from 5 to 1 to indicate where you stood on each component at the beginning of the semester (5 = poor rating, 1 = excellent or ideal rating).
2. Color in blue a second number from 5 to 1 to indicate where you stand on each component at the present time.
3. Select one or two components that you intend to work on in the next two months. Start with components in which you think you will have a high chance for success. Color in yellow the intended goal (number) to accomplish by the end of the two months. Once you achieve your goal, you later may color another number, also in yellow, to indicate your next goal.

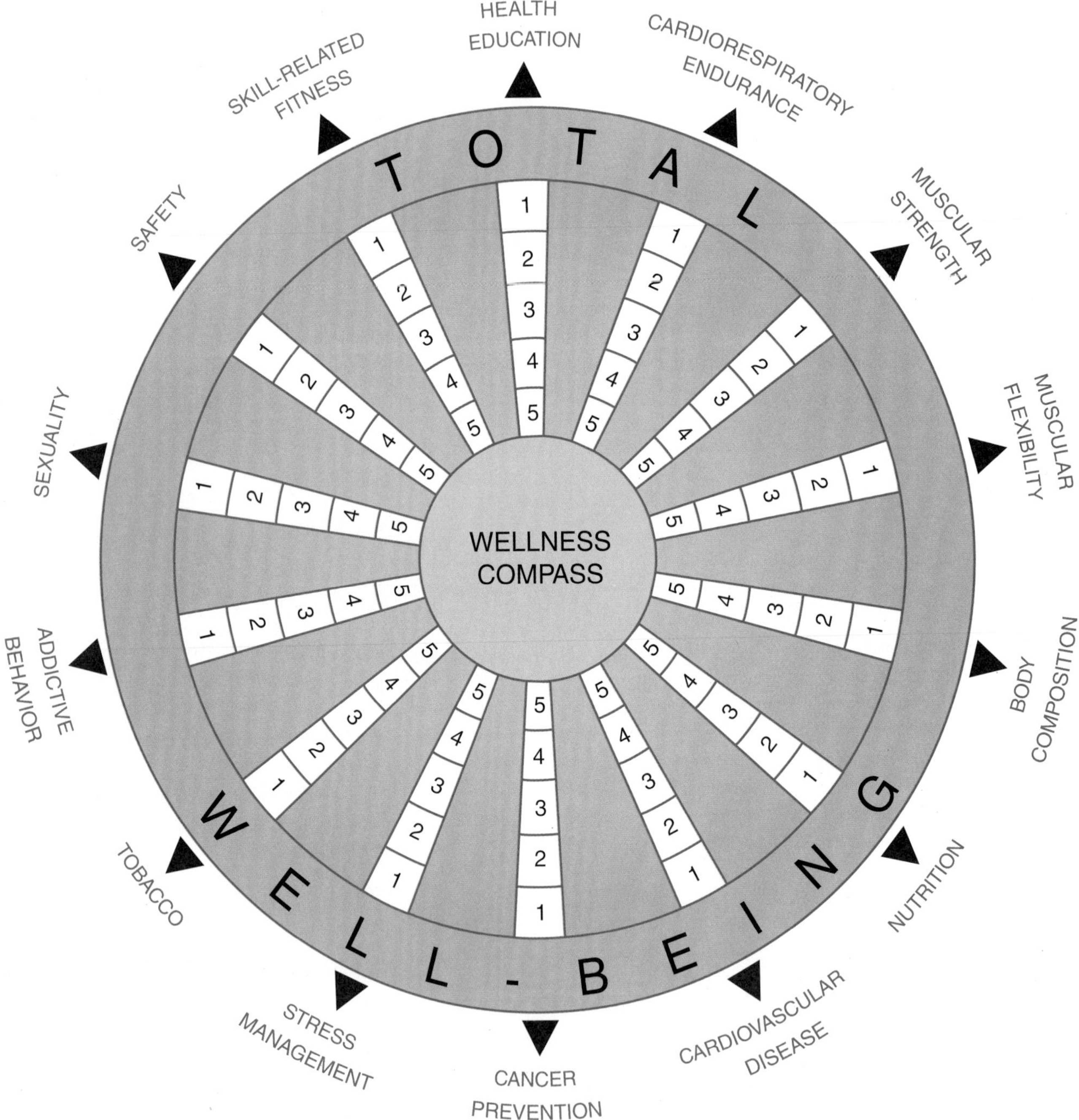

III. Behavioral Goals for the Future

Identify one or two SMART goals you will work on during the next couple of months and write specific objectives that you will use to accomplish each goal (you may not need six objectives; write only as many as needed).

Goal: ______________________________

Objectives:

1. ______________________________
2. ______________________________
3. ______________________________
4. ______________________________
5. ______________________________
6. ______________________________

Goal: ______________________________

Objectives:

1. ______________________________
2. ______________________________
3. ______________________________
4. ______________________________
5. ______________________________
6. ______________________________

IV. This Course and Your Future Lifestyle

1. Briefly evaluate this course and its impact on your quality of life. Indicate what you feel will be needed for you to continue to adhere to an active and healthy lifestyle.

____

____

____

____

____

____

____

____

____

2. Explain the exercise program that you implemented in this course, indicate your feelings about the outcomes of this program, and evaluate how well you accomplished your fitness goals.

3. List nutritional or dietary changes that you were able to implement this term and the effects of these changes on your body composition and personal wellness.

4. List other lifestyle changes that you were able to make this term that may decrease your risk for disease. In a few sentences, explain how you feel about these changes and their impact on your overall well-being.

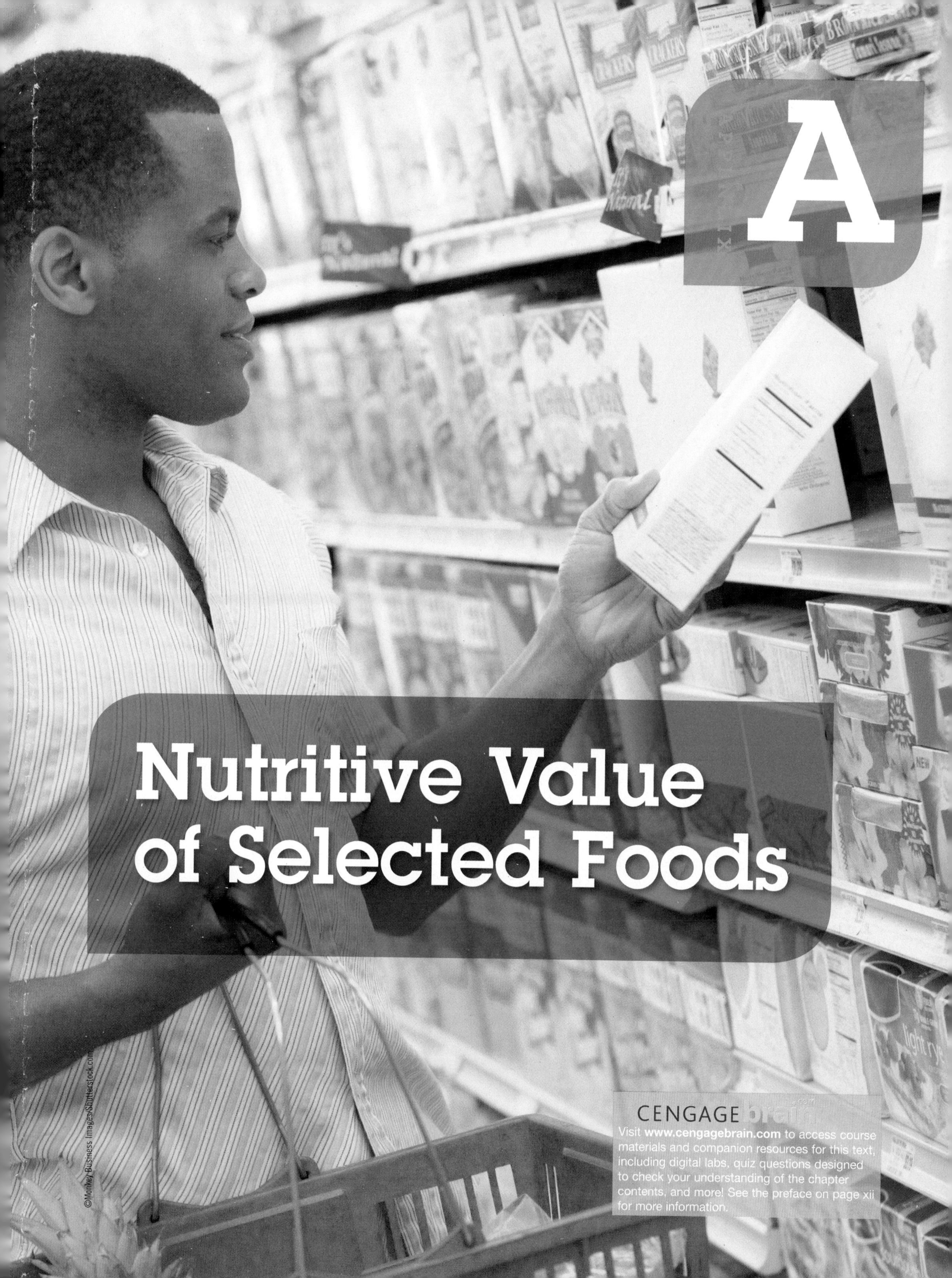

A

Nutritive Value of Selected Foods

CENGAGEbrain

Visit **www.cengagebrain.com** to access course materials and companion resources for this text, including digital labs, quiz questions designed to check your understanding of the chapter contents, and more! See the preface on page xii for more information.

Food Description	Qty	Measure	Wt (g)	Ener (cal)	Prot (g)	Carb (g)	Dietary Fiber (g)	Fat (g)	Fat Breakdown (g) Sat	Mono	Poly	Trans	Chol (mg)	Calc (mg)	Iron (mg)	Sodi (mg)	Vit E (mg)	Folate (mcg)	Vit C (mg)	Sele-nium (mcg)
Almonds, dry roasted, no salt added	¼	cup(s)	35	206	8	7	4	18	1.40	11.61	4.36	—	0	92	1.56	<1	8.97	11	0	1
Apple juice, unsweetened, canned	½	cup(s)	124	58	<1	14	<1	<1	0.02	0.01	0.04	—	0	9	0.46	4	0.01	0	1	<1
Apples, raw medium, w/peel	1	item(s)	138	72	<1	19	3	<1	0.04	0.01	0.07	—	0	8	0.17	1	—	4	6	0
Applesauce, sweetened, canned	½	cup(s)	128	97	<1	25	2	<1	0.04	0.01	0.07	—	0	5	0.45	4	0.27	1	2	<1
Apricot, fresh w/o pits	4	item(s)	140	67	2	16	3	1	0.04	0.24	0.11	—	0	18	0.55	1	1.25	13	14	<1
Apricot, halves w/skin, canned in heavy syrup	½	cup(s)	129	107	1	28	2	<1	0.01	0.04	0.02	—	0	12	0.39	5	0.77	3	4	<1
Asparagus, boiled, drained	½	cup(s)	90	20	2	4	2	0.19	0.06	0	0.12	—	0	20.7	0.81	12.6	1.35	134.1	6.92	5.48
Avocado, California, whole, w/o skin or pit	1	item(s)	170	284	3	15	12	26	3.59	16.61	3.42	—	0	22	1.00	14	3.35	105	15	1
Bacon, cured, broiled, pan fried, or roasted	2	slice(s)	13	68	5	<1	0	5	1.73	2.33	0.57	0	14	1	0.18	291	0.04	<1	0	8
Bagel chips, plain	3	item(s)	29	130	3	19	1	5	0.50	—	—	—	0	0	0.72	70	—	—	0	—
Bagel, plain, enriched, toasted	1	item(s)	66	195	7	38	2	1	0.16	0.09	0.49	0	0	53	2.52	379	0.08	64	0	23
Banana, fresh whole, w/o peel	1	item(s)	118	105	1	27	3	<1	0.13	0.04	0.09	—	0	6	0.31	1	0.12	24	10	1
Beans, black, boiled	½	cup(s)	86	114	8	20	7	<1	0.12	0.04	0.20	—	0	23	1.81	1	—	128	0	1
Beans, Fordhook lima, frozen, boiled, drained	½	cup(s)	85	88	5	16	5	<1	0.07	0.02	0.14	—	0	26	1.55	59	0.25	18	11	1
Beans, mung, sprouted, boiled, drained	½	cup(s)	62	13	1	3	<1	<1	0.02	0.00	0.02	—	0	7	0.40	6	0.04	18	7	<1
Beans, red kidney, canned	½	cup(s)	128	109	7	20	8	<1	0.06	0.03	0.24	—	0	31	1.61	436	0.77	65	1	2
Beans, refried, canned	½	cup(s)	127	119	7	20	7	2	0.60	0.71	0.19	—	10	44	2.10	378	0.00	14	8	2
Beans, yellow snap, string or wax, boiled, drained	½	cup(s)	62	22	1	5	2	<1	0.04	0.00	0.09	—	0	29	0.80	2	0.28	21	6	<1
Beef, chuck, arm pot roast, lean & fat, ¼" fat, braised	3	ounce(s)	85	282	23	0	0	20	7.97	8.68	0.77	—	84	9	2.64	51	0.19	8	0	21
Beef, corned, canned	3	ounce(s)	85	213	23	0	0	13	5.25	5.07	0.54	—	73	10	1.77	855	0.13	8	0	36
Beef, ground, lean, broiled, well	3	ounce(s)	85	238	24	0	0	15	5.89	6.56	0.56	—	86	10	2.08	76	—	9	0	22
Beef, ground, regular, broiled, medium	3	ounce(s)	85	246	20	0	0	18	6.91	7.70	0.65	—	77	9	2.07	71	—	8	0	16
Beef, liver, pan fried	3	ounce(s)	85	149	23	4	0	4	1.27	0.56	0.49	0.17	324	5	5.24	65	0.39	221	1	28
Beef, rib steak, small end, lean, ¼" fat, broiled	3	ounce(s)	85	188	24	0	0	10	3.84	4.01	0.27	—	68	11	2.18	59	0.12	7	0	19
Beef, rib, whole, lean & fat, ¼" fat, roasted	3	ounce(s)	85	320	19	0	0	27	10.71	11.42	0.94	—	72	9	1.96	54	—	6	0	19
Beef, short loin, T-bone steak, lean, ¼" fat, broiled	3	ounce(s)	85	174	23	0	0	9	3.05	4.23	0.26	—	50	5	3.11	65	0.12	7	0	9
Beer	12	fluid ounce(s)	356	118	1	6	<1	<1	0.00	0.00	0.00	0	0	18	0.07	14	0.00	21	0	2
Beer, light	12	fluid ounce(s)	354	99	1	5	0	0	0.00	0.00	0.00	0	0	18	0.14	11	0.00	14	0	2
Beets, sliced, canned, drained	½	cup(s)	85	26	1	6	1	<1	0.02	0.02	0.04	—	0	13	1.55	165	0.03	26	3	<1
Biscuits	1	item(s)	41	121	3	16	1	5	1.40	1.41	1.82	0	<1	33	1.01	205	0.01	26	0	7
Blueberries, raw	½	cup(s)	72	41	1	10	2	<1	0.02	0.03	0.11	—	0	4	0.20	1	0.41	4	7	<1
Bologna, beef	1	slice(s)	28	90	3	1	0	8	3.50	4.26	0.31	—	20	0	0.36	310	—	4	0	—
Bologna, turkey	1	slice(s)	28	50	3	1	0	4	1.00	1.09	0.98	—	20	40	0.36	270	—	—	0	—
Brazil nuts, unblanched, dried	¼	cup(s)	35	230	5	4	3	23	5.30	8.59	7.20	—	0	56	0.85	1	2.01	8	<1	671
Bread, cracked wheat	1	slice(s)	25	65	2	12	1	1	0.23	0.48	0.17	—	0	11	0.70	135	—	15	0	6
Bread, French	1	slice(s)	25	69	2	13	1	1	0.16	0.30	0.17	—	0	19	0.63	152	0.08	37	0	8
Bread, mixed grain	1	slice(s)	26	65	3	12	2	1	0.21	0.40	0.24	—	0	24	0.90	127	0.09	31	<1	8
Bread, pita	1	item(s)	60	165	5	33	1	1	0.10	0.06	0.32	—	0	52	1.57	322	0.18	64	0	16
Bread, pumpernickel	1	slice(s)	32	80	3	15	2	1	0.14	0.30	0.40	—	0	22	0.92	215	0.13	30	0	8
Bread, rye	1	slice(s)	32	83	3	15	2	1	0.20	0.42	0.26	—	0	23	0.91	211	0.11	35	<1	10
Bread, white	1	slice(s)	25	67	2	13	1	1	0.18	0.17	0.34	—	0	38	0.94	170	0.05	28	0	4
Bread, whole wheat	1	slice(s)	46	128	4	24	3	2	0.37	0.53	1.35	—	0	15	1.43	159	0.35	30	0	18
Broccoli, chopped, boiled, drained	½	cup(s)	78	27	2	6	3	<1	0.06	0.03	0.13	—	0	31	0.52	32	1.13	84	51	1
Brownie, prepared from mix	1	item(s)	24	112	1	12	1	7	1.76	2.60	2.26	—	18	14	0.44	82	—	7	<1	3
Brussels sprouts, boiled, drained	½	cup(s)	78	28	2	6	2	<1	0.08	0.03	0.20	—	0	28	0.94	16	0.34	47	48	1
Bulgur, cooked	½	cup(s)	91	76	3	17	4	<1	0.04	0.03	0.09	—	0	9	0.87	5	0.01	16	0	1
Buns, hamburger, plain	1	item(s)	43	120	4	21	1	2	0.47	0.48	0.85	—	0	59	1.43	206	0.03	48	0	8
Butter	1	tablespoon(s)	15	108	<1	<1	0	12	6.13	5.00	0.43	—	32	4	0.00	86	0.35	<1	0	<1
Buttermilk, low fat	1	cup(s)	245	98	8	12	0	2	1.34	0.62	0.08	—	10	284	0.12	257	0.12	12	2	5
Cabbage, boiled, drained, no salt added	1	cup(s)	150	33	2	7	3	1	0.08	0.05	0.29	—	0	47	0.26	12	0.18	30	30	1
Cabbage, raw, shredded	1	cup(s)	70	17	1	4	2	<1	0.01	0.01	0.04	—	0	33	0.41	13	0.10	30	23	1

Cake, angel food, from mix	1	slice(s)	50	129	3	29	<1	<1	0.02	0.01	0.06	—	0	42	0.12	255	0.00	10	0	8
Cake, butter pound, ready to eat, commercially prepared	1	slice(s)	75	291	4	37	<1	15	8.67	4.43	0.80	—	166	26	1.04	299	—	0	<1	—
Cake, carrot, cream cheese frosting, from mix	1	slice(s)	111	484	5	52	1	29	5.43	7.24	15.10	—	60	28	1.39	273	—	13	1	—
Cake, chocolate, chocolate icing, commercially prepared	1	slice(s)	64	235	3	35	2	10	3.05	5.61	1.18	—	27	28	1.41	214	—	11	<1	2
Cake, devil's food cupcake, chocolate frosting	1	item(s)	35	120	2	20	1	4	1.80	1.60	0.60	—	19	21	0.70	92	—	2	0	2
Cake, white, coconut frosting, from mix	1	slice(s)	112	399	5	71	1	12	4.36	4.14	2.42	—	1	101	1.30	318	0.13	35	<1	12
Candy, Almond Joy bar	1	item(s)	49	240	2	29	2	13	9.00	3.63	0.74	0	3	20	0.36	70	—	—	0	—
Candy, Life Savers	1	item(s)	2	8	0	2	0	<1	0.00	—	—	0	0	<1	0.04	1	—	—	0	0
Candy, M&M's peanut chocolate candy, small bag	1	item(s)	49	250	5	30	2	13	5.00	5.42	2.07	—	5	40	0.36	25	—	17	1	2
Candy, M&M's plain chocolate candy, small bag	1	item(s)	48	240	2	34	1	10	6.00	3.30	0.30	—	5	40	0.36	30	—	3	1	1
Candy, milk chocolate bar	1	item(s)	91	483	8	53	2	28	16.69	7.20	0.63	—	22	228	0.83	92	—	11	2	—
Candy, Milky Way bar	1	item(s)	58	270	2	41	1	10	5.00	3.50	0.35	—	5	60	0.18	95	—	6	1	3
Candy, Reese's peanut butter cups	2	piece(s)	45	250	5	25	1	14	5.00	6.17	2.34	0	3	20	0.36	140	—	25	0	2
Candy, Special Dark chocolate bar	1	item(s)	41	220	2	24	3	13	8.00	4.59	0.41	0	3	0	0.72	0	—	1	0	1
Candy, Starburst fruit chews, original fruits	1	package	59	240	0	48	0	5	1.00	2.10	1.83	—	0	10	0.18	0	—	0	30	<1
Candy, York peppermint patty	1	item(s)	42	170	1	34	1	3	2.00	1.32	0.12	0	0	0	0.36	10	—	2	0	—
Cantaloupe	½	cup(s)	80	27	1	7	1	<1	0.04	0.00	0.07	—	0	7	0.17	13	0.04	17	30	<1
Carrots, raw	½	cup(s)	61	25	1	6	2	<1	0.02	0.01	0.06	0	0	20	0.18	42	0.40	12	4	<1
Carrots, sliced, boiled, drained	½	cup(s)	78	27.29	0.59	6.41	2.33	0.14	0.02	0	0.08	—	0	23.39	0.26	45.24	0.80	10.92	2.8	0.54
Cashews, dry roasted	¼	cup(s)	34	197	5	11	1	16	3.14	9.36	2.68	—	0	15	2.06	5	0.32	24	0	4
Catsup/ketchup	1	tablespoon(s)	15	14	<1	4	<1	<1	0.01	0.01	0.04	—	0	3	0.08	167	0.22	2	2	<1
Cauliflower, boiled, drained	½	cup(s)	62	14	1	3	2	<1	0.04	0.02	0.13	—	0	10	0.20	9	0.04	27	27	<1
Celery, stalk	2	item(s)	80	11	1	2	1	<1	0.03	0.03	0.06	—	0	32	0.16	64	0.22	29	2	<1
Cereal, All-Bran	1	cup(s)	62	160	8	46	20	2	0.00	0.00	1.00	0	0	300	9.00	160	—	800	12	6
Cereal, All-Bran Buds	1	cup(s)	91	212	6	73	42	3	—	—	—	0	0	0	13.64	606	—	1212	18	26
Cereal, Bran Flakes, Post	1	cup(s)	40	133	4	32	7	1	0.00	0.00	0.71	—	0	0	10.77	293	—	133	0	—
Cereal, Cap'n Crunch	1	cup(s)	36	144	2	30	1	2	0.53	0.39	0.27	—	0	5	6.00	269	—	133	0	7
Cereal, Cheerios	1	cup(s)	30	110	3	22	3	2	0.00	0.50	0.50	—	0	100	8.10	280	—	200	6	11
Cereal, Complete wheat bran flakes	1	cup(s)	39	120	4	31	7	1	—	—	—	0	0	0	23.94	279	—	532	80	4
Cereal, Corn Flakes	1	cup(s)	28	100	2	24	1	0	0.00	0.00	0.00	0	0	0	8.10	200	—	100	6	1
Cereal, Corn Pops	1	cup(s)	31	120	1	28	0	0	0.00	0.00	0.00	0	0	0	1.80	120	—	100	6	2
Cereal, Cracklin' Oat Bran	1	cup(s)	65	266	5	47	7	9	2.70	4.70	1.33	0	0	27	2.38	186	—	218	20	14
Cereal, Cream of Wheat, instant, prepared	½	cup(s)	121	61	2	13	<1	<1	0.01	0.01	0.04	0	0	27	8.60	1	—	357	0	—
Cereal, Frosted Flakes	1	cup(s)	41	160	1	37	1	0	0.00	0.00	0.00	0	0	0	5.99	200	—	133	8	2
Cereal, Frosted Mini-Wheats	5	item(s)	51	180	5	41	5	1	0.00	0.00	0.50	0	0	0	15.30	5	—	100	0	2
Cereal, granola, prepared	½	cup(s)	61	299	9	32	5	15	2.76	4.7	6.53	—	0	48	2.59	13	3.59	51	1	16.95
Cereal, Kashi puffed	1	cup(s)	25	70	3	13	2	1	0.00	—	—	—	0	0	0.72	0	—	—	0	—
Cereal, Life	1	cup(s)	43	160	4	33	3	2	0.35	0.64	0.61	—	0	124	11.92	218	—	142	0	11
Cereal, Multi-Bran Chex	1	cup(s)	58	200	4	49	7	2	0.00	0.00	0.00	0	0	100	16.20	390	—	100	6	5
Cereal, Nutri-Grain golden wheat	1	cup(s)	40	133	4	31	5	1	0.00	0.00	0.67	—	0	0	1.46	279	—	133	20	9
Cereal, oatmeal, cooked w/water	½	cup(s)	117	74	3	13	2	1	0.19	0.37	0.44	—	0	9	0.80	1	0.12	5	0	9
Cereal, Product 19	1	cup(s)	30	100	2	25	1	0	0.00	0.00	0.00	0	0	0	18.00	210	—	400	60	4
Cereal, Raisin Bran	1	cup(s)	59	190	4	47	8	1	0.00	0.10	0.36	—	0	20	10.80	300	—	140	0	—
Cereal, Rice Chex	1	cup(s)	25	96	2	22	<1	0	0.00	0.00	0.00	0	0	80	7.20	232	—	160	5	1
Cereal, Rice Krispies	1	cup(s)	26	96	2	23	0	0	0.00	0.00	0.00	0	0	0	1.44	256	—	80	5	4
Cereal, Shredded Wheat	1	cup(s)	25	88	3	20	3	1	0.04	0.01	0.10	—	0	10	1.08	2	—	12	0	1
Cereal, Smacks	1	cup(s)	36	133	3	32	1	1	0.00	0.00	0.00	—	0	0	0.48	67	—	133	8	17
Cereal, Special K	1	cup(s)	31	110	7	22	1	0	0.00	0.00	0.00	0	0	0	8.70	220	—	400	15	7
Cereal, Total whole grain	1	cup(s)	40	146	3	31	4	1	0.00	0.00	0.00	—	0	1330	23.94	253	31.24	532	80	2
Cereal, Wheaties	1	cup(s)	30	110	3	24	3	1	0.00	0.00	0.00	—	0	0	8.10	220	2.26	200	6	1
Cheese, American, processed	1	ounce(s)	28	106	6	<1	0	9	5.58	2.54	0.28	—	27	156	0.05	422	0.08	2	0	4
Cheese, blue, crumbled	1	ounce(s)	28	100	6	1	0	8	5.29	2.21	0.23	—	21	150	0.09	395	0.07	10	0	4
Cheese, cheddar, shredded	¼	cup(s)	28	114	7	<1	0	9	5.96	2.65	0.27	—	30	204	0.19	175	0.08	5	0	4
Cheese, feta	1	ounce(s)	28	74	4	1	0	6	4.18	1.29	0.17	—	25	138	0.18	312	0.05	9	0	4
Cheese, Monterey jack	1	ounce(s)	28	104	7	<1	0	8	5.34	2.45	0.25	—	25	209	0.20	150	0.07	5	0	4

Food Description	Qty	Measure	Wt (g)	Ener (cal)	Prot (g)	Carb (g)	Dietary Fiber (g)	Fat (g)	Fat Breakdown (g) Sat	Mono	Poly	Trans	Chol (mg)	Calc (mg)	Iron (mg)	Sodi (mg)	Vit E (mg)	Folate (mcg)	Vit C (mg)	Sele-nium (mcg)
Cheese, mozzarella, part skim milk	1	ounce(s)	28	71	7	1	0	4	2.83	1.26	0.13	—	18	219	0.06	173	0.04	3	0	4
Cheese, Parmesan, grated	1	tablespoon(s)	5	22	2	<1	0	1	0.87	0.42	0.06	—	4	55	0.05	76	0.01	1	0	1
Cheese, ricotta, part skim milk	¼	cup(s)	62	85	7	3	0	5	3.03	1.42	0.16	—	19	167	0.27	77	0.04	8	0	10
Cheese, Swiss	1	ounce(s)	28	106	8	2	0	8	4.98	2.04	0.27	—	26	221	0.06	54	0.11	2	0	5
Cherries, sweet, raw	½	cup(s)	73	46	1	12	2	<1	0.03	0.03	0.04	—	0	9	0.26	0	0.05	3	5	0
Chicken, broiler breast, meat & skin, flour coated, fried	3	ounce(s)	85	189	27	1	<.1	8	2.08	2.98	1.67	—	76	14	1.01	65	—	5	0	20
Chicken, broiler drumstick, meat & skin, flour coated, fried	3	ounce(s)	85	208	23	1	<.1	12	3.11	4.61	2.75	—	77	10	1.14	76	—	9	0	16
Chicken, light meat, roasted	3	ounce(s)	85	130	23	0	0	3	0.92	1.29	0.79	—	64	11	0.92	43	0.23	3	0	22
Chicken, roasted (meat only)	3	ounce(s)	85	142	21	0	0	6	1.54	2.13	1.28	—	64	10	1.03	64	—	4	0	21
Chickpeas or bengal gram, garbanzo beans, boiled	½	cup(s)	82	134	7	22	6	2	0.22	0.48	0.95	—	0	40	2.37	6	0.29	141	1	3
Chocolate milk, low fat	1	cup(s)	250	158	8	26	1	3	1.54	0.75	0.09	—	8	288	0.60	153	0.05	13	2	5
Cilantro	1	teaspoon(s)	2	<1	<.1	<.1	<.1	<.1	0.00	0.00	0.00	—	0	1	0.03	1	—	1	1	<.1
Cocoa, hot, prepared w/milk	1	cup(s)	250	193	9	27	3	6	3.58	1.69	0.09	0.18	20	263	1.20	110	0.08	13	1	7
Coconut, dried, not sweetened	¼	cup(s)	60	393	4	14	10	38	34.06	1.63	0.42	—	0	15	1.98	22	0.26	5	1	11
Cod, Atlantic cod or scrod, baked or broiled	3	ounce(s)	44	46	10	0	0	<1	0.07	0.05	0.13	—	24	6	0.22	35	—	5	<1	17
Coffee, brewed	8	fluid ounce(s)	237	9	<1	0	0	0	0.00	0.00	0.00	0	0	2	0.02	2	0.02	5	0	0
Collard greens, boiled, drained	½	cup(s)	95	25	2	5	3	<1	0.04	0.02	0.16	—	0	133	1.10	15	0.84	88	17	<1
Cookies, animal crackers	12	piece(s)	30	134	2	22	<1	4	1.03	2.29	0.56	—	0	13	0.82	1118	0.04	50	0	—
Cookies, chocolate chip	1	item(s)	30	140	2	16	1	8	2.09	3.26	2.09	0	13	11	0.70	109	0.54	16	<.1	4
Cookies, chocolate sandwich, extra crème filling	1	item(s)	13	65	<1	9	<1	3	0.50	1.39	1.22	1.10	0	3	0.37	64	0.25	6	0	<1
Cookies, Fig Newtons	1	item(s)	16	55	1	10	1	1	0.50	0.50	0.00	0.50	0	5	0.36	60	—	—	<1	—
Cookies, oatmeal	1	item(s)	69	234	6	45	3	4	0.70	1.28	1.85	0	<.1	26	1.94	311	0.23	30	<1	17
Cookies, peanut butter	1	item(s)	35	163	4	17	1	9	1.65	4.72	2.43	0	13	28	0.67	157	0.74	21	<.1	5
Cookies, sugar	1	item(s)	16	61	1	7	<1	3	0.63	1.27	0.87	0	18	5	0.32	50	0.28	8	<.1	3
Corn, yellow sweet, frozen, boiled, drained	½	cup(s)	82	66	2	16	2	1	0.08	0.16	0.26	—	0	2	0.39	1	0.06	29	3	1
Cornbread	1	piece(s)	55	141	5	18	1	5	2.09	1.44	1.50	0	21	88	1.01	209	0.33	36	2	6
Cornmeal, yellow whole grain	½	cup(s)	61	221	5	47	4	2	0.31	0.58	1.00	—	0	4	2.10	21	0.26	15	0	9
Cottage cheese, low fat, 1% fat	½	cup(s)	113	81	14	3	0	1	0.73	0.33	0.04	—	5	69	0.16	459	0.01	14	0	10
Cottage cheese, low fat, 2% fat	½	cup(s)	113	102	16	4	0	2	1.38	0.62	0.07	—	9	78	0.18	459	0.02	15	0	12
Crab, blue, canned	2	ounce(s)	57	56	12	0	0	1	0.14	0.12	0.25	—	50	57	0.48	189	1.04	24	2	18
Crackers, cheese (mini)	30	item(s)	30	151	3	17	1	8	2.81	3.63	0.74	—	4	45	1.43	299	0.66	46	0	3
Crackers, honey graham	4	item(s)	28	118	2	22	1	3	0.43	1.14	1.07	—	0	7	1.04	169	0.09	13	0	3
Crackers, matzo, plain	1	item(s)	28	112	3	24	1	<1	0.06	0.04	0.17	—	0	4	0.90	1	0.02	5	0	10
Crackers, Ritz	5	item(s)	16	80	1	10	1	4	0.50	1.50	0.00	—	0	20	0.72	135	—	10	1	—
Crackers, rye crispbread	1	item(s)	10	37	1	8	2	<1	0.01	0.02	0.06	—	0	3	0.24	26	0.08	5	0	4
Crackers, saltine	5	item(s)	15	65	1	11	<1	2	0.44	0.96	0.25	0.54	0	18	0.81	195	0.15	19	0	2
Crackers, wheat	10	item(s)	30	142	3	19	1	6	1.55	3.43	0.84	—	0	15	1.32	239	0.15	35	0	2
Cranberry juice cocktail	½	cup(s)	127	72	0	18	<1	<1	0.01	0.02	0.06	—	0	4	0.19	3	0.28	0	45	0
Cream cheese	2	tablespoon(s)	29	101	2	1	0	10	6.37	2.85	0.37	—	32	23	0.35	86	0.09	4	0	1
Cream, heavy whipping, liquid	1	tablespoon(s)	15	52	<1	<1	0	6	3.45	1.60	0.21	—	21	10	0.00	6	0.16	1	<.1	<.1
Cream, light whipping, liquid	1	tablespoon(s)	15	44	<1	<1	0	5	2.90	1.36	0.13	—	17	10	0.00	5	0.13	1	<.1	<.1
Croissant, butter	1	item(s)	57	231	5	26	1	12	6.59	3.15	0.62	—	38	21	1.16	424	—	35	<1	13
Cucumber	¼	item(s)	75	11	<1	3	<1	<.1	0.03	0.00	0.04	—	0	12	0.21	2	0.02	5	2	<1
Danish pastry, nut	1	item(s)	65	280	5	30	1	16	3.78	8.90	2.78	—	30	61	1.17	236	0.53	54	1	9
Dates, domestic, whole	¼	cup(s)	44.5	126	1	33	4	<1	0.01	0.01	0	—	0	17	0.45	1	0.02	9	<1	1
Distilled alcohol, 90 proof	1	fluid ounce(s)	28	73	0	0	0	0	0.00	0.00	0.00	0	0	0	0.01	<1	0.00	0	0	0
Doughnut, cake	1	item(s)	47	198	2	23	1	11	1.70	4.37	3.70	—	17	21	0.92	257	—	22	<.1	0
Doughnut, glazed	1	item(s)	60	242	4	27	1	14	3.49	7.72	1.74	—	4	26	0.36	205	—	13	<.1	5
Egg substitute, Egg Beaters	¼	cup(s)	61	30	6	1	0	0	0.00	0.00	0.00	0	0	20	1.08	115	—	60	0	—
Eggs, fried	1	item(s)	46	92	6	<1	0	7	1.98	2.92	1.22	—	210	27	0.91	94	0.56	23	0	16
Eggs, hard boiled	1	item(s)	50	78	6	1	0	5	1.63	2.04	0.71	—	212	25	0.60	62	0.51	22	0	15

Eggs, poached	1	item(s)	50	74	6	<1	0	5	1.54	1.90	0.68	—	211	27	0.92	147	0.48	24	0	16
Eggs, raw, white	1	item(s)	33	17	4	<1	0	<.1	0.00	0.00	0.00	—	0	2	0.03	55	0.00	1	0	7
Eggs, raw, whole	1	item(s)	50	74	6	<1	0	5	1.55	1.91	0.68	—	212	27	0.92	70	0.49	24	0	16
Eggs, raw, yolk	1	item(s)	17	53	3	1	0	4	1.59	1.95	0.70	—	205	21	0.45	8	0.43	24	0	9
Eggs, scrambled, prepared w/milk & butter	2	item(s)	122	203	14	3	0	15	4.49	5.82	2.62	—	429	87	1.46	342	1.04	37	<1	27
Figs, raw, medium	2	item(s)	101	74	1	19	3	<1	0.06	0.07	0.14	—	0	35	0.37	1	0.11	6	2	<1
Fish fillets, batter coated or breaded, fried	3	ounce(s)	85	197.19	12.46	14.42	0.42	10.44	2.39	2.19	5.32	—	28.89	15.3	1.79	452.2	—	17	0	7.73
Flounder, baked	3	ounce(s)	85	114	15	<1	<.1	6	1.15	2.17	1.44	0	44	19	0.35	281	0.41	7	3	34
Flour, all purpose, white, bleached, enriched	½	cup(s)	63	228	6	48	2	1	0.10	0.05	0.26	—	0	9	2.90	1	0.04	114	0	21
Flour, whole wheat	½	cup(s)	60	203	8	44	7	1	0.19	0.14	0.47	—	0	20	2.33	3	0.49	26	0	42
Frankfurter, beef & pork	1	item(s)	57	174	7	1	1	16	6.14	7.79	1.56	—	29	6	0.66	638	0.14	2	0	8
Frankfurter, beef	1	item(s)	45	149	5	2	0	13	5.26	6.44	0.53	—	24	6	0.68	513	0.09	2	0	4
Frankfurter, turkey	1	item(s)	45	102	6	1	0	8	2.65	2.51	2.25	—	48	48	0.83	642	0.28	4	0	7
Frozen yogurt, chocolate, soft serve	½	cup(s)	72	115	3	18	2	4	2.61	1.26	0.16	—	4	106	0.90	71	—	8	<1	2
Frozen yogurt, vanilla, soft serve	½	cup(s)	72	117	3	17	0	4	2.46	1.14	0.15	—	1	103	0.22	63	0.08	4	1	2
Fruit cocktail, canned in heavy syrup	½	cup(s)	124	91	<1	23	1	<.1	0.01	0.02	0.04	—	0	7	0.36	7	0.50	4	2	1
Fruit cocktail, canned in juice	½	cup(s)	119	55	1	14	1	<.1	0.00	0.00	0.00	—	0	9	0.25	5	0.47	4	3	1
Granola bar, plain, hard	1	item(s)	25	115	2	16	1	5	0.58	1.07	2.95	—	0	15	0.72	72	—	6	<1	4
Grape juice, sweetened, added vitamin C, from frozen concentrate	½	cup(s)	125	64	<1	16	<1	<1	0.04	0.01	0.03	—	0	5	0.13	3	0.00	1	30	<1
Grapefruit juice, pink, sweetened, canned	½	cup(s)	125	58	1	14	<1	<1	0.02	0.02	0.03	—	0	10	0.45	3	0.05	13	34	<1
Grapefruit juice, white	½	cup(s)	124	48	1	11	<1	<1	0.02	0.02	0.03	—	0	11	0.25	1	0.27	12	47	<1
Grapefruit, raw, pink or red	½	cup(s)	115	48	1	12	2	<1	0.02	0.02	0.04	—	0	25	0.09	0	0.15	15	36	<1
Grapes, European, red or green, adherent skin	½	cup(s)	80	55	1	14	1	<1	0.04	0.01	0.04	—	0	8	0.29	2	0.15	2	9	<.1
Haddock, baked or broiled	3	ounce(s)	44	50	11	0	0	<1	0.07	0.07	0.14	—	33	19	0.60	39	—	4	0	18
Halibut, Atlantic & Pacific, cooked, dry heat	3	ounce(s)	85	119	23	0	0	2	0.35	0.82	0.80	—	35	51	0.91	59	—	12	0	40
Ham, cured, boneless, 11% fat, roasted	3	ounce(s)	85	151	19	0	0	8	2.65	3.77	1.20	—	50	7	1.14	1275	0.26	3	0	17
Ham, deli sliced, cooked	1	slice(s)	28	30	5	1	0	1	0.50	0.39	0.11	—	15	0	0.00	240	—	—	0	—
Honey	1	tablespoon(s)	21	64	<.1	17	<.1	0	0.00	0.00	0.00	0	0	1	0.09	1	0.00	<1	<1	<1
Honeydew melon	½	cup(s)	89	32	<1	8	1	<1	0.03	0.00	0.05	—	0	5	0.15	16	0.02	17	16	1
Ice cream, chocolate	½	cup(s)	66	143	3	19	1	7	4.49	2.12	0.27	—	22	72	0.61	50	0.20	11	<1	2
Ice cream, chocolate, soft serve	½	cup(s)	87	177	3	24	1	8	5.17	2.43	0.31	—	22	103	0.33	44	0.22	5	1	—
Ice cream, light vanilla	½	cup(s)	66	109	4	18	<1	3	1.71	0.57	0.10	—	17	77	0.05	49	0.08	3	<1	1
Jams, jellies, preserves, all flavors	1	tablespoon(s)	20	56	<.1	14	<1	<.1	0.00	0.01	0.00	—	0	4	0.10	6	0.00	2.20	1.76	—
Jams, jellies, preserves, all flavors, low sugar	1	tablespoon(s)	18	25	<.1	6	<1	<.1	0.00	0.01	0.02	—	0	2	0.05	<1	0.01	—	4.93	—
Kale, frozen, chopped, boiled, drained	½	cup(s)	65	20	2	3	1	<1	0.04	0.02	0.15	—	0	90	0.61	10	0.60	9	16	1
Kiwifruit	1	item(s)	77	53	1	11	3	1	0.02	0.03	0.19	—	0	30	0.38	2	—	<.1	74	—
Lamb, chop, loin, domestic, lean & fat, ¼" fat, broiled	3	ounce(s)	85	269	21	0	0	20	8.36	8.25	1.43	—	85	17	1.54	65	0.11	15	0	23
Lamb, leg, domestic, lean & fat, ¼" fat, cooked	3	ounce(s)	85	250	21	0	0	18	7.51	7.50	1.28	—	82	14	1.60	61	0.12	15	0	22
Lemon juice	1	tablespoon(s)	15	4	<.1	1	<.1	0	0.00	0.00	0.00	—	0	1	0.00	<1	0.02	2	7	<.1
Lemonade, from frozen concentrate	8	fluid ounce(s)	248	131	<1	34	<1	<1	0.02	0.00	0.04	—	0	10	0.52	7	0.02	2	13	<1
Lentils, boiled	½	cup(s)	99	115	9	20	8	<1	0.05	0.06	0.17	—	0	19	3.30	2	0.11	179	1	3
Lentils, sprouted	1	cup(s)	77	82	7	17	0	<1	0.04	0.08	0.17	—	0	19	2.47	8	—	77	13	<1
Lettuce, butterhead, Boston, or bibb	1	cup(s)	55	7	1	1	1	<1	0.02	0.00	0.06	—	0	19	0.69	3	0.10	40	2	<1
Lettuce, romaine, shredded	1	cup(s)	56	10	1	2	1	<1	0.02	0.01	0.09	—	0	19	0.55	5	0.07	77	14	<1
Lobster, northern, cooked, moist heat	3	ounce(s)	85	83	17	1	0	1	0.09	0.14	0.08	—	61	52	0.33	323	0.85	9	0	36
Macadamias, dry roasted, no salt added	¼	cup(s)	34	241	3	4	3	25	4.00	19.86	0.50	—	0	23	0.89	1	0.19	3	<1	1
Mayonnaise w/soybean oil	1	tablespoon(s)	14	99	<1	1	0	11	1.64	2.70	5.89	0.04	5	2	0.07	78	0.72	1	0	<1
Mayonnaise, low calorie	1	tablespoon(s)	16	37	<.1	3	0	3	0.53	0.72	1.70	—	4	<.1	0.00	80	0.32	0	0	—
Milk, fat free, nonfat, or skim	1	cup(s)	245	83	8	12	0	<1	0.29	0.12	0.02	—	5	223	1.23	108	0.02	12	0	8
Milk, fat free, nonfat, or skim, w/nonfat milk solids	1	cup(s)	245	91	9	12	0	1	0.40	0.16	0.02	—	5	316	0.12	130	0.00	12	2	5
Milk, low fat, 1%	1	cup(s)	244	102	8	12	0	2	1.54	0.68	0.09	—	12	264	0.85	122	0.02	12	0	8
Milk, low fat, 1%, w/nonfat milk solids	1	cup(s)	245	105	9	12	0	2	1.48	0.69	0.09	—	10	314	0.12	127	—	12	2	6
Milk, reduced fat, 2%	1	cup(s)	244	122	8	11	0	5	2.35	2.04	0.17	—	20	271	0.24	115	0.07	12	<1	6
Milk, reduced fat, 2%, w/nonfat milk solids	1	cup(s)	245	125	9	12	0	5	2.93	1.36	0.17	—	20	314	0.12	127	—	12	2	6
Milk, whole, 3.3%	1	cup(s)	244	146	8	11	0	8	4.55	1.98	0.48	—	24	246	0.07	105	0.15	12	0	9

Food Description	Qty	Measure	Wt (g)	Ener (cal)	Prot (g)	Carb (g)	Dietary Fiber (g)	Fat (g)	Fat Breakdown (g) Sat	Mono	Poly	Trans	Chol (mg)	Calc (mg)	Iron (mg)	Sodi (mg)	Vit E (mg)	Folate (mcg)	Vit C (mg)	Selenium (mcg)
Milk, whole, evaporated, canned	2	tablespoon(s)	32	42	2	3	0	2	1.45	0.74	0.08	—	9	82	0.06	33	0.04	3	1	1
Milkshakes, chocolate	1	cup(s)	227	270	7	48	1	6	3.81	1.77	0.23	—	25	299	0.70	252	0.11	11	0	4
Muffin, English, plain, enriched	1	item(s)	57	134	4	26	2	1	0.15	0.17	0.51	—	0	30	1.43	264	—	42	0	—
Muffin, English, wheat	1	item(s)	57	127	5	26	3	1	0.16	0.16	0.48	—	0	101	1.64	218	0.26	36	0	17
Muffins, blueberry	1	item(s)	63	160	3	23	1	6	0.87	1.48	3.25	0	20	50	1.15	288	0.76	29	<1	9
Mushrooms, raw	½	cup(s)	35	8	1	1	<1	<1	0.02	0.00	0.05	—	0	1	0.18	1	0.00	6	1	3
Mustard greens, frozen, boiled, drained	½	cup(s)	75	14	2	2	2	<1	0.01	0.08	0.04	—	0	76	0.84	19	1.01	53	10	<1
Oil, canola	1	tablespoon(s)	14	120	0	0	0	14	0.97	8.01	4.03	—	0	0	0.00	0	2.33	0	0	0
Oil, corn	1	tablespoon(s)	14	120	0	0	0	14	1.73	3.29	7.98	0.04	0	0	0.00	0	1.94	0	0	0
Oil, olive	1	tablespoon(s)	14	119	0	0	0	14	1.82	9.98	1.35	—	0	<1	0.09	<1	1.94	0	0	0
Oil, peanut	1	tablespoon(s)	14	119	0	0	0	14	2.28	6.24	4.32	—	0	0	0.00	0	2.12	0	0	0
Oil, safflower	1	tablespoon(s)	14	120	0	0	0	14	0.84	10.15	1.95	—	0	0	0.00	0	4.64	0	0	0
Oil, soybean w/cottonseed oil	1	tablespoon(s)	14	120	0	0	0	14	2.45	4.01	6.54	—	0	0	0.00	0	1.65	0	0	0
Okra, sliced, boiled, drained	½	cup(s)	80	18	1	4	2	<1	0.04	0.02	0.04	—	0	62	0.22	5	0.22	37	13	<1
Onions, chopped, boiled, drained	½	cup(s)	106	47	1	11	1	<1	0.03	0.03	0.08	—	0	23	0.26	3	0.02	16	6	1
Orange juice, unsweetened, from frozen concentrate	½	cup(s)	125	56	1	13	<1	<.1	0.01	0.01	0.01	—	0	11	0.12	1	0.25	55	48	<1
Orange, raw	1	item(s)	131	62	1	15	3	<1	0.02	0.03	0.03	—	0	52	0.13	0	0.24	39	70	1
Oysters, eastern, farmed, raw	3	ounce(s)	85	50	4	5	0	1	0.38	0.13	0.50	—	21	37	4.91	151	—	15	4	54
Oysters, eastern, wild, cooked, moist heat	3	ounce(s)	85	116	12	7	0	4	1.31	0.53	1.65	—	89	77	10.19	359	—	12	5	61
Pancakes, blueberry, from recipe	3	item(s)	114	253	7	33	1	10	2.26	2.64	4.74	—	64	235	1.96	470	—	41	3	16
Pancakes, from mix w/egg & milk	3	item(s)	114	249	9	33	2	9	2.33	2.36	3.33	—	81	245	1.48	576	—	105	1	—
Papaya, raw	½	cup(s)	70	27	<1	7	1	<.1	0.03	0.03	0.02	—	0	17	0.07	2	0.51	27	43	<1
Pasta, egg noodles, enriched, cooked	½	cup(s)	80	106	4	20	1	1	0.25	0.34	0.33	0.02	26	10	1.27	6	0.14	51	0	17
Pasta, macaroni, enriched, cooked	½	cup(s)	70	99	3	20	1	<1	0.07	0.06	0.19	—	0	5	0.98	1	0.04	54	0	15
Pasta, spaghetti, al dente, cooked	½	cup(s)	65	95	4	20	1	1	0.05	0.05	0.15	—	0	7	1.00	1	0.04	8	0	40
Pasta, spaghetti, whole wheat, cooked	½	cup(s)	70	87	4	19	3	<1	0.07	0.05	0.15	—	0	11	0.74	2	0.21	4	0	18
Pasta, tricolor vegetable macaroni, enriched, cooked	½	cup(s)	67	86	3	18	3	<.1	0.01	0.01	0.03	—	0	7	0.33	4	0.06	44	0	13
Peach, halves, canned in heavy syrup	½	cup(s)	131	97	1	26	2	<1	0.01	0.05	0.06	—	0	4	0.35	8	0.64	4	4	<1
Peach, halves, canned in water	½	cup(s)	122	29	1	7	2	<.1	0.01	0.03	0.03	—	0	2	0.39	4	0.60	4	4	<1
Peach, raw, medium	1	item(s)	98	38	1	9	1	<1	0.02	0.07	0.08	—	0	6	0.25	0	0.72	4	6	<.1
Peanut butter, smooth	1	tablespoon(s)	16	96	4	3	1	8	1.60	3.96	2.38	—	0	8	0.30	80	1.44	12	0	1
Peanuts, oil roasted, salted	¼	cup(s)	36	216	10	5	3	19	3.12	9.33	5.49	—	0	22	0.54	115	2.50	43	<1	1
Pear, halves, canned in heavy syrup	½	cup(s)	133	98	<1	25	2	<1	0.01	0.04	0.04	—	0	7	0.29	7	0.11	1	1	0
Pear, raw	1	item(s)	166	96	1	26	5	<1	0.01	0.04	0.05	—	0	15	0.28	2	0.20	12	7	<1
Peas, green, canned, drained	½	cup(s)	85	59	4	11	3	<1	0.05	0.03	0.14	—	0	17	0.81	214	0.03	37	8	1
Peas, green, frozen, boiled, drained	½	cup(s)	80	62	4	11	4	<1	0.04	0.02	0.10	—	0	19	1.22	58	0.02	47	8	1
Pecans, dry roasted, no salt added	¼	cup(s)	57	403	5	8	5	42	3.56	24.92	11.66	—	0	41	1.59	1	0.74	9	<1	2
Pepperoni, beef & pork	1	slice(s)	11	55	2	<1	0	5	1.77	2.32	0.48	—	9	1	0.15	224	—	<1	0	—
Peppers, green bell or sweet, raw	½	cup(s)	75	15	1	3	1	<1	0.04	0.01	0.05	—	0	7	0.25	2	0.28	8	60	0
Pickle relish, sweet	1	tablespoon(s)	15	20	<.1	5	<1	<.1	0.01	0.03	0.02	—	0	<1	0.13	122	0.06	<1	<1	0
Pickle, dill	1	ounce(s)	28	5	<1	1	<1	<.1	0.01	0.00	0.02	—	0	3	0.15	363	0.03	<1	1	0
Pie crust, frozen, ready to bake, enriched, baked	1	slice(s)	16	82	1	8	<1	5	1.69	2.51	0.65	—	0	3	0.36	104	0.42	9	0	<1
Pie crust, prepared w/water, baked	1	slice(s)	20	100	1	10	<1	6	1.54	3.46	0.77	—	0	12	0.43	146	—	20	0	—
Pie, apple, from home recipe	1	slice(s)	155	411	4	58	2	19	4.73	8.36	5.17	—	0	11	1.74	327	—	37	3	12
Pie, pecan, from home recipe	1	slice(s)	122	503	6	64	0	27	4.87	13.64	6.97	—	106	39	1.81	320	—	32	<1	15
Pie, pumpkin, from home recipe	1	slice(s)	155	316	7	41	0	14	4.92	5.73	2.81	—	65	146	1.97	349	—	33	3	11
Pineapple, canned in extra heavy syrup	½	cup(s)	130	108	<1	28	1	<1	0.01	0.02	0.05	—	0	18	0.49	1	—	7	9	—
Pineapple, canned in juice	½	cup(s)	125	75	1	20	1	<.1	0.01	0.01	0.04	—	0	17	0.35	1	0.01	6	12	<1
Pineapple, raw, diced	½	cup(s)	78	37	<1	10	1	<.1	0.01	0.01	0.03	—	0	10	0.22	1	0.02	12	28	<.1
Pinto beans, boiled, drained, no salt added	½	cup(s)	114	25	2	5	0	<1	0.04	0.03	0.21	—	0	17	0.75	58	—	146	7	1
Pomegranate	1	item(s)	154	105	1	26	1	<1	0.06	0.07	0.10	—	0	5	0.46	5	0.92	9	9	1
Popcorn, air popped	1	cup(s)	8	31	1	6	1	<1	0.05	0.09	0.15	—	0	1	0.22	<1	0.02	2	0	1
Popcorn, popped in oil	1	cup(s)	33	165	3	19	3	9	1.61	2.70	4.43	—	0	3	0.92	292	—	6	<.1	2

Pork, ribs, loin, country style, lean & fat, roasted	3	ounce(s)	85	279	20	0	0	22	7.83	9.36	1.71	—	78	21	0.90	44	—	4	<1	32
Potato chips, salted	20	item(s)	28	152	2	15	1	10	3.11	2.79	3.46	—	0	7	0.46	169	1.91	13	9	2
Potatoes, au gratin mix, prepared w/water, whole milk, & butter	½	cup(s)	114	106	3	15	1	5	2.94	1.34	0.15	—	17	94	0.36	499	—	8	4	3
Potatoes, baked, flesh & skin	1	item(s)	202	220	5	51	4	<1	0.05	0.00	0.09	—	0	20	2.75	16	—	22	26	2
Potatoes, baked, flesh only	½	cup(s)	61	57	1	13	1	<.1	0.02	0.00	0.03	—	0	3	0.21	3	0.02	5	8	<1
Potatoes, hashed brown	½	cup(s)	78	207	2	27	2	10	1.11	3.13	2.78	—	0	11	0.43	267	0.01	12	10	<1
Potatoes, mashed, from dehydrated granules w/milk, water, & margarine	½	cup(s)	105	122	2	17	1	5	1.27	2.05	1.41	—	2	34	0.22	181	0.54	8	7	6
Pretzels, plain, hard, twists	5	item(s)	30	114	3	24	1	1	0.23	0.41	0.37	—	0	11	1.30	515	—	51	0	2
Prune juice, canned	1	cup(s)	256	182	2	45	3	<.1	0.01	0.05	0.02	—	0	31	3.02	10	0.31	0	10	2
Prunes, dried	2	item(s)	17	40	<1	11	1	<.1	0.01	0.06	0.02	—	0	9	0.42	1	0.00	1	1	<1
Pudding, chocolate	½	cup(s)	144	154	5	23	1	5	2.78	1.94	0.23	0	35	138	1.04	135	0.00	7	<1	5
Pudding, tapioca, ready to eat	1	item(s)	142	169	3	28	<1	5	0.85	2.24	1.93	—	1	119	0.33	226	0.43	4	1	2
Pudding, vanilla	½	cup(s)	136	116	5	17	<.1	3	1.31	1.21	0.16	0	35	133	0.25	134	0.00	6	<1	5
Quinoa, dry	½	cup(s)	85	318	11	59	5	5	0.50	1.30	1.99	—	0	51	7.86	18	—	42	0	—
Raisins, seeded, packed	¼	cup(s)	41	122	1	32	3	<1	0.07	0.01	0.07	—	0	12	1.07	12	—	1	2	<1
Raspberries, raw	½	cup(s)	62	32	1	7	4	<1	0.01	0.04	0.23	—	0	15	0.42	1	0.54	13	16	<1
Raspberries, red, sweetened, frozen	½	cup(s)	125	129	1	33	6	<1	0.01	0.02	0.11	—	0	19	0.81	1	0.90	33	21	<1
Rice, brown, long grain, cooked	½	cup(s)	98	108	3	22	2	1	0.18	0.32	0.31	—	0	10	0.41	5	0.03	4	0	10
Rice, white, long grain, boiled	½	cup(s)	79	103	2	22	<1	<1	0.06	0.07	0.06	—	0	8	0.95	1	0.03	46	0	6
Rice, wild brown, cooked	½	cup(s)	82	82.81	3.27	17.49	1.47	0.27	0.04	0.04	0.17	—	0	2.46	0.49	2.46	—	21.31	0	0.65
Roll, hard	1	item(s)	57	167	6	30	1	2	0.35	0.65	0.98	—	0	54	1.87	310	0.24	54	0	22
Salad dressing, blue cheese	2	tablespoon(s)	31	154	1	2	0	16	3.03	3.76	8.51	—	5	25	0.06	335	1.84	9	1	<1
Salad dressing, French	2	tablespoon(s)	31	143	<1	5	0	14	1.76	2.63	6.56	—	0	7	0.25	261	1.56	0	0	0
Salad dressing, French, low fat	2	tablespoon(s)	33	76	<1	10	<1	4	0.36	1.92	1.64	—	0	4	0.28	262	0.10	1	0	1
Salad dressing, Italian	2	tablespoon(s)	29	86	<1	3	0	8	1.32	1.86	3.80	—	0	2	0.19	486	1.47	0	0	1
Salad dressing, Italian, diet	2	tablespoon(s)	30	23	<1	1	0	2	0.14	0.66	0.51	—	2	3	0.20	410	0.06	0	0	2
Salad dressing, ranch	2	tablespoon(s)	30	146	<1	2	<.1	16	2.32	3.85	8.92	—	1	4	0.03	354	1.85	<1	<.1	—
Salad dressing, thousand island	2	tablespoon(s)	31	115	<1	5	<1	11	1.59	2.46	5.68	—	8	5	0.37	269	1.25	0	0	<1
Salad dressing, thousand island, low calorie	2	tablespoon(s)	31	62	<1	7	<1	4	0.23	1.98	0.82	—	<1	5	0.28	254	0.31	0	0	0
Salami, pork, dry or hard	1	slice(s)	13	52	3	<1	0	4	1.52	2.05	0.48	—	10	2	0.17	289	—	<1	0	3
Salmon, broiled or baked w/butter	3	ounce(s)	85	155	23	0	0	6	1.16	2.29	2.33	—	40	15	1.02	99	1.15	4	2	41
Salmon, smoked chinook (lox)	2	ounce(s)	57	66	10	0	0	2	0.52	1.14	0.56	—	13	6	0.48	1134	—	1	0	22
Salsa	2	tablespoon(s)	16	4	<1	1	<1	<.1	0.00	0.00	0.02	—	0	5	0.16	69	0.19	3	2	<.1
Sardines, Atlantic, with bones, canned in oil	2	item(s)	24	50	6	0	0	3	0.36	0.92	1.23	—	34	108	0.70	121	0.49	3	0	13
Sauerkraut, canned	½	cup(s)	114	22	1	5	3	<1	0.04	0.01	0.07	—	0	34	1.67	751	0.11	27	17	1
Sausage, Italian, pork, cooked	1	item(s)	68	220	14	1	0	17	6.14	8.13	2.23	—	53	16	1.02	627	—	3	1	15
Sausage, smoked, pork link	1	piece(s)	76	295	17	2	—	24	8.58	11.09	2.85	—	52	23	0.88	1137	—	4	0	16
Scallops, mixed species, breaded, fried	3	item(s)	47	100	8	5	0	5	1.24	2.09	1.32	—	28	20	0.38	216	—	23	1	13
Seaweed, spirulina, dried	½	cup(s)	8	22	4	2	<1	1	0.20	0.05	0.16	—	0	9	2.14	79	0.38	7	1	1
Shrimp, mixed species, breaded, fried	3	ounce(s)	85	205.69	18.18	9.74	0.34	10.43	1.77	3.24	4.32	—	150.44	56.95	1.07	292.39	—	20.39	1.27	35.44
Shrimp, mixed species, cooked, moist heat	3	ounce(s)	85	84	18	0	0	1	0.25	0.17	0.37	—	166	33	2.63	190	1.17	3	2	34
Soda, Coca-Cola Classic cola	12	fluid ounce(s)	360	146	0	41	0	0	0.00	0.00	0.00	0	0	—	—	50	—	—	0	—
Soda, Coke diet cola	12	fluid ounce(s)	360	2	0	<1	0	0	0.00	0.00	0.00	0	0	—	—	42	—	—	0	—
Soda, cola	12	fluid ounce(s)	426	179	<1	46	0	0	0.00	0.00	0.00	—	0	13	0.09	17	0.00	0	0	<1
Soda, ginger ale	12	fluid ounce(s)	366	124	0	32	0	0	0.00	0.00	0.00	0	0	11	0.66	26	0.00	0	0	<1
Soda, lemon-lime	12	fluid ounce(s)	368	147	0	38	0	0	0.00	0.00	0.00	—	0	7	0.26	41	0.00	0	0	0
Soda, root beer	12	fluid ounce(s)	370	152	0	39	0	0	0.00	0.00	0.00	0	0	18	0.18	48	0.00	0	0	<1
Sour cream	2	tablespoon(s)	24	51	1	1	0	5	3.13	1.45	0.19	—	11	28	0.01	13	0.14	3	<1	1
Sour cream, fat free	2	tablespoon(s)	32	24	1	5	0	0	0.00	0.00	0.00	0	3	40	0.00	45	0.00	4	0	—
Soy sauce	1	tablespoon(s)	18	10	1	2	0	<.1	0.00	0.00	0.01	—	0	3	0.36	1029	0.00	3	0	—
Spinach, canned, drained	½	cup(s)	108	25	3	4	3	1	0.09	0.02	0.23	—	0	138	2.49	29	2.10	106	16	2
Spinach, chopped, boiled, drained	½	cup(s)	90	21	3	3	2	<1	0.04	0.01	0.10	—	0	122	3.21	63	1.87	131	9	1
Spinach, raw, chopped	1	cup(s)	30	7	1	1	1	<1	0.02	0.00	0.05	—	0	30	0.81	24	0.61	58	8	<1
Squash, acorn, baked	½	cup(s)	103	57	1	15	5	<1	0.03	0.01	0.06	—	0	45	0.95	4	—	19	11	1
Squash, summer, all varieties, sliced, boiled, drained	½	cup(s)	90	18	1	4	1	<1	0.06	0.02	0.12	—	0	24	0.32	1	0.13	18	5	<1

Food Description	Qty	Measure	Wt (g)	Ener (cal)	Prot (g)	Carb (g)	Dietary Fiber (g)	Fat (g)	Fat Breakdown (g) Sat	Mono	Poly	Trans	Chol (mg)	Calc (mg)	Iron (mg)	Sodi (mg)	Vit E (mg)	Folate (mcg)	Vit C (mg)	Sele-nium (mcg)
Squash, winter, all varieties, baked, mashed	½	cup(s)	103	38	1	9	3	<1	0.13	0.05	0.27	—	0	23	0.45	1	0.12	21	10	<1
Squid, mixed species, fried	3	ounce(s)	85	149	15	7	0	6	1.60	2.34	1.82	—	221	33	0.86	260	—	12	4	44
Strawberries, raw	½	cup(s)	72	23	<1	6	1	<1	0.01	0.03	0.11	—	0	12	0.30	1	0.21	17	42	<1
Strawberries, sweetened, frozen, thawed	½	cup(s)	128	99	1	27	2	<1	0.01	0.02	0.09	—	0	14	0.60	1	0.31	5	50	1
Sugar, brown, packed	1	teaspoon(s)	5	17	0	4	0	0	0.00	0.00	0.00	0	0	4	0.09	2	0.00	<.1	0	<.1
Sugar, white, granulated	1	teaspoon(s)	4	15	0	4	0	0	0.00	0.00	0.00	—	0	<.1	0.00	0	0.00	0	0	<.1
Sweet potatoes, baked, peeled	½	cup(s)	100	90	2	21	3	<1	0.03	0.00	0.06	—	0	38	0.69	36	0.71	6	20	<1
Syrup, maple	¼	cup(s)	80	209	0	54	0	<1	0.03	0.05	0.08	—	0	54	0.96	7	0.00	0	0	<1
Taco shell, hard	1	item(s)	13	62	1	8	1	3	0.43	1.19	1.13	—	0	21	0.33	49	0.22	17	0	2
Tangerine, raw	1	item(s)	84	37	1	9	2	<1	0.02	0.03	0.03	—	0	12	0.08	1	0.17	17	26	<1
Tea, decaffeinated, prepared	8	fluid ounce(s)	237	2	0	1	0	0	0.00	0.00	0.01	0	0	0	0.05	7	0.00	12	0	0
Tea, herbal, prepared	8	fluid ounce(s)	237	2	0	<1	0	0	0.00	0.00	0.01	0	0	5	0.19	2	0.00	2	0	0
Tea, prepared	8	fluid ounce(s)	237	2	0	1	0	0	0.00	0.00	0.01	0	0	0	0.05	7	0.00	12	0	0
Teriyaki sauce	1	tablespoon(s)	18	15	1	3	<.1	0	0.00	0.00	0.00	0	0	5	0.31	690	0.00	4	0	<1
Tofu, firm	3	ounce(s)	79	80	8	2	1	4	0.50	0.87	2.17	—	0	60	1.08	0	—	—	0	—
Tomato juice, canned	½	cup(s)	122	21	1	5	<1	<.1	0.01	0.01	0.03	—	0	12	0.52	328	0.39	24	22	<1
Tomato sauce	½	cup(s)	112	46	2	8	2	1	0.18	0.29	0.72	0	0	21	1.08	199	0.39	15	15	1
Tomatoes, fresh, ripe, red	1	item(s)	123	22.13	1.08	4.82	1.47	0.24	0.05	0.06	0.16	—	0	12.3	0.33	6.15	0.66	18.45	15.62	0
Tomatoes, stewed, canned, red	½	cup(s)	128	33	1	8	1	<1	0.03	0.04	0.10	—	0	43	1.70	282	1.06	6	10	1
Tortilla chips, plain	6	item(s)	28	142	2	18	2	7	1.43	4.39	1.03	—	0	44	0.43	150	1	3	0	2
Tortillas, corn, soft	1	item(s)	26	58	1	12	1	1	0.09	0.17	0.29	—	0	46	0.36	42	0.07	26	0	1
Tortillas, flour	1	item(s)	32	104	3	18	1	2	0.56	1.21	0.34	—	0	40	1.06	153	0.06	33	0	7
Tuna, light, canned in oil, drained	2	ounce(s)	57	113	17	0	0	5	0.87	1.68	1.64	—	10	7	0.79	202	0.50	3	0	43
Tuna, light, canned in water, drained	2	ounce(s)	57	66	14	0	0	<1	0.13	0.09	0.19	—	17	6	0.87	192	0.19	2	0	46
Turkey, breast, processed, oven roasted, fat free	1	slice(s)	28	25	4	1	0	0	0.00	0.00	0.00	0	10	0	0.00	330	—	—	0	—
Turkey, breast, processed, traditional carved	2	slice(s)	45	40	9	0	0	1	0.00	0.07	0.14	—	20	0	0.72	540	—	—	0	—
Turkey, roasted, dark meat, meat only	3	ounce(s)	85	159	24	0	0	6	2.06	1.39	1.84	—	72	27	1.98	67	0.54	8	0	35
Turkey, roasted, light meat, meat only	3	ounce(s)	85	133	25	0	0	3	0.88	0.48	0.73	—	59	16	1.15	54	0.08	5	0	27
Turnip greens, chopped, boiled, drained	½	cup(s)	72	14	1	3	3	<1	0.04	0.01	0.07	—	0	99	0.58	21	1.35	85	20	1
Turnips, cubed, boiled, drained	½	cup(s)	78	17	1	4	2	<.1	0.01	0.00	0.03	—	0	26	0.14	12	0.02	7	9	<1
Vegetables, mixed, canned, drained	½	cup(s)	82	40	2	8	2	<1	0.04	0.01	0.10	—	0	22	0.86	121	0.28	20	4	<1
Vinegar, balsamic	1	tablespoon(s)	15	10	0	2	0	0	0.00	0.00	0.00	0	0	0	0.00	0	—	—	0	—
Waffle, plain, frozen, toasted	2	item(s)	66	174	4	27	2	5	0.95	2.12	1.84	—	16	153	2.95	519	0.65	36	0	11
Walnuts, dried black, chopped	¼	cup(s)	31	193	8	3	2	18	1.05	4.69	10.96	—	0	19	0.98	1	0.56	10	1	5
Watermelon	½	cup(s)	77	23	<1	6	<1	<1	0.01	0.03	0.04	—	0	5	0.19	1	0.04	2	6	<1
Wheat germ, crude	2	tablespoon(s)	14	52	3	7	2	1	0.24	0.20	0.86	—	0	6	0.90	2	—	40	0	11
Wine cooler	10	fluid ounce(s)	300	150	<1	18	<.1	<.1	0.01	0.00	0.02	—	0	17	0.81	25	0.02	5	<.1	
Wine, red, California	5	fluid ounce(s)	150	125	<1	4	0	0	0.00	0.00	0.00	0	0	12	1.43	15	0.00	1	0	—
Wine, sparkling, domestic	5	fluid ounce(s)	150	105	<1	4	0	0	0.00	0.00	0.00	0	0	—	—	—	—	—	—	—
Wine, white	5	fluid ounce(s)	148	100	<1	1	0	0	0.00	0.00	0.00	0	0	13	0.47	7	—	0	0	<1
Yogurt, custard style, fruit flavors	6	ounce(s)	170	190	7	32	0	4	2.00	—	—	—	15	200	0.00	90	—	—	0	—
Yogurt, fruit, low fat	1	cup(s)	245	243	10	46	0	3	1.82	0.77	0.08	—	12	338	0.15	130	0.05	22	1	7
Yogurt, fruit, nonfat, sweetened w/low calorie sweetener	1	cup(s)	241	122	11	19	1	<1	0.21	0.10	0.04	—	3	370	0.62	139	0.17	26	1	—
Yogurt, plain, low fat	1	cup(s)	245	154	13	17	0	4	2.45	1.04	0.11	—	15	448	0.20	172	0.05	27	2	8
VEGETARIAN FOODS																				
Prepared																				
Macaroni & cheese (lacto)	8	ounce(s)	226	181	8	17	<1	9	4.37	2.88	0.89	0	22	187	0.77	768	0.29	39	<.1	16
Steamed rice & vegetables (vegan)	8	ounce(s)	228	265	5	40	3	10	1.84	3.91	4.07	0	0	41	1.43	1403	3.05	28	13	8
Vegan spinach enchiladas (vegan)	1	piece(s)	82	93	5	15	2	2	0.34	0.55	1.27	—	0	117	1.13	134	—	46	1	5
Vegetable chow mein (vegan)	8	ounce(s)	227	166	6	22	2	6	0.65	2.66	2.47	0	0	190	3.65	371	0.06	47	7	6
Vegetable lasagna (lacto)	8	ounce(s)	225	177	12	25	2	4	1.92	0.93	0.34	0	10	144	1.91	637	0.05	64	15	19

Vegetarian chili (vegan)	8	ounce(s)	227	116	6	21	7	2	0.24	0.29	0.74	0	<1	68	2.42	383	0.15	58	16	5
Vegetarian vegetable soup (vegan)	8	ounce(s)	226	92	3	14	2	4	0.77	1.67	1.30	0	0	37	1.32	503	0.55	38	24	1
Boca burger																				
All American flamed grilled patty	1	item(s)	71	110	14	6	4	4	1.00	—	—	0	3	150	1.80	370	—	—	0	—
Boca meatless ground burger	½	cup(s)	57	70	11	7	4	1	0.00	—	—	—	0	80	1.44	220	—	—	0	—
Breakfast links	2	item(s)	45	100	10	6	5	4	0.00	—	—	0	0	60	1.44	330	—	—	0	—
Breakfast patties	1	item(s)	38	80	8	5	3	4	0.00	—	—	0	0	60	1.44	260	—	—	0	—
Vegan original patty	1	item(s)	71	90	13	4	0	1	0.00	—	—	0	0	80	1.80	350	—	—	1	—
Gardenburger																				
Black bean burger	1	item(s)	71	80	8	11	4	2	0.00	—	—	0	0	40	1.44	330	—	—	0	—
Chik'n grill	1	item(s)	71	100	13	5	3	3	0.00	—	—	0	0	60	3.60	360	—	—	0	—
Meatless breakfast sausage	1	item(s)	43	50	5	2	2	4	0.00	—	—	0	0	20	0.72	120	—	—	0	—
Meatless meatballs	6	item(s)	85	110	12	8	4	5	1.00	—	—	0	0	60	1.80	400	—	—	0	—
Original	3	ounce(s)	85	132	7	19	4	4	1.80	1.80	0.60	0	24	72	0.00	672	—	12	0	8
Morningstar Farms																				
America's Original Veggie Dog links	1	item(s)	57	80	11	6	1	1	0.00	0.00	0.00	0	0	0	0.72	580	—	—	0	—
Better n Eggs egg substitute	¼	cup(s)	57	20	5	0	0	0	0.00	0.00	0.00	0	0	20	0.63	90	—	24	0	—
Breakfast links	2	item(s)	45	80	9	3	2	3	0.50	0.50	2.00	0	0	0	1.44	320	—	—	0	—
Breakfast strips	2	item(s)	16	60	2	2	1	5	0.50	1.00	3.00	0	0	0	0.27	220	—	—	0	—
Garden veggie patties	1	item(s)	67	100	10	9	4	3	0.50	0.50	1.50	0	0	40	0.72	350	—	—	0	—
Spicy black bean veggie burger	1	item(s)	78	150	11	16	5	5	0.50	1.50	2.50	0	0	40	1.80	470	—	—	0	—
MIXED FOODS, SOUPS, SANDWICHES																				
Mixed Dishes																				
Bean burrito	1	item(s)	149	327	17	33	6	15	8.30	4.73	0.85	0	38	331	2.95	514	0.01	115	4	18
Beef & vegetable fajita	1	item(s)	223	397	23	35	3	18	5.50	7.53	3.45	—	45	84	3.74	757	0.80	23	27	—
Chicken & vegetables w/broccoli, onion, bamboo shoots in soy based sauce	1	cup(s)	162	287	22	6	1	19	5.13	7.65	4.68	—	84	22	1.38	962	1.12	13	8	—
Chicken cacciatore	1	cup(s)	230	266	28	5	1	14	3.98	5.78	3.11	0	103	45	2.21	451	0.00	15	8	22
Chicken waldorf salad	½	cup(s)	100	178	14	6	1	11	1.76	3.18	5.05	0	42	20	0.78	246	0.62	15	2	11
Fettuccine alfredo	1	cup(s)	222	247	11	42	1	3	1.61	0.79	0.43	0	9	153	1.88	386	0.00	103	1	35
Hummus	½	cup(s)	123	218	6	25	5	11	1.38	6.04	2.56	—	0	60	1.93	298	0.92	73	10	3
Lasagna w/ground beef	1	cup(s)	237	288	18	22	2	15	7.47	4.84	0.84	0	68	222	2.33	493	0.22	50	10	22
Macaroni & cheese	1	cup(s)	200	393	15	40	1	19	8.18	6.72	2.66	—	30	323	2.26	800	0.72	12	<1	—
Meat loaf	1	slice(s)	115	244	17	7	<1	16	6.15	6.89	0.83	0	85	54	2.09	423	0.00	20	<1	17
Potato salad	½	cup(s)	125	179	3	14	2	10	1.79	3.10	4.67	—	85	24	0.81	661	—	9	13	5
Spaghetti & meatballs w/tomato sauce, prepared	1	cup(s)	248	330	19	39	3	12	3.90	4.40	2.20	—	89	124	3.70	1009	—	—	22	22
Spicy Thai noodles (pad thai)	8	ounce(s)	231	222	9	36	3	6	0.83	3.33	1.83	0	37	32	1.58	598	0.36	44	22	3
Sushi w/vegetables in seaweed	6	piece(s)	156	182	3	41	1	<1	0.10	0.11	0.11	—	0	20	1.54	153	0.12	10	2	—
Tuna salad	½	cup(s)	103	192	16	10	0	9	1.58	2.96	4.23	0	13	17	1.03	412	0.00	8	2	42
Soups																				
Chicken noodle, condensed, prepared w/water	1	cup(s)	241	75	4	9	1	2	0.65	1.11	0.55	—	7	17	0.77	1106	0.10	22	<1	6
Cream of chicken, condensed, prepared w/milk	1	cup(s)	248	191	7	15	<1	11	4.64	4.46	1.64	—	27	181	0.67	1047	—	7	1	8
Cream of mushroom, condensed, prepared w/milk	1	cup(s)	248	203	6	15	<1	14	5.13	2.98	4.61	—	20	179	0.60	918	1.24	10	2	4
Manhattan clam chowder, condensed, prepared w/water	1	cup(s)	244	78	2	12	1	2	0.38	0.38	1.29	—	2	27	1.63	578	0.34	10	4	9
Minestrone, condensed, prepared w/water	1	cup(s)	241	82	4	11	1	3	0.55	0.70	1.11	—	2	34	0.92	911	—	36	1	8
New England clam chowder, condensed, prepared w/milk	1	cup(s)	248	164	9	17	1	7	2.95	2.26	1.09	—	22	186	1.49	992	0.45	10	3	13
Split pea	1	cup(s)	165	85	4	19	2	<1	0.07	0.03	0.18	0	0	30	1.25	608	0.00	61	9	<1
Tomato, condensed, prepared w/milk	1	cup(s)	248	161	6	22	3	6	2.90	1.61	1.12	—	17	159	1.81	744	1.24	17	68	2
Tomato, condensed, prepared w/water	1	cup(s)	244	85	2	17	<1	2	0.37	0.44	0.95	—	0	12	1.76	695	2.32	15	66	<1
Vegetable beef, condensed, prepared w/water	1	cup(s)	244	78	6	10	<1	2	0.85	0.81	0.12	—	5	17	1.12	791	0.37	10	2	4
Vegetarian vegetable, condensed, prepared w/water	1	cup(s)	241	72	2	12	—	2	0.29	0.82	0.72	—	0	22	1.08	822	—	10	1	4

Food Description	Qty	Measure	Wt (g)	Ener (cal)	Prot (g)	Carb (g)	Dietary Fiber (g)	Fat (g)	Fat Breakdown (g) Sat	Mono	Poly	Trans	Chol (mg)	Calc (mg)	Iron (mg)	Sodi (mg)	Vit E (mg)	Folate (mcg)	Vit C (mg)	Sele-nium (mcg)
Sandwiches																				
Bacon, lettuce, & tomato w/mayonnaise	1	item(s)	164	349	11	34	2	19	4.54	7.22	6.07	—	20	76	2.54	837	1.16	31	15	—
Cheeseburger, large, plain	1	item(s)	185	609	30	47	0	33	14.84	12.74	2.44	—	96	91	5.46	1589	—	74	0	39
Cheeseburger, large, w/bacon, vegetables, & condiments	1	item(s)	195	608	32	37	2	37	16.24	14.49	2.71	—	111	162	4.74	1043	—	86	2	33
Club w/bacon, chicken, tomato, lettuce, & mayonnaise	1	item(s)	246	555	31	48	3	26	5.94	—	—	—	72	116	4.05	855	1.53	48	9	—
Cold cut submarine w/cheese & vegetables	1	item(s)	228	456	22	51	2	19	6.81	8.23	2.28	—	36	189	2.51	1651	—	87	12	31
Egg salad	1	item(s)	126	278	10	29	1	13	2.96	3.97	4.79	—	217	107	2.60	494	0.13	82	1	24
Hamburger, double patty, large, w/condiments & vegetables	1	item(s)	226	540	34	40	0	27	10.52	10.33	2.80	—	122	102	5.85	791	—	77	1	26
Hamburger, large, plain	1	item(s)	137	426	23	32	2	23	8.38	9.88	2.14	—	71	74	3.58	474	—	60	0	27
Hot dog w/bun, plain	1	item(s)	98	242	10	18	2	15	5.11	6.85	1.71	—	44	24	2.31	670	—	48	<.1	26
Pastrami	1	item(s)	134	331	14	27	2	18	6.18	8.74	1.02	—	51	68	2.64	1335	0.27	21	2	—
Peanut butter & jelly	1	item(s)	93	330	11	42	3	15	3.00	6.87	3.82	—	1	68	2.11	409	2.02	37	<1	—
FAST FOOD																				
Arby's																				
Au jus sauce	1	serving(s)	85	5	<1	1	<.1	<.1	0.02	—	—	—	0	0	0.00	386	—	—	0	—
Beef 'n cheddar sandwich	1	item(s)	198	480	23	43	2	24	8.00	—	—	—	90	100	3.60	1240	—	—	1	—
Curly fries, medium	1	serving(s)	128	400	5	50	4	20	5.00	—	—	—	0	0	1.80	990	—	—	15	—
Market Fresh grilled chicken Caesar salad w/o dressing	1	serving(s)	338	230	33	8	3	8	3.50	—	—	—	80	200	1.80	920	—	—	42	—
Roast beef deluxe sandwich, light	1	item(s)	182	296	18	33	6	10	3.00	5.00	2.00	—	42	130	4.50	826	—	—	8	—
Roast beef sandwich, giant	1	item(s)	228	480	32	41	3	23	10.00	—	—	—	110	60	5.40	1440	—	—	0	—
Roast beef sandwich, regular	1	item(s)	157	350	21	34	2	16	6.00	—	—	—	85	60	3.60	950	—	—	0	—
Roast chicken deluxe sandwich, light	1	item(s)	194	260	23	33	3	5	1.00	—	—	—	40	100	2.70	1010	—	—	2	—
Burger King																				
BK Broiler chicken sandwich	1	item(s)	258	550	30	52	3	25	5.00	—	—	—	105	60	3.60	1110	—	—	6	—
Croissanwich w/sausage, egg, & cheese	1	item(s)	157	520	19	24	1	39	14.00	—	—	1.93	210	300	4.50	1090	—	—	0	—
Fish Fillet sandwich	1	item(s)	185	520	18	44	2	30	8.00	—	—	1.12	55	150	2.70	840	—	—	1	—
French fries, medium, salted	1	item(s)	117	360	4	46	4	18	5.00	—	—	4.50	0	20	0.72	640	—	—	9	—
Onion rings, medium	1	serving(s)	91	320	4	40	3	16	4.00	—	—	3.50	0	97	0.00	460	—	—	0	—
Whopper	1	item(s)	291	710	31	52	4	43	13.00	—	—	1	85	150	6.30	980	—	—	9	—
Whopper w/cheese	1	item(s)	316	800	36	53	4	50	18.00	—	—	2	110	250	6.30	1420	—	—	9	—
Chick-Fil-A																				
Chargrilled chicken garden salad	1	item(s)	275	180	22	9	3	6	3.00	—	—	0	70	150	0.72	660	—	—	30	—
Chargrilled deluxe chicken sandwich	1	item(s)	195	290	27	31	2	7	1.50	—	—	0	70	80	1.80	990	—	—	5	—
Chicken biscuit w/cheese	1	item(s)	151	450	19	43	2	23	7.00	—	—	2.85	45	150	2.70	1430	—	—	0	—
Chicken salad sandwich	1	item(s)	153	350	20	32	5	15	3.00	—	—	0	65	150	1.80	880	—	—	0	—
Chick-n-Strips	4	item(s)	127	290	29	14	1	13	2.50	—	—	0	65	20	0.36	730	—	—	1	—
Coleslaw	1	item(s)	105	210	1	14	2	17	2.50	—	—	0	20	40	0.36	180	—	—	27	—
Dairy Queen																				
Banana split	1	item(s)	369	510	8	96	3	12	8.00	3.00	0.50	0	30	250	1.80	180	—	—	15	—
Chocolate chip cookie dough blizzard, small	1	item(s)	319	720	12	105	0	28	14.00	—	—	2.50	50	350	2.70	370	—	—	1	—
Chocolate malt, small	1	item(s)	418	650	15	111	0	16	10.00	—	—	0.50	55	450	1.80	370	—	—	2	—
Vanilla soft serve	½	cup(s)	94	140	3	22	0	5	3.00	—	—	0	15	150	0.72	70	—	—	0	—
Domino's																				
Classic hand-tossed pizza																				
America's favorite feast, 12"	2	slice(s)	205	508	22	57	4	22	9.20	—	—	—	49	202	3.70	1221	—	—	1	—
Pepperoni feast, extra pepperoni & cheese, 12"	2	slice(s)	196	534	24	56	3	25	10.92	—	—	—	57	279	3.36	1349	—	—	<1	—
Vegi feast, 12"	2	slice(s)	203	439	19	57	4	16	7.09	—	—	—	34	279	3.44	987	—	—	1	—
Thin crust pizza																				
Extravaganzza, 12"	¼	item(s)	159	425	20	34	3	24	9.41	—	—	—	53	245	1.95	1408	—	—	1	—
Pepperoni, extra pepperoni & cheese, 12"	¼	item(s)	159	420	20	32	2	24	10.46	—	—	—	54	316	1.34	1362	—	—	<1	—
Vegi, 12"	¼	item(s)	159	338	16	34	3	17	7.08	—	—	—	34	317	1.42	1047	—	—	1	—

Ultimate deep dish pizza																				
America's favorite, 12"	2	slice(s)	235	617	26	59	4	33	12.88	—	—	—	58	334	4.43	1573	—	—	1	—
Pepperoni, extra pepperoni & cheese, 12"	2	slice(s)	235	629	26	57	4	34	13.57	—	—	—	61	332	4.25	1650	—	—	1	—
Vegi, 12"	2	slice(s)	235	547	22	59	4	26	10.19	—	—	—	41	333	4.33	1334	—	—	2	—
In-n-Out Burger																				
Cheeseburger w/mustard & ketchup	1	item(s)	268	400	22	41	3	18	9.00	—	—	—	55	200	3.60	1080	—	—	15	—
Chocolate shake	1	item(s)	425	690	9	83	0	36	24.00	—	—	—	95	300	0.72	350	—	—	0	—
Double-Double cheeseburger w/mustard & ketchup	1	item(s)	328	590	37	42	3	32	17.00	—	—	—	115	350	5.40	1510	—	—	15	—
French fries	1	item(s)	125	400	7	54	2	18	5.00	—	—	—	0	20	1.80	245	—	—	0	—
Hamburger w/mustard & ketchup	1	item(s)	243	310	16	41	3	10	4.00	—	—	—	35	40	3.60	720	—	—	15	—
Jack in the Box																				
Chicken club salad	1	item(s)	535	310	28	15	5	16	6.00	—	—	0	65	300	3.60	890	—	—	54	—
Hamburger	1	item(s)	104	250	12	30	2	9	3.50	—	—	0.88	30	100	3.60	610	—	—	0	—
Jack's Spicy Chicken sandwich	1	item(s)	253	580	24	53	3	31	6.00	—	—	2.81	60	150	1.80	950	—	—	9	—
Jumbo Jack hamburger w/cheese	1	item(s)	294	690	26	60	3	38	16.00	—	—	1.55	75	250	4.50	1360	—	—	9	—
Sourdough Jack	1	item(s)	244	700	30	36	3	49	16.00	—	—	2.98	80	200	4.50	1220	—	—	9	—
Jamba Juice																				
Banana berry smoothie	24	fluid ounce(s)	719	470	5	112	5	2	0.50	—	—	—	5	200	1.08	85	0.32	33	15	0
Chocolate mood smoothie	24	fluid ounce(s)	612	690	16	142	2	8	4.50	—	—	—	25	500	1.08	280	0.00	9	6	4
Jamba powerboost smoothie	24	fluid ounce(s)	730	440	6	103	7	2	0.00	—	—	—	0	1100	1.44	40	17.71	640	294	70
Orange juice, freshly squeezed	16	fluid ounce(s)	496	220	3	52	1	1	0.00	—	—	—	0	60	1.08	0	—	160	246	0
Protein berry pizzaz smoothie	24	fluid ounce(s)	710	440	20	92	6	2	0.00	—	—	—	0	1100	2.62	240	0.31	58	60	4
Kentucky Fried Chicken (KFC)																				
Extra Crispy chicken, breast	1	item(s)	162	470	34	19	0	28	8.00	—	—	4.50	135	19	1.44	1230	—	—	1	—
Hot & spicy chicken, whole wing	1	item(s)	55	180	11	9	0	11	3.00	—	—	0	60	10	0.72	420	—	—	1	—
Original Recipe chicken, drumstick	1	item(s)	59	140	14	4	0	8	2.00	—	—	1	75	10	0.70	440	—	—	1	—
Long John Silver's																				
Baked cod	1	serving(s)	101	120	22	1	0	5	1.00	—	—	—	90	20	0.72	240	—	—	0	—
Batter dipped fish sandwich	1	item(s)	177	440	17	48	3	20	5.00	—	—	—	35	60	3.60	1120	—	—	9	—
Clam chowder	1	item(s)	227	220	9	23	0	10	4.00	—	—	—	25	150	0.72	810	—	—	0	—
Crunchy shrimp basket	21	item(s)	114	340	12	32	2	19	5.00	—	—	—	105	500	1.80	720	—	—	1	—
McDonald's																				
Big Mac hamburger	1	item(s)	216	590	24	47	3	34	11.00	—	—	1.48	85	300	4.50	1090	—	—	4	—
Cheeseburger	1	item(s)	121	330	15	36	2	14	6.00	—	—	1.02	45	250	2.70	830	—	—	2	—
Chicken McNuggets	4	item(s)	72	210	10	12	1	13	2.50	—	—	1.13	35	20	0.72	460	—	—	1	—
Egg McMuffin	1	item(s)	138	300	18	29	2	12	4.50	—	—	0.42	235	300	2.70	830	0.72	—	1	—
Filet-o-fish sandwich	1	item(s)	156	470	15	45	1	26	5.00	—	—	1.11	50	200	1.80	890	—	—	1	—
French fries, small	1	serving(s)	68	210	3	26	2	10	1.50	—	—	2.30	0	10	0.36	135	—	—	9	—
Fruit n' yogurt parfait	1	item(s)	338	380	10	76	2	5	2.00	—	—	0.18	15	300	1.80	240	—	—	24	—
Hash browns	1	item(s)	53	130	1	14	1	8	1.50	—	—	2	0	10	0.36	330	—	—	2	—
Honey sauce	1	item(s)	14	45	0	12	0	0	0.00	0.00	0.00	—	0	10	0.18	0	—	—	1	—
McSalad Shaker garden salad	1	item(s)	149	100	7	4	2	6	3.00	—	—	—	75	150	1.08	120	—	—	15	—
McSalad Shaker grilled chicken caesar salad	1	item(s)	163	100	17	3	2	3	1.50	—	—	—	40	100	1.08	240	—	—	12	—
Newman's Own creamy Caesar salad dressing	1	item(s)	59	190	2	4	0	18	3.50	—	—	0.29	20	60	0.18	500	15.40	—	1	—
Plain hotcakes w/syrup & margarine	3	item(s)	228	600	9	104	0	17	3.00	—	—	4	20	100	4.50	770	—	—	1	—
Quarter Pounder hamburger	1	item(s)	172	430	23	37	2	21	8.00	—	—	1.01	70	200	4.50	840	—	—	2	—
Quarter Pounder hamburger w/cheese	1	item(s)	200	530	28	38	2	30	13.00	—	—	1.51	95	350	4.50	1310	—	—	2	—
Sausage McMuffin w/egg	1	item(s)	164	450	20	29	2	28	10.00	—	—	0.59	255	300	2.70	930	0.72	—	1	—
Vanilla milkshake	8	fluid ounce(s)	227	254	9	40	0	7	4.28	1.98	0.26	—	27	331	0.23	215	0.11	16	0	5
Pizza Hut																				
Pepperoni Lovers stuffed crust pizza	1	slice(s)	171	480	23	44	3	24	11.00	—	—	1.05	65	300	2.70	1300	—	—	4	—
Pepperoni Lovers thin 'n crispy pizza	1	slice(s)	94	270	13	22	2	14	7.00	—	—	0.51	40	200	1.44	700	—	—	2	—
Personal Pan supreme pizza	1	slice(s)	73	170	8	19	1	7	3.00	—	—	0.95	15	80	1.86	400	—	—	4	—
Veggie Lovers stuffed crust pizza	1	slice(s)	181	370	17	45	3	14	7.00	—	—	0.53	35	250	2.70	980	—	—	12	—
Veggie Lovers thin 'n crispy pizza	1	slice(s)	110	190	8	23	2	7	3.00	—	—	0.54	15	150	1.44	480	—	—	12	—

Food Description	Qty	Measure	Wt (g)	Ener (cal)	Prot (g)	Carb (g)	Dietary Fiber (g)	Fat (g)	Fat Breakdown (g) Sat	Mono	Poly	Trans	Chol (mg)	Calc (mg)	Iron (mg)	Sodi (mg)	Vit E (mg)	Folate (mcg)	Vit C (mg)	Selenium (mcg)
Starbucks																				
Cappuccino, tall	12	fluid ounce(s)	360	120	7	10	0	6	4.00	—	—	—	25	250	0.00	95	—	—	1	—
Cinnamon spice mocha, tall nonfat w/o whipped cream	12	fluid ounce(s)	360	170	11	32	0	0	0.50	0.00	0.00	0	5	300	0.72	150	—	—	0	—
Frappuccino, tall chocolate	12	fluid ounce(s)	360	290	13	52	1	5	1.00	—	—	—	3	400	1.80	300	—	—	5	—
Latte, tall w/nonfat milk	12	fluid ounce(s)	360	123	12	17	0	1	0.40	0.16	0.02	0	6	420	0.18	174	—	18	4	—
Latte, tall w/whole milk	12	fluid ounce(s)	360	212	11	17	0	11	6.90	3.24	0.42	—	46	400	0.18	165	—	17	3	—
Macchiato, tall caramel w/whole milk	12	fluid ounce(s)	360	190	6	27	0	7	4.00	—	—	—	25	200	0.36	105	—	—	1	—
Tazo chai black tea, tall nonfat	12	fluid ounce(s)	360	170	6	37	0	0	0.00	0.00	0.00	0	5	200	0.36	95	—	—	0	—
Subway																				
Chocolate chip cookie	1	item(s)	48	209	3	29	1	10	3.50	—	—	1.07	12	0	1.00	135	—	—	0	—
Classic Italian B.M.T. sandwich, 6", white bread	1	item(s)	250	453	21	40	3	24	8.00	—	—	0	56	100	2.70	1740	—	—	24	—
Meatball sandwich, 6", white bread	1	item(s)	284	501	23	46	4	25	10.00	—	—	0.75	56	100	3.60	1350	—	—	24	—
Roast beef sandwich, 6", white bread	1	item(s)	220	264	18	39	3	5	1.00	—	—	0	20	40	3.60	840	—	—	24	—
Roasted chicken breast sandwich, 6", white bread	1	item(s)	234	311	25	40	3	6	1.50	—	—	0	48	60	3.60	880	—	—	24	—
Tuna sandwich, 6", white bread	1	item(s)	252	419	18	39	3	21	5.00	—	—	—	42	100	2.70	1180	—	—	24	—
Turkey breast sandwich, 6", white bread	1	item(s)	220	254	16	39	3	4	1.00	—	—	0	15	40	2.70	1000	—	—	24	—
Taco Bell																				
7-layer burrito	1	item(s)	283	530	18	67	10	22	8.00	—	—	3	25	300	3.59	1360	—	—	5	—
Beef burrito supreme	1	item(s)	248	440	18	51	7	18	8.00	—	—	2	40	200	2.70	1330	—	—	9	—
Grilled chicken burrito	1	item(s)	198	390	19	49	3	13	4.00	—	—	—	40	151	1.44	1240	—	—	2	—
Taco	1	item(s)	78	170	8	13	3	10	4.00	—	—	0.50	25	60	1.08	350	—	—	2	—
Veggie fajita wrap supreme	1	item(s)	255	470	11	55	3	22	7.00	—	—	—	30	150	1.44	990	—	—	6	—
CONVENIENCE MEALS																				
Budget Gourmet																				
Cheese manicotti w/meat sauce	1	item(s)	284	420	18	38	4	22	11.00	6.00	1.34	—	85	300	2.70	810	—	31	0	—
Chicken w/fettuccine	1	item(s)	284	380	20	33	3	19	10.00	—	—	—	85	100	2.70	810	—	—	0	—
Light beef stroganoff	1	item(s)	248	290	20	32	3	7	4.00	—	—	—	35	40	1.80	580	—	19	2	—
Light sirloin of beef in herb sauce	1	item(s)	269	260	19	30	5	7	4.00	2.30	0.31	—	30	40	1.80	850	—	38	6	—
Light vegetable lasagna	1	item(s)	298	290	15	36	5	9	1.79	0.89	0.60	—	15	283	3.03	780	—	75	59	—
Healthy Choice																				
Chicken enchilada suprema meal	1	item(s)	320	360	13	59	8	7	3.00	2.00	2.00	—	30	40	1.44	580	—	—	4	—
Lemon pepper fish meal	1	item(s)	303	280	11	49	5	5	2.00	1.00	2.00	—	30	40	0.36	580	—	—	30	—
Traditional salisbury steak meal	1	item(s)	354	360	23	45	5	9	3.50	4.00	1.00	—	45	80	2.70	580	—	—	21	—
Traditional turkey breasts meal	1	item(s)	298	330	21	50	4	5	2.00	1.50	1.50	—	35	40	1.44	600	—	—	0	—
Zucchini lasagna	1	item(s)	383	280	13	47	5	4	2.50	—	—	—	10	200	1.80	310	—	—	0	—
Stouffers																				
Cheese enchiladas with Mexican rice	1	serving(s)	276	370	12	48	5	14	5.00	—	—	—	25	200	1.44	890	—	—	12	—
Chicken pot pie	1	item(s)	284	740	23	56	4	47	18.00	12.41	10.48	—	65	150	2.70	1170	—	—	2	—
Homestyle beef pot roast & potatoes	1	item(s)	252	270	16	25	3	12	4.50	—	—	—	35	20	1.80	820	—	—	6	—
Homestyle roast turkey breast w/stuffing & mashed potatoes	1	item(s)	273	300	16	34	2	11	3.00	—	—	—	35	40	0.72	1190	—	—	0	—
Lean Cuisine Everyday Favorites chicken chow mein w/rice	1	item(s)	255	210	12	33	2	3	1.00	1.00	0.50	0	30	20	0.36	620	—	—	0	—
Lean Cuisine Everyday Favorites lasagna w/meat sauce	1	item(s)	291	300	19	41	3	8	4.00	2.00	0.50	0	30	200	1.08	650	—	—	5	—
Weight Watchers																				
Smart Ones chicken enchiladas suiza entree	1	serving(s)	255	270	15	33	2	9	3.50	—	—	—	50	250	1.08	660	—	—	4	—
Smart Ones garden lasagna entree	1	item(s)	312	270	14	36	5	7	3.50	—	—	—	30	350	1.80	610	—	—	6	—
Smart Ones pepperoni pizza	1	item(s)	158	390	23	46	4	12	4.00	—	—	—	45	450	1.80	650	—	—	5	—
Smart Ones spicy penne pasta & ricotta	1	item(s)	289	280	11	45	4	6	2.00	—	—	—	5	150	2.70	400	—	—	6	—
Smart Ones spicy Szechuan style vegetables & chicken	1	item(s)	255	220	11	39	3	2	0.50	—	—	—	10	150	1.80	730	—	—	2	—

glossary

Acquired immune deficiency syndrome (AIDS) Any of a number of diseases that arise when the body's immune system is compromised by HIV; the final stage of HIV infection.

Action stage Stage of change in the transtheoretical model in which the individual is actively changing a negative behavior or adopting a new, healthy behavior.

Activities of daily living Everyday behaviors that people normally do to function in life (cross the street, carry groceries, lift objects, do laundry, sweep floors, etc.).

Acupuncture A Chinese medical system that requires body piercing with fine needles during therapy to relieve pain and treat ailments and diseases.

Addiction Compulsive and uncontrollable behavior(s) or use of substance(s).

Adenosine triphosphate (ATP) A high-energy chemical compound that the body uses for immediate energy.

Adequate Intake (AI) The recommended amount of a nutrient intake when sufficient evidence is not available to calculate the EAR and subsequent RDA.

Adipose tissue Fat cells in the body.

Advanced glycation end products (AGEs) Derivatives of glucose–protein and glucose–lipid interactions that are linked to aging and chronic diseases.

Aerobic Exercise that requires oxygen to produce the necessary energy (ATP) to carry out the activity.

Agility The ability to quickly and efficiently change body position and direction.

Air displacement Technique to assess body composition by calculating the body volume from the air replaced by an individual sitting inside a small chamber.

Alcohol Ethyl alcohol, a depressant drug that affects the brain, slows central nervous system activity, and has strong addictive properties.

Alcoholism A disease in which an individual loses control over drinking alcoholic beverages.

Altruism Unselfish concern for the welfare of others.

Alveoli Air sacs in the lungs where gas exchange (oxygen and carbon dioxide) takes place.

Amenorrhea Cessation of regular menstrual flow.

Amino acids Chemical compounds that contain nitrogen, carbon, hydrogen, and oxygen; the basic building blocks the body uses to build different types of protein.

Amphetamines A class of powerful central nervous system stimulants.

Amotivational syndrome A condition characterized by loss of motivation, dullness, apathy, and no interest in the future.

Anabolic steroids Synthetic versions of the male sex hormone testosterone, which promotes muscle development and hypertrophy.

Anaerobic Exercise that does not require oxygen to produce the necessary energy (ATP) to carry out the activity.

Anaerobic threshold The highest percentage of VO_{2max} at which an individual can exercise (maximal steady state) for an extended time without accumulating significant amounts of lactic acid, which forces an individual to reduce exercise intensity or stop exercising.

Android obesity Obesity pattern seen in individuals who tend to store fat in the trunk or abdominal area.

Angiogenesis The formation of blood vessels (capillaries).

Angina pectoris Chest pain associated with CHD.

Angioplasty A procedure in which a balloon-tipped catheter is inserted and then inflated to widen the inner lumen of the artery.

Anorexia nervosa An eating disorder characterized by self-imposed starvation to lose and maintain very low body weight.

Anthropometric measurement Techniques to measure body girths at different sites.

Antibodies Substances produced by the white blood cells in response to an invading agent.

Antioxidants Compounds such as vitamins C and E, beta-carotene, and selenium that prevent oxygen from combining with other substances in the body to form harmful compounds.

Aquaphobic Having a fear of water.

Arrhythmias Irregular heart rhythms.

Arterial–venous oxygen difference ($a\text{-}vO2_{diff}$) Amount of oxygen removed from the blood as determined by the difference in oxygen content between arterial and venous blood.

Atherosclerosis Fatty or cholesterol deposits in the walls of the arteries leading to formation of plaque.

Atrophy Decrease in the size of a cell.

Autogenic training A stress management technique using a form of self-suggestion, wherein an individual is able to place himself or herself in an autohypnotic state by repeating and concentrating on feelings of heaviness and warmth in the extremities.

Ayurveda A Hindu system of medicine based on herbs, diet, massage, meditation, and yoga to help the body boost its natural healing process.

Balance The ability to maintain the body in proper equilibrium.

Ballistic (dynamic) stretching Stretching exercises performed with jerky, rapid, and bouncy movements.

Basal metabolic rate (BMR) The lowest level of oxygen consumption (and energy requirement) necessary to sustain life.

Behavior modification The process of permanently changing negative behaviors to positive behaviors that will lead to better health and well-being.

Benign Noncancerous.

Binge-eating disorder An eating disorder characterized by uncontrollable episodes of eating excessive amounts of food within a relatively short time.

Bioelectrical impedance Technique to assess body composition by running a weak electrical current through the body.

Biofeedback A stress management technique in which a person learns to influence physiological responses that are not typically under voluntary control or responses that typically are regulated but for which regulation has broken down as a result of injury, trauma, or illness.

Blood lipids (fats) Cholesterol and triglycerides.

Blood pressure A measure of the force exerted against the walls of the vessels by the blood flowing through them.

Bod Pod Commercial name of the equipment used to assess body composition through the air displacement technique.

Body composition The fat and non-fat components of the human body; important in assessing recommended body weight.

Body mass index (BMI) Technique to determine thinness and excessive fatness that incorporates height and weight to estimate critical fat values at which the risk for disease increases.

Bradycardia Slower heart rate than normal.

Breathing exercises A stress management technique wherein the individual concentrates on "breathing away" the tension and inhaling fresh air to the entire body.

Bulimia nervosa An eating disorder characterized by a pattern of binge eating and purging in an attempt to lose weight and maintain low body weight.

C-reactive protein (CRP) A protein whose blood levels increase with inflammation, at times hidden deep in the body; elevation of this protein is an indicator of potential cardiovascular events.

Calorie The amount of heat necessary to raise the temperature of one gram of water 1°C; used to measure the energy value of food and cost (energy expenditure) of physical activity.

Cancer A group of diseases characterized by uncontrolled growth and spread of abnormal cells.

Capillaries Smallest blood vessels carrying oxygenated blood to the tissues in the body.

Carbohydrates A classification for nutrients containing carbon, hydrogen, and oxygen; the major source of energy for the human body.

Carbohydrate loading Increasing intake of carbohydrates during heavy aerobic training or prior to aerobic endurance events that last longer than 90 minutes.

Carcinogens Substances that contribute to the formation of cancers.

Carcinoma in situ An encapsulated malignant tumor that has not spread.

Cardiac output Amount of blood pumped by the heart in one minute.

Cardiomyopathy A disease affecting the heart muscle.

Cardiorespiratory endurance The ability of the lungs, heart, and blood vessels to deliver adequate amounts of oxygen to the cells to meet the demands of prolonged physical activity.

Cardiorespiratory (CR) training zone Recommended TI range, in terms of exercise heart rate, to obtain adequate CR endurance development.

Cardiovascular disease (CVD) The array of conditions that affect the heart and the blood vessels.

Carotenoids Pigment substances in plants that are often precursors to vitamin A. More than 600 carotenoids are found in nature, about 50 of which are precursors to vitamin A, the most potent one being beta-carotene.

Catecholamines Fight-or-flight hormones, including epinephrine and norepinephrine.

Cellulite Term frequently used in reference to fat deposits that "bulge out," caused by the herniation of subcutaneous fat within fibrous connective tissue and giving the tissue a padded appearance.

Chiropractics A health care system that proposes many diseases and ailments are related to misalignments of the vertebrae and emphasizes manipulation of the spinal column.

Chlamydia An STI, caused by a bacterial infection, that can significantly damage the reproductive system.

Cholesterol A waxy substance, technically a steroid alcohol, found only in animal fats and oil and used in making cell membranes, as a building block for some hormones, in the fatty sheath around nerve fibers, and in other necessary substances.

Chronic diseases Illnesses that develop as a result of an unhealthy lifestyle and last a long time.

Chronological age Calendar age.

Chylomicrons Triglyceride-transporting molecules.

Circuit training Alternating exercises by performing them in a sequence of three to six or more.

Cirrhosis A disease characterized by scarring of the liver.

Clinical study A research study in which the investigator intervenes (makes certain changes or uses certain interventions or programs) to prevent or treat a disease.

Cocaine 2-beta-carbomethoxy-3-betabenozoxytropane, the primary psychoactive ingredient derived from coca plant leaves.

Cold turkey Eliminating a negative behavior all at once.

Complementary and alternative medicine (CAM) A group of diverse medical and health care systems, practices, and products that are not presently considered part of conventional medicine; also called unconventional, nonallopathic, or integrative medicine.

Complex carbohydrates Carbohydrates formed by three or more simple sugar molecules linked together; also referred to as polysaccharides.

Concentric Shortening of a muscle during muscle contraction.

Contemplation stage Stage of change in the transtheoretical model in which the individual is considering changing behavior within the next six months.

Contraindicated exercises Exercises that are not recommended because they may cause injury to a person.

Controlled ballistic stretching Exercises done with slow, short, gentle, and sustained movements.

Conventional Western medicine A traditional medical practice based on methods that are tested through rigorous scientific trials; also called allopathic medicine.

Cooldown Tapering off an exercise session slowly.

Coordination The integration of the nervous and muscular systems to produce correct, graceful, and harmonious body movements.

Core strength training A program designed to strengthen the abdominal, hip, and spinal muscles (the core of the body).

Coronary heart disease (CHD) A condition in which the arteries that supply the heart muscle with oxygen and nutrients are narrowed by fatty deposits, such as cholesterol and triglycerides.

Creatine An organic compound derived from meat, fish, and amino acids that combines with inorganic phosphate to form CP.

Creatine phosphate (CP) A high-energy compound that the cells use to resynthesize ATP during all-out activities of very short duration.

Cross-training A combination of aerobic activities that contribute to overall fitness.

Cruciferous vegetables Plants that produce cross-shaped leaves (cauliflower, broccoli, cabbage, Brussels sprouts, and kohlrabi), which seem to have a protective effect against cancer.

Daily Values (DVs) Reference values for nutrients and food components used in food labels.

Dentists Practitioners who specialize in diseases of the teeth, gums, and oral cavity.

Deoxyribonucleic acid (DNA) The genetic substance of which genes are made; the molecule that contains a cell's genetic code.

Diabetes mellitus A disease in which the body doesn't produce or utilize insulin properly.

Diastolic blood pressure (DBP) Pressure exerted by the blood against the walls of the arteries during the relaxation phase (diastole) of the heart.

Dietary fiber A complex carbohydrate in plant foods that is not digested but is essential to digestion.

Dietary Reference Intakes (DRIs) A general term that describes four types of nutrient standards that establish adequate amounts and maximum safe nutrient intakes in the diet: EAR, RDA, AI, and UL.

Disaccharides Simple carbohydrates formed by two monosaccharide units linked together, one of which is glucose. The major disaccharides are sucrose, lactose, and maltose.

Distress Negative stress; unpleasant or harmful stress under which health and performance begin to deteriorate.

Dopamine A neurotransmitter that affects emotional, mental, and motor functions.

Dual energy x-ray absorptiometry (DXA) Method to assess body composition that uses very low-dose beams of x-ray energy to measure total body fat mass, fat distribution pattern, and bone density.

Dynamic constant external resistance (DCER) See fixed resistance.

Dynamic stretching Stretching exercises that require speed of movement, momentum, and active muscular effort to help increase the range of motion around a joint or group of joints.

Dynamic training Strength-training method referring to a muscle contraction with movement.

Dysmenorrhea Painful menstruation.

Eccentric Lengthening of a muscle during muscle contraction.

Elastic elongation Temporary lengthening of soft tissue.

Electrocardiogram (ECG or EKG) A recording of the electrical activity of the heart.

Electrolytes Substances that become ions in solution and are critical for proper muscle and neuron activation (include sodium, potassium, chloride, calcium, magnesium, phosphate, and bicarbonate).

Emotional eating The consumption of large quantities of food to suppress negative emotions.

Emotional wellness The ability to understand your own feelings, accept your limitations, and achieve emotional stability.

Endorphins Morphinelike substances released from the pituitary gland (in the brain) during prolonged aerobic exercise and thought to induce feelings of euphoria and natural well-being.

Energy-balancing equation A principle holding that as long as caloric input equals caloric output, the person does not gain or lose weight. If caloric intake exceeds output, the person gains weight; when output exceeds input, the person loses weight.

Environmental wellness The capability to live in a clean and safe environment that is not detrimental to health.

Enzymes Catalysts that facilitate chemical reactions in the body.

Epigenetics The study of differences in an organism caused by changes in gene expression rather than changes in the genome itself.

Essential fat Minimal amount of body fat needed for normal physiological functions; constitutes about 3 percent of total weight in men and 12 percent in women.

Estimated Average Requirement (EAR) The amount of a nutrient that meets the dietary needs of half the people in a specific age and gender group.

Estimated Energy Requirement (EER) The average dietary energy (caloric) intake that is predicted to maintain energy balance in a healthy adult of defined age, gender, weight, height, and level of physical activity, consistent with good health.

Estrogen Female sex hormone essential for bone formation and conservation of bone density.

Eustress Positive stress; health and performance continue to improve even as stress increases.

Exercise A type of physical activity that requires planned, structured, and repetitive bodily movement with the intent of improving or maintaining one or more components of physical fitness.

Exercise intolerance The inability to function during exercise because of excessive fatigue or extreme feelings of discomfort.

Explanatory style The way people perceive the events in their lives, from an optimistic or a pessimistic perspective.

Fast-twitch fibers Muscle fibers with greater anaerobic potential and fast speed of contraction.

Fats A classification for nutrients containing carbon, hydrogen, some oxygen, and sometimes other chemical elements.

Ferritin Iron stored in the body.

Fight-or-flight mechanism The physiological response of the body to stress that prepares the individual to take action by stimulating the body's vital defense systems.

Fighting spirit Determination; the open expression of emotions, whether negative or positive.

FITT Acronym used to describe the four CR exercise prescription variables: frequency, intensity, type (mode), and time (duration).

Fixed resistance Type of exercise in which a constant resistance is moved through a joint's full range of motion (dumbbells, barbells, and machines using a constant resistance).

Flexibility The achievable range of motion at a joint or group of joints without causing injury.

Folate One of the B vitamins.

Fortified foods Foods that have been modified by the addition or increase of nutrients that either were not present or were present in insignificant amounts, with the intent of preventing nutrient deficiencies.

Free weights Barbells and dumbbells.

Frequency Number of times per week a person engages in exercise.

Functional capacity The ability to perform ordinary and unusual demands of daily living without limitations and excessive fatigue or injury.

Functional foods Foods or food ingredients containing physiologically active substances that provide specific health benefits beyond those supplied by basic nutrition.

Functional independence The ability to carry out activities of daily living without assistance from other individuals.

General adaptation syndrome (GAS) A theoretical model that explains the body's adaptation to sustained stress. It includes three stages: alarm reaction, resistance, and exhaustion and recovery.

Genetically modified (GM) food Food whose basic genetic material (DNA) is manipulated by inserting genes with desirable traits from one plant, animal, or microorganism into another one to either introduce new traits or enhance existing ones.

Genital herpes An STI caused by a viral infection of HSV-1 or HSV-2. The virus can attack different areas of the body but typically causes blisters on the genitals.

Genital warts An STI caused by a viral infection.

Girth measurements Technique to assess body composition by measuring circumferences at specific body sites.

Glucose intolerance A condition characterized by slightly elevated blood glucose levels.

Glycemic index A measure used to rate the plasma glucose response of carbohydrate-containing foods, comparing it with the response produced by the same amount of carbohydrates from a standard source, usually glucose or white bread.

Glycogen Form in which glucose is stored in the body.

Goals The ultimate aims toward which effort is directed.

Gonorrhea An STI caused by a bacterial infection.

Gynoid obesity Obesity pattern seen in people who store fat primarily around the hips and thighs.

Hatha yoga A form of yoga that incorporates specific sequences of static-stretching postures to help induce the relaxation response.

Health State of complete well-being—not just the absence of disease or infirmity.

Health fitness standards The lowest fitness requirements for maintaining good health, decreasing the risk for chronic diseases, and lowering the incidence of muscular–skeletal injuries.

Health promotion The science and art of enabling people to increase control over their lifestyle to move toward a state of wellness.

Health-related fitness Fitness programs prescribed to improve the individual's overall health.

Heart rate reserve (HRR) The difference between the MHR and the RHR.

Heat cramps Muscle spasms caused by heat-induced changes in electrolyte balance in muscle cells.

Heat exhaustion Heat-related fatigue.

Heat stroke An emergency situation resulting from the body being subjected to high atmospheric temperatures.

Hemoglobin Protein–iron compound in red blood cells that transports oxygen in the blood.

Hepatitis B (HBV) An STI caused by a viral infection that affects the liver.

Herbal medicine An unconventional system that uses herbs to treat ailments and disease.

Heroin A potent drug that is a derivative of opium.

High-density lipoproteins (HDLs) Cholesterol-transporting molecules in the blood ("good" cholesterol) that help clear cholesterol from the blood.

High-intensity interval training (HIIT) A training program that involves high- to very high-intensity (80 to 90 percent of maximal capacity) intervals, each followed by a low- to moderate-intensity recovery interval. Usually, a 1:3 or lower work-to-recovery ratio is used.

Homeopathy A system of treatment based on the use of minute quantities of remedies that in large amounts produce effects similar to the disease being treated.

Homeostasis A natural state of equilibrium, which the body attempts to maintain by constantly reacting to external forces that attempt to disrupt this fine balance.

Homocysteine An amino acid that, when allowed to accumulate in the blood, may lead to plaque formation and blockage of arteries.

Human immunodeficiency virus (HIV) A virus that leads to AIDS.

Human papillomavirus (HPV) A group of viruses that can cause STIs.

Hydrostatic weighing Underwater technique to assess body composition; considered the most accurate of the body composition assessment techniques.

Hypertension Chronically elevated blood pressure.

Hypertrophy An increase in the size of the cell, as in muscle hypertrophy.

Hypokinetic diseases *Hypo* denotes "lack of"; therefore, illnesses related to lack of physical activity.

Hyponatremia A low sodium concentration in the blood caused by overhydration with water.

Hypotension Low blood pressure.

Hypothermia A breakdown in the body's ability to generate heat; a drop in body temperature below 95°F.

Imagery Mental visualization of relaxing images and scenes to induce body relaxation in times of stress or as an aid in the treatment of certain medical conditions, such as cancer, hypertension, asthma, chronic pain, and obesity.

Immunity The function that guards the body from invaders, both internal and external.

Insulin A hormone secreted by the pancreas; essential for proper metabolism of blood glucose (sugar) and maintenance of blood glucose level.

Insulin resistance The inability of the cells to respond appropriately to insulin.

Integrative medicine The combination of the practices and methods of alternative medicine with conventional Western medicine.

Intensity In CR exercise, how hard a person has to exercise to improve or maintain fitness. In flexibility exercise, the degree of stretch.

International unit (IU) Measure of nutrients in food.

Isokinetic training Strength-training method in which the speed of the muscle contraction is kept constant because the equipment (machine) provides an accommodating resistance to match the user's force (maximal) through the range of motion.

Isometric training Strength-training method referring to a muscle contraction that produces little or no movement, such as pushing or pulling against an immovable object.

Iyengar yoga A form of yoga that aims to develop flexibility, strength, balance, and stamina using props (belts, blocks, blankets, and chairs) to aid in the correct performance of asanas, or yoga postures.

Lactic acid End product of anaerobic glycolysis (metabolism).

Lactovegetarians Vegetarians who consume foods from the milk group.

Lapse (v.) To slip or fall back temporarily into unhealthy behavior(s); (n.) short-term failure to maintain healthy behaviors.

Lean body mass Body weight without body fat.

Learning theories Behavioral modification perspective stating that most behaviors are learned and maintained under complex schedules of reinforcement and anticipated outcomes.

Life expectancy Number of years a person is expected to live based on the person's birth year.

Lipoproteins Lipids covered by proteins, which transport fats in the blood. Types are LDL, HDL, and VLDL.

Locus of control A concept examining the extent to which a person believes he or she can influence the external environment.

Low-density lipoproteins (LDLs) Cholesterol-transporting molecules in the blood ("bad" cholesterol) that tend to increase blood cholesterol.

Lymphocytes Immune system cells responsible for waging war against disease or infection.

MDMA 3,4-methylenedioxymethamphetamine, a synthetic hallucinogen drug with a chemical structure that closely resembles MDA and methamphetamine; also known as Ecstasy.

Magnetic therapy Unconventional treatment that relies on magnetic energy to promote healing.

Maintenance stage Stage of change in the transtheoretical model in which the individual maintains behavioral change for up to five years.

Malignant Cancerous.

Mammogram Low-dose x-rays of the breasts used as a screening technique for the early detection of breast tumors.

Marijuana A psychoactive drug prepared from a mixture of crushed leaves, flowers, small branches, stems, and seeds from the hemp plant *Cannabis sativa;* also called pot, grass, or weed.

Massage therapy The rubbing or kneading of body parts to treat ailments.

Maximal heart rate (MHR) Highest heart rate for a person, related primarily to age.

Maximal oxygen uptake (VO_{2max}) Maximum amount of oxygen the body is able to utilize per minute of physical activity, commonly expressed in milliliters per kilogram per minute (mL/kg/min); the best indicator of CR or aerobic fitness.

Meditation A stress management technique used to gain control over attention by clearing the mind and blocking out the stressor(s) responsible for the increased tension.

Mediterranean diet Typical diet of people around the Mediterranean region, focusing on olive oil, red wine, fish, grains, legumes, vegetables, and fruits, with limited amounts of red meat, fish, milk, and cheese.

Megadose For most vitamins, 10 times the RDA or more; for vitamin A, five times the RDA.

Melanoma The most virulent, rapidly spreading form of skin cancer.

Mental wellness A state in which your mind is engaged in lively interaction with the world around you.

Metabolic equivalent (MET) Rate of energy expenditure at rest; 1 MET is the equivalent of a VO_2 of 3.5 mL/kg/min.

Metabolic profile A measurement of plasma insulin, glucose, lipid, and lipoprotein levels to assess risk for diabetes and cardiovascular disease.

Metabolic syndrome An array of metabolic abnormalities that contribute to the development of atherosclerosis triggered by insulin resistance. These conditions include low HDL cholesterol, high triglycerides, high blood pressure, and an increased blood-clotting mechanism.

Metabolism All energy and material transformations that occur within living cells and are necessary to sustain life.

Metastasis The movement of cells from one part of the body to another.

Methamphetamine A potent form of amphetamine; also called meth.

Methylenedioxyamphetamine (MDA) A hallucinogenic drug that is structurally similar to amphetamines.

Minerals Inorganic nutrients essential for normal body functions and found in the body and in food.

Mitochondria Structures within the cells where energy transformations take place.

Mode Form or type of exercise.

Moderate-intensity exercise CR exercise that noticeably increases heart rate and breathing, one that requires an intensity level of approximately 50 percent of capacity.

Moderate physical activity Activity that uses 150 calories of energy per day, or 1,000 calories per week.

Monogamous A sexual relationship in which two people have sexual relations only with each other.

Monosaccharides The simplest carbohydrates (sugars), formed by five- or six-carbon skeletons. The three most common monosaccharides are glucose, fructose, and galactose.

Morbidity A condition related to or caused by illness or disease.

Motivation The desire and will to do something.

Motor neurons Nerves connecting the central nervous system to the muscle.

Motor unit The combination of a motor neuron and the muscle fibers that neuron innervates.

Muscular endurance The ability of a muscle to exert submaximal force repeatedly over time.

Muscular strength The ability of a muscle to exert maximum force against resistance (e.g., 1 repetition maximum [or 1 RM] on the bench press exercise).

Myocardial infarction Heart attack; damage to or death of an area of the heart muscle as a result of an obstructed artery to that area.

Myocardium Heart muscle.

Myofibrillar hypertrophy Muscle hypertrophy as a result of increased protein synthesis in the myosin and actin myofibrils.

Naturopathic medicine An unconventional system of medicine that relies exclusively on natural remedies to treat disease and ailments.

Negative resistance The lowering or eccentric phase of a repetition during a strength-training exercise.

Neustress Neutral stress; stress that is neither harmful nor helpful.

New psychoactive substances (NPS) Unregulated substances of abuse whose effects are made to mimic that of controlled drugs.

Nicotine An addictive compound found in tobacco leaves.

Nitrosamines Potentially cancer-causing compounds formed when nitrites and nitrates, which prevent the growth of harmful bacteria in processed meats, combine with other chemicals in the stomach.

Nonexercise activity thermogenesis (NEAT) Energy expended doing everyday activities not related to exercise.

Nonresponders Individuals who exhibit small or no improvements in fitness compared to others who undergo the same training program.

Nurses Health care practitioners who assist in the diagnosis and treatment of health problems and provide many services to patients in a variety of settings.

Nutrients Substances found in food that provide energy, regulate metabolism, and help with growth and repair of body tissues.

Nutrient density A measure of the amount of nutrients and calories in various foods.

Nutrition Science that studies the relationship of foods to optimal health and performance.

Obesity An excessive accumulation of body fat, usually at least 30 percent above recommended body weight.

Objectives Steps required to reach a goal.

Observational study A research study in which the investigator does not intervene to make changes but only observes the outcomes based on a particular lifestyle pattern.

Occupational wellness The ability to perform your job skillfully and effectively under conditions that provide personal and team satisfaction and adequately reward each individual.

Oligomenorrhea Irregular menstrual cycles.

Omega-3 fatty acids Polyunsaturated fatty acids found primarily in cold-water seafood, flaxseed, and flaxseed oil and thought to lower blood cholesterol and triglycerides.

Omega-6 fatty acids Polyunsaturated fatty acids found primarily in corn and sunflower oils and most oils in processed foods.

Oncogenes Genes that initiate cell division.

One repetition maximum (1 RM) The maximum amount of resistance an individual is able to lift in a single effort.

Ophthalmologists Medical specialists concerned with diseases of the eye and prescription of corrective lenses.

Opportunistic infections Infections that arise in the absence of a healthy immune system, which would fight them off in healthy people.

Optometrists Health care practitioners who specialize in the prescription and adaptation of lenses.

Oral surgeons Dentists who specialize in surgical procedures of the oral–facial complex.

Orthodontists Dentists who specialize in the correction and prevention of tooth irregularities.

Osteopath A medical practitioner with specialized training in musculoskeletal problems who uses diagnostic and therapeutic methods of conventional medicine, in addition to manipulative measures.

Osteoporosis A condition of softening, deterioration, or loss of bone mineral density that leads to disability, bone fractures, and even death from medical complications.

Overload principle Training concept that the demands placed on a system (cardiorespiratory or muscular) must be increased systematically and progressively over time to cause physiological adaptation (development or improvement).

Overtraining An emotional, behavioral, and physical condition marked by increased fatigue, decreased performance, persistent muscle soreness, mood disturbances, and feelings of "staleness" or "burnout" as a result of excessive physical training.

Overweight An excess amount of weight against a given standard, such as height or recommended percent body fat.

Ovolactovegetarians Vegetarians who include eggs and milk products in their diet.

Ovovegetarians Vegetarians who allow eggs in their diet.

Oxygen free radicals Substances formed during metabolism that attack and damage proteins and lipids, in particular the cell membrane and DNA, leading to diseases such as heart disease, cancer, and emphysema.

Oxygen uptake (VO_2) The amount of oxygen the human body uses.

Passive stretching Stretching exercises performed with the aid of an external force applied by either another individual or an external apparatus.

Pedometer An electronic device that senses body motion and counts footsteps. Some pedometers also record distance, calories burned, speeds, "aerobic steps," and time spent being physically active.

Pelvic inflammatory disease (PID) An overall designation referring to the effects of other STIs, primarily chlamydia and gonorrhea.

Percent body fat Proportional amount of fat in the body based on the person(s total weight; includes both essential fat and storage fat; also termed fat mass.

Periodization A training approach that divides the season into three cycles (macrocycles, mesocycles, and microcycles) using systematic variation in intensity and volume of training to enhance fitness and performance.

Peripheral vascular disease Narrowing of the peripheral blood vessels.

Peristalsis Involuntary muscle contractions of intestinal walls that facilitate excretion of wastes.

Personal trainer A health or fitness professional who evaluates, motivates, educates, and trains clients to help them meet individualized, healthy, lifestyle goals.

Physical activity Bodily movement produced by skeletal muscles, which requires expenditure of energy and produces progressive health benefits. Examples include walking, taking the stairs, dancing, gardening, working in the yard, cleaning the house, shoveling snow, washing the car, and all forms of structured exercise.

Physical activity perceived exertion (or H-PAPE) scale A perception scale to monitor or interpret the intensity of aerobic exercise.

Physical fitness The ability to meet the ordinary, as well as unusual, demands of daily life safely and effectively without being overly fatigued and still have energy left for leisure and recreational activities.

Physical fitness standards A fitness level that allows a person to sustain moderate-to-vigorous physical activity without undue fatigue and the ability to closely maintain this level throughout life.

Physical wellness Good physical fitness and confidence in your personal ability to take care of health problems.

Physician assistants Health care practitioners trained to treat most standard cases of care.

Physiological age The biological and functional capacity of the body as it should be in relation to the person's maximal potential at any given age in the lifespan.

Phytonutrients Compounds found in fruits and vegetables that block formation of cancerous tumors and disrupt the progress of cancer.

Phytonutrients Compounds thought to prevent and fight cancer and found in large quantities in fruits and vegetables.

Pilates A training program that uses exercises designed to help strengthen the body's core by developing pelvic stability and abdominal control; exercises are coupled with focused breathing patterns.

Plastic elongation Permanent lengthening of soft tissue.

Plyometric exercise Explosive jump training, incorporating speed and strength training to enhance explosiveness.

Positive resistance The lifting, pushing, or concentric phase of a repetition during a strength-training exercise.

Power The ability to produce maximum force in the shortest time.

Prayer Sincere and humble communication with a higher power.

Precontemplation stage Stage of change in the transtheoretical model in which an individual is unwilling to change behavior.

Preparation stage Stage of change in the transtheoretical model in which the individual is getting ready to make a change within the next month.

Primary care physician A medical practitioner who provides routine treatment of ailments; typically, the patient's first contact for health care.

Primordial prevention Prevention of the development of risk factors for disease.

Principle of individuality Training concept holding that genetics plays a major role in individual responses to exercise training and these differences must be considered when designing exercise programs for different people.

Probiotics Healthy microbes (bacteria) that help break down foods and prevent disease-causing organisms from settling in the intestines.

Problem solving model Behavioral modification model proposing that many behaviors are the result of making decisions as the individual seeks to solve the problem behavior.

Processed foods Includes all agricultural commodities that undergo processing (cooking, canning, freezing, dehydration, or milling) or addition of another ingredient.

Processes of change Actions that help you achieve change in behavior.

Progressive muscle relaxation A stress management technique that involves sequential contraction and relaxation of muscle groups throughout the body.

Progressive resistance training A gradual increase of resistance used during strength training over a period of time.

Proprioceptive neuromuscular facilitation (PNF) A mode of stretching that uses reflexes and neuromuscular principles to relax the muscles being stretched.

Proteins A classification for nutrients consisting of complex organic compounds containing nitrogen and formed by combinations of amino acids; the main substances used in the body to build and repair tissues.

Quackery and fraud The conscious promotion of unproven claims for profit.

Range of motion Entire arc of movement of a given joint.

Reaction time The time required to initiate a response to a given stimulus.

Recommended body weight Body weight at which there seems to be no harm to human health; healthy weight.

Recommended Dietary Allowance (RDA) The daily amount of a nutrient (statistically determined from the EAR) that is considered adequate to meet the known nutrient needs of almost 98 percent of all healthy people in the United States.

Recovery time Amount of time that the body takes to return to resting levels after exercise.

Registered dietitian (RD) A person with a college degree in dietetics who meets all certification and continuing education requirements of the American Dietetic Association or Dietitians of Canada.

Relapse (v.) To slip or fall back into unhealthy behavior(s) over a longer time; (n.) longer-term failure to maintain healthy behaviors.

Relapse prevention model Behavioral modification model based on the principle that high-risk situations can be anticipated through the development of strategies to prevent lapses and relapses.

Repetitions The number of times a given resistance is performed.

Resistance Amount of weight lifted.

Resistance training See strength training.

Responders Individuals who exhibit improvements in fitness as a result of exercise training.

Resting heart rate (RHR) Heart rate after a person has been sitting quietly for 15 to 20 minutes.

Resting metabolic rate (RMR) The energy requirement to maintain the body's vital processes in the resting state.

Resting metabolism Amount of energy (expressed in milliliters of oxygen per minute or total calories per day) an individual requires during resting conditions to sustain proper body function.

Reverse cholesterol transport A process in which HDL molecules attract cholesterol and carry it to the liver, where it is changed to bile and eventually excreted in the stool.

Ribonucleic acid (RNA) The genetic material that guides the formation of cell proteins.

RICE An acronym used to describe the standard treatment procedure for acute sports injuries: *r*est, *i*ce (cold application), *c*ompression, and *e*levation.

Risk factors Lifestyle and genetic variables that may lead to disease.

Sarcopenia Age-related loss of lean body mass, strength, and function.

Sarcoplasm The equivalent of the cytoplasm in other cells—a semifluid substance that contains myosin and actin filaments, as well other muscle cell organelles.

Sarcoplasmic hypertrophy Muscle hypertrophy as a result of an increase in sarcoplasm.

Sedentary Description of a person who is relatively inactive and whose lifestyle is characterized by a lot of sitting.

Sedentary death syndrome (SeDS) Cause of deaths attributed to a lack of regular physical activity.

Self-efficacy One's belief in the ability to perform a given task.

Self-esteem A sense of positive self-regard and self-respect.

Semivegetarians Vegetarians who include milk products, eggs, and fish and poultry in their diet.

Set A fixed number of repetitions; one set of bench presses might be 10 repetitions.

Setpoint Weight control theory that the body has an established weight and strongly attempts to maintain that weight.

Sexually transmitted infections (STIs) Communicable diseases spread through sexual contact.

Side stitch A sharp pain in the side of the abdomen.

Shin splints Injury to the lower leg characterized by pain and irritation in the shin region of the leg.

Simple carbohydrates Formed by simple or double sugar units with little nutritive value; divided into monosaccharides and disaccharides.

Skill-related fitness Fitness components important for success in skillful activities and athletic events; encompasses agility, balance, coordination, reaction time, speed, and power.

Skinfold thickness Technique to assess body composition by measuring a double thickness of skin at specific body sites.

Slow-twitch fibers Muscle fibers with greater aerobic potential and slow speed of contraction.

SMART (goals) An acronym used in reference to specific, measurable, attainable, realistic, and time-specific goals.

Social cognitive theory Behavioral modification model holding that behavior change is influenced by the environment, self-efficacy, and characteristics of the behavior itself.

Social wellness The ability to relate well to others, both within and outside the family unit.

Specific adaptation to imposed demand (SAID) training Training principle stating that, for improvements to occur in a specific activity, the exercises performed during a strength-training program should resemble as closely as possible the movement patterns encountered in that particular activity.

Specificity of training Principle that training must be done with the specific muscle(s) the person is attempting to improve.

Speed The ability to rapidly propel the body or a part of the body from one point to another.

Sphygmomanometer Inflatable bladder contained within a cuff and a mercury gravity manometer (or aneroid manometer) from which blood pressure is read.

Spiritual wellness The sense that life is meaningful and has purpose and that some power brings all humanity together; the ethics, values, and morals that guide you and give meaning and direction to life.

Spontaneous remission Inexplicable recovery from incurable disease.

Spot reducing Fallacious theory proposing that exercising a specific body part results in significant fat reduction in that area.

Static stretching (slow-sustained stretching) Exercises in which the muscles are lengthened gradually through a joint's complete range of motion.

Sterols Derived fats, of which cholesterol is the best-known example.

Storage fat Body fat in excess of essential fat; stored in adipose tissue.

Strength training A program designed to improve muscular strength and/or endurance through a series of progressive resistance (weight) training exercises that overload the muscular system and cause physiological development.

Stress The mental, emotional, and physiological response of the body to any situation that is new, threatening, frightening, or exciting.

Stress electrocardiogram An exercise test during which the workload is increased gradually until the individual reaches maximal fatigue, with blood pressure and 12-lead electrocardiographic monitoring throughout the test; also known as graded exercise stress test or maximal exercise tolerance test.

Stress events scale A questionnaire used to assess sources of stress in life.

Stressor A stress-causing event.

Stretching Moving the joints beyond the accustomed range of motion.

Stroke A condition in which a blood vessel that feeds the brain is clogged, leading to blood flow disruption to the brain.

Stroke volume Amount of blood pumped by the heart in one beat.

Structured interview An assessment tool used to determine behavioral patterns that define type A and type B personalities.

Subcutaneous fat Deposits of fat directly under the skin.

Subluxation Partial dislocation of a joint.

Substrates Substances acted upon by an enzyme (e.g., carbohydrates and fats).

Sun protection factor (SPF) The degree of protection offered by ingredients in sunscreen lotion; at least SPF 15 is recommended.

Supplements Tablets, pills, capsules, liquids, or powders containing vitamins, minerals, antioxidants, amino acids, herbs, or fiber that individuals take to increase their intake of these nutrients.

Suppressor genes Genes that deactivate the process of cell division.

Synergistic action The effect of mixing two or more drugs, which can be much greater than the sum of two or more drugs acting by themselves.

Synergy A reaction in which the result is greater than the sum of its two parts.

Syphilis An STI caused by a bacterial infection.

Systolic blood pressure (SBP) Pressure exerted by blood against walls of arteries during forceful contraction (systole) of the heart.

Tachycardia Faster-than-normal heart rate.

Tai chi A self-paced form of exercise often described as "meditation in motion," because it promotes serenity through gentle, balanced, low-impact movements that bring together the mind, body, and emotions.

Tar A chemical compound that forms during the burning of tobacco leaves.

Techniques of change Methods or procedures used during each process of change.

Telomerase An enzyme that allows cells to reproduce indefinitely.

Telomeres A strand of molecules at both ends of a chromosome.

Termination/adoption stage Stage of change in the transtheoretical model in which the individual has eliminated an undesirable behavior or maintained a positive behavior for more than five years.

Thermogenic response The amount of energy required to digest food.

Tolerable Upper Intake Level (UL) The highest level of nutrient intake that seems safe for most healthy people, beyond which exists an increased risk of adverse effects.

Trans-fatty acid Solidified fat formed by adding hydrogen to monounsaturated and polyunsaturated fats to increase shelf life.

Transtheoretical model Behavioral modification model proposing that change is accomplished through a series of progressive stages in keeping with a person's readiness to change.

Trichomoniasis An STI caused by a parasitical infection.

Triglycerides Fats formed by glycerol and three fatty acids; also called free fatty acids.

Type 1 diabetes Insulin-dependent diabetes mellitus, a condition in which the pancreas produces little or no insulin; also known as juvenile diabetes.

Type 2 diabetes Non-insulin-dependent diabetes mellitus, a condition in which insulin is not processed properly; also known as adult-onset diabetes.

Type A The behavior pattern characteristic of a hard-driving, overambitious, aggressive, and at times hostile and overly competitive person.

Type B The behavior pattern characteristic of a calm, casual, relaxed, and easygoing individual.

Type C The behavior pattern of individuals who are just as highly stressed as the type A but do not seem to be at higher risk for disease than the type B individuals.

Ultraviolet B (UVB) rays Ultraviolet rays that cause sunburn and lead to skin cancers.

Ultraviolet A (UVA) rays Ultraviolet rays that pass deeper into the skin and are believed to cause skin damage and skin cancers.

Underweight Extremely low body weight.

Variable resistance Training using special machines equipped with mechanical devices that provide differing amounts of resistance through the range of motion.

Vegans Vegetarians who eat no animal products.

Vegetarians Individuals whose diet is of vegetable or plant origin.

Very low-calorie diet A diet that allows an energy intake (consumption) of only 800 calories or less per day.

Very low-density lipoproteins (VLDLs) Triglyceride, cholesterol, and phospholipid-transporting molecules in the blood.

Vigorous activity Any exercise that requires a metabolic equivalent task (MET) level equal to or greater than 6 METs (21 mL/kg/min). One MET is the energy expenditure at rest (3.5 mL/kg/min), and METs are defined as multiples of this resting metabolic rate (examples of activities that require a 6-MET level include aerobics, walking uphill at 3.5 mph, cycling at 10 to 12 mph, playing doubles in tennis, and vigorous strength training).

Vigorous exercise CR exercise that requires an intensity level of approximately 70 percent of capacity.

Vitamins Organic nutrients essential for normal metabolism, growth, and development of the body.

Volume (of training) The total amount of training performed in a given work period (day, week, month, or season).

Volume (in strength training) The sum of all repetitions performed multiplied by resistances used during a strength-training session.

Waist circumference (WC) A waist girth measurement to assess potential risk for disease based on intra-abdominal fat content.

Warm-up Starting a workout slowly.

Water The most important classification for essential body nutrients, involved in almost every vital body process.

Weight-regulating mechanism (WRM) A feature of the hypothalamus of the brain that controls how much the body should weigh.

Wellness The constant and deliberate effort to stay healthy and achieve the highest potential for well-being. It encompasses seven dimensions—physical, emotional, mental, social, environmental, occupational, and spiritual—and integrates them all into a quality life.

Whole grains Foods that contain all three major parts of a seed grain: the germ, the bran, and the endosperm. Each part contains essential nutrients and plant chemicals that work in synergy to provide optimal health and prevent disease.

Workload Load (or intensity) placed on the body during physical activity.

Yoga A school of thought in the Hindu religion that seeks to help the individual attain a higher level of spirituality and peace of mind.

Answers to Assess Your Knowledge

1	2	3	4	5	6	7	8	9	10	11	12	13	14	15
1. c	1. a	1. b	1. e	1. b	1. a	1. c	1. b	1. d	1. a	1. e	1. b	1. e	1. c	1. e
2. e	2. a	2. e	2. b	2. c	2. d	2. d	2. e	2. a	2. c	2. b	2. a	2. a	2. b	2. c
3. d	3. e	3. c	3. d	3. e	3. c	3. a	3. a	3. b	3. c	3. a	3. a	3. c	3. e	3. b
4. a	4. d	4. d	4. a	4. a	4. c	4. b	4. a	4. e	4. e	4. e	4. e	4. d	4. e	4. d
5. e	5. c	5. d	5. b	5. b	5. c	5. d	5. b	5. d	5. e	5. e	5. e	5. d	5. d	5. e
6. d	6. d	6. a	6. e	6. e	6. e	6. a	6. e	6. b	6. e	6. e	6. e	6. d	6. a	6. a
7. c	7. a	7. a	7. b	7. a	7. b	7. c	7. c	7. a	7. a	7. e	7. b	7. d	7. a	7. e
8. b	8. b	8. c	8. b	8. c	8. d	8. c	8. b	8. e	8. a	8. e	8. e	8. e	8. d	8. c
9. a	9. e	9. a	9. e	9. d	9. c	9. e	9. e	9. a	9. b	9. e	9. b	9. e	9. e	9. e
10. b	10. e	10. e	10. e	10. e	10. c	10. e	10. d	10. e	10. c	10. a	10. e	10. e	10. c	10. a

index

A

Abdominal-crunch
on stability ball, 301
with weights, 291
without weights, 287
Abdominal-crunch test, 265–266 (Figure 7.3)
Acceptable goals, 66
Accidents, 6–7
ACSM. *See* American College of Sports Medicine (ACSM)
Action stage, 59
Activities of daily living (ADL), 260–261
Acupuncture, 553
Addiction. *See also* Drug abuse
behavior assessment, 518
behavior questionnaires, 521–522 (Lab 13A)
defined, 492
FAQs, 493
knowledge assessment, 518–519
my profile, 493
risk factors for, 494–495
symptoms of, 493
tobacco, 511
treatment of, 493, 506
types of, 492–493
Adductor stretch, 331
Adenosine triphosphate (ATP)
cardiovascular endurance and, 218
defined, 117
strength training and, 275
Adequate intake (AI), 94–95
Adipose tissue, 83
Adolescents
drug use among, 494
physical activity guidelines for, 10
STIs and, 528 (Figure 14.1)
Advanced glycation end products (AGEs), 106–107
Aerobic, 219
Aerobic exercise
apps for, 235–236
asthmatics and, 351–352
benefits of, 220–222
blood pressure management with, 446, 447 (Table 11.12)
body composition and, 156 (Figure 4.12)
cardiovascular benefits of, 216–217
cooldown, 238
CR endurance and, 219–220
duration recommendation, 237–238
energy drinks for, 217
examples of, 219–220
fitness benefits of, 240–242
fluid replacement during, 357
frequency of, 238–239
guidelines, 240 (Figure 6.11)
H-PAPE in, 236
hard-intensity intervals, 368
heart rate, assessment, 249–252 (Lab 6B)
mode of, 236–237
periodization in, 369
physical high from, 351
prescription for, 255–256 (Lab 6D)
principles of, 232–233
progression rate for, 239–240
readiness questionnaire, 253–254 (Lab 6C)
recommended pattern for, 235 (Figure 6.7)
record form for, 243 (Figure 6.12)
responders/nonresponders, 222–223
selected activities, ratings of, 241 (Table 6.10)
starting and committing to, 242, 244–245
stepwise intensity interval, 368
training zone, 234
warm-up, 238
weight-maintenance benefits, 184
African Americans
CAM use by, 555
cancer risk, 460
CVD among, 447
diets of, 108
hypertension among, 443–447
STI risk for, 535
Agility tests, 346–347
Aging
activity recommendations based on, 9–10
BMR and, 181
CVD and, 449
exercise and, 361
functional capacity, lifestyles and, 550 (Figure 15.1)
mental decline and, 387
muscle fitness and, 260–263
physical activity and, 548
process of, 550
types of, 548
AIDS. *See* HIV/AIDS
Alarm reaction, 387
Alcohol
caloric values of, 99 (Figure 3.7)
cancer and, 466–467
defined, 503
reducing use, 505–506
social acceptance of, 502–503
standard drink, 503
Alcohol abuse
behavior questionnaire, 522 (Lab 13A)
college students use of, 504–505, 505 (Figure 13.3)
consequences of, 503–504
long-term risks, 504 (Figure 13.2)
prevalence of, 503
Alcoholism, 503
All-out interval training, 368
Allopathic medicine. *See* Conventional western medicine
Alpha-linoleic acid (ALA), 88
Alternating bent leg sit-ups, 322 (Figure 8.5)
Altruism, 17–18
Alveoli
defined, 219
function of, 218
normal and diseased, 508 (Figure 13.5)
Alzheimer's disease, 384
Ambulatory activities, 190
Amenorrhea
defined, 123
exercise and, 354
osteoporosis risk and, 122
American College of Sports Medicine (ACSM), 559
Amino acids
characterization of, 89
classification of, 90 (Table 3.3)
defined, 89
levels, strength training and, 277
Amotivational syndrome, 496–497
Amphetamines, 498–499
Anabolic steroids, 262
Anaerobic
defined, 219
exercise, CR endurance and, 219–220
threshold, 239
Anaerobic acid system, 117
Android obesity, 151
Anger management, 392
Angina pectoris, 431
Angiogenesis, 459
Angioplasty, 425
Anorexia athletica, 177
Anorexia nervosa, 174–175
Antibiotics, 79
Antibodies, 384
Antioxidants
effectiveness of, 110
food sources of, 113
polynutrients *vs.*, 81
protection of, 111 (Figure 3.13)
Apps, 235–236
Aquaphobic, 139
Arm circles, 329
Arm curl, 288, 295
Arrhythmias, 448–449
Arterial–venous oxygen difference, 223–224
Arteries, 432 (Figure 11.6)
Arthritis, 352
Ashwell shape chart, 153 (Figure 4.10)
Asian Americans
CAM use by, 555
CVD among, 447
diets of, 109
Aspirin therapy, 450, 457
Asthma, 351–352
Astrand-Rhyming test
administration of, 227–228
benefits of, 226
estimates, 230 (Table 6.5)
Atherosclerosis
cholesterol profile and, 431–432
defined, 431
process of, 431 (Figure 11.5)
vitamin E and C effects on, 434
Athletes. *See also* Sports
carbohydrate loading by, 118–119
creatine for, 119
eating disorders and, 177
HIIT training for, 363–366
supplementation for, 117–118
Atkins diet, 171
ATP-CP system, 117
Atrophy, 268
Autogenic training, 402
Ayurveda, 553

B

Back extension, 300
Back extension stretch, 334
Back pain. *See* Lower back pain
Back stretch, 333
Balance test, 347
Ballistic stretching, 318
Barefoot running, 355–356
Basal metabolic rate (BMR)
aging and, 181
defined, 179
function of, 178
muscle mass and, 184
slowing of, 179
Behavior
addictive, 60
fitness and wellness goals, 562
HIV/AIDs and, 537–538
patterns, 389
supportive, 60 (Figure 2.4)
values and, 50–51
Behavior modification. *See also* Change
behavior assessment, 67
defined, 61
knowledge assessment, 67–68
my profile, 45
self-efficacy in, 54
theories of, 57–61
weight management adherence and, 195–196
Behavior modification planning
anger management tips, 392
blood chemistry test guidelines, 437
for cancer prevention, 463, 470, 481
change log, 73–74 (Lab 2B)
common time killers, 393
diabetes prevention, 442
drinking on dates, 505
eating on the run, 180
exercise compliance tips, 244
fast food fat content lists for, 98–99
financial fitness, 21–22
five-minute destress technique, 400
healthy diet guidelines, 115
healthy lifestyle habits, 28
hypertension prevention guidelines, 447
increasing physical activity tips, 222
lifestyle guidelines, 557
lower back pain prevention, 325
minimizing food contamination, 116
nutritious food selection, 104
overtraining symptoms, 367
for previously inactive people, 238

Behavior modification planning (continued)
restaurant eating strategies, 108
smoking cessation tips, 516–517
STI protection, 540
strategies, 196–199
strength training, 279
stress management characteristics, 401
stress symptoms, 395
successful, steps for, 62
thirty-second body scan, 397
type A personality changes, 391
for weight management
breakfast choices, 193
exercise guidelines, 183
lifetime, 155, 184
log for, 205 (Lab 5B)
physical activity guidelines, 183
Behavioral analysis
defined, 61
process of, 61–62
techniques for, 65 (Table 2.2)
Beliefs, 52
Bench (chest) press, 291
Bench-jump test, 265 (Figure 7.3)
Benign tumors, 456
Bent-arm pullover, 299
Bent-leg curl-up, 287
Bent-leg curl-up test, 265 (Figure 7.3)
Bent-over lateral raise, 292
Best life diet, 171
Beta-carotene, 111
Bias, Len, 497
Bicycle commuting, 364–365
Binge-eating disorder, 176
Bioelectric impedance, 142–143, 148
Bladder cancer, 479
Blood
cancer of, 480
chemistry test guidelines, 427
oxygen removed from, 223–224
vessels of, 426 (Figure 11.2)
Blood pressure. *See also* Hypertension
aerobic exercise effects on, 446
assessment of, 29–30
categories of, 29
defined, 443
guidelines, 443 (Table)
log for, 41–42 (Lab C)
mean, 29
measurement of, 443
BMR. *See* Basal metabolic rate (BMR)
Bod Pod, 140–141
Body composition
assessments for
accuracy of, 137
air displacement, 140–141
behavior, 156
bioelectric impedance, 142–143, 148
BMI, 137, 149–150, 150 (Table)
disease risk, 161–162 (Lab 4B)
DXA, 138–139
girth measurements, 142, 145–148 (Table 4.4–4.5)
hydrostatic weighing, 139–140, 159–160 (Lab 4A)
regular, importance of, 155–156
skinfold thickness, 141–142, 143–144 (Table 4.1–4.3)
WC, 150–152
WHtR, 137, 152–154
changes
exercise and, 155
frequent diet/without exercise and, 181 (Figure 5.7)
typical, 156 (Figure 4.11)
classification, 153 (Table 4.10)
defined, 136
FAQ, 137
knowledge assessment, 157
my profile, 136
personal fitness program and, 372
typical composition, 138 (Figure 4.1)
Body fat
burning, 217, 230
calorie intake for, 193 (Table 5.5)
classification of, 138
desired percentages of, 154
excessive, CHD risk from, 447–448
exercise and, 184
lean, 136
loss of, diets and, 181 (Figure 5.6)
loss of, HIIT and, 186
mass-obesity gene and, 187
percentage of, 136
risk factors, 151
storage, 138–139, 150
subcutaneous, 141, 151 (Figure 4.9)
supplies, 117
swimming and, 189
visceral, 151 (Figure 4.9)
Body mass index (BMI)
calculation of, 149
cancer incidence and, 461
defined, 149
determination of, 149 (Table 4.6)
disease risk and, 149–150, 150 (Table 4.7), 152 (Table 4.9)
limitations of, 137
use of, 148–149
WC *vs.*, 151
Body rotation, 330
Body temperatures, 356
Body weight. *See also* Obesity; Overweight; Recommended body weight
-physical activity, heart failure and, 448 (Table 11.13)
excessive, health consequences of, 167
ideal, 137
lifetime management of, 155
monitoring, 182
tolerable, 168–169
Body-based practices, 553
Bone health, 120–122
Boot camp. *See* Fitness boot camp
Bounce back ratings, 552
Bradycardia, 29
Brain functions
emotions and, 384
habits and, 51–52
physical exercise and, 24–25
Brain-derived neurotrophic factor (BDNF), 24
Brazil nut, 111
BRCA1/BRCA2 genes, 475
Breast cancer
mammograms, 477
risk factors, 475–477
self-exams, 470, 476 (Figure 12.12)
Breastfeeding, 124
Breathing techniques, 399–400
Bulimia nervosa, 174–176

C

C-reactive protein (CRP), 439–340
Caffeine
addiction to, 492
in energy drinks, 492, 494
performance enhancement and, 217
Calcium
food rich in, 121 (Table 3.14)
intake recommendations, 121 (Table 3.13)
osteoporosis prevention with, 120–121
sources for vegetarians, 105
Calf press, 293
Calories
balancing, 124
defined, 83
expenditures, in selected activities, 192 (Table 5.4)
expenditures, predicting, 230–233
fat intake for, 193 (Table 5.5)
food values, 99 (Figure 3.7)
in nuts, 105
requirements, computing, 203 (Lab 5A)
restricted diet plans, 208–211 (Lab 5C)
setpoint for, 179
CAM. *See* Complementary and alternative medicine (CAM)
Cancer
development of, 459
incidence of, 460–461
metastasis, 459 (Figure 12.4)
mortality, 461 (Figure 12.5), 461 (Figure 12.7), 469 (Figure 12.8)
prevention of
behavior assessment, 481
early detection, 470
estimated cases, 467 (Table 12.2)
FAQs, 457
fiber for, 464
guidelines for, 460–462, 485 (Lab 12A)
knowledge assessment, 482
lifestyles, 481
my profile, 456
physical activity for, 469–470
phytonutrients, 464
soy products, 466
spices for, 465
tea for, 464–465
vegetables for, 462–463
vitamin C for, 465
vitamin D for, 463–464
process of, 456–457
risk factors for
alcohol use, 466–467
dietary, 433, 465–467
environmental, 459–460, 462
excessive sun exposure, 468–469
genetic, 459–460
profile, 489–490 (Lab 12C)
questionnaire, 472–473 (Figure 12.9)
reduction of, 457
relative role of, 461 (Figure 12.6)
for specific-sites, 471, 474–480
tobacco use, 467–468
warning signs, 470, 487 (Lab 12B)
Capillaries, 220–221
Capsaicin, 464 (Table 12.1)
Carbohydrate loading
body weight/timing of, 345
defined, 118
function of, 118
Carbohydrates
caloric values of, 99 (Figure 3.7)
complex, 84
defined, 83
exercise needs, 345
major types of, 83 (Figure 3.2)
total calories, RDA percentages, 94 (Figure 3.7)
vigorous PA and, 118–119
Carcinogens, 464–465
Carcinoma in situ, 459
Cardiac output, 220–221
Cardio/resistance training program, 368
Cardiomyopathy, 504–505
Cardiorespiratory (CR) endurance. *See also* Maximal oxygen uptake (VOinf2max/inf)
assessment, 247–248 (Lab 6A)
behavior assessment, 245
CVD risk based on, 236 (Figure 6.8)
defined, 21
exercises for (*See* Aerobic exercise)
FAQs, 217–218
in highly trained males, 221 (Table 6.1)
importance of, 216
improvements in older adults, 361–362
knowledge assessment, 245–246
my profile, 218
physiology of, 218–219
programming example, 370–371
selected benefits of, 221 (Figure 6.1)
tests for, 224–229
Cardiorespiratory (CR) training zone, 235
Cardiovascular disease (CVD). *See also* Coronary heart disease (CHD); Stroke
alcohol-related, 504
behavior assessment, 450
CR endurance and, 236 (Figure 6.8)
ECG/EKG for, 428–429
ethnicity factors, 447
family/personal history and, 449
incidences of, 425 (Figure 11.1)
knowledge assessment, 450
my profile, 422
prevalence of, 424
prevention of
antioxidants, 434
aspirin therapy, 450
FAQs, 423–424
medications, 438
risk factors
age, 449
cholesterol levels, 429, 431–434
cigarette smoking, 448
diabetes, 440–442
elevated homocysteine, 438–439
elevated triglycerides, 438

endurance based, 236 (Figure 6.8)
high-GI foods, 442
hypertension, 443–447
inflammation, 439–440
low-birth rate, 450
metabolic syndrome, 442–443
reduction of, 450
Carotenoids, 462–463
Cat stretch, 334
Catecholamines, 448–449
Cell division
abnormal process, 458
normal *vs.* abnormal, 458 (Figure 12.1)
process of, 456–457
Cellulite, 188, 189
Cellulose, 85
Cervical cancer, 477
Change. *See also* Behavior modification
barriers to, 52–54
body composition
aerobic exercise only, 155, 156 (Figure 4.11)
strength training only, 262–263
strength/aerobic combined, 263 (Figure 7.1)
dietary habits, 165, 263–264
goal setting in, 60 (Figure 2.4)
identification, 66 (Figure 2.6)
motivation and, 54–56
my profile, 45
process of, 61–62
stages of, 58–61, 65 (Table 2.3)
stress-inducing, 389
techniques of, 64–67
willful, steps to, 56
willpower and, 52
CHD. *See* Coronary heart disease (CHD)
Chemical tags, 460
Chest fly, 297
Chest stretch, 330
Chewing tobacco, 468
Children
healthy dietary habits for, 125
physical activity guidelines for, 10
physical inactivity among, 48
weight management in, 155
Chiropractics, 553
Chlamydia, 529–530
Chlorogenic acids, 464 (Table 12.1)
Chocolate, 423–424
Cholesterol. *See also* specific lipoproteins
abnormal profile of, 429, 431–434
counteracting, 433–434
defined, 429
guidelines, 432 (Table 11.3)
numeric targets, 430
reverse transport of, 432
selected food content of, 433
trans-fats and, 434
Chromosome erosion, 458 (Figure 12.2)
Chronic diseases
BMI and, 149–150
body fat risks to, 151 (Figure 4.9)
defined, 5
genetic factors in, 7
life style-related risk factors, 6 (Figure 1.5)
percentage of deaths related to, 4
stress factors in, 384
Chronic lower respiratory disease, 6
Chronological age, 548, 550
Chylomicrons, 431, 438
Cigarette smoking. *See also* Tobacco
addiction/dependency, 511
cancer-induced by, 460, 508
cardiovascular effects of, 507–508
cessation of
cold turkey approach, 511, 514
cutting down approach, 514
questionnaire for, 523–526 (Lab 13B)
relationship support for, 63
steps, 512–514
substitution products for, 514–515
test for, 512
tips for, 516–517
costs of, 510
electric, 515
exercise and, 354–355
health effects of, 508 (Figure 13.6)
life after, 515
morbidity/mortality of, 507
prevalence of, 506
reasons for, 510–511
secondhand, 471, 508–509
social attitudes toward, 510
Circuit training, 275, 363–364
Cirrhosis, 503
Classical periodization, 270
Clinical study, 107
Clothing, 355, 358
Cocaine, 497–498
Cold turkey, 511, 514
Cold weather, 358
Colon cancer, 471
Commitment, 61
Competence, 55
Complacency, 52
Complementary and alternative medicine (CAM), 553
characterization of, 548
conventional providers referrals to, 555
costs of, 554
healing philosophies of, 53
herbs used in, 554–555
integrative approach, 555–556
promotion of, 556
quackery and fraud in, 556–558
reasons for, 552
scrutiny of, 553
shortcomings, 554
therapy classification, 552–553
use by age, 552 (Figure 15.2)
use by race and ethnicity, 555
Complete natural breathing, 400
Complex carbohydrates
defined, 85
examples of, 84
fiber as, 84–86
major groups, 83 (Figure 3.2)
Complexity, 53
Comprehensive fitness program
economic benefits of, 25–26
health benefits of, 23–25
types, benefits based on, 23 (Figure 1.14)
Computed tomography (CT), 139
Concentric resistance, 271
Conditioning programs
comprehensive, 23–26
interval, 368
periodization, 369–370
Confident consumers
"get fit fast" gimmick, 237
HIIT programs, 366
mastering stress, 390
self-confidence development and, 55
strength training equipment, 273
stretching exercise claims, 321
weight-loss gut check claims, 185
Consciousness-raising, 61, 65 (Table 2.2)
Contemplation stage, 58–59
Control. *See* Locus of control
Controlled ballistic stretching, 318
Conventional western medicine
advances in, 550
CAM *vs.*, 548
defined, 551
effectiveness of, 552
hospitals, 551–552
practitioners of, 550–551
scrutiny of, 553
Cooldowns, 238
Coordination tests, 347–349
Core strength training, 279, 363
Core values, 51–52
Coronary heart disease (CHD)
characterization of, 425
incidences of, 425
premature, 449
prevention
fiber intake and, 84
moderate-intensity activity for, 427–428
vitamin C and E for, 434
yoga for, 404
risk factors for
excessive body fat, 447–448
fat intake and, 436
gum disease, 450
hypertension, 444
leading, 425–427
red meat consumption, 91
salt intake and, 81
stress and, 384, 388
type A behavior and, 390
self-assessment, 453–454 (Lab 11A)
Cortisol, 384
p-Coumaric, 464 (Table 12.1)
Countering, 62, 65 (Table 2.2)
Crack cocaine, 497
Cradle, 322 (Figure 8.5)
Creatine phosphate (CP)
defined, 119
stores, benefits of, 120
strength training and, 275
supplementation of, 119–120
CRP. *See* C-reactive protein (CRP)
Cruciferous vegetables, 462–463
Culture
CVD risk and, 447
diet and, 108–109
drug abuse and, 495
food choices and, 107–109
osteoporosis risk and, 120
preconditioned beliefs and, 52
CVD. *See* Cardiovascular disease (CVD)

D

Daily values
bases of, 96
defined, 95
on food labels, 97 (Table 3.6)
uses of, 94
Dairy products, 82 (Figure 3.1)
DASH diet, 171, 447
Death
cancer-associated, 460
leading causes of, 6 (Figure 1.4)
life-style related, 6
selected causes of, 4 (Figure 1.1)
Deep breathing, 400
Dentists, 551
Deoxyribonucleic acid (DNA)
alteration of, 456–457
chemical tags, 460
defined, 457
duplication of, 458
function of, 456
Desk ergonomics, 326
Dextrins, 84
Diabetes mellitus
characterization of, 440
diseases associated with, 440–441
incidence of, 440
prevention of
aerobic exercise for, 352–353, 441
diets for, 441–442
exercise guidelines, 353–354, 442
strength training for, 353
types of, 352, 441–443
Diastolic blood pressure, 29–30, 443
Diet books, 170
Dietary fats
caloric values of, 99 (Figure 3.7)
cancer and, 465
in chocolate, 423–424
compound, 89
content, food label listing, 100 (Figure 3.8)
defined, 87
derived, 89
function of, 86
intake recommendations, 435
major type of, 86 (Figure 3.3)
oils, 100
saturated, 86–87
in selected foods, 101 (Figure 3.9)
simple, chemistry, 86
total calories, RDA percentages, 94 (Figure 3.7)
unsaturated fats, 87–89
Dietary fiber
cancer prevention and, 464
foods rich in, 84 (Table 3.1)
function of, 84
increase, modification plan for, 85
intake recommendations, 435
recommended intake, 85
types of, 85–86
Dietary Guidelines for Americans 2010, 123
Diets
calorie-restricted plans
1,200 per day, 207 (Lab 5C)
1,500 per day, 208 (Lab 5C)
1,800 per day, 209 (Lab 5C)
2,000 per day, 210 (Lab 5C)
cancer fighting, 462–464
fad, 169–170, 173
fat loss and, 181 (Figure 5.6)
hypertension lowering, 171, 447
low-fat, 436
metabolism and, 180–181
moderate-fat intake, 435
percentage of population on, 167
popular, 171–172
weight management and, 165
yo-yo, 169
Dips, 287, 299
Disaccharides, 83
Docosahexaenoic acid (DHA), 88

Donkey kicks, 322 (Figure 8.5)
Dopamine, 51, 499
Double-knee-to-chest stretch, 333
Double-leg lift, 322 (Figure 8.5)
Dramatic release. *See* Emotional arousal
Drug abuse
  characterization of, 495
  prescriptions, 495–496
  racial/ethic disparities in, 495
  types of
    amphetamines, 498–499
    cocaine, 497–498
    heroin, 500–501
    inhalants, 496
    marijuana, 496–497
    MDMA, 499–500
    methamphetamine, 498–499
    NPS, 501–502
Drunkorexia, 177
Dual energy X-ray absorptiometry (DXA), 138–139
Duration principle, 237–238
DXA. *See* Dual energy X-ray absorptiometry (DXA)
Dynamic balance, 344–345
Dynamic external resistance (DCER), 272–273
Dynamic stretching, 318
Dynamic training
  action phases in, 271–272
  advantage of, 271
  equipment for, 272
  machine *vs.* free weights in, 272–273
  muscle contractions in, 270
Dysmenorrhea, 310, 354

E

Eating. *See also* Diets
  cultural differences, 107–109
  environmental influence on, 48–50
  before exercise, 345
  habits, changing, 165
  healthy breakfast, 193
  healthy patterns for, 124
  low-fat entree, 194–195
  on the run, 180
  vigorous exercise and, 355
Eating disorders
  anorexia nervosa, 174–175
  binge-eating, 176
  defined, 174
  development of, 174–175
  emotional eating, 176
  not otherwise specified, 177
  treatment of, 177
Eccentric resistance, 271
ECG/EKG. *See* Electrocardiogram (ECG/EKG)
Ecstasy, 499–500
Eicosapentaenoic acid (EPA), 88
Elastic elongation, 313
Elastic-band resistive exercise, 280, 281 (Figure 7.8)
Electrocardiogram (ECG/EKG)
  abnormal, 429 (Figure 11.4)
  defined, 429
  normal, 429 (Figure 11.3)
  procedure for, 428–429
  purpose of, 428
Electrolytes, 119
Electronic cigarettes, 515
Elongation, 313
Emotional arousal, 61, 65 (Table 2.2)
Emotional eating, 176
Emotional wellness
  behavior and, 382
  benefits of, 16
  defined, 15
Emotions
  brain produced, 384
  healthy expression of, 388
  physiologic responses to, 382–383
Endomentrial cancer, 477
Endomondo, 235
Endorphins, 351, 396–397
Energy drinks
  addiction and, 494
  caffeine in, 494
  health concerns and, 80
  performance enhancement and, 217
Energy expenditures, 189 (Figure 5.9)
Energy substrates, 117
Energy-balancing equation, 177–178
Environment
  animal protein consumption and, 90
  cancer and, 459–460, 469
  control of, 63, 65 (Table 2.2)
  diet/nutrition and, 48–50
  exercising control over, 71–72 (Lab 2A)
  for meditation, 402
  physical activity and, 46–48
  tobacco smoke in, 508
  toxic elements, 44–46
Environmental wellness, 16–17
Enzymes, 89
Epigallocatechin gallate (EGCG), 464–465
Epigenetics, 460–461
Ergonomics. *See* Desk ergonomics
Esophageal cancer, 479
Essential fat, 138–139
Estimated average requirement, 94–95
Estimated energy requirement (EER)
  age, weight and height based, 191 (Table 5.3)
  calculation of, 190
  computing, 203 (Lab 5A)
  defined, 96
  setting of, 94–95
  weight loss and, 177–178
Estrogen, 120, 469
Ethnic diets
  African American, 108
  guide for, 109 (Table 3.10)
  healthfulness of, 107–108
  Hispanic, 108
Eustress, 387
Exercise. *See also* Aerobic exercise; Strength training; *specific intensity*
  aging and, 361
  arthritis and, 352
  best time for, 356
  cigarette smoking and, 354–355
  clothing for, 355
  in cold weather, 358
  with cold/flu, 358–359
  contraindications
    older people, 362
    pregnancy, 355
    stretching, 321, 322 (Figure 8.5)
    yoga, 322 (Figure 8.5)
  defined, 9
  dropout cycle, 44 (Figure 2.1)
  for dysmenorrhea, 354
  eating before, 345
  equipment, 561
  in hot weather, 355–356
  immediate benefits of, 23 (Table 1.4)
  injuries related to, 359
  intensity levels, and calories burned, 187 (Table 5.2)
  long-term benefits of, 25 (Table 1.5)
  losing weight with, 165
  as medicine, 10
  menstruation and, 354
  osteoporosis prevention with, 122
  primary fuel for, 345
  readiness for, 232–233, 253–254 (Lab 6C)
  requirements of, 8
  safety in, 27
  specific considerations for, 351–358
  stress reducing, 396
  weight management with
    benefits of, 182–185
    intensity/duration in, 185–187
    lifetime aerobic, 184
Exercise volume, 239
Exercise-induced asthma (EIA), 351–352
Explanatory styles, 388

F

Fartlek training, 368
Fast-twitch fibers, 269
Fat. *See* Body fat; Dietary fat
Fatty acids
  benefits of, 433–434
  elevated, CVD and, 438
  energy from, 117
  storage of, 438
  types of, 88–89
Ferritin, 122–123
Fiber. *See* Dietary fiber
50-yard dash test, 350
Fight-or-flight mechanism, 395, 396 (Figure 10.4)
Fighting spirit, 388
Fish, 80, 88 (Table 3.2)
Fitness. *See* Physical fitness
Fitness boot camp, 363
FITT (frequency, intensity, time, type)
  defined, 233
  for diabetics, 352–353
  duration component, 237–238
  frequency component, 238–239
  intensity component, 233–234
Five-minute destress technique, 400
Fixed-resistance machines, 272–274
Flavonoids, 423, 464 (Table 12.1)
Flexibility. *See also* Stretching
  assessment of
    body posture, 313, 316–318
    categories, 317 (Tables 8.4–8.5)
    interpreting results, 313–318
    log for, 337–338 (Lab 8A)
    shoulder rotation test, 315 (Figure 8.3), 317 (Table 8.3)
    sit-and-reach test, 313 (Figure 8.1), 315 (Figure 8.1)
    specificity of, 312–313
    total body rotation test, 314 (Figure 8.2), 316 (Table 8.2)
  behavior assessment, 327
  benefits of, 310–312
  defined, 310
  development, 320 (Figure 8.4), 341–342 (Lab 8C)
  knowledge assessment, 327
  my profile, 310
  in older adults, 312
  personal program for, 371–372
  principles of, 318
  sports specific, 365
  strength training and, 310
  test results, interpretation of, 313–318
Fluid replacement solutions, 357–358
Folate, 113, 439
Food labels
  daily values on, 96, 97 (Table 3.6)
  fat content on, 100 (Figure 3.8)
  trans fats listed on, 434
Food logs, 194
Foods. *See also* Diets; Nutrition; *specific products*
  addiction to, 492
  antioxidant
    rich, 113, 114 (Table 3.12)
  benefits of, 113–114
  beta carotene rich, 111
  calcium rich, 121 (Table 3.14)
  caloric needs and, 124
  choices, effects of, 195
  contamination of, 116
  ethnic, 108–109
  fats in, 101 (Figure 3.9)
  fiber-rich, 84 (Table 3.1)
  folate rich, 113
  fortified, 114–115
  functional, 114–115
  genetically modified, 115–117
  glycemic load of, 81, 172 (Table 5.1)
  healthy, choosing, 103
  iron rich, 123 (Table 3.15)
  low-fat, 194–195
  meal choice examples, 191 (Figure 5.10)
  nutritious, selection of, 104
  omega-3 rich, 88
  organic, 114–115
  potassium rich, 445 (Table 11.11)
  potential risks in, 79–81
  pregnancy and, 124
  probiotic rich, 106
  processed, 87, 434, 465–466
  PUFA rich, 87
  restaurant, 49
  selenium rich, 111
  sodium rich, 445 (Table 11.11)
  sugar in, 79–80
  trans-fats in, 423
  vitamin C rich, 111
  vitamin D rich, 112
  water in, 91–92
Fortified foods, 114–115
Fraud. *See* Quackery and fraud
Free radicals. *See* Oxygen free radicals
Free weights, 272–273
Frequency principle, 238–239
Fructose, 83
Fruits
  antioxidants in, 113
  cardiovascular benefits of, 439
  recommended daily amounts, 82 (Figure 3.1)
FTO gene, 187
Full squat, 322 (Figure 8.5)

Functional capacity, 549, 550 (Figure 15.1)
Functional fitness, 364
Functional foods, 114–115
Functional independence, 362

G

Gender differences
- eating disorders, 174
- life expectancy, 5
- in muscle fitness, 261–262
- obesity rates, 167 (Figure 5.3)
- osteoporosis risk, 120
- recommended body weight, 154

General adaptation syndrome (GAS)
- body's response to, 387 (Figure 10.2)
- defined, 387
- stages of, 387–388

Genes
- breast cancer, 475
- cancer, 457–460
- obesity, 187
- suppressor, 456–457

Genetic deposition
- cancer, 459–460, 475
- eating disorders, 174
- fat mass, 187
- LDL, 432

Genetically modified (GM) food
- avoidance of, 116–117
- defined, 115
- introduction of, 116
- purpose of, 115
- safety of, 115–117

Genistein, 464 (Table 12.1)
Genital herpes, 533–534
Genital warts, 532–533
"Get fit fast" gimmick, 237
Ghrelin, 181
GI. *See* Glycemic index (GI)
Girth measurement technique
- conversion constants, 145–147 (Table 4.4–4.5)
- defined, 142
- procedure for, 148 (Table 4.5)

Glucocorticoid hormones, 384
Glucolipids, 89
Glucose
- blood levels
  - GI effects on, 173
  - guidelines for, 441 (Table 11.9)
  - tests for, 442
- defined, 83
- energy from, 117
- in sports drinks, 357

Gluteal stretch, 333
Gluten sensitivity, 79
Glycemic index (GI)
- blood glucose levels and, 173 (Figure 5.4)
- CVD risk and, 442
- diet based on, 170–171
- selected foods, 172 (Table 5.1)

Glycemic load, 81
Glycogen
- defined, 85
- function of, 84
- storage of, 118, 170

Goals
- defined, 65
- evaluation of, 67
- fitness and wellness, 562, 573–576 (Lab 15C)
- measurable, 66
- Pilates system, 280
- setting, 60 (Figure 2.4), 62
- SMART, 64–67
- time specific, 415–418 (Lab 10D)
- written, 62–63

Golgi tendon organ, 319
Gonorrhea, 531
Gore-Tex, 358
Gratification, 52
Group personal training, 363
Gums, 86
"Gut check claims," 185
Gwynn, Tony, 468
GymPact, 235
Gyms. *See* Health and fitness facilities
Gynoid obesity, 151

H

H-PAPE. *See* Physical activity perceived exertion (H-PAPE)
Habits
- dietary, changing, 165, 263–264
- environmental influences in, 51
- healthy lifestyle, 28
- neurological factors in, 51–52
- smoking, 511–514

Hamstring roll, 303
Hand grip strength tests, 264
Hatha yoga, 404
Head rolls, 322 (Figure 8.5)
Health
- apps for, 235–236
- bone, 120–122
- defined, 3
- factors impacting, 4 (Figure 1.2)
- history questionnaires, 39–40 (Lab C)
- mindful meditation for, 403
- objectives for 2020, 11 (Figure 1.7)
- perceptions and, 388
- reliable information on, 558, 560
- self-esteem, 388
- stress/performance relationship to, 386 (Figure 10.1)

Health and fitness facilities
- ACSM standards, 559 (Figure 15.3)
- memberships, 559–560
- personal trainers at, 560

Health care costs
- country-based comparisons, 26 (Figure 1.16), 26 (Figure 1.17)
- increments of, 26 (Figure 1.15)
- tobacco use, 509–510

Health fitness
- components of, 19
- defined, 21
- standards of, 20–21

Health newsletters, 560
Healthy breakfasts, 193
Healthy lifestyles
- for CVD prevention, 430
- habits for, 28
- lifetime, guidelines, 557

Heart attack. *See* Myocardial infarctions
Heart rate. *See also* Maximal heart rate; Resting heart rate
- assessment, 249–252 (Lab 6B)
- monitoring, 235–236

Heart rate reserve (HRR), 233
Heart vessels, 426 (Figure 11.2)
Heat cramps, 356
Heat exhaustion, 356–357
Heat stroke, 357
Heel cord stretch, 331
Heel raise, 289
Helping relationships, 63, 65 (Table 2.2)
Helplessness, 53
Hemicellulose, 86
Hemoglobin
- defined, 123, 219
- function of, 218
- iron in, 122

Hepatitis B virus (HBV), 534
Herbal medicine
- defined, 553
- safety of, 554
- side effects of, 554–555

Heroin, 500–501
The hero, 322 (Figure 8.5)
Heterocyclic amines (HCAs), 465–466
High-density lipoproteins (HDL), 87
- benefits of, 433
- cigarette smoking and, 507
- decrease, arrhythmias from, 448
- defined, 431
- dietary modification of, 435–436
- protein components of, 423
- subgroups of, 432–433

High-fructose corn syrup (HFCS), 79–80
HIIT (high-intensity intermittent training)
- for athletes, 363–364, 366
- body fat loss and, 186
- defined, 367
- sample programs, 368

Hip flexor stretch, 332
Hispanic Americans. *See* Latino Americans
Histones, 460
HIV/AIDS
- data on, 538 (Figure 14.4)
- immune system damage, 530
- incidences of, 536–537 (Figure 14.2–14.3)
- myths, 537–538
- risk reduction, 541–543
- risky behavior for, 537–538
- self-quiz, 545–546 (Lab 14A)
- symptoms of, 535–536
- test for, 535, 539
- transmission of, 530
- treatments for, 536, 539–540
- trends in, 538–539
- virus transmission, 536–538

Homeopathy, 553
Homeostasis, 387
Homocysteine
- defined, 439
- elevated, CVD and, 438–439
- function of, 438–439
- guidelines, 439 (Table 11.7)
- measurement of, 439

Hormone replacement therapy (HRT), 475
Hormones
- appetite regulation and, 181
- in emotional response, 382
- estrogen, 120, 469
- sleep deprivation and, 182
- stress-related, 384

Hospitals, 551–552
Hostility assessment, 411–412 (Lab 10B)
Hot weather, 355–356
Hot5, 235
Human papilloma virus (HPV)
- cervical cancer and, 477
- health risks from, 532–533
- prevention of, 533
- treatment of, 533
- types of, 532

Humanistic theory of change, 57
Hurdler stretch, 322 (Figure 8.5)
Hydrostatic weighing technique
- defined, 159–160 (Lab 4A)
- drawbacks of, 139
- log for, 159–160 (Lab 4A)
- procedure for, 140 (Figure 4.2)

Hypertension. *See also* Blood pressure
- CHD and, 444
- diagnosis of, 443
- incidents of, 443–444
- medications for, 444, 447
- prevention of
  - dietary, 444–445, 447
  - exercise, 446
  - guidelines for, 447
- sodium intake and, 444–445

Hypertrophy, 261, 268
Hypokinetic disease
- defined, 21
- premature, 20
- types of, 215

Hypokinetic diseases, 239
Hyponatremia, 119
Hypotension, 443

I

Immune system
- cells of, 384
- explanatory styles and, 388
- HIV damage to, 530
- sleep deprivation and, 384

Immunity, 382
Indifference, 53
Inhalant abuse, 496
Injuries
- common, 359–360
- exercise-related, 359
- prevention, stretching for, 310
- RICE for, 359

Insulin, 441
Insulin resistance, 440–442
Insulin-dependent diabetes mellitus (IDDM), 352, 441
Integral yoga, 404
Integrative medicine, 555–556
Intensity. *See also* Moderate-intensity exercise; Vigorous-intensity exercise
- defined, 233
- duration and, 185–186
- intervals, 368
- levels, and calories burned, 187 (Table 5.2)
- measurement of, 242
- principle of, 233–234
- stretching, 319–320

Intermediate-density lipoproteins, 432
International units, 110–111
Interval training, 368
Invincibility, 53–54
Iron
- deficiency, 122–123
- foods rich in, 123 (Table 3.15)
- sources for vegetarians, 105
- supplements, 110

Isoflavones, 106
Isokinetic training, 272–273
Isometric training, 270–271
Iyengar yoga, 325, 404

J

Jackknives, 303
Jogging. *See* Running

K

Kidney cancer, 479
Knee to chest, 322 (Figure 8.5)

L

Lactic acid, 117
Lactobacillus spp., 106
Lactovegetarians, 103
Lapse, 57
Lat pull-down, 294
Lateral trunk extension, 300
Latino Americans
  CAM use by, 555
  CVD risks for, 447
  diets of, 108
  STI risk for, 535
Lean body fat, 136
Lean body mass, 99 (Figure 3.7)
Learning theories, 57
Leg abduction/adduction, 289, 294–295
Leg curl, 287, 292
Leg extension, 296
Leg press, 291
Leptin, 181
Leukemia, 480
Life expectancy
  at birth, 4 (Figure 1.3)
  defined, 5
  gender differences in, 5
  increase in, 4
  physiological age and, 550
  prediction questionnaire, 567–570 (Lab 15A)
Life time fitness and wellness
  behavior assessment, 564
  behavioral goals for, 562, 573–576 (Lab 15C)
  benefits of, 548
  CAM for, 552–555
  challenge for future, 562–564
  community resources, 571–572
  conventional medicine for, 550–552
  equipment for, 561
  FAQs, 548
  fraudulent products in, 556–557
  gym membership and, 559–560
  integrative medicine for, 555–556
  knowledge assessment, 564–565
  my profile, 549
  objectives of, 561–562
  self-evaluation of, 562, 573–576 (Lab 15C)
Lifestyles. *See also* Healthy lifestyles; Sedentary lifestyles
  cancer fighting, 481
  cancer risk and, 461 (Figure 12.7)
  cardiac death risk and, 427
  functional capacity, aging and, 550 (Figure 15.1)
  patterns, energy expenditure and, 189 (Figure 5.9)
Linoleic acid (LA), 88
Lipids. *See* Dietary fats
Lipoprotein-a, 432
Lipoproteins, 89
Liver cancer, 480
Locus of control
  defined, 55
  exercising, 71–72 (Lab 2A)
  motivation and, 54–56
Longevity, 18–19
Low-birth weight, 450
Low-carbohydrate/high-protein (LCHP) diets
  blood
    glucose levels, 173 (Figure 5.4)
  characteristics of, 170
  disease risks from, 173
  popular, 171
  weight loss in, 172–174
Low-density lipoproteins (LDL)
  characterization of, 86–87
  defined, 431
  lowering
    dietary approach to, 435–436
    guidelines for, 437
    medication for, 438
    niacin for, 438
  nut consumption and, 105
  phenotype B, 438
  protein components of, 423
  types of, 432
  vitamin E and C effects on, 434
Lower back pain
  assessment of, 323
  causes of
    posture/mechanics, 323
    stress, 326
    trauma, 323
  incidence of, 321
  muscle strength and, 321, 323
  prevention of
    behavior modification tips, 325
    conditioning program for, 326
    core strengthening, 325
    exercises for, 332–336
    good posture for, 324 (Figure 8.7)
    yoga for, 325–326
  reduction of, 323, 325
  rehabilitation
    conditioning for, 341–342 (Lab 8C)
    core strengthening, 325
    rest/medication, 323
Lung cancer, 467–468, 471
Lymphocytes, 384
Lymphoma, 480–481

M

Machines. *See* Fixed-resistance machines
Magnetic resonance imaging (MRI), 139
Magnetic therapy, 553
Maintenance stage, 60–61
Malignant tumors, 456
Mammograms, 477–478
Manipulative practices, 553
Marijuana
  characterization of, 496
  long-term effects of, 496–497
  synthetic, 502
Massage therapy, 553
Maximal heart rate, 223
Maximal oxygen uptake (VO_{2max})
  aged-base correction factors, 231 (Table 6.6)
  ATP generation and, 117
  components of, 223
  defined, 221
  estimation of
    Astrand-Rhyming test, 226, 228, 230 (Table 6.5)
    interpretation of, 229–230
    onef1.5-mile run, 225, 226 (Table 6.2)
    onem1.0-mile walk, 225, 227 (Figure 6.3)
    pulse beats conversion for, 229 (Table 6.4)
    step-test, 225, 227 (Figure 6.4)
    12-minute swim test, 228, 229 (Figure 6.6)
  fitness classification according to, 231 (Table 6.8)
  increasing, benefits of, 220
  for jogging/walking, predicting, 230–233
  for older adults, 361
  in physical inactivity people, 427
MDMA, 499–500
Measurable goals, 66
Meat
  processed, 465–466
  red, consumption, 90–91
Medicine. *See* Complementary and alternative medicine (CAM); Conventional western medicine; Integrative medicine
Meditation
  environment for, 402
  mechanisms of, 402
  mindful, 403–404
  mindless, 402–404
Mediterranean diet, 107, 172
Megadose, 109
Melanoma, 468–469
Menopausal hormone therapy (MHT), 122
Menstruation, 354
Mental wellness, 16–17
Metabolic equivalents (METs), 242
Metabolic profile, 21
Metabolic syndrome
  characterization of, 443
  defined, 443
  diagnosis of, 442
Metabolism
  defined, 261
  diets and, 180–181
  resting, 261
  strength levels and, 261
Metastasis, 459
Methamphetamine, 498–499
Methyl groups, 460
Methylenedioxyamphetamine (MDA), 500
Mind-body connection, 382
Mind-body medicine, 553
Mindful meditation, 403–404
Mindfulness, 62
Mindless meditation
  pain relief with, 402–403
  routine for, 402
  steps for, 403
Minerals
  defined, 91
  major functions of, 93 (Table 3.6)
  ULs for adults, 96 (Table 3.9)
Mitochondria, 220, 221
Mode, 236–237
Moderate physical activity
  defined, 9
  insulin sensitivity and, 441
  recommendations for, 8–9
Moderate-intensity exercise
  CVD prevention with, 427–428
  defined, 233
  vigorous-intensity *vs.*, 234
Modified dip, 287
Modified push-up test, 265 (Figure 7.3)
Modified-dip test, 265 (Figure 7.3)
Mole appearance, 474 (Figure 12.10)
Monitoring
  function of, 62–63
  studies on, 63
  techniques, 65 (Table 2.2)
Monogamous relationships, 540–541
Monosaccharides, 83
Monosaturated fats, 86 (Figure 3.4)
Morbidity. *See also* Death
  cigarette smoking, 507
  defined, 7
Mortality
  cancer, 461 (Figure 12.5), 469 (Figure 12.8)
  cigarette smoking, 507
  lifestyle and, 461 (Figure 12.7)
  red meat consumption and, 91
Motivation
  defined, 55
  locus of control and, 54–56
  problems of, 56
Motor skills, 20 (Figure 1.13)
Motor unit, 269
Mucilages, 86
Multivitamins, 111–112
Muscle mass, 184
Muscles
  basic structure of, 268 (Figure 7.5)
  cramps, 361
  fiber types, 268–269
  heart, 428–429
  lower back pain and, 321, 323
  major, 278 (Figure 7.7)
  progressive relaxation of, 398–399
  soreness/stiffness, 275, 359
  spindle, 319
Muscular strength and endurance
  aging and, 260–263
  assessment of, 263–268, 305–306 (Lab 7A)
  benefits of, 259
  defined, 262
  dietary guidelines for, 277–279
  factors affecting, 269
  FAQs, 259
  gender differences in, 261–262
  muscle fiber density and, 268–269
  my profile, 258
  in older adults, 362
  periodization program for, 370 (Table 9.7), 371 (Table 9.4)
  personal program for, 371–372
  scoring table, 266–267 (Table 7.2–7.3)
MyFitnessPal, 235
Myocardial infarctions
  body weight/physical activity and, 448
  CRP risk, 440
  defined, 431
  energy drink-induced, 217
  physiological results of, 426 (Figure 11.2)
  warning signs of, 424
Myocardium, 428–429
Myofibrillar hypertrophy, 268
MyPlate food plan
  recommendations in, 82 (Figure 3.1)
  record form, 133–134 (Lab 3B)
  for vegetarians, 105

N

National Activity Plan, 11
National initiatives to promote healthy and active lifestyles, 9–11
Naturopathic medicine, 553
NEAT. *See* Nonexercise activity thermogenesis (NEAT)
Neck stretches, 329
Negative resistance, 271
Neural function, 269
Neuropeptide Y (NPY), 384
Neustress, 389
New psychoactive substances (NPS), 501–502
Niacin, 438
Nicotine
- addictive properties of, 511
- defined, 507
- release of, 506
- substitution products, 514–515

Nitrosamines, 464–465
Nonexercise activity thermogenesis (NEAT), 14, 239
Noninsulin-dependent diabetes mellitus (NIDDM), 352, 441
Nonmelanoma skin cancer, 463
Nonresponders, 223
Nonsteroidal anti-inflammatory drugs (NSAIDs), 457
NPS. *See* New psychoactive substances (NPS)
Nurses, 551
Nutrient density, 83
Nutrients
- analysis of, 96, 98, 129 (LAB 3A)
- approximate proportions of, 94 (Figure 3.5)
- caloric needs and, 124
- carbohydrates, 83–86
- daily intake log, 130–131 (Lab 3A.1–3A.2)
- deficient in vegetarian diets, 105
- defined, 81
- essential, 81–83
- fats, 86–89
- proteins, 89–91
- setpoint for, 179
- variety in, 81

Nutrition
- AGEs and, 106
- for athletes, 117–120
- behavior assessment, 125
- cultural differences, 107–109
- defined, 81
- environmental influences, 48–50
- exercising control over, 71–72 (Lab 2A)
- FAQ, 79–81
- food plan for, 82 (Figure 3.1)
- information, reliable sources for, 560
- knowledge assessment, 125–126
- lifetime prescription for, 124–125
- for muscular strength and endurance, 277–279
- my profile, 78
- probiotics and, 106
- specific recommendations for, 123
- standards, 94–96
- vegetarianism and, 103, 105

Nuts, 105–106

O

Obesity
- android, 151
- cancer risk, 467
- defined, 139
- determination of, 138
- epidemic, 164, 166
- fat mass gene, 187
- fight against, 165
- gynoid, 151
- overweight *versus,* 168
- percentages in U.S., 164 (Figure 5.1)
- prescriptions for, 430
- prevalence based on gender/education, 167 (Figure 5.3)
- prevalence of, 150 (Figure 4.8)
- racial/ethnic disparities in, 169
- sleep deprivation and, 182
- trends in, 150 (Figure 4.7), 166 (Figure 5.2)

Observational study, 107
Occupational wellness, 17
Oils, 100
Older adults
- dietary recommendations for, 124
- exercise contraindications, 362
- flexibility in, 312
- muscle fitness in, 260–261
- osteoporosis risk and, 120
- physical activity guidelines for, 10
- physical training for, 361–362
- vitamin D deficiency in, 113

Oligomenorrhea, 122–123
Omega-9-fatty acids, 89
Omega-6-fatty acids, 88–89
Omega-3-fatty acids
- cardiac death risk and, 434 (Figure 11.7)
- defined, 87
- health benefits of, 87

Oncogenes, 457
One repetition maximum (1 RM), 263, 274 (Table 7.4)
One-foot stand test, 347
1.0 Mile walk, 225, 227 (Figure 6.3)
1.5-Mile run test
- estimated V0inf2max/inf for, 225 (Figure 6.2)
- procedure for, 225 (Figure 6.2)
- use of, 225

1RM. *See* One repetition maximum (1 RM)
Ophthalmologists, 551
Opportunistic infections, 535
Optometrists, 551
Oral cancer, 479
Oral surgeons, 551
Organic foods, 114–115
Ornish diet, 171
Orthotic, 177
Osteopath, 551
Osteoporosis
- process of, 120
- risks for, 121 (Figure 3.15), 122
- treatments for, 122

Outdoor training, 363
Ovarian cancer, 479–480
Overload principle, 269
Overtraining
- effects of, 368–369
- prevention of, 270
- symptoms of, 367

Overweight
- cancer risk, 467
- defined, 139
- determination of, 138
- and fit debate, 187–188
- obesity *versus,* 168
- trends in, 150 (Figure 4.7)

Ovolactovegetarians, 103
Ovovegetarians, 103
Oxygen free radicals, 110
Oxygen removal, 223–224
Oxygen uptake (VO2). *See also* Maximal oxygen uptake (VOinf2max/inf)
- CR system and, 219
- defined, 219
- for walking/jogging speeds, 232 (Table 6.0)

P

Pain. *See* Lower back pain
Pancreatic cancer, 478
Passive stretching, 318
Pectins, 86
Pedometer, 12–13
Peer support, 63
PEITC, 464 (Table 12.1)
Pelvic clock, 335
Pelvic inflammatory disease (PID), 531
Pelvic tilt, 290, 334
Performance
- –stress/health relationship to, 386 (Figure 10.1)
- caffeine effects on, 217
- energy drinks effects on, 217
- tai chi effects on, 362

Performance tests
- cardiorespiratory, 223–234
- muscular strength, 263–268
- for skill-related fitness, 346–349

Periodization
- contraindications for, 370
- cycles in, 369
- defined, 370
- for strength, 369, 370 (Table 9.7), 371 (Table 9.4)
- types of, 270
- use of, 369–370

Peripheral vascular disease, 424
Peristalsis muscle, 85
Personal fitness plan
- base conditioning, 365–366
- example, 370–372
- log for, 377–380 (Lab 9B)
- overtraining precautions, 368–369
- periodization, 369–370

Personal trainers, 560–561
Personal training
- group, 363
- at gyms, 560–561
- outdoor, 363

Pesticides, 116
Phenethy isothiocyanate (PEITC), 464 (Table 12.1)
Phospholipids, 89
Physical activity
- aging and, 548
- body weight, heart failure and, 448 (Table 11.13)
- blood pressure management with, 446
- cancer prevention and, 457
- CVD risk based on, 236 (Figure 6.8)
- federal guidelines for, 237
- in hot weather, 355–356
- for older adults, 361–362
- weight management guidelines, 183

Physical activity (PA). *See also* Moderate physical activity; Vigorous-intensity exercise
- benefits of, 8
- body weight decrease based on, 183 (Figure 5.8)
- daily log for, 33–34 (Lab 1A)
- decline in, 216–217
- defined, 9
- duration/intensity recommendations, 8 (Table 1.1)
- energy substrates for, 117
- environmental influences, 46–48
- exercising control over, 71–72 (Lab 2A)
- increasing, tips for, 222
- longevity and, 18–19
- monitoring, 11–13
- national plan for, 11
- protein needs for, 90 (Table 3.4)
- requirements of, 8
- steps per day-based, 12 (Table 1.2)
- technology and, 2–3
- weight management guidelines, 183

Physical activity perceived exertion (H-PAPE), 236, 354
Physical activity pyramid, 240 (Figure 6.10)
Physical fitness
- aerobics and, 240–242
- apps for, 235–236
- assessment of, 222
- behavior assessment, 30
- classification of, 19
- defined, 19
- FAQs, 3
- information, reliable sources for, 560
- knowledge assessment, 30
- motor-skills in, 20 (Figure 1.13)
- my profile, 3
- and overweight debate, 187–188
- standards of, 21
- types of, 19–20

Physical inactivity
- breast cancer risk and, 475
- CVD risk and, 427–428
- environmental influences, 47–48
- epidemic of, 3
- leptin resistance and, 181
- sitting disease and, 13–14
- VOinf2max/inf and, 427

Physical wellness, 15
Physical stillness, 239{
Physician assistants, 551
Physiological age
- defined, 549
- physical activity and, 548
- prediction questionnaire, 567–570 (Lab 15A)

Phytonutrients
- antioxidants *vs.,* 81
- cancer prevention and, 173, 464
- defined, 100

PID. *See* Pelvic inflammatory disease (PID)
Pilates system
- creation of, 279–280
- defined, 279
- goals of, 280

Plank, 290, 300
Plastic elongation, 313
Plyometric exercise, 276–277
Polycyclic aromatic hydrocarbons (PAHs), 465–466
Polyphenols, 464–465
Polyunsaturated fatty acids (PUFA)
- chemical structure of, 86 (Figure 3.4)

Polyunsaturated fatty acids (PUFA) (continued)
- foods rich in, 87
- types of, 87–89

Positive outlook commitment, 61, 65 (Table 2.2)
Positive resistance, 271
Postpartum women, 10–11
Posture
- assessment of
  - photographs for, 316–318
  - rating chart for, 316, 339–340 (Lab 8B)
  - result interpretation, 313
- correct, 324 (Figure 8.7)
- desk ergonomics, 326
- elongation in, 313
- evaluation standards for, 317 (Table 8.6)
- mechanics of, 313, 316
- pelvic alignment, 323 (Figure 8.6)
- rating chart for, 316
- role of, 313

Potassium, 445 (Table 11.11)
Power test, 349
Power yoga, 404
Prayer, 17
Precontemplation stage, 58–59
Prefrontal cortex, 52
Pregnancy
- dietary needs, 124
- exercise guidelines, 354–355
- folate needs in, 113
- physical activity guidelines for, 10–11

Pregorexia, 177
Preparation stage, 59
Prescription drugs
- nonmedical use of, 495–496
- research, evaluation of, 558

Primary care physician, 550–551
Primordial prevention, 14–15
Principle of individuality, 223
Probiotics, 106–107
Problem-solving model, 57
Processed foods, 87, 434
Procrastination, 52
Programmed cell death, 458
Progression model, 60 (Figure 2.5)
Progressive muscle relaxation, 398–399
Prohibition, 502
Proprioceptive neuromuscular facilitation (PNF), 318–319
Prostate cancer, 477–478
Proteins
- caloric values of, 99 (Figure 3.7)
- cholesterol lowering, 423
- complementing, 103, 104 (Figure 3.11)
- complete, 89–90
- daily intake, importance of, 90
- daily intake, recommended, 90 (Table 3.4)
- deficiency, 90
- defined, 89
- grains rich in, 86
- in nuts, 106
- osteoporosis prevention with, 121
- recommended daily amounts, 82 (Figure 3.1)
- sources of, 90–91
- strength training and, 119
- total calories, RDA percentages, 94 (Figure 3.7)
- vigorous PA and, 119

Psyllium, 435–436
PUFA. *See* Polyunsaturated fatty acids (PUFA)
Pull-up, 288
Push-up, 286, 302

Q

Quackery and fraud
- consumer protection against, 557–558
- defined, 557
- innocent, 557
- precautions against, 556–557
- rise in, 556

Quad stretch, 331
Questionnaires
- addictive behavior, 521–522 (Lab 13A)
- cancer risk assessment, 472–473 (Figure 12.9)
- exercise readiness, 253–254 (Lab 6C)
- health history, 39–40 (Lab C)
- life expectancy/physiological age, 567–570 (Lab 15A)
- smoking cessation, 523–526 (Lab 13B)
- wellness lifestyle, 35–37 (Lab 1B)

Quinoa, 86

R

Radiation risks, 469
Radon gas exposure, 471
Range of motion, 271
Rationalization, 53
RDA. *See* Recommended dietary allowances (RDA)
Reaction tests, 349–350
Realistic goals, 66–67
Recommended body weight
- computation of, 154–15
- defined, 136
- metrics for, 148–149

Recommended dietary allowances (RDA)
- age-specific, 95 (Table 3.8)
- folate, 95 (Table 3.8)
- use of, 94

Recovery stress stage, 387–388
Recovery time, 220–221
Rectum cancer, 471
Refined grains, 100
Registered dietitian, 114
Relapse
- defined, 57
- model of, 60 (Figure 2.5)
- prevention of, 57

Relaxation techniques. *See also* Stress management
- autogenic training, 402
- benefits of, 397
- biofeedback, 397–398
- breathing exercises, 399–400
- five-minute destress, 400
- meditation, 402–404
- progressive muscle, 398–399
- visual imagery, 400–402

Repetitions
- maximum, 263
- number of, 274 (Table 7.4)
- stretching, 320

Resistance
- defined, 275
- fixed, 272–273
- function of, 274
- to stress, 387
- variable, 272

Responders, 223
Restaurants, 49, 108
Resting heart rate
- assessment of, 29–30
- decrease in, 220
- energy drink consumption and, 217
- guidelines for, 29 (Table 1.7)
- log for, 41–42 (Lab C)

Resting metabolic rate (RMR), 178–179
Resting metabolism, 261
Resveratrol, 423
Reverse cholesterol transport, 432
Reverse crunch, 289
Reverse periodization, 270
Reverse supine bridge, 301
Rewards, 63–64, 65 (Table 2.2)
Riboflavin, 105
Ribonucleic acid (RNA), 456–457
RICE treatment, 359
Risk assessment, 430
Risk complacency, 52
Risk factors
- assessment of, 430
- body fat as, 151
- cancer, 433
  - alcohol use, 466–467
  - dictary, 433, 465–467
  - environmental, 459–460, 462
  - excessive sun exposure, 468–469
  - genetic, 459–460
  - profile, 489–490 (Lab 12C)
  - questionnaire, 472–473 (Figure 12.9)
  - reduction of, 457
  - relative role of, 461 (Figure 12.6)
  - for specific-sites, 471, 474–480
  - tobacco use, 467–468
- CHD
  - analysis of, 425–426
  - self-assessment for, 453–454 (Lab 11A)
  - very low category, 426
  - weighting system for, 426 (Table 11.2)
- chronic diseases, 6 (Figure 1.5)
- CVD
  - activity volume-based, 236 (Figure 6.8)
  - age, 449
  - cholesterol levels, 429, 431–434
  - cigarette smoking, 448
  - elevated homocysteine, 438–439
  - elevated triglycerides, 438
  - endurance based, 236 (Figure 6.8)
  - excessive body fat, 447–448
  - gum disease, 450
  - inflammation, 439–440
  - low-birth weight, 450
  - reduction of, 450
- defined, 7
- osteoporosis, 120, 122

Rogers, Don, 497
Rotary Torso, 294
Rowing torso, 286, 292
RunKeeper, 235
Running
- barefoot, 355–356
- speeds, estimated VOinf2/inf requirements, 232 (Table 6.9)
- VOinf2max/inf for, predicting, 230–233

S

Safe sex, 530
SAID. *See* Specific adaptation to imposed demand (SAID)
Sarcopenia, 260–261
Sarcoplasm, 268
Sarcoplasmic hypertrophy, 268
Saturated fats
- chemical structure of, 86 (Figure 3.4)
- classification of, 86–87
- foods rich in, 433
- selected food content of, 433

Seated back, 293
Seated leg curl, 299
Secondhand smoke, 471, 508–509
Sedentary, 5
Sedentary death syndrome (SeDS), 3
Sedentary lifestyles
- daily energy expenditure and, 189 (Figure 5.9)
- economic effects of, 25–26
- hypokinetic diseases and, 239

Selective estrogen receptor modulators (SERMs), 122
Selenium, 111
Self-analysis, 61, 65 (Table 2.2)
Self-confidence, 54–56
Self-control. *See* Willpower
Self-efficacy, 54–55, 57
Self-esteem, 388
Self-reevaluation, 62, 65 (Table 2.2)
Semivegetarians, 103
SEMO agility test, 346–347
Setpoint
- defined, 179
- example of, 179
- lowering, 179–180
- recommendations, 179
- theory of, 178–179

Sets
- defined, 275
- multiple, 274
- time factors, 274–275

Sexually transmitted diseases (STDs), 530
Sexually transmitted infections (STIs)
- adolescents with, 528 (Figure 14.1)
- behavior assessment, 543
- FAQs, 530
- knowledge assessment, 543–544
- my profile, 530
- prevalence of, 528
- prevention of
  - guidelines, 529
  - monogamous relationships, 540–541
  - wise dating, 540
- risk reduction, 541–543
- STD *vs.*, 530
- types of
  - chlamydia, 529–530
  - genital herpes, 533–534
  - gonorrhea, 531
  - hepatitis, 534
  - HPV, 477, 532–533
  - PDI, 531
  - syphilis, 531–532
  - trichomoniasis, 532

Shin-splints, 360–361
Shoes, 355, 355–356
Shoulder hyperextension, 330
Shoulder press, 297
Shoulder rotation stretch, 330

Shoulder rotation test
  indicators of, 312
  percentile ranks for, 317 (Table 8.3)
  procedure for, 315 (Figure 8.3)
Side plank, 290
Side stitch, 360
Side stretch, 329
Sighing, 400
Simple carbohydrates, 83
Single-knee-to-chest stretch, 333
Sit-and-reach stretch, 332
Sit-and-reach-test
  indicators of, 312
  percentile ranks for, 315 (Table 8.1)
  procedures for, 313 (Figure 8.1)
Sit-ups, 322 (Figure 8.5)
Sitting adductor stretch, 331
Sitting disease, 13–14
Skill-related fitness
  assessment, 375–376 (Lab 9A)
  behavior assessment, 372
  categories, 350 (Table 9.3)
  components of, 20, 351 (Table 9.4)
  contributions of, 345
  defined, 21
  FAQs, 345
  knowledge assessment, 373
  learning rate in, 346
  my profile, 344
  need for, 344–345
  percentile rank for, 350 (Table 9.1)
  performance tests for, 346–349
  principles of, 345–346
  for team sports, 350–351
Skin cancer
  melanoma, 468–469
  nonmelanoma, 463
  risk factors, 471
  self-examination, 474 (Figure 12.11)
  warning signs, 474 (Figure 12.10)
Skinfold thickness technique
  defined, 141
  fat percentage estimates, 143–144 (Table 4.1–4.3)
  landmarks for, 141 (Figure 4.3)
  procedure for, 141–142, 142 (Figure 4.4)
Sleep
  amount needed, 385
  disorders, 385
  enhancing quality of, 385
  weight management and, 182
  wellness and, 384–385
Slow-twitch fibers, 269
SMART goals
  components of, 64–67
  defined, 65
  setting, 74–75 (Lab 2C)
Smokeless tobacco, 466–467
Social cognitive theory, 57
Social liberation, 61, 65 (Table 2.2)
Social wellness, 16, 17
Soda consumption, 79–80
Soda test, 347–348
Sodium
  CHD and, 81
  foods high in, 445 (Table 11.11)
  hypertension and, 444–445
Soluble fiber, 85
South Beach diet, 171
Soy products, 106, 466
Specific adaptation to imposed demand (SAID), 270
Specific goals, 64–66
Speed tests, 350
Sphygmomanometer, 29
Spinning, 364
Spiritual wellness, 17–18
Spontaneous remission, 388
Sports. *See also* Athletes
  conditioning for
    base fitness, 365–366
    HIIT programs, 366
    overtraining risk in, 368–369
    periodization, 369–370
  injuries in, 359, 360 (Table 9.5)
  preactivity screening for, 365–366
  preparing for, 363–365
  skill-related components of, 351 (Table 9.4)
  specific stretching for, 320
  team, fitness for, 350–351
Sports drinks, 357
Spot reducing, 188, 189
Squat, 298
Stability exercise balls
  abdominal-crunch, 301
  for athletes, 363
  guidelines for, 280
  hamstring roll, 303
  jackknives, 303
  plank on, 300
  push-up on, 301
  reverse supine bridge, 301
  wall squat, 302
Standing long jump test, 349
Standing toe touch, 322 (Figure 8.5)
Starch, 84
Static stretching, 318
Statin drugs, 438, 440
Stearic acid, 423
Step test
  estimated V0inf2max/inf for, 227 (Figure 6.3)
  procedure for, 227 (Figure 6.4)
  use of, 225–226
Step-up, 286
Steps per day, 12 (Table 1.2), 13 (Table 1.3)
Sterol regulatory element-binding proteins (SRBPs), 423
Sterols, 89
STIs. *See* Sexually transmitted infections (STIs)
Stomach cancer, 479
Storage fat, 138–139, 150
Straight-let sit-ups, 322 (Figure 8.5)
Strength training. *See also* Muscular strength and endurance; specific exercises
  for athletes, 363
  behavior assessment, 284
  benefits of, 260
  blood pressure management with, 446
  body composition changes, 262–263
  defined, 259
  diabetes and, 353
  dynamic, 271–273
  exercises, guidelines for, 276–277
  flexibility and, 310
  frequency of, 275–276
  gains, observation of, 276
  guidelines, 276 (Table 7.6)
  healthy, 279
  knowledge assessment, 284
  machines for, 272–274
  mode of, 270–272
  overload principle in, 269
  periodization in, 369
  Pilates system, 279–280
  plyometrics, 276
  prescription for, 268–269
  principles of, 270–276
  protein needs and, 119
  recovery time in, 275
  resistance in, 274
  safety guidelines, 280–282
  sets in, 274–275
  specificity of, 270
  sport of, 262
  sports specific, 365
  stability balls for, 280
  steroid use for, 262
  volume in, 270–271
  weight management and, 184
  with weights, 291–300
  without weights, 286–290
Strength training programs
  guidelines for, 276 (Table 7.5)
  ideal, 273–274
  log for, 307–308 (Lab 7B)
  record form, 283 (Figure 7.9)
  setting up, 282–283
Streptococcus salivarius thermophilus, 106
Stress
  -performance/health relationship to, 386 (Figure 10.1)
  adaptation to, 387–388
  behavior patterns in, 389
  common symptoms of, 395
  CVD and, 448–449
  defined, 385–386
  FAQs, 383
  hormones and, 384
  illness and, 384
  knowledge assessment, 406
  lower back pain and, 326
  mastering, 390
  perception of, 394–395
  physiological response to, 396 (Figure 10.4)
  smoking and, 511
  sources of, 388–389
  vulnerability questionnaire, 413–414 (Lab 10C)
  vulnerability to, 392
Stress electrocardiogram, 428–429
Stress events scale, 389, 409–410 (10A)
Stress management. *See also* Relaxation techniques
  behavior assessment, 406
  evaluation log for, 419–420 (Lab 10E)
  good, characteristics of, 401
  individuality of, 405
  knowledge assessment, 406
  my profile, 383
  physical activity for, 395–397
  tai chi for, 405
  thirty-second body scan for, 397
  time management for, 392–394, 415–418 (Lab 10D)
  yoga for, 404–405
Stressors, 387, 389 (Figure 10.3)
Stretching. *See also* Flexibility
  basic, 329–332
  behavior assessment, 327
  contraindicated, 321, 322 (Figure 8.5)
  defined, 310
  for dysmenorrhea, 310
  FAQ, 310
  frequency, 320
  guidelines for, 320 (Figure 8.4)
  intensity of, 319–320
  knowledge assessment, 327
  for low-back pain, 332–336
  modes of, 318–319
  physiological response to, 319
  repetitions in, 320
  sports specific, 320
  stage changes, 341–342 (Lab 8C)
  warm-up and, 320
  weight loss and, 321
Stroke
  consequences of, 424
  risk, diet and, 423
  warning signs of, 424
Stroke volume
  defined, 221
  lower RHR and, 220
  ranges of, 223
Structured interview, 389
Subcutaneous fat, 141, 151 (Figure 4.9)
Subluxation, 310
Substance Abuse and Mental Health Services Administration, 506
Substrates, 81
Sugar
  cancer and, 465
  in chocolate, 423–424
  excessive intake, risk of, 79–80
  in sports drinks, 357
Sulforaphane, 464 (Table 12.1)
Sun exposure, 468–469
Sun protection factor (SPF), 468–469
Supine bridge, 335
Supplementation
  antioxidants, 110
  athletes. need for, 117–118
  beta-carotene, 111
  calcium, 120–121
  cancer risk from, 467
  creatine phosphate, 119–120
  defined, 109
  dietary needs of, 118
  folate, 113
  Iron, 110
  megadose risks of, 109–110
  multivitamins, 111–112
  selenium, 111
  vitamin C, 111
  Vitamin D, 112
Suppressor genes, 456–457
Supramaximal interval training, 368
Swan stretch, 322 (Figure 8.5)
Swimming, 189
Synergistic action, 503
Synergy, 114
Synthetic Drug Abuse Prevention Act, 502
Synthetic marijuana, 502
Syphilis, 531–532
Systolic blood pressure, 29, 443

T

Tachycardia, 496
Tai chi
  defined, 397
  health benefits of, 405
  performance-related benefits, 362
  stress reduction with, 396
Tar, 506–507
Tea consumption, 464–465
Television viewing, 47
Telomerase, 458

Telomeres, 458–459
Tempo training, 368
Termination/adoption stage, 60–61
Testicular cancer, 470, 478, 478 (Figure 12.13)
Tests. *See* Performance tests
delta-9-Tetrahydrocannabional (THC), 496
Thermogenic response, 357
Thirty-second body scan, 397
Thyroid cancer, 480
Time killers, 416 (Lab 10D)
Time management
  evaluation of, 418 (Lab 10D)
  goals and skills, 415–418 (Lab 10D)
  skills, 394
  steps, 392–393
Time-specific goals, 67
Tobacco. *See also* Cigarette smoking
  adolescent use, 507 (Figure 13.4)
  cancer-induced by, 460, 467–468
  CVD risk and, 448
  environmental, 508
  health care costs of, 509–510
  products, 506
  smokeless, 466–467, 509
  trends in, 510
Tolerable upper intake levels (ULs)
  defined, 95
  function of, 96
  selected, 96 (Table 3.9)
  use of, 94
Total body electric conductivity (TOBEC), 139
Total body rotation test
  indicators of, 312
  percentile ranks for, 316 (Table 8.2)
  procedure for, 314 (Figure 8.2)
Total daily energy requirement, 178 (Figure 5.5)
Training volume, 270
Trans-fatty acids
  characterization of, 87
  cholesterol elevation by, 434
  foods containing, 423, 435 (Table 11.5)
Transtheoretical model
  applicable processes of, 59 (Table 2.1)
  defined, 57
  stages of, 58–59
Triceps extension, 295
Triceps stretch, 332
Trichomoniasis, 532
Triglycerides. *See* Fatty acids
Trimethylamine-*N*-oxide, 90
Trunk rotation/lower back stretch, 334
Tumors
  benign, 456
  forms of, 456
  malignant, 456
  mutations for, 458
12-Minute swim test
  fitness categories, 231 (Table 6.7)
  procedure for, 229 (Figure 6.6)
  use of, 228
Type A behavior
  assessment, 411–412 (Lab 10B)
  changing, 391
  characteristics of, 389
Type B behavior, 389
Type C behavior, 389

U

U.S. Pharmacopoeia standards, 114
ULs. *See* Tolerable upper intake levels (ULs)
Ultraviolet A (UVA) rays, 468, 471
Ultraviolet B (UVB) rays, 468
Underweight, 149
Undulating periodization, 270
Unilateral eccentric knee flexion, 296
Unsaturated fats
  foods rich in, 433–434
  omega-3, 87–89
  omega-9, 89
Upper and lower back stretch, 333
Upright double-leg lift, 322 (Figure 8.5)
Upright rowing, 298
Urge surfing. *See* Mindfulness

V

V-sits, 322 (Figure 8.5)
Values
  caloric, 99
  core, 51–52
  daily, 95–97
  establishment of, 50–51
Vegans, 103
Vegetables
  antioxidants in, 113
  cardiovascular benefits of, 439
  cruciferous, 462–463
  recommended daily amounts, 82 (Figure 3.1)
Vegetarianism
  defined, 103
  nutrient concerns in, 103–105, 105
  soy products and, 106
  types of, 103
Very low-calorie diet, 179
Very low-density proteins, 431
Vigorous-intensity exercise
  daily energy expenditure and, 189 (Figure 5.9)
  defined, 19
  eating before, recommendations, 355
  energy formation mechanisms in, 117 (Figure 3.14)
  insulin sensitivity and, 441
  moderate-intensity *vs.*, 234
  protein needs and, 119
Viny yoga, 404
Visceral fat, 151 (Figure 4.9)
Visual imagery
  defined, 401
  procedure for, 400–402
  research on, 400
Vitamin A, 91
Vitamin Binf12/inf, 439
Vitamin Binf6/inf, 439
Vitamin C
  cardiac benefits of, 434
  function of, 91
  supplements, 111
Vitamin D
  cancer prevention with, 462–464
  deficiency, 113
  foods rich in, 112 (Table 3.11)
  sources for vegetarians, 105
  sources of, 91
  supplements, 112
Vitamin E, 110–111, 434
Vitamins
  classification of, 91
  defined, 91
  major functions of, 92 (Table 3.5)
  Uls for adults, 96 (Table 3.9)
VOinf2max/inf. *See* Maximal oxygen uptake (VOinf2max/inf)
Volume
  CVD risk based on, 236 (Figure 6.8)
  exercise, 239
  increasing, 368–369
  strength training, 270–271
  stroke, 220–221, 223
  training, 270
Volumetrics eating plan, 171

W

Waist circumference (WC) technique
  defined, 151
  disease risks based on, 151–152 (Table 4.8–4.9)
  procedure for, 150
  use of, 137
Waist-to-height ratio (WHtR)
  Ashwell shape chart, 153 (Figure 4.10)
  guidelines for, 152–153
  procedure for, 152
  use, 137
  use of, 154
Walking, 230–233, 232 (Table 6.9)
Wall squat, 302
Warm-ups, 238, 320
Water
  during exercise, 357
  in food, 91–92
  function of, 91
WC. *See* Waist circumference (WC) technique
Weight gain, 188, 211–212 (Lab 5D)
Weight management
  adherence, behavior modification and, 195–196
  appetite regulation in, 181
  balancing calories for, 124
  behavior assessment, 199
  behavior modification log for, 205 (Lab 5B)
  BMR and, 184
  daily food logs for, 194–195
  dilemma, 169
  exercise for
    benefits of, 182–185
    intensity/duration in, 185–187
    lifetime aerobic, 184
  fad diets for, 169–170, 173
  FAQ, 165
  healthy plan for, 211–212 (Lab 5D)
  knowledge assessment, 199–200
  measuring progress in, 213–214 (Lab 5E)
  my profile, 166
  myths, 188
  nutrition and, 180
  physical activity guidelines for, 183
  physiology of, 177–180
  sensible, 188–194
  setpoint theory of, 178–180
  sleep and, 182
  strategies for, 196–199
  strength training and, 184
  stretching and, 321
Weight Watchers diet, 171
Weight-regulating mechanism (WRM), 178
Wellness
  behavior assessment, 30
  challenges, 26–27
  continuum of, 16 (Figure 1.6)
  defined, 15
  dimensions of, 15–18
  evaluation, 574 (Lab 15C)
  health promotion and, 15
  information, reliable sources for, 560
  knowledge assessment, 30
  lifestyle questionnaire, 35–37 (Lab 1B)
  longevity and, 18–19
  my profile, 3
  personalized approach to, 27
  sleep and, 384–385
Whole grains
  defined, 81
  protein rich, 86
  recommended daily amounts, 82 (Figure 3.1)
  refined grains *versus,* 100
Willpower, 52
Windmill, 322 (Figure 8.5)
Workload, 220
Written goals, 62–63

Y

Yoga
  for athletes, 364
  for CHD prevention, 404
  contraindicated, 322 (Figure 8.5)
  defined, 397
  for stress reduction, 396
  types of, 325, 404
Yogalates, 404
Yogarobics, 404
Yogurts, 106

Z

Zinc, 105
Zocor, 438
Zone diet, 171
Zumba, 364–365

HEALTH-RELATED COMPONENTS OF PHYSICAL FITNESS

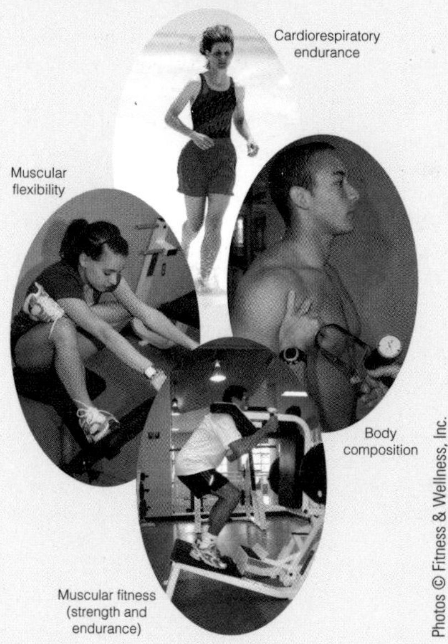

Photos © Fitness & Wellness, Inc.

Cardiorespiratory endurance The ability of the lungs, heart, and blood vessels to deliver adequate amounts of oxygen to the cells to meet the demands of prolonged physical activity.
Body composition The fat and non-fat components of the human body; important in assessing recommended body weight.
Muscular strength The ability of a muscle to exert maximum force against resistance (for example, 1 repetition maximum [or 1 RM] on the bench press exercise).
Muscular endurance The ability of a muscle to exert submaximal force repeatedly over time.
Flexibility The achievable range of motion at a joint or group of joints without causing injury.

HEALTHY LIFESTYLE HABITS

Research indicates that adhering to the following 12 lifestyle habits will significantly improve health and extend life.

I PLAN TO	I DID IT	
❑	❑	1. Participate in a lifetime physical activity program.
❑	❑	2. Do not smoke cigarettes.
❑	❑	3. Eat right.
❑	❑	4. Avoid snacking.
❑	❑	5. Maintain recommended body weight through adequate nutrition and exercise.
❑	❑	6. Sleep 7 to 8 hours each night.
❑	❑	7. Lower your stress levels.
❑	❑	8. Be wary of alcohol.
❑	❑	9. Surround yourself with healthy friendships.
❑	❑	10. Be informed about the environment.
❑	❑	11. Increase education.
❑	❑	12. Take personal safety measures.

TRY IT

Look at the list above and indicate which habits are already a part of your lifestyle. What changes could you make to incorporate some additional healthy habits into your daily life?

ESTIMATED NUMBER OF STEPS TO WALK, JOG, OR RUN A MILE BASED ON PACE, HEIGHT, AND GENDER

	Pace (min/mile)											
	Walking								Jogging/Running			
	20		18		16		15		12	10	8	6
Height	Women	Men	Women	Men	Women	Men	Women	Men	(both men and women)			
5'0"	2,371	2,338	2,244	2,211	2,117	2,084	2,054	2,021	1,997	1,710	1,423	1,136
5'2"	2,343	2,310	2,216	2,183	2,089	2,056	2,026	1,993	1,970	1,683	1,396	1,109
5'4"	2,315	2,282	2,188	2,155	2,061	2,028	1,998	1,965	1,943	1,656	1,369	1,082
5'6"	2,286	2,253	2,160	2,127	2,033	2,000	1,969	1,937	1,916	1,629	1,342	1,055
5'8"	2,258	2,225	2,131	2,098	2,005	1,872	1,941	1,908	1,889	1,602	1,315	1,028
5'10"	2,230	2,197	2,103	2,070	1,976	1,943	1,913	1,880	1,862	1,575	1,288	1,001
6'0"	2,202	2,169	2,075	2,042	1,948	1,915	1,885	1,852	1,835	1,548	1,261	974
6'2"	2,174	2,141	2,047	2,014	1,920	1,887	1,857	1,824	1,808	1,521	1,234	947

Prediction equations (pace in min/mile and height in inches):
Walking
Women: Steps/mile = 1,949 + [(63.4 x pace) – (14.1 x height)]
Men: Steps/mile = 1,916 + [(63.4 x pace) – (14.1 x height)]
Jogging
Women and Men: Steps/mile = 1,084 + [(63.4 x pace) – (14.1 x height)]

Adapted from Werner W. K. Hoeger et al., "One-Mile Step Count at Walking and Running Speeds," *ACSM's Health & Fitness Journal*, Vol 12(1):14-19, 2008.

Physical activity Bodily movement produced by skeletal muscles; requires expenditure of energy and produces progressive health benefits. Examples include walking, taking the stairs, dancing, gardening, yard work, house cleaning, snow shoveling, washing the car, and all forms of structured exercise.
Exercise A type of physical activity that requires planned, structured, and repetitive bodily movement with the intent of improving or maintaining one or more components of physical fitness.
Moderate physical activity Activity that uses 150 calories of energy per day, or 1,000 calories per week.
Vigorous activity Any exercise that requires an MET level equal to or greater than 6 METs (21 mL/kg/min). 1 MET is the energy expenditure at rest, 3.5 mL/kg/min, and METs are defined as multiples of this resting metabolic rate (examples of activities that require a 6-MET level include aerobics, walking uphill at 3.5 mph, cycling at 10 to 12 mph, playing doubles in tennis, and vigorous strength training).
Physical fitness The ability to meet the ordinary as well as the unusual demands of daily life safely and effectively without being overly fatigued and still have energy left for leisure and recreational activities.
Wellness The constant and deliberate effort to stay healthy and achieve the highest potential for well-being. It encompasses seven dimensions—physical, emotional, mental, social, environmental, occupational, and spiritual—and integrates them all into a quality life.
Health-related fitness Fitness programs that are prescribed to improve the individual's overall health.
Health A state of complete well-being—not just the absence of disease or infirmity.
Risk factors Lifestyle and genetic variables that may lead to disease.

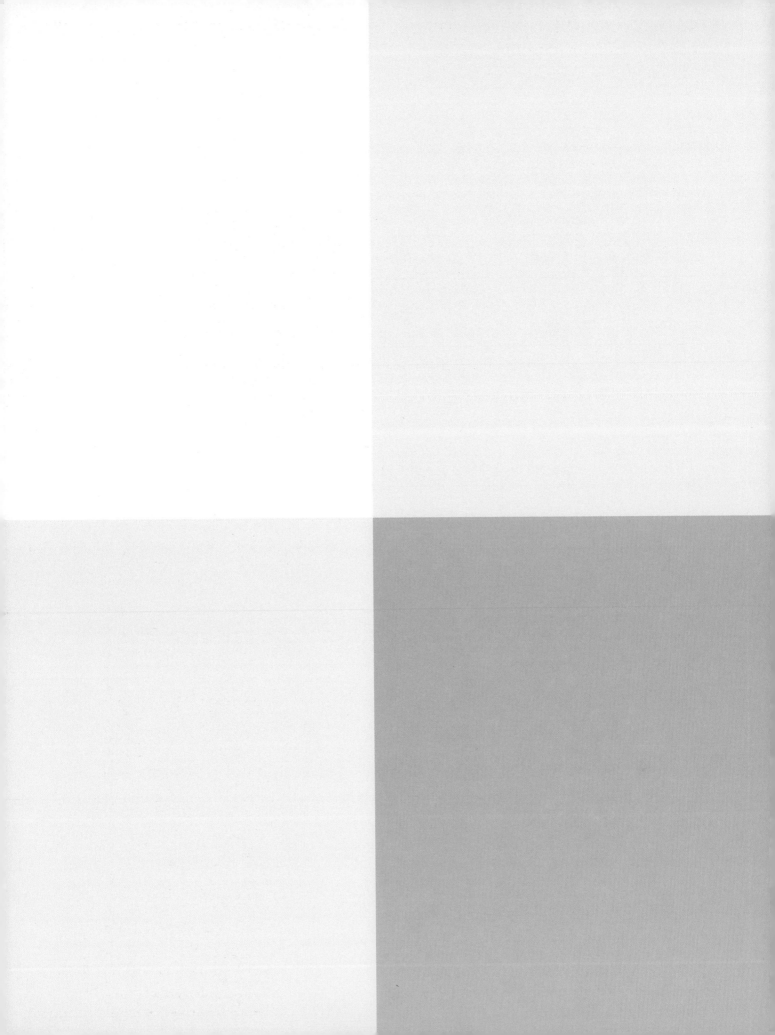

STAGES OF CHANGE: MODEL OF PROGRESSION AND RELAPSE

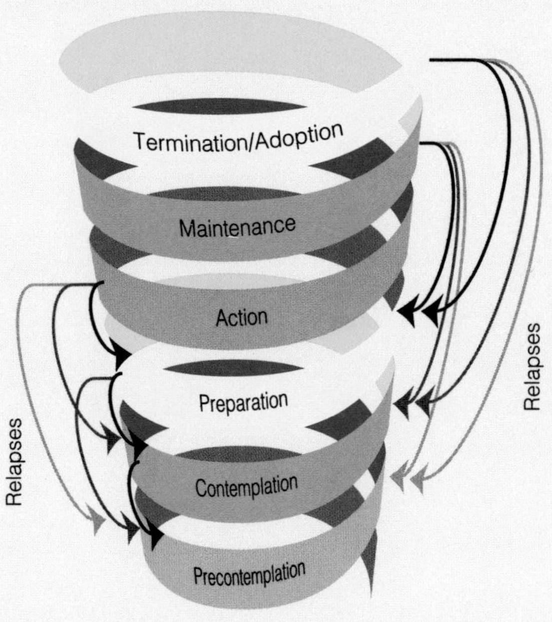

Behavior modification The process of permanently changing negative behaviors to positive behaviors that will lead to better health and well-being.
Motivation The desire and will to do something.
Transtheoretical model Behavioral modification model proposing that change is accomplished through a series of progressive stages in keeping with a person's readiness to change.
Precontemplation stage Stage of change in the transtheoretical model in which an individual is unwilling to change behavior.
Contemplation stage Stage of change in the transtheoretical model in which the individual is considering changing behavior within the next 6 months.
Preparation stage Stage of change in the transtheoretical model in which the individual is getting ready to make a change within the next month.
Action stage Stage of change in the transtheoretical model in which the individual is actively changing a negative behavior or adopting a new, healthy behavior.
Maintenance stage Stage of change in the transtheoretical model in which the individual maintains behavioral change for up to 5 years.
Termination/adoption stage Stage of change in the transtheoretical model in which the individual has eliminated an undesirable behavior or maintained a positive behavior for more than 5 years.
Processes of change Actions that help a person achieve change in behavior.
Self-efficacy One's belief in the ability to perform a given task.
Goals The ultimate aims toward which effort is directed.
SMART An acronym used in reference to Specific, Measurable, Attainable, Realistic, and Time-specific goals.
Objectives Steps required to reach a goal.

STEPS FOR SUCCESSFUL BEHAVIOR MODIFICATION

I PLAN TO	I DID IT	
❑	❑	1. Acknowledge that you have a problem.
❑	❑	2. Describe the behavior to change (increase physical activity, stop overeating, quit smoking).
❑	❑	3. List advantages and disadvantages of changing the specified behavior.
❑	❑	4. Decide positively that you will change.
❑	❑	5. Identify your stage of change.
❑	❑	6. Set a realistic goal (SMART goal), completion date, and sign a behavioral contract.
❑	❑	7. Define your behavioral change plan: List processes of change, techniques of change, and objectives that will help you reach your goal.
❑	❑	8. Implement the behavior change plan.
❑	❑	9. Monitor your progress toward the desired goal.
❑	❑	10. Periodically evaluate and reassess your goal.
❑	❑	11. Reward yourself when you achieve your goal.
❑	❑	12. Maintain the successful change for good.

TRY IT

In your Online Journal or class notebook, record your answers to the following questions:

Have you consciously attempted to incorporate a healthy behavior into or eliminate a negative behavior from your lifestyle? If so, what steps did you follow, and what helped you achieve your goal?

COMPUTATION FOR FAT CONTENT IN FOOD

Nutrition Facts

Serving Size 1 cup (240 ml)
Servings Per Container 4

Amount Per Serving

Calories 120	Calories from Fat 45
	% Daily Value*
Total Fat 5g	**8%**
Saturated Fat 3g	**15%**
Trans Fat 0g	**0%**
Cholesterol 20mg	**7%**
Sodium 120mg	**5%**
Total Carbohydrate 12g	**4%**
Dietary Fiber 0g	**0%**
Sugars 12g	
Protein 8g	

Vitamin A	10%	Vitamin C	4%
Calcium	30%	Iron	0%

* Percent Daily Values are based on a 2,000 calorie diet. Your daily values may be higher or lower depending on your calorie needs:

	Calories	2,000	2,500
Total Fat	Less than	65g	80g
Sat Fat	Less than	20g	25g
Cholesterol	Less than	300mg	300mg
Sodium	Less than	2,300mg	2,300mg
Total Carbohydrate		300g	375g
Fiber		25g	30g

Calories per gram:
Fat 9 • Carbohydrate 4 • Protein 4

Percent fat calories = (grams of fat × 9) ÷ calories per serving × 100

5 grams of fat × 9 calories per grams of fat = 45 calories from fat

45 calories from fat ÷ 120 calories per serving × 100 = 38% fat

THE AMERICAN DIET: CURRENT AND RECOMMENDED CARBOHYDRATE, FAT, AND PROTEIN INTAKE EXPRESSED AS A PERCENTAGE OF TOTAL CALORIES

	Current Percentage	Recommended Percentage*
Carbohydrates	50	45–65
Simple	26	<25
Complex	24	20–40
Fat	34	20–30**
Monounsaturated	11	≤20
Polyunsaturated	10	≤10
Saturated	13	<7
Protein	16	10–35

*Adapted from the 2002 recommended guidelines by the National Academy of Sciences.
**Less than 30% is recommended by most major national health organizations. Up to 35% is allowed for individuals with metabolic syndrome who may need additional fat in the diet.

CALORIC AND FAT CONTENT OF SELECTED FAST FOODS

	Calories	Total Fat	Saturated Fat (grams)	Percent Fat Calories
Subway Steak & Cheese	390	14	5	32
Subway Cold Cut Trio	440	21	7	43
Subway Tuna	450	22	6	44
Mexican				
Taco Bell Crunchy Taco	170	10	4	53
Taco Bell Taco Supreme	220	14	6	57
Taco Bell Soft Chicken Taco	190	7	3	33
Taco Bell Bean Burrito	370	12	4	29
Taco Bell Fiesta Steak Burrito	370	12	4	29
Taco Bell Grilled Steak Soft Taco	290	17	4	53
Taco Bell Double Decker Taco	340	14	5	37
French Fries				
Wendy's, biggie (5 ½ oz)	440	19	7	39
McDonald's, large (6 oz)	540	26	9	43
Burger King, large (5 ½ oz)	500	25	13	45

Continued on back

CALORIC AND FAT CONTENT OF SELECTED FAST FOODS

	Calories	Total Fat	Saturated Fat (grams)	Percent Fat Calories
Burgers				
McDonald's Big Mac	590	34	11	52
McDonald's Big N' Tasty with Cheese	590	37	12	56
McDonald's Quarter Pounder with Cheese	530	30	13	51
Burger King Whopper	760	46	15	54
Burger King Bacon Double Cheeseburger	580	34	18	53
Burger King BK Smoke-house Cheddar Griller	720	48	19	60
Burger King Whopper with Cheese	850	53	22	56
Burger King Double Whopper	1,060	69	27	59
Burger King Double Whopper with Cheese	1,150	76	33	59
Wendy's Baconator	830	51	22	55

Continued on back

"SUPER" FOODS

The following "super" foods that fight disease and promote health should be included often in the diet. Are you eating these foods regularly?

I PLAN TO	I DID IT		I PLAN TO	I DID IT	
❑	❑	Acai berries	❑	❑	Salmon (wild)
❑	❑	Avocados	❑	❑	Soy
❑	❑	Bananas	❑	❑	Oats and oatmeal
❑	❑	Barley	❑	❑	Olives and olive oil
❑	❑	Beans	❑	❑	Onions
❑	❑	Beets	❑	❑	Oranges
❑	❑	Blueberries	❑	❑	Peppers
❑	❑	Broccoli	❑	❑	Pomegranates
❑	❑	Butternut squash	❑	❑	Quinoa
❑	❑	Carrots	❑	❑	Spinach
❑	❑	Goji berries	❑	❑	Strawberries
❑	❑	Grapes	❑	❑	Sweet potatoes
❑	❑	Kale	❑	❑	Tea (green, black, red)
❑	❑	Kiwifruit			
❑	❑	Flaxseeds	❑	❑	Tomatoes
❑	❑	Lentils	❑	❑	Walnuts
❑	❑	Nuts (Brazil, walnuts)	❑	❑	Watermelon

	Calories	Total Fat	Saturated Fat (grams)	Percent Fat Calories
Shakes				
Wendy's Frosty, medium (16 oz)	440	11	7	23
McDonald's McFlurry, small (12 oz)	610	22	14	32
Burger King, Old Fashioned Ice Cream Shake, medium (22 oz)	760	41	29	49
Hash Browns				
McDonald's Hash Browns (2 oz)	130	8	4	55
Burger King, Hash Browns, small (2 ½ oz)	230	15	9	59

* 6-inch sandwich with no mayo

TRY IT

Using the information in the table, record in your Online Journal or class notebook ways you can restructure fast-food consumption to decrease caloric value and fat and saturated fat content in your diet.

SOURCE: Adapted from Restaurant Confidential Copyright © 2002 by the Center for Science in the Public Interest. Used by permission of Workman Publishing Co., Inc, New York.

I PLAN TO	I DID IT	
❑	❑	Yogurt

TRY IT

Using the above list, make a list of which super foods you can add to your diet and when you can eat them (snacks/meals). List meals that you can add these foods to.

	Calories	Total Fat	Saturated Fat (grams)	Percent Fat Calories
Sandwiches				
Arby's Regular Roast Beef	350	16	6	41
Arby's Super Roast Beef	470	23	7	44
Arby's Roast Chicken Club	520	28	7	48
Arby's Market Fresh Roast Beef & Swiss	810	42	13	47
McDonald's Crispy Chicken	430	21	8	43
McDonald's Filet-O-Fish	470	26	5	50
McDonald's Chicken McGrill	400	17	3	38
Wendy's Chicken Club	470	19	4	36
Wendy's Breast Fillet	430	16	3	34
Wendy's Grilled Chicken	300	7	2	21
Burger King Specialty Chicken	560	28	6	45
Subway Veggie Delight*	226	3	1	12
Subway Turkey Breast	281	5	2	16
Subway Sweet Onion Chicken Teriyaki	374	5	2	12

SELECTING NUTRITIOUS FOODS

Do you regularly follow the habits below?

To select nutritious foods:

I PLAN TO	I DID IT		
❑	❑	1.	Given the choice between whole foods and refined, processed foods, choose the former (apples rather than apple pie, potatoes rather than potato chips). No nutrients have been refined out of the whole foods, and they contain less fat, salt, and sugar.
❑	❑	2.	Choose the leaner cuts of meat. Select fish or poultry often, beef seldom. Ask for broiled, not fried, to control your fat intake.
❑	❑	3.	Use both raw and cooked vegetables and fruits. Raw foods offer more fiber and vitamins, such as folate and thiamin, that are destroyed by cooking. Cooking foods frees other vitamins and minerals for absorption.
❑	❑	4.	Include milk, milk products, or other calcium sources for the calcium you need. Use low-fat or non-fat items to reduce fat and calories.
❑	❑	5.	Learn to use margarine, butter, and oils sparingly. A little gives flavor, a lot overloads you with fat, calories, and increases disease risk.
❑	❑	6.	Vary your choices. Eat broccoli today, carrots tomorrow, and corn the next day. Eat Chinese today, Italian

Continued on back

GUIDELINES FOR A HEALTHY DIET

I PLAN TO	I DID IT	
❑	❑	Exercise portion control (keep portions moderate).
❑	❑	Base your diet on a large variety of foods.
❑	❑	Consume ample amounts of green, yellow, and orange fruits and vegetables.
❑	❑	Eat foods high in complex carbohydrates, including at least three 1-ounce servings of whole-grain foods per day.
❑	❑	Obtain most of your vitamins and minerals from food sources.
❑	❑	Eat foods rich in vitamin D.
❑	❑	Maintain adequate calcium intake and consider a vitamin D_3 supplement during the winter months (or throughout the year if you don't regularly get "safe sun exposure").
❑	❑	Consume protein in moderation.
❑	❑	Limit daily fat, trans fat, and saturated fat intake.
❑	❑	Limit cholesterol consumption to less than 300 mg per day.
❑	❑	Limit sodium intake to 2,300 mg per day.

Continued on back

Specific Nutrition Recommendations in the *Dietary Guidelines for Americans 2010*

Increase consumption of

- Fruits and vegetables
- Whole grains
- Low-fat dairy products
- Various lean protein choices
- Seafood
- Healthy fats
- Foods high in fiber, calcium, potassium, and vitamin D

Decrease intake of

- Saturated fats
- Trans fats
- Dietary cholesterol
- Sodium
- Refined grains
- Alcohol

Nutrition Science that studies the relationship of foods to optimal health and performance.

Nutrients Substances found in food that provide energy, regulate metabolism, and help with growth and repair of body tissues.

Glycemic index (GI) A measure that is used to rate the plasma glucose response of carbohydrate-containing foods with the response produced by the same amount of carbohydrate from a standard source, usually glucose or white bread.

Glycemic load A numeric value calculated by multiplying the GI of a particular food by its carbohydrate content in grams and dividing by 100. The usefulness of the glycemic load is based on the theory that a high-glycemic-index food eaten in small quantities provides a similar effect in blood sugar rise as a consumption of a larger quantity of a low-glycemic food.

Trans fatty acid Solidified fat formed by adding hydrogen to monounsaturated and polyunsaturated fats to increase shelf life.

Omega-3 fatty acids Polyunsaturated fatty acids found primarily in cold-water seafood, flaxseed, and flaxseed oil; thought to lower blood cholesterol and triglycerides.

Vitamins Organic nutrients essential for normal metabolism, growth, and development of the body.

Minerals Inorganic nutrients essential for normal body functions; found in the body and in food.

Dietary Reference Intakes (DRI) A general term that describes four types of nutrient standards that establish adequate amounts and maximum safe nutrient intakes in the diet: Estimated Average Requirements (EAR), Recommended Dietary Allowances (RDA), Adequate Intakes (AI), and Tolerable Upper Intake Levels (UL).

Estimated Average Requirement (EAR) The amount of a nutrient that meets the dietary needs of half the people.

Recommended Dietary Allowance (RDA) The daily amount of a nutrient (statistically determined from the EARs) that is considered adequate to meet the known nutrient needs of almost 98 percent of all healthy people in the United States.

Adequate Intake (AI) The recommended amount of a nutrient intake when sufficient evidence is not available to calculate the EAR and subsequent RDA.

Upper Intake Level (UL) The highest level of nutrient intake that seems safe for most healthy people, beyond which exists an increased risk of adverse effects.

Daily Values (DVs) Reference values for nutrients and food components used in food labels.

Continued on back

- ❑ ❑ Limit sugar intake.
- ❑ ❑ If you drink alcohol, do so in moderation (one daily drink for women and two for men).

TRY IT

Carefully analyze the above guidelines and note the areas where you can improve your diet.

Work on one guideline each week until you are able to adhere to all of the above guidelines.

tomorrow, and broiled fish with brown rice and steamed vegetables the third day.

- ❑ ❑ 7. Load your plate with vegetables and unrefined starchy foods. A small portion of meat or cheese is all you need for protein.
- ❑ ❑ 8. When choosing breads and cereals, choose the whole-grain varieties.

To select nutritious fast foods:

- ❑ ❑ 9. Choose the broiled sandwich with lettuce, tomatoes, and other goodies—and hold the mayo—rather than the fish or chicken patties coated with breadcrumbs and cooked in fat.
- ❑ ❑ 10. Select a salad—and use more plain vegetables than those mixed with oily or mayonnaise-based dressings.
- ❑ ❑ 11. Order chili with more beans than meat. Choose a soft bean burrito over tacos with fried shells.
- ❑ ❑ 12. Drink low-fat milk rather than a cola beverage.

When choosing from a vending machine:

- ❑ ❑ 13. Choose cracker sandwiches over chips and pork rinds (virtually pure fat). Choose peanuts, pretzels, and popcorn over cookies and candy.
- ❑ ❑ 14. Choose milk and juices over cola beverages.

TRY IT

Based on what you have learned, list strategies you can use to increase food variety, enhance the nutritive value of your diet, and decrease fat and caloric content in your meals.

Phytonutrients Compounds thought to prevent and fight cancer; found in large quantities in fruits and vegetables.

Supplements Tablets, pills, capsules, liquids, or powders that contain vitamins, minerals, antioxidants, amino acids, herbs, or fiber that individuals take to increase their intake of these nutrients.

Antioxidants Compounds such as vitamins C and E, beta-carotene, and selenium that prevent oxygen from combining with other substances in the body to form harmful compounds.

Registered dietitian (RD) A person with a college degree in dietetics who meets all certification and continuing education requirements of the American Dietetic Association or Dietitians of Canada.

DISEASE RISK ACCORDING TO BODY MASS INDEX (BMI)

BMI	Disease Risk	Classification
<18.5	Increased	Underweight
18.5–21.99	Low	Acceptable
22.0–24.99	Very Low	Acceptable
25.0–29.99	Increased	Overweight
30.0–34.99	High	Obesity I
35.0–39.99	Very High	Obesity II
≥40.00	Extremely High	Obesity III

Continued on back

Body composition The fat and non-fat components of the human body; important in assessing recommended body weight.
Percent body fat Proportional amount of fat in the body based on the person's total weight; includes both essential fat and storage fat; also termed fat mass.
Lean body mass Body weight without body fat.
Essential fat Minimal amount of body fat needed for normal physiological functions; constitutes about 3 percent of total weight in men and 12 percent in women.
Storage fat Body fat in excess of essential fat; stored in adipose tissue.
Dual energy X-ray absorptiometry (DXA) Method to assess body composition that uses very low-dose beams of X-ray energy to measure total body fat mass, fat distribution pattern, and bone density.
Hydrostatic weighing Underwater technique to assess body composition; considered the most accurate of the body composition assessment techniques.
Skinfold thickness Technique to assess body composition by measuring a double thickness of skin at specific body sites.
Body mass index (BMI) Technique to determine thinness and excessive fatness that incorporates height and weight to estimate critical fat values at which the risk for disease increases.
Android obesity Obesity pattern seen in individuals who tend to store fat in the trunk or abdominal area.
Gynoid obesity Obesity pattern seen in people who store fat primarily around the hips and thighs.
Waist circumference (WC) A waist girth measurement to assess potential risk for disease based on intra-abdominal fat content.

TIPS FOR LIFETIME WEIGHT MANAGEMENT

Maintenance of recommended body composition is one of the most significant health issues of the 21st century. If you are committed to lifetime weight management, the following strategies will help:

I PLAN TO	I DID IT	
❏	❏	Accumulate 60 to 90 minutes of physical activity daily.
❏	❏	Exercise at a vigorous aerobic pace (high intensity) for a minimum of 20 minutes three times per week.
❏	❏	Strength train two to three times per week.
❏	❏	Use common sense and moderation in your daily diet.
❏	❏	Consume primarily a nutrient dense/low calorie diet (fruits, vegetables, whole grains, moderate protein, and low fat products—see chapter 5).
❏	❏	"Junior-size" instead of "super-size."
❏	❏	Regularly monitor body weight, body composition, body mass index, and waist circumference.

Continued on back

PHYSICAL ACTIVITY GUIDELINES FOR WEIGHT MANAGEMENT

The following physical activity guidelines are recommended to effectively manage body weight:

I PLAN TO	I DID IT	
❏	❏	30 minutes of physical activity on most days of the week if you do not have difficulty maintaining body weight (more minutes and/or higher intensity if you choose to reach a high level of physical fitness).
❏	❏	60 minutes of daily activity if you want to prevent weight gain.
❏	❏	Between 60 and 90 minutes each day if you are trying to lose weight or attempting to keep weight off following extensive weight loss (30 pounds of weight loss or more). Be sure to include some high-intensity/low-impact activities at least twice a week in your program.

Continued on back

DISEASE RISK ACCORDING TO BODY MASS INDEX (BMI) AND WAIST CIRCUMFERENCE (WC)

		Disease Risk Relative to Normal Weight and WC	
Classification	BMI (kg/m²)	Men ≤40″ (102 cm) Women ≤35″ (88 cm)	Men >40″ (102 cm) Women >35″ (88 cm)
Underweight	<18.5	Increased	Low
Normal	18.5–24.9	Very low	Increased
Overweight	25.0–29.9	Increased	High
Obesity Class I	30.0–34.9	High	Very high
Obesity Class II	35.0–39.9	Very high	Very high
Obesity Class III	≥40.0	Extremely high	Extremely high

Adapted from Expert Panel, *Executive Summary of the Clinical Guidelines on the Identification, Evaluation, and Treatment of Overweight and Obesity in Adults,* Archives of Internal Medicine 158:1855–1867, 1998.

TRY IT

In your Behavior Change Planner Progress Tracker, Online Journal, or class notebook, record how many minutes of daily physical activity you accumulate on a regular basis and record your thoughts on how effectively your activity has helped you manage your body weight. Is there one thing you could do today to increase your physical activity?

❑ | ❑ Do not allow increases in body weight (percent fat) to accumulate; deal immediately with the problem through moderate reductions in caloric intake and maintenance of physical activity and exercise habits.

TRY IT

In your Online Journal or your class notebook, note which of these tips you are already using and which ones you can incorporate into your daily habits right away.

Estimated energy requirement (EER) The average dietary energy (caloric) intake that is predicted to maintain energy balance in a healthy adult of defined age, gender, weight, height, and level of physical activity, consistent with good health.

Resting metabolic rate (RMR) The energy requirement to maintain the body's vital processes in the resting state.

Basal metabolic rate (BMR) The lowest level of oxygen consumption necessary to sustain life.

Weight-regulating mechanism (WRM) A feature of the hypothalamus of the brain that controls how much the body should weigh.

Setpoint Weight control theory that the body has an established weight and strongly attempts to maintain that weight.

Spot reducing Fallacious theory proposing that exercising a specific body part will result in significant fat reduction in that area.

Cellulite Term frequently used in reference to fat deposits that "bulge out"; these deposits are nothing but enlarged fat cells from excessive accumulation of body fat.

CARDIORESPIRATORY EXERCISE PRESCRIPTION GUIDELINES

Mode: Moderate- or vigorous-intensity aerobic activity (examples: walking, jogging, stair climbing, elliptical activity, aerobics, water aerobics, cycling, swimming, cross-country skiing, racquetball, basketball, and soccer)

Intensity: 30% to 85% of heart rate reserve (the training intensity is based on age, health status, initial fitness level, exercise tolerance, and exercise program goals)

Duration: Be active 20 to 90 minutes. At least 20 minutes of continuous vigorous-intensity or 30 minutes of moderate-intensity aerobic activity (the latter may be accumulated in segments of at least 10 minutes in duration each over the course of the day)

Frequency: 3 to 5 days per week for vigorous-intensity aerobic activity to accumulate at least 75 minutes per week, or 5 days per week of moderate-intensity aerobic activity for a minimum total of 150 minutes weekly

Rate of progression:

- Start with three training sessions per week of 15 to 20 minutes
- Increase the duration by 5 to 10 minutes per week and the frequency so that by the fourth or fifth week you are exercising five times per week
- Progressively increase frequency, duration, and intensity of exercise until you reach your fitness goal prior to exercise maintenance

Source: American College of Sports Medicine, *ACSM's Guidelines for Exercise Testing and Prescription* (Philadelphia: Lippincott Williams & Wilkins, 2010).

CARDIORESPIRATORY EXERCISE PRESCRIPTION

Intensity of Exercise

1. Estimate your own maximal heart rate (MHR)

   MHR = 207 − (.70 × age)

   MHR = 207 − (.70 × [ ]) = [ ] bpm

2. Resting Heart Rate (RHR). Determine your RHR by counting your pulse for a full minute in the evening after you have been sitting quietly, reading or watching a relaxing TV show.

   (RHR) = [ ] bpm

3. Heart Rate Reserve (HRR) = MHR − RHR

   HRR = [ ] − [ ] = [ ] beats

Continued on back

Cardiorespiratory (CR) endurance The ability of the lungs, heart, and blood vessels to deliver adequate amounts of oxygen to the cells to meet the demands of prolonged physical activity.

Aerobic Describes exercise that requires oxygen to produce the necessary energy (ATP) to carry out the activity.

Anaerobic Describes exercise that does not require oxygen to produce the necessary energy (ATP) to carry out the activity.

Oxygen uptake (VO_2) The amount of oxygen the human body uses.

Maximal oxygen uptake (VO_{2max}) Maximum amount of oxygen the body is able to utilize per minute of physical activity, commonly expressed in mL/kg/min; the best indicator of CR or aerobic fitness.

Cardiac output Amount of blood pumped by the heart in one minute.

Stroke volume Amount of blood pumped by the heart in one beat.

Principle of individuality Training concept holding that genetics plays a major role in individual responses to exercise training and these differences must be considered when designing exercise programs for different people.

Arterial-venous oxygen difference ($a\text{-}vO_{2diff}$) The amount of oxygen removed from the blood as determined by the difference in oxygen content between arterial and venous blood.

Vigorous exercise CR exercise that requires an intensity level of approximately 70% of capacity.

Heart rate reserve (HRR) The difference between maximal heart rate and resting heart rate.

Cardiorespiratory training zone Recommended training intensity range, in terms of exercise heart rate, to obtain adequate cardiorespiratory endurance development.

Rate of perceived exertion (RPE) A perception scale to monitor or interpret the intensity of aerobic exercise.

Anaerobic threshold The highest percentage of the VO_{2max} at which an individual can exercise (maximal steady state) for an extended time without accumulating significant amounts of lactic acid (accumulation of lactic acid forces an individual to slow down the exercise intensity or stop altogether).

MET Short for metabolic equivalent, the rate of energy expenditure at rest; 1 MET is the equivalent of a VO_2 of 3.5 mL/kg/min.

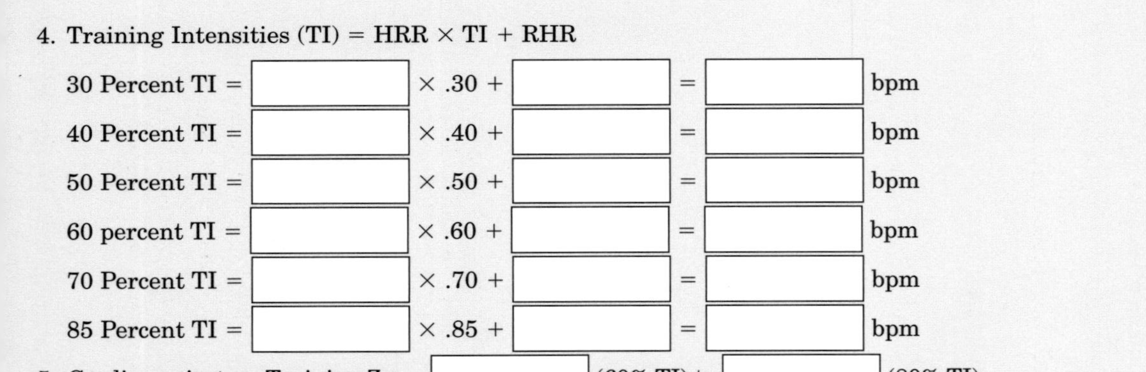

4. Training Intensities (TI) = HRR × TI + RHR

30 Percent TI = ______ × .30 + ______ = ______ bpm

40 Percent TI = ______ × .40 + ______ = ______ bpm

50 Percent TI = ______ × .50 + ______ = ______ bpm

60 percent TI = ______ × .60 + ______ = ______ bpm

70 Percent TI = ______ × .70 + ______ = ______ bpm

85 Percent TI = ______ × .85 + ______ = ______ bpm

5. Cardiorespiratory Training Zone: ______ (60% TI) to ______ (80% TI)

STRENGTH-TRAINING GUIDELINES

Mode: Select 8 to 10 dynamic strength-training exercises that involve the body's major muscle groups and include opposing muscle groups (chest and upper back, abdomen and lower back, front and back of the legs).

Resistance: Sufficient resistance to perform 8 to 12 repetitions maximum for muscular strength and 15 to 25 repetitions to near fatigue for muscular edurance. Older adults and injury prone individuals should use 10 to 15 repetitions with moderate resistance (50% to 60% of their 1 RM).

Sets: 2 to 4 sets per exercise with 2 to 3 minutes recovery between sets for optimal strength development. Less than 2 minutes per set if exercises are alternated that require different muscle groups (chest and upper back) or between muscular endurance sets.

Frequency: 2 to 3 days per week on nonconsecutive days. More frequent training can be done if different muscle groups are exercised on different days. (Allow at least 48 hours between strength-training sessions of the same muscle group.)

Source: Adapted from American College of Sports Medicine, ACSM's Guidelines for Exercise Testing and Prescription (Philadelphia: Wolters Kluwer / Lippincott Williams & Wilkins, 2010).

EXERCISE 15 Bench (Chest) Press

MACHINE From a seated position, grasp the bar handles (a) and press forward until the arms are completely extended (b), then return to the original position. Do not arch the back during this exercise.

FREE WEIGHTS Lie on the bench with arms extended and have one or two spotters help you place the barbell directly over your shoulders (a). Lower the weight to your chest (b) and then push it back up until you achieve full extension of the arms. Do not arch the back during this exercise.

MUSCLES DEVELOPED Pectoralis major, triceps, and deltoid

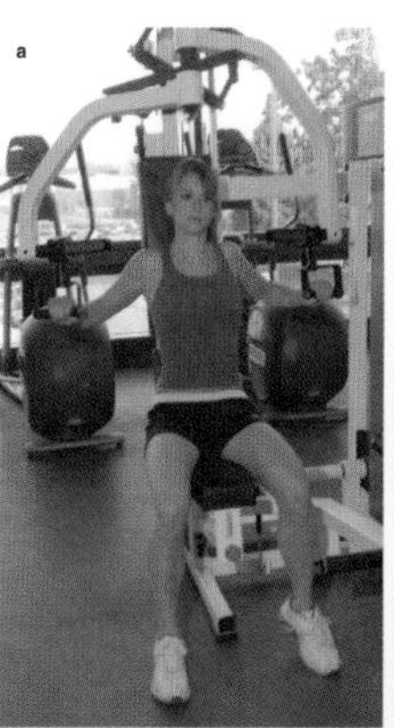

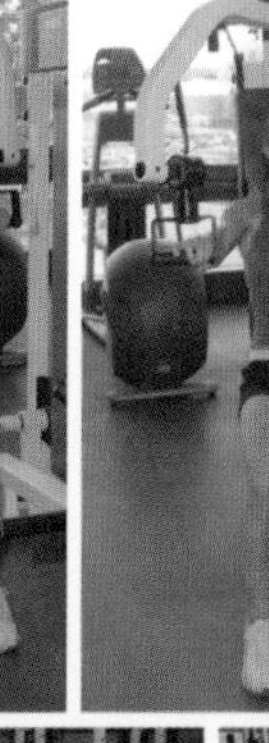

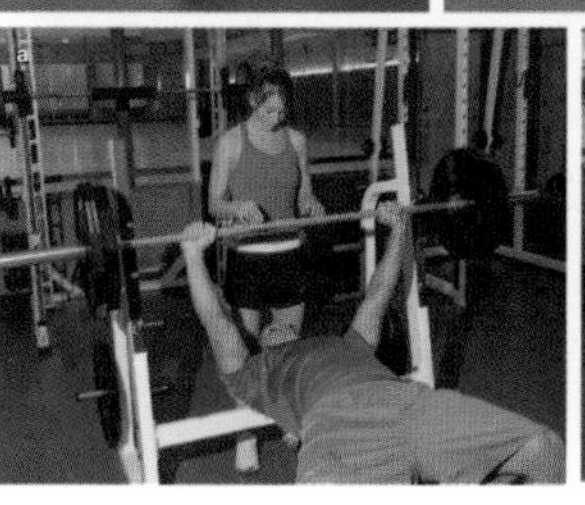

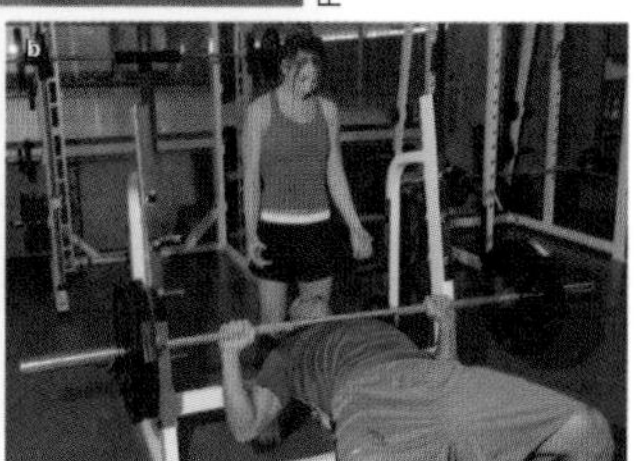

Photos © Fitness & Wellness, Inc.

Continued on back

HEALTHY STRENGTH TRAINING

I PLAN TO	I DID IT	
❑	❑	Make a progressive resistance strength-training program a priority in your weekly schedule.
❑	❑	Strength-train at least once a week; even better, twice a week.
❑	❑	Find a facility where you feel comfortable training and where you can get good professional guidance.
❑	❑	Learn the proper technique for each exercise.
❑	❑	Train with a friend or group of friends.
❑	❑	Consume a pre-exercise snack consisting of a combination of carbohydrates and some protein about 30 to 60 minutes before each strength-training session.
❑	❑	Use a minimum of 8 to 10 exercises that involve all major muscle groups of your body.
❑	❑	Perform at least one set of each exercise to near muscular fatigue.
❑	❑	To enhance protein synthesis, consume one post-exercise snack with a 4-to-l gram ratio of carbohydrates to protein immediately following strength training and a second snack 1 hour thereafter.

Continued on back

EXERCISE 16 Leg Press

ACTION From a sitting position with the knees flexed at about 90° and both feet on the footrest (a), extend the legs fully (b), then return slowly to the starting position.

MUSCLES DEVELOPED Quadriceps and gluteal muscles

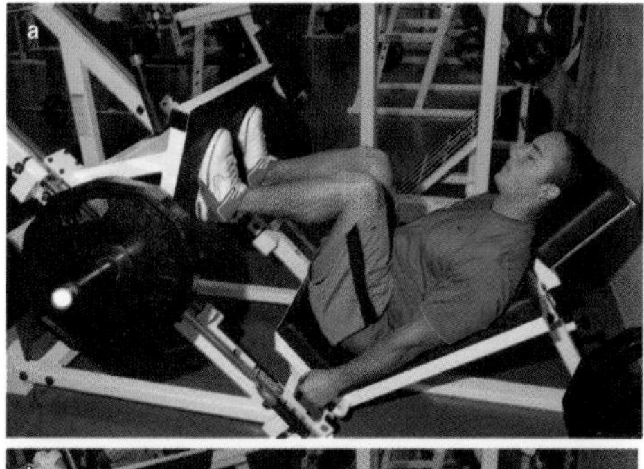

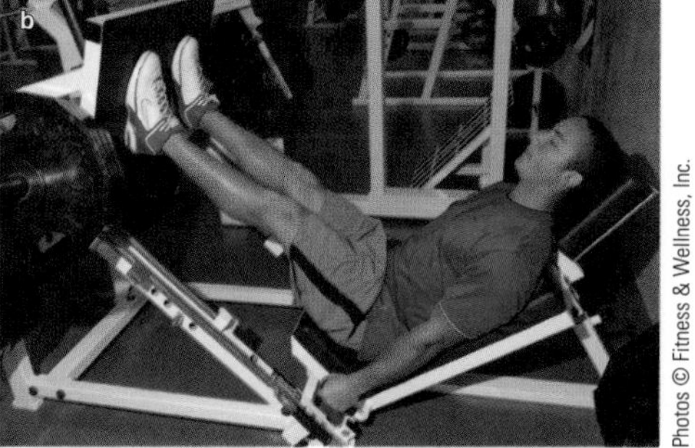

Photos © Fitness & Wellness, Inc.

Continued on back

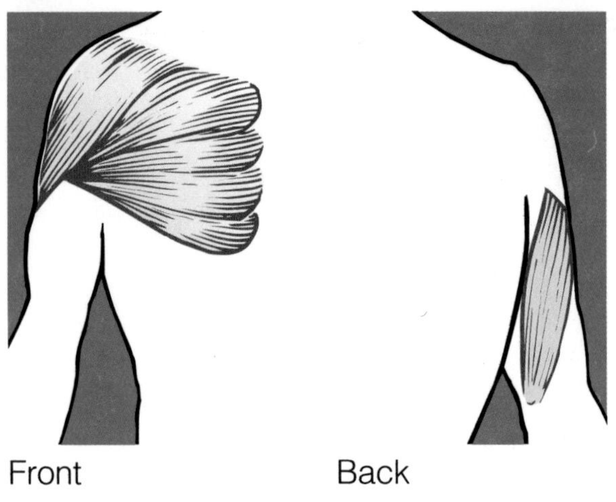

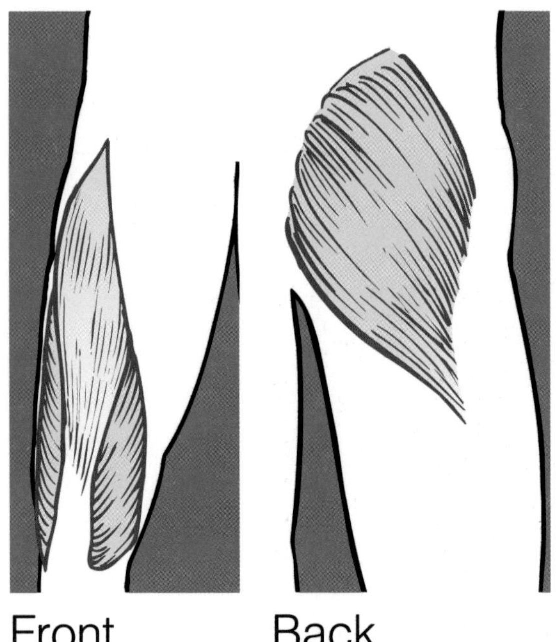

❑ | ❑ Allow at least 48 hours between strength-training sessions that involve the same muscle groups.

TRY IT

Attend the school's fitness or recreation center and have an instructor or fitness trainer help you design a progressive resistance strength-training program. Train twice a week for the next 4 weeks. Thereafter, evaluate the results and write down your feelings about the program.

EXERCISE 17 Abdominal Crunch

ACTION Sit in an upright position. Grasp the handles in front of you and crunch forward. Return slowly to the original position.

MUSCLES DEVELOPED Abdominals

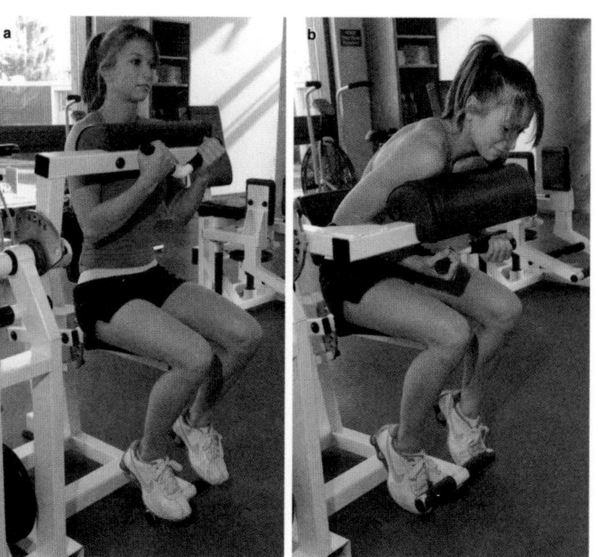

Photos © Fitness & Wellness, Inc.

Continued on back

EXERCISE 18-cont'd Bent-Over Lateral Raise

ACTION Bend over with your back straight and knees bent at about 5 to 10° (a). Hold one dumbbell in each hand. Raise the dumbbells laterally to about shoulder level (b) and then slowly return them to the starting position.

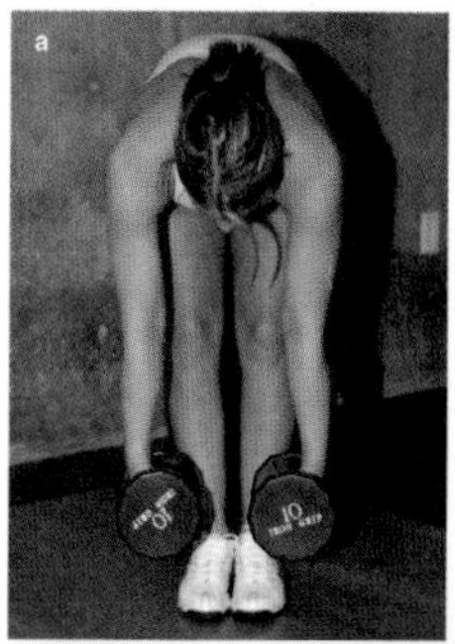

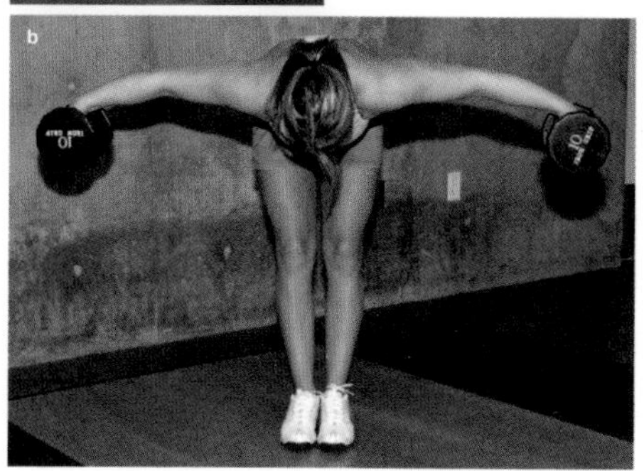

Continued on back

EXERCISE 18 Rowing Torso

ACTION Sit in the machine and grasp the handles in front of you (a). Press back as far as possible, drawing the shoulder blades together (b). Return to the original position.

MUSCLES DEVELOPED

Posterior deltoid, rhomboids, and trapezius

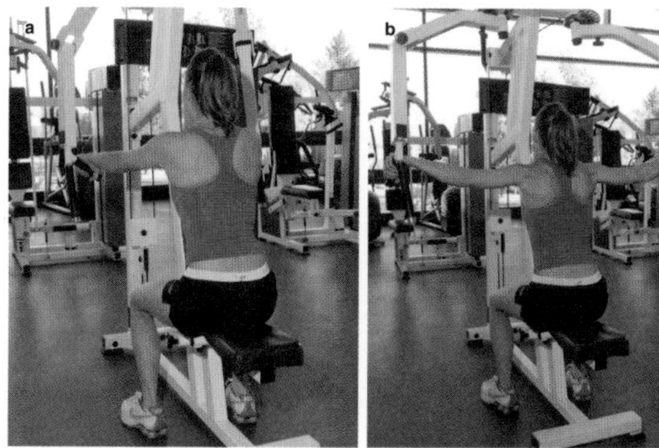

Photos © Fitness & Wellness, Inc.

Continued on back

EXERCISE 19 Leg Curl

ACTION Lie face down on the bench, legs straight, and place the back of the feet under the padded bar (a). Curl up to at least 90° (b), and return to the original position.

MUSCLES DEVELOPED Hamstrings

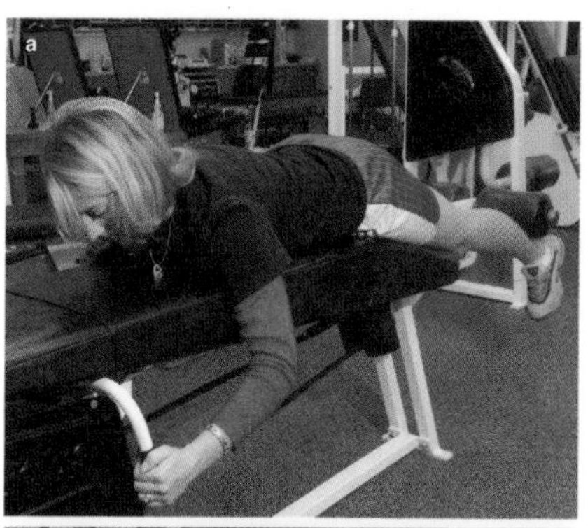

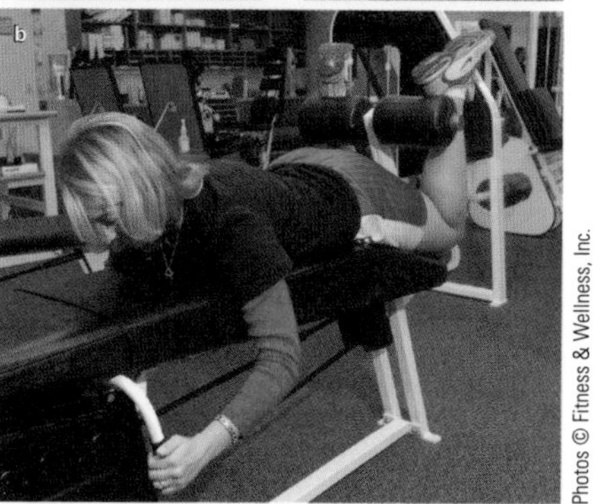

Photos © Fitness & Wellness, Inc.

Continued on back

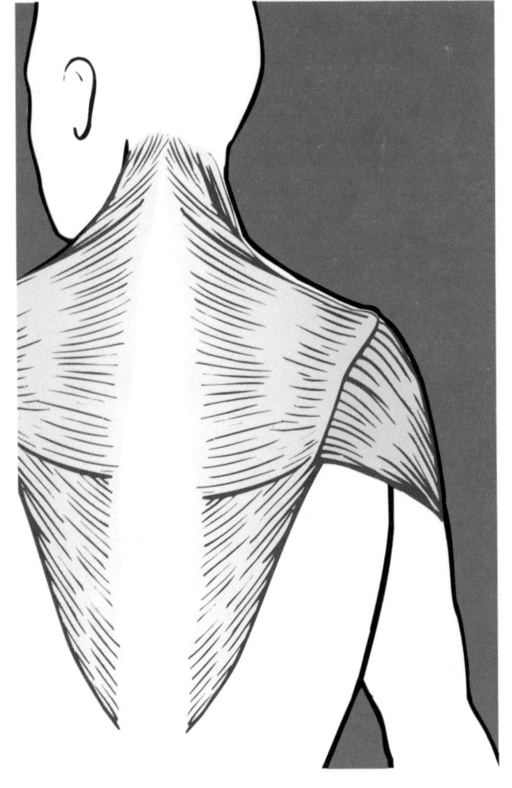

Back

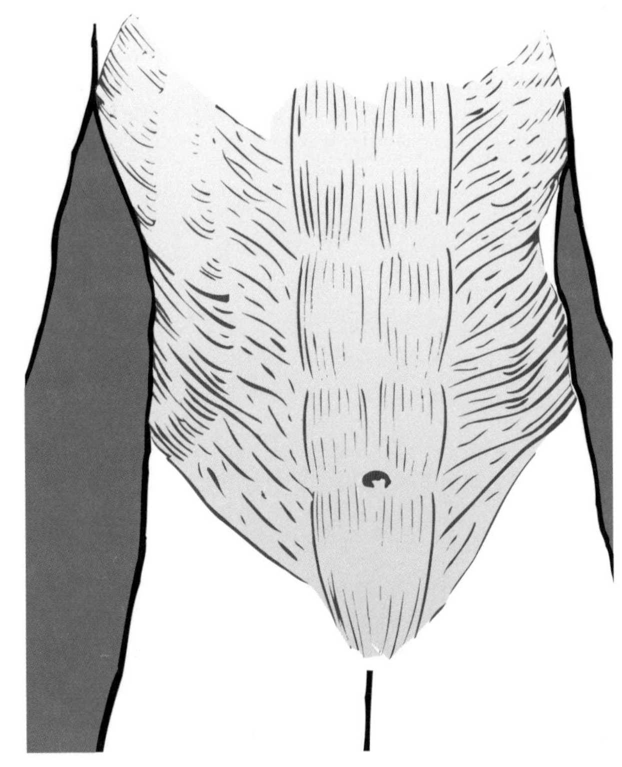

Front

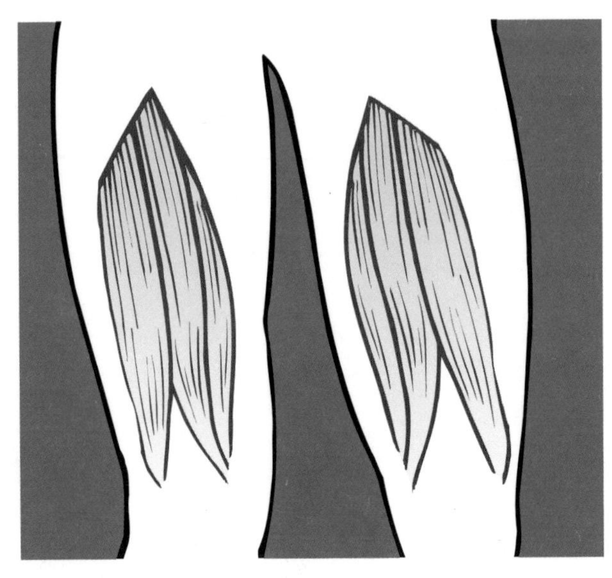

Back

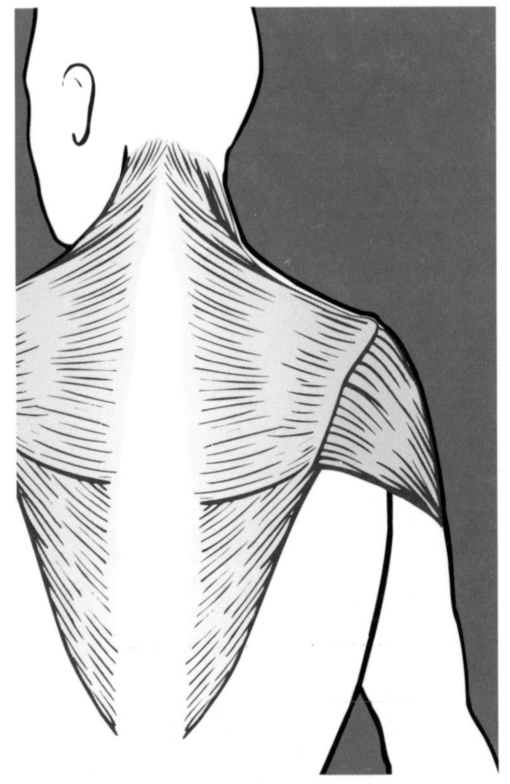

Back

EXERCISE 20 Seated Back

ACTION Sit in the machine with your trunk flexed and the upper back against the shoulder pad. Place the feet under the padded bar and hold on with your hands to the bars on the sides (a). Start the exercise by pressing backward, simultaneously extending the trunk and hip joints (b). Slowly return to the original position.

MUSCLES DEVELOPED Erector spinae and gluteus maximus

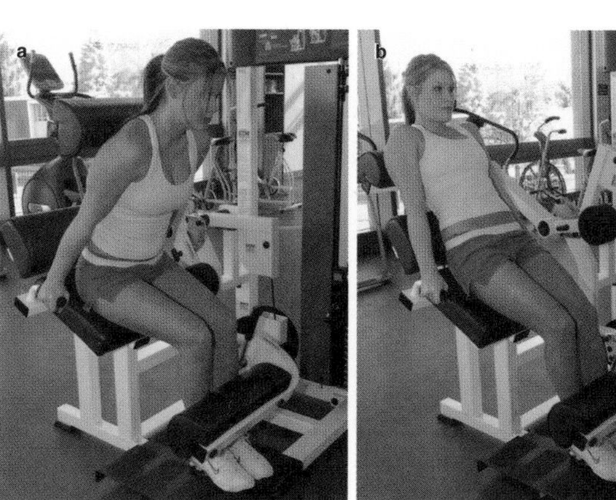

Photos © Fitness & Wellness, Inc.

Continued on back

EXERCISE 21 Calf Press

FREE WEIGHTS In a standing position, place a barbell across the shoulders and upper back. Grip the bar by the shoulders (a). Raise your heels off the floor or step box as far as possible (b) and then slowly return them to the starting position.

MACHINE Start with your feet flat on the plate (a). Now extend the ankles by pressing on the plate with the balls of your feet (b).

MUSCLES DEVELOPED Gastrocnemius, soleus

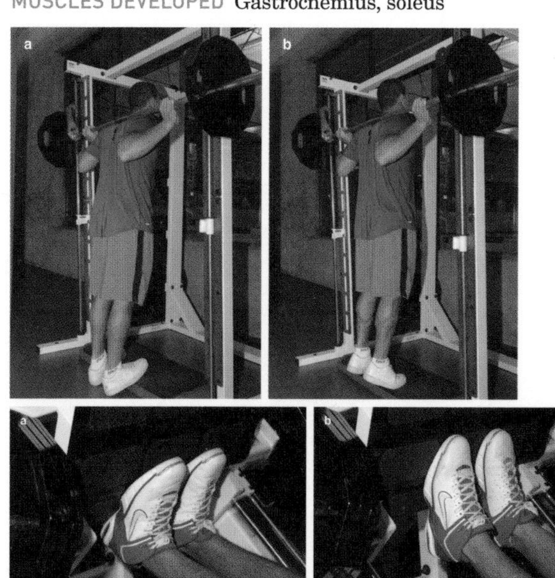

Photos © Fitness & Wellness, Inc.

Continued on back

EXERCISE 22 Leg (Hip) Adduction

ACTION Adjust the pads on the inside of the thighs as far out as the desired range of motion to be accomplished during the exercise (a). Press the legs together until both pads meet at the center (b). Slowly return to the starting position.

MUSCLES DEVELOPED Hip adductors (pectineus, gracilis, adductor magnus, adductor longus, and adductor brevis)

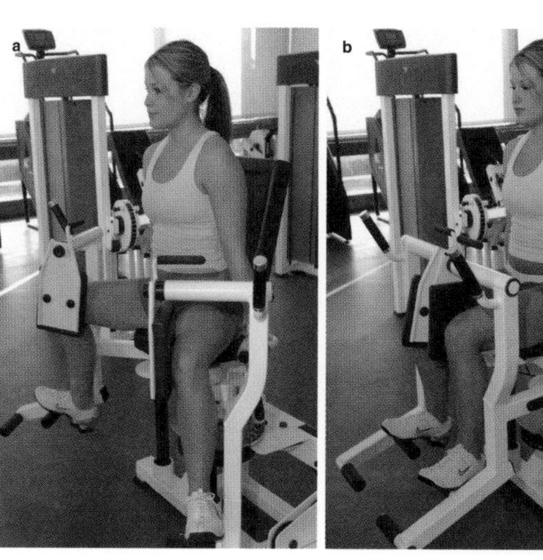

Photos © Fitness & Wellness, Inc.

Continued on back

EXERCISE 23 Leg (Hip) Abduction

ACTION Place your knees together with the pads directly outside the knees (a). Press the legs laterally out as far as possible (b). Slowly return to the starting position.

MUSCLES DEVELOPED
Hip abductors (rectus femoris, sartori, gluteus medius and minimus)

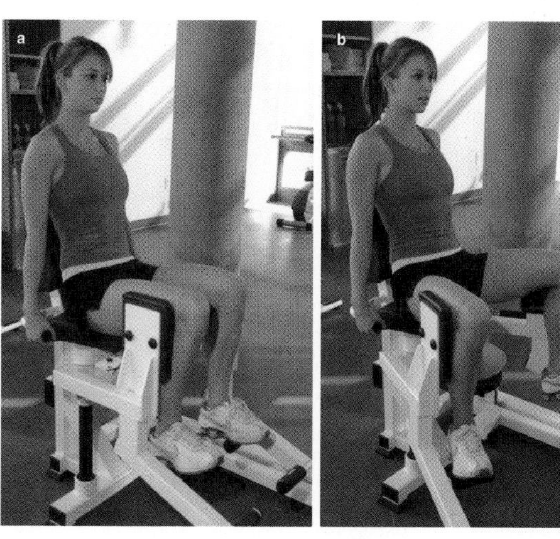

Photos © Fitness & Wellness, Inc.

Continued on back

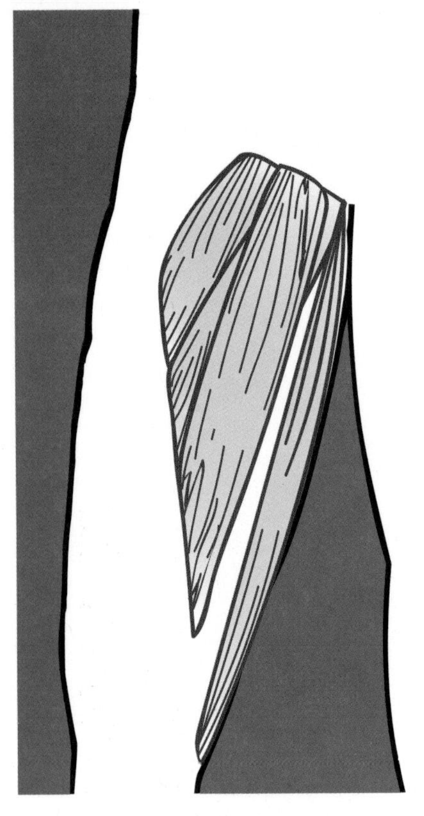

Front

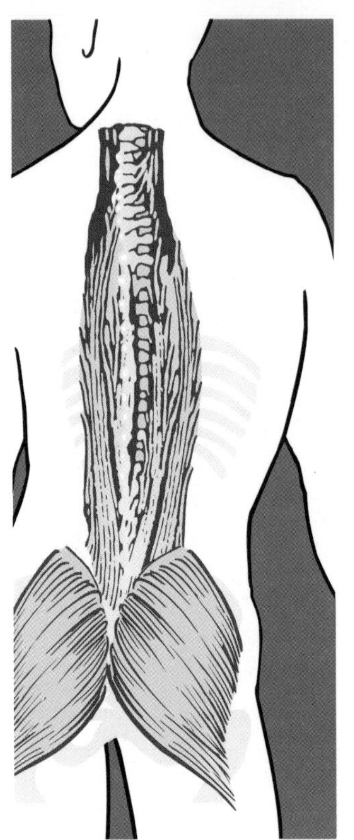

Back

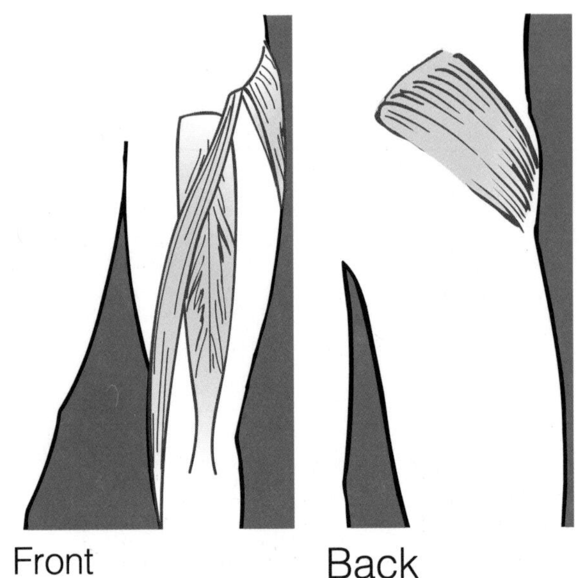

Front

Back

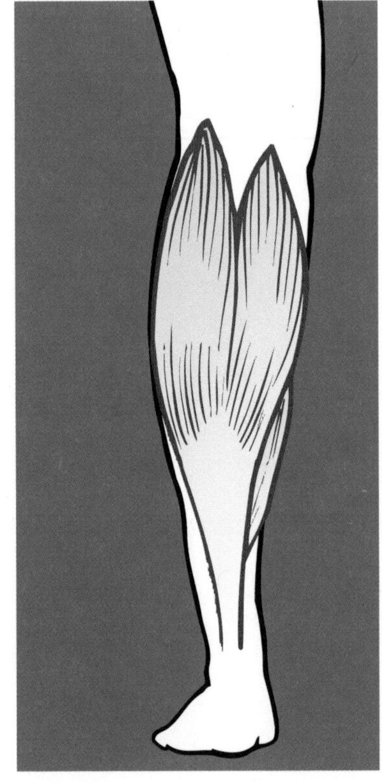

Back

EXERCISE 24 Lat Pull-Down

ACTION Starting from a sitting position, hold the exercise bar with a wide grip (a). Pull the bar down in front of you until it reaches the upper chest (b), then return to the starting position.

MUSCLES DEVELOPED Latissimus dorsi, pectoralis major, and biceps

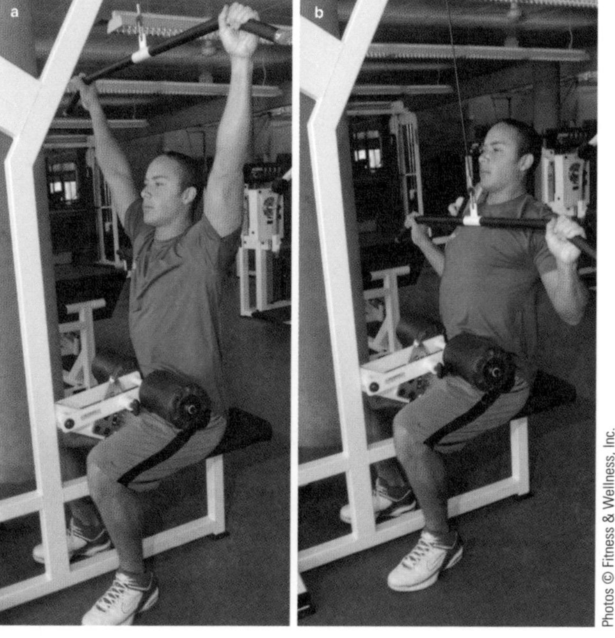

Photos © Fitness & Wellness, Inc.

Continued on back

EXERCISE 25 Rotary Torso

FREE WEIGHTS Stand with your feet slightly apart. Place a barbell across your shoulders and upper back, holding on to the sides of the barbell. Now gently, and in a controlled manner, twist your torso to one side as far as possible and then do so in the opposite direction.

MUSCLES DEVELOPED Internal and external obliques (abdominal muscles)

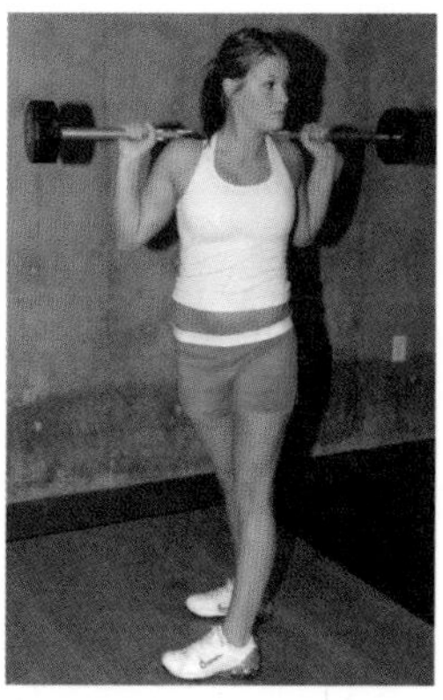

Continued on back

EXERCISE 26 Triceps Extension

MACHINE Sit in an upright position and grasp the bar behind the shoulders (a). Fully extend the arms (b) and then return to the original position.

MACHINE Using a palms-down grip, grasp the bar slightly closer than shoulder-width and start with the elbows almost completely bent (a). Extend the arms fully (b), then return to starting position.

FREE WEIGHTS In a standing position, hold a barbell with both hands overhead and with the arms in full extension (a). Slowly lower the barbell behind your head (b) and then return it to the starting position.

MUSCLES DEVELOPED Triceps

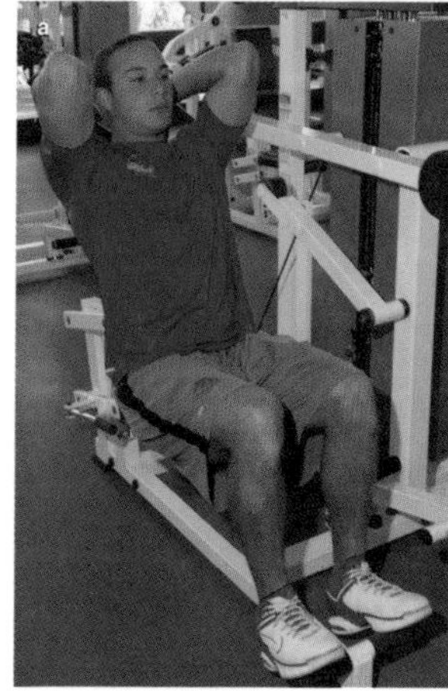

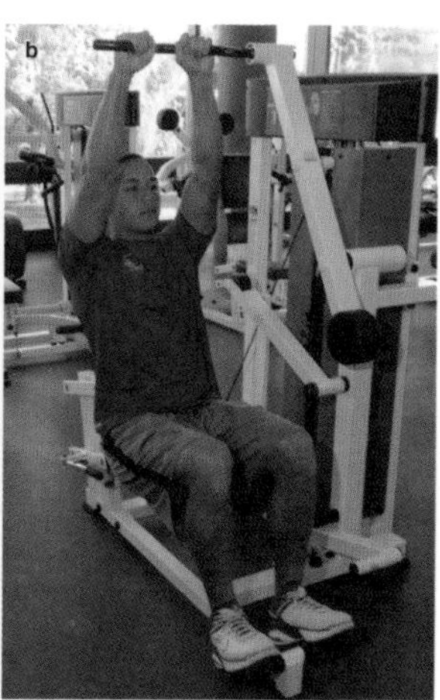

Photos © Fitness & Wellness, Inc.

Continued on back

EXERCISE 27 Arm Curl

MACHINE Using a supinated (palms-up) grip, start with the arms almost completely extended (a). Curl up as far as possible (b), then return to the starting position.

FREE WEIGHTS Standing upright, hold a barbell in front of you at about shoulder width with arms extended and the hands in a thumbs-out position (supinated grip) (a). Raise the barbell to your shoulders (b) and slowly return it to the starting position.

MUSCLES DEVELOPED Biceps, brachioradialis, and brachialis

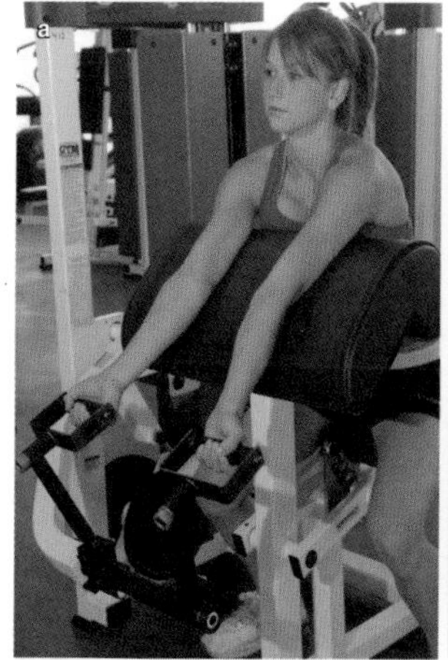

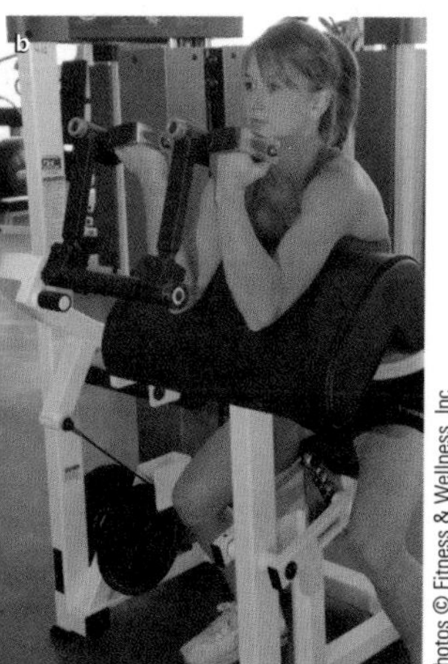

Photos © Fitness & Wellness, Inc.

Continued on back

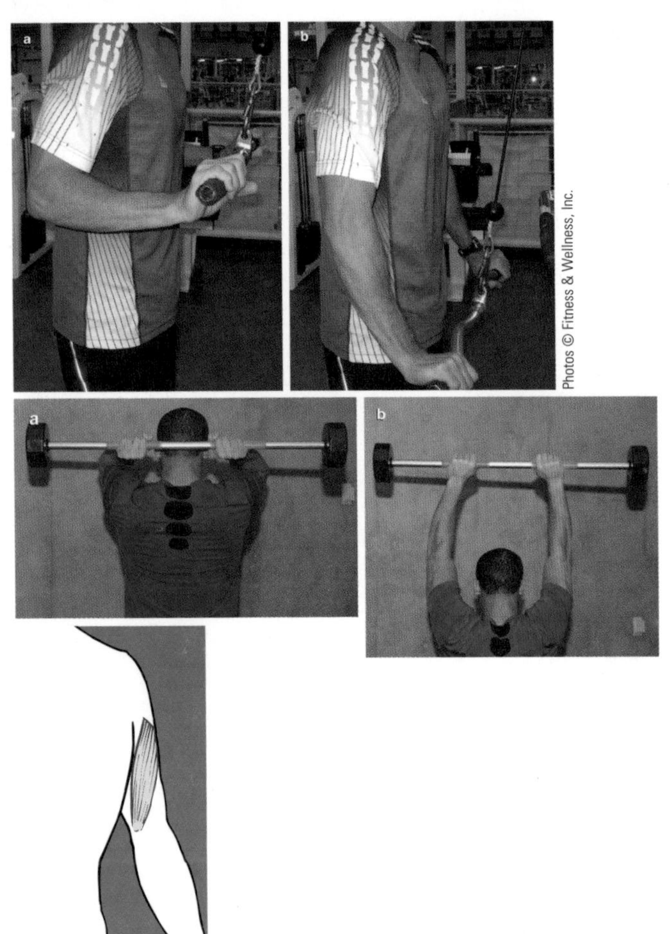
a
b
Photos © Fitness & Wellness, Inc.
a
b

Back

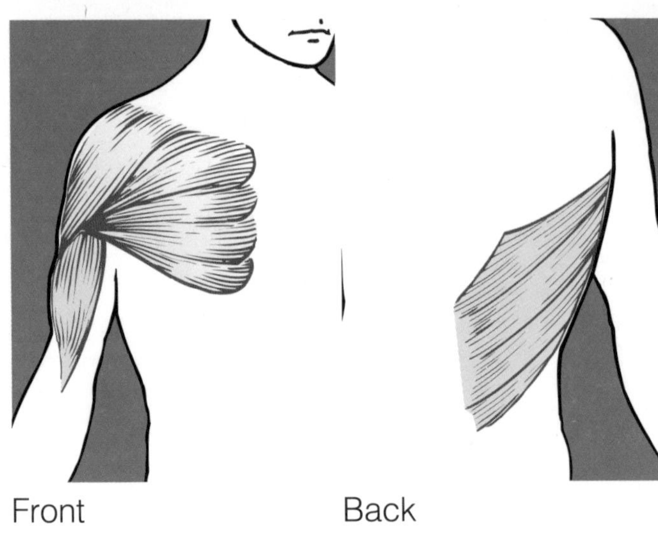
Front
Back

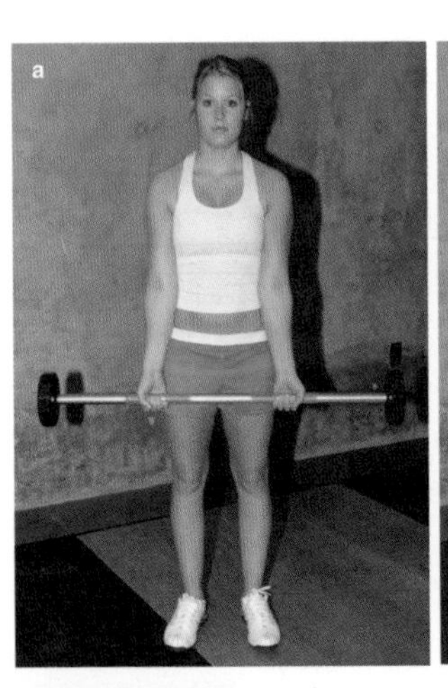
a

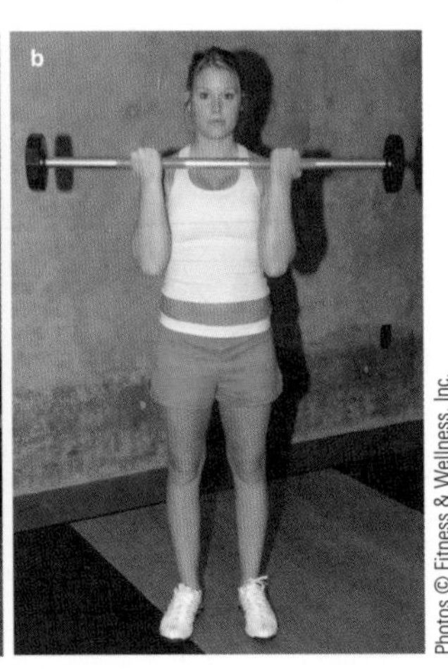
b
Photos © Fitness & Wellness, Inc.

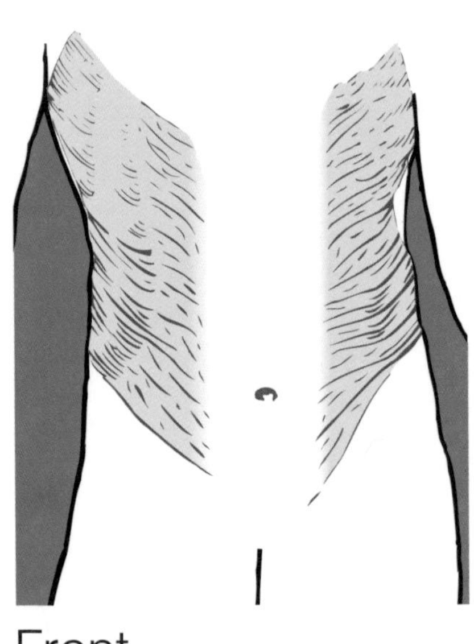
Front

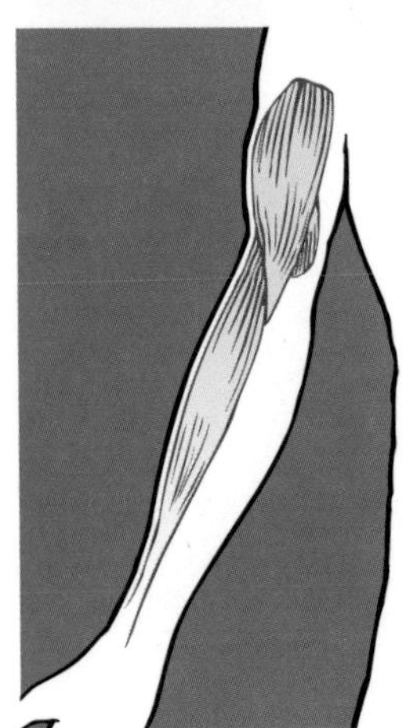
Front

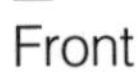

Strength training A program designed to improve muscular strength and/or endurance through a series of progressive resistance (weight) training exercises that overload the muscle system and cause physiological development.
Metabolism All energy and material transformations that occur within living cells; necessary to sustain life.
Muscular strength The ability of a muscle to exert maximum force against resistance (for example, 1 repetition maximum [or 1 RM] on the bench press exercise).
Muscular endurance The ability of a muscle to exert submaximal force repeatedly over time.
Hypertrophy An increase in the size of the cell, as in muscle hypertrophy.
Atrophy Decrease in the size of a cell.
Slow-twitch fibers Muscle fibers with greater aerobic potential and slow speed of contraction.
Fast-twitch fibers Muscle fibers with greater anaerobic potential and fast speed of contraction.
Overload principle Training concept that the demands placed on a system (cardiorespiratory or muscular) must be increased systematically and progressively over time to cause physiological adaptation (development or improvement).
Specificity of training Principle that training must be done with the specific muscle the person is attempting to improve.
Isometric training Strength-training method referring to a muscle contraction that produces little or no movement, such as pushing or pulling against an immovable object.
Dynamic training Strength-training method referring to a muscle contraction with movement.
Concentric Describes shortening of a muscle during muscle contraction.
Eccentric Describes lengthening of a muscle during muscle contraction.
Negative resistance The lowering or eccentric phase of a repetition during a strength-training exercise.
Fixed resistance Type of exercise in which a constant resistance is moved through a joint's full range of motion (dumbbells, barbells, machines using a constant resistance).
Variable resistance Training using special machines equipped with mechanical devices that provide differing amounts of resistance through the range of motion.
Isokinetic training Strength-training method in which the speed of the muscle contraction is kept constant because the equipment (machine) provides an ac-

Continued on back

TIPS TO PREVENT LOW BACK PAIN

I PLAN TO	I DID IT	
❑	❑	Be physically active.
❑	❑	Maintain recommended body weight (excess weight strains the back).
❑	❑	Stretch often using spinal exercises through a functional range of motion.
❑	❑	Regularly strengthen the core of the body using sets of 10 to 12 repetitions to near fatigue with isometric contractions when applicable.
❑	❑	Lift heavy objects by bending at the knees and carry them close to the body. Place one foot forward and keep your knees slightly bent while standing.
❑	❑	Avoid sitting (over 50 minutes) or standing in one position for lengthy periods of time.
❑	❑	Maintain correct posture.
❑	❑	Sleep on your back with a pillow under the knees or on your side with the knees drawn up and a small pillow between the knees.
❑	❑	Try out different mattresses of firm consistency before selecting a mattress.

Continued on back

GUIDELINES FOR FLEXIBILITY DEVELOPMENT

Mode: Static, dynamic, or proprioceptive neuromuscular facilitation (PNF) stretching to include all major muscle/tendon groups of the body
Intensity: To the point of mild tension or limits of discomfort
Repetitions: Repeat each exercise 2 to 4 times, holding the final position between 10 and 30 seconds per repetition, with a cumulative goal of 60 seconds per exercise
Frequency: At least 2 or 3 days per week
Ideally, 5 to 7 days per week
When: Following cardiorespiratory or strength-training exercises, or as a stand-alone program

CONTRAINDICATED EXERCISES

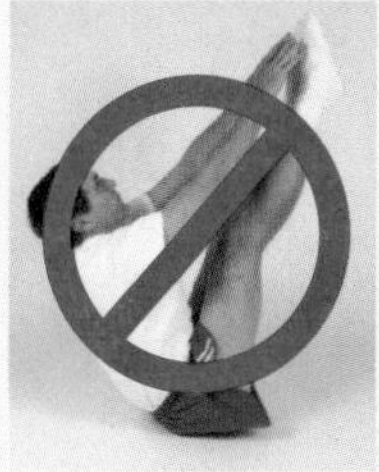

V-Sits

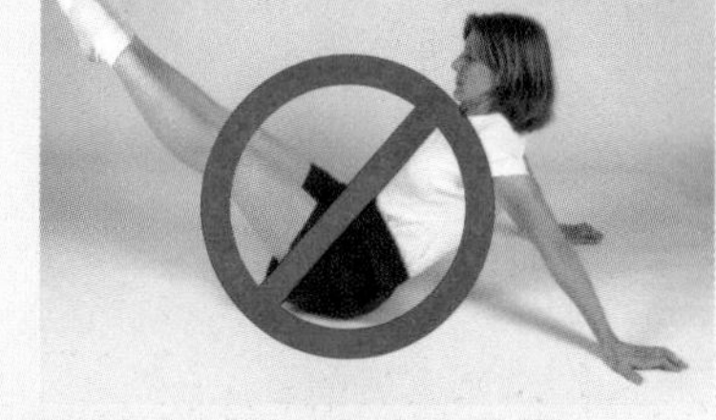

Upright Double-Leg Lifts

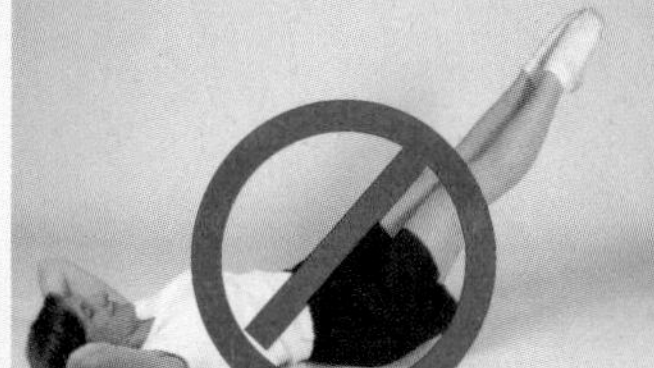

Double-Leg Lift

All three of these exercises cause excessive strain on the spine and may harm disks.

Alternatives: Strength Exercises 4 and 17, pages 287 and 291

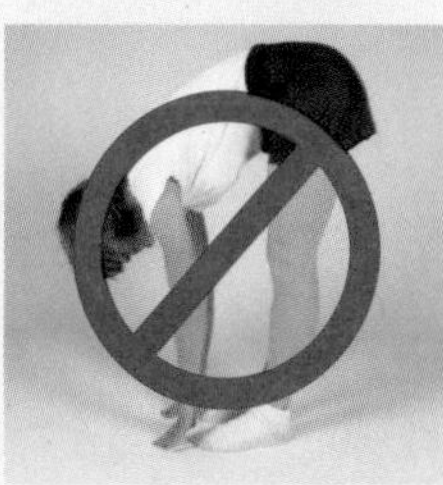

Standing Toe Touch
Excessive strain on the knee and lower back.
Alternative: Flexibility Exercise 12, page 332

Continued on back

- ❑ ❑ Warm up properly using mild stretches before engaging in physical activity.
- ❑ ❑ Practice adequate stress management techniques.
- ❑ ❑ Don't smoke (it reduces blood flow to the spine, increasing back pain risk).

TRY IT

In your class notebook, record how many of the above actions are a regular part of your healthy low back program. If you are not using all of them, what is necessary to incorporate these behaviors into your lifestyle?

commodating resistance to match the user's force (maximal) through the range of motion.

Progressive resistance training A gradual increase of resistance over a period of time.

Volume The sum of all the repetitions performed multiplied by the resistances used during a strength-training session.

Periodization A training approach that divides the season into cycles using a systematic variation in intensity and volume of training to enhance fitness and performance.

Plyometric exercise Explosive jump training, incorporating speed and strength training to enhance explosiveness.

Core strength training A program designed to strengthen the abdominal, hip, and spinal muscles (the core of the body).

Pilates A training program that uses exercises designed to help strengthen the body's core by developing pelvic stability and abdominal control; exercises are coupled with focused breathing patterns.

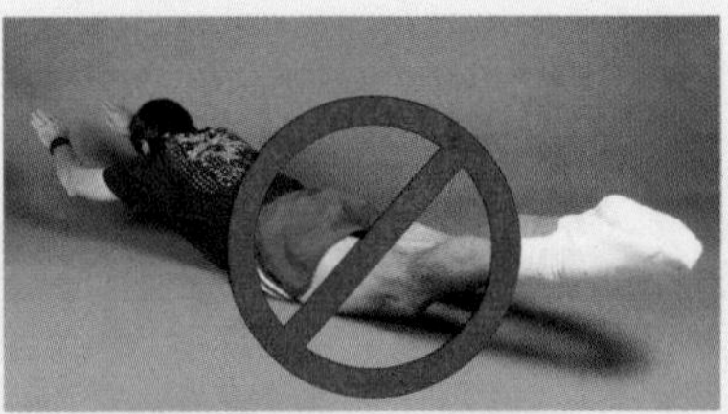

Swan Stretch
Excessive strain on the spine; may harm intervertebral disks.
Alternative: Flexibility Exercise 20, page 334

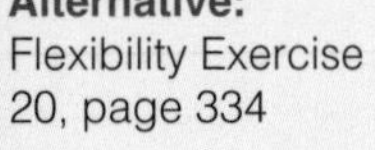

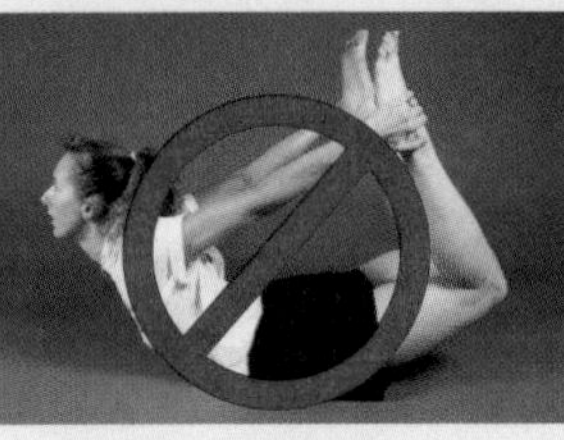

Cradle
Excessive strain on the spine, knees, and shoulders.
Alternatives: Flexibility Exercises 20, 8, and 6, pages 334, 331, and 330

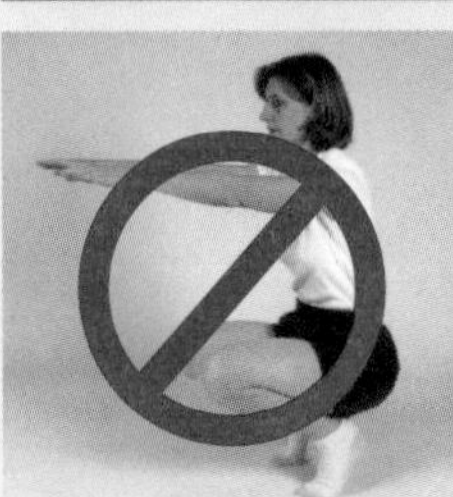

Full Squat
Excessive strain on the knees.
Alternatives: Flexibility Exercise 8, page 316; Strength Exercises 1, 16, 28A, and 28B, pages 186, 291, and 296

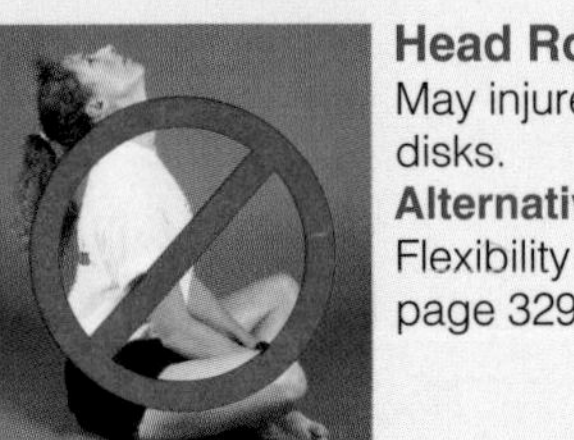

Head Rolls
May injure neck disks.
Alternative: Flexibility Exercise 1, page 329

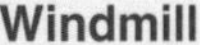

Windmill
Excessive strain on the spine and knees.
Alternatives: Flexibility Exercises 12 and 21, pages 332 and 333

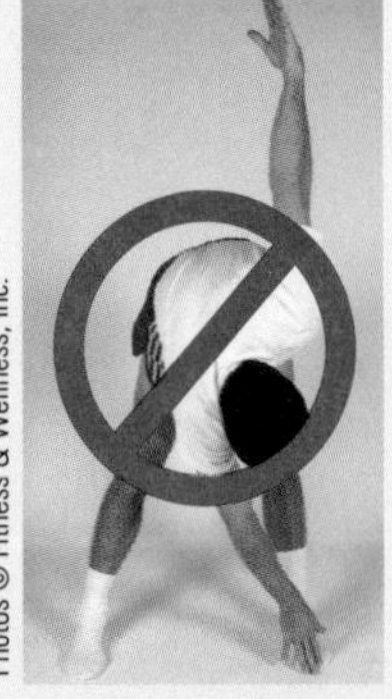

Photos © Fitness & Wellness, Inc.

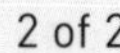

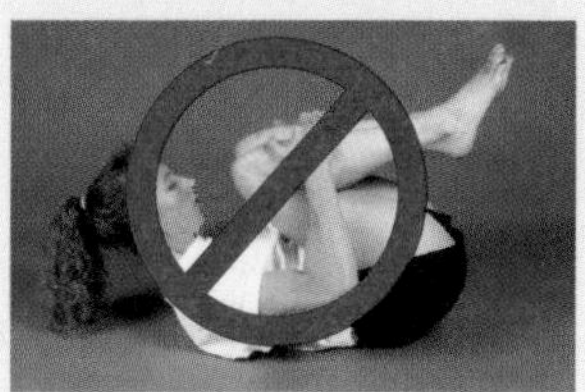

Knee to Chest
(with hands over the shin)
Excessive strain on the knee.

Alternative: Flexibility Exercises 15 and 16, page 333

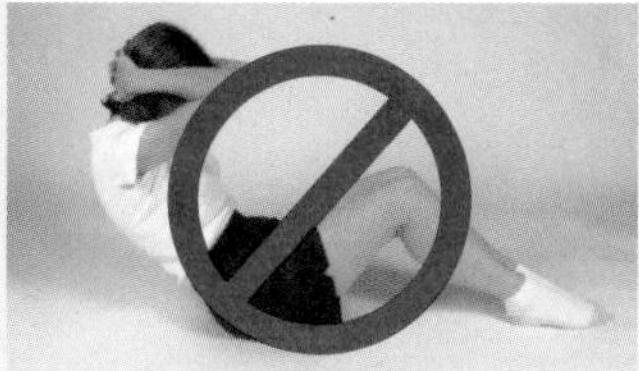

Sit-Ups with Hands Behind the Head
Excessive strain on the neck.

Alternatives: Strength Exercises 4 and 17, pages 287 and 291

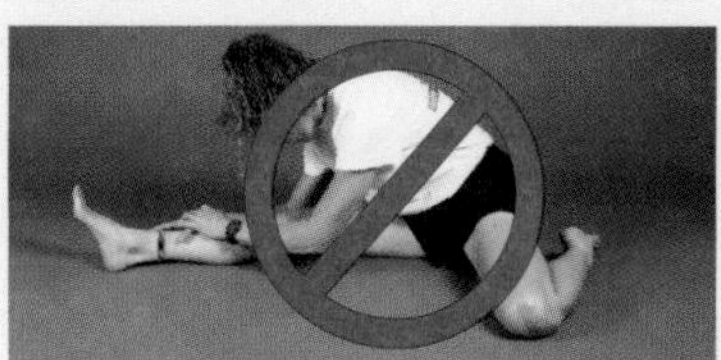

Hurdler Stretch
Excessive strain on the bent knee.

Alternatives:
Flexibility Exercises 8 and 12, pages 331 and 332

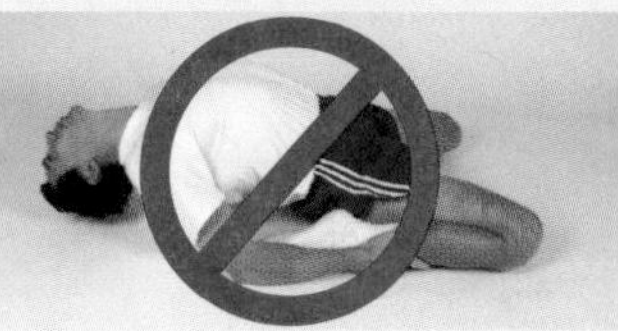

The Hero
Excessive strain on the knees.

Alternatives:
Flexibility Exercises 8 and 14, pages 331 and 332

Continued on back

Contraindications to Exercise during Pregnancy

Stop exercise and seek medical advice if you experience any of the following symptoms:

- Unusual pain or discomfort, especially in the chest or abdominal area
- Cramping, primarily in the pelvic or lower back areas
- Muscle weakness, excessive fatigue, or shortness of breath
- Abnormally high heart rate or a pounding (palpitations) heart rate
- Decreased fetal movement
- Insufficient weight gain
- Amniotic fluid leakage
- Nausea, dizziness, or headaches
- Persistent uterine contractions
- Vaginal bleeding or rupture of the membranes
- Swelling of ankles, calves, hands, or face

Flexibility The achievable range of motion at a joint or group of joints without causing injury.
Subluxation Partial dislocation of a joint.
Plastic elongation Permanent lengthening of soft tissue.
Elastic elongation Temporary lengthening of soft tissue.
Static stretching (slow-sustained stretching) Exercises in which the muscles are lengthened gradually through a joint's complete range of motion.
Passive stretching Stretching exercises performed with the aid of an external force applied by either another individual or an external apparatus.
Ballistic (dynamic) stretching Stretching exercises performed with jerky, rapid, and bouncy movements.
Dynamic Stretching Stretching exercises that require speed of movement, momentum, and active muscular effort to help increase the range of motion about a joint or group of joints.
Controlled ballistic stretching Exercises done with slow, short, gentle, and sustained movements.
Proprioceptive neuromuscular facilitation (PNF) Mode of stretching that uses reflexes and neuromuscular principles to relax the muscles being stretched.
Contraindicated exercises Exercises that are not recommended because they may cause injury to a person.

Skill-related fitness Fitness components important for success in skillful activities and athletic events; encompasses agility, balance, coordination, power, reaction time, and speed.
Heat cramps Muscle spasms caused by heat-induced changes in electrolyte balance in muscle cells.
Heat exhaustion Heat-related fatigue.
Heat stroke Emergency situation resulting from the body being subjected to high atmospheric temperatures.
Hypothermia A breakdown in the body's ability to generate heat; a drop in body temperature below 95°F.
Exercise intolerance Inability to function during exercise because of excessive fatigue or extreme feelings of discomfort.
Interval training A system of exercise in which a short period of intense effort is followed by a specified recovery period according to a prescribed ratio; for instance, a 1:3 work-to-recovery ratio.
Overtraining An emotional, behavioral, and physical condition marked by increased fatigue, decreased performance, persistent muscle soreness, mood disturbances, and feelings of "staleness" or "burnout" as a result of excessive physical training.
Periodization A training approach that divides the season into three cycles (macrocycles, mesocycles, and microcycles) using a systematic variation in intensity and volume of training to enhance fitness and performance.
Cross-training A combination of aerobic activities that contribute to overall fitness.

Yoga Plow
Excessive strain on the spine, neck, and shoulders.

Alternatives: Flexibility Exercises 12, 15, 16, 17, and 19, pages 332 and 333

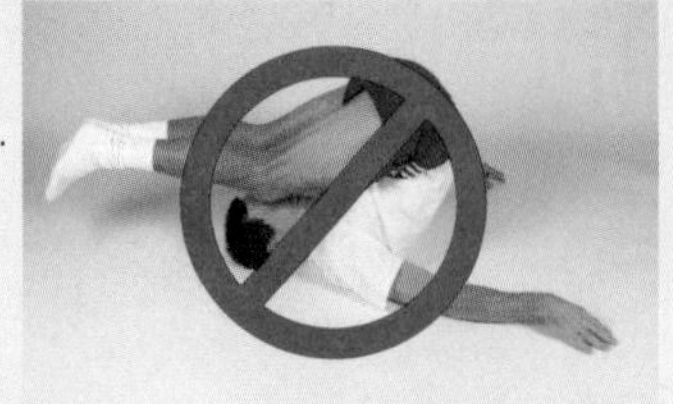

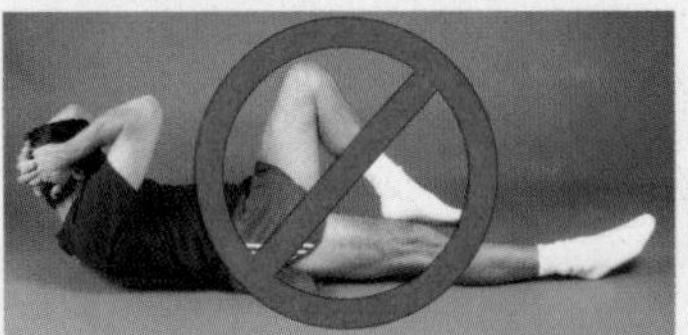

Alternating Bent-Leg Sit-Ups

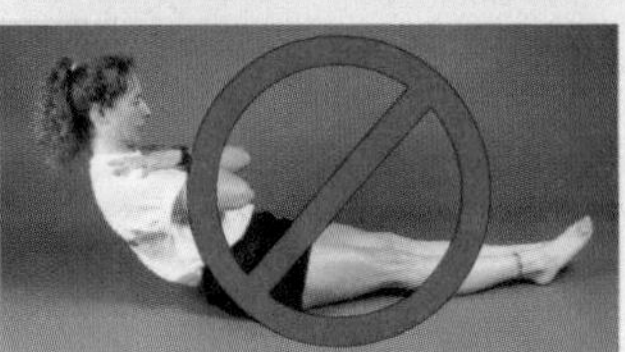

Straight-Leg Sit-Ups

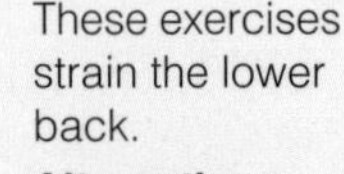

These exercises strain the lower back.

Alternatives: Strength Exercises 4 and 17, pages 287 and 291

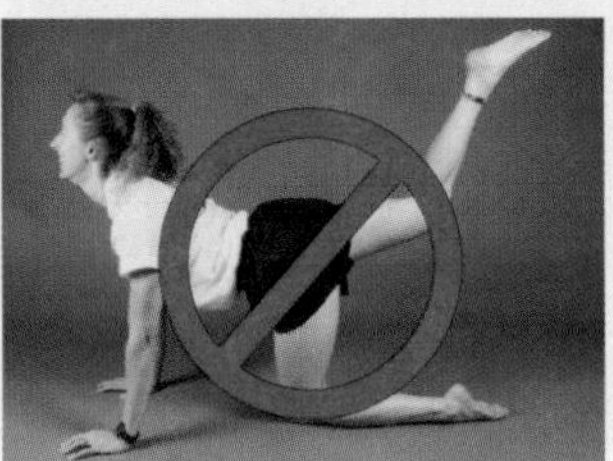

Donkey Kicks
Excessive strain on the back, shoulders, and neck.

Alternatives: Flexibility Exercises 20, 14, and 1, pages 334, 332, and 329

STRESSORS IN THE LIVES OF COLLEGE STUDENTS

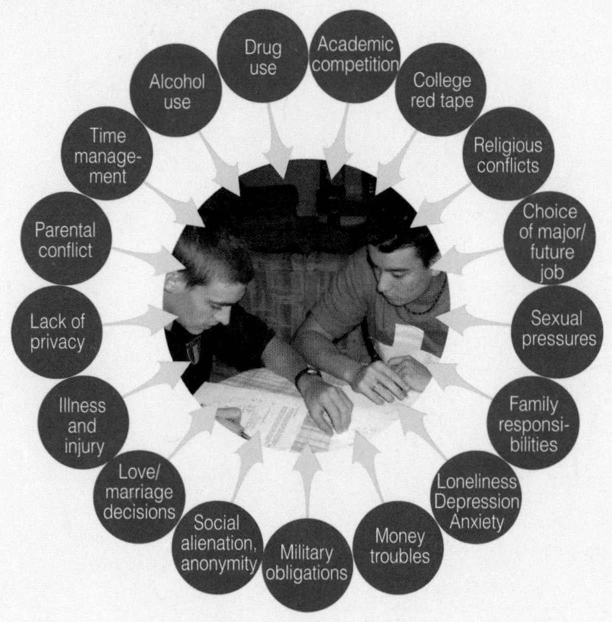

Adapted from W. W. K. Hoeger, L. W. Turner, and B. Q. Hafen. *Wellness Guidelines for a Healthy Lifestyle.* Wadsworth/Thomson Learning, 2007.

Stress The mental, emotional, and physiological response of the body to any situation that is new, threatening, frightening, or exciting.
Stressor Stress-causing event.
Eustress Positive stress: Health and performance continue to improve, even as stress increases.
Distress Negative stress: Unpleasant or harmful stress under which health and performance begin to deteriorate.
General adaptation syndrome (GAS) A theoretical model that explains the body's adaptation to sustained stress that includes three stages: alarm reaction, resistance, and exhaustion/recovery.
Structured interview Assessment tool used to determine behavioral patterns that define Type A and B personalities.
Fight or flight Physiological response of the body to stress that prepares the individual to take action by stimulating the body's vital defense systems.
Endorphins Morphine-like substances released from the pituitary gland in the brain during prolonged aerobic exercise, thought to induce feelings of euphoria and natural well-being.
Autogenic training A stress management technique using a form of self-suggestion, wherein an individual is able to place himself or herself in an autohypnotic state by repeating and concentrating on feelings of heaviness and warmth in the extremities.
Meditation A stress management technique used to gain control over one's attention by clearing the mind and blocking out the stressor(s) responsible for the increased tension.
Hatha yoga A form of yoga that incorporates specific sequences of static-stretching postures to help induce the relaxation response.

TIPS TO MANAGE ANGER

I PLAN TO	I DID IT	
❏	❏	Commit to change and gain control over the behavior.
❏	❏	Remind yourself that chronic anger leads to illness and disease and may eventually kill you.
❏	❏	Recognize when feelings of anger are developing and ask yourself the following questions: • Is the matter really that important? • Is the anger justified? • Can I change the situation without getting angry? • Is it worth risking my health over it? • How will I feel about the situation in a few hours?
❏	❏	Tell yourself, "Stop, my health is worth it" every time you start to feel anger.

Continued on back

CHOLESTEROL GUIDELINES

	Amount	Rating
Total cholesterol	<200 mg/dL	Desirable
	200–239 mg/dL	Borderline high
	≥240 mg/dL	High risk
LDL cholesterol	<100 mg/dL	Optimal
	100–129 mg/dL	Near or above optimal
	130–159 mg/dL	Borderline high
	160–189 mg/dL	High
	≥190 mg/dL	Very high
HDL cholesterol	<40 mg/dL	Low (high risk)
	≥60 mg/dL	High (low risk)

From National Cholesterol Education Program.

TRIGLYCERIDES GUIDELINES

Amount	Rating
<150 mg/dL	Desirable
150–199 mg/dL	Borderline high
200–499 mg/dL	High
≥500 mg/dL	Very high

Source: National Heart, Lung and Blood Institute.

Continued on back

BLOOD GLUCOSE GUIDELINES

Amount	Rating
≤100 mg/dL	Normal
101–125 mg/dL	Pre-diabetes
≥126 mg/dL	Diabetes*

*Confirmed by two tests on different days.

BLOOD PRESSURE GUIDELINES

Rating	Systolic	Diastolic
Normal	<120	<80
Prehypertension	121–139	81–89
Stage 1 hypertension	140–159	90–99
Stage 2 hypertension	≥160	≥100

Source: National High Blood Pressure Education Program.

- ❑ | ❑ Prepare for a positive response: Ask for an explanation or clarification of the situation, walk away and evaluate the situation, exercise, or use appropriate stress management techniques (breathing, meditation, imagery) before you become angry and hostile.
- ❑ | ❑ Manage anger at once; do not let it build up.
- ❑ | ❑ Never attack anyone verbally or physically.
- ❑ | ❑ Keep a journal and ponder the situations that cause you to be angry.
- ❑ | ❑ Seek professional help if you are unable to overcome anger by yourself: You are worth it.

TRY IT

If you and others feel that anger is disrupting your health and relationships, the above management strategies are critical to help restore a sense of well-being in your life. In your Online Journal or class notebook, list all of the strategies on a separate sheet of paper, study them each morning, and then evaluate yourself every night for the next week. If you gain control over the behavior, continue with the exercise until it becomes a healthy behavior. If you still struggle, professional help is recommended. "You are worth it."

Signs of Heart Attack and Stroke

Time is extremely critical when suffering a heart attack or stroke. Any or all of the following signs may occur during a heart attack or a stroke. **If you experience any of these and they last longer than a few minutes, call 911 and seek medical attention immediately.** Failure to do so may cause irreparable damage and even result in death.

Warning Signs of a Heart Attack

- Chest pain, discomfort, pressure, or squeezing that lasts for several minutes. These feelings may go away and return later.
- Pain or discomfort in the shoulders, neck, or arms or between the shoulder blades
- Chest discomfort with shortness of breath, lightheadedness, cold sweats, nausea and/or vomiting, a feeling of indigestion, sudden fatigue or weakness, fainting, or sense of impending doom

HEART DISEASE AND STROKE PREVENTION GUIDELINES

These guidelines by the American Heart Association (AHA) and the American College of Cardiology target four high-risk groups for whom statin drugs are recommended:

1. People with pre-existing CVD (those who have suffered angina, a heart attack, stroke, a transient ischemic attack or mini stroke, and anyone who has had a cardiovascular procedure such as angioplasty to widen arteries).
2. Type 2 diabetics between 40 and 75 years of age.
3. People with very high LDL cholesterol (190 mg/dl or above).
4. People between 40 and 75 without CVD or diabetes who have a 10-year risk of CVD of at least 7.5 percent based on a new *online risk calculator* (see AHA website).

AMERICAN HEART ASSOCIATION DIET AND LIFESTYLE RECOMMENDATIONS FOR CARDIOVASCULAR DISEASE RISK REDUCTION

❑ I PLAN TO	❑ I DID IT	
❑	❑	Balance caloric intake and physical activity to achieve or maintain a healthy body weight.
❑	❑	Consume a diet rich in vegetables and fruits.
❑	❑	Consume whole-grain, high-fiber foods.
❑	❑	Consume fish, especially oily fish, at least twice a week.
❑	❑	Limit your intake of saturated fat to less than 7 percent and trans fat to less than 1 percent of total daily caloric intake.
❑	❑	Limit cholesterol intake to less than 300 mg per day.
❑	❑	Minimize your intake of beverages and foods with added sugars.
❑	❑	Choose and prepare foods with little or no salt.
❑	❑	If you consume alcohol, do so in moderation.

Continued on back

Cardiovascular disease (CVD) The array of conditions that affect the heart and the blood vessels.
Stroke Condition in which a blood vessel that feeds the brain ruptures or is clogged, leading to blood flow disruption to the brain.
Coronary heart disease (CHD) Condition in which the arteries that supply the heart muscle with oxygen and nutrients are narrowed by fatty deposits, such as cholesterol and triglycerides.
Cholesterol A waxy substance, technically a steroid alcohol, found only in animal fats and oil; used in making cell membranes, as a building block for some hormones, in the fatty sheath around nerve fibers, and other necessary substances.
High-density lipoproteins (HDLs) Cholesterol-transporting molecules in the blood ("good" cholesterol) that help clear cholesterol from the blood.
Low-density lipoproteins (LDLs) Cholesterol-transporting molecules in the blood ("bad" cholesterol) that tend to increase blood cholesterol.
Very low-density lipoproteins (VLDLs) Triglyceride, cholesterol, and phospholipid-transporting molecules in the blood that tend to increase blood cholesterol.
Atherosclerosis Fatty/cholesterol deposits in the walls of the arteries leading to formation of plaque.
Myocardial infarction Heart attack; damage to or death of an area of the heart muscle as a result of an obstructed artery to that area.
Triglycerides Fats formed by glycerol and three fatty acids; also called free fatty acids.
Homocysteine An amino acid that, when allowed to accumulate in the blood, may lead to plaque formation and blockage of arteries.
C-reactive protein (CRP) A protein whose blood levels increase with inflammation, at times hidden deep in the body; elevation of this protein is an indicator of potential cardiovascular events.
Diabetes mellitus A disease in which the body doesn't produce or utilize insulin properly.
Insulin A hormone secreted by the pancreas; essential for proper metabolism of blood glucose (sugar) and maintenance of blood glucose level.
Insulin resistance Inability of the cells to respond appropriately to insulin.

Continued on back

Warning Signs of Stroke

The acronym FAST is commonly used to help recognize and enhance responsiveness for a stroke victim.

- **F**acial dropping. Part of the face is dropping, weak, numb, or hard to move.
- **A**rm weakness. An inability to completely raise one arm.
- **S**peech difficulties. The inability to understand or repeat a simple sentence.
- **T**ime. Time is often the essence when suffering a stroke.
- Other symptoms may include a sudden headache, confusion, dizziness, difficulty walking, loss of balance or coordination, sudden visual difficulty.

Type 1 diabetes Insulin-dependent diabetes mellitus (IDDM), a condition in which the pancreas produces little or no insulin; also known as juvenile diabetes.
Type 2 diabetes Non-insulin-dependent diabetes mellitus (NIDDM), a condition in which insulin is not processed properly; also known as adult-onset diabetes.
Metabolic syndrome An array of metabolic abnormalities that contribute to the development of atherosclerosis triggered by insulin resistance. These conditions include low HDL-cholesterol, high triglycerides, high blood pressure, and an increased blood-clotting mechanism.

❑ | ❑ When you eat food that is prepared outside of the home, follow the above recommendations.

❑ | ❑ Avoid use of and exposure to tobacco products.

TRY IT

In your Online Journal or class notebook, record which of the above recommendations you fall short on and propose at least one thing you could do to improve.

Reducing Environmental Contaminants that May Cause Cancer

Since its creation in 1971, the U. S. President's Cancer Panel monitors exposure by the public to potential environmental cancer risks in daily life. The public remains by and large unaware of most of these widespread and underestimated risks, factors that are critical in any cancer prevention efforts. Exposure to environmental contaminants poses a threat to health because they may alter or interfere with a variety of biologic processes. Among the recommendations released in 2010 by the presidential panel are:

1. Filter tap water or well water and whenever possible use filtered water instead of commercially bottled water.
2. Properly dispose of pharmaceuticals, household chemicals, paints, and other products to minimize drinking water and soil contamination.
3. Eliminate exposure to secondhand smoke (and tobacco use in general).
4. Use stainless steel, glass, or BPA-free plastic water bottles.
5. Microwave in ceramic or glass instead of plastic containers.
6. Remove shoes before entering a home to avoid bringing in toxic chemicals, including pesticides.

Continued on back

LIFESTYLE FACTORS THAT DECREASE CANCER RISK

Do you have these healthy lifestyle factors working in your favor?

I PLAN TO	I DID IT	Factor	Function
❑	❑	Physical activity	Controls body weight, may influence hormone levels, strengthens the immune system.
❑	❑	Fiber	Contains anti-cancer substances, increases stool movement, blunts insulin secretion.
❑	❑	Fruits and vegetables	Contain phytonutrients and vitamins that thwart cancer.
❑	❑	Recommended weight	Helps control hormones that promote cancer.
❑	❑	Healthy grilling	Prevents formation of heterocyclic amines (HCAs) and polycyclic aromatic hydrocarbons (PAHs), both carcinogenic substances.

Continued on back

TIPS FOR A HEALTHY CANCER-FIGHTING DIET

I PLAN TO	I DID IT	
		I. Increase intake of antioxidants and phytonutrients, fiber, and cruciferous vegetables by:
❑	❑	Eating a predominantly vegetarian diet
❑	❑	Eating more fruits and vegetables every day (six to eight servings per day maximize anticancer benefits)
❑	❑	Increasing the consumption of broccoli, cauliflower, kale, turnips, cabbage, kohlrabi, Brussels sprouts, hot chili peppers, red and green peppers, carrots, sweet potatoes, winter squash, spinach, garlic, onions, strawberries, tomatoes, pineapple, and citrus fruits in your regular diet
❑	❑	Eating vegetables raw or quickly cooked by steaming or stir-frying
❑	❑	Substituting tea and fruit and vegetable juices for coffee and soda
❑	❑	Eating whole-grain breads
❑	❑	Including calcium in the diet (or from a supplement)
❑	❑	Including soy products in the diet

Continued on back

Benign Noncancerous.
Malignant Cancerous.
Cancer Group of diseases characterized by uncontrolled growth and spread of abnormal cells.
Carcinoma in situ Encapsulated malignant tumor that has not spread.
Angiogenesis Formation of blood vessels (capillaries).
Metastasis The movement of cells from one part of the body to another.
Nonmelanoma skin cancer Cancer that spreads or grows at the original site but does not metastasize to other regions of the body.
Carcinogens Substances that contribute to the formation of cancers.
Melanoma The most virulent, rapidly spreading form of skin cancer.
Ultraviolet B (UVB) rays Ultraviolet rays that cause sunburn and lead to skin cancers.
Ultraviolet A (UVA) rays Ultraviolet rays that pass deeper into the skin and are believed to cause skin damage and skin cancers.
Mammogram Low-dose X-rays of the breasts used as a screening technique for the early detection of breast tumors.

❑	❑ Tea	Contains polyphenols that neutralize free radicals, including epigallocatechin gallate (EGCG), which protects cells and the DNA from damage believed to cause cancer.
❑	❑ Spices	Provide phytonutrients and strengthen the immune system.
❑	❑ Vitamin D	Disrupts abnormal cell growth.
❑	❑ Monounsaturated fat	May contribute to cancer cell destruction.

TRY IT

In your Online Journal or class notebook, note ways you can incorporate all of these factors into your everyday lifestyle.

7. Limit the consumption of food that is grown with pesticides and meats from animals raised with antibiotics and growth hormones.
8. Limit the consumption of processed, charred, or well-done meats, which are high in heterocyclic amines and polyaromatic hydrocarbons.
9. Practice safe-sun exposure and avoid overexposure to ultraviolet light when the sunlight is most intense.
10. Reduce radiation exposure (X-rays) from medical sources.
11. Avoid exposure to three highly carcinogenic chemicals: formaldehyde, benzene, and radon.*
12. Use headsets and text, instead of talking on cell phones, and keep cell-phone calls brief to reduce exposure to electromagnetic energy. Although not scientifically proven, there is concern that frequent exposure to electromagnetic energy from cell phone use increases cancer risk.
13. Contaminant exposure in children is of significant concern because per pound of body weight they take in more food, water, air, and other substances than adults do. Toxic chemicals remain active longer in their developing brain and organs, placing them at far greater risk through chemical exposure.

*Formaldehyde is used in particle board, plywood, carpet, draperies, foam insulation, furniture, toiletries, and permanent press fabrics. Exposure is highest when newly installed. Benzene exposure is widespread and found primarily in vehicle exhaust. Radon exposure, which forms naturally and collects in homes, should be checked on a regular basis.

❑	❑	Using whole-wheat flour instead of refined white flour in baking
❑	❑	Using brown (unpolished) rice instead of white (polished) rice
		II. Limit saturated and trans fats by
❑	❑	Using primarily unsaturated fats (olive oil, canola oil, nuts, seeds, avocado, fish, flaxseeds, and flaxseed oil)
		III. Balancing caloric input
❑	❑	Balancing caloric input with caloric output to maintain recommended body weight

TRY IT

Make a copy of these "Cancer-Fighting Diet" tips and each week incorporate into your lifestyle two additional dietary behaviors from the above list.

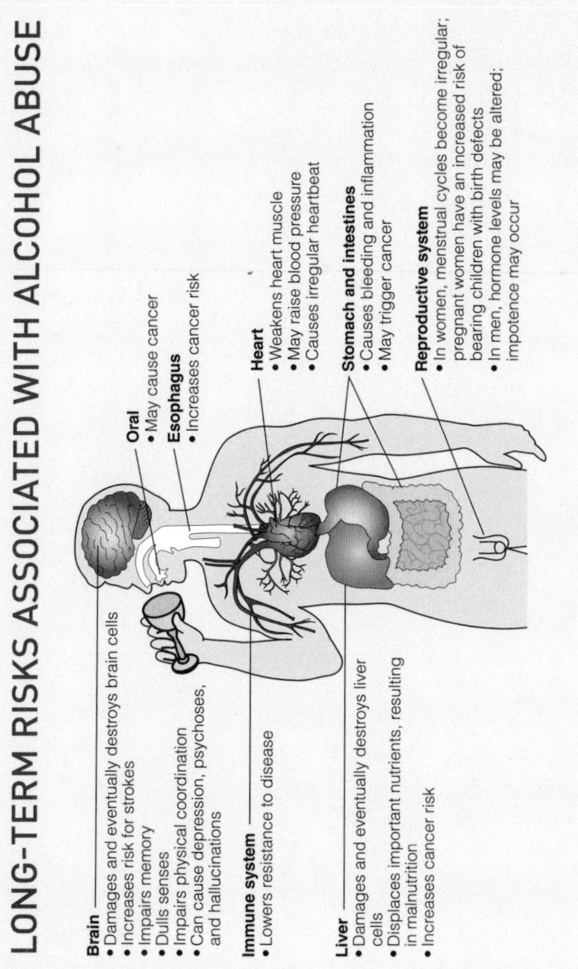
LONG-TERM RISKS ASSOCIATED WITH ALCOHOL ABUSE
Brain
• Damages and eventually destroys brain cells
• Increases risk for strokes
• Impairs memory
• Dulls senses
• Impairs physical coordination
• Can cause depression, psychoses, and hallucinations
Immune system
• Lowers resistance to disease
Liver
• Damages and eventually destroys liver cells
• Displaces important nutrients, resulting in malnutrition
• Increases cancer risk
Oral
• May cause cancer
Esophagus
• Increases cancer risk
Heart
• Weakens heart muscle
• May raise blood pressure
• Causes irregular heartbeat
Stomach and intestines
• Causes bleeding and inflammation
• May trigger cancer
Reproductive system
• In women, menstrual cycles become irregular; pregnant women have an increased risk of bearing children with birth defects
• In men, hormone levels may be altered; impotence may occur

HEALTHY LIFESTYLE GUIDELINES

❑ I PLAN TO	❑ I DID IT	
❑	❑	1. Accumulate a minimum of 30 minutes of moderate-intensity physical activity at least five days per week.
❑	❑	2. Exercise aerobically in the proper cardiorespiratory training zone at least three times per week for a minimum of 20 minutes.
❑	❑	3. Accumulate at least 10,000 steps on a daily basis.
❑	❑	4. Strength train at least once a week (preferably twice a week) using a minimum of eight exercises that involve all major muscle groups of the body.
❑	❑	5. Perform flexibility exercises that involve all major joints of the body at least two to three times per week.
❑	❑	6. Avoid excessive sitting throughout the day: Take intermittent 10-minute breaks for every hour that you are sitting (at the computer, studying, playing table games, or watching television).
❑	❑	7. Eat a healthy diet that is rich in whole-wheat grains, fruits, and vegetables and is low in saturated and trans fats.
❑	❑	8. Eat a healthy breakfast every day.
❑	❑	9. Do not use tobacco in any form, avoid secondhand smoke, and avoid all other forms of substance abuse.

Continued on back

PROTECTING YOURSELF AND OTHERS FROM STIs

Are you sexually active? If you are not, read the following items to better educate yourself regarding intimacy. If you are sexually active, continue through all the questions below.

- ❑ Do you plan ahead before you get into a sexual situation?
- ❑ Do you know whether your partner now has or has ever had an STI? Are you comfortable asking your partner this question?
- ❑ Are you in a mutually monogamous sexual relationship and you know that your partner does not have an STI?
- ❑ Do you have multiple sexual partners? If so, do you *always* practice safe sex?
- ❑ Do you avoid alcohol and drugs in situations where you may end up having planned or unplanned sex?
- ❑ Do you abstain from sexual activity if you know or suspect that you have an STI? Do you seek medical care and advice as to when you can safely resume sexual activity?

TRY IT

Taking chances during sexual contact is not worth the risk of an STI. Sex lasts a few minutes; the STI can last a lifetime, with potentially fatal consequences. Think ahead, know the facts, and don't place yourself in a situation where you may no longer be able to or have the desire to say no. Keep in mind that more than half of all Americans will acquire at least one STI in their lifetime. A few minutes of sexual pleasure can easily have consequences that you may regret for the rest of your life.

Addiction Compulsive and uncontrollable behavior(s) or use of substance(s).
Synergistic action The effect of mixing two or more drugs, which can be much greater than the sum of two or more drugs acting by themselves.
Sexually transmitted infections (STIs) Communicable diseases spread through sexual contact.
HIV (Human immunodeficiency virus) Virus that leads to acquired immunodeficiency syndrome (AIDS).
AIDS (Acquired immunodeficiency syndrome) Any of a number of diseases that arise when the body's immune system is compromised by HIV; the final stage of HIV infection.
Physiological age The biological and functional capacity of the body as it should be in relation to the person's maximal potential at any given age in the lifespan.
Functional capacity The ability to perform the ordinary and unusual demands of daily living without limitations and excessive fatigue or injury.
Conventional Western medicine Traditional medical practice based on methods that are tested through rigorous scientific trials; also called allopathic medicine.

- ☐ | ☐ 10. Maintain healthy body weight (achieve a range between the high-physical fitness and health-fitness standards for percent body fat).
- ☐ | ☐ 11. Get 7 to 8 hours of sleep per night.
- ☐ | ☐ 12. Practice safe sex every time you have sex and don't have sexual contact with anyone who doesn't practice safe sex.
- ☐ | ☐ 13. Get 10 to 20 minutes of safe sun exposure on most days of the week.
- ☐ | ☐ 14. Manage stress effectively.
- ☐ | ☐ 15. Limit daily alcohol intake to two or less drinks per day if you are a man or one drink or less per day if you are a woman (or do not consume any alcohol at all).
- ☐ | ☐ 16. Have at least one close friend or relative in whom you can confide and to whom you can express your feelings openly.
- ☐ | ☐ 17. Be aware of your surroundings and take personal safety measures at all times.
- ☐ | ☐ 18. Seek continued learning on a regular basis.
- ☐ | ☐ 19. Subscribe to a reputable health/fitness/nutrition newsletter to stay up-to-date on healthy lifestyle guidelines.
- ☐ | ☐ 20. Seek proper medical evaluations as necessary.

TRY IT

Now that you are about to complete this course, evaluate how many of the above healthy lifestyle guidelines have become part of your personal wellness program. Prepare a list of those that you still need to work on and use Lab 15C to write SMART goals and specific objectives that will help you achieve the desired behaviors. Remember that each one of the above guidelines will lead to a longer, healthier, and happier life.